Hg	mercury		
Hgb	hemoglobi...		
HIV	human im... virus		...ter
HMG-CoA	3-hydroxy... coenzyr...		
HR	heart rate		...olled analgesia
h.s.	at bedtime	per	through, by
H.S.	half-strength	P.O.	by mouth
I.M.	intramuscular	P.R.	by rectum
INR	International Normalized Ratio	p.r.n.	as needed
		PT	prothrombin time
IPPB	intermittent positive-pressure breathing	PTT	partial thromboplastin time
		PVC	premature ventricular contraction
IU	international unit	q	every
I.V.	intravenous	Q.D.	every day
K	potassium	q.i.d.	four times daily
kg	kilogram	Q.O.D.	every other day
KVO	keep vein open	RBC	red blood cell
L	liter	RDA	recommended dietary allowance
lb	pound		
LD	lactate dehydrogenase	RNA	ribonucleic acid
LDL	low-density lipoprotein	RSV	respiratory syncytial virus
m	meter	SA	sinoatrial
m^2	square meters	S.C.	subcutaneous
MAO	monoamine oxidase	SI	International System of Units
mcg	microgram		
MDI	metered-dose inhaler	SIADH	syndrome of inappropriate antidiuretic hormone secretion
mEq	milliequivalent		
mg	milligram		
$MgSO_4$	magnesium sulfate		
ml	milliliter	S.L.	sublingual
mm	millimeter	S.Q.	subcutaneous
mm^3	cubic millimeters	SSRI	selective serotonin reuptake inhibitor
mm Hg	millimeters of mercury		
mmol	millimole	T_3	triiodothyronine
MS	morphine sulfate	T_4	thyroxine
MSO_4	magnesium sulfate	TCA	tricyclic antidepressant
µg	microgram	t.i.d.	three times daily
Na	sodium	T.I.W.	three times a week
NA	not applicable	tRNA	transfer ribonucleic acid
NaCl	sodium chloride	tsp	teaspoon
ng	nanogram	VMA	vanillylmandelic acid
NG	nasogastric	USP	United States Pharmacopeia
N.P.O.	nothing by mouth	WBC	white blood cell
NSAID	nonsteroidal anti-inflammatory drug		

Clinical alert. **Do not use.**

Premier **2005** *Edition*

Nursing Spectrum
DRUG
Handbook

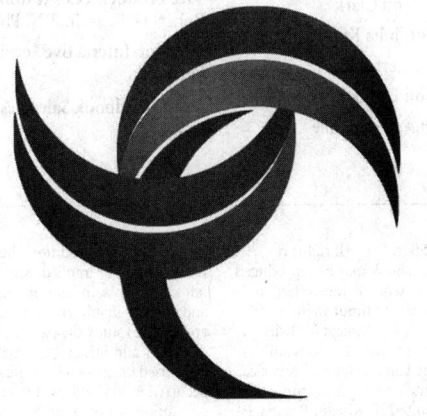

Patricia Dwyer Schull, RN, MSN

www.nursesdrughandbook.com

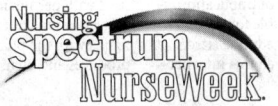

This book was developed by MedVantage Publishing, LLC, and published by Nursing Spectrum.

MedVantage Publishing Staff

Director: Patricia Dwyer Schull, RN, MSN

Clinical Manager: Minnie Bowen Rose, BSN, MEd

Editorial Manager: Kathy E. Goldberg

Design Manager: Stephanie Peters

Website Development Manager: Don Saul

Clinical Editors: Julia Gerhart, PharmD; Collette Hendler, RN, BS, CCRN; Sandy Keefe, RN, MSN; Jeannette Wick, RPh

Editors: Mary Lou Ambrose, Alison T. Kelley, Julie Munden, Jessica Baskin Taylor

Copy Editors: Karen Comerford; Ellen K. Weil, MS, RPh, ELS; Doris Weinstock

Designer: Joseph John Clark

Editorial Assistant: Julia Knipe

Indexer: Karen Comerford

Cover Design: John Hubbard

Illustrator: Kevin A. Somerville

Nursing Spectrum Staff

President and Publisher: Patti McCook Rager, RN, MSN, MBA

Executive Vice President, Professional Services: Fred J. DiCostanzo RN, MA

Executive Vice President, Editorial: Cynthia L. Saver, RN, MS

Executive Vice President, Advertising, Marketing & Interactive Services: Steven H. Hauber

Executive Vice President, Operations: Melyni Serpa

Executive Vice President, Finance: Jim Filiaggi

Senior Vice President, Marketing and Research: John Leggett

Vice President, Continuing Education: Robert G. Hess, Jr., RN, PhD

Director, Interactive Services: Doug Jankowski

Drug Handbook Sales Associate: Lesley McGerald

ISSN: 1550-0543
ISBN: 1-930745-01-X

The author, editors, and publisher have made every effort to verify the accuracy of the information in this book and to ensure that it mirrors currently accepted medical recommendations and practices at the time of publication. However, they are not responsible for inadvertent errors or omissions or for adverse effects stemming from the way in which this information is applied. In addition, they make no warranty, express or implied, with respect to the book's contents. In light of ongoing research and changes in government regulation, readers are urged to study the package insert for each drug they administer—especially new or seldom-used drugs—to determine if changes have occurred in indications, dosage requirements, precautions, or other aspects of drug use.

This book covers some drugs that the Food and Drug Administration (FDA) has approved for limited use in restricted settings, such as research. It is the reader's responsibility to identify the FDA status of each drug before using it in a clinical setting.

Photographs on pages P1-P16 are licensed and used with permission from Sigler and Flanders, Inc. However, copyright of the photographs remains with the pharmaceutical company that produces and owns each drug.

A note from the publisher

I am delighted to introduce *2005 Nursing Spectrum Drug Handbook,* the premier edition of our medication administration manual for nurses. Nursing Spectrum's mission has always been to educate, recognize, and support nurses through our magazines, website, educational programs, and involvement in the nursing community. If you have read *Nursing Spectrum* or *NurseWeek* magazines lately or visited our websites (www.nursingspectrum.com and www.nurseweek.com), you'll know we offer articles and continuing education modules on pharmacology and drug administration.

Because drug administration is such a critical nursing activity, we decided to go one step further in helping nurses carry out their professional responsibilities with competence and confidence. *2005 Nursing Spectrum Drug Handbook* reflects our ongoing commitment to nursing education. It offers accurate, in-depth information on approximately 1,000 generic-name and 3,000 trade-name drugs.

2005 Nursing Spectrum Drug Handbook can help you face the challenge of one of the most demanding aspects of clinical nursing. It presents practical, reliable drug information in an attractive format that's easy to use. The handbook is small enough to carry in your pocket and durable enough to withstand the heavy use it's likely to get. It's jam-packed with must-have features and written in a concise style that makes it a snap to use and understand.

As you know, pharmacology is a rapidly changing field. To keep up with the steady flow of new drug information, *Nursing Spectrum Drug Handbook* will be updated and published annually. Its companion website, www.nursesdrughandbook.com, will be updated often throughout the year to keep you informed of ongoing developments in the pharmacology world.

Like everything else we publish, *2005 Nursing Spectrum Drug Handbook* was written for nurses by nurses. We're delighted to be working with our author, Patricia Dwyer Schull, RN, MSN, the director of MedVantage Publishing. Pat has more that 20 years' experience in publishing drug information products for nurses. She has assembled a first-rate team of clinical experts, text editors, and designers with extensive experience in developing nursing drug reference products. Content, contributions, and reviews have been acquired from more than 40 practicing pharmacists, nurses, and consultants. An advisory board of highly respected nurse leaders and pharmacists with expertise in clinical practice, management, and publishing has been assembled.

The result of all this hard work is a reference book that you simply can't afford to be without. Thank you for purchasing *2005 Nursing Spectrum Drug Handbook* and for allowing us to demonstrate, once again, our commitment to serving nurses.

Patti Rager, RN, MSN, MBA
President & Publisher
Nursing Spectrum

Contents

Foreword

When it comes to administering drugs, the nurse serves as the final "safety officer." No matter how many error-reducing protocols and processes your facility may use to promote safe drug administration, you're responsible for keeping your patient safe from untoward drug effects. Human error is always possible—and your knowledge and skills can help prevent such error.

The goal of reducing medication errors may sound overwhelming. Roughly 1 in every 15 patients experiences an adverse drug event (ADE)—an injury caused by a medication error or an adverse drug reaction. In fact, medication errors cause more than 7,000 deaths each year. In 1999, the Institute of Medicine reported that medication errors account for 1 in every 854 inpatient deaths and 1 in every 131 outpatient deaths. What's more, half of ADEs were found to be preventable.

To reduce ADEs, health care facilities are trying everything from bar code labeling of drug containers and electronic real-time medication charting, to "smart" drug drawers that open only when certain criteria are met. Others use wireless medication scanners and automated drug alerts and reminders. In addition, The Joint Commission on Accreditation of Healthcare Organizations now requires the use of constraints and "forcing functions" to prevent certain actions until the right conditions are met.

Ultimately, though, effective drug administration relies on the basics of medication safety that we learned in nursing school, namely the "five rights"—right patient, drug, time, dosage, and administration route. To help prevent medication errors, we must increase our understanding of each drug we administer. *2005 Nursing Spectrum Drug Handbook* is the ideal resource for any nurse who gives hands-on care or teaches patients about drugs. Besides providing such basic information as indications and dosages, it presents key aspects of administration and patient monitoring, emphasizing the vital information you must have to give drugs safely and effectively.

Along with other health-care team members, nurses must continue to search for ways to reduce medication errors and promote appropriate practice changes. And they must keep their knowledge, judgment, and skills current. *2005 Nursing Spectrum Drug Handbook* helps you meet these challenges. Whether you're administering a familiar drug you've given hundreds of times or a new medication you've never heard of, this book will boost your confidence. I recommend it without reservation.

Linda Groah, RN, MS, CNOR, CNAA, FAAN
Director of Hospital Operations
Kaiser Permanente Medical Center
San Francisco

Advisors

Ann M. Barrow, RN, MSN
Publishing Consultant
Coordinator of College Relations
College of Nursing
Villanova University
Villanova, Pa

Vicki L. Buchda, RN, MS
Director of Nursing
Mayo Clinic in Scottsdale
Scottsdale, AZ

Pamela R. Dellinger, RN, BC, PhD
President-Elect, National Association
    for Healthcare Recruitment
Director of Recruitment
Lincoln Medical Center
Lincolnton, NC

Gloria F. Donnelly, RN, PhD, FAAN
Dean and Professor
College of Nursing and Health
    Professions
Drexel University
Philadelphia

Harriet R. Feldman, RN, PhD, FAAN
Dean and Professor
Lienhard School of Nursing
Pace University
Pleasantville, NY

**Linda Groah, RN, MS, CNOR, CNAA,
    FAAN**
Director of Hospital Operations
Kaiser Permanente Medical Center
San Francisco

David Hawkins, PharmD
Professor and Senior Associate Dean
    of Pharmacy
Mercer University
Southern School of Pharmacy
Atlanta

**Peggy Kalowes, RN, MSN, CNRN,
    CNS**
Assistant Professor
School of Nursing
California State University
Los Angeles

Terris E. Kennedy, RN, PhD
Vice President and Chief Nursing
    Officer
Shore Memorial Hospital
Nassawadox, Va

James A. Koestner, BS, PharmD
Director of Pharmaceutical Care
Vanderbilt University Medical Center
Franklin, Tenn

Claire M. Young, RN, MBA
Chief Nursing Officer
Chair, Division of Nursing
The Cleveland Clinic Foundation
Cleveland

Contributors and reviewers

Sue Apple, RN, DNSc
Instructor
School of Nursing and Health Studies
Georgetown University
Washington, D.C.

Cathy L. Bartels, PharmD
Associate Professor
Department of Pharmacy Practice
Creighton University
Omaha

Melanie Boock, RN, BSN
Administrative Supervisor
Emergency Room Staff Nurse
Vail Valley Medical Center
Vail, Colo

Vicky Borders-Hemphill, PharmD
Medical Writer
Clinton, Md

Cheryl A. Bozman, RRT, RN, BSN
Clinical Educator
Oakwood Hospital and Medical Center
Dearborn, Mich

Susan C. Braun, RN, MS, CS
Family Nurse Practitioner
University of Illinois
Chicago

Jason D. Buckway, RN, BSN
Nurse Manager
McKay-Dee Hospital Center
Intermountain Health Care System
Ogden, Utah

Linda Carman Copel, RN, CS, PhD, DAPA
Associate Professor
College of Nursing
Villanova University
Villanova, Pa

Joseph T. Catalano, RN, PhD
Professor and Chairman
Department of Nursing
East Central University
Ada, Okla

Justin G. Dalton, RN, BSN
Clinical Nurse Educator
McKay-Dee Hospital Center
Intermountain Health Care System
Ogden, Utah

Teresa Dowdell, BS, RPh
Visiting Instructor
College of Nursing
University of South Florida
Tampa

Julie M. Gerhart, BS, RPh
Staff Pharmacist
Ambler Care Pharmacy
Ambler, Pa

Cheryl A. Grandinetti, PharmD
Senior Clinical Research Pharmacist
Cancer Therapy Evaluation Program
Division of Cancer Treatment and
    Diagnosis
National Cancer Institute
Clarksburg, Md

Franklin R. Grollman, PharmD
Clinical Pharmacist
National Naval Medical Center
Bethesda, Md

Helena M. Hardin, RN
Assistant Clinical Manager
Coronary Intensive Care Unit
Oakwood Hospital and Medical Center
Dearborn, Mich

Collette B. Hendler, RN, BS, CCRN
Clinical Leader
Medical Intensive Care Unit
Abington Memorial Hospital
Abington, Pa

Monica Holmberg, PharmD
Phoenix Indian Medical Center
Phoenix

Sandy Keefe, RN, MSN
Health Care Manager
Freelance Writer
Camp Costanoan
Cupertino, Calif

Nancy L. Laplante, RN, MSN
Instructor
Nursing Department
Neumann College
Aston, Pa

Mary Jane J. McDevitt, RN, BS
Home Care Nurse
Delaware County Memorial Hospital
Drexel Hill, Pa

Miranda L. Moyer, RN, BSN
Staff Nurse
Nursing Care Services
Colmar, Pa

Keith M. Olsen, PharmD, FCCP, FCCM
Associate Professor of Pharmacy
College of Pharmacy
University of Nebraska Medical Center
Omaha

Lois A. Piano, RN, MSN, EdD
Senior Research Associate
Curtis Analytic Partners
Philadelphia

Christine A. Price, PharmD
Clinical Coordinator
Morton Plant Mease Health Care
Clearwater, Fla

Barbara J. Putrycus, RN, MSN, CCRN
Director
Preoperative Holding and
    Post-Anesthesia Care Unit
Oakwood Hospital and Medical Center
Dearborn, Mich

Melinda K. Schott, RPh, PharmD
Staff Pharmacist
Stop & Shop Pharmacy
Wallingford, Conn

Ann Marie Smith, RN, BSN, MA
Clinical Instructor
Department of Nursing Education
    and Research
Cleveland Clinic Foundation
Cleveland

Mary E. Stassi, RNC
Health Occupations Coordinator
St. Charles Community College
St. Peters, Mo

Tracey R. Troop, RN
Nurse
Intensive Care Unit
Abington Memorial Hospital
Abington, Pa

Ellen K. Weil, MS, RPh, ELS
Drug Information Consultant
New York City

Jeannette Y. Wick, RPh, MBA
Senior Clinical Research Pharmacist
Pharmaceutical Management Branch
Cancer Therapy Evaluation Program
National Cancer Institute
Bethesda, Md

Preface and user's guide

The average nurse spends at least a third of her time giving drugs and managing patients' drug regimens—a proportion that accurately reflects the central role of drug therapy in patient care.

Medical science has developed new approaches to drug therapy, creating powerful medications whose advanced pharmacologic features hold out the promise of faster and more effective cures. Not only are many patients receiving more powerful drugs; they're receiving *more* drugs than ever. The sickest patients—those in intensive care—typically receive anywhere from 20 to 40 different drugs. These patients may be the most vulnerable to adverse reactions and drug interactions, as well as the life-threatening consequences of a medication error. Consequently, patient protection and advocacy related to drug therapy has become one of the major challenges in our everyday practice.

Over the past few years, medication errors have drawn increasing attention, especially since a 1999 report by the Institute of Medicine suggested that preventable drug errors and other adverse events account for more deaths than motor vehicle accidents, breast cancer, and AIDS. For nurses, this intense scrutiny, along with the common use of multidrug regimens, underscores the need for a thorough understanding of the drugs we give and for expertise in administering them. *2005 Nursing Spectrum Drug Handbook* will enhance your understanding of drugs and help you meet the many challenges of safe and effective drug administration.

How this book and companion website evolved

Nursing Spectrum's mission is to provide nurses with relevant continuing education products—and what could be more relevant than a drug reference?

When we first set out to create this book, we traveled around the country to discover firsthand exactly what nurses want in a compact, portable drug handbook. As we met with staff nurses and nurse-managers from a wide range of practice settings, it became clear that your primary concern is to keep patients safe from harm while protecting your professional well-being. This concern inspired us to make *safety* the book's major theme. When we asked which specific features you value most in a drug handbook, "ease of use" was by far the leading response.

From the initial stages of developing *2005 Nursing Spectrum Drug Handbook*, we based every decision on nurses' concerns about promoting drug safety and their desire for a user-friendly format. We've made the book the perfect size for carrying with you on the job. We've designed the page for maximum legibility and kept the writing simple and succinct. We've even built in a ribbon bookmark to help you keep your place throughout your workday.

To ensure accuracy, a concise editorial process was developed and implemented by a team of managers, each with many years of experience in publishing nursing drug books. Material was contributed by practicing nurses and pharmacists throughout the country, and reviewed by a team of drug information experts and consultants, including an advisory board of well-known nurse-leaders and pharmacists with expertise in education, clinical practice, pharmacology, management, and publishing.

Outstanding features

Here's a preview of what you'll find in this premier edition:
• individual monographs for approximately 1,000 generic drugs and 3,000 trade drugs, arranged in alphabetical order
• "Clinical Alert" logos in eye-catching red to call your attention to critical considerations
• dosages highlighted with a scored tablet icon for quick identification
• detailed administration guidelines for every drug, with specific instructions on oral, I.M., and I.V. routes when applicable
• monitoring guidelines, including ongoing patient assessment, follow-up laboratory tests to identify adverse reactions, and warning signs of an untoward event
• life-threatening adverse reactions shown in **boldface**
• interactions with other drugs, diagnostic tests, foods, herbal remedies and supplements, and behaviors
• more than 30 pages of drug safety guidelines throughout the book, including numerous appendices and 16 pages in the full-color "Safe drug administration" insert—all marked with a red and black "safety guidelines" logo
• photogallery of common tablets and capsules
• appendices that sharpen your perspective on drugs and their use
• companion website with drug updates, drug news, and other valuable features.

General drug administration guidelines

From the time the prescriber orders a drug to the time the patient receives it, the process of drug administration may involve anywhere from 80 to 200 individual steps. Missteps can happen at any point in this process—but you can help prevent certain missteps long before the dose is prepared. During initial patient evaluation, for instance, check the patient's current drug regimen, obtain drug allergy information, and collect baseline assessment data to help determine the risk for an adverse reaction.

The "five rights" of drug administration

Nurses are legally responsible for applying the "five rights" of drug administration. Although these rights have been probably etched into your mind since your nursing school days, I'd feel remiss if I didn't review them here to refresh your memory.
• **Right patient.** Always confirm the patient's identity before administering a drug. Check the patient's ID bracelet and ask him to state his name; then confirm his name, age, and allergies. The Joint Commission on Accreditation of Healthcare Organizations requires use of two identifiers, such as the patient number, his telephone number, or his Social Security number. Ideally, match the ordered treatment to the patient using his name bracelet and ID number, comparing it to the drug order transcribed in the medication administration record (MAR).
• **Right drug.** Giving the wrong drug is the most common type of medication error. It typically results from such factors as look-alike and sound-alike drug names, similar drug labels and packaging, and poor communication. Never try to decipher an illegible drug order, and never give a drug if you're not sure

why it was prescribed. To make sure the right drug is given, match the drug label against the order in the MAR *three times*—once when you remove the container from the patient's drug drawer, again before you remove the dose from the container, and finally, before you return the container to the drawer or discard it. Never give a drug from a container that is unlabeled or has an unreadable label.

• **Right dosage.** Check the dosage against the order in the MAR. Determine if the dosage is appropriate based on the patient's age, size, and vital signs. If the dose needs to be measured, use appropriate equipment—for instance, an oral syringe rather than a parenteral syringe to measure an oral liquid drug. When giving a high-risk drug, such as I.V. insulin or heparin, or when giving an infusion to an infant or a child, double-check the dosage and pump settings; then verify these with a colleague.

• **Right time.** Usually, a dose should be given within 30 minutes before or after the time specified in the order. Administer each dose as it's prepared. To maximize the drug's therapeutic efficacy, check whether it should be given with or without food or whether it could interact with or impede the absorption of concurrently administered drugs. If the patient's scheduled for diagnostic testing, determine whether to withhold the dose until after the test.

• **Right route.** Many drugs can be given by multiple routes. The prescriber chooses the route based on such factors as the patient's condition and the desired onset of action. In turn, the prescribed dosage is based on the administration route. Generally, oral dosages of a given drug are greater than injected dosages, so a serious overdose may occur if a dose intended for oral administration is given by injection instead.

Additional nursing responsibilities

Of course, nursing responsibilities don't stop with these five rights. Documentation, monitoring, and patient teaching are also crucial to drug administration.

After giving the drug, always document that it was administered. Document the dose as soon as it is given—never before. When documenting, use only accepted abbreviations and avoid those that could be misread. If the patient refuses a medication, report this to the prescriber immediately. Then record his refusal on both the MAR and the patient's record; include your initials, full name, and credentials on both records.

During the course of drug therapy, monitor the patient to determine drug efficacy and detect signs and symptoms of an adverse reaction or interaction. Teach the patient the name of the prescribed drug, its dosage, administration route, dosing frequency and times, and duration of therapy. Make sure he knows how to recognize the drug's therapeutic effects, adverse reactions, and interactions with other drugs, foods, herbs, or behaviors.

User's guide to *Nursing Spectrum Drug Handbook*

This book is organized in three main parts.

Part 1: A to Z drug monographs

Part 1 presents individual drug monographs in alphabetical order by generic name. Each monograph starts with basic information, including dosages and administration guidelines. Next come adverse reactions, interactions, nursing care to provide during drug therapy, and teaching points to review with the patient. Within each monograph, information is presented in the following order:

Understanding pregnancy risk categories

Whenever possible, pregnant women should avoid drug therapy. The risks of taking drugs during pregnancy range from relatively minor fetal defects (such as ear tags or extra digits) to fetal death.

When drug therapy is considered, the drug's benefits to the mother must be weighed against the risk to the fetus. Ideally, the drug should provide clear benefits to the mother without harming the fetus. To help prescribers and pregnant patients assess a drug's risk-to-benefit ratio, the Food and Drug Administration assigns one of five pregnancy risk categories to each drug. In addition, certain drugs are not rated.

Category A: No evidence of risk exists. Adequate, well-controlled studies in pregnant women don't show an increased risk of fetal abnormalities during any trimester.

Category B: The risk of fetal harm is possible but remote. Animal studies show no fetal risk; however, controlled studies haven't been done in humans. Or animal studies do show a risk to the fetus, but adequate studies in pregnant women haven't shown such a risk.

Category C: Fetal risk can't be ruled out. Although animal studies show risks, adequate, well-controlled human studies are lacking. Despite the potential fetal risks, use of the drug may be acceptable because of benefits to the mother.

Category D: Positive evidence of fetal risk exists. Nevertheless, potential benefits from the drug may outweigh the risk. For example, the drug may be acceptable in a life-threatening situation or serious disease if safer drugs can't be used or are ineffective.

Category X: Contraindicated during pregnancy. Studies in animals or humans or reports of adverse reactions show evidence of fetal risk that clearly outweighs any possible benefit to the patient.

Category NR: Not rated.

Generic name. A drug's generic name is the nonproprietary name, typically assigned by the manufacturer. When more than one therapeutic form of the drug is available, generic names of these forms are listed alphabetically.

Trade names. A drug's common trade, or brand, name is the proprietary, trademarked name under which it's marketed. Trade-name and generic drugs are therapeutically equivalent in strength, quality, performance, and use; when interchanged, they have the same effects and no differences. However, they may vary in preservatives, color, shape, labeling, and, possibly, scoring. In the monograph, trade names available only in Canada are followed by a maple leaf for easy identification.

Pharmacologic and therapeutic classes. This section specifies the drug's pharmacologic class (based on its pharmacologic properties and action—for example, sulfonamide or corticosteroid) and therapeutic class (based on approved therapeutic uses of the drug—for instance, antineoplastic or antihypertensive). Many drugs fall into multiple therapeutic classes.

Pregnancy risk category. This section lists the category assigned by the Food and Drug Administration (FDA) to indicate the drug's potential danger to the fetus when taken during pregnancy. (See *Understanding pregnancy risk categories*.)

Controlled substance schedule. Narcotics, stimulants, and certain other drugs fall under the Controlled Substances Act. The Drug Enforcement Agency assigns each of these drugs a category, or schedule, based on its abuse potential and other factors. (See *Schedules of controlled substances*.) When applicable, this section lists the drug's assigned schedule.

Action. This section summarizes how the drug achieves its therapeutic effect—the action that takes place when it reaches its target site and combines with cellular drug receptors to cause certain physiologic responses. When a drug's action isn't known or when researchers have proposed theories for the action but haven't clarified it definitively, we state this fact.

Availability. This section lists the physical forms in which the drug is produced and dispensed, plus available strengths (the amount of active ingredient present) for each form.

Indications and dosages. Marked with a red scored tablet icon 🔴 for quick identification, this section details the drug's FDA-approved indications for adults, children, infants, and neonates (when appropriate), along with recommended dosages, administration routes, and dosing frequency for each indication. The indications and dosages shown reflect current clinical trends, not unequivocal standards, and must be considered in light of the patient's condition and diagnosis. (*Note:* Although we've made every effort to ensure the accuracy of all dosages, we urge you to become familiar with the official package insert for each drug you administer.)

Dosage adjustment. This section tells which patient groups (such as children or elderly patients), diseases, or disorders (such as renal or hepatic dysfunction) may necessitate dosage adjustment.

Off-label uses. Here you'll find a list of off-label (unlabeled or unapproved) uses of the drug, when applicable. Off-label use has become increasingly common as clinical research moves ahead of the FDA's approval process. In some cases, off-label use has become the standard of care.

Contraindications. This section lists conditions that contraindicate use of the drug, such as preexisting diseases or other conditions. As a rule, never

Schedules of controlled substances

The Controlled Substances Act of 1970 regulates the production and distribution of stimulants, narcotics, depressants, hallucinogens, and anabolic steroids. Drugs regulated by this law fall into five categories, or schedules, based on their abuse potential, medicinal value, and harmfulness. Schedule I drugs are the most hazardous; schedule V drugs, the least hazardous.

Schedule I: High potential for abuse; no currently accepted medical use in the United States. Using the drug even under medical supervision is thought to be unsafe.

Schedule II: High potential for abuse; currently accepted medical use in the United States (or currently accepted medical use with severe restrictions). Abuse may lead to severe psychological or physical dependence. Emergency telephone orders for limited quantities may be authorized, but the prescriber must provide a written, signed prescription order.

Schedule III: Lower abuse potential than schedule I and II drugs; currently accepted medical use in the United States. Abuse may lead to a moderate or low degree of physical dependence or high psychological dependence. Telephone orders are permitted.

Schedule IV: Lower abuse potential than schedule I, II, or III drugs; currently accepted medical use in the United States. Abuse may lead to limited physical dependence or psychological dependence. Telephone orders are permitted.

Schedule V: Low abuse potential compared to drugs in other schedules; currently accepted medical use in the United States. Abuse may lead to limited physical dependence or to psychological dependence. Some schedule V drugs may be available in limited quantities without a prescription (if permitted under state law).

High-alert drugs

SAFETY
GUIDELINES

Certain drugs expose patients to an increased risk of significant harm when used in error. The Institute for Safe Medication Practices (ISMP) has created a list of high-alert drugs based on voluntary medication error reports, harmful medication errors described in the literature, practitioner feedback, and expert reviews. The ISMP has identified both high-alert drug classes (or categories) and specific high-alert drugs.

High-alert drug classes and categories

- adrenergic agonists, I.V.
- adrenergic antagonists, I.V.
- cardioplegic solutions
- chemotherapeutic agents
- dextrose (20% or greater)
- dialysis solutions
- epidural and intrathecal drugs
- general anesthetics
- glycoprotein IIb/IIIa inhibitors
- hypoglycemics, oral
- inotropic drugs, I.V.
- liposomal drug forms
- moderate sedation agents, I.V. (or oral agents for children)
- narcotics and opioids
- neuromuscular blocking agents
- thrombolytics and fibrinolytics, I.V.
- total parenteral nutrition solutions

Specific high-alert drugs

- amiodarone, I.V.
- colchicine, injection
- heparin, low molecular weight
- heparin, unfractionated, I.V.
- insulin, subcutaneous and I.V.
- lidocaine, I.V.
- magnesium sulfate injection
- methotrexate, oral nononcologic use
- nesiritide
- potassium chloride for injection
- potassium phosphates injection
- sodium chloride injection
- sodium nitroprusside for injection
- warfarin

give a drug to a patient who has a history of hypersensitivity to that drug. Drugs commonly implicated in hypersensitivity reactions include antibiotics, histamines, iodides, phenothiazines, tranquilizers, anesthetics, diagnostic agents (such as iodinated contrast media), and biological agents (such as insulin, vaccines, and antitoxins).

Administration. Here you'll find information to help you prepare the drug and administer it correctly and safely, regardless of the route—including whether to give it with or without food, how to mix it for I.V. or I.M. use, and what flow rate to use.

Route, onset, peak, and duration. Presented in table form, this section provides a pharmacokinetic profile—onset of action, peak blood level, and duration of action—for each route by which the drug is administered.

Adverse reactions. Occurring in roughly 30% of hospital patients, adverse reactions are undesirable and unintended drug effects that can range from mild to life-threatening. They may arise immediately and suddenly, or they may take weeks or even months to develop. Adverse reactions may be especially dangerous if a medication error occurs in a patient who's receiving a high-alert drug. *(See High-alert drugs.)* In this section, we list the most commonly reported adverse reactions by body system. Life-threatening reactions appear in **boldface**.

Interactions. With Americans taking more prescription and nonprescription drugs than ever, you're likely to encounter patients experiencing the effects of drug interactions. Many people also take herbs and supplements that can interact with drugs to cause dangerous effects or to impede a drug's intended effect. This section presents documented and clinically significant interactions that may occur if the drug is used concurrently with other drugs, specific foods, and certain herbs or supplements or if it's combined with certain behaviors (for instance, smoking or alcohol use). It also describes the drug's effects on diagnostic test results, which can be especially important with hospital patients.

Precautions. For some patients, a specific drug may pose an increased risk of untoward effects—yet the doctor prescribes it because, in his judgment, the potential benefits outweigh the risks. For instance, many drugs can be dangerous for elderly patients, pregnant or breastfeeding women, young children, and patients with renal or hepatic dysfunction. This section tells you which patients to whom you must administer the drug cautiously.

Patient monitoring. To help gauge whether the drug is effective and to detect untoward reactions or interactions, your patient must be monitored closely during drug therapy (and in some cases, even after therapy ends). Early assessment of troublesome side effects or drug inefficacy allows timely adjustments in therapy and may prevent patient injury or avoid a treatment delay. This section discusses important nursing assessments and interventions to perform, such as monitoring blood drug levels to help determine the correct dosage and to prevent toxicity.

Patient teaching. The nurse's responsibility for teaching patients about their care has never been greater. What's more, patients are now demanding more information about their treatment. This section describes key teaching points to cover with a patient who's receiving the drug, including essential information needed to create a patient teaching plan and to protect your patient even after discharge. Topics include how and when the patient should take the drug, which symptoms he should report immediately, and which drugs, foods, herbs, or behaviors he should avoid during drug therapy.

Part 2: Ophthalmic drugs, drug classes, vitamins and minerals, herbs and supplements

Part 2 presents abbreviated monographs for common ophthalmic drugs, vitamins, minerals, herbs, and supplements, as well as collective monographs on therapeutic drug classes. The use of herbal remedies and supplements is soaring—yet many users and health care practitioners are in the dark about these products' adverse effects and potential interactions with prescription and over-the-counter drugs. This section gives basic information that may help your patient use herbs more safely.

Monographs on therapeutic drug classes familiarize you with the overall attributes of an entire drug class and the individual drugs within that class. These monographs also list other drugs the prescriber may substitute if a particular drug in the same class is unsuitable for your patient.

Part 3: Appendices, selected references, and index

Appendices serve as handy references on drug safety topics and related issues—everything from managing overdoses and reporting adverse events to monitoring for therapeutic and toxic drug levels. One appendix even presents a sampling of drug imprint codes, with instructions on how to access additional imprint codes on the book's companion website.

The book's comprehensive index allows you to look up a drug by its generic name, trade name, or indications.

Website and other bonuses

Our website, www.nursesdrughandbook.com, gives you 24-hour access to hundreds of drug imprint codes, online versions of all the book's safety guidelines, drug news (including new approvals and indications), downloadable monographs of the top 50 most commonly prescribed drugs, continuing education modules that focus on drug administration, and patient teaching aids on common drugs (which you can customize and give to patients). We'll keep adding more features to the website, so visit often.

Acknowledgments

A project of this size and scope could not have been initiated or completed without the support, contributions, and dedication of many individuals. My thanks to the entire Nursing Spectrum team, especially my friends and colleagues Patti Rager and Steven Hauber, who championed this project from the start (and without whom this project wouldn't exist), and to Cindy Saver for her generous assistance with acquisitions and her valuable editorial critiques.

I'm particularly indebted to the exceptional MedVantage team—Minnie Rose, clinical manager; Kathy Goldberg, editorial manager; Stephanie Peters, design manager; and Julia Knipe, editorial assistant—for their generosity, expertise, and tireless efforts to make this book the best it can be. I also wish to thank Don Saul, Karen Comerford, and Joe Clark; if it weren't for their diligence and hard work, we might not have met our deadline.

Thanks also to the many nurses and pharmacists who so generously shared their expertise by serving as advisors, contributors, and reviewers.

Special thanks to my immediate family for their love and support, especially my husband Bill for his patience, support, and willingness to go that extra mile.

Finally, I'd like to acknowledge nurses everywhere for your inspiration, commitment, and dedication to providing the best patient care. I'm proud to be one of you.

I'm certain *2005 Nursing Spectrum Drug Handbook* will enhance your practice and help you make drug therapy safer and more effective for your patients. No matter how complex the drug or the drug regimen, this book will serve as a reliable resource that will help you master the demands of drug administration.

Patricia Dwyer Schull, RN, MSN
Author

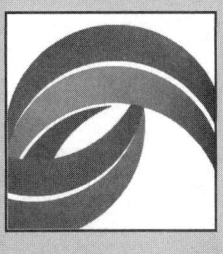

Part 1

Drugs A to Z

Photogallery of common tablets and capsules

Safe drug administration

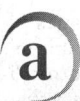

abacavir sulfate
Ziagen

Pharmacologic class: Carbocyclic nucleoside reverse transcriptase
Therapeutic class: Antiretroviral
Pregnancy risk category C

Action
Inhibits activity of human immunodeficiency virus-1 (HIV-1) reverse transcriptase; interferes with DNA and RNA synthesis, thereby inhibiting viral reproduction

Availability
Oral solution: 20 mg/ml
Tablets: 300 mg

Indications and dosages
➤ HIV-1 infection (in combination with other antiretrovirals)
Adults: 300 mg P.O. b.i.d.
Children ages 3 months to 16 years: 8 mg/kg P.O. b.i.d., to a maximum dosage of 300 mg b.i.d.

Contraindications
- Hypersensitivity to drug
- Liver disease, lactic acidosis
- Breastfeeding
- Children younger than age 3 months

Administration
◀€ Be aware that drug may cause fatal hypersensitivity reactions.
- Give with food if GI upset occurs.
- Always give in combination with other antiretrovirals.

Route	Onset	Peak	Duration
P.O.	Unknown	0.5-1.7 hr	Unknown

Adverse reactions
CNS: headache, weakness, insomnia
GI: nausea, vomiting, diarrhea, poor appetite, pancreatitis
Hematologic: neutropenia, severe anemia
Hepatic: liver failure
Metabolic: mild hyperglycemia, **lactic acidosis**
Skin: rash, erythema multiforme, **toxic epidermal necrolysis**
Other: body fat redistribution, **Stevens-Johnson syndrome, fatal hypersensitivity reaction**

Interactions
Drug-diagnostic tests. *Alanine aminotransferase, aspartate aminotransferase, creatine phosphokinase, gammaglutamyltransferase, glucose, triglycerides:* increased levels
Drug-herb. *St. John's wort:* decreased drug blood level and reduced drug effect
Drug-behaviors. *Alcohol use:* increased drug half-life and concentration

Precautions
Use cautiously in:
- impaired renal function, bone marrow suppression
- risk factors for liver disease
- elderly patients
- pregnant patients.

Patient monitoring
◀€ Assess for severe lactic acidosis, especially in women and obese patients.
◀€ Evaluate closely for signs and symptoms of hypersensitivity reaction, which can be fatal. These include fever, rash, fatigue, nausea, vomiting, diarrhea, and abdominal pain.
◀€ Never restart therapy if patient has experienced previous hypersensitivity reaction.
- Check for liver enlargement.

• Monitor complete blood count, serum electrolytes, and liver and kidney function test results.

Patient teaching

🔈 Teach patient to recognize hypersensitivity reaction. Instruct him to stop taking drug and contact prescriber immediately if signs or symptoms of a reaction occur.

🔈 Tell patient to contact prescriber if he develops a rash (possible sign of Stevens-Johnson syndrome).

• Tell patient to take with food to minimize GI upset.

• Inform patient that drug doesn't cure HIV but lowers viral count.

• Instruct patient to obtain medication guide and warning card with each refill.

• Instruct patient to refrigerate drug but not to freeze it.

• Tell patient that he'll undergo frequent blood and urine testing during therapy.

abciximab
c7E3 Fab, ReoPro♣

Pharmacologic class: Platelet aggregation inhibitor
Therapeutic class: Antithrombotic, antiplatelet drug
Pregnancy risk category C

Action

Inhibits fibrinogen binding and platelet-platelet interaction by impeding fibrinogen binding to platelet's receptor sites, thereby prolonging bleeding time

Availability

Injection: 2 mg/ml (5-ml vials containing 10 mg)

Indications and dosages

➤ Adjunct to aspirin and heparin to prevent acute cardiac ischemic complications in patients undergoing percutaneous coronary intervention (PCI)
Adults: 0.25 mg/kg I.V. bolus given 10 to 60 minutes before start of PCI, followed by an infusion of 0.125 mcg/kg/minute for 12 hours. Maximum dosage is 10 mcg/minute.

➤ Adjunct to aspirin and heparin in patients with unstable angina who haven't responded to conventional medical therapy and will undergo PCI within 24 hours
Adults: 0.25 mg/kg I.V. bolus, followed by 18- to 24-hour infusion of 10 mcg/minute, ending 1 hour after PCI

Contraindications

• Hypersensitivity to drug
• Active internal bleeding
• Severe, uncontrolled hypertension
• Thrombocytopenia
• Neutropenia
• Aneurysm
• Arteriovenous malformation
• History of cerebrovascular accident
• Oral anticoagulant therapy within past 7 days

Administration

🔈 Stop continuous infusion after failed PCI.

• Give through separate I.V. line with no other drugs.

• Avoid noncompressible I.V. sites, such as subclavian or jugular vein.

• Restrict patient to bed rest for 6 to 8 hours after drug withdrawal, or 4 hours after heparin withdrawal (whichever occurs first).

• After catheter removal, apply pressure to femoral artery for at least 30 minutes.

Route	Onset	Peak	Duration
I.V.	Rapid	30 min	48 hr

Adverse reactions

CNS: dizziness, anxiety, agitation, abnormal thinking, hypoesthesia, difficulty speaking, confusion, weakness, cerebral ischemia, **coma**
CV: pseudoaneurysm, palpitations, vascular disorders, arteriovenous fistula, hypotension, peripheral edema, weak pulse, intermittent claudication, bradycardia, **ventricular or supraventricular tachycardia, atrial fibrillation or flutter, atrioventricular block, nodal arrhythmias, pericardial effusion, embolism, thrombophlebitis**
EENT: abnormal or double vision
GI: nausea, vomiting, diarrhea, constipation, dyspepsia, ileus, gastroesophageal reflux, dry mouth, enlarged abdomen
GU: urinary tract infection, urine retention or urinary incontinence, painful urination, frequent voiding, abnormal renal function, cystalgia, prostatitis
Hematologic: anemia, **leukocytosis, thrombocytopenia, bleeding**
Metabolic: hyperkalemia, diabetes mellitus
Musculoskeletal: myopathy, myalgia, increased muscle tension, reduced muscle stretching ability
Respiratory: pneumonia, crackles, rhonchi, bronchitis, pleurisy, **pleural effusion, bronchospasm, pulmonary edema, pulmonary embolism**
Skin: pallor, cellulitis, petechiae, pruritus, bullous eruptions, diaphoresis
Other: abscess, peripheral coldness, development of human antichimeric antibodies

Interactions

Drug-drug. *Drugs that affect hemostasis (such as aspirin, dextran, dipyridamole, heparin, nonsteroidal antiinflammatory drugs, oral anticoagulants, thrombolytics, ticlopidine):* increased bleeding risk
Drug-diagnostic tests. *Activated partial thromboplastin time (APTT), clotting time, prothrombin time (PT):* increased values
Platelets: decreased count

Precautions

Use cautiously in:
• patients receiving drugs that affect hemostasis (such as thrombolytics, anticoagulants, or antiplatelet drugs)
• pregnant or breastfeeding patients.

Patient monitoring

🔊 Monitor catheter insertion site frequently for bleeding.
• Assess platelet count before, during, and after therapy.
• During catheter insertion and for 6 hours after catheter removal, frequently monitor digital pulse in leg where catheter is inserted.
• Monitor complete blood count, PT, APTT, and International Normalized Ratio.
• Minimize arterial or venous punctures, automatic blood pressure cuff use, I.M. injections, nasotracheal intubation, nasogastric tube placement, and urinary catheterization.
• Use indwelling venipuncture device, such as heparin lock, to draw blood.

Patient teaching

• Tell patient what to expect during and after drug administration.
• Teach patient to minimize GI upset by eating small, frequent servings of food and drinking plenty of fluids.
• Instruct patient to report unusual bleeding or bruising.
• Caution patient to avoid activities that may cause injury; advise him to use soft toothbrush and electric razor to avoid gum and skin injury.
• Notify patient that he'll undergo regular blood testing during therapy.

acarbose
Prandase♣, Precose

Pharmacologic class: Alpha-glucosidase inhibitor
Therapeutic class: Hypoglycemic
Pregnancy risk category B

Action
Improves blood glucose control by slowing carbohydrate digestion in intestine and prolonging conversion of carbohydrates to glucose

Availability
Tablets: 25 mg, 50 mg, 100 mg

⚠ Indications and dosages
➤ Treatment of type 2 (non-insulin-dependent) diabetes mellitus when diet alone doesn't control blood glucose (used alone or in combination with insulin, metformin, or sulfonylureas, such as glipizide, glyburide, or glimepiride)
Adults: Initially, 25 mg P.O. t.i.d. with first bite of each meal. Increase q 4 to 8 weeks as needed until maintenance dosage is reached. Maximum dosage is 100 mg P.O. t.i.d. for adults weighing more than 60 kg (132 lb); 50 mg P.O. t.i.d. for adults weighing 60 kg or less.

Contraindications
• Hypersensitivity to drug
• Renal dysfunction
• Type 1 diabetes mellitus, diabetic ketoacidosis
• GI disease
• Cirrhosis
• Colonic ulceration
• Pregnancy or breastfeeding

Administration
• Give daily with first bite of patient's three main meals.

• Know that drug prevents breakdown of table sugar (sucrose); thus, mild hypoglycemia must be corrected with oral glucose (such as dextrose or D-glucose), and severe hypoglycemia may warrant I.V glucose or glucagon injection.

Route	Onset	Peak	Duration
P.O.	Rapid	1 hr	Unknown

Adverse reactions
GI: diarrhea, abdominal pain, flatulence
Metabolic: hypoglycemia (when used with insulin or sulfonylureas)

Interactions
Drug-drug. *Activated charcoal, calcium channel blockers, corticosteroids, digestive enzymes, diuretics, estrogen, hormonal contraceptives, isoniazid, nicotinic acid, phenothiazines, phenytoin, sympathomimetics, thyroid products:* decreased therapeutic effect of acarbose
Insulin, sulfonylureas: hypoglycemia
Digoxin: decreased blood digoxin level and reduced therapeutic effect
Drug-diagnostic tests. *Alanine aminotransferase, aspartate aminotransferase:* increased levels
Calcium, vitamin B_6: decreased levels
Hematocrit: decreased value

Precautions
Use cautiously in:
• patients receiving concurrent hypoglycemics
• children.

Patient monitoring
• Monitor patient for hypoglycemia if he is taking drug concurrently with insulin or sulfonylureas.
• Stay alert for hyperglycemia during periods of increased stress.
• Assess GI signs and symptoms to differentiate drug effects from those caused by paralytic ileus.

• Check 1-hour postprandial glucose level to gauge drug's efficacy.
• Monitor liver function test results; report abnormalities so that dosage adjustments may be made as needed.

Patient teaching
• Inform patient that drug may cause serious interactions with many common medications, so he should tell all prescribers he's taking drug.
• Instruct patient about other ways to control blood glucose level, such as following recommendations regarding diet, exercise, weight reduction, and stress management.
• Stress importance of testing urine and blood glucose regularly.
• Teach patient about signs and symptoms of hypoglycemia. Tell him that although this drug doesn't cause hypoglycemia when used alone, hypoglycemic symptoms may arise if he takes it with other hypoglycemics.
• Urge patient to keep oral glucose on hand to correct mild hypoglycemia; inform him that sugar in candy won't correct hypoglycemia.
• Inform patient that GI symptoms such as flatulence may result from delayed digestion of carbohydrate in intestine.
• Advise patient to obtain medical alert identification and to carry or wear it at all times.

acebutolol hydrochloride
Monitan✿, Rhotral✿, Sectral

Pharmacologic class: Beta-adrenergic blocker (selective)

Therapeutic class: Antihypertensive, antiarrhythmic (class II)

Pregnancy risk category B

Action
At low doses, selectively inhibits response to adrenergic stimulation by blocking cardiac beta$_1$-adrenergic receptors (with little effect on beta$_2$-adrenergic receptors of bronchial and vascular smooth muscle). At high doses, inhibits both beta$_1$- and beta$_2$-adrenergic receptors, causing airway resistance.

Availability
Capsules: 200 mg, 400 mg
Tablets: 100 mg, 200 mg, 400 mg

💊 Indications and dosages
➤ Hypertension
Adults: Initially, 400 mg P.O. daily or 200 mg b.i.d. Optimal response usually occurs at 400 to 800 mg daily. For severe hypertension, increase dosage gradually to a maximum of 1,200 mg daily in two divided doses.
➤ Premature ventricular arrhythmias
Adults: Initially, 200 mg P.O. b.i.d. Increase dosage gradually until optimum response occurs, usually at 600 to 1,200 mg daily.
Dosage adjustment
• Renal impairment
• Elderly patients

Off-label uses
• Acute phase of myocardial infarction (MI)
• Stable angina

Contraindications
• Hypersensitivity to drug
• Heart failure or cardiogenic shock
• Second- or third-degree heart block
• Severe bradycardia
• Obstructive airway disease
• Breastfeeding

Administration
◀€ Withhold drug and notify prescriber if patient's apical pulse is below 60 beats/minute.

• Before surgery, notify anesthesiologist that patient is receiving drug.

Route	Onset	Peak	Duration
P.O. (blood pressure effect)	1-1.5 hr	2-8 hr	12-24 hr
P.O. (antiarrhythmic effect)	1 hr	4-6 hr	Up to 10 hr

Adverse reactions

CNS: fatigue, lethargy, insomnia, dizziness, depression, short-term memory loss, emotional lability, anxiety, confusion, headache, partial sensation loss, hemiparesis

CV: hypotension, chest pain, palpitations, peripheral vascular insufficiency, peripheral vasodilation, worsening arterial insufficiency, claudication, **bradycardia, heart failure, intensified atrioventricular nodal block**

EENT: dry burning eyes, abnormal or blurred vision, eye irritation and pain, conjunctivitis, tinnitus, pharyngitis

GI: nausea, vomiting, diarrhea, constipation, dyspepsia, abdominal pain, dry mouth, anorexia, **mesenteric arterial thrombosis, ischemic colitis**

GU: frequent or difficult urination, nocturia, diminished libido, impotence, Peyronie's disease

Hematologic: agranulocytosis, nonthrombocytopenic purpura

Hepatic: elevations in serum transaminase, alkaline phosphatase (ALP), low-density lipoproteins, and bilirubin

Metabolic: type 2 diabetes mellitus, hypoglycemia in nondiabetic patients, increased hypoglycemic response to insulin

Musculoskeletal: joint, back, or muscle pain

Respiratory: dyspnea, wheezing, cough, shortness of breath, **bronchospasm, bronchoconstriction**

Skin: rash, pruritus, diaphoresis

Other: fever, thirst, edema, pneumonitis, pleurisy, lupus erythematosus–like illness, **hypersensitivity reaction, pulmonary granuloma, pleuropulmonary fibrosis**

Interactions

Drug-drug. *Alpha agonists (such as nasal decongestants and other beta-adrenergic blockers):* increased risk of severe hypertension

Aluminum salts, barbiturates, calcium salts, cholestyramine, colestipol, indomethacin, nonsteroidal anti-inflammatory drugs, penicillin, rifampin, salicylates, sulfinpyrazone: decreased antihypertensive effect

Anticholinergics, hydralazine, methyldopa, prazosin: increased risk of bradycardia and hypotension

Beta$_2$-agonists (such as theophylline): decreased beta-$_2$ agonist effect, possibly leading to bronchoconstriction

Calcium channel blockers (nondihydropyridine): synergistic effects

Cardiac glycosides: additive negative effect on sinoatrial (SA) or atrioventricular node conduction, slowing or completely suppressing SA node activity

Catecholamine-depleting drugs: marked bradycardia, hypertension, vertigo, syncope, and orthostatic blood pressure changes

Diuretics: increased hypotensive effect

Epinephrine: increased risk of blocked sympathomimetic effects

Ergot alkaloids: increased risk of peripheral ischemia and gangrene

Glyburide in patients with type 2 diabetes: decreased hypoglycemic effect

Lidocaine: increased blood lidocaine level and possible drug toxicity

Drug-diagnostic tests. *Glucose tolerance test:* altered tolerance

ALP, antinuclear antibody titers, bilirubin, blood urea nitrogen, lactate dehydrogenase: increased levels

Transaminases: markedly increased levels

Drug-herb. *Aloe, buckthorn bark or berry, cascara bark, rhubarb root, senna leaf or fruit:* increased acebutolol effect

Ephedra: arrhythmias

Precautions

Use cautiously in:

- renal or hepatic impairment, inadequate cardiac function, peripheral or mesenteric vascular disease, hyperthyroidism, diabetes mellitus
- elderly patients
- pregnant patients
- children.

Patient monitoring

- Carefully monitor blood pressure during initial dosage titration; notify prescriber of significant or abrupt blood pressure decrease.
- Observe for orthostatic hypotension, especially when giving acebutolol with other antihypertensives.
- Watch closely for marked bradycardia or hypotension if giving drug with reserpine or other catecholamine-depleting agents.
- Be aware that drug may mask signs and symptoms of hypoglycemia in patients with diabetes mellitus or hyperthyroidism.

◀╚ Taper dosage gradually over 2 weeks when discontinuing. Be aware that abrupt withdrawal may exacerbate angina or precipitate MI, especially in patients with coronary artery disease.

Patient teaching

- Teach patient how to take his pulse; tell him to notify prescriber if pulse rate is below 60 beats/minute.
- Instruct patient to avoid driving and other hazardous activities until he knows how drug affects concentration, alertness, and vision.
- Teach patient to watch for and report hypoglycemia signs and symptoms.
- Instruct patient with bronchospastic disease to keep bronchodilator on hand at all times.
- Instruct patient to store drug in tight container at room temperature and protected from light.

a

acetaminophen

Abenol✤, Acephen, Aceta, Acetaminophen, Actimol, Aminofen, Apacet, Apo-Acetaminophen✤, Arthritis Foundation Pain Reliever, Aspirin Free, Aspirin Free Anacin, Aspirin Free Pain Relief, Atasol✤, Banesin, Children's Pain Reliever, Children's Tylenol Soft Chews, Dapa, Dolono, Datril, Dynafed✤, Dynafed E.X., Exdol✤, Feverall, Genapap, Genebs, Halenol, Halenol Children's, Infant's Pain Reliever, Liquiprin, Mapap, Maranox, Neopap, Oraphen-PD, Panadol, Redutemp, Ridenol, Robigesic✤, Silapap, St. Joseph Aspirin-Free Drops, Tapanol, Tempra, Tylenol, Tylenol Arthritis, Uni-Ace

Pharmacologic class: Synthetic nonopioid p-aminophenol derivative

Therapeutic class: Analgesic, antipyretic

Pregnancy risk category B

Action

Unclear; pain relief may occur through blocking of pain impulses (perhaps via inhibition of prostaglandin synthesis in CNS). Fever reduction may occur through action on heat-regulating center in hypothalamus.

Availability

Caplets, capsules: 160 mg, 500 mg, 650 mg (extended-release)
Drops: 100 mg/ml
Elixir: 80 mg/2.5 ml, 80 mg/5 ml, 120 mg/5 ml, 160 mg/5 ml
Gelcaps: 500 mg
Liquid: 160 mg/5 ml, 500 mg/15 ml
Solution: 80 mg/1.66 ml, 100 mg/1 ml, 120 mg/2.5 ml, 160 mg/5 ml, 167 mg/5 ml

Suppositories: 80 mg, 120 mg, 125 mg, 300 mg, 325 mg, 650 mg
Suspension: 32 mg/ml, 160 mg/5 ml
Syrup: 160 mg/5 ml
Tablets (chewable): 80 mg, 160 mg
Tablets (extended-release): 160 mg, 325 mg, 500 mg, 650 mg
Tablets (film-coated): 160 mg, 325 mg, 500 mg

🖊 Indications and dosages

➤ Mild to moderate pain caused by headache, muscle ache, backache, minor arthritis, common cold, toothache, or menstrual cramps; fever
Adults: 325 to 650 mg P.O. q 4 to 6 hours, or 1,000 mg three or four times daily. Or two extended-release caplets or tablets P.O. q 8 hours, to a maximum dosage of 4,000 mg/day. Or 650 mg P.R. q 4 to 6 hours, to a maximum dosage of 4,000 mg/day.

Oral use

Age	Usual dosage	Maximum dosage
11-12 years	480 mg q 4 hr	5 doses in 24 hr
9-10 years	400 mg q 4 hr	5 doses in 24 hr
6-8 years	320 mg q 4 hr	5 doses in 24 hr
4-5 years	240 mg q 4 hr	5 doses in 24 hr
2-3 years	160 mg q 4 hr	5 doses in 24 hr
1 year	120 mg q 4 hr	5 doses in 24 hr
4-11 months	80 mg q 4 hr	5 doses in 24 hr
0-3 months	40 mg q 4 hr	5 doses in 24 hr

Rectal use

Age	Usual dosage	Maximum dosage
6-12 years	325 mg q 4 to 6 hr	2,600 mg/day
3-6 years	120-125 mg q 4-6 hr	720 mg/day
1-3 years	80 mg q 4 hr	
3-11 months	80 mg q 6 hr	

Dosage adjustment
• Renal or hepatic impairment

Contraindications
• Hypersensitivity to drug

Administration
• Be aware that although most patients tolerate acetaminophen well, toxicity can occur with a single dose.
• Know that acetylcysteine may be ordered to treat acetaminophen toxicity, depending on patient's blood drug level. Activated charcoal is used to treat acute, recent acetaminophen overdose (within 1 hour of ingestion).
• Determine overdose severity by measuring blood acetaminophen level no sooner than 4 hours after overdose ingestion (to ensure that peak concentration has been reached).

Route	Onset	Peak	Duration
P.O.	0.5-1 hr	10-60 min	3-8 hr (dose dependent)
P.R.	0.5-1 hr	10-60 min	3-4 hr

Adverse reactions
Hematologic: hemolytic anemia, **neutropenia, leukopenia, pancytopenia, thrombocytopenia**
Hepatic: jaundice, **hepatotoxicity**
Metabolic: hypoglycemic coma
Skin: rash, urticaria
Other: hypersensitivity reactions (such as fever)

Interactions
Drug-drug. *Activated charcoal, cholestyramine, colestipol:* decreased acetaminophen absorption
Barbiturates, carbamazepine, diflunisal, hydantoins, isoniazid, rifabutin, rifampin, sulfinpyrazone: increased risk of hepatotoxicity
Hormonal contraceptives: decreased acetaminophen efficacy
Oral anticoagulants: increased anticoagulant effect
Phenothiazines (such as chlorpromazine, fluphenazine, thioridazine): severe hypothermia

Zidovudine: increased risk of granulocytopenia

Drug-diagnostic tests. *Home blood glucose measurement systems, urine 5-hydroxyindole acetic acid:* false-positive results

Drug-behaviors. *Alcohol use:* increased risk of hepatotoxicity

Precautions

Use cautiously in:
• anemia, hepatic or renal disease
• elderly patients
• pregnant or breastfeeding patients
• children younger than age 2.

Patient monitoring

• Observe for acute toxicity and overdose. Signs and symptoms of acute toxicity are as follows—*Phase 1:* nausea, vomiting, anorexia, malaise, diaphoresis. *Phase 2:* right upper quadrant pain or tenderness, liver enlargement, elevated bilirubin and liver enzyme levels, prolonged prothrombin time, oliguria (occasional). *Phase 3:* recurrent anorexia, nausea, vomiting, and malaise; jaundice; hypoglycemia; coagulopathy; encephalopathy; possible renal failure and cardiomyopathy. *Phase 4:* either recovery or progression to fatal complete liver failure.

Patient teaching

• Caution parents or other caregivers not to give acetaminophen to children younger than age 2 without consulting prescriber first.
• Tell patient, parents, or other caregivers not to use drug concurrently with other acetaminophen-containing products.
• Teach patient, parents, or other caregivers to contact prescriber if fever or other symptoms persist despite taking recommended amount of drug.
• Inform patient with chronic alcoholism that drug may increase risk of severe liver damage.

a

acetazolamide

Acetazolam♣, AK-Zol, Apo-Acetazolamide♣, Dazamide, Diamox, Diamox Sequels, Storzolamide

Pharmacologic class: Carbonic anhydrase inhibitor

Therapeutic class: Diuretic, antiglaucoma drug, anticonvulsant, altitude agent, urinary alkalinizer

Pregnancy risk category C

Action

Inhibits carbonic anhydrase in kidneys, decreasing reabsorption of water, sodium, potassium, and bicarbonate. Lowers intraocular pressure by decreasing aqueous humor. May raise seizure threshold by reducing carbonic anhydrase in CNS, thereby decreasing neuronal conduction.

Availability

Capsules (sustained-release): 500 mg
Injection: 500 mg/vial
Tablets: 125 mg, 250 mg

🖊 Indications and dosages

➤ Open-angle (chronic simple) glaucoma (given with miotics)
Adults: 250 mg P.O. one to four times daily, or 500-mg extended-release capsule P.O. once or twice daily. Don't exceed total daily dosage of 1 g.
➤ Preoperative treatment of closed-angle (secondary) glaucoma
Adults: 250 mg P.O. q 4 hours or 250 mg P.O. b.i.d.; in acute cases only, 500 mg P.O. followed by 125 to 250 mg P.O. q 4 hours. For rapid relief of increased intraocular pressure, 500 mg I.V., repeated in 2 to 4 hours; then 125 to 250 mg P.O. q 4 to 6 hours.
Children: 10 to 15 mg/kg/day P.O. in divided doses q 6 to 8 hours, or 5 to 10 mg/kg I.V. q 6 hours

---

♣ Canada ◀€ Clinical alert Reactions in **bold** are life-threatening

➤ Seizure disorder (given with other anticonvulsants)

Adults and children: 250 mg P.O. daily when given with another anticonvulsant, or 8 to 30 mg/kg daily P.O. in one to four divided doses. Usual dosage range is 375 mg to 1 g daily.

➤ Drug-induced edema or edema secondary to heart failure

Adults: Initially, 250 to 375 mg P.O. daily. If diuresis fails, give dose on alternate days, or give for 2 days alternating with day of rest.

Children: 5 mg/kg P.O. daily, or 150 mg/m² P.O. or I.V. once daily in morning

➤ Acute high-altitude (mountain) sickness

Adults: 500 mg to 1 g P.O. daily in divided doses, or sustained-release capsule q 12 to 24 hours. Begin dosing 24 to 48 hours before ascent, give during ascent, and continue giving for 48 hours after reaching desired altitude. For rapid ascent, 1-g P.O. dose is recommended.

Dosage adjustment
• Mild renal failure

Off-label uses
• Acute pancreatitis
• Alkalosis after open-heart surgery
• Hereditary ataxia
• Peptic ulcer
• Periodic paralysis
• Renal calculi
• Phenobarbital or lithium overdose
• Hydrocephalus in infants

Contraindications
• Hypersensitivity to drug or sulfonamides
• Adrenocortical insufficiency
• Closed-angle glaucoma
• Severe pulmonary obstruction
• Severe renal disease, hypokalemia, hyponatremia
• Hepatic disease

Administration
◀ Before giving, ask if patient is pregnant; drug may cause fetal toxicity.
• Direct I.V. administration is preferred. When giving by direct I.V. route, reconstitute 500-mg vial with more than 5 ml of sterile water for injection; administer over 1 minute.
• When giving drug intermittently, further dilute with normal saline solution or dextrose solution and infuse over 4 to 8 hours.
• Be aware that I.M. administration is painful because solution is alkaline.
• If necessary, crush tablets and mix in nonsweet, nonalcoholic syrup or nonglycerin solution.

Route	Onset	Peak	Duration
P.O.	1 hr	2-4 hr	8-12 hr
P.O. (sustained)	2 hr	8-12 hr	18-24
I.V., I.M.	1-2 min	15-18 min	4-5 hr

Adverse reactions
CNS: weakness, nervousness, irritability, drowsiness, confusion, dizziness, depression, tremor, headache, paresthesia, flaccid paralysis, **seizures**
EENT: transient myopia, tinnitus, hearing dysfunction, sensation of lump in throat, altered taste and smell
GI: nausea, vomiting, diarrhea, constipation, melena, abdominal distention, dry mouth, anorexia
GU: dysuria, hematuria, glycosuria, polyuria, crystalluria, renal colic, renal calculi, **uremia, sulfonamide-like renal lesions, renal failure**
Hematologic: hemolytic anemia, **leukopenia, agranulocytosis, thrombocytopenia, thrombocytopenic purpura, pancytopenia, bone marrow depression with aplastic anemia**
Hepatic: elevated bilirubin level, **hepatic insufficiency**
Metabolic: hypokalemia, hyperchloremic acidosis, hyperglycemia and

glycosuria, hyperuricemia and gout, metabolic acidosis
Respiratory: hyperpnea
Skin: rash, pruritus, urticaria, photosensitivity, hirsutism, cyanosis
Other: weight loss, fever, excessive thirst, pain at I.M. injection site, **hypersensitivity reactions, Stevens-Johnson syndrome**

Interactions

Drug-drug. *Amphetamines, procainamide, quinidine, tricyclic antidepressants:* decreased excretion and enhanced or prolonged effect of these drugs, leading to toxicity
Amphotericin B, corticosteroids, corticotrophin, other diuretics: increased risk of hypokalemia
Lithium, phenobarbital, salicylates: increased excretion of these drugs, possibly reducing their efficacy
Methenamine compounds: inactivation of these drugs
Phenytoin, primidone: severe osteomalacia
Salicylates: increased risk of salicylate toxicity
Drug-diagnostic tests. *Ammonia, bilirubin, glucose, chloride, uric acid, calcium:* increased levels
Thyroid iodine uptake: decreased uptake in patients with hyperthyroidism or normal thyroid function
Urinary protein (with some reagents): false-positive result
Drug-behaviors. *Sun exposure:* increased risk of photosensitivity

Precautions

Use cautiously in:
• respiratory disease, renal disease, hepatic disease, diabetes mellitus, hypercalcemia, gout, adrenocortical insufficiency
• pregnant or breastfeeding patients.

Patient monitoring

◀◉ Evaluate for signs and symptoms of sulfonamide sensitivity; drug can cause fatal hypersensitivity.
◀◉ Monitor laboratory test results for hematologic changes; blood glucose, potassium, bicarbonate, and chloride levels; and hepatic and renal function changes.
• Observe for signs and symptoms of bleeding tendency.
• Monitor fluid intake and output.

Patient teaching

• Advise patient to take drug with food if GI upset occurs.
• Teach patient to avoid driving and other hazardous activities until he knows how drug affects concentration and alertness.
• Tell patient to eat potassium-rich foods (such as seafood, bananas, and oranges) if taking drug long term or receiving other potassium-depleting drugs.
• Teach patient to avoid activities that can cause injury. Advise him to use soft toothbrush and electric razor to avoid gum and skin injury.
• Tell patient to report significant numbness or tingling.
• Inform patient that he'll undergo regular blood testing during therapy.

acetylcysteine
(*N*-acetylcysteine)
Mucomyst✤, Mucomyst 10, Mucosil-10, Mucosil-20, Parvolex✤

Pharmacologic class: *N*-acetyl derivative of naturally occurring amino acid (L-cysteine)
Therapeutic class: Mucolytic, acetaminophen antidote
Pregnancy risk category B

Action

Decreases viscosity of secretions; promotes secretion removal through coughing, postural drainage, and mechanical means. Also maintains and restores hepatic glutathione (needed to inactivate toxic metabolites in acetaminophen overdose).

Availability

Injection: 200 mg/ml
Solution: 10%, 20%

⏰ Indications and dosages

➤ Mucolytic agent in adjunctive treatment of abnormal, thick, viscid mucus secretions in acute and chronic bronchopulmonary disease (bronchitis, bronchiectasis, chronic asthmatic bronchitis, emphysema, pneumonia, primary amyloidism of lungs, tuberculosis, tracheobronchitis), pulmonary complications of cystic fibrosis, atelectasis caused by mucus obstruction, or pulmonary complications related to surgery, anesthesia, posttraumatic chest conditions, or tracheostomy care
Adults, children, elderly patients: 2 to 10 ml of 10% solution or 1 to 10 ml of 20% solution by nebulization into face mask three or four times daily
Adults and children: 1 to 2 ml of 10% or 20% solution q 1 to 4 hours by direct instillation into tracheostomy
➤ Diagnostic bronchial studies
Adults and children: Two to three doses of 1 to 2 ml of 20% solution or 2 to 4 ml of 10% solution by nebulization or intratracheal instillation
➤ Acetaminophen overdose
Adults, children, elderly patients: Give immediately if 24 hours or less have elapsed since acetaminophen ingestion. Use the following protocol: Empty stomach by lavage or by inducing emesis with ipecac syrup, then have patient drink copious amounts of water; if no emesis occurs within 20 minutes, repeat ipecac dose. Draw blood for acetaminophen plasma assay, pro-

thrombin time, and bilirubin, blood glucose, and creatinine clearance levels. If ingested acetaminophen dose is in toxic range, give acetylcysteine 140 mg/kg P.O. as loading dose from 20% solution. Administer 17 maintenance doses of 70 mg/kg P.O. q 4 hours, starting 4 hours after loading dose. Repeat procedure until acetaminophen blood level is safe.

Off-label uses

• Unstable angina

Contraindications

• Hypersensitivity to drug (except with antidotal use)
• Status asthmaticus (except with antidotal use)

Administration

• Separate administration times of this drug and antibiotics.
• Use plastic, glass, or stainless steel container when giving by nebulizer because solution discolors on contact with rubber and some metals.
• Once solution is exposed to air, use within 96 hours.

Route	Onset	Peak	Duration
P.O.	30-60 min	1-2 hr	Unknown
Instillation, inhalation	1 min	5-10 min	2-3 hr

Adverse reactions

CNS: dizziness, drowsiness, headache
CV: hypotension, hypertension, tachycardia
EENT: severe rhinorrhea, tooth damage
GI: nausea, vomiting, stomatitis, constipation, anorexia
Hepatic: abnormal liver function test results, **hepatotoxicity**
Respiratory: hemoptysis, tracheal and bronchial irritation, increased secretions, wheezing, chest tightness, **bronchospasm**

Skin: urticaria, rash, clamminess, angioedema
Other: chills, fever

Interactions
Drug-drug. *Activated charcoal:* increased absorption and decreased efficacy of acetylcysteine
Nitroglycerine: increased nitroglycerine effects, causing hypotension and headache
Drug-diagnostic tests. *Alanine aminotransferase, aspartate aminotransferase:* increased levels

Precautions
Use cautiously in:
• renal or hepatic disease, Addison's disease, alcoholism, brain tumor, bronchial asthma, seizure disorders, hypothyroidism, respiratory insufficiency, psychosis
• elderly patients
• pregnant or breastfeeding patients.

Patient monitoring
• Monitor respirations, cough, and character of secretions.

Patient teaching
• Instruct patient to report worsening cough and other respiratory symptoms.
• Advise patient to mix oral form with juice or cola to mask bad taste and odor.

a

acetylsalicylic acid (aspirin)
Acuprin, Apo-Asa✦, Apo–ASEN✦, Arthrinol✦, Arthrisin✦, Arthritis Foundation Pain Reliever, Artria S.R.✦, ASA, Aspergum, Aspirin✦, Aspir-Low, Aspirtab, Astrin✦, Bayer, Coryphen✦, Easprin, Ecotrin, Empirin, Entrophen✦, Genprin, Halfprin, Headache Tablet✦, Healthprin, Heartline, Norwich, Novasen✦, PMS-ASA✦, Sal-Adult✦, Sal-Infant✦, Sloprin, St. Joseph, Supasa✦, Sureprin, ZORprin

Pharmacologic class: Nonsteroidal anti-inflammatory drug (NSAID)
Therapeutic class: Nonopioid analgesic, antipyretic, antiplatelet drug
Pregnancy risk category C (with full dose in third trimester: *D*)

Action
Reduces pain and inflammation by inhibiting prostaglandin production. Fever reduction mechanism unknown; may be linked to decrease in endogenous pyrogens in hypothalamus resulting from prostaglandin inhibition. Exerts antiplatelet effect by inhibiting synthesis of prostacyclin and thromboxane A_2.

Availability
Gum (chewable): 227 mg
Suppositories: 60 mg, 120 mg, 200 mg, 300 mg, 325 mg, 600 mg, 650 mg
Tablets: 81 mg, 325 mg, 500 mg, 650 mg (extended-release)
Tablets (chewable): 81 mg
Tablets (enteric-coated, delayed-release): 81 mg, 162 mg, 325 mg, 500 mg, 650 mg, 975 mg
Tablets (extended-release): 800 mg
Tablets (film-coated): 325 mg, 500 mg

❶ Indications and dosages

➣ Mild pain or fever
Adults: 325 to 500 mg P.O. q 3 hours, or 325 to 650 mg P.O. q 4 hours, or 650 to 1,000 mg P.O. q 6 hours, to a maximum dosage of 4,000 mg/day. Extended-release tablets—650 mg q 8 hours, or 800 mg q 12 hours.

Children: 65 mg/kg/24 hours in two to six divided doses, not to exceed total daily dosage of 3.6 g. See chart below.

Age (years)	Dosage (q 4 hr)
11-12	486 mg
9-10	405 mg
6-8	324 mg
4-5	243 mg
2-3	162 mg

➣ Mild to moderate pain caused by inflammation (as in rheumatoid arthritis or osteoarthritis)
Adults: 3.2 to 6 g/day P.O. in divided doses, to a maximum dosage of 6 g/day
Children: 10 to 15 mg/kg/day P.O. in divided doses q 4 to 6 hours, to a maximum dosage of 80 mg/kg/day
➣ Juvenile rheumatoid arthritis
Children: 60 to 110 mg/kg/day P.O. or P.R. in divided doses q 6 to 8 hours
➣ Acute rheumatic fever
Adults: 5 to 8 g/day P.O. in divided doses
Children: Initially, 100 mg/kg/day in individual doses for first 2 weeks; then maintenance dosage of 75 mg/kg/day in divided doses for next 4 to 6 weeks
➣ To reduce the risk of transient ischemic attacks (TIAs) or cerebrovascular accident in men with a history of TIAs caused by emboli
Adults: 650 mg P.O. b.i.d or 325 mg P.O. q.i.d.
➣ To reduce the risk of myocardial infarction (MI) in patients with a history of MI or unstable angina
Adult: 75 to 325 mg/day P.O. or P.R.

➣ Kawasaki disease
Children: Initially, 80 to120 mg/kg/day P.O. in four divided doses. Maintenance dosage is 3 to 8 mg/kg/day in a single dose for up to 8 weeks.
➣ Thromboembolic disorders
Adults: 325 to 650 P.O. mg once or twice daily

Contraindications

• Hypersensitivity to salicylates, other NSAIDs, or tartrazine
• Impaired renal function
• Severe hepatic impairment
• Hemorrhagic states or blood coagulation defects
• Vitamin K deficiency caused by dehydration
• Concurrent anticoagulant use
• Pregnancy (third trimester) or breastfeeding

Administration

◀€ Never administer to child or adolescent who has signs or symptoms of chickenpox or flulike illness.
◀€ Don't give within 6 weeks after administration of live varicella virus vaccine because of risk of Reye's syndrome.
• Give with food or large amounts of water or milk to minimize GI irritation.
• Know that extended-release or enteric-coated forms are best for long-term therapy.
• Be aware that aspirin should be discontinued at least 1 week before surgery because it may inhibit platelet aggregation.

Route	Onset	Peak	Duration
P.O. (tablets)	15-30 min	1-2 hr	4-6 hr
P.O. (chewable)	Rapid	Unknown	1-4 hr
P.O. (enteric-coated)	5-30 min	2-4 hr	8-12 hr
P.O. (extended)	5-30 min	1-4 hr	3-6 hr
P.R.	5-30 min	3-4 hr	1-4 hr

Adverse reactions

EENT: hearing loss, tinnitus, oto-toxicity

GI: nausea, vomiting, abdominal pain, dyspepsia, epigastric distress, heartburn, anorexia, **GI bleeding**

Hematologic: hemolytic anemia, prolonged bleeding time, prolonged prothrombin time, prolonged activated partial thromboplastin time (APTT), **leukopenia, agranulocytosis, thrombocytopenia, shortened red blood cell life span**

Hepatic: hepatotoxicity

Metabolic: hypoglycemia, hyponatremia, hypokalemia

Respiratory: wheezing, hyperpnea, **pulmonary edema with toxicity**

Skin: rash, urticaria, bruising, angioedema

Other: hypersensitivity reactions, **salicylism or acute toxicity** (signs and symptoms include diplopia, electrocardiogram abnormalities, generalized seizures, hallucinations, hyperthermia, oliguria, acute renal failure, incoherent speech, irritability, restlessness, tremor, vertigo, confusion, disorientation, mania, lethargy, laryngeal edema, anaphylaxis, and coma)

Interactions

Drug-drug. *Acidifying drugs (such as ammonium chloride):* increased salicylate blood level

Activated charcoal: decreased salicylate absorption

Alkalinizing drugs (such as antacids): decreased salicylate blood level

Angiotensin-converting enzyme (ACE) inhibitors: decreased antihypertensive effect

Anticoagulants, NSAIDs, thrombolytics: increased bleeding risk

Carbonic anhydrase inhibitors (such as acetazolamide): salicylism

Corticosteroids: increased salicylate excretion and decreased blood level

Furosemide: increased diuretic effect

Live varicella virus vaccine: increased risk of Reye's syndrome

Methotrexate: decreased methotrexate excretion and increased blood level, causing greater risk of toxicity

Nizatidine: increased salicylate blood level

Spironolactone: decreased spironolactone effect

Sulfonylureas (chlorpropamide, tolbutamide): enhanced sulfonylurea effects

Tetracycline (oral): decreased absorption of tetracycline (with buffered aspirin)

Drug-diagnostic tests. *Alanine aminotransferase, alkaline phosphatase, amylase, aspartate aminotransferase, coagulation studies, $PaCO_2$, uric acid:* increased values

Cholesterol, glucose, potassium, protein-bound iodine, sodium, thyroxine, triiodothyronine: decreased levels

Pregnancy test, protirelin-induced thyroid stimulating hormone, radionuclide thyroid imaging, serum theophylline (Schack and Waxler method), urine catecholamines, urine glucose, urine hydroxyindoleacetic acid, urine ketones (ferric chloride method), urine vanillylmandelic acid: test interference

Tests using phenosulfonphthalein as diagnostic agent: decreased urinary excretion of phenosulfonphthalein

Urine protein: increased level

Drug-food. *Urine-acidifying foods:* increased salicylate blood level

Drug-herb. *Anise, arnica, cayenne, chamomile, clove, fenugreek, feverfew, garlic, ginger, ginkgo biloba, ginseng, horse chestnut, kelpware, licorice:* increased bleeding risk

Drug-behaviors. *Alcohol use:* increased bleeding risk

Precautions

Use with extreme caution, if at all, in:
• hepatic disorders, anemia, asthma, gastritis, Hodgkin's disease

• heart failure or other conditions in which high sodium content is harmful (buffered aspirin)
• patients receiving other salicylates or NSAIDs concurrently
• elderly patients
• children and adolescents.

Patient monitoring

◀€ Watch for signs and symptoms of hypersensitivity and other adverse reactions, especially bleeding tendency.
• Monitor elderly patients carefully; they're at greater risk for salicylate toxicity.
• With prolonged therapy, frequently assess hemoglobin, hematocrit, International Normalized Ratio, and kidney function test results.
• Check salicylate blood levels frequently.
• Evaluate patient for signs and symptoms of ototoxicity (hearing loss, tinnitus, ataxia, and vertigo).

Patient teaching

• Tell patient to report ototoxicity symptoms, unusual bleeding, and bruising.
• Caution patient to avoid activities that may cause injury; advise him to use soft toothbrush and electric razor to avoid gum and skin injury.
• Instruct patient to tell all prescribers he's taking drug, because it may cause serious interactions with many common medications.
• Teach patient not to take other over-the-counter preparations containing aspirin.
• Inform patient that he may need to undergo regular blood testing during therapy.

acitretin
Soriatane

Pharmacologic class: Second-generation retinoid
Therapeutic class: Antipsoriatic
Pregnancy risk category X

Action

Unknown; promotes normal growth cycle of skin cells, possibly by targeting retinoid receptors in these cells and adjusting factors that affect epidermal proliferation and synthesis of RNA and DNA

Availability

Capsules: 10 mg, 25 mg

🚫 Indications and dosages

➤ Severe psoriasis, including erythrodermic and generalized pustule types
Adults and elderly patients: Initially, 25 to 50 mg/day P.O. as a single dose with main meal; if initial response is satisfactory, give maintenance dosage of 25 to 50 mg/day P.O.

Off-label uses

• Darier's disease (keratosis follicularis)
• Lamellar ichthyosis (in children)
• Lichen planus
• Nonbullous and bullous ichthyosiform erythroderma
• Palmoplantar pustulosis
• Sjögren-Larsson syndrome

Contraindications

• Hypersensitivity to drug or paraben (used as preservative in gelatin capsule)
• Pregnancy or anticipated pregnancy within 3 years after drug discontinuation (drug has teratogenic and embryotoxic effects)

- Women of childbearing age who may not use reliable contraception during therapy and for at least 3 years after discontinuing drug
- Breastfeeding

Administration

🔊 Verify that patient isn't pregnant before giving drug.
- Give as a single dose with main meal.

Route	Onset	Peak	Duration
P.O.	Unknown	Unknown	Unknown

Adverse reactions

CNS: headache, depression, insomnia, drowsiness, fatigue, migraine, rigors, abnormal gait, nerve inflammation, hyperesthesia, paresthesia, pseudotumor cerebri
EENT: abnormal or blurred vision, dry eyes, eye irritation, eyebrow and eyelash loss, eyelid inflammation, cataract, papilledema, conjunctivitis, corneal epithelial abnormality, reduced night vision, photophobia, recurrent styes, earache, tinnitus, hearing loss, epistaxis, rhinitis, sinusitis
GI: nausea, vomiting, diarrhea, constipation, abdominal pain, gastritis, stomatitis, glossitis, tongue ulcers, gingival bleeding, gingivitis, esophagitis, melena, painful straining at stool, pancreatitis, lip inflammation and cracking, dry mouth, abnormal taste, anorexia
GU: abnormal urine, dysuria, atrophic vaginitis, leukorrhea
Hepatic: abnormal hepatic function, jaundice, **hepatitis**
Metabolic: poor blood glucose control
Musculoskeletal: joint, muscle, back, and bone pain; arthritis; bone disorders; spinal bone overgrowth; increased muscle tone or rigidity; tendinitis
Respiratory: coughing, increased sputum, laryngitis
Skin: dry skin, pruritus, skin atrophy, skin peeling, abnormal skin odor, sticky skin, seborrhea, dermatitis, diaphoresis, cold clammy skin, skin infection, rash, pyrogenic granuloma, skin ulcers, skin fissures, sunburn, flushing, purpura, nail disorder, inflammation of tissue surrounding nails, abnormal hair texture, alopecia
Other: edema, thirst, hot flashes

Interactions

Drug-drug. *Glyburide:* increased blood glucose clearance
Methotrexate: increased risk of hepatotoxicity
Oral contraceptives ("minipill"): decreased contraceptive efficacy
Drug-diagnostic tests. *Low-density lipoproteins:* decreased level
Alanine aminotransferase, aspartate aminotransferase, triglycerides: increased levels
Drug-behaviors. *Alcohol use:* interference with acitretin elimination, possible drug toxicity

Precautions

Use cautiously in:
- hepatic or renal impairment, diabetes mellitus, obesity
- elevated cholesterol or triglyceride levels
- elderly patients.

Patient monitoring

- Monitor patient with early signs or symptoms of pseudotumor cerebri, such as headache, nausea, vomiting, and visual disturbances; discontinue drug immediately if papilledema occurs.
- Check blood lipid levels before therapy begins and every 1 to 2 weeks during therapy.
- Monitor blood glucose levels and kidney and liver function test results.
- If acitretin causes open skin lesions resulting from dermatitis or blisters, watch for signs and symptoms of infection.

• Assess for pain, stinging, and itching; apply cool compresses as needed for relief.

◀€ Be aware that women taking this drug must avoid alcohol-containing foods, beverages, medications, and over-the-counter products during therapy and for 2 months afterward.

Patient teaching
• Instruct patient to take drug with main meal to minimize GI upset.
• Teach patient to avoid driving and other hazardous activities until he knows how drug affects concentration, alertness, and vision.
• Caution patient not to drink alcohol during therapy.
◀€ Advise female to use effective contraception for at least 1 month before starting drug, throughout entire course of therapy, and for 3 years after discontinuing drug.
• Explain that disease may seem to worsen at start of therapy.
• Tell contact lens wearers that intolerance to lenses may develop.

activated charcoal
Actidose, Actidose-Aqua, CharcoAid, CharcoAid 2000, Charco Caps, Liqui-Char

Pharmacologic class: Carbon residue
Therapeutic class: Antiflatulent, antidote
Pregnancy risk category C

Action
Binds to poisons, toxins, irritants, and drugs; forms barrier between remaining particulate material and GI mucosa, thereby inhibiting GI absorption of drugs and chemicals. As an antiflatulent, reduces intestinal gas volume and relieves related discomfort.

Availability
Capsules: 260 mg
Granules: 15 g/120 ml
Liquid: 15 g/120 ml, 50 g/240 ml, 208 mg/1 ml
Oral suspension: 12.5 g/60 ml, 15 g/75 ml, 25 g/120 ml, 30 g/120 ml, 50 g/240 ml
Powder: 15, 30, 40, 130, 240 g/container

ⓘ Indications and dosages
➤ Poisoning
Adults: 25 to 100 g P.O. (or 1 g/kg, or about 10 times the amount of poison ingested) as a suspension in 120 to 240 ml (4 to 8 oz) of water
Children: Initially, 1 to 2 g/kg P.O. (or 10 times the amount of poison ingested) as a suspension in 120 to 240 ml (4 to 8 oz) of water
➤ Flatulence
Adults: 600 mg to 5 g P.O. as a single dose, or 975 mg to 3.9 g in divided doses

Off-label uses
• Diarrhea
• GI distress
• Hypercholesterolemia

Contraindications
None

Administration
◀€ Don't try to give activated charcoal to semiconscious patient.
◀€ If signs of aspiration occur, stop giving drug immediately to avoid fatal airway obstruction or infection.
• Administer by large-bore nasogastric tube after gastric lavage, as needed.
• Give within 30 minutes of poison ingestion when possible.
• Mix powder with tap water to form thick syrup. Add fruit juice or flavoring to improve taste.
• Be aware that drug inactivates ipecac syrup.

• Know that drug is ineffective in poisoning from ethanol, methanol, and iron salts.

• Don't give children more than one dose of drug product containing sorbitol (sweetener).

• When used for indications other than as antidote, give at least 2 hours before or 1 hour after other drugs.

Route	Onset	Peak	Duration
P.O.	Immediate	Unknown	Unknown

Adverse reactions

GI: nausea, vomiting, diarrhea, constipation, black stools, **intestinal obstruction**

Interactions

Drug-drug. *Acetaminophen, barbiturates, carbamazepine, digitoxin, digoxin, furosemide, glutethimide, hydantoins, methotrexate, nizatidine, phenothiazines, phenylbutazones, propoxyphene, salicylates, sulfonamides, sulfonylurea, tetracycline, theophyllines, tricyclic antidepressants, valproic acid:* decreased absorption of these drugs
Syrup of ipecac: ipecac absorption and inactivation
Drug-food. *Milk, ice cream, sherbet:* decreased absorptive activity of drug

Precautions

Use cautiously in:
• patients who have aspirated corrosives or hydrocarbons and are vomiting.

Patient monitoring

• Monitor patient for constipation.
• If patient vomits soon after receiving dose, contact prescriber about repeating dose.

Patient teaching

• Instruct patient to drink six to eight glasses of fluid daily to prevent constipation.

• Tell patient that stools will be black when charcoal is excreted from body.

a

acyclovir

acyclovir sodium

Alti-Acyclovir✤, Avirax✤, Zovirax

Pharmacologic class: Acyclic purine nucleoside analogue
Therapeutic class: Antiviral
Pregnancy risk category B

Action

Inhibits viral DNA polymerase, thereby inhibiting replication of viral DNA. Specific for herpes simplex types 1 (HSV-1) and 2 (HSV-2), varicella-zoster virus, Epstein-Barr virus, and cytomegalovirus (CMV)

Availability

Capsules: 200 mg
Injection: 50 mg/ml
Powder for injection: 500 mg/vial, 1,000 mg/vial
Suspension: 200 mg/5 ml
Tablets: 400 mg, 800 mg

✪ Indications and dosages

➤ Acute treatment of herpes zoster (shingles)
Adults: 800 mg P.O. q 4 hours while awake (5 times/day) for 7 to 10 days
➤ Initial episode of genital herpes
Adults: 200 mg P.O. q 4 hours while awake (1,000 mg/day) for 10 days
➤ Chronic suppressive therapy for recurrent genital herpes episodes
Adults: 400 mg P.O. b.i.d., or 200 mg P.O. three to five times daily for up to 12 months
➤ Intermittent therapy for recurrent genital herpes episodes
Adults: 200 mg P.O. q 4 hours while awake (5 times/day) for 5 days, initiat-

ed at first sign or symptom of recurrence

➤ Varicella (chickenpox)

Adults and children weighing more than 40 kg (88 lb): 800 mg P.O. q.i.d. for 5 days

Children older than age 2: 20 mg/kg P.O. q.i.d. for 5 days

➤ Mucosal and cutaneous herpes simplex infections (HSV-1 and HSV-2) in immunocompromised patients

Adults and children older than age 12: 5 mg/kg I.V. infusion over 1 hour given q 8 hours for 7 days

Children younger than age 12: 10 mg/kg I.V. infusion over 1 hour given q 8 hours for 7 days

➤ Herpes simplex encephalitis

Adults and children older than age 12: 10 mg/kg I.V. over 1 hour given q 8 hours for 10 days

Children ages 3 months to 12 years: 20 mg/kg I.V. over 1 hour given q 8 hours for 10 days

Children from birth to 3 months: 10 mg/kg I.V. over 1 hour given q 8 hours for 10 days

➤ Varicella zoster infections in immunocompromised patients

Adults and adolescents older than age 12: 10 mg/kg I.V. over 1 hour given q 8 hours for 7 days

Children younger than age 12: 20 mg/kg I.V. over 1 hour given q 8 hours for 7 days

Dosage adjustment
• Renal impairment
• Obesity (adult dosage based on ideal weight)
• Elderly patients

Off-label uses
• Herpes zoster encephalitis
• CMV and HSV infection after bone marrow or kidney transplantation
• Infectious mononucleosis
• Varicella pneumonia

Contraindications
• Hypersensitivity to drug or valacyclovir

Administration
• Make sure patient is adequately hydrated before starting therapy.
• Give I.V. infusion over at least 1 hour to minimize renal damage.
• Don't give by I.V. bolus or by I.M. or S.C. route.

Route	Onset	Peak	Duration
P.O.	Variable	1.5-2 hr	4 hr
I.V.	Immediate	1 hr	8 hr

Adverse reactions
CNS: aggressive behavior, dizziness, malaise, weakness, paresthesia, headache; with I.V. use—**encephalopathic changes** (lethargy, tremors, obtundation, confusion, hallucinations, agitation, seizures, coma)
CV: peripheral edema
EENT: vision abnormalities
GI: nausea, vomiting, diarrhea, gingival hyperplasia
GU: proteinuria, hematuria, crystalluria, elevated blood urea nitrogen (BUN) and creatinine levels, vaginitis, candidiasis, changes in menses, vulvitis, oliguria, **renal failure, glomerulonephritis**
Hematologic: anemia, lymphadenopathy, **thrombotic thrombocytopenic purpura/hemolytic uremic syndrome (in immunocompromised patients), thrombocytopenia, disseminated intravascular coagulation, hemolysis, leukopenia, leukoclastic vasculitis**
Hepatic: elevated liver function test results, hyperbilirubinemia, jaundice, **hepatitis**
Musculoskeletal: myalgia
Skin: photosensitivity rash, pruritus, angioedema, alopecia, urticaria, severe local inflammatory reactions with I.V. extravasation, **toxic epidermal necrolysis, erythema multiforme**

Other: fever, excessive thirst, pain at injection site, **anaphylaxis, Stevens-Johnson syndrome**

Interactions

Drug-drug. *Interferon:* additive effect
Nephrotoxic drugs: increased risk of nephrotoxicity
Probenecid: increased acyclovir blood level
Zidovudine: increased CNS effects, especially drowsiness
Drug-diagnostic tests. *Alanine aminotransferase, aspartate aminotransferase, BUN, creatinine:* increased levels

Precautions

Use cautiously in:
• preexisting serious neurologic, hepatic, pulmonary, or fluid or electrolyte abnormalities
• renal impairment
• obesity
• pregnant or breastfeeding patients.

Patient monitoring

• Monitor fluid intake and output.
• Assess for signs and symptoms of encephalopathy.
• Evaluate patient frequently for adverse reactions, especially bleeding tendency.
• Monitor complete blood count with white cell differential and kidney function test results.

Patient teaching

• Advise patient to drink enough fluids to ensure adequate urinary output.
• Teach patient to monitor urine output and report significant changes.
• Instruct patient to report unusual bleeding or bruising.
• Instruct patient to avoid driving and other hazardous activities until he knows how acyclovir affects concentration and alertness.
• Teach patient to minimize GI upset by eating small, frequent servings of food and drinking plenty of fluids.

• Tell patient to use soft toothbrush and electric razor to avoid injury to gums and skin.
• Advise patient to avoid sexual intercourse when visible herpes lesions are present.
• Advise patient that he may need to undergo regular blood testing during therapy.

adalimumab
Humira

Pharmacologic class: Biological modifier

Therapeutic class: Antirheumatic (disease-modifying), immunomodulator

Pregnancy risk category B

Action

Human immunoglobulin (Ig) G1 monoclonal antibody that binds to human tumor necrosis factor (TNF), which plays a role in inflammation and immune responses. Also modulates biological responses induced or modulated by TNF.

Availability

Injection (preservative-free): 40 mg/0.8 ml
Prefilled syringes: 40 mg/ml

🖊 Indications and dosages

➤ To reduce signs and symptoms of moderately to severely active rheumatoid arthritis and slow disease progression in patients ages 18 and older who don't respond adequately to disease-modifying antirheumatics
Adults: 40 mg S.C. every other week. Patients not receiving methotrexate concurrently may benefit from dosage increase to 40 mg weekly.

Contraindications
- Hypersensitivity to drug
- Active infection, including chronic or localized infection

Administration
- Give S.C.; rotate injection sites.
- Store in refrigerator and protect from light.

Route	Onset	Peak	Duration
S.C.	Slow	75-187 hr	Unknown

Adverse reactions
CNS: headache, **demyelinating disease**
CV: arrhythmias, hypertension
EENT: sinusitis
GI: nausea, vomiting, abdominal pain
GU: urinary tract infection, hematuria
Metabolic: hyperlipidemia, hypercholesterolemia, increased alkaline phosphatase level
Musculoskeletal: back pain
Respiratory: upper respiratory tract infection
Skin: rash
Other: accidental injury, pain and swelling at injection site, flulike symptoms, lupuslike syndrome, fungal infection, allergic reactions, **tuberculosis (TB) reactivation, malignancies**

Interactions
Drug-drug. *Immunosuppressants (including corticosteroids):* serious infection
Live-virus vaccines: serious illness

Precautions
Use cautiously in:
- preexisting or recent onset of demyelinating disorders, immunosuppression, or lymphoma
- elderly patients
- pregnant or breastfeeding patients
- children.

Patient monitoring
- Monitor complete blood count.

◀€ Monitor for signs and symptoms of infection if patient's receiving concurrent corticosteroids or other immunosuppressants (because of risk that infection may progress).

Patient teaching
- Teach patient to recognize and report signs and symptoms of allergic response and other adverse reactions.
- Tell patient that drug lowers resistance to infection; instruct him to immediately report fever, cough, breathing problems, and other infection symptoms.
- Teach patient to minimize GI upset by eating small, frequent servings of healthy food and drinking plenty of fluids.

adefovir dipivoxil
Hepsera

Pharmacologic class: Nucleotide reverse transcriptase inhibitor
Therapeutic class: Antiviral
Pregnancy risk category C

Action
Inhibits hepatitis B virus (HBV) DNA polymerase and suppresses HBV replication

Availability
Tablets: 10 mg

🖊 Indications and dosages
➢ Chronic HBV with active viral replication, plus persistent elevations in alanine aminotransferase (ALT) or aspartate aminotransferase (AST) or histologically active disease
Adults: 10 mg P.O. daily
Dosage adjustment
- Renal impairment

Contraindications
• Hypersensitivity to drug

Administration
• Offer human immunodeficiency virus (HIV) testing before starting therapy (drug may increase resistance to antiretrovirals in HIV patients).
• Give with or without food.

Route	Onset	Peak	Duration
P.O.	Rapid	0.6-4 hr	Unknown

Adverse reactions
CNS: headache
GI: nausea, vomiting, diarrhea, abdominal pain, flatulence, dyspepsia, anorexia, **pancreatitis**
GU: increasd blood urea nitrogen, **renal dysfunction**
Hepatic: elevated liver enzyme levels, **severe hepatomegaly with steatosis, hepatitis exacerbation** (if therapy is withdrawn)
Metabolic: elevated creatinine kinase, amylase, lipase, and blood glucose levels; **lactic acidosis**
Respiratory: pneumonia
Other: fever, infection, pain, resistance to antiretrovirals in patients with unrecognized HIV

Interactions
Drug-drug. *Acetaminophen, aspirin, indomethacin:* granulocytopenia
Acyclovir, adriamycin, amphotericin B, benzodiazepines, cimetidine, dapsone, doxorubicin, experimental nucleotide analogue, fluconazole, flucytosine, ganciclovir, indomethacin, interferon, morphine, phenytoin, probenecid, sulfonamide, trimethoprim, vinblastine, vincristine: increased risk of nephrotoxicity

Precautions
Use cautiously in:
• lactic acidosis, renal or hepatic impairment
• elderly patients
• pregnant or breastfeeding patients
• children.

Patient monitoring
• Monitor fluid intake and output.
• Watch for hematuria.
• Assess for signs and symptoms of lactic acidosis, especially in women and overweight patients.
• Check for liver enlargement.
• Monitor liver and kidney function test results.
• After therapy ends, monitor patient for evidence of serious hepatitis exacerbation.

Patient teaching
• Advise patient to take drug with or without food.
• Instruct patient to drink plenty of fluids to ensure adequate urine output.
• Teach patient to monitor urine output and color and to report significant changes.
• Tell patient that drug may cause weakness; discuss appropriate lifestyle adjustments.
• Caution patient not to take over-the-counter analgesics without prescriber's approval.
• Inform patient that he'll undergo regular blood testing during therapy.

adenosine
Adenocard, Adenoscan

Pharmacologic class: Endogenous nucleoside
Therapeutic class: Antiarrhythmic
Pregnancy risk category C

Action
Converts paroxysmal supraventricular tachycardia (PSVT) to normal sinus rhythm by slowing conduction through atrioventricular (AV) node and interrupting reentry pathway; also

used as a diagnostic agent in thallium scanning

Availability
Injection: 3 mg/ml

Indications and dosages
Adenocard—
➤ PSVT, including that associated with Wolff-Parkinson-White syndrome, after attempting vagal maneuvers when appropriate
Adults and children weighing more than 50 kg (110 lb): Initially, 6 mg by rapid I.V. bolus over 1 to 2 seconds. If desired effect isn't achieved within 1 to 2 minutes, give 12 mg by rapid I.V. bolus; may repeat 12-mg I.V. bolus dose as needed. Maximum single dose is 12 mg.
Children weighing less than 50 kg (110 lb): 0.05 to 0.1 mg/kg by rapid I.V. bolus. If this dosage proves ineffective, increase by 0.05mg/kg q 2 minutes, to a maximum single dosage of 0.3 mg/kg. Maximum single dose is 12 mg.
Adenoscan—
➤ Diagnosis of coronary artery disease in conjunction with thallium-201 myocardial perfusion scintigraphy in patients unable to exercise adequately during testing
Adults: 140 mcg/kg/minute by I.V. infusion over 6 minutes, for a total dosage of 0.84 mg/kg. Required dose of thallium-201 is injected at midpoint (after first 3 minutes) of Adenoscan infusion.

Off-label uses
• Diagnosis of supraventricular arrhythmias
• Pulmonary hypertension

Contraindications
• Hypersensitivity to drug
• Second- or third-degree AV block, sinus node disease
• Bronchoconstrictive lung disease

Administration
• Administer I.V. injection as rapid bolus directly into vein whenever possible.
• Flush I.V. line immediately with normal saline solution to drive drug into bloodstream.
• Don't give more than 12 mg as a single dose.
• In adults, don't administer through central line (may cause prolonged asystole).

Route	Onset	Peak	Duration
I.V.	Immediate	10 sec	20-30 sec

Adverse reactions
CNS: light-headedness, dizziness, tingling in arms, headache, numbness, apprehension
CV: first- or second-degree AV block, ST-segment depression, chest pain, palpitations, hypotension, **atrial tachyarrhythmias, other arrhythmias**
EENT: blurred vision, tightness in throat
GI: nausea, metallic taste, pressure in groin
Musculoskeletal: discomfort in neck, jaw, and arms
Respiratory: chest pressure, dyspnea and urge to breathe deeply, hyperventilation
Skin: burning sensation, facial flushing, sweating

Interactions
Drug-drug. *Carbamazepine:* worsening of progressive heart block
Digoxin, verapamil: increased risk of ventricular fibrillation
Dipyridamole: increased adenosine effect
Theophylline: decreased adenosine effect
Drug-food. *Caffeine:* decreased adenosine effect
Drug-herb. *Aloe, buckthorn bark or berry, cascara sagrada, rhubarb root,*

senna leaf or fruits: increased adenosine effect
Guarana: decreased adenosine effect
Drug-behaviors. *Smoking:* increased risk of tachycardia

Precautions
Use cautiously in:
• asthma, angina
• elderly patients
• pregnant patients
• children.

Patient monitoring
• Monitor heart rhythm for new arrhythmias after administering dose.
• Check vital signs; assess for chest pain or pressure, dyspnea, and sweating.
• Watch for bronchoconstriction in patient with asthma, emphysema, or bronchitis.
• Ask patient if he's recently used aloe, buckthorn, cascara sagrada, guarana, rhubarb root, or senna. If he has, notify prescriber.

Patient teaching
• Advise patient to report problems at infusion site.
• Tell patient he may experience 1 to 2 minutes of flushing, chest pain, chest pressure, and breathing difficulty during administration. Assure him that these effects will subside quickly.
• Teach patient to minimize GI upset by eating small, frequent servings of healthy food and drinking plenty of fluids.

a

agalsidase beta
Fabrazyme, Fibrazyme

Pharmacologic class: Homodimeric glycoprotein

Therapeutic class: Recombinant human alpha-galactosidase enzyme

Pregnancy risk category B

Action
Provides exogenous source of alpha-galactosidase A (deficient in Fabry disease) and reduces deposits of globotriaosylceramide in kidneys and other body tissues

Availability
Powder for reconstitution: 35 mg

Indications and dosages
➢ Fabry disease
Adults: 1 mg/kg I.V. q 2 weeks. Infuse no faster than 0.25 mg/minute; if tolerated, increase rate by 0.05 to 0.08 mg/minute in subsequent infusions. Pretreat with antipyretics, as prescribed.

Contraindications
None

Administration
• To reconstitute, slowly inject 7.2 ml of sterile water for injection into vial, then roll and tilt vial gently to mix drug.
• Don't shake drug, and don't use filter needles.
• Dilute reconstituted solution with normal saline injection to final volume of 500 ml.
• Infuse through separate I.V. line; don't mix with other drugs.

Route	Onset	Peak	Duration
I.V.	End of infusion	90 min	Up to 5 hr

Adverse reactions
CNS: anxiety, depression, dizziness, paresthesias, pain
CV: dependent edema, chest pain, cardiomegaly
EENT: pharyngitis, rhinitis, sinusitis
GI: nausea, dyspepsia
GU: testicular pain
Musculoskeletal: arthrosis, bone pain
Respiratory: bronchitis, bronchospasm, laryngitis
Skin: pallor
Other: allergic reactions, **infusion reactions** (hypertension, chest tightness, dyspnea, fever, rigors, hypotension, abdominal pain, pruritus, myalgia, headache, urticaria)

Interactions
Drug-drug. *Amiodarone, chloroquine, gentamicin, monobenzone:* inhibition of intracellular agalsidase activity

Precautions
Use cautiously in:
• cardiac dysfunction
• pregnant or breastfeeding patients
• children.

Patient monitoring
• Watch closely for signs and symptoms of allergic reaction or infusion reaction.
• Monitor vital signs and fluid intake and output; stay alert for dependent edema, blood pressure changes, and chest pain.
• Measure temperature; watch for signs and symptoms of infection (particularly EENT and respiratory infections).
• Evaluate patient's mood; report significant depression or anxiety.

Patient teaching
• Teach patient to recognize and immediately report signs and symptoms of allergic or infusion reaction.
• Instruct patient to avoid driving and other hazardous activities until he knows how drug affects mood, balance, and blood pressure.
• Advise patient to report signs and symptoms of infection (particularly EENT and respiratory infections).
• Caution patient that drug can cause depression and anxiety; instruct him to notify prescriber if these effects occur.

albumin (human normal serum)

5%: Albumarc, Albuminar-5, Albunex, Albutein 5%, Buminate 5%, Plasbumin-5
25%: Albumarc, Albuminar-25, Albutein 25%, Buminate 25%, Plasbumin-25

Pharmacologic class: Blood product, colloid
Therapeutic class: Volume expander
Pregnancy risk category C

Action
Provides colloidal oncotic pressure, increases circulating plasma volume, regulates fluid balance, and helps maintain normal blood volume; also acts as carrier for intermediate metabolites in transport

Availability
Albumin 5% injection: 50-ml, 250-ml, 500-ml, and 1,000-ml vials
Albumin 25% injection: 20-ml, 50-ml, and 100-ml vials

⚕ Indications and dosages
➤ Hypovolemia with shock
Adults: Initially, 500 ml of 5% solution by rapid I.V. infusion, repeated in 30 minutes if desired effect isn't achieved
Children: 50 ml of 5% solution by I.V. infusion, repeated in 15 to 30 minutes if desired effect isn't achieved, or 2.5 to 5 ml of 25% solution/kg by I.V. infu-

sion, repeated after 10 to 30 minutes. Total dosage shouldn't exceed 20 ml/kg.

Neonates and infants: 10 to 20 ml/kg by I.V. infusion based on response, delivered at 25% to 50% of adult rate. Total dosage shouldn't exceed 20 ml/kg.

➤ Severe burns (to maintain plasma volume and prevent intravascular hemoconcentration)

Adults: For initial therapy, give large volumes of crystalloids and lesser amounts of 5% solution I.V. to maintain plasma volume. After 24 hours, may increase 5% albumin I.V. to maintain plasma albumin level of about 2.5 g +/- 0.5 g/100 ml, or total serum protein level of about 5.2 g/100 ml.

➤ Acute hypoproteinemia

Adults: 200 to 300 ml of 25% solution I.V. (if edema is present or considerable albumin has been lost); not to exceed 3 ml/minute.

➤ Hyperbilirubinemia/erythroblastosis fetalis

Infants: 1 g/kg (4 ml/kg of 25% solution) I.V. within 1 to 2 hours before exchange transfusion

➤ Acute nephrosis

Adults: Initially, 100 ml of 25% solution I.V., repeated daily for 7 days if needed (given concurrently with loop diuretic)

Contraindications

• Hypersensitivity to drug
• Cardiac failure, hypervolemia, or pulmonary edema
• Severe anemia

Administration

• Make sure patient is well hydrated before giving drug.
• Adhere to prescribed infusion rate, which varies with patient's age, clinical condition, and diagnosis. Don't administer too rapidly.
• Administer by I.V. infusion with no further dilution.

• Withhold angiotensin-converting enzyme (ACE) inhibitors 24 hours before giving albumin, if possible.

Route	Onset	Peak	Duration
I.V.	Immediate	End of infusion	Several hr

Adverse reactions

CNS: headache, light-headedness, dizziness
CV: tachycardia, hypotension, **fluid overload**
EENT: blurred vision, throat tightness
GI: nausea, vomiting, metallic taste, increased salivation
Musculoskeletal: back pain
Respiratory: respiratory changes, hyperventilation, dyspnea, chest pressure, **pulmonary edema**
Skin: rash, urticaria, flushing
Other: chills, fever, groin pressure

Interactions

Drug-drug. *ACE inhibitors:* increased risk of atypical reactions
Drug-diagnostic tests. *Alkaline phosphatase:* false increase

Precautions

Use cautiously in:
• dehydration, renal failure, hepatic disease, hypertension, low cardiac reserve, pulmonary disease
• pregnant patients.

Patient monitoring

• Monitor for hemorrhage and shock after injury or surgery; rapid postinfusion blood pressure increase may cause bleeding from severed vessels.
• Check vital signs frequently.
• Monitor for signs and symptoms of heart failure and pulmonary edema.
• Evaluate fluid intake and output.
• Monitor hemoglobin, hematocrit, protein, and electrolyte levels.

Patient teaching

• Inform patient that he'll undergo regular blood testing during therapy.

albuterol (salbutamol)
Proventil, Ventolin

albuterol sulfate (salbutamol sulfate)
AccuNeb, Airet, Asmol✿, Gen-Salbutamol✿, Novo-Salmol✿, Proventil HFA, Proventil Repetabs, Ventodisk, Ventolin HFA, Volmax

Pharmacologic class: Sympathomimetic (beta₂-adrenergic agonist)
Therapeutic class: Bronchodilator, antiasthmatic
Pregnancy risk category C

Action

Relaxes smooth muscles by stimulating beta₂-receptors, causing bronchodilation and vasodilation

Availability

Oral solution: 2 mg/5 ml
Syrup: 2 mg/5 ml
Tablets: 2 mg, 4 mg
Tablets (extended-release): 4 mg, 8 mg

🕖 Indications and dosages

➤ To prevent and relieve bronchospasm in patients with reversible obstructive airway disease
Adults and children ages 12 and older: *Tablets*—2 to 4 mg P.O. three or four times daily, not to exceed 32 mg daily. *Extended-release tablets*—4 to 8 mg P.O. q 12 hours, not to exceed 32 mg daily in divided doses. *Syrup*—2 to 4 mg (1 to 2 tsp or 5 to 10 ml) three or four times daily, not to exceed 8 mg q.i.d.
Children ages 6 to 12: *Tablets*—2 mg P.O. three or four times daily; maxi-

mum daily dosage is 24 mg, given in divided doses. *Extended-release tablets*—4 mg q 12 hours; maximum daily dosage is 24 mg/kg given in divided doses. *Syrup*—2 mg (1 tsp or 5 ml) three or four times daily, not to exceed 24 mg.
Children ages 2 to 6: *Syrup*—Initially, 0.1 mg/kg P.O. t.i.d., not to exceed 2 mg (1 tsp) t.i.d. Maximum dosage is 4 mg (2 tsp) t.i.d.
Dosage adjustment
• Sensitivity to beta-adrenergic stimulants
• Elderly patients

Off-label uses

• Chronic obstructive pulmonary disease
• Hyperkalemia with renal failure
• Preterm labor management

Contraindications

• Hypersensitivity to drug

Administration

• Give extended-release tablets whole; don't crush or mix with food.

Route	Onset	Peak	Duration
P.O.	15-30 min	2-3 hr	6-12 hr
P.O. (extended)	30 min	2-3 hr	12 hr

Adverse reactions

CNS: dizziness, excitement, headache, hyperactivity, insomnia
CV: hypertension, palpitations, tachycardia, chest pain
EENT: conjunctivitis, dry and irritated throat, pharyngitis, tooth discoloration
GI: nausea, vomiting, anorexia, heartburn, GI distress, dry mouth
Metabolic: hypokalemia
Musculoskeletal: muscle cramps
Respiratory: cough, dyspnea, wheezing, **paradoxical bronchospasm**
Skin: pallor, urticaria, rash, angioedema, flushing, sweating

Other: increased appetite, **hypersensitivity reaction**

Interactions

Drug-drug. *Beta blockers:* inhibited albuterol action, possibly causing severe bronchospasm in asthmatic patients
Digoxin: decreased digoxin level
Monoamine oxidase inhibitors: increased cardiovascular adverse effects
Oxytoxics: severe hypotension
Potassium-wasting diuretics: electrocardiogram changes, hypokalemia
Theophylline: increased risk of theophylline toxicity

Drug-food. *Caffeine-containing foods and beverages (such as coffee, green or black tea, chocolate):* increased stimulant effect

Drug-herb. *Cola nut, ephedra, guarana, yerba maté:* increased stimulant effect

Precautions

Use cautiously in:
• cardiac disease, hypertension, diabetes mellitus, glaucoma, seizure disorder, hyperthyroidism, exercise-induced bronchospasm, prostatic hypertrophy
• elderly patients
• pregnant or breastfeeding patients
• children.

Patient monitoring

◀≶ Stay alert for hypersensitivity reactions and paradoxical bronchospasm; stop drug immediately if these occur.
• Monitor serum electrolyte levels.

Patient teaching

◀≶ Teach patient signs and symptoms of hypersensitivity reaction and paradoxical bronchospasm; tell him to stop taking drug immediately and contact prescriber if these occur.
• Tell patient to swallow extended-release tablets whole and not to mix them with food.

• Instruct patient to avoid driving and other hazardous activities until he knows how drug affects concentration and alertness.
• Advise patient to establish effective bedtime routine and to take drug well before bedtime to minimize insomnia.

aldesleukin
(interleukin-2, IL-2)
Proleukin

Pharmacologic class: Interleukin-2 (IL-2), human recombinant (cytokine)
Therapeutic class: Antineoplastic (miscellaneous)
Pregnancy risk category C

Action

Activates cellular immunity and inhibits tumor growth by increasing lymphocytes, cytokines, and platelets

Availability

Injection: 22 million IU/vial
Powder for injection: 22×10^6 IU/vial

⚱ Indications and dosages

➤ Metastatic renal cell carcinoma
Adults older than age 18: 600,000 IU/kg given I.V. over 15 minutes q 8 hours for a maximum of 14 doses, followed by 9 days of rest. Repeat for another 14 doses, for a maximum of 28 doses per course.

Off-label uses

• Colorectal cancer
• Kaposi's sarcoma
• Metastatic melanoma
• Non-Hodgkin's lymphoma

Contraindications

• Hypersensitivity to drug
• Arrhythmias, cardiac tamponade, coma or toxic psychosis lasting more

than 48 hours, seizures, severe GI
bleeding
• Organ allograft
• Abnormal thallium stress test or pulmonary function test results

Administration

• Make sure patient's thallium stress test and pulmonary function test results are normal before giving.
• Don't give if patient is drowsy or severely lethargic; contact prescriber immediately.
• Reconstitute drug according to label directions with 1.2 ml of sterile water for injection by injecting diluent against side of vial (to prevent excessive foaming).
• Further dilute reconstituted dose with 50 ml of 5% dextrose injection.
• Administer I.V. infusion over 15 minutes.
• Don't use in-line filter to administer.

Route	Onset	Peak	Duration
I.V.	5 min	13 min	3-4 hr

Adverse reactions

CNS: dizziness, mental status changes, syncope, sensory or motor dysfunction, headache, fatigue, weakness, malaise, poor memory, depression, sleep disturbances, hallucinations, rigors
CV: myocardial ischemia, bradycardia, arrhythmias, premature atrial complexes, premature ventricular contractions, sinus tachycardia, **cardiac arrest, capillary leak syndrome and severe hypotension, myocardial infarction**
EENT: reversible visual changes, conjunctivitis
GI: nausea, vomiting, constipation, diarrhea, dyspepsia, abdominal pain, stomatitis, anorexia, **intestinal perforation, ileus, GI bleeding**
GU: hematuria, proteinuria, dysuria, **renal failure, oliguria** or **anuria**
Hematologic: anemia, purpura, eosinophilia, **coagulation disorders,**

thrombocytopenia, leukopenia, leukocytosis
Hepatic: jaundice, ascites
Metabolic: acidosis, alkalosis, hypoglycemia, hyperglycemia
Musculoskeletal: joint and back pain, myalgia
Respiratory: tachypnea, wheezing, dyspnea, pulmonary congestion, cough, chest pain, **pulmonary edema, respiratory failure, apnea, pleural effusion**
Skin: erythema, pruritus, rash, dry skin, petechiae, urticaria, **exfoliative dermatitis**
Other: weight gain or loss, fever, chills, edema, infection, pain or reaction at injection site, hypersensitivity reaction

Interactions

Drug-drug. *Aminoglycosides, asparaginase, cytotoxic chemotherapy agents, doxorubicin, indomethacin, methotrexate:* increased toxicity
Antihypertensives: increased hypotensive effect
Glucocorticoids: reduced antitumor effects
Drug-diagnostic tests. *Alkaline phosphatase, bilirubin, glucose, blood urea nitrogen, creatinine, potassium, transaminases:* increased levels
Calcium, glucose, magnesium, phosphorus, potassium, protein sodium, uric acid: decreased levels

Precautions

Use cautiously in:
• anemia, bacterial infections, heart disease, CNS metastases, hepatic disease, pulmonary disease, renal disease, thrombocytopenia
• pregnant or breastfeeding patients
• children.

Patient monitoring

• Monitor heart rate and rhythm, vital signs, and fluid intake and output.
• Assess for signs and symptoms of hypersensitivity reaction and infection.

• Monitor for adverse CNS effects; report these immediately.
• Evaluate chest X-rays.
• Monitor complete blood count, electrolyte levels, and liver and kidney function test results.

Patient teaching
• Teach patient that drug lowers resistance to infections. Advise him to immediately report fever, cough, breathing problems, and other signs or symptoms.
• Instruct patient to minimize GI upset by eating small, frequent servings of food and drinking plenty of fluids.
• Provide dietary counseling; refer patient to dietitian if adverse GI effects significantly limit food intake.
• Notify patient that he'll undergo blood testing and have chest X-rays taken during therapy.

alemtuzumab
Campath

Pharmacologic class: Monoclonal antibody
Therapeutic class: Antineoplastic
Pregnancy risk category C

Action
Binds to CD52 antigen on surface of B- and T-lymphocytes, as well as most monocytes, macrophages, "natural killer" cells, and granulocytes. Lyses leukemic cells and reduces tumor size.

Availability
Solution for injection: 30 mg/3 ml

Indications and dosages
➤ Chronic lymphocytic (B-cell) leukemia when fludarabine therapy fails
Adults: Initially, 3 mg/day I.V. given over 2 hours; if tolerated, increase to 10 mg/day, to a maximum single dosage of 30 mg/day. Then give a maintenance dosage of 30 mg three times weekly on nonconsecutive days (such as Monday, Wednesday, Friday) for up to 12 weeks.
Dosage adjustment
• Hematologic toxicity

Contraindications
• Type I hypersensitivity or anaphylactic reaction to drug or its components
• Active systemic infection
• Immunodeficiency (such as human immunodeficiency virus infection)

Administration
◀€ Withhold drug and contact prescriber if patient has signs or symptoms of systemic infection at time of scheduled infusion.
◀€ Don't give by I.V. push or bolus.
• Withdraw dose from ampule and filter with sterile, low-protein-binding, 5-micron filter.
• Dilute with 100 ml of normal saline solution or dextrose 5% in water.
• Infuse over 2 hours.
• Protect I.V. solution from light.

Route	Onset	Peak	Duration
I.V.	Unknown	Unknown	Unknown

Adverse reactions
CNS: tremor, malaise, dizziness, depression, insomnia, drowsiness, weakness, headache, abnormal sensations, fatigue
CV: peripheral edema, chest pain, hypotension, hypertension, tachycardia, **supraventricular tachycardia**
EENT: rhinitis, pharyngitis, epistaxis
GI: nausea, vomiting, constipation, diarrhea, dyspepsia, abdominal pain, stomatitis, anorexia
Hematologic: bone marrow depression, anemia, **pancytopenia**, **bone marrow hypoplasia**, **neutropenia**, **thrombocytopenia**

Metabolic: hypokalemia, hypomagnesemia

Musculoskeletal: myalgia, bone or back pain

Respiratory: cough, bronchitis, dyspnea, pneumonitis, rhinitis, **bronchospasm**

Skin: herpes simplex infection, urticaria, pruritus, diaphoresis

Other: edema, fever, candidiasis, infection, **infusion-related reactions, sepsis**

Interactions

Drug-drug. *Live-virus vaccines:* decreased drug efficacy and increased adverse effects

Drug-diagnostic tests. *CD4+ T lymphocytes, hematocrit, hemoglobin, lymphocytes, neutrophils platelets, red blood cells, white blood cells:* decreased levels

Precautions

Use cautiously in:
• pregnant or breastfeeding patients
• children.

Patient monitoring

• Assess for hypotension during infusion.
• Monitor vital signs frequently throughout entire course of therapy.
• Monitor complete blood count, CD4+ level, electrolyte levels, and platelet counts.

Patient teaching

• Teach patient that drug lowers resistance to infection. Instruct him to report fever, cough, breathing problems, sore throat, and other signs or symptoms immediately.
• Caution patient to avoid driving and other hazardous activities until he knows how drug affects concentration and alertness.
• Advise patient to minimize GI upset by eating small, frequent servings of food and drinking plenty of fluids.

• Instruct patient to follow regular bedtime routine and avoid bedtime stimulants.
• Encourage patient to discuss activity recommendations and pain management with prescriber.
• Inform patient that he'll undergo regular blood testing during therapy.

alendronate sodium
Fosamax

Pharmacologic class: Bisphosphonate

Therapeutic class: Bone-resorption inhibitor

Pregnancy risk category C

Action

Impedes bone resorption by inhibiting osteoclast activity, absorbing calcium phosphate crystal in bone, and directly blocking dissolution of hydroxyapatite crystal of bone, without inhibiting bone formation or mineralization

Availability

Tablets: 5 mg, 10 mg, 35 mg, 40 mg, 70 mg

🕖 Indications and dosages

➤ Paget's disease of bone

Adults: 40 mg P.O. daily for 6 months. Then administer only with water at least a half hour before first oral intake of day.

➤ Prevention of osteoporosis in postmenopausal women

Adults: 5 mg P.O. daily or 35 mg P.O. once weekly. Then administer only with water at least a half hour before first oral intake of day.

➤ Glucocorticoid-induced osteoporosis in adults with low bone mineral density who are receiving daily glucocorticoid doses equivalent to 7.5 mg or more of prednisone

Adults: 5 mg P.O. daily. Then administer only with water at least a half hour before patient's first oral intake or medication of day.

➤ Osteoporosis in postmenopausal women

Adults: 10 mg P.O. daily. Then administer only with water at least a half hour before first oral intake or medication of day.

➤ Osteoporosis in postmenopausal woman; to increase bone mass in men with osteoporosis

Adults: 10 mg P.O. daily or 70 mg P.O. once weekly. Then administer only with water at least a half hour before first oral intake or medication of day.

Contraindications
• Hypersensitivity to bisphosphonates
• Hypocalcemia
• Renal insufficiency
• Esophageal abnormalities

Administration
• Give with 6 to 8 oz of water before first food, beverage, or medication of day.
• Don't give food, other beverages, or oral drugs for at least 30 minutes after giving dose.
• Keep patient upright for at least 30 minutes after administering dose to avoid serious esophageal irritation.
• Be aware that aspirin and non-steroidal anti-inflammatory drugs (NSAIDs) may worsen GI upset. Discuss alternative analgesics with prescriber.

Route	Onset	Peak	Duration
P.O.	1 mo	3-6 mo	3 wk-7 mo

Adverse reactions
CNS: headache
CV: hypertension
GI: nausea, vomiting, diarrhea, constipation, abdominal pain, acid regurgitation, esophageal ulcer, flatulence, dyspepsia, abdominal distention, dysphagia, abnormal taste
GU: urinary tract infection
Hematologic: anemia
Metabolic: hypomagnesemia, hypophosphatemia, hypokalemia, fluid overload
Musculoskeletal: bone or muscle pain
Skin: rash, redness, photosensitivity

Interactions
Drug-drug. *Antacids, calcium supplements:* decreased alendronate absorption
NSAIDs, salicylates: increased risk of GI upset
Ranitidine: increased alendronate effect
Drug-diagnostic tests. *Calcium, phosphate:* decreased levels
Drug-food. *Any food, caffeine (coffee, tea, cocoa), mineral water, orange juice:* decreased drug absorption

Precautions
Use cautiously in:
• renal insufficiency, esophageal disease, GI ulcers, gastritis
• pregnant or breastfeeding women
• children.

Patient monitoring
• Monitor for signs and symptoms of GI irritation, including ulcers.
• Monitor blood pressure.
• Evaluate blood calcium and phosphate levels.

Patient teaching
◀€ Tell patient to immediately report serious vomiting, severe chest or abdominal pain, difficulty swallowing, or abdominal swelling.
• Instruct patient to take drug first thing in morning on an empty stomach, with 6 to 8 oz of water only.
• Tell patient not to lie down for at least 30 minutes after taking drug.
• Instruct patient not to eat, drink, or take other oral medications for 30 minutes after taking dose.

• Teach patient to take only those pain relievers suggested by prescriber. Inform him that some over-the-counter pain medicines (such as aspirin and NSAIDs) may worsen adverse effects.

allopurinol

Alloprim, Apo-Allopurinol✤, Lopurin, Purinol, Zyloprim

Pharmacologic class: Xanthine oxidase inhibitor
Therapeutic class: Antigout drug
Pregnancy risk category C

Action
Inhibits conversion of xanthine to uric acid, decreasing serum and urine levels

Availability
Injection: 500 mg/30-ml vial
Tablets: 100 mg, 300 mg

🖋 Indications and dosages
➤ Gout in patients with frequent disabling attacks, or resulting from hyperuricemia, acute or chronic leukemia, psoriasis, or multiple myeloma
Adults: 200 to 300 mg P.O. daily in mild cases, and 400 to 600 mg P.O. daily in severe cases to a maximum dosage of 800 mg/day, or 200 to 400 mg/m²/day I.V. as a single infusion or in equally divided doses q 6, 8, or 12 hours. Divide doses larger than 300 mg.
Children ages 6 to 10: 300 mg P.O. daily
Children younger than age 6: 150 mg P.O. daily
➤ To prevent acute gouty attacks
Adults: 100 mg P.O. daily; increase by 100 mg at weekly intervals, without exceeding maximum dosage of 800 mg, until uric acid level falls to 6 mg/dl or less

➤ Recurrent calcium oxalate calculi
Adults: 200 to 300 mg P.O. daily in single dose or divided doses
➤ To prevent uric acid nephropathy during cancer chemotherapy
Adults: 600 to 800 mg P.O. daily for 2 to 3 days, accompanied by high fluid intake
Dosage adjustment
• Renal impairment

Off-label uses
• Hematemesis caused by gastritis induced by nonsteroidal anti-inflammatory drugs
• Pain from acute pancreatitis
• Seizures refractory to standard therapy

Contraindications
• Hypersensitivity to drug
• Idiopathic hemochromatosis

Administration
• Don't mix I.V. form with other drugs or give through same I.V. port as drugs that may be incompatible.
• Give I.V. solution within 10 hours of reconstitution.
• Don't refrigerate reconstituted I.V. solution.
• Give oral form with or right after meals.
• Don't give oral form with mineral water, orange juice, or beverages containing caffeine.

Route	Onset	Peak	Duration
P.O.	2-3 days	0.5-2 hr	1-2 wk
I.V.	Unknown	0.5 hr	Unknown

Adverse reactions
CNS: drowsiness, dizziness, headache, peripheral neuropathy, neuritis, paresthesia
CV: necrotizing vasculitis, hypersensitivity vasculitis
EENT: retinopathy, cataract, epistaxis

GI: nausea, vomiting, diarrhea, abdominal pain, dyspepsia, gastritis, abnormal taste, loss of taste

GU: uremia, exacerbation of gout and renal calculi, **renal failure**

Hematologic: leukocytosis, eosinophilia, anemia, **bone marrow depression, agranulocytosis, aplastic anemia, thrombocytopenia, leukopenia**

Hepatic: hyperbilirubinemia, **hepatomegaly, cholestatic jaundice, hepatitis, hepatic necrosis**

Musculoskeletal: myopathy, joint pain

Skin: rash; alopecia; maculopapular, urticarial, or purpuric lesions; severe furunculosis of nose; ichthyosis; bruising; **scaly or exfoliative erythema multiforme; toxic epidermal necrolysis**

Other: fever, chills

Interactions

Drug-drug. *Amoxicillin, ampicillin, bacampicillin:* increased risk of rash
Anticoagulants (except warfarin): increased anticoagulant effect
Antineoplastics: increased risk of myelosuppression
Azathioprine, mercaptopurine: inhibition of allopurinol metabolism
Chlorpropamide: increased hypoglycemic effects
Diazoxide, diuretics, mecamylamine, pyrazinamide: increased uric acid levels
Ethacrynic acid, thiazide diuretics: increased risk of allopurinol toxicity
Uricosurics: increased uric acid excretion
Urine-acidifying drugs (ammonium chloride, ascorbic acid, potassium or sodium phosphate): increased risk of renal calculi
Xanthines: increased theophylline levels

Drug-diagnostic tests. *Alanine aminotransferase, alanine phosphatase, aspartate aminotransferase, bilirubin, eosinophils:* increased levels
Granulocytes, hemoglobin, platelets, white blood cells: decreased levels

Drug-food. *Caffeine-containing beverages and foods, mineral water, orange juice:* decreased drug absorption, increased uric acid level

Drug-behaviors. *Alcohol use:* increased uric acid level

Precautions

Use cautiously in:
• acute gout attack, renal insufficiency, dehydration
• pregnant or breastfeeding women.

Patient monitoring

• Assess fluid intake and output; intake should be sufficient to yield daily output of at least 2 L of slightly alkaline urine.
• Monitor uric acid levels to help evaluate drug efficacy.

Patient teaching

◀€ Instruct patient to promptly report painful urination, bloody urine, rash, eye irritation, or swelling of lips and mouth.
• Tell patient to take drug with food or milk, exactly as prescribed.
• Explain that gouty attacks may not ease significantly until 2 to 6 weeks of therapy.
• Instruct patient to avoid driving and other hazardous tasks until he knows how drug affects concentration and alertness.

almotriptan malate
Axert

Pharmacologic class: Serotonin (5-hydroxytryptamine [5-HT]) receptor agonist

Therapeutic class: Vascular headache suppressant, antimigraine drug

Pregnancy risk category C

Action
Promotes vascular constriction and relieves migraine by stimulating specific 5-HT receptors in intracranial blood vessels and sensory trigeminal nerves

Availability
Tablets: 6.25 mg, 12.5 mg

Indications and dosages
➤ Acute migraine with or without aura
Adults: Single dose of 6.25 to 12.5 mg P.O. at first sign or symptom of migraine; may repeat if symptoms reappear within 2 hours. Don't exceed two doses in 24-hour period.

Contraindications
- Hypersensitivity to drug
- Ischemic heart disease, myocardial infarction (MI), cerebrovascular accident
- Uncontrolled hypertension
- Ischemic bowel disease
- Basilar or hemiplegic migraine
- Monoamine oxidase (MAO) inhibitor use within past 14 days
- Children

Administration
- Give with or without food.
- Wait at least 2 hours after initial dose before giving repeat dose.
- Don't exceed two doses in 24 hours.
- Don't give within 14 days of MAO inhibitor therapy.

Route	Onset	Peak	Duration
P.O.	Variable	1-3 hr	Unknown

Adverse reactions
CNS: headache, anxiety, fatigue, malaise, weakness, cold or hot sensations, sedation, dizziness, numbness, burning or tingling sensations
CV: blood pressure changes, palpitations, tachycardia, **coronary artery vasospasm, MI, ventricular fibrillation, ventricular tachycardia**

EENT: vision changes; throat, mouth, and nasal discomfort
GI: nausea, dry mouth, abdominal distress, dysphagia
Musculoskeletal: weakness, neck stiffness, muscle pain
Respiratory: chest tightness or pressure
Skin: sweating, flushing

Interactions
Drug-drug. *CYP2D6 inhibitors (erythromycin, itraconazole, ritonavir):* increased almotriptan effect
Ergot derivatives, other 5-HT agonists: prolonged vasoactive action
Ketoconazole and other CYP3A inhibitors: increased almotriptan blood level, leading to toxicity
MAO inhibitors: increased risk of severe adverse effects when taken within 14 days of almotriptan
Selective serotonin reuptake inhibitors: weakness, hyperreflexia, poor coordination

Precautions
Use cautiously in:
- impaired renal or hepatic function
- cardiovascular risk factors
- pregnant or breastfeeding patients
- children younger than age 18.

Patient monitoring
- Assess patient's cardiovascular status; especially note chest tightness or pressure.
- Monitor vital signs.

Patient teaching
◀€ Tell patient to report chest tightness or pressure immediately.
- Inform patient that he may take drug with or without food.
- If second dose is needed, advise patient to wait at least 2 hours after initial dose.
- Caution patient not to take more than two doses in 24 hours.

---

a

• Instruct patient to avoid driving and other hazardous activities until he knows how drug affects concentration and alertness.

alprazolam
Apo-Alpraz✤, Novo-Alprazol✤, Nu-Alpraz✤, Xanax, Xanax TS✤

Pharmacologic class: Benzodiazepine
Therapeutic class: Anxiolytic
Controlled substance schedule IV
Pregnancy risk category D

Action
Unclear; thought to act at limbic, thalamic, and hypothalamic levels of CNS, producing sedative, anxiolytic, skeletal muscle relaxant, and anticonvulsant effects

Availability
Oral solution: 0.5 mg/5 ml
Solution: 1 mg/ml
Tablets (extended-release): 0.5 mg, 1 mg, 2 mg, 3 mg
Tablets (immediate-release): 0.25 mg, 0.5 mg, 1 mg, 2 mg

🖊 Indications and dosages
➤ Anxiety disorders
Adults: Initially, 0.25 to 0.5 mg P.O. t.i.d; maximum dosage is 4 mg daily in divided doses.
Elderly patients: Initially, 0.25 mg P.O. two or three times daily; maximum dosage is 4 mg daily in divided doses.
➤ Panic disorders
Adults: Initially, 0.5 mg P.O. t.i.d; increase by a maximum of 1 mg at intervals of 3 to 4 days. Maximum dosage is 10 mg daily in divided doses.
Dosage adjustment
• Hepatic impairment

Off-label uses
• Agoraphobia
• Depression
• Premenstrual syndrome

Contraindications
• Hypersensitivity to benzodiazepines
• Narrow-angle glaucoma
• Psychosis
• Shock
• Coma
• Labor and delivery
• Pregnancy or breastfeeding

Administration
• Don't give with grapefruit juice.
• Make sure patient swallows extended-release tablets whole without chewing or crushing.
◀€ Don't withdraw drug suddenly; seizures and other withdrawal symptoms may occur unless dosage is tapered carefully.

Route	Onset	Peak	Duration
P.O.	30 min	1-2 hr	4-6 hr

Adverse reactions
CNS: dizziness, drowsiness, depression, fatigue, light-headedness, disorientation, anger, hostility, euphoria, hypomanic episodes, restlessness, confusion, crying, delirium, headache, stupor, rigidity, tremor, paresthesia, vivid dreams, extrapyramidal symptoms
CV: bradycardia, tachycardia, hypertension, hypotension, palpitations, **CV collapse**
EENT: blurred or double vision, nystagmus, nasal congestion, dry mouth
GI: gastric disorders, dysphagia, anorexia, increased salivation
GU: menstrual irregularities, urinary retention, urinary incontinence, libido changes, gynecomastia
Hematologic: blood dyscrasias, such as eosinophilia, **agranulocytosis, leukopenia, and thrombocytopenia**
Hepatic: elevated alanine aminotransferase (ALT), alkaline phosphatase

---

(ALP), aspartate aminotransferase (AST), and lactate dehydrogenase (LDH) levels; **hepatic dysfunction** (including **hepatitis**)

Musculoskeletal: muscle rigidity, joint pain

Skin: dermatitis, rash, pruritus, urticaria, increased sweating

Other: weight gain or loss, hiccups, fever, edema, psychological drug dependence, drug tolerance

Interactions

Drug-drug. *Antidepressants, antihistamines, other benzodiazepines, opioids:* increased CNS depression

Barbiturates, rifampin: increased metabolism and decreased efficacy of alprazolam

Cimetidine, disulfiram, erythromycin, fluoxetine, hormonal contraceptives, isoniazid, ketoconazole, metoprolol, propoxyphene, propranolol, valproic acid: decreased metabolism and increased action of alprazolam

Digoxin: increased risk of digoxin toxicity

Levodopa: decreased antiparkinsonian effect

Theophylline: increased sedative effect

Tricyclic antidepressants (TCAs): increased blood TCA levels

Drug-diagnostic tests. *ALP, ALT, AST, LDH:* increased levels

Drug-food. *Grapefruit juice:* decreased drug metabolism and increased blood level

Drug-herb. *Chamomile, hops, kava, skullcap, valerian:* increased CNS depression

Drug-behaviors. *Alcohol use:* increased CNS depression

Smoking: decreased alprazolam efficacy

Precautions

Use cautiously in:
• hepatic dysfunction
• history of attempted suicide or drug dependence
• elderly patients.

Patient monitoring

• Watch for excessive CNS depression if patient is concurrently taking antidepressants, other benzodiazepines, antihistamines, or opioids.

• If patient is taking TCAs concurrently, watch for increase in adverse TCA effects.

• Monitor complete blood count and liver and kidney function test results.

• Monitor vital signs and weight.

• Report signs of drug abuse, including frequent requests for early refills.

Patient teaching

◀€ Tell patient that drug may make him more depressed, angry, or hostile. Urge him to contact prescriber immediately if he thinks he's dangerous to himself or others.

• Instruct patient to swallow extended-release tablets whole without crushing or chewing.

• Advise patient to avoid driving and other hazardous activities until he knows how drug affects concentration and alertness.

• Inform patient that drug may cause tremors, muscle rigidity, and other movement problems; advise him to report these effects to prescriber.

◀€ Caution patient not to stop taking drug suddenly. Withdrawal symptoms, including seizures, may occur if drug isn't tapered carefully.

alprostadil

Caverject, Edex, Muse, Prostin VR Pediatric

Pharmacologic class: Prostaglandin E_1

Therapeutic class: Impotence agent, ductus arteriosus patency adjunct

Pregnancy risk category NR

Action
Produces vasodilation, inhibits platelet aggregation, and stimulates intestinal and uterine smooth muscles. In ductus arteriosus, relaxes smooth muscle of ductus arteriosus. In erectile dysfunction, promotes erection by relaxing trabecular smooth muscle and dilating cavernosal arteries.

Availability
Injection: 5 mcg/ml, 10 mcg/ml, 20 mcg/ml, 40 mcg/ml, 500 mcg/ml
Pellets: 124 mcg
Powder for injection: 6.15 mcg (5 mg/ml), 11.9 mcg (10 mcg/ml), 23.2 mcg (20 mcg/ml)

⚕ Indications and dosages
➤ Palliative therapy for infants to temporarily maintain patency of ductus arteriosus
Infants: 0.05 to 0.1 mcg/kg/minute I.V. (Prostin VR Pediatric). Once therapeutic response occurs, reduce infusion to lowest dosage required to maintain response. Maximum dosage is 0.4 mcg/kg/minute.
➤ Erectile dysfunction of vasculogenic, psychogenic, or mixed etiology
Adults: Initially, 2.5 mcg intracavernously (Caverject, Edex, Muse). If adequate response occurs, give second 2.5-mcg dose; then increase in increments of 5 to 10 mcg until patient achieves suitable erection that lasts no more than 1 hour. If no response occurs, may increase second dose to 7.5 mcg within 1 hour; then increase in 5- to 10-mcg increments until patient achieves suitable erection. Don't repeat for at least 24 hours.

Off-label uses
• Angiography of penile vasculature
• Atherosclerosis
• Gangrene and pain due to vascular disease

Contraindications
• Hypersensitivity to drug
• Penile deformity or implant
• Respiratory distress syndrome
• Men who engage in sexual intercourse with pregnant women (unless condoms are used)
• Women and children (intracavernous use)

Administration
• Inject concentrate into diluent in infusion chamber; don't let concentrate touch plastic side of chamber.
• Infuse at 0.05 to 0.1 mcg/kg/minute. When therapeutic response occurs, reduce to lowest dosage that maintains response.
• Don't give faster than 0.4 mcg/kg/minute.
• Don't give by direct injection or intermittent infusion. Use infusion pump for continuous infusion.
• In infants, use large peripheral vein or central vein or give through umbilical artery catheter at ductus level.

Route	Onset	Peak	Duration
I.V.	20 min	1-2 hr	Length of infusion
Intra-cavernous	5-20 min	5-20 min	1-6 hr

Adverse reactions
Unless otherwise noted, adverse effects below pertain to Prostin VR Pediatric.
CNS: dizziness, headache (intracavernous use); **seizures**
CV: hypertension (intracavernous use); tachycardia, edema, hypotension, **bradycardia, cardiac arrest**
EENT: nasal congestion (intracavernous use)
GI: diarrhea
GU: (all with intracavernous use) penile, urethral, or testicular pain; urethral burning; trauma; prolonged erection; priapism; penile fibrosis; penile edema; penile disorders; prostate enlargement, hypertrophy, or pain

Hematologic: disseminated intravascular coagulation, inhibited platelet aggregation
Metabolic: hypokalemia
Musculoskeletal: cortical proliferation of long bones (long-term infusions), back pain (intracavernous use)
Respiratory: respiratory tract infection, cough (intracavernous use); **apnea**
Skin: flushing; hematoma or bruising at injection site; penile rash (intracavernous use)
Other: flulike symptoms (intracavernous use); fever, **sepsis**

Interactions
Drug-drug. *Anticoagulants:* increased risk of bleeding
Cyclosporine: decreased cyclosporine blood level
Vasoactive agents: safety and efficacy not established
Drug-diagnostic tests. *Potassium:* decreased level

Precautions
Use cautiously in:
- bleeding tendencies
- neonates.

Patient monitoring
🔊 Monitor infant's cardiopulmonary status and be prepared to provide respiratory support for apnea (most likely to occur during first hour of infusion).
🔊 Evaluate infant for adverse cardiovascular effects (especially bradycardia) and adverse CNS reactions (especially seizures), which are more common in smaller infants and after 48 hours of infusion.
🔊 Monitor infant's arterial pressure with umbilical artery catheter, auscultation, or Doppler transducer.
🔊 Assess infant for signs of sepsis and for bleeding caused by disseminated intravascular coagulation.
- Monitor blood oxygenation, systemic blood pressure, and blood pH to evaluate drug efficacy.
- Monitor infant's clotting studies and serum electrolyte levels.
- With intracavernous use, monitor patient for hypotension.

Patient teaching
- Explain reason for drug use to parents and provide updates on its effectiveness.
- Tell parents about adverse effects and subsequent nursing interventions as appropriate.
- If patient's using drug to treat erectile dysfunction, review administration guidelines (after initial treatment) to ensure proper use.
- Tell patient with erectile dysfunction to report signs and symptoms of infection (such as foul penile discharge), other adverse reactions, and prolonged erection (more than 6 hours).
- Advise patient with erectile dysfunction not to have sexual intercourse with a pregnant woman without using a condom.

alteplase (tissue plasminogen activator, recombinant)
Activase, Activase rt-PA✤, Cathflo Activase, Lysatec rt-PA✤

Pharmacologic class: Plasminogen activator
Therapeutic class: Thrombolytic
Pregnancy risk category C

Action
Converts plasminogen to plasmin, which in turn breaks down fibrin and fibrinogen, thereby dissolving thrombus

Availability

Injection: 2-mg single-patient vials; 20-mg, 50-mg, 100-mg vials

Indications and dosages

➤ Lysis of thrombi obstructing coronary arteries in acute myocardial infarction (MI)

3-hour infusion—

Adults: 100 mg I.V. over 3 hours as follows: 60 mg in first hour (give 6 to 10 mg as bolus over first 1 to 2 minutes), then 20 mg I.V. over second hour, then 20 mg I.V. over third hour

Adults weighing less than 65 kg (143 lb): 1.25 mg/kg I.V. in divided doses over 3 hours, not to exceed 100 mg

Accelerated infusion—

Adults weighing more than 67 kg (147 lb): Give total dosage of 100 mg as follows: 15 mg I.V. bolus over 1 to 2 minutes, then 50 mg I.V. over next 30 minutes, then 35 mg I.V. over next 60 minutes

Adults weighing 67 kg (147 lb) or less: 15 mg I.V. bolus over 1 to 2 minutes, followed by 0.75 mg/kg I.V. over next 30 minutes (not to exceed 50 mg), followed by 0.5 mg/kg I.V. over the next hour

➤ Acute ischemic cerebrovascular accident (CVA)

Adults: 0.9 mg/kg I.V. over 1 hour, to a maximum dosage of 90 mg, with 10% of total dosage given as I.V. bolus in first minute

➤ Acute massive pulmonary embolism

Adults: 100 mg I.V. over 2 hours, followed by heparin

Off-label uses

• Blocked venous catheter (2-mg bolus injected into catheter for adults and children ages 2 years and older)
• Small-vessel occlusion by microthrombi
• Peripheral arterial thromboembolism

Contraindications

• Active MI or pulmonary embolism in patient with increased bleeding risk
• Previous CVA, history of intracranial hemorrhage, uncontrolled hypertension, seizures, active internal bleeding

Administration

◀€ Be aware that intracranial hemorrhage must be ruled out before therapy begins.
• Give I.V. only, using controlled-infusion device.
◀€ To treat acute ischemic CVA, give within 3 hours of initial signs or symptoms.
◀€ If uncontrolled bleeding occurs, stop infusion and notify prescriber immediately.
• Reconstitute only with unpreserved sterile water for injection, using large-bore needle to shoot diluent stream directly into powder. Wait a few minutes for foam to settle, and then draw up dose and administer right away.

Route	Onset	Peak	Duration
I.V.	Unknown	Unknown	Unknown

Adverse reactions

CNS: cerebral hemorrhage, cerebral edema, CVA (with accelerated infusion)
CV: electromechanical dissociation, hypotension, bradycardia, recurrent ischemia, mitral regurgitation, pericardial effusion, pericarditis, **arrhythmias, cardiogenic shock, heart failure, cardiac arrest, cardiac tamponade, myocardial rupture, embolization, venous thrombosis**
GI: nausea, vomiting, **GI bleeding**
GU: increased blood urea nitrogen, GU tract bleeding
Hematologic: bone marrow depression, spontaneous bleeding
Musculoskeletal: musculoskeletal pain
Respiratory: pulmonary edema
Skin: bruising, flushing

Other: fever, edema, phlebitis or bleeding at I.V. site, hypersensitivity reaction (including rash, **anaphylactic reaction, laryngeal edema**), **sepsis**

Interactions
Drug-drug. *Aspirin, drugs affecting platelet activity (such as abciximab, heparin, dipyridamole, oral anticoagulants, vitamin K antagonists):* increased risk of bleeding

Precautions
Use cautiously in:
• hypersensitivity to anistreplase or streptokinase
• GI or genitourinary bleeding, ophthalmic hemorrhage, organ biopsy, severe hepatic or renal disease
• elderly patients
• pregnant or breastfeeding patients
• children.

Patient monitoring
• Monitor vital signs, electrocardiogram, and neurologic status.
• Maintain strict bed rest.
• Watch for signs and symptoms of bleeding tendency and hemorrhage.
• Monitor patient on Cathflo Activase for GI bleeding, venous thrombosis, and sepsis.
• Evaluate results of clotting studies.

Patient teaching
◀€ Instruct patient to immediately report adverse reactions, especially unusual bleeding or bruising.
• Stress importance of strict bed rest.
• Tell patient to avoid activities that can cause injury. Advise him to use soft toothbrush and electric razor to avoid gum and skin injury.
• Advise patient that he'll undergo regular blood testing during therapy.

aluminum hydroxide
AlternaGEL, Alu-Cap, Alugel♣, Alu-Tab, Amphojel, Basaljel, Dialume

Pharmacologic class: Inorganic salt
Therapeutic class: Antacid
Pregnancy risk category NR

Action
Dissolves in acidic gastric secretions, releasing anions that partially neutralize gastric hydrochloric acid. Also elevates gastric pH, inhibiting the action of pepsin, an effect important to peptic ulcer disease.

Availability
Capsules: 400 mg, 475 mg, 500 mg
Oral suspension: 320 mg/5 ml, 450 mg/5 ml, 600 mg/5 ml, 675 mg/5 ml
Tablets: 300 mg, 500 mg, 600 mg

⚠ Indications and dosages
➤ Hyperacidity
Adults: 500 to 1,500 mg (tablet or capsule) P.O. 1 hour after meals and at bedtime; or 300 or 600 mg (tablet) five to six times daily after meals and at bedtime; or 5 to 30 ml (oral suspension) between meals and at bedtime, as needed or directed

Off-label uses
• Bleeding from stress ulcers
• Gastroesophageal reflux disease

Contraindications
None

Administration
• Give 1 hour after meals and at bedtime.
• Administer 20 to 40 minutes after meals and at bedtime in reflux esophagitis.

• Don't give within 1 to 2 hours of antibiotics, histamine$_2$-blockers, iron preparations, corticosteroids, or enteric-coated drugs.
• Administer drug with water or fruit juice.
• Provide care as appropriate if patient becomes constipated.

Route	Onset	Peak	Duration
P.O. (hypo-phosph.)	Variable	Days-wks	Days-wks
P.O. (antacid)	15-30 min	30 min	30 min-3 hr

Adverse reactions
CNS: encephalopathy, aluminum build-up and neurotoxicity, malaise (with prolonged use)
GI: constipation, anorexia (with prolonged use), **intestinal obstruction**
Metabolic: hypophosphatemia (with prolonged use)
Musculoskeletal: osteomalacia and chronic phosphate deficiency with bone pain, malaise, muscle weakness (with prolonged use)
Other: aluminum toxicity

Interactions
Drug-drug. *Allopurinol, antibiotics (including quinolones, tetracyclines), corticosteroids, diflunisal, digoxin, ethambutol, histamine$_2$-blockers, hydantoins, iron salts, isoniazid, penicillamine, phenothiazines, salicylates, thyroid hormone, ticlopidine:* decreased effects of these drugs
Enteric-coated drugs: premature release of these drugs in stomach
Drug-diagnostic tests. *Gastrin:* increased level
Phosphate: decreased level
Some imaging studies: test interference
Drug-food. *Milk, other foods high in vitamin D:* milk-alkali syndrome (headache, confusion, distaste for food, nausea, vomiting, hypercalcemia, hypercalciuria)

Precautions
Use cautiously in:
• gastric outlet obstruction, hypercalcemia, hypophosphatemia, and massive upper GI hemorrhage
• patients using other aluminum products concurrently
• patients on dialysis
• pregnant or breastfeeding patients.

Patient monitoring
• Monitor long-term use of high doses if patient is on sodium-restricted diet (drug contains sodium).
• Assess for GI bleeding.
• Watch for constipation.
• With long-term use, monitor blood phosphate level and assess for signs and symptoms of hypophosphatemia (anorexia, malaise, muscle weakness). Also monitor bone density.

Patient teaching
• Teach patient to take drug 1 hour after meals and at bedtime.
• Caution patient not to take drug within 1 to 2 hours of antibiotics, histamine$_2$-blockers, iron, corticosteroids, or enteric-coated drugs.
• Advise patient to take drug with water or fruit juice.
• Instruct patient to report signs and symptoms of GI bleeding and hypophosphatemia (appetite loss, malaise, muscle weakness).
• Teach patient to increase fiber and fluid intake and get regular physical activity to help ease constipation.
• Inform patient that drug contains sodium, so he should discuss drug therapy with health care providers if he's later told to eat low-sodium diet.
• Advise patient that he will need to undergo periodic blood testing and bone mineral density tests if he's receiving long-term therapy.

amantadine hydrochloride
Symmetrel

Pharmacologic class: Anticholinergic-like agent
Therapeutic class: Antiviral, antiparkinsonian
Pregnancy risk category C

Action
Antiviral action unclear; may prevent penetration of influenza A virus into host cell. Antiparkinson action unknown; may ease parkinsonian symptoms by increasing dopamine release, preventing dopamine reuptake into presynaptic neurons, stimulating dopamine receptors, or enhancing dopamine sensitivity.

Availability
Capsules (liquid-filled): 100 mg
Syrup: 50 mg/5 ml
Tablets: 100 mg

💊 Indications and dosages
➤ Symptomatic treatment or prophylaxis of influenza type A virus in patients with respiratory conditions
Adults over age 65 with normal renal function: 100 mg P.O. once daily
Adults to age 64 with normal renal function: 200-mg tablet or 4 tsp of syrup P.O. daily in a single dose, or 100-mg tablet or 2 tsp of syrup P.O. b.i.d.
Children ages 9 to 12: 100 mg P.O. q 12 hours
Children ages 10 and older weighing less than 45 kg (99 lb): 2.2 mg/kg P.O. q 12 hours
Children ages 1 to 9 or weighing less than 45 kg (99 lb): 100-mg tablet P.O. b.i.d., not to exceed 200 mg daily; or 2.2 to 4.4 mg/kg/day of syrup P.O. q 12 hours, not to exceed 150 mg daily

➤ Parkinson's disease
Adults: Initially, 100 mg P.O. daily, increased to 100 mg b.i.d. if needed. If patient doesn't respond adequately, give 200 mg b.i.d., up to 400 mg/day.
➤ Drug-induced extrapyramidal reactions
Adults: 100 mg to 300 mg P.O. daily in divided doses
Dosage adjustment
• Renal impairment

Contraindications
• Hypersensitivity to drug
• Untreated closed-angle glaucoma

Administration
• For antiviral use, start therapy within 24 to 48 hours of symptom onset and continue for 24 to 48 hours after symptoms resolve.
• When giving as prophylactic antiviral, start therapy as soon as possible and continue for at least 10 days after exposure to virus.
• When giving with influenza vaccine, continue drug for 2 to 3 weeks while patient develops antibody response to vaccine.

Route	Onset	Peak	Duration
P.O.	48 hr	2 wk	Unknown

Adverse reactions
CNS: stupor, delirium, depression, dizziness, drowsiness, insomnia, lightheadedness, anxiety, irritability, hallucinations, confusion, ataxia, headache, nervousness, abnormal dreams, agitation, fatigue, delusions, aggressive behavior, manic reaction, psychosis, slurred speech, euphoria, abnormal thinking, amnesia, increased or decreased motor activity, paresthesia, tremor, abnormal gait, **coma**
CV: orthostatic hypotension, tachycardia, peripheral edema, **heart failure, cardiac arrest, arrhythmias**

EENT: blurred vision, mydriasis, keratitis, photosensitivity, optic nerve palsy, nasal congestion
GI: nausea, vomiting, diarrhea, constipation, dry mouth, dysphagia, anorexia
GU: urine retention, decreased libido
Hematologic: leukocytosis
Musculoskeletal: involuntary muscle contractions
Respiratory: tachypnea, **acute respiratory failure, pulmonary edema**
Skin: purplish skin discoloration, rash, pruritus, diaphoresis
Other: edema, fever, allergic reactions, including **anaphylaxis**

Interactions
Drug-drug. *Anticholinergics, antihistamines, phenothiazines, quinidine, tricyclic antidepressants:* increased atropine-like adverse effects
CNS stimulants: increased CNS stimulation
Hydrochlorothiazide, triamterene: increased amantadine effects
Drug-diagnostic tests. *Alanine aminotransferase, alkaline phosphatase, aspartate aminotransferase, bilirubin, blood urea nitrogen, creatine phosphokinase, creatinine, gamma-glutamyltransferase, lactate dehydrogenase:* increased levels
Drug-herb. *Angel's trumpet, jimsonweed, scopolia:* increased cardiac and anticholinergic-like drug effects
Drug-behaviors. *Alcohol use:* increased CNS adverse reactions

Precautions
Use cautiously in:
• cardiac disease, hepatic disease, renal impairment, seizure disorder, psychiatric problems
• elderly patients
• pregnant or breastfeeding patients.

Patient monitoring
• Monitor patient for depression and suicidal ideation.
• Watch for mental status changes, especially in elderly patients.

• Stay alert for worsening of psychiatric problems if patient has a history of such problems or substance abuse.
• Monitor for orthostatic hypotension.
• Evaluate for signs and symptoms of fluid overload.
• Monitor renal and liver function test results.

Patient teaching
◀€ Caution patient that taking more than prescribed dosage may lead to serious adverse reactions or even death.
• Instruct patient to avoid driving and other hazardous activities until he knows how drug affects concentration and alertness.
• Advise patient to establish effective bedtime routine and to take drug several hours before bedtime to minimize insomnia.
• Teach patient to minimize GI upset by eating small, frequent servings of foods and drinking plenty of fluids.
• Instruct patient to contact prescriber if he develops signs or symptoms of depression.

amifostine
Ethyol

Pharmacologic class: Organic thiophosphate cytoprotective drug
Therapeutic class: Antineoplastic
Pregnancy risk category C

Action
Undergoes conversion to free thiol, an active metabolite that reduces toxic effects of cisplatin on renal tissue

Availability
Powder for injection: 500-mg anhydrous base and 500 mg mannitol in 10-ml vials

✐ Indications and dosages

➤ To reduce cumulative renal toxicity of cisplatin administration in patients with ovarian cancer or non-small-cell lung cancer

Adults: 910 mg/m² I.V. daily as a 15-minute infusion, starting 30 minutes before chemotherapy

➤ To reduce moderate to severe xerostomia in patients undergoing postoperative radiation treatment for head or neck cancer

Adults: 200 mg/m² I.V. daily as a 3-minute infusion, starting 15 to 30 minutes before standard fraction radiation therapy

Off-label uses

- Protection of lung fibroblasts from damaging effects of paclitaxel

Contraindications

- Hypersensitivity to drug
- Hypotension
- Concurrent antihypertensive therapy that can't be discontinued for 24 hours before amifostine treatment
- Definitive radiotherapy

Administration

- Ensure that patient is adequately hydrated before starting drug.
- Give antiemetics before and during therapy.
- Reconstitute single-dose vial with 9.7 ml of sterile normal saline injection.
- Know that drug also can be prepared in polyvinyl chloride bags.
- Don't mix with other drugs or solutions.
- Don't infuse longer than 15 minutes; doing so increases risk of adverse reactions.

◀€ Keep patient supine during administration.

Route	Onset	Peak	Duration
I.V.	5-8 min	Unknown	Unknown

Adverse reactions

CNS: dizziness, drowsiness, rigors
CV: hypotension
GI: nausea, vomiting
Metabolic: hypocalcemia
Respiratory: dyspnea, sneezing
Skin: erythema multiforme, flushing, rash, urticaria
Other: chills, warm sensation, hiccups, allergic reactions

Interactions

Drug-drug. *Antihypertensives:* increased risk of hypotension
Drug-diagnostic tests. *Calcium:* decreased level

Precautions

Use cautiously in:
- arrhythmias, heart failure, ischemic heart disease, renal impairment, hearing impairment, hypocalcemia, myasthenia gravis, nausea, vomiting, hypotension, obesity
- history of cerebrovascular accident or transient ischemic attacks
- elderly patients
- pregnant patients (safety and efficacy not established)
- breastfeeding patients
- children (safety and efficacy not established).

Patient monitoring

- Monitor blood pressure.
- Assess for severe nausea and vomiting.
- Monitor fluid intake and output.
- Monitor calcium blood level; give calcium supplements as needed.

Patient teaching

- Emphasize importance of remaining supine during drug administration to prevent hypotension.
- Caution patient to avoid driving and other hazardous activities until he knows how drug affects concentration and alertness.

• Teach patient to minimize GI upset by eating small, frequent servings of food and drinking plenty of fluids.
• Provide dietary counseling; refer patient to dietitian if adverse GI effects significantly limit food intake.
• Inform patient that sneezing is a normal effect of drug.

amikacin sulfate
Amikin

Pharmacologic class: Aminoglycoside
Therapeutic class: Anti-infective
Pregnancy risk category D

Action
Interferes with protein synthesis in bacterial cells by binding to 30S ribosomal subunit, leading to bacterial cell death

Availability
Injection: 50 mg/ml, 250 mg/ml

Indications and dosages
➤ Uncomplicated urinary tract infections caused by organisms not susceptible to other drugs
Adults: 250 mg I.M. or I.V. b.i.d.
➤ Severe systemic infections caused by sensitive strains of *Pseudomonas aeruginosa, Escherichia coli,* or *Proteus, Klebsiella, Serratia, Enterobacter, Actinobactor, Providencia, Citrobactor,* or *Staphylococcus* species
Adults, children, and older infants: 15 mg/kg/day I.V. or I.M. in two to three divided doses q 8 to 12 hours in 100 to 200 ml of dextrose 5% in water (D₅W) over 30 to 60 minutes; maximum dosage is 1.5 g/day.
Neonates: Initially, 10 mg/kg I.M.; then 7.5 mg/kg I.M. q 12 hours
Dosage adjustment
• Renal impairment (adults)
• Patients undergoing hemodialysis

Off-label uses
• *Mycobacterium avium-intracellulare* infection

Contraindications
• Hypersensitivity to aminoglycosides
• Renal or hepatic disease
• Myasthenia gravis
• Parkinsonism
• Breastfeeding

Administration
• Don't physically mix amikacin with other drugs. Administer separately.
• For I.V. use, dilute in 100 to 200 ml of normal saline solution or D₅W and give over 30 to 60 minutes.
• Ensure adequate fluid intake to avoid dehydration.
• Draw peak blood levels 1 hour after I.M. infusion or 30 to 60 minutes after I.V. infusion.
• Draw trough blood levels just before next dose.

Route	Onset	Peak	Duration
I.V.	Immediate	30 min	8-12 hr
I.M.	Variable	1 hr	8-12 hr

Adverse reactions
CNS: dizziness, vertigo, tremor, numbness, depression, confusion, lethargy, headache, paresthesia, **neuromuscular blockade, convulsions, neurotoxicity**
CV: hypotension, hypertension, palpitations
EENT: nystagmus and other visual disturbances, ototoxicity, deafness, tinnitus
GI: nausea, vomiting, splenomegaly, stomatitis, increased salivation, anorexia
GU: azotemia, increased urinary excretion of casts, polyuria, painful urination, impotence, **nephrotoxicity**
Hematologic: purpura, leukemoid reaction, eosinophilia, increased or decreased reticulocyte count, **aplastic anemia, neutropenia, agranulocyto-**

sis, **leukopenia, thrombocytopenia, pancytopenia, hemolytic anemia**
Hepatic: elevated alanine aminotransferase (ALT), aspartate aminotransferase (AST), and bilirubin; **hepatomegaly; hepatic necrosis; hepatotoxicity**
Musculoskeletal: joint pain, muscle twitching
Respiratory: apnea
Skin: rash, alopecia, urticaria, itching, exfoliative dermatitis
Other: weight loss, superinfection, pain and irritation at I.M. site

Interactions

Drug-drug. *Acyclovir, amphotericin B, cephalosporin, cisplatin, diuretics, vancomycin:* increased risk of ototoxicity and nephrotoxicity
Depolarizing and nondepolarizing neuromuscular junction blockers, general anesthetics: increased aminoglycoside effect, possibly leading to respiratory depression
Dimenhydrinate: masking of ototoxicity signs and symptoms
Indomethacin: increased trough and peak amikacin levels
Parenteral penicillin: amikacin inactivation
Drug-diagnostic tests. *ALT, AST, alkaline phosphatase, bilirubin, blood urea nitrogen, lactate dehydrogenase, creatinine, nonprotein nitrogen, nitrogen compounds (such as urea):* increased levels
Calcium, potassium, magnesium, sodium: decreased levels

Precautions

Use cautiously in:
• decreased renal function, neuromuscular disorders
• elderly patients
• pregnant patients.

Patient monitoring

• Monitor kidney function test results, urine cultures, urine output, and urine specific gravity.
• Monitor results of peak and trough drug blood levels.
• Evaluate for signs and symptoms of ototoxicity (hearing loss, tinnitus, ataxia, vertigo).
• Assess for secondary superinfections, particularly upper respiratory tract infections.

Patient teaching

◀€ Inform patient that drug may cause hearing loss, seizures, and other neurologic problems. Tell him to report these symptoms immediately.
• Tell patient to report fever, cough, breathing problems, sore throat, and other signs and symptoms of infection immediately.
• Advise patient to avoid driving and other hazardous activities until he knows how drug affects concentration and alertness.
• Instruct patient to notify prescriber if he's urinating much more or much less than normal.
• Advise patient to minimize GI upset by eating small, frequent servings of food and drinking plenty of fluids.
• Inform patient that he'll undergo regular blood and urine testing during therapy.

amiloride hydrochloride
Midamor

Pharmacologic class: Pyrazine-carbonyl-guanidine
Therapeutic class: Potassium-sparing diuretic
Pregnancy risk category B

Action
Inhibits sodium reabsorption at distal convoluted renal tubule, cortical collecting tubule, and collecting duct, thereby causing sodium and fluid loss and potassium retention

Availability
Tablets: 5 mg

⚠ Indications and dosages
➢ Heart failure or hypertension in patients receiving concurrent thiazides or other potassium-wasting diuretics
Adults: 5 mg P.O. daily as adjunct to usual antihypertensive or potassium-wasting diuretic; may increase to 20 mg daily with careful electrolyte monitoring
➢ Single-drug therapy in patients with heart failure or hypertension
Adults: Initially, 5 mg P.O. daily; if needed, increase to 10 mg P.O. daily. In persistent hypokalemia, may increase to 15 to 20 mg P.O. daily with careful electrolyte monitoring.

Contraindications
• Hypersensitivity to drug
• Impaired renal function
• Concurrent use or ingestion of potassium supplements
• Children

Administration
• Give with meals.
• Never give to patient concurrently taking potassium supplements or other potassium-sparing diuretics.

Route	Onset	Peak	Duration
P.O.	2 hr	6-10 hr	24 hr

Adverse reactions
CNS: headache, weakness, fatigue, dizziness, encephalopathy, paresthesia
GI: nausea, vomiting, constipation, abdominal pain, flatulence, appetite changes
GU: polyuria, impotence
Metabolic: hyperkalemia, electrolyte imbalances (when used with other diuretics)
Musculoskeletal: muscle cramps
Respiratory: cough, dyspnea
Skin: rash

Interactions
Drug-drug. *Angiotensin-converting enzyme (ACE) inhibitors, cyclosporine, potassium supplements, other potassium-sparing diuretics, tacrolimus:* increased risk of severe hyperkalemia
Digoxin: decreased digoxin efficacy
Lithium: reduced lithium clearance and increased risk of lithium toxicity
Nonsteroidal anti-inflammatory drugs: reduced diuretic and antihypertensive effects of amiloride
Drug-diagnostic tests. *Blood urea nitrogen (BUN), potassium:* increased levels
Chloride, hemoglobin, magnesium, neutrophils, sodium: decreased levels
Liver function tests: decreased values
Drug-food. *Foods high in potassium, salt substitutes containing potassium:* hyperkalemia
Drug-herb. *Licorice:* increased risk of hypokalemia

Precautions
Use cautiously in:
• hepatic insufficiency, cardiopulmonary disease, diabetes mellitus, renal disease
• elderly patients
• pregnant patients.

Patient monitoring
• Monitor blood chemistry and liver and kidney function test results, complete blood count, and electrolyte levels (especially potassium).
• Assess for signs and symptoms of hyperkalemia, especially in patients also taking ACE inhibitors or indomethacin.
• Evaluate patient for orthostatic hypertension.

♣ Canada   ◀︎€ Clinical alert   Reactions in **bold** are life-threatening

Patient teaching

• Tell patient to immediately report signs and symptoms of hyperkalemia (tingling, fatigue, muscle weakness or paralysis).
• Caution patient to avoid driving or other hazardous activities until he knows how the drug affects concentration and alertness.
• Tell patient to avoid high-potassium salt substitutes and foods.
• Teach patient to minimize GI upset by taking drug with meals; eating small, frequent servings of healthy food; and drinking plenty of fluids.
• Encourage patient to discuss activity recommendations and pain management with prescriber. Advise him to avoid NSAIDs, which interfere with drug's action.
• Inform patient that he'll undergo regular blood testing during therapy.

amino acids

high metabolic stress formulations
Aminosyn-HBC, BranchAmin 4%, FreAmine-HBC

renal failure formulations
Aminess 5.2%, Aminosyn-RF 5.2%, 5.4% NephrAmine, RenAmin

hepatic failure or hepatic encephalopathy formulations
HepatAmine

amino acid injection
FreAmine, HepatAmine, Primene♣, Vamin N♣

crystalline amino acid infusions
Aminosyn, FreAmine III, Novamine, Travasol, TrophAmine

crystalline amino acid infusions with dextrose
Aminosyn (various strengths), Travasol (various strengths)

crystalline amino acid infusions with electrolytes
Aminosyn (various strengths), FreAmine (various strengths), ProcalAmine, Travasol (various strengths)

crystalline amino acid infusions with electrolytes in dextrose
Aminosyn (various strengths)

Pharmacologic class: Protein substrate
Therapeutic class: Caloric drug, nitrogen product
Pregnancy risk category C

Action
Provides substrate for protein synthesis (anabolism) or helps conserve existing body protein (protein-sparing effect)

Availability
Injection: Many strengths and concentrations available. Specific formulation to use depends on patient's status, underlying disease or disorder, and duration of therapy.

🖋 Indications and dosages
Indications and dosages given below are limited to those used in common nutritional therapies.
➤ Total parenteral nutrition (TPN) supplement for patients with negative nitrogen balance secondary to inability

of GI tract to absorb protein; patients unable to receive adequate nutrition through tube feedings; and patients requiring bowel rest

Adults: 1 to 1.7 g/kg/day of amino acids I.V. (by peripheral vein) with low concentration of dextrose solution as required, or 500 ml amino acids I.V. injection (by central vein), mixed with 500 ml of concentrated dextrose injection, electrolytes, and vitamins, given over 8 hours

Children: Follow manufacturer's directions and use with caution.

➤ Nutritional supplement for patients with high metabolic stress

Adults: With adequate calories, 1.5 g/kg/day of amino acids I.V. May be mixed with other solutions, as directed, and given by peripheral vein if amino acid solution contains minimal calories and central route isn't indicated

➤ Nutritional supplement for patients with renal failure

Adults: 250 to 600 ml of Aminosyn I.V. daily, depending on formulation. May necessitate mixing formulations with other solutions before infusing.

Children: Initially, start with low dosage, following manufacturer's directions; increase to maximum daily dosage of 0.5 to 1g/kg I.V. May necessitate mixing formulations with other solutions before infusing.

➤ Nutritional supplement in patients with hepatic failure or hepatic encephalopathy

Adults: 80 to 120 g of amino acids (12 to 18 g of nitrogen) I.V. daily, mixed with other solutions as required. May be given by peripheral vein if central route isn't indicated.

Contraindications

• Hypersensitivity to amino acids
• Intracranial or intraspinal hemorrhage
• Severe renal or hepatic disease
• Metabolic disorders

Administration

• Don't give by I.V. push or bolus.
• Don't give hypertonic solutions via peripheral vein.
◀€ Begin I.V. infusion slowly. Control infusion rate carefully with infusion pump; monitor infusion rate closely.
• Don't stop therapy abruptly; rebound hypoglycemia may occur.
• For subclavian administration, infuse drug into midsuperior vena cava.
• Use strict aseptic technique when mixing and preparing solution. Replace all I.V. equipment every 24 hours.
• Check infusion site often for infection, phlebitis, and tissue damage.
• Change dressing every 24 hours.

Route	Onset	Peak	Duration
I.V.	Immediate	Immediate	Unknown

Adverse reactions

CNS: headache, dizziness, confusion, **loss of consciousness**
CV: hypertension, tachycardia, **heart failure, venous thrombosis, circulatory overload**
GI: nausea, vomiting, abdominal pain
GU: osmotic diuresis, glycosuria
Hepatic: jaundice, **fatty liver, hepatic impairment**
Metabolic: rebound hypoglycemia (with abrupt cessation of long-term infusion), hyperglycemia, excessive urea buildup, fatty acid deficiency, electrolyte imbalances, hyperosmolar syndrome, hyperammonemia, hypophosphatemia, hypocalcemia, metabolic acidosis and alkalosis, dehydration, **hyperosmolar hyperglycemic nonketotic syndrome**
Musculoskeletal: osteoporosis
Respiratory: pulmonary edema
Skin: rash, generalized flushing, warm sensation, papular eruptions, chills, urticaria, extravasation necrosis, phlebitis or tissue sloughing at injection site
Other: hypersensitivity reaction, fever, chills, pain, **catheter sepsis**

✚ Canada   ◀€ Clinical alert   Reactions in **bold** are life-threatening

Interactions
Drug-drug. *Tetracycline:* reduced protein-sparing effects of amino acid

Precautions
Use cautiously in:
- heart failure, hypertension, diabetes mellitus, hepatic or renal impairment
- elderly patients
- pregnant patients
- children.

Patient monitoring
- When initiating therapy, monitor blood glucose level frequently until stabilized; then monitor daily.
- Monitor serum electrolyte levels; report unusual electrolyte losses (for instance, from nasogastric tube, vomiting, drainage, or diarrhea).
- Watch for circulatory overload in patient with cardiac insufficiency.
- Monitor blood urea nitrogen level.
- Evaluate fractional urine regularly for glycosuria, which may signal glucose intolerance and sepsis onset.
- Assess for sepsis continually, such as by checking temperature every 4 hours.
- Evaluate patient's nutritional status regularly.

Patient teaching
- Caution patient to avoid driving and other hazardous activities until he knows how drug affects concentration and alertness.
- Tell patient that TPN infusion may increase risk of infection; advise him to report fever, chills, and other signs and symptoms.
- Instruct patient to report unusual pain, redness, swelling, and other changes at infusion site.
- Instruct patient to notify prescriber of vomiting or diarrhea.

aminocaproic acid
Amicar, EACA

Pharmacologic class: Carboxylic acid derivative
Therapeutic class: Antihemorrhagic, antifibrinolytic
Pregnancy risk category C

Action
Interferes with plasminogen activator substances; also blocks antiplasmin activity, resulting in breakdown of blood clots

Availability
Injection: 250 mg/ml
Syrup: 250 mg/ml
Tablets: 500 mg

Indications and dosages
➤ Excessive bleeding caused by fibrinolysis
Adults: 5 g P.O. during first hour, then 1 to 1.25 g/hour until bleeding is controlled. Or, 4 to 5 g I.V. over 1 hour, followed by continuous infusion of 1 g per hour. Continue for 8 hours or until bleeding stops. Maximum daily dosage is 30 g.

Off-label uses
- Dental extractions
- Hemorrhage

Contraindications
- Hypersensitivity to drug
- Upper urinary tract bleeding
- Disseminated intravascular coagulation
- Neonates (injectable form)

Administration
- Dilute I.V. form in sterile water for injection, normal saline solution, dextrose 5% in water, or Ringer's solu-

tion for injection. Give at prescribed rate.

• Know that oral and I.V. doses are the same.

Route	Onset	Peak	Duration
P.O.	1 hr	2 hr	Unknown
I.V.	1 hr	Unknown	3 hr

Adverse reactions

CNS: dizziness, malaise, headache, delirium, hallucinations, weakness, **seizures**

CV: hypotension, cardiomyopathy, elevated creatine kinase (CK) level, ischemia, thrombophlebitis, **bradycardia, arrhythmias**

EENT: conjunctival suffusion, tinnitus, nasal congestion

GI: nausea, vomiting, diarrhea, abdominal pain, dyspepsia

GU: elevated blood urea nitrogen (BUN), intrarenal obstruction, **renal failure**

Hematologic: generalized thrombosis, **agranulocytosis, leukopenia, thrombocytopenia**

Hepatic: elevated aspartate aminotransferase (AST) level

Musculoskeletal: myopathy, rhabdomyolysis

Respiratory: dyspnea, **pulmonary embolism**

Skin: rash, pruritus

Other: elevated serum aldolase and potassium levels

Interactions

Drug-drug. *Estrogens, hormonal contraceptives:* increased risk of hypercoagulation

Activated prothrombin, prothrombin complex concentrates: increased signs of active intravascular clotting

Drug-diagnostic tests. *Alanine aminotransferase, AST, BUN, creatinine, CK:* increased levels

Drug-herb. *Alfalfa, anise, arnica, astragalus, bilberry, black currant seed oil, capsaicin, cat's claw, celery, chaparral, clove oil, dandelion, dong quai, evening primrose oil, feverfew, garlic, ginger, ginkgo, papaya extract rhubarb, safflower oil, skullcap:* increased anticoagulant effect

Coenzyme Q10, St. John's wort: reduced anticoagulant effect

Precautions

Use cautiously in:

• heart, hepatic, or renal failure.

Patient monitoring

• Monitor vital signs, fluid intake and output, and electrocardiogram.

• Assess for signs and symptoms of thrombophlebitis and pulmonary embolism.

• Monitor neurologic status, especially for signs of impending seizure.

• Monitor kidney and liver function test results, serum electrolyte levels, and complete blood count with white cell differential.

• Evaluate for blood dyscrasias, particularly bleeding tendencies.

Patient teaching

• Tell patient that drug may significantly affect many body systems; assure him that he'll be monitored closely.

• Instruct patient to immediately report signs and symptoms of thrombophlebitis, pulmonary embolism, or unusual bleeding.

• Tell patient he'll undergo frequent blood testing during therapy.

aminophylline (theophylline, ethylenediamine)
Phyllocontin, Phyllocontin-350, Truphylline

Pharmacologic class: Xanthine
Therapeutic class: Bronchodilator
Pregnancy risk category C

Action
Unknown; thought to directly relax smooth muscle of bronchial airways and increase pulmonary blood flow by inhibiting phosphodiesterase

Availability
Injection: 250 mg/10 ml, 500 mg/20 ml, 100 mg/100 ml in half-normal saline solution, 200 mg/100 ml in half-normal saline solution
Oral liquid: 105 mg/5 ml
Suppositories: 250 mg, 500 mg
Tablets: 100 mg, 200 mg
Tablets (extended-release): 225 mg, 350 mg

🕐 Indications and dosages
➤ Symptomatic relief of bronchospasm in patients with acute symptoms requiring rapid theophyllinization
Adults (nonsmokers): 0.7 mg/kg/hour I.V. for first 12 hours; maintenance dosage is 0.5 mg/kg/hour I.V.
Children ages 9 to 16: 1 mg/kg/hour I.V. for first 12 hours; maintenance dosage is 0.8 mg/kg/hour I.V.
Children ages 6 months to 9 years: 1.2 mg/kg/hour I.V. for first 12 hours; maintenance dosage is 1 mg/kg/hour I.V.
➤ Chronic bronchial asthma
Adults and children: Dosage is highly individualized. Common initial dosage is 16 mg/kg/24 hours I.V. or 400 mg/24 hours I.V. in divided doses at 6- or 8-hour intervals. If needed, dosage may be increased 25% at 3-day intervals.
Dosage adjustment
• Heart failure
• Hepatic disease
• Elderly patients
• Smokers

Off-label uses
• Dyspnea in patients with chronic obstructive pulmonary disease (COPD)

Contraindications
• Hypersensitivity to xanthine compounds or ethylenediamine
• GI disease
• Seizure disorders

Administration
• For I.V. use, dilute according to label directions and infuse at no more than 25 mg/minute.
• Don't give in I.V. solutions containing invert sugar, fructose, or fat emulsions.
• Give oral form at meals with 8 oz of water.

Route	Onset	Peak	Duration
P.O. (extended)	Variable	Variable	Variable
P.O. (liquid)	15-60 min	1-7 hr	Variable
I.V.	Immediate	Immediate	6-8 hr
P.R.	Unknown	Unknown	Unknown

Adverse reactions
CNS: irritability, dizziness, nervousness, restlessness, headache, insomnia, stammering speech, abnormal behavior, mutism, unresponsiveness alternating with hyperactivity, **seizures**
CV: palpitations, marked hypotension, sinus tachycardia, extrasystoles, **arrhythmias, circulatory failure**
GI: nausea, vomiting, diarrhea, epigastric pain, hematemesis, gastroesophageal reflux, anorexia

GU: urine retention (in men with enlarged prostate), diuresis, increased excretion of renal tubular cells and red blood cells, proteinuria

Hepatic: elevated aspartate aminotransferase (AST) level

Metabolic: hyperglycemia

Musculoskeletal: muscle twitching

Respiratory: tachypnea, **respiratory arrest**

Skin: flushing

Other: fever, hypersensitivity reactions (including exfoliative dermatitis and urticaria)

Interactions

Drug-drug. *Adenosine:* decreased antiarrhythmic effect of adenosine

Barbiturates, nicotine, phenytoin, rifampin: decreased aminophylline blood level

Beta blockers: antagonism of aminophylline effects

Calcium channel blockers, cimetidine, ciprofloxacin, disulfiram, erythromycin, hormonal contraceptives, influenza vaccine, interferon, methotrexate: elevated aminophylline blood level

Carbamazepine, isoniazid, loop diuretics (such as furosemide): increased or decreased aminophylline blood level

Ephedrine, other sympathomimetics: toxicity, arrhythmias

Lithium: increased lithium excretion

Drug-diagnostic tests. *AST, glucose:* increased levels

Drug-herb. *Cayenne:* increased risk of aminophylline toxicity

Drug-behaviors. *Smoking:* increased aminophylline elimination

Precautions

Use cautiously in:

• COPD, diabetes mellitus, glaucoma, renal or hepatic disease, heart failure or other cardiac or circulatory impairment, hypertension, hyperthyroidism, peptic ulcer, severe hypoxemia

• elderly patients

• neonates, infants, and young children.

Patient monitoring

◀€ Monitor aminophylline blood level; adjust dosage if signs or symptoms of toxicity appear (tachycardia, headache, anorexia, nausea, vomiting, diarrhea, restlessness, and irritability).

• Assess for arrhythmias, especially after giving loading dose.

• Check vital signs and fluid intake and output.

• Monitor patient's response to drug and assess pulmonary function test results.

Patient teaching

• Advise patient to take oral doses at meals with 8 oz of water.

• Caution patient to avoid driving and other hazardous activities until he knows how drug affects concentration and alertness.

• Teach patient to minimize GI upset by eating small, frequent servings of food and drinking plenty of fluids.

• Advise patient to establish an effective bedtime routine to minimize insomnia.

• Caution patient not to change aminophylline brands.

• If patient smokes, tell him to notify prescriber if he stops smoking; aminophylline dosage may need adjustment.

amiodarone hydrochloride
Cordarone, Pacerone

Pharmacologic class: Adrenergic blocker

Therapeutic class: Antiarrhythmic (class III)

Pregnancy risk category D

Action
Prolongs duration and refractory period of action potential; slows electrical conduction, electrical impulse generation from sinoatrial node, and conduction through accessory pathways. Also dilates blood vessels.

Availability
Injection: 50 mg/ml in 3-ml ampules
Tablets: 200 mg, 400 mg

⏀ Indications and dosages
➢ Life-threatening ventricular arrhythmias
Adults: 150 mg by rapid I.V. infusion over 10 minutes, followed by 360 mg by slow I.V. infusion over the next 6 hours; then 540-mg I.V. maintenance infusion over next 18 hours. Or 800 to 1,600 mg P.O. daily in one to two doses for 1 to 3 weeks; then 600 to 800 mg P.O. daily in one to two doses for 1 month; then 400-mg P.O. daily maintenance dosage.

Off-label uses
• Atrioventricular (AV) nodal reentry tachycardia (with parenteral use)
• Conversion of atrial fibrillation to normal sinus rhythm

Contraindications
• Hypersensitivity to drug
• Cardiogenic shock
• Second- or third-degree AV block
• Marked sinus bradycardia
• Neonates
• Breastfeeding

Administration
◣€ Give loading dose in hospital setting with continuous electrocardiographic (ECG) monitoring.
• Administer oral loading dose in two equal doses with meals. Give maintenance dose daily or in two divided doses to minimize GI upset.

• Don't give I.V. unless patient is on continuous ECG monitoring.
• Dilute I.V. drug with dextrose 5% in water and use in-line filter; drug isn't compatible with normal saline solution.
• Use central venous catheter when giving repeated doses; if possible, use dedicated catheter for drug.

Route	Onset	Peak	Duration
P.O.	Variable	3-7 hr	Wks-mos
I.V.	Hrs	Unknown	Variable

Adverse reactions
CNS: dizziness, fatigue, headache, insomnia, paresthesia, peripheral neuropathy, poor coordination, involuntary movements, tremor, sleep disturbances
CV: hypotension, heart failure, **worsening arrhythmia, AV block, sinoatrial node dysfunction, bradycardia, asystole, cardiac arrest, cardiogenic shock, electromechanical dissociation, ventricular tachycardia**
EENT: corneal microdeposits, corneal or macular degeneration, visual disturbances, dry eyes, eye discomfort, optic neuritis or neuropathy, scotoma, lens opacities, photophobia, visual halos, abnormal smell, **papilledema**
GI: nausea, vomiting, constipation, abdominal pain, abnormal taste, abnormal salivation, anorexia
GU: abnormal kidney function tests, decreased libido
Hematologic: coagulation abnormalities, thrombocytopenia
Hepatic: hepatic function abnormalities, nonspecific hepatic disorders
Metabolic: hypothyroidism, hyperthyroidism
Respiratory: cough, **adult respiratory distress syndrome, pulmonary inflammation or fibrosis, pulmonary edema**
Skin: flushing, photosensitivity, toxic epidermal necrolysis

Other: edema, fever, **Stevens-Johnson syndrome**

Interactions

Drug-drug. *Anticoagulants:* increased prothrombin time (PT)
Beta blockers: increased risk of bradycardia and hypotension
Calcium channel blockers: increased risk of AV block (with verapamil, diltiazem) or hypotension (with any calcium channel blocker)
Cholestyramine: decreased amiodarone blood level
Cimetidine, ritonavir: increased amiodarone blood level
Class I antiarrhythmics (disopyramide, flecainide, lidocaine, mexiletine, procainamide, quinidine): increased blood levels of these drugs, leading to toxicity
Cyclosporine: elevated cyclosporine and creatinine blood levels
Dextromethorphan: impaired dextromethorphan metabolism (with amiodarone therapy of 2 weeks or longer)
Digoxin: increased digoxin blood level, leading to toxicity
Fentanyl: increased bradycardia, hypotension
Fluoroquinolones: increased risk of life-threatening arrhythmias
Methotrexate: impaired methotrexate metabolism, possibly causing toxicity (with amiodarone use longer than 2 weeks)
Phenytoin: decreased amiodarone blood level or increased phenytoin blood level (with amiodarone use longer than 2 weeks)
Theophylline: increased theophylline blood level (with amiodarone use longer than 1 week)

Precautions

Use cautiously in:
• electrolyte imbalances, severe pulmonary or hepatic disease, thyroid disorders
• history of heart failure
• elderly patients
• pregnant patients
• children.

Patient monitoring

◀€ Monitor patient closely; drug may cause serious or life-threatening adverse reactions.
◀€ Watch for slow onset of life-threatening arrhythmias, especially after giving loading dose.
◀€ Monitor ECG continuously during loading dose and when dosage is changed.
• Check patient's blood pressure, pulse, and heart rhythm regularly.
• Assess for signs and symptoms of lung inflammation.
• Monitor baseline and subsequent chest X-rays, as well as pulmonary, liver, and thyroid function test results.
• Closely monitor patient who's receiving other drugs concurrently because amiodarone can interact with many drugs. Check digoxin blood levels if patient is receiving digoxin; monitor PT or International Normalized Ratio if patient is receiving anticoagulants.

Patient teaching

◀€ Teach patient that drug may cause serious adverse reactions; instruct him to report these immediately.
• Instruct patient to take oral doses with meals; advise him to divide daily dose into two doses if drug causes GI upset.
• Tell patient that adverse reactions are most common with high doses and may grow more frequent after 6 months of therapy.
• Inform patient that he'll undergo regular blood testing, chest X-rays, and pulmonary function tests during therapy.

amitriptyline hydrochloride

Apo-Amitriptyline, Elavil, Endep, Levate✢, Novotriptyn✢

Pharmacologic class: Tricyclic compound
Therapeutic class: Antidepressant
Pregnancy risk category D

Action

Unknown; inhibits norepinephrine and serotonin reuptake at presynaptic neuron, increasing levels of these neurotransmitters in brain; also has sedative, anticholinergic, and mild peripheral vasodilating effects

Availability

Injection: 10 mg/ml
Syrup: 10 mg/5 ml
Tablets: 10 mg, 25 mg, 50 mg, 75 mg, 100 mg, 150 mg

⃠ Indications and dosages

➤ Depression (often given in conjunction with psychotherapy)
Adults: 75 mg P.O. daily in divided doses; may increase gradually to 150 mg/day. Or start with 50 to 100 mg P.O. at bedtime, and increase by 25 to 50 mg as needed to a total dosage of 150 mg. Hospitalized patients initially may receive 100 mg P.O. daily, with gradual increases as needed to a total dosage of 300 mg P.O. With I.M. use, give 20 to 30 mg q.i.d.
Dosage adjustment
• Adolescents
• Elderly patients
• Outpatients

Off-label uses

• Analgesic adjunct for phantom limb pain or chronic pain

Contraindications

• Hypersensitivity to drug or other tricyclic antidepressants (TCAs)
• Monoamine oxidase (MAO) inhibitor use within past 14 days
• Impaired renal or hepatic function
• Children younger than age 12

Administration

• Administer full dose at bedtime to minimize orthostatic hypotension.
• Give injectable form by I.M. route only.
• Don't withdraw drug suddenly; instead, taper dosage gradually.
• If patient is scheduled for surgery, discuss dosage tapering with prescriber.

Route	Onset	Peak	Duration
P.O.	2-4 wk	2-6 wk	Unknown
I.M.	2-3 wk	2-6 wk	Unknown

Adverse reactions

CNS: headache, fatigue, agitation, numbness, paresthesia, peripheral neuropathy, weakness, restlessness, panic, anxiety, dizziness, drowsiness, difficulty speaking, excitement, hypomania, psychosis exacerbation, extrapyramidal effects, poor coordination, fatigue, hallucinations, insomnia, nightmares, **seizures, coma**
CV: electrocardiogram changes, MI, tachycardia, hypertension, orthostatic hypotension, **arrhythmias, heart block**
EENT: blurred vision, dry eyes, mydriasis, abnormal visual accommodation, increased intraocular pressure, tinnitus
GI: nausea, vomiting, constipation, dry mouth, epigastric pain, anorexia, **paralytic ileus**
GU: urine retention, delayed voiding, urinary tract dilation, gynecomastia
Hematologic: blood dyscrasias, agranulocytosis, thrombocytopenia, thrombocytopenic purpura, leukopenia

---

Metabolic: changes in blood glucose level

Skin: photosensitivity rash, urticaria, flushing, diaphoresis

Other: increased appetite, weight gain, high fever, edema, hypersensitivity reaction

Interactions

Drug-drug. *Activated charcoal:* decreased amitriptyline absorption

Adrenergics, anticholinergics, anticholinergic-like drugs: increased anticholinergic effects

Amiodarone, cimetidine, quinidine, ritonavir: increased amitriptyline effects

Barbiturates: decreased amitriptyline blood level, increased CNS and respiratory effects

Clonidine: hypertensive crisis

CNS depressants (including alcohol, antihistamines, opioids, sedativehypnotics): increased CNS depression

Drugs metabolized by cytochrome P450 enzyme 2D6 (such as other antidepressants, phenothiazines, carbamazepine, class 1C antiarrhythmics): decreased amitriptyline clearance, possibly causing toxicity

Guanethidine: antagonism of antihypertensive action

Levodopa: delayed or decreased levodopa absorption, hypertension

MAO inhibitors: hypotension, tachycardia, potentially fatal reactions

Rifabutin, rifampin, rifapentine: decreased amitriptyline blood level and effects

Selective serotonin reuptake inhibitors: increased risk of toxicity

Sympathomimetics: increased pressor effect of direct-acting sympathomimetics (epinephrine, norepinephrine), possibly causing arrhythmias; decreased pressor effect of indirect-acting sympathomimetics (ephedrine, metaraminol)

Drug-diagnostic tests. *Eosinophils, liver function tests:* increased values

Glucose, granulocytes, platelets, white blood cells: increased or decreased levels

Drug-herb. *Angel's trumpet, jimsonweed, scopolia:* increased anticholinergic effects

Chamomile, hops, kava, skullcap, valerian: increased CNS depression

St. John's wort: decreased drug blood level and reduced efficacy

Drug-behaviors. *Alcohol use:* increased CNS sedation

Smoking: increased drug metabolism and altered effects

Sun exposure: increased risk of photosensitivity reactions

Precautions

Use cautiously in:

• seizures, cardiovascular disease, renal or hepatic impairment, urine retention, hyperthyroidism, increased intraocular pressure, closed-angle glaucoma, prostatic hypertrophy, bipolar disorder, schizophrenia, paranoia

• elderly patients

• pregnant or breastfeeding patients.

Patient monitoring

• Evaluate for signs and symptoms of psychosis; if present, discuss possible dosage change with prescriber.

• Assess for changes in patient's mood or mental status.

• Monitor for signs and symptoms of depression and assess for suicidal ideation.

• Check blood pressure for orthostatic hypertension.

• Monitor complete blood count with white cell differential, glucose levels, and liver function test results.

Patient teaching

• Instruct patient to contact prescriber if he experiences severe mood changes or suicidal thoughts.

• Caution patient to avoid driving and other hazardous activities until he knows how drug affects concentration and alertness.

• Tell patient that drug may cause temporary blood pressure decrease if he stands up suddenly. Advise him to rise slowly and carefully.
• Tell patient to minimize GI upset by eating small, frequent servings of food and drinking plenty of fluids.
• Inform patient that he'll undergo frequent blood testing during therapy.

amlodipine besylate
Norvasc L

Pharmacologic class: Calcium channel blocker

Therapeutic class: Antihypertensive

Pregnancy risk category C

Action
Inhibits influx of extracellular calcium ions, which decreases myocardial contractility, relaxes coronary and vascular muscles, and decreases peripheral resistance

Availability
Tablets: 2.5 mg, 5 mg, 10 mg

Indications and dosages
➤ Essential hypertension, chronic stable angina pectoris, and vasospastic angina (Prinzmetal's angina), given alone or with other drugs
Adults: 5 to 10 mg P.O. once daily
Dosage adjustment
• Hepatic impairment
• Elderly patients

Off-label uses
• Pulmonary hypertension
• Raynaud's disease

Contraindications
• Hypersensitivity to drug

Administration
• Be aware that this drug may be given concurrently with other antihypertensives and antianginals.

Route	Onset	Peak	Duration
P.O.	Unknown	6-9 hr	24 hr

Adverse reactions
CNS: headache, dizziness, drowsiness, light-headedness, fatigue, weakness, lethargy
CV: peripheral edema, angina, bradycardia, hypotension, palpitations
GI: nausea, abdominal discomfort
Musculoskeletal: muscle cramps, muscle pain or inflammation
Respiratory: shortness of breath, dyspnea, wheezing
Skin: rash, pruritus, urticaria, flushing

Interactions
Drug-drug. *Beta blockers:* increased risk of adverse effects
Fentanyl, nitrates, other antihypertensives, quinidine: additive hypotension
Drug-behaviors. *Acute alcohol ingestion:* additive hypotension

Precautions
Use cautiously in:
• aortic stenosis, severe hepatic impairment, heart failure
• elderly patients
• pregnant or breastfeeding patients.
• children.

Patient monitoring
◀€ Monitor patient for worsening angina.
• Monitor heart rate and rhythm and blood pressure, especially at start of therapy.
• Assess for heart failure; report signs and symptoms (peripheral edema, dyspnea) to prescriber promptly.
• Give sublingual nitroglycerin, as prescribed, if patient has signs or symptoms of acute myocardial infarction, especially when dosage is increased.

Patient teaching
• Instruct patient to avoid driving and other hazardous activities until he knows how drug affects concentration and alertness.
• If patient also uses sublingual nitroglycerin, tell him he can take nitroglycerin as needed for acute angina.

amoxapine
Asendin

Pharmacologic class: Tricyclic compound
Therapeutic class: Antidepressant
Pregnancy risk category C

Action
Unclear; inhibits reuptake of norepinephrine or serotonin at presynaptic neuron, enhancing levels of these neurotransmitters in brain. Also has sedative, anticholinergic, and mild peripheral vasodilatory properties.

Availability
Tablets: 25 mg, 50 mg, 100 mg, 150 mg

⚠ Indications and dosages
➤ Depression accompanied by anxiety or agitation
Adults: Initially, 50 mg P.O. two or three times daily, increased to 100 mg two or three times daily by end of first week. If starting dosage (up to 300 mg/day) is tolerated but ineffective for at least 2 weeks, dosage may be increased. For outpatients, maximum suggested dosage is 400 mg/day; for hospitalized patients, 600 mg/day.
Dosage adjustment
• Elderly patients

Off-label uses
• Analgesic adjunct for phantom limb pain or chronic pain

Contraindications
• Hypersensitivity to drug or tricyclic antidepressants (TCA)
• Monoamine oxidase (MAO) inhibitor use within past 14 days
• Patients younger than age 16

Administration
• Don't give drug if patient has taken MAO inhibitors within past 14 days.
• If desired, give daily dose up to 300 mg at bedtime.
• If patient is scheduled for surgery, discuss need for dosage tapering with prescriber.

Route	Onset	Peak	Duration
P.O.	Unknown	2-4 hr	2-4 wk

Adverse reactions
CNS: agitation, restlessness, fatigue, panic, anxiety, dizziness, drowsiness, difficulty articulating words, excitement, hypomania, psychosis exacerbation, extrapyramidal effects, tardive dyskinesia, poor coordination, hallucinations, headache, insomnia, nightmares, numbness, paresthesia, peripheral neuropathy, weakness, **neuroleptic malignant syndrome, seizures, coma**
CV: ECG changes, hypertension, orthostatic hypotension, **arrhythmias, heart block, myocardial infarction, tachycardia,**
EENT: blurred vision, dry eyes, mydriasis, abnormal visual accommodation, increased intraocular pressure, tinnitus
GI: nausea, vomiting, constipation, anorexia, epigastric pain, dry mouth, **paralytic ileus**
Hematologic: blood dyscrasias, agranulocytosis, thrombocytopenia, thrombocytopenic purpura, leukopenia
GU: urine retention, delayed voiding, urinary tract dilation, gynecomastia
Metabolic: changes in blood glucose level
Skin: photosensitivity rash, urticaria, flushing, diaphoresis

Other: increased appetite, weight gain, high fever, edema, **hypersensitivity reactions**

Interactions
Drug-drug. *Adrenergics, anticholinergics, anticholinergic-like drugs:* increased anticholinergic effects
Amiodarone, cimetidine, quinidine, ritonavir: increased amoxapine effects
Barbiturates: reduced amoxapine blood level, increased CNS and respiratory effects
Clonidine: hypertensive crisis
CNS depressants (including antihistamines, opioids, sedative-hypnotics): increased CNS depression
Drugs metabolized by cytochrome P450 enzyme 2D6 (such as other antidepressants, carbamazepine, class IC antiarrhythmics, phenothiazines): decreased amoxapine clearance, possible toxicity
Guanethidine: antagonism of antihypertensive action
Levodopa: delayed or decreased levodopa absorption, hypertension
MAO inhibitors: hypotension, tachycardia, fever, extreme excitation, hyperpyrexia, seizures
Rifabutin, rifampin, rifapentine: decreased amoxapine blood level and effects
Selective serotonin reuptake inhibitors: increased toxicity
Sympathomimetics: increased pressor effects of direct-acting sympathomimetics (epinephrine, norepinephrine), possibly causing arrhythmias; decreased pressor effects of indirect-acting sympathomimetics (ephedrine, metaraminol)
Valproic acid: increased valproic acid blood level, greater risk of adverse effects
Drug-diagnostic tests. *Eosinophils, liver function tests:* increased values
Glucose, granulocytes, platelets, white blood cells: increased or decreased values

Drug-herb. *Evening primrose:* lower seizure threshold, increased risk of seizures
Drug-behaviors. *Alcohol use:* increased CNS sedation
Smoking: increased metabolism and altered drug effects
Sun exposure: increased risk of photosensitivity reactions

Precautions
Use cautiously in:
• renal or hepatic impairment, prostatic hypertrophy, hyperthyroidism, closed-angle glaucoma, bipolar disorder, schizophrenia
• elderly patients
• pregnant or breastfeeding patients.

Patient monitoring
◀≶ Watch for signs and symptoms of neuroleptic malignant syndrome (high fever, rapid pulse and breathing, profuse sweating).
• Monitor patient for signs and symptoms of psychosis; if these occur, consult prescriber.
• Evaluate patient for development of tardive dyskinesia (involuntary movements of face, arms, legs, and trunk).
• Assess for changes in mood and mental status.
• Check blood pressure for orthostatic hypertension.
• Watch for signs and symptoms of depression, and assess for suicidal ideation.
• Monitor complete blood count with white cell differential, glucose levels, and kidney and liver function test results.

Patient teaching
◀≶ Tell patient to contact prescriber immediately if he develops high fever, rapid pulse and breathing, profuse sweating, changes in mental status, or involuntary movements.

• Instruct patient to promptly report severe mood changes or suicidal thoughts.

• Teach patient to avoid driving and other hazardous activities until he knows how drug affects concentration and alertness.

• Tell patient that stopping drug suddenly can cause withdrawal symptoms.

• Inform patient that drug may cause temporary blood pressure decrease if he stands up suddenly. Advise him to rise slowly and carefully.

• Teach patient that drug may cause serious interactions with many common drugs; instruct him to tell all prescribers he's taking drug.

• Advise patient to minimize GI upset by eating small, frequent servings of food and drinking plenty of fluids.

• Tell patient he'll undergo frequent blood testing during therapy.

amoxicillin

amoxycillin trihydrate
Amoxil, Amoxil Pediatric Drops, Apo-Amoxil✦, Novamoxin✦, Nu-Amoxil✦, Trimox, Trimox Pediatric Drops, Wymox

Pharmacologic class: Aminopenicillin
Therapeutic class: Anti-infective
Pregnancy risk category B

Action
Inhibits cell-wall synthesis during bacterial multiplication, leading to cell death. Shows enhanced activity toward gram-negative bacteria compared to natural and penicillinase-resistant penicillins.

Availability
Capsules: 250 mg, 500 mg
Powder for oral suspension: 50 mg/ml and 125 mg/5 ml (pediatric), 200 mg/5 ml, 250 mg/5 ml, 400 mg/5 ml
Tablets: 500 mg, 875 mg
Tablets (chewable): 125 mg, 200 mg, 250 mg, 400 mg

⚕ Indications and dosages
➤ Uncomplicated gonorrhea
Adults and children weighing at least 40 kg (88 lb): 3 g P.O. as single dose
Children ages 2 and older weighing less than 40 kg (88 lb): 50 mg/kg P.O. given with probenecid 25 mg/kg P.O. as a single dose
➤ Bacterial endocarditis prophylaxis for dental, GI, and GU procedures
Adults: 2 g P.O. 1 hour before procedure
Children: 50 mg/kg P.O. 1 hour before procedure
➤ Lower respiratory tract infections caused by streptococci, pneumococci, non-penicillinase-producing staphylococci, and *Haemophilus influenzae*
Adults and children weighing more than 20 kg (44 lb): 500 mg P.O. q 8 hours
Children weighing less than 20 kg (44 lb): 40 mg/kg P.O. in divided doses q 8 hours
➤ Ear, nose, and throat infections caused by streptococci, pneumococci, non-penicillinase-producing staphylococci, and *H. influenzae*; GU infections caused by *Escherichia coli, Proteus mirabilis,* and *Streptococcus faecalis*; skin and soft-tissue infections caused by streptococci, susceptible staphylococci, and *E. coli*
Adults and children weighing more than 20 kg (44 lb): 250 to 500 mg P.O. q 8 hours
Children weighing less than 20 kg (44 lb): 20 to 40 mg/kg P.O. in divided doses q 8 hours
➤ Postexposure anthrax prophylaxis
Adults: 500 mg P.O. t.i.d. for 60 days
Children: 80 mg/kg/day P.O. t.i.d. for 60 days

Dosage adjustment
• Renal impairment
• Hemodialysis

Off-label uses
• *Chlamydia trachomatis* infection in pregnant patients

Contraindications
• Hypersensitivity to drug or to penicillins or cephalosporins
• History of jaundice or hepatic dysfunction

Administration
• Give with or without food.
• Store liquid form in refrigerator when possible.

Route	Onset	Peak	Duration
P.O.	30 min	1-2 hr	8-12 hr

Adverse reactions
CNS: lethargy, hallucinations, anxiety, confusion, agitation, depression, dizziness, fatigue, hyperactivity, insomnia, behavioral changes, **seizures** (with high doses)
GI: nausea, vomiting, diarrhea, bloody diarrhea, abdominal pain, gastritis, stomatitis, glossitis, black "hairy" tongue, furry tongue, enterocolitis, **pseudomembranous colitis**
GU: nephropathy, vaginitis, **interstitial nephritis**
Hematologic: eosinophilia, anemia, **thrombocytopenia, thrombocytopenic purpura, leukopenia,** hemolytic anemia, agranulocytosis, bone narrow depression
Hepatic: hepatic cholestasis, **cholestatic hepatitis, nonspecific hepatitis, cholestatic jaundice**
Respiratory: wheezing
Skin: rash
Other: superinfections (oral and rectal candidiasis), fever, **anaphylaxis**

Interactions
Drug-drug. *Allopurinol:* increased risk of rash
Chloramphenicol, macrolides, sulfonamides, tetracycline: decreased amoxicillin efficacy
Hormonal contraceptives: decreased contraceptive efficacy
Probenecid: decreased renal excretion
Drug-diagnostic tests. *Alanine aminotransferase, alkaline phosphatase, eosinophils, lactate dehydrogenase:* increased levels
Granulocytes, hemoglobin, platelets, white blood cells: decreased values
Direct Coombs' test, urine glucose, urine protein: false-positive results
Drug-food. *Any food:* delayed or reduced drug absorption
Drug-herb. *Khat:* decreased antimicrobial efficacy

Precautions
Use cautiously in:
• severe renal insufficiency, infectious mononucleosis
• pregnant patients
• children.

Patient monitoring
• Monitor for signs and symptoms of hypersensitivity reaction.
◀€ Evaluate for seizures when giving high doses.
• Monitor patient's temperature and watch for other signs and symptoms of superinfection (especially oral or rectal candidiasis).

Patient teaching
• Instruct patient to immediately report signs and symptoms of hypersensitivity reactions, such as rash, fever, or chills.
• Tell patient he may take drug with or without food.
• Advise patient to minimize GI upset by eating small, frequent servings of food and drinking plenty of fluids.

- Tell patient taking hormonal contraceptives that drug may reduce contraceptive efficacy; suggest she use alternative birth control method.
- Inform patient that drug lowers resistance to other types of infections. Instruct him to report new signs and symptoms of infection, especially in mouth or rectum.
- Tell parents they may give liquid form of drug directly to child or may mix it with food or beverages.

amoxicillin and clavulanate potassium
Augmentin, Augmentin ES-600, Augmentin XR, Clavulin✚

Pharmacologic class: Aminopenicillin
Therapeutic class: Anti-infective
Pregnancy risk category B

Action
Amoxicillin inhibits transpeptidase, preventing cross-linking of bacterial cell wall and leading to cell death. Addition of clavulanate (a beta-lactam) increases drug's resistance to beta-lactamase (an enzyme produced by bacteria that may inactivate amoxicillin).

Availability
Oral suspension: 125 mg amoxicillin with 31.25 mg clavulanic acid/5 ml, 200 mg amoxicillin with 28.5 mg clavulanic acid/5 ml, 250 mg amoxicillin with 62.5 mg clavulanic acid/5 ml, 400 mg amoxicillin with 57 mg clavulanic acid/5 ml
Tablets (chewable): 125 mg amoxicillin with 31.25 mg clavulanate, 200 mg amoxicillin with 28.5 mg clavulanate, 250 mg amoxicillin with 62.5 mg clavulanate, 400 mg amoxicillin with 57 mg clavulanate

Tablets (extended-release): 1,000 mg amoxicillin with 62.5 mg clavulanate
Tablets (film-coated): 250 mg amoxicillin with 125 mg clavulanate, 500 mg amoxicillin with 125 mg clavulanate, 875 mg amoxicillin with 125 mg clavulanate

Indications and dosages
➤ Lower respiratory tract infections, otitis media, sinusitis, skin and skin-structure infections, and urinary tract infections (UTIs) caused by susceptible strains of gram-negative and gram-positive organisms
Adults and children weighing more than 40 kg (88 lb): 250 mg P.O. based on amoxicillin component q 8 hours, or 500 mg q 12 hours. For severe infections, 500 mg P.O. q 8 hours, or 875 mg P.O. q 12 hours.
➤ Serious infections and community-acquired pneumonia
Adults and children weighing more than 40 kg (88 lb): 875 mg P.O. q 12 hours or 500 mg P.O. q 8 hours
Infants and children ages 3 months and older weighing less than 40 kg (88 lb): 20 to 40 mg/kg/day in divided doses q 8 hours, or 20 to 45 mg/kg/day P.O. in divided doses q 12 hours, based on severity of infection and amoxicillin component (125 mg/5 ml or 250 mg/5 ml suspension)
Infants younger than age 3 months: 30 mg/kg/day P.O. divided q 12 hours based on amoxicillin component (125 mg/5 ml oral suspension is recommended)
➤ Recurrent or persistent acute otitis media caused by *Streptococcus pneumoniae, Haemophilus influenzae,* or *Moraxella catarrhalis* in children ages 2 and younger and in children who received antibiotic therapy within last 3 months
Children ages 3 months to 12 years: 90 mg/kg/day of Augmentin ES-600 P.O. q 12 hours for 10 days

Dosage adjustment
• Renal impairment
• Hemodialysis

Contraindications
• Hypersensitivity to penicillin or clavulanate
• Phenylketonuria
• History of cholestatic jaundice or hepatic dysfunction associated with drug use

Administration
◀₤ Ask about history of allergies to penicillin or cephalosporins before giving.
• Give with or without food.
• Refrigerate oral suspension when possible, or store at room temperature for up to 7 days.

Route	Onset	Peak	Duration
P.O.	Unknown	1-2.5 hr	6-8 hr
P.O. (extended)	Unknown	1-4 hr	Unknown

Adverse reactions
CNS: lethargy, hallucinations, anxiety, confusion, agitation, depression, dizziness, fatigue, hyperactivity, insomnia, behavioral changes, **seizures** (with high doses)
GI: nausea, vomiting, diarrhea, abdominal pain, stomatitis, glossitis, gastritis, black "hairy" tongue, furry tongue, enterocolitis, **pseudomembranous colitis**
GU: nephropathy, vaginitis, **interstitial nephritis**
Hematologic: anemia, **thrombocytopenia, thrombocytopenic purpura, leukopenia, hemolytic anemia, agranulocytosis, bone narrow depression, eosinophilia**
Hepatic: cholestatic hepatitis
Respiratory: wheezing
Skin: rash
Other: superinfections (oral and rectal candidiasis), fever, **anaphylaxis**

Interactions
Drug-drug. *Allopurinol:* increased risk of rash
Chloramphenicol, macrolides, sulfonamides, tetracycline: decreased amoxicillin effect
Hormonal contraceptives: decreased contraceptive efficacy
Probenecid: decreased renal excretion and increased blood level of amoxicillin
Drug-food. *Any food:* delayed or reduced drug absorption
Drug-herb. *Khat:* decreased antimicrobial effect

Precautions
Use cautiously in:
• severe renal insufficiency, infectious mononucleosis
• pregnant patients
• children.

Patient monitoring
• Monitor patient carefully for signs and symptoms of hypersensitivity reaction.
◀₤ Monitor for seizures when giving high doses.
• Check patient's temperature and watch for other signs and symptoms of superinfection, especially oral or rectal candidiasis.

Patient teaching
• Instruct patient to immediately report signs or symptoms of hypersensitivity reaction, such as rash, fever, or chills.
• Tell patient he can take drug with or without food.
• Inform patient that drug lowers resistance to some types of infections. Instruct him to report new signs or symptoms of infection, especially of mouth or rectum.
• Teach patient to minimize GI upset by eating small, frequent servings of food and drinking plenty of fluids.

• Tell patient taking hormonal contraceptives that drug may reduce contraceptive efficacy; suggest that she use alternative birth control method.

• Inform parents they may give liquid form of drug directly to child or may mix it with food or drink.

amphotericin B

amphotericin B cholesteryl sulfate
Amphotec

amphotericin B desoxycholate
Amphocin, Fungizone Intravenous

amphotericin B, lipid-based
Abelcet, AmBisome, Amphotec

Pharmacologic class: Systemic polyene antifungal
Therapeutic class: Antifungal
Pregnancy risk category B

Action
Binds to sterols in fungal cell membrane, increasing permeability; this allows potassium to exit the cell, causing fungal impairment or death

Availability
Amphotericin B cholesteryl sulfate—
Injection: 50 mg/20 ml, 100 mg/50 ml
Amphotericin B desoxycholate—
Injection: 50-mg vial
Oral suspension: 100 mg/ml in 24-ml bottles
Amphotericin B, lipid based—
Powder for injection: 50 mg/vial
Suspension for injection: 100 mg/20-ml vials

⦿ Indications and dosages
➤ Invasive aspergillosis in patients with renal impairment or unacceptable toxicity who can't tolerate or don't respond to amphotericin B desoxycholate in effective doses
Adults and children: Perform following test before giving first dose—Infuse 10 ml of final preparation containing 1.6 to 8.3 mg of amphotericin B cholesteryl sulfate I.V. over 15 to 30 minutes; monitor patient for next 30 minutes. If dose is tolerated, give 3 to 4 mg/kg/day I.V. Dilute in dextrose 5% in water (D_5W) and give by continuous infusion at 1 mg/kg/hour.
➤ Systemic fungal infections in histoplasmosis, coccidioidomycosis, blastomycosis, cryptoccocosis, phycomycosis, disseminated candidiasis, zygomycosis, and meningitis
Adults: Initially, give test dose of 1 mg amphotericin B desoxycholate in 20 ml D_5W I.V. over 20 to 30 minutes. If dose is tolerated, give 0.25 to 0.3mg/kg daily by slow I.V. infusion (0.1 mg/ml over 2 to 6 hours). Gradually increase to maximum dosage of 1.5 mg/kg/day in potentially fatal infection. If drug is discontinued for 1 week or longer, start again with initial dosage.
➤ GI tract infections caused by *Candida albicans*
Adults: 100 mg amphotericin B desoxycholate P.O. q.i.d for 2 weeks
➤ Visceral leishmaniasis in immunocompetent patients
Adults and children: 3 mg/kg lipid-based amphotericin B given I.V. over 2 hours on days 1 through 5, 14, and 21. Repeat course if initial treatment fails to clear parasites.
➤ Visceral leishmaniasis in immunosuppressed patients
Adults and children: 4 mg/kg lipid-based amphotericin B given I.V. over 2 hours on days 1 through 5, 10, 17, 24, 31, and 38

➤ Cryptococcal meningitis in patients with human immunodeficiency virus (HIV)

Adults and children: 6 mg/kg/day lipid-based amphotericin B given I.V. over 2 hours. Increase or decrease infusion time as needed.

➤ Empiric therapy for presumed fungal infection in febrile, neutropenic patients

Adults: 3 mg/kg/day lipid-based amphotericin B given I.V. over 120 minutes

➤ Systemic fungal infections caused by *Aspergillis, Candida,* or *Cryptococcus* species

Adults: 3 to 5 mg/kg/day lipid-based amphotericin B given I.V. at rate of 2.5 mg/kg/hour

Off-label uses

• Chemoprophylaxis in immunocompromised patients
• Coccidioidal arthritis
• Prophylaxis of fungal infections in bone marrow transplant recipients, patients with primary amoebic meningoencephalitis caused by *Naegleria fowleri*, and patients with ocular aspergillosis

Contraindications

• Hypersensitivity to drug
• Renal dysfunction
• Breastfeeding

Administration

• Pretreat with antihistamines, antipyretics, or corticosteroids, as prescribed.
• Give through separate I.V. line, using infusion pump and in-line filter larger than 1 micron.
• Choose distal vein for I.V. site; alternate sites regularly.
• Mix with 10 ml of sterile water to reconstitute. Don't mix with sodium chloride, other electrolytes, or bacteriostatic products.

• Flush I.V. line with 5% dextrose injection before and after infusion.
• Keep dry form of drug away from light. Once mixed with fluid, solution can be kept in light for up to 8 hours.

Route	Onset	Peak	Duration
P.O.	Unknown	Unknown	Unknown
I.V.	Rapid	End of infusion	24 hr

Adverse reactions

CNS: anxiety, confusion, headache, insomnia, weakness, depression, dizziness, drowsiness, hallucinations, speech difficulty, stupor, psychosis, **seizures**
CV: hypotension, hypertension, tachycardia, phlebitis, chest pain, orthostatic hypotension, vasodilation, **asystole, atrial fibrillation, bradycardia, cardiac arrest, shock, supraventricular tachycardia**
EENT: double or blurred vision, amblyopia, eye hemorrhage, hearing loss, tinnitus, epistaxis, rhinitis, sinusitis, pharyngitis
GI: nausea, vomiting, diarrhea, melena, abdominal pain, abdominal distention, dry mouth, gingivitis, mouth inflammation, oral candidiasis, anorexia, **GI hemorrhage**
GU: hematuria, albuminuria, painful urination, glycosuria, oliguria, excessive urea buildup, urine of low specific gravity, nephrocalcinosis, **renal failure, renal tubular acidosis, anuria**
Hematologic: eosinophilia, leukocytosis, normochromic anemia, normocytic anemia, hypochromic anemia, **thrombocytopenia, leukopenia, agranulocytosis, coagulation disorders**
Hepatic: hyperbilirubinemia, jaundice, abnormal liver function test results, **acute liver failure, hepatitis**
Metabolic: hypomagnesemia, hypokalemia, hypocalcemia, hypernatremia, hyperglycemia, acidosis, dehydration, hypoproteinemia, hypervolemia, hyperlipidemia

---

Musculoskeletal: muscle, joint, neck, or back pain

Respiratory: increased cough, hypoxia, lung disorders, hyperventilation, asthma, dyspnea, hemoptysis, wheezing, tachypnea, **bronchospasm, respiratory failure, pulmonary edema, pleural effusion**

Skin: discoloration, bruising, flushing, pruritus, acne, rash, sweating, nodules, skin ulcers, urticaria, alopecia, **maculopapular rash**

Other: fever, infection, peripheral or facial edema, weight changes, pain or reaction at injection site, tissue damage with extravasation, hypersensitivity reaction

Interactions

Drug-drug. *Antineoplastics (such as mechlorethamine):* renal toxicity, bronchospasm, hypotension

Cardiac glycosides: increased risk of digitalis toxicity (in potassium-depleted patient)

Corticosteroids: increased potassium depletion

Cyclosporine, tacrolimus: increased creatinine levels

Flucytosine: increased flucytosine toxicity

Imidazoles (clotrimazole, fluconazole, ketoconazole, miconazole): antagonism of amphotericin B effect

Leukocyte transfusion: pulmonary reactions

Nephrotoxic drugs (such as antibiotics, pentamidine): increased risk of renal toxicity

Thiazides: increased electrolyte depletion

Skeletal muscle relaxants: increased skeletal muscle relaxation

Zidovudine: increased myelotoxicity and nephrotoxicity

Drug-diagnostic tests. *Alanine aminotransferase, alkaline phosphatase, aspartate aminotransferase, bilirubin, blood urea nitrogen, creatinine, gamma-glutamyltransferase, lactate dehydrogenase, nitrogenous compounds (urea), uric acid:* increased levels

Calcium, hemoglobin, magnesium, platelets, potassium, protein: decreased levels

Eosinophils, glucose, white blood cells: increased or decreased levels

Prothrombin time: prolonged

Drug-herb. *Gossypol:* increased risk of renal toxicity

Precautions

Use cautiously in:
• renal impairment, electrolyte abnormalities
• pregnant patients
• children.

Patient monitoring

◀€ Monitor for infusion-related reactions (fever, chills, hypotension, GI symptoms, breathing difficulties, and headache). Stop infusion and notify prescriber immediately if reaction occurs.

• Monitor vital signs and temperature every 30 minutes for at least 4 hours after giving test dose.

• Assess fluid intake and output.

• Monitor kidney and liver function test results and serum electrolyte levels.

• Evaluate for signs and symptoms of ototoxicity (hearing loss, tinnitus, ataxia, vertigo).

Patient teaching

◀€ Advise patient to contact prescriber immediately if he has fever, chills, headache, vomiting, diarrhea, cough, or breathing problems.

• Teach patient to report hearing loss, dizziness, or unsteady gait.

• Tell patient to avoid driving and other hazardous activities until he knows how drug affects concentration, alertness, and vision.

• Instruct patient to drink plenty of fluids.

• Teach patient to monitor urine output and notify prescriber of significant changes.
• Advise patient to minimize GI upset by eating small, frequent servings of food and drinking plenty of fluids.

ampicillin sodium
Ampicin✦, Apo-Ampi✦, Marcillin, Novo-Ampicillin✦, Nu-Ampi✦, Omnipen, Omnipen-N, Penbritin✦, Polycillin, Principen, Totacillin

Pharmacologic class: Aminopenicillin
Therapeutic class: Anti-infective
Pregnancy risk category B

Action
Destroys bacteria by inhibiting bacterial cell-wall synthesis during microbial multiplication

Availability
Capsules: 250 mg, 500 mg
Oral suspension: 125 mg/5 ml, 250 mg/5 ml
Powder for injection: 125 mg, 250 mg, 500 mg, 1 g, 2 g, 10 g

Indications and dosages
➢ Respiratory tract, skin, and soft-tissue infections
Adults and children weighing 40 kg (88 lb) or more: 250 to 500 mg I.V. or I.M. q 6 hours
Adults and children weighing less than 40 kg (88 lb): 25 to 50 mg/kg/day I.M. or I.V. in divided doses q 6 to 8 hours
Children weighing 20 kg (44 lb) or less: 50 mg/kg/day P.O. in divided doses q 6 to 8 hours
➢ Bacterial meningitis caused by *Haemophilus influenzae, Staphylococcus pneumoniae, Neisseria meningitidis,* or septicemia

Adults: 150 to 200 mg/kg/day by continuous I.V. infusion or I.M. injection in equally divided doses q 3 to 4 hours, to a maximum dosage of 14 g
Children: 100 to 200 mg/kg/day I.V. in divided doses q 3 to 4 hours; after 3 days, switch to I.M. route.
➢ GI or urinary tract infections, including *Neisseria gonorrhoeae* infection in women
Adults and children weighing more than 40 kg (88 lb): 500 mg I.M. or I.V. q 6 hours
Adults and children weighing 40 kg (88 lb) or less: 50 to 100 mg/kg/day I.M. or I.V. in equally divided doses q 6 to 8 hours
Children weighing less than 20 kg (44 lb): 100 mg/kg/day P.O. in equally divided doses q 6 to 8 hours
➢ Endocarditis prophylaxis for dental, oral, or upper respiratory tract procedures
Adults: 2 g I.M. or I.V. within 30 minutes before procedure
Children: 50 mg/kg I.V. or I.M. within 30 minutes before procedure
➢ Prevention of bacterial endocarditis before GI or GU surgery or instrumentation
Adults: 2 g I.M. or I.V. with gentamicin 1.5 mg/kg I.M. or I.V. within 30 minutes before procedure; 6 hours later, give 1 g I.M. or I.V., or 1 g of amoxicillin P.O.
Children: 50 mg/kg I.M. or I.V. with 1.5 mg/kg of gentamicin I.M. or I.V. within 30 minutes before procedure; 6 hours later, give 25 mg/kg I.M. or I.V. or 25 mg/kg amoxicillin P.O.
➢ *N. gonorrhoeae* infections
Adults: 3.5 g P.O. with l g probenecid
Children weighing 40 kg (88 lb) or more: 500 mg I.M. or I.V. q 6 hours
Children weighing less than 40 kg (88 lb): 50 mg/kg/day in divided doses q 6 to 8 hours

➤ Urethritis caused by *N. gonorrhoeae* (in males)

Adults and children weighing 40 kg (88 lb) or more: 500 mg I.V. or I.M., repeated 8 to 12 hours later

➤ Prophylaxis against sexually transmitted diseases in adult rape victims

Adults: 3.5 g P.O. with 1 g of probenecid as a single dose

Dosage adjustment
• Renal impairment

Contraindications

• Hypersensitivity to penicillins, cephalosporins, imipenem, or other beta-lactamase inhibitors

Administration

• For I.V. use, mix powder with bacteriostatic water for injection in amount listed on label.
• For direct I.V. injection, give over 10 to 15 minutes. Don't exceed 100 mg/minute.
• For intermittent I.V. infusion, mix with 50 to 100 ml of normal saline solution and give over 15 to 30 minutes.
• Change I.V. site every 48 hours.
• Give oral doses 1 hour before or 2 hours after meals.

Route	Onset	Peak	Duration
P.O.	30 min	2 hr	6-8 hr
I.V.	Immediate	5 min	6-8 hr
I.M.	15 min	1 hr	6-8 hr

Adverse reactions

CNS: lethargy, hallucinations, anxiety, confusion, agitation, depression, fatigue, dizziness, **seizures**

CV: vein irritation, thrombophlebitis, heart failure

EENT: blurred vision, itchy eyes

GI: nausea, vomiting, diarrhea, abdominal pain, enterocolitis, gastritis, stomatitis, glossitis, black "hairy" tongue, furry tongue, oral or rectal candidiasis, **pseudomembranous colitis**

GU: nephropathy, vaginitis, **interstitial nephritis**

Hematologic: anemia, eosinophilia, **agranulocytosis, hemolytic anemia, leukopenia, thrombocytopenic purpura, thrombocytopenia, blood dyscrasias, neutropenia**

Hepatic: nonspecific hepatitis

Musculoskeletal: arthritis exacerbation

Respiratory: wheezing, dyspnea, hypoxia, **apnea**

Skin: rashes, urticaria, fever, diaphoresis

Other: pain at injection site, superinfections, hyperthermia, **hypersensitivity reaction, anaphylaxis, serum sickness**

Interactions

Drug-drug. *Allopurinol:* increased risk of rashes

Chloramphenicol: synergistic or antagonistic effects

Hormonal contraceptives: decreased contraceptive effect, increased risk of breakthrough bleeding

Probenecid: decreased renal excretion of ampicillin, increased ampicillin blood level

Tetracyclines: reduced bactericidal effect

Drug-diagnostic tests. *Conjugated estrone, estradiol, estriol-glucuronide, total conjugated estriols:* increased levels in pregnant patients

Granulocytes, hemoglobin, platelets, white blood cells: decreased counts

Coombs' test, urine glucose: false-positive results

Eosinophils: increased count

Drug-food. *Any food:* reduced ampicillin efficacy

Precautions

Use cautiously in:
• severe renal insufficiency, infectious mononucleosis
• pregnant or breastfeeding patients.

Patient monitoring

• Watch for signs and symptoms of hypersensitivity reaction.

◀≣ Monitor for seizures when giving high doses.

• Frequently measure patient's temperature and check for other signs and symptoms of superinfection, especially oral or rectal candidiasis.

• Monitor for bleeding tendency or hemorrhage.

Patient teaching

• Instruct patient to immediately report signs and symptoms of hypersensitivity reaction, such as rash, fever, or chills.

• Tell patient to take oral dose with 8 oz of water 1 hour before or 2 hours after a meal.

• Inform patient that drug lowers resistance to certain other infections. Tell him to report new signs or symptoms of infection, especially in mouth or rectum.

• Advise patient to minimize GI upset by eating small, frequent servings of food and drinking plenty of fluids.

• Instruct patient to report unusual bleeding or bruising to prescriber.

• Tell patient to avoid activities that can cause injury. Advise him to use soft toothbrush and electric razor to avoid gum and skin injury.

• Inform patient taking hormonal contraceptives that drug may reduce contraceptive efficacy; advise her to use alternative birth control method.

ampicillin sodium and sulbactam sodium
Unasyn

Pharmacologic class: Aminopenicillin, beta-lactamase inhibitor

Therapeutic class: Anti-infective

Pregnancy risk category B

Action

Destroys bacteria by inhibiting bacterial cell-wall synthesis during microbial multiplication. Addition of sulbactam enhances drug's resistance to beta-lactamase, an enzyme produced by bacteria that may inactivate ampicillin.

Availability

Injection: Vials, piggyback vials containing 1.5 g (l g ampicillin sodium and 0.5 g sulbactam sodium), 3 g (2 g ampicillin sodium and l g sulbactam sodium), and 15 g (10 g ampicillin sodium and 5 g sulbactam sodium)

Indications and dosages

➤ Intra-abdominal, gynecologic, and skin-structure infections caused by susceptible beta-lactamase-producing strains

Adults and children weighing 40 kg (88 lb) or more: 1.5 to 3 g (l g ampicillin and 0.5 g sulbactam to 2 g ampicillin and l g sulbactam) I.M. or I.V. q 6 hours. Maximum dosage is 4 g sulbactam daily.

Children ages 1 year and older: 75 mg (50 mg ampicillin and 25 mg sulbactam)/kg I.V. q 6 hours

Dosage adjustment

• Renal impairment

Contraindications

• Hypersensitivity to penicillins, cephalosporins, imipenem, or other beta-lactamase inhibitors

Administration
- Let vial stand several minutes until foam has evaporated before administering drug.
- Give 1 hour before bacteriostatic antibodies.
- Don't mix I.V. form with other I.V. drugs.
- Give direct I.V. dose over 10 to 15 minutes.
- Give intermittent infusion in 50 to 100 ml of compatible solution over 15 to 30 minutes.
- Change I.V. site every 48 hours.
- Don't give to children by I.M. route.

Route	Onset	Peak	Duration
I.V.	Immediate	End of infusion	6-8 hr
I.M.	Rapid	1 hr	6-8 hr

Adverse reactions
CNS: lethargy, hallucinations, anxiety, confusion, agitation, depression, fatigue, dizziness, **seizures**
CV: vein irritation, thrombophlebitis, **heart failure**
EENT: blurred vision, itchy eyes
GI: nausea, vomiting, diarrhea, abdominal pain, enterocolitis, gastritis, stomatitis, glossitis, black "hairy" tongue, furry tongue, oral and rectal candidiasis, **pseudomembranous colitis**
GU: nephropathy, hematuria, hyaline casts in urine, vaginitis, **interstitial nephritis**
Hematologic: anemia, **agranulocytosis, hemolytic anemia, leukopenia, thrombocytopenic purpura, thrombocytopenia, blood dyscrasias, neutropenia, eosinophilia**
Hepatic: nonspecific hepatitis
Musculoskeletal: arthritis exacerbation
Respiratory: wheezing, dyspnea, hypoxia, **apnea**
Skin: rashes, urticaria, diaphoresis
Other: pain at injection site, fever, hyperthermia, superinfections, hypersensitivity reactions, **anaphylaxis, serum sickness**

Interactions
Drug-drug. *Allopurinol:* increased risk of rashes
Chloramphenicol: synergistic or antagonistic effects
Hormonal contraceptives: decreased contraceptive efficacy, increased risk of breakthrough bleeding
Probenecid: decreased renal excretion and increased blood level of ampicillin
Tetracyclines: reduced bactericidal effects
Drug-diagnostic tests. *Alanine aminotransferase, alkaline phosphatase, aspartate aminotransferase, bilirubin, blood urea nitrogen, creatine kinase, creatinine, gamma-glutamyltransferase, eosinophils, lactate dehydrogenase:* increased levels
Estradiol, estriol-glucuronide, granulocytes, hemoglobin, lymphocytes, neutrophils, platelets, white blood cells: decreased levels
Coombs' test: false-positive result
Urinalysis: red blood cells, hyaline casts

Precautions
Use cautiously in:
- severe renal insufficiency, infectious mononucleosis
- pregnant or breastfeeding patients.

Patient monitoring
- Monitor for signs and symptoms of hypersensitivity reaction.
- Check for signs of infection at injection site.
- ◄⏑ Monitor for seizures when giving high doses.
- Watch for bleeding tendency and hemorrhage.
- Check patient's temperature and watch for other signs and symptoms of superinfection, especially oral or rectal candidiasis.
- Monitor complete blood count and liver function test results.

Patient teaching

• Instruct patient to immediately report signs and symptoms of hypersensitivity reaction, such as rash, fever, or chills.

• Teach patient to report signs and symptoms of infection or other problems at injection site.

• Advise patient to minimize GI upset by eating small, frequent servings of food and drinking plenty of fluids.

• Inform patient that drug lowers resistance to certain infections. Instruct him to report new signs or symptoms of infection, especially in mouth or rectum.

• Tell patient to report unusual bleeding or bruising.

• Inform patient taking hormonal contraceptives that drug may reduce contraceptive efficacy; advise her to use alternative birth control method.

• Teach patient to avoid activities that can cause injury. Advise him to use soft toothbrush and electric razor to avoid gum and skin injury.

• Inform patient that he may need to undergo regular blood testing during therapy.

---

amprenavir
Agenerase

Pharmacologic class: Protease inhibitor
Therapeutic class: Antiretroviral
Pregnancy risk category C

Action

Inhibits replication of human immunodeficiency virus-1 (HIV-1) by interfering with HIV-1 protease blocking maturation of virus and causing formation of nininfectious virions

Availability

Capsules: 50 mg, 150 mg

Oral solution: 15 mg/ml

Indications and dosages

➤ Treatment of HIV-1 infection (in combination with other antiretrovirals)

Adults and children ages 13 to 16 weighing more than 50 kg (110 lb): 1,200 mg P.O. b.i.d.

Children ages 13 to 16 weighing 50 kg (110 lb) or less: 1,200 mg P.O. b.i.d.

Children ages 4 to 12 and children ages 13 to 16 weighing less than 50 kg (110 lb): *Capsules*—20 mg/kg P.O. b.i.d. or 15 mg/kg P.O. t.i.d., to a maximum dosage of 2,400 mg/day, given with other antiretrovirals. *Oral solution*—22.5 mg/kg P.O. b.i.d. or 17 mg/kg P.O. t.i.d., to a maximum dosage of 2,800 mg/day (given with other antiretrovirals)

Dosage adjustment

• Renal or hepatic impairment

Contraindications

• Hypersensitivity to drug
• Renal failure
• Pregnancy
• Children younger than age 4

Administration

◀€ Stop drug if patient develops signs or symptoms of Stevens-Johnson syndrome.

• Don't give with meals or grapefruit juice or within 1 hour of antacids.

• Be aware that capsules and oral solution aren't interchangeable on a milligram-to-milligram basis.

Route	Onset	Peak	Duration
P.O.	Rapid	1-2 hr	8-12 hr

Adverse reactions

CNS: depression, dizziness, mood disorders, headache, anxiety, peripheral paresthesia, oral and perioral paresthesia, mood disorders

GI: nausea, vomiting, diarrhea, abdominal pain, abnormal taste

---

Hematologic: acute hemolytic anemia, spontaneous bleeding (in patients with hemophilia A or B)
Metabolic: hyperglycemia, hypertriglyceridemia, hypercholesterolemia, cushingoid appearance (moon face, buffalo hump)
Skin: rash, pruritus
Other: fat redistribution, peripheral wasting, breast enlargement, **Stevens-Johnson syndrome**

Interactions

Drug-drug. *Abacavir, cimetidine, pimozide, ritonavir:* increased amprenavir blood level
Amiodarone, bepridil, dihydroergotamine, ergotamine, lidocaine (systemic), midazolam, quinidine, tricyclic antidepressants, triazolam: life-threatening reactions
Antacids: interference with amprenavir absorption
Anticonvulsants: decreased amprenavir blood level; increased carbamazepine blood level (with carbamazepine)
Antihistamines, dapsone, lovastatin, simvastatin: increased levels of these drugs, possibly leading to toxicity
Azole antifungals (itraconazole, ketoconazole): changes in blood level of amprenavir or antifungal
Benzodiazepines, calcium channel blockers, cisapride, ergot alkaloids: competitive interference, resulting in life-threatening reactions
Clozapine: increased clozapine blood level
Erythromycin: increased amprenavir and erythromycin blood levels
Hormonal contraceptives: reduced contraceptive efficacy
Indinavir: increased amprenavir blood level, decreased indinavir blood level
Rifampin: decreased amprenavir blood level, increased rifampin blood level
Saquinavir: decreased amprenavir blood level, increased saquinavir blood level

Sildenafil: increased sildenafil blood level
Warfarin: inhibition of warfarin metabolism, possibly resulting in life-threatening effects
Zidovudine: increased levels of both drugs
Drug-diagnostic tests. *Cholesterol, glucose, triglyceride:* increased levels
Drug-food. *Fatty foods, grapefruit juice:* interference with drug absorption
Drug-herb. *St. John's wort:* more than 50% reduction in amprenavir blood level

Precautions

Use cautiously in:
• hepatic or renal impairment, diabetes mellitus, hemophilia
• patients receiving concurrent amiodarone, parenteral lidocaine, tricyclic antidepressants, or quinidine
• pregnant patients.

Patient monitoring

• Watch for signs and symptoms of depression; assess for suicidal ideation.
• Monitor blood glucose, triglyceride, and cholesterol levels.
• Monitor clotting functions in patients with hemophilia.
• Evaluate body fat distribution throughout course of therapy.
• Assess dental hygiene and monitor oral health in patients with oral or perioral paresthesia.

Patient teaching

• Teach patient to contact prescriber if rash or signs or symptoms of depression occur.
• Instruct patient not to take drug with fatty foods, grapefruit juice, or antacids, which interfere with drug absorption.
• Caution patient to avoid driving and other hazardous activities until he knows how drug affects concentration and alertness.

• Teach patient to minimize GI upset by eating small, frequent servings of foods and drinking plenty of fluids.
• Inform patient that drug may interfere with hormonal contraceptive use; suggest she use alternative birth control measure.
• Teach patient that he'll undergo regular blood testing during therapy.

amyl nitrite
Amyl Nitrite, Aspirols, Vaporole

Pharmacologic class: Coronary vasodilator
Therapeutic class: Antianginal
Pregnancy risk category C

Action
Relaxes vascular smooth muscle, thereby dilating large coronary vessels, decreasing systemic vascular resistance, reducing afterload, decreasing cardiac output, and relieving angina

Availability
Ampules: 0.3 ml

ⓘ Indications and dosages
➤ Acute angina attack
Adults: 0.18 to 0.3 ml by inhalation, repeated in 3 to 5 minutes if needed
➤ Antidote for cyanide poisoning
Adults and children: 0.3 ml by inhalation for 15 to 60 seconds q 5 minutes until sodium nitrite infusion is available

Contraindications
• Hypersensitivity to drug

Administration
• Crush ampule and wave under patient's nose one to six times; if needed, repeat in 3 to 5 minutes.

Route	Onset	Peak	Duration
Inhalation	30 sec	Unknown	3-5 min

Adverse reactions
CNS: headache, dizziness, weakness, syncope, restlessness
CV: orthostatic hypotension, flushing, palpitations, **tachycardia**
EENT: increased intraocular pressure
GI: nausea, vomiting, fecal incontinence
GU: urinary incontinence
Hematologic: hemolytic anemia, methemoglobinemia
Skin: cutaneous vasodilation, rash, pallor, facial and neck flushing

Interactions
Drug-drug. *Aspirin:* increased amyl nitrite blood level and action
Calcium channel blockers: increased risk of symptomatic orthostatic hypotension
Sildenafil: increased risk of hypotension
Sympathomimetics: decreased antianginal effects, hypotension, tachycardia
Drug-behaviors. *Alcohol use:* severe hypotension, cardiovascular collapse

Precautions
Use cautiously in:
• glaucoma, hypotension, hyperthyroidism, severe anemia, early myocardial infarction
• elderly patients
• pregnant or breastfeeding patients.

Patient monitoring
• Monitor vital signs; stay alert for tachycardia and orthostatic hypotension.
• Assess for bowel and bladder incontinence.
• Monitor neurologic response; watch closely for dizziness and syncope.
• Assess level of headache pain.
• In long-term therapy, monitor complete blood count.

Patient teaching

• Teach patient to crush capsule and wave it under his nose until angina is relieved (usually requires one to six inhalations).

• Tell patient that drug often causes dizziness, orthostatic hypotension, and syncope; advise him to sit or lie down until these effects subside.

• Inform patient that drug often causes headache; encourage him to follow prescriber's recommendations for pain relief.

• Tell patient that drug may cause fecal or urinary incontinence; encourage him to use bathroom frequently to avoid accidents.

anagrelide hydrochloride
Agrylin

Pharmacologic class: Hematologic drug
Therapeutic class: Antiplatelet drug
Pregnancy risk category C

Action
Unclear; may reduce platelet production by decreasing megakaryocytic hypermaturation, thereby decreasing platelet count and inhibiting platelet aggregation (at higher doses)

Availability
Capsules: 0.5 mg, 1 mg

Indications and dosages

➤ Essential thrombocythemia
Adults: 0.5 mg P.O. q.i.d. or 1 mg P.O. b.i.d. for 1 week. Adjust dosage as needed to lowest effective dosage that maintains platelet count below 600,000/mm^3. Maximum dosage is 10 mg daily or 2.5 mg as a single dose.
Dosage adjustment
• Hepatic or renal disease

Contraindications
None

Administration
• Give 1 hour before or 2 hours after meals.

Route	Onset	Peak	Duration
P.O.	Immediate	1 hr	48 hr

Adverse reactions
CNS: amnesia, confusion, depression, dizziness, drowsiness, weakness, headache, syncope, insomnia, migraine, nervousness, pain, paresthesia, malaise, **seizures**
CV: angina, chest pain, hypertension, palpitations, orthostatic hypotension, peripheral edema, vasodilation, **arrhythmias, tachycardia, heart failure, hemorrhage, myocardial infarction, cardiomyopathy, cardiomegaly, atrial fibrillation, complete heart block, pericarditis, cerebrovascular accident**
EENT: amblyopia, abnormal or double vision, visual field abnormalities, tinnitus, epistaxis, rhinitis, sinusitis
GI: nausea, vomiting, diarrhea, constipation, abdominal pain, melena, gastric or duodenal ulcers, dyspepsia, aphthous stomatitis, anorexia, flatulence, gastritis, **pancreatitis, GI hemorrhage**
GU: painful urination, hematuria
Hematologic: bleeding tendency, **anemia, thrombocytopenia, lymphadenoma**
Hepatic: elevated hepatic enzyme levels
Metabolic: dehydration
Musculoskeletal: leg cramps; joint, back, muscle, neck pain
Respiratory: asthma, bronchitis, dyspnea, pneumonia, respiratory disease, **pulmonary infiltrates, pulmonary fibrosis, pulmonary hypertension**
Skin: bruising, photosensitivity reaction, pruritus, rash, alopecia, urticaria, skin disease
Other: chills, fever, flulike symptoms, edema

Interactions

Drug-drug. *Sucralfate:* interference with absorption of anagrelide

Drug-diagnostic tests. *Hemoglobin, platelets:* decreased values

Hepatic enzymes: elevated levels

Drug-food. *Any food:* decreased drug bioavailability

Drug-herb. *Evening primrose oil, feverfew, garlic, ginger, ginkgo biloba, ginseng, grapeseed:* increased antiplatelet effect

Precautions

Use cautiously in:
• renal, hepatic, or cardiac dysfunction
• pregnant or breastfeeding patients
• children younger than age 16.

Patient monitoring

◀€ Watch for signs and symptoms of vasodilation, heart failure, and arrhythmias in patients with cardiovascular disease.

• For first 2 weeks, monitor complete blood count and liver and kidney function test results.

• Monitor platelet counts regularly until maintenance dosage is established.

• Check regularly for adverse reactions, especially bleeding tendency.

• Monitor blood pressure for orthostatic hypertension.

Patient teaching

• Teach patient to take drug 1 hour before or 2 hours after meals.

• Caution patient to avoid driving and other hazardous activities until he knows how drug affects concentration, alertness, and vision.

• Inform patient that drug may cause a temporary blood pressure decrease if he stands or sits up suddenly. Tell him to rise slowly and carefully.

• Instruct patient to report unusual bleeding or bruising.

• Inform patient using hormonal contraceptives that drug may interfere with contraceptive efficacy; advise her to use alternative birth control method.

• Tell patient to avoid activities that may cause injury. Tell him to use soft toothbrush and electric razor to avoid gum and skin injury.

• Teach patient to minimize GI upset by eating small, frequent servings of food and drinking plenty of fluids.

• Notify patient that he'll undergo regular blood testing during therapy.

anakinra
Kineret

Pharmacologic class: Interleukin-1 blocker

Therapeutic class: Immunomodulator, antirheumatic

Pregnancy risk category B

Action

Inhibits binding of interleukin-1 (IL-1) with IL type I receptors, thereby mediating immunologic, inflammatory, and other physiologic responses

Availability

Prefilled glass syringes: 100 mg/ml

🕛 Indications and dosages

➤ Moderately to severely active rheumatoid arthritis in patients ages 18 and older who don't respond to disease-modifying antirheumatics alone

Adults: 100 mg/day S.C. given at same time each day

Contraindications

• Hypersensitivity to drug or *Escherichia coli*–derived protein
• Serious infections
• Children

Administration

• Withhold drug and notify prescriber if patient shows signs or symptoms of active infection.

◀❃ Use extreme caution if patient is concurrently receiving drugs that block tumor necrosis factor (TNF), because of increased risk of serious infection.

• Give entire dose from prefilled syringe.

• Don't freeze or shake syringe.

Route	Onset	Peak	Duration
S.C.	Slow	3-7 hr	Unknown

Adverse reactions

CNS: headache
EENT: sinusitis
GI: nausea, diarrhea, abdominal pain
Hematologic: neutropenia, thrombocytopenia
Respiratory: upper respiratory tract infection
Skin: rash, pruritus, injection site reaction or bruising, rash, erythema, inflammation
Other: flulike symptoms, infections

Interactions

Drug-drug. *Etanercept, infliximab, other drugs that block TNF:* increased risk of serious infection
Live-virus vaccines: ineffectiveness of vaccine
Drug-diagnostic tests. *Neutrophils:* decreased level

Precautions

Use cautiously in:
• immunosuppression, active infection, chronic illness, renal impairment
• elderly patients
• pregnant or breastfeeding patients
• children.

Patient monitoring

• Monitor complete blood count with white cell differential.
• Assess injection site for reactions.

Patient teaching

• Tell patient to immediately report signs or symptoms of infection.
• Teach patient to report signs and symptoms of allergic response.
• Instruct patient to take drug at same time each day for best response.
• Teach patient about proper drug disposal (in puncture-resistant container). Caution him against reusing needles, syringes, and drug product.
• Tell patient not to freeze or shake drug.

anastrozole
Arimidex

Pharmacologic class: Nonsteroidal aromatase inhibitor
Therapeutic class: Antineoplastic
Pregnancy risk category D

Action

Reduces serum estradiol levels with no significant effect on adrenocorticoid or aldosterone level; decreases stimulating effect of estrogen on tumor growth

Availability

Tablets: 1 mg

ⓥ Indications and dosages

➤ Postmenopausal women with hormone receptor-unknown or hormone receptor-positive advanced breast cancer or with advanced breast cancer after tamoxifen therapy; adjuvant treatment for hormone receptor-positive breast cancer
Adults: 1 mg P.O. daily

Contraindications

• Pregnancy
• Children

Administration
• Verify that patient isn't pregnant before giving drug.

Route	Onset	Peak	Duration
P.O.	>24 hr	Unknown	<6 days

Adverse reactions
CNS: headache, weakness, dizziness, depression, paresthesia, lethargy
CV: chest pain, thromboembolic disease, peripheral edema, vasodilation, hypertension
EENT: pharyngitis
GI: nausea, vomiting, diarrhea, constipation, abdominal pain, anorexia, dry mouth, food distaste
GU: vaginal bleeding, leukorrhea, vaginal dryness, pelvic pain
Hepatic: elevated hepatic enzyme levels
Musculoskeletal: bone or back pain, muscle weakness
Respiratory: dyspnea, cough
Skin: rash
Other: weight gain, swelling, hot flashes, flulike symptoms, tumor flare, increased high-density lipoprotein and low-density lipoprotein levels

Interactions
Drug-diagnostic tests. *Cholesterol:* increased levels

Precautions
Use cautiously in:
• women of childbearing age
• breastfeeding patients.

Patient monitoring
◀€ Check regularly for signs and symptoms of thromboembolic disease, especially dyspnea and chest pain.
• Monitor for circulatory overload (suggested by peripheral edema, cough, and dyspnea).
• Assess for signs and symptoms of depression; evaluate patient for suicidal ideation.
• Monitor liver function test results.

Patient teaching
◀€ Teach patient to immediately report signs and symptoms of thromboembolic disease and circulatory overload.
◀€ Emphasize importance of preventing pregnancy during therapy.
• Tell patient to contact prescriber if she develops signs or symptoms of depression.
• Instruct patient to avoid driving and other hazardous activities until she knows how drug affects concentration and alertness.
• Teach patient to minimize GI upset by eating small, frequent servings of food and drinking plenty of fluids.
• Inform patient that she'll undergo regular blood testing during therapy.

anistreplase (anisoylated plasminogen streptokinase activator complex, APSAC)
APSAC, Eminase

Pharmacologic class: Plasminogen activator
Therapeutic class: Thrombolytic enzyme
Pregnancy risk category C

Action
Combines with plasminogen to form activated complex, which converts plasminogen to plasmin and causes lysis of thrombi in arteries

Availability
Powder for injection: 30 units/vial

⟊ Indications and dosages
➤ Management of acute myocardial infarction (MI), including lysis of thrombi obstructing coronary arteries, reduction of infarct size, improvement

of ventricular function, and prevention of death

Adults: 30 units by direct I.V. injection given over 2 to 5 minutes, starting as soon as possible after onset of acute MI symptoms

Contraindications

• Hypersensitivity to anistreplase or streptokinase
• Active or recent internal bleeding
• Cerebrovascular accident within past 2 months
• Aneurysm
• Uncontrolled hypertension
• Hepatic disease
• Breastfeeding

Administration

• Don't further dilute reconstituted solution before giving drug or adding to infusion fluids.
• Don't add other medications to vial or syringe.
• Gently roll vial to mix. To minimize foaming, don't shake.

Route	Onset	Peak	Duration
I.V.	Immediate	45 min	4-6 hr

Adverse reactions

CNS: dizziness, fever, headache, **intracranial hemorrhage**
CV: conduction disorders, hypotension, **arrhythmias**
EENT: gum or mouth hemorrhages, epistaxis
GI: nausea, vomiting, abdominal pain, constipation, **GI hemorrhage**
GU: hematuria, proteinuria, vaginal bleeding
Hematologic: eosinophilia, **bleeding tendency**
Musculoskeletal: joint pain or stiffness, myalgia, back or bone pain
Respiratory: hemoptysis, dyspnea, **bronchospasm**
Skin: hematoma, urticaria, pruritus, flushing, angioedema, delayed purpuric rash

Other: bleeding at puncture site, ankle edema, chills, fever, **shock, anaphylaxis**

Interactions

Drug-drug. *Drugs that alter platelet function (such as aspirin, dipyridamole, heparin, oral anticoagulants):* increased bleeding risk
Drug-diagnostic tests. *Alpha$_2$-antiplasmin, factor V, factor VIII, fibrinogen and plasminogen activity, hematocrit, hemoglobin:* decreased values
Eosinophils, International Normalized Ratio, partial thromboplastin time, prothrombin time: increased values

Precautions

Use cautiously in:
• hemorrhagic conditions, severe hepatic or renal disease
• patients receiving warfarin concurrently
• elderly patients
• pregnant patients
• children.

Patient monitoring

◀▓ Monitor patient for signs and symptoms of anaphylaxis.
◀▓ Watch for bleeding tendency and hemorrhaging.
• Assess neurologic status and vital signs regularly.
• Evaluate patient for arrhythmias, conduction disorders, and hypotension.
• Monitor complete blood count and blood coagulation studies.

Patient teaching

• Teach patient to report signs and symptoms of allergic reaction.
• Instruct patient to report unusual bleeding or bruising.
• Caution patient to avoid activities that can cause injury. Advise him to use soft toothbrush and electric razor to avoid gum and skin injury.
• Explain to patient that he will be on bed rest during entire course of

---

♣ Canada   ◀▓ Clinical alert   Reactions in **bold** are life-threatening

treatment and will be monitored closely.

• Teach patient to minimize GI upset by eating small, frequent servings of food and drinking plenty of fluids.

• Caution patient not to use aspirin during therapy.

• Inform patient that he'll undergo regular blood testing during therapy.

antihemophilic factor (AHF, factor VIII)
Alphanate, Bioclate, HelixateFS, Hemofil M, Humate-P, Hyate:C, Koate-DVI, Kogenate, Kogenate FS, Monarc-M, Monoclate-P, Recombinate, ReFacto

Pharmacologic class: Hemostatic
Therapeutic class: Antihemophilic
Pregnancy risk category C

Action
Promotes conversion of prothrombin to thrombin (needed for blood coagulation), thereby increasing clotting time. Replaces deficient clotting factors, stopping or preventing bleeding episodes.

Availability
I.V. injection: 250 IU/vial, 500 IU/vial, 1,000 IU/vial, 1,500 IU/vial in numerous preparations

⟡ Indications and dosages
➤ Spontaneous hemorrhage in patients with hemophilia A (factor VIII deficiency)
Adults and children: Dosage is highly individualized, calculated as follows: AHF required (IU) equals weight (kg) times desired factor VIII increase (% of normal) times 0.5

To control bleeding, desired factor VIII level is 20% to 40% of normal for

minor hemorrhage; 30% to 60% of normal for moderate hemorrhage; or 60% to 100% of normal for severe hemorrhage. To prevent spontaneous hemorrhage, desired factor is 5% of normal.
➤ To prevent bleeding in patients with hemophilia who are scheduled for surgery
Adults: 25 to 30 IU/kg I.V. 1 hour before surgery, plus oral antifibrinolytics within 1 hour of surgery. Titrate dosage to achieve AHF level that's 80% to 100% of normal; maintain at 30% to 60% of normal for at least 10 to 14 days postoperatively.

Contraindications
• Hypersensitivity to drug or mouse, hamster, or bovine protein

Administration
• Before giving, verify that patient has no history of hypersensitivity to drug or to mouse, hamster, or bovine protein.
• Follow prescriber's instructions regarding hepatitis B prophylaxis before starting therapy.
• Refrigerate concentrate until ready to reconstitute drug.
• Warm bottles of concentrate and diluent to room temperature before mixing.
• Roll bottle gently between hands until drug is well-mixed.
• After drug is reconstituted, don't refrigerate, shake, or store near heat.
• Don't mix with other I.V. solutions.
• Use plastic (not glass) syringe and filter.

Route	Onset	Peak	Duration
I.V.	Immediate	1-2 hr	Unknown

Adverse reactions
CNS: headache; lethargy; fatigue; dizziness; jitteriness; drowsiness; depersonalization; tingling in arms, ears, and face

CV: chest tightness, angina pectoris, tachycardia, slight hypotension, **increased bleeding tendency, thrombosis**

EENT: blurred or abnormal vision, eye disorder, otitis media, epistaxis, rhinitis, sore throat

GI: nausea, vomiting, diarrhea, constipation, stomachache, abdominal pain, gastroenteritis, anorexia, taste changes

Hematologic: forehead bruises, infected hematoma, **hemolytic anemia, thrombocytopenia, intravascular hemolysis, hyperfibrinogenemia**

Hepatic: hepatitis B transmission

Musculoskeletal: myalgia, muscle weakness, bone pain, finger pain

Respiratory: dyspnea, coughing, wheezing, **bronchospasm**

Skin: rash, acne, flushing, diaphoresis, urticaria

Other: allergic reaction, fever, chills, cold feet, cold sensations, stinging at injection site, **anaphylaxis, human immunodeficiency virus transmission**

Interactions

Drug-diagnostic tests. *Bilirubin, creatine kinase:* increased levels
Hemoglobin, platelets: decreased values

Precautions

Use cautiously in:
• hepatic disease
• blood types A, B, and AB
• patients receiving factor VIII inhibitors
• pregnant patients
• neonates and infants.

Patient monitoring

◀€ Monitor for signs and symptoms of anaphylaxis and hemolysis.

◀€ Watch for bleeding tendency and hemorrhage.

• Check vital signs regularly.

• Monitor complete blood count and coagulation studies.

• Monitor urine color; report orange or red urine.

• Assess for severe headache (may indicate intracranial hemorrhage).

Patient teaching

• Teach patient to immediately report signs and symptoms of allergic response or bleeding tendency.

• Advise patient to monitor urine color and to report orange or red urine.

• Instruct patient to avoid driving and other hazardous activities until he knows how drug affects concentration, alertness, and vision.

• Teach patient to minimize GI upset by eating small, frequent servings of food and drinking plenty of fluids.

• Caution patient not to use aspirin during therapy.

• Instruct patient to contact prescriber if drug becomes less effective.

• Teach patient to report signs or symptoms of hepatitis B.

• Notify patient that he'll undergo regular blood testing during therapy.

antithrombin III, human (AT-III, heparin cofactor 1)
Thrombate III

Pharmacologic class: Blood derivative, coagulation inhibitor
Therapeutic class: Antithrombin
Pregnancy risk category B

Action

Inactivates thrombin and activated forms of factors IXa, Xa, XIa, and XIIa, thereby inhibiting coagulation and thromboembolism formation

Availability

Injection: 500 IU, 1,000 IU

⬤ Indications and dosages
➤ Thromboembolism related to AT-III deficiency

Adults: Initial dosage is individualized to amount required to increase AT-III activity to 120% of normal (determined 20 minutes after administration). Usual infusion rate is 50 to a maximum of 100 IU/minute I.V. Dosage calculation is based on anticipated 1.4% increase in plasma AT-III activity produced by 1 IU/kg body weight.

Use this formula:

Required dosage (IU) equals desired activity (%) minus baseline AT-III activity (%) times weight (kg) divided by 1.4 (IU/kg).

Maintenance dosage is individualized to amount required to maintain AT-III activity at 80% of normal.

Contraindications
• Children (safety and efficacy not established)

Administration
• Mix powder with 10 ml of sterile water, normal saline solution, or dextrose 5% in water.
• Use filter needle provided by manufacturer to draw up solution.
• Don't shake vial.
• Know that drug may be diluted further in same solution if desired.
• Don't mix with other solutions.
• Infuse over 10 to 20 minutes.
• Administer within 3 hours of reconstituting.
◀€ If adverse reactions occur, decrease infusion rate or, if indicated, stop infusion until symptoms disappear.

Route	Onset	Peak	Duration
I.V.	Immediate	Unknown	4 days

Adverse reactions
CNS: dizziness, light-headedness, headache
CV: vasodilation, reduced blood pressure, chest pain
EENT: perception of "film" over eyes
GI: nausea, sensation of intestinal fullness, foul taste
GU: diuresis
Musculoskeletal: muscle cramps
Respiratory: dyspnea, shortness of breath
Skin: urticaria, oozing lesions, hives, hematoma
Other: chills, fever

Interactions
Drug-drug. *Heparin:* increased anticoagulant effect

Precautions
Use cautiously in:
• pregnant or breastfeeding patients
• children.

Patient monitoring
• Monitor AT-III activity levels regularly.
• Watch for signs and symptoms of too-rapid infusion, such as dyspnea and hypertension.
• Monitor vital signs and temperature.
• Assess fluid intake and output to detect dehydration.

Patient teaching
• Instruct patient to immediately report chest tightness, dizziness, and fever.
• Caution patient to avoid driving and other hazardous activities until he knows how drug affects concentration and alertness.
• Teach patient to minimize GI upset and unpleasant taste by eating small, frequent servings of healthy food and drinking plenty of fluids.
• Tell patient that he'll undergo regular blood testing during therapy.

aprepitant
Emend

Pharmacologic class: Substance P and neurokinin-1 antagonist
Therapeutic class: Adjunctive antiemetic
Pregnancy risk category B

Action
Unknown; augments antiemetic activity of ondansentron (a 5-hydroxytryptamine$_3$-receptor antagonist) and dexamethasone; also inhibits cisplatin-induced emesis.

Availability
Capsules: 80 mg, 125 mg

⚕ Indications and dosages
➤ To prevent acute and delayed nausea and vomiting caused by highly emetogenic cancer chemotherapy
Adults: 125 mg P.O. 1 hour before chemotherapy on day 1; then 80 mg P.O. once daily in morning on days 2 and 3. Give with 12 mg dexamethasone P.O. and 32 mg ondansetron I.V. on day 1 and with 8 mg dexamethasone P.O. on days 2 to 4.

Contraindications
• Hypersensitivity to drug
• Concurrent pimozide, terfenadine, astemizole, or cisapride therapy
• Breastfeeding

Administration
• Give 1 hour before chemotherapy on day 1, together with other antiemetics as prescribed.
• Give on mornings of days 2 and 3.

Route	Onset	Peak	Duration
P.O.	Unknown	Unknown	Unknown

Adverse reactions
CNS: dizziness, neuropathy, headache, insomnia, asthenia, fatigue
EENT: tinnitus
GI: nausea, vomiting, constipation, diarrhea, epigastric discomfort, gastritis, heartburn, abdominal pain, anorexia
Hematologic: neutropenia
Other: fever, dehydration, hiccups

Interactions
Drug-drug. *CYP3A4 inducers (carbamazepine, phenytoin, rifampin):* decreased aprepitant blood level
CYP3A4 inhibitors (azole antifungals, clarithromycin, nefazodone, ritonavir): increased aprepitant blood level
Dexamethasone, methylprednisolone: increased steroid exposure
Docetaxel, etoposide, ifosfamide, imatinib, irinotecan, paclitaxel, vinblastine, vincristine, vinorelbine: increased blood levels of these drugs
Hormonal contraceptives: decreased contraceptive efficacy
Paroxetine: decreased efficacy of either drug
Pimozide: increased blood level and toxic effects of aprepitant
Tolbutamide, warfarin: CYP2C9 induction, decreased efficacy of these drugs

Precautions
Use cautiously in:
• patients receiving warfarin or CYP3A4 inhibitors concurrently
• pregnant patients.

Patient monitoring
• Monitor neurologic status; institute measures to prevent injury.
• Assess nutritional and hydration status.
• Monitor complete blood count.

Patient teaching
• Tell patient that drug may cause CNS effects; reassure him he'll be monitored to ensure his safety.

• Teach patient to minimize GI upset by eating small, frequent servings of foods and drinking plenty of fluids.
• Instruct patient to avoid driving and other hazardous activities until he knows how drug affects concentration, hearing, strength, balance, and alertness.

argatroban
Acova

Pharmacologic class: L-arginine–derived thrombin inhibitor
Therapeutic class: Anticoagulant
Pregnancy risk category B

Action
Binds rapidly to site of thrombi, neutralizing conversion of fibrinogen to fibrin, activation of coagulation factors, and platelet aggregation, necessary for formation of clotting

Availability
Injection: 100 mg/ml in 2.5-ml vials

🕖 Indications and dosages
➤ Treatment or prophylaxis of thrombosis in patients with heparin-induced thrombocytopenia
Adults: 2 mcg/kg/minute as a continuous I.V. infusion, to a maximum dosage of 10 mcg/kg/minute. Adjust dosage as needed to maintain activated partial thromboplastin time (APTT) 1.5 to 3 times initial baseline value (not to exceed 100 seconds).
➤ Anticoagulation during percutaneous coronary intervention in patients who have or are at risk for heparin-induced thrombocytopenia
Adults: Start a continuous I.V. infusion at 25 mcg/kg/minute and give 350 mcg/kg I.V. bolus over 3 to 5 minutes. Check activated clotting time (ACT) 5 to 10 minutes after bolus dose is given;

adjust dosage until ACT is between 300 and 450 seconds.
Dosage adjustment
• Hepatic impairment

Contraindications
• Hypersensitivity to drug
• Breastfeeding

Administration
• Stop all parenteral anticoagulants before starting argatroban.
• Dilute in normal saline solution, dextrose 5% in water, or lactated Ringer's solution to a concentration of 1 mg/ml.
• Inject contents of 2.5-ml vial into 250-ml bag of diluent.
• Protect solution from direct sunlight.

Route	Onset	Peak	Duration
I.V.	Rapid	1-3 hr	Duration of infusion

Adverse reactions
CNS: headache
CV: hypotension, unstable angina, **atrial fibrillation, cardiac arrest, ventricular tachycardia, cerebrovascular disorders**
GI: nausea, vomiting, diarrhea, abdominal pain, anorexia, **GI bleeding**
GU: abnormal renal function, urinary tract infection, minor GU tract bleeding and hematuria
Hematologic: groin bleeding, brachial bleeding, decreased hemoglobin and hematocrit values, **hypoprothrombinemia, thrombocytopenia, bleeding or hemorrhage**
Respiratory: cough, dyspnea, pneumonia, hemoptysis
Skin: rash, bleeding at puncture site
Other: allergic reaction, pain, infection, fever, **sepsis, anaphylaxis**

Interactions
Drug-drug. *Oral anticoagulants:* prolonged prothrombin time, increased

---

International Normalized Ratio, increased risk of bleeding
Thrombolytics: increased risk of intracranial bleeding
Drug-diagnostic tests. *Hematocrit, hemoglobin:* decreased values

Precautions
Use cautiously in:
• hepatic impairment or disease, intracranial bleeding
• pregnant or breastfeeding patients
• children younger than age 18.

Patient monitoring
• Monitor patient for signs and symptoms of anaphylaxis.
◄€ Evaluate patient for bleeding tendency and hemorrhage.
• Assess neurologic status and vital signs frequently.
• Monitor complete blood count and coagulation studies, especially partial thromboplastin time.
• Check for signs and symptoms of arrhythmias and hypotension.

Patient teaching
• Teach patient to immediately report allergic reaction and unusual bleeding or bruising.
• Tell patient to avoid activities that can cause injury. Advise him to use a soft toothbrush and electric razor to avoid gum and skin injury.
• Advise patient to minimize GI upset by eating small, frequent servings of food and drinking plenty of fluids.
• Tell patient that he'll undergo regular blood testing during therapy.

a

aripiprazole
Abilify

Pharmacologic class: Quinolone-derived atypical antipsychotic agent

Therapeutic class: Antipsychotic, neuroleptic

Pregnancy risk category C

Action
Unclear; thought to exert partial agonist activity at central dopamine D_2 and type 1A serotonin (5-HT_{1A}) receptors and antagonistic activity at serotonin 5-HT_{2A} receptors. Also has alpha-adrenergic and histamine$_1$-blocking properties.

Availability
Tablets: 10 mg, 15 mg, 20 mg, 30 mg

Indications and dosages
➤ Schizophrenia
Adults: 10 to 15 mg P.O. daily. If needed, increase to 30 mg daily after 2 weeks.
Dosage adjustment
• Concurrent use of potent CYP3A4 inhibitors (such as ketoconazole), CYP2D6 inhibitors (such as fluoxetine, paroxetine, quinidine), or CYP3A4 inducers (such as carbamazepine)

Contraindications
• Hypersensitivity to drug

Administration
• Give with or without food.
• Don't administer with grapefruit juice.

Route	Onset	Peak	Duration
P.O.	Slow	3-5 hr	Unknown

Adverse reactions
CNS: drowsiness, insomnia, akathisia, agitation, anxiety, headache, light-

headedness, drowsiness, tremor, tardive dyskinesia, **seizures, neuroleptic malignant syndrome, increased suicide risk**

CV: orthostatic hypotension, hypertension, peripheral edema, chest pain, **bradycardia, tachycardia**

EENT: rhinitis

GI: nausea, vomiting, diarrhea, constipation, jaundice, abdominal pain, esophageal motility disorders

Respiratory: cough

Skin: rash

Other: fever

Interactions

Drug-drug. *CNS depressants:* increased sedation

Drugs that induce CYP3A4 (such as carbamazepine): decreased aripiprazole effect

Drugs that inhibit CYP3A4 (such as ketoconazole) or CYP2D6 (such as fluoxetine, paroxetine, quinidine): serious toxic effects

Other antipsychotic agents: increased extrapyramidal effects

Drug-herb. *Kava:* increased CNS depression

Drug-behaviors. *Alcohol use:* increased sedation

Precautions

Use cautiously in:

• cerebrovascular disease, hypotension, seizure disorder, suicidal ideation

• pregnant or breastfeeding patients

• children.

Patient monitoring

• Watch for signs and symptoms of depression, and evaluate patient for suicidal ideation.

• Monitor neurologic status closely; watch for tardive dyskinesia.

• Evaluate patient for neuroleptic malignant syndrome (fever, altered mental status, rigid muscles, arrhythmia, tachycardia, sweating). Stop drug and notify prescriber if these signs and symptoms occur.

• Monitor blood pressure, pulse, and weight.

Patient teaching

• Inform patient that symptoms will subside slowly over several weeks.

• Tell patient he can take drug with or without food.

• Caution patient to avoid driving and other hazardous activities until he knows how drug affects concentration and alertness.

• Instruct patient to contact prescriber if he experiences depression or has suicidal thoughts.

• Advise patient to establish effective bedtime routine to minimize insomnia.

• Tell patient to minimize GI upset by eating small, frequent servings of food and drinking plenty of fluids.

• Teach patient to avoid strenuous exercise and hot environments whenever possible.

arsenic trioxide
Trisenox

Pharmacologic class: Nonmetallic element, white arsenic

Therapeutic class: Antineoplastic

Pregnancy risk category D

Action

Unclear; may cause morphologic changes and DNA fragmentation in promyelocytic leukemia cells, causing cell death and degradation of or damage to PML/RAR alpha (a fusion protein).

Availability

Injection: 1 mg/ml

✔ Indications and dosages

➤ Acute promyelocytic leukemia (APL) in patients who relapse or are refractory to retinoid and anthracycline chemotherapy

Adults and children ages 5 and older: *Induction phase*—0.15 mg/kg I.V. daily until bone marrow remission occurs, to a maximum of 60 doses. *Consolidation phase*—0.15 mg/kg I.V. daily for 25 doses over 5 weeks, starting 3 to 6 weeks after completion of induction phase.

Contraindications

- Hypersensitivity to drug
- Pregnancy

Administration

◀€ Know that drug is carcinogenic; follow facility policy for preparing and handling antineoplastics.

- Dilute in 100 to 250 ml of dextrose 5% in water or normal saline solution.
- Don't mix with other drugs.
- Infuse over 1 to 2 hours (may infuse over 4 hours if patient has vasomotor reaction).

Route	Onset	Peak	Duration
I.V.	Unknown	Unknown	Unknown

Adverse reactions

CNS: headache, insomnia, paresthesia, dizziness, tremor, drowsiness, anxiety, confusion, agitation, rigors, weakness, **seizures, coma**

CV: electrocardiogram (ECG) abnormalities, tachycardia, palpitations, chest pain, hypotension, hypertension, **prolonged QT interval, torsades de pointes**

EENT: blurred vision, painful red eye, dry eyes, eye irritation, swollen eyelids, tinnitus, earache, nasopharyngitis, postnasal drip, epistaxis, sinusitis, sore throat

GI: nausea, vomiting, constipation, diarrhea, abdominal pain, fecal incontinence, dyspepsia, dry mouth, mouth blisters, oral candidiasis, anorexia, **GI hemorrhage**

GU: renal impairment, urinary incontinence, oliguria, intermenstrual bleeding, **renal failure, vaginal hemorrhage**

Hematologic: leukocytosis, anemia, lymphadenopathy, **thrombocytopenia, neutropenia, disseminated intravascular coagulation, hemorrhage**

Hepatic: elevated alanine aminotransferase (ALT) and aspartate aminotransferase (AST) levels

Metabolic: hypokalemia, hypomagnesemia, hyperglycemia, acidosis, hypoglycemia, **hyperkalemia**

Musculoskeletal: joint, muscle, bone, back, neck, or limb pain

Respiratory: dyspnea, cough, hypoxia, wheezing, crackles, tachypnea, decreased breath sounds, crepitation, hemoptysis, rhonchi, upper respiratory tract infection, **pleural effusion**

Skin: flushing, erythema, pallor, bruising, petechiae, pruritus, dermatitis, dry skin, hyperpigmentation, urticaria, skin lesions, herpes simplex infection, local exfoliation, diaphoresis, night sweats

Other: fever, facial edema, weight gain or loss, bacterial infection, pain and edema at injection site, **hypersensitivity reaction, sepsis**

Interactions

Drug-drug. *Drugs that can cause electrolyte abnormalities (such as amphotericin B, diuretics):* increased risk of electrolyte abnormalities

Drugs that can prolong QT interval (antiarrhythmics, thioridazines, some quinolones): increased QT interval prolongation

Drug-diagnostic tests. *ALT, AST, calcium, magnesium, white blood cells:* increased levels

Glucose, potassium: altered levels

Hemoglobin, neutrophils, platelets: decreased values

Precautions
Use cautiously in:
- renal impairment, cardiac abnormalities
- elderly patients
- breastfeeding patients
- children.

Patient monitoring
◀℥ Watch for signs and symptoms of APL differentiation syndrome (fever, dyspnea, weight gain, pulmonary infiltrates, and pleural or pericardial effusions).
- Evaluate vital signs and neurologic status.
◀℥ Obtain baseline ECG; monitor ECG at least weekly.
- Assess for arrhythmias and conduction disorders.
◀℥ Discontinue drug and notify prescriber if patient develops syncope, tachycardia, or arrhythmias.
- Monitor serum electrolyte levels, complete blood count (CBC), and coagulation studies.
- Assess for hypoglycemia and hyperglycemia if patient is diabetic.

Patient teaching
- Instruct patient to immediately report signs and symptoms of allergic responses, fever, breathing problems, and seizures.
- Tell patient that drug increases risk of serious infection; instruct him to immediately report signs or symptoms of infection.
- Caution patient to avoid driving and other hazardous activities until he knows how drug affects concentration and alertness.
◀℥ Emphasize importance of avoiding pregnancy during therapy.
- Teach patient to minimize GI upset by eating small, frequent servings of food and drinking plenty of fluids.
- Advise patient to establish effective bedtime routine to minimize insomnia.

- Notify patient that he'll undergo regular blood testing during therapy.

asparaginase
Elspar, Kidrolase✚

Pharmacologic class: Enzyme
Therapeutic class: Antineoplastic (miscellaneous)
Pregnancy risk category C

Action
Hydrolyzes asparagine (amino acid needed for malignant cell growth in acute lymphocytic leukemia), resulting in leukemic cell death

Availability
Injection: 10,000 IU-vial (with mannitol)

🕖 Indications and dosages
➤ Acute lymphocytic leukemia, given with other drugs as part of antineoplastic regimen
Children: 1,000 IU/kg I.V. daily for 10 successive days, with asparaginase initiated on day 22 of regimen
➤ Sole agent used to induce remission of acute lymphocytic leukemia
Adults and children: 200 IU/kg I.V. daily for 28 days
➤ Drug desensitization regimen
Adults and children: Initially, 1 IU I.V.; then double the dosage q 10 minutes until total planned daily dosage has been given.

Contraindications
- Hypersensitivity to drug
- Pancreatitis or history of pancreatitis
- Impaired hepatic function
- Bone marrow depression
- Pregnancy or breastfeeding

Administration

◀€ Administer intradermal skin test as ordered at start of therapy and when drug hasn't been given for 1 week or more.

• Follow prescriber's orders for drug desensitization when indicated (usually before therapy starts and again during retreatment).

◀€ Know that drug may be carcinogenic, mutagenic, or teratogenic; follow appropriate facility policy for handling and preparing.

• Before starting drug, give allopurinol as prescribed to lower risk of neuropathy.

• Add sterile water or normal saline solution (5 ml for I.V. dose, 2 ml for I.M. dose) to powdered drug in vial.

• Filter through 5-micron filter.

• For I.V. use, inject into normal saline solution or dextrose 5% in water and infuse over 30 minutes.

• For I.M. use, give a maximum of 2 ml at any one site.

• Don't use solution unless it's clear.

• If drug touches skin or mucous membranes, rinse with copious amounts of water for at least 15 minutes.

• Provide adequate fluid intake to prevent tumor lysis.

Route	Onset	Peak	Duration
I.V.	Immediate	Immediate	23-33 days
I.M.	Immediate	14-24 hr	23-33 days

Adverse reactions

CNS: confusion, drowsiness, depression, hallucinations, fatigue, agitation, headache, lethargy, irritability, **seizures, coma**

GI: nausea, vomiting, anorexia, abdominal cramps, stomatitis, **hemorrhagic pancreatitis, fulminant pancreatitis**

GU: azotemia, glycosuria, polyuria, uric acid nephropathy, **renal failure**

Hematologic: anemia, **leukopenia, hypofibrinogenemia, depression of clotting factor synthesis, bone marrow depression, intracranial hemorrhage and fatal bleeding**

Hepatic: fatty liver changes, **hepatotoxicity**

Metabolic: hypoglycemia, hyperglycemia, hyperuricemia, hypocalcemia, hyperammonemia

Musculoskeletal: joint pain

Skin: rash, urticaria

Other: chills, fever, weight loss, hypersensitivity reactions, **anaphylaxis, fatal hyperthermia**

Interactions

Drug-drug. *Methotrexate:* decreased methotrexate efficacy

Prednisone: hyperglycemia, increased drug toxicity

Vincristine: hyperglycemia, increased drug toxicity, increased risk of neuropathy

Drug-diagnostic tests. *Alanine aminotransferase, ammonia, aspartate aminotransferase, blood urea nitrogen, glucose, uric acid:* increased levels

Calcium, hemoglobin, white blood cells: decreased levels

Thyroid function tests: interference with test interpretation

Precautions

Use cautiously in:

• hepatic or renal disease, CNS depression, clotting abnormalities, infection

• women of childbearing age.

Patient monitoring

• Observe for signs and symptoms of anaphylaxis.

◀€ Monitor for bleeding tendency and hemorrhage.

• Assess vital signs, temperature, and neurologic status.

• Monitor complete blood count, blood and urine glucose levels, and liver, kidney, and bone marrow function study results.

- Monitor fluid intake and output.

Patient teaching

- Instruct patient to immediately report allergic response and unusual bleeding or bruising.
- Caution patient to avoid driving and other hazardous activities until he knows how drug affects concentration and alertness.
- Advise patient to drink plenty of fluids to ensure adequate urine output.
- Teach patient to monitor urine output and report significant changes.
- Instruct patient to avoid activities that can cause injury. Tell him to use soft toothbrush and electric razor to avoid injury to gums and skin.
- Teach patient to minimize GI upset by eating small, frequent servings of food and drinking plenty of fluids.
- Tell patient that he'll undergo regular blood testing during therapy.

atenolol

Apo-Atenolol✤, Novo-Atenol✤, Tenormin

Pharmacologic class: Beta-adrenergic blocker (selective)
Therapeutic class: Antianginal, antihypertensive
Pregnancy risk category D

Action

Selectively blocks $beta_1$-adrenergic receptors (myocardial); decreases cardiac output, peripheral resistance, and myocardial oxygen consumption. Also depresses renin secretion without affecting $beta_2$-adrenergic receptors (pulmonary, vascular, uterine).

Availability

Injection: 5 mg/10 ml
Tablets: 25 mg, 50 mg, 100 mg

Indications and dosages

➤ Hypertension
Adults: Initially, 50 mg P.O. once daily, increased to 100 mg after 7 to 14 days if needed

➤ Angina pectoris
Adults: Initially, 50 mg P.O. once daily, increased to 100 mg after 7 days if needed. Some patients may require up to 200 mg daily.

➤ Acute myocardial infarction
Adults: Initially, 5 mg I.V. over 5 minutes, followed by 5 mg I.V. 10 minutes later; 10 minutes after last I.V. dose, give 50-mg tablet P.O., then give 50 mg P.O. in 12 hours. Maintenance dosage is 100 mg P.O. daily or 50 mg b.i.d. for 6 to 9 days.

Dosage adjustment
- Renal impairment
- Elderly patients

Contraindications

- Cardiogenic shock
- Sinus bradycardia
- Greater than first-degree heart block

Administration

◀ᛟ If apical pulse is below 60 beats/minute, withhold dose and call prescriber.
- Mix I.V. dose with dextrose or sodium chloride injection solution.
- For I.V. use, administer slowly (no faster than 1 mg/minute).
- Use I.V. solution within 48 hours of mixing.
- Don't discontinue drug suddenly; instead, taper dosage over 2 weeks.

Route	Onset	Peak	Duration
P.O.	1 hr	2 hr	24 hr
I.V.	5 min	5 min	12 hr

Adverse reactions

CNS: fatigue, lethargy, vertigo, drowsiness, dizziness, depression, disorientation, short-term memory loss

---

CV: hypertension, intermittent claudication, cold arms and legs, orthostatic hypotension, **bradycardia, heart failure, cardiogenic shock, myocardial reinfarction, arrhythmias**
EENT: blurred vision, dry eyes, eye irritation, conjunctivitis, stuffy nose, rhinitis, pharyngitis, **laryngospasm**
GI: nausea, vomiting, diarrhea, constipation, gastric pain, flatulence, anorexia, **ischemic colitis, retroperitoneal fibrosis, acute pancreatitis, mesenteric arterial thrombosis**
GU: impotence, decreased libido, dysuria, nocturia, Peyronie's disease, **renal failure**
Hematologic: agranulocytosis
Hepatic: elevated alanine aminotransferase (ALT) and aspartate aminotransferase (AST) levels, **hepatomegaly**
Metabolic: hypoglycemia, increased lactate dehydrogenase level
Musculoskeletal: muscle cramps, back and joint pain
Respiratory: dyspnea, wheezing, respiratory distress, **bronchospasm, bronchial obstruction, pulmonary emboli**
Other: fever, decreased exercise tolerance, allergic reaction, fever, development of antinuclear antibodies, hypersensitivity reaction

Interactions
Drug-drug. *Amiodarone, cardiac glycosides, diltiazem, verapamil:* increased myocardial depression, causing excessive bradycardia and heart block
Amphetamines, cocaine, ephedrine, norepinephrine, phenylephrine, pseudoephedrine: excessive hypertension, bradycardia
Ampicillin, calcium salts: decreased antihypertensive and antianginal effects
Aspirin, bismuth subsalicylate, magnesium salicylate, nonsteroidal antiinflammatory drugs: decreased antihypertensive effect
Clonidine: life-threatening blood pressure increase after clonidine withdrawal

or after simultaneous withdrawal of both drugs
Dobutamine, dopamine: decrease in beneficial beta-cardiovascular effects
Lidocaine: increased lidocaine levels, greater risk of toxicity
Monoamine oxidase inhibitors: bradycardia
Prazosin: increased risk of orthostatic hypotension
Reserpine: increased hypotension, marked bradycardia
Theophylline: decreased theophylline elimination
Drug-diagnostic tests. *Alkaline phosphatase, ALT, AST, antinuclear antibody titers, blood urea nitrogen, creatinine, lactate dehydrogenase, platelets, potassium, uric acid:* increased levels
Glucose: increased or decreased level
Insulin tolerance test: false results
Drug-behaviors. *Alcohol use:* increased hypotension

Precautions
Use cautiously in:
• renal failure, hepatic impairment, pulmonary disease, diabetes mellitus, thyrotoxicosis
• pregnant or breastfeeding patients
• children.

Patient monitoring
• Watch for signs and symptoms of hypersensitivity reaction.
• Monitor vital signs (especially blood pressure), electrocardiogram, and exercise tolerance.
• Check closely for hypotension if patient is receiving hemodialysis.
• Monitor blood glucose level regularly if patient is diabetic; drug may mask signs and symptoms of hypoglycemia.

Patient teaching
• Instruct patient to immediately report signs and symptoms of allergic response, breathing problems, and chest pain.

• Caution patient to avoid driving and other hazardous activities until he knows how drug affects concentration and alertness.

• Teach patient to take drug at same time every day.

• Inform patient that he may experience serious reactions if he stops taking drug suddenly. Advise him to consult prescriber before discontinuing drug.

• Tell patient that drug may cause a temporary blood pressure decrease if he stands or sits up suddenly. Teach him to rise slowly and carefully.

◀≣ Inform women that drug can't be taken during pregnancy; urge them to report planned or suspected pregnancy.

• Tell men that drug may cause erectile dysfunction (impotence); advise them to discuss this issue with prescriber.

atomoxetine hydrochloride
Strattera

Pharmacologic class: Selective norepinephrine reuptake inhibitor
Therapeutic class: Antipsychotic agent
Pregnancy risk category C

Action
Unclear; may block norepinephrine reuptake at neuronal synapse.

Availability
Capsules: 10 mg, 18 mg, 25 mg, 40 mg, 60 mg

⭕ Indications and dosages
➤ Attention deficit hyperactivity disorder (ADHD)
Adults and children weighing more than 70 kg (154 lb): Initially, 40 mg P.O. daily. After 3 days, may increase to target total daily dosage of 80 mg P.O. given either as a single dose in morning or in evenly divided doses in morning and late afternoon or early evening. If desired response isn't reached, may increase dosage after 2 to 4 more weeks, to a maximum dosage of 100 mg P.O. daily.

Adults and children weighing 70 kg (154 lb) or less: Initially, 0.5 mg/kg/day P.O. Increase after at least 3 days to target daily dosage of 1.2 mg/kg, given either as single daily dose in morning or as evenly divided doses in morning and late afternoon or early evening.
Dosage adjustment
• Hepatic impairment
• Concurrent use of potent CYP2D6 inhibitors (such as paroxetine, fluoxetine, quinidine) in children weighing less than 70 kg (154 lb)

Contraindications
• Hypersensitivity to drug
• Closed-angle glaucoma
• Monoamine oxidase (MAO) inhibitor use within past 14 days

Administration
• Give as a single dose in morning, or give half of total daily dose in morning and other half in late afternoon or early evening.
• Don't give to patient who has taken MAO inhibitors within past 14 days.

Route	Onset	Peak	Duration
P.O.	Rapid	1-2 hr	Unknown

Adverse reactions
CNS: aggression, insomnia, dizziness, drowsiness, headache, irritability, crying, mood swings, fatigue, rigors
CV: orthostatic hypotension, palpitations, **tachycardia**
EENT: rhinorrhea, sinusitis
GI: nausea, vomiting, constipation, upper abdominal pain, flatulence, dyspepsia, dry mouth, decreased appetite
GU: urine retention, urinary hesitancy, dysmenorrhea, erectile problems, ejaculation failure, impotence, prostatitis
Musculoskeletal: muscle pain

Respiratory: cough
Skin: dermatitis, sweating
Other: fever, hot flashes, growth retardation, weight loss

Interactions
Drug-drug. *Albuterol:* increased cardiovascular effects
MAO inhibitors: hyperthermia, myoclonus, rapid changes in vital signs
Potent CYP2D6 inhibitors (such as fluoxetine, paroxetine, quinidine) in children weighing less than 70 kg (154 lb): increased atomoxetine effects
Vasopressors: hypertensive crisis

Precautions
Use cautiously in:
• impaired renal, cardiac, cerebrovascular, hepatic, or endocrine function; hypotension
• pregnant or breastfeeding patients
• children younger than age 6.

Patient monitoring
• Monitor growth in children.
• Assess for weight loss.
• Check blood pressure and pulse, especially after dosage changes.
• Monitor for changes in mood, sleep patterns, and behavior.
• Evaluate for urinary hesitancy or urinary retention and sexual dysfunction.
• Provide dietary counseling: refer patient to dietitian if adverse GI effects significantly limit food intake.

Patient teaching
• Instruct patient to avoid driving and other hazardous activities until he knows how drug affects concentration and alertness.
• To minimize insomnia, advise patient to establish effective bedtime routine and to take drug in single morning dose or in divided half-doses in morning and late afternoon or early evening.
• Teach patient to minimize GI upset by eating small, frequent servings of food and drinking plenty of fluids.

a

atorvastatin calcium
Lipitor

Pharmacologic class: 3-hydroxy-3-methylglutaryl-coenzyme A (HMG-CoA) reductase inhibitor
Therapeutic class: Lipid-lowering agent
Pregnancy risk category X

Action
Inhibits HMG-CoA reductase, which catalyzes first step in cholesterol synthesis pathway; this action reduces concentrations of serum cholesterol and low-density lipoproteins (LDLs), linked to higher risk of coronary artery disease (CAD). Also increases concentration of high-density lipoproteins (HDLs), linked to decreased CAD risk.

Availability
Tablets: 10 mg, 20 mg, 40 mg, 80 mg

🖊 Indications and dosages
➢ Adjunct to diet for controlling LDL, total cholesterol, apo-lipoprotein B, and triglyceride levels and to increase HDL levels in patients with primary hypercholesterolemia and mixed dyslipidemia; primary dysbetalipoproteinemia in patients unresponsive to diet alone. Adjunct to diet to reduce elevated triglyceride levels.
Adults: Initially, 10 mg P.O. daily; increase to 80 mg P.O. daily if needed. Adjust dosage according to patient's cholesterol level.
➢ Adjunct to other lipid-lowering treatments in patients with homozygous familial hypercholesterolemia
Adults: 10 to 80 mg P.O. daily
➢ Adjunct to diet to decrease total cholesterol, LDL, and apo-lipoprotein B levels in boys and postmenarchal girls ages 10 to 17 who have familial

and nonfamilial heterozygous hyper-cholesterolemia
Boys and girls: Initially, 10 mg P.O. daily; adjust dosage upward or downward based on lipid levels. Maximum dosage is 20 mg daily.

Off-label uses
• To lower total cholesterol levels

Contraindications
• Hypersensitivity to drug
• Active hepatic disease
• Females of childbearing age
• Pregnancy or breastfeeding

Administration
• Give with or without food.
• Don't give with grapefruit juice or antacids.

Route	Onset	Peak	Duration
P.O.	Unknown	1-2 hr	Unknown

Adverse reactions
CNS: amnesia, abnormal dreams, emotional lability, headache, hyperactivity, poor coordination, malaise, paresthesia, peripheral neuropathy, drowsiness, syncope, weakness
CV: arrhythmias, orthostatic hypotension, palpitations, phlebitis, vasodilation, increased creatine kinase level
EENT: amblyopia, altered refraction, glaucoma, dry eyes, eye hemorrhage, hearing loss, tinnitus, epistaxis, sinusitis, pharyngitis
GI: nausea, vomiting, diarrhea, constipation, abdominal cramps, abdominal or biliary pain, colitis, indigestion, dyspepsia, flatulence, stomach ulcers, gastroenteritis, melena, tenesmus, rectal hemorrhage, glossitis, mouth sores, gingival bleeding, dry mouth, taste loss, dysphagia, esophagitis, appetite changes, **pancreatitis**
GU: hematuria, nocturia, dysuria, urinary frequency or urgency, urinary retention, nephritis, renal calculi, abnor-mal ejaculation, cystitis, decreased libido, impotence, epididymitis
Hematologic: thrombocytopenia, anemia
Hepatic: jaundice, **hepatic failure, hepatitis**
Metabolic: hyperglycemia, hypoglycemia
Musculoskeletal: bursitis, joint pain, back pain, leg cramps, gout, muscle pain or aches, myositis, myasthenia gravis, neck rigidity, torticollis
Respiratory: dyspnea, pneumonia, bronchitis
Skin: alopecia, acne, contact dermatitis, eczema, dry skin, pruritus, rash, urticaria, skin ulcers, seborrhea, photosensitivity, diaphoresis
Other: allergic reaction, fever, facial paralysis, facial or generalized edema, flulike symptoms, infection, weight gain

Interactions
Drug-drug. *Antacids, colestipol:* decreased atorvastatin level
Azole antifungals, cyclosporine, erythromycin, fibric acid derivatives, niacin, other HMG-CoA inhibitors: increased risk of myopathy
Digoxin: increased digoxin level, greater risk of toxicity
Hormonal contraceptives: increased estrogen level
Drug-diagnostic tests. *Alanine aminotransferase, aspartate aminotransferase:* increased levels
Drug-food. *Grapefruit juice:* increased drug level, greater risk of adverse effects
Drug-herb. *Red yeast rice:* increased risk of adverse effects

Precautions
Use cautiously in:
• renal impairment, hypotension, uncontrolled seizures, myopathy, alcoholism

---

• severe metabolic, endocrine, or electrolyte disorders
• women of childbearing age
• children younger than age 18.

Patient monitoring
• Monitor patient for signs and symptoms of allergic response.
• Evaluate for muscle weakness, a symptom of myositis.
• Monitor liver function test results and lipid blood levels.

Patient teaching
• Teach patient to immediately report allergic response.
• Tell patient he may take drug with or without food.
• Caution patient to avoid driving and other hazardous activities until he knows how drug affects concentration, alertness, and vision.
• Instruct patient to avoid grapefruit juice during therapy.
• Teach patient to minimize GI upset by eating small, frequent servings of food and drinking plenty of fluids.
• Inform patient taking hormonal contraceptives that drug increases estrogen levels; instruct her to tell all prescribers she's taking drug.
• Inform men that drug may cause erectile dysfunction and abnormal ejaculation; encourage them to discuss these issues with prescriber.
• Tell patient he'll undergo regular blood testing during therapy.

atracurium besylate
Tracrium

Pharmacologic class: Nondepolarizing neuromuscular blocker
Therapeutic class: Skeletal muscle relaxant
Pregnancy risk category C

Action
Prevents binding of acetylcholine with receptor sites on motor end-plate

Availability
Injection: 10 mg/ml

Indications and dosages
➤ Adjunct to general anesthesia to facilitate endotracheal intubation and relax skeletal muscles during surgery
Adults and children ages 2 and older: Initially, 0.4 to 0.5 mg/kg by I.V. bolus. With prolonged surgery, maintenance dosage of 0.08 to 0.1 mg/kg is given within 20 to 45 minutes; may repeat q 15 to 25 minutes, as needed. During prolonged procedure, may administer constant infusion of 5 to 9 mcg/kg/minute.
Children ages 1 month to 2 years: 0.3 to 0.4 mg/kg I.V.; repeat if needed.

Off-label uses
• Myasthenia gravis

Contraindications
• Hypersensitivity to drug

Administration
• Use only under direct supervision of trained medical staff who can maintain patent airway.
• Before giving drug, make sure emergency respiratory equipment is at hand.
• Ensure that patient receives sedative or general anesthetic before giving atracurium.
• Give I.V. only (bolus, intermittent infusion, or continuous infusion); never give I.M.
• Be aware that patient can hear while drug is in effect. Provide ongoing reassurance.
• Be ready to reverse drug's effects with anticholinesterase drug once spontaneous recovery begins.
• Store in refrigerator without freezing.

Route	Onset	Peak	Duration
I.V.	2 min	3-5 min	35-70 min

Adverse reactions

CNS: inadequate neuromuscular blockade, **prolonged neuromuscular blockade, seizures**

CV: hypotension, tachycardia, **bradycardia**

Respiratory: wheezing, dyspnea, **apnea, bronchospasm, laryngospasm**

Skin: flushing, rash, urticaria, erythema, pruritus

Other: injection site reaction, **anaphylaxis**

Interactions

Drug-drug. *Acetylcholinesterase inhibitors:* inhibition of muscle relaxation and reversal of neuromuscular blockade

Aminoglycosides, enflurane, halothane, isoflurane, lithium, procainamide, trimethaphan, verapamil: increased muscle relaxation

Carbamazepine, phenytoin, theophylline: resistance to or reversal of neuromuscular blockade

Clindamycin, lithium, magnesium salt, opioids, polymyxin antibiotics (colistin, polymyxin B sulfate), procainamide, quinine, thiazide and loop diuretics: enhanced neuromuscular blockade

Corticosteroids: prolonged weakness

Edrophonium, neostigmine, pyridostigmine: atracurium inhibition, reversal of neuromuscular blockade

Succinylcholine: faster atracurium onset, increased depth of muscle relaxation

Precautions

Use cautiously in:
• elderly patients
• pregnant or breastfeeding patients
• children.

Patient monitoring

◀€ Monitor patient for anaphylaxis and injection site reaction.

• Check vital signs and airway patency until patient recovers completely from drug effects.

• Assess for pain and give analgesics as needed. Be aware that patient may be unable to express pain while drug is in effect.

• Evaluate patient's recovery with muscle strength tests, nerve stimulation, and train-of-four monitoring.

• While drug is in effect, explain events to patient as they occur.

Patient teaching

• Before giving, carefully describe drug effects to patient, explaining that he will be able to hear but won't be able to move.

atropine sulfate
AtroPen, Atropine-1, Atropisol, Isopto-Atropine

Pharmacologic class: Anticholinergic (antimuscarinic)

Therapeutic class: antiarrhythmic

Pregnancy risk category C

Action

Inhibits acetylcholine at parasympathetic neuroeffector junction of smooth muscle and cardiac muscle, blocking sinoatrial (SA) and atrioventricular (AV) nodes; these actions increase impulse conduction and raise heart rate

Availability

Injection: 0.05 mg/ml, 0.1 mg/ml, 0.3 mg/ml, 0.4 mg/ml, 0.5 mg/ml, 0.8 mg/ml, 1 mg/ml

Tablets: 0.4 mg

⚕ Indications and dosages

➤ Bradyarrhythmias, symptomatic bradycardia

Adults: 0.5 to 1 mg by I.V. push repeated every 3 to 5 minutes as needed, to a maximum dosage of 2 mg

Children: 0.01 mg/kg I.V. to a maximum dosage of 0.4 mg or 0.3 mg/m². May repeat I.V. dose q 4 to 6 hours.

➤ Antidote for anticholinesterase insecticide poisoning

Adults: 2 to 3 mg I.V. repeated every 5 to 10 minutes until symptoms disappear or a toxic level is reached; for severe poisoning, 6 mg q hour

Children: 0.05 mg/kg I.M. or I.V. repeated every 10 to 30 minutes until symptoms disappear or a toxic level is reached

➤ Preoperatively to diminish secretions and block cardiac vagal reflexes

Adults and children weighing at least 20 kg (44 lb): 0.4 to 0.6 mg I.M., S.C., or I.V. 30 to 60 minutes before anesthesia

Children weighing 12 to 16 kg (26 to 35 lb): 0.3 mg I.M. or S.C. 30 to 60 minutes before anesthesia

Children weighing 7 to 9 kg (15 to 20 lb): 0.2 mg I.M. or S.C. 30 to 60 minutes before anesthesia

Children weighing 3 kg (6.5 lb): 0.1 mg I.M. or S.C. 30 to 60 minutes before anesthesia

➤ Peptic ulcer disease, functional GI disorders (such as hypersecretory states)

Adults: 0.4 to 0.6 mg P.O. q 4 to 6 hours

Children: 0.01 mg/kg or 0.3/m² P.O. q 4 to 6 hours

➤ Parkinsonism

Adults: 0.1 to 0.25 mg P.O. q.i.d.

➤ Antidote for mushroom toxicity from muscarine

Adults: 1 to 2 mg/hour I.M. or I.V. until respiratory function improves

Off-label uses
• Cholinergic-mediated bronchial asthma

Contraindications
• Hypersensitivity to drug
• Acute angle-closure glaucoma
• Obstructive GI tract disease
• Unstable cardiovascular status
• Asthma
• Myasthenia gravis
• Thyrotoxicosis
• Infants ages 3 months and younger

Administration
• For I.V. dose, infuse directly into large vein or I.V. tubing over at least 1 minute.
• Be aware that slow I.V. infusion may cause slowing of heart rate.
• Don't administer oral dose within 1 hour of giving antacids.
• Be aware that patients with Down syndrome may be unusually sensitive to drug.

Route	Onset	Peak	Duration
P.O.	0.5-2 hr	1-2 hr	4-6 hr
I.V.	Immediate	2-4 min	4-6 hr
I.M., S.C.	Rapid	15-50 min	4-6 hr

Adverse effects
CNS: headache, restlessness, ataxia, disorientation, delirium, insomnia, dizziness, drowsiness, agitation, nervousness, confusion, excitement
CV: palpitations, bradycardia, **tachycardia**
EENT: photophobia, blurred version, increased intraocular pressure, mydriasis, cycloplegia, nasal congestion, dry mouth
GI: nausea, vomiting, constipation, bloating, dyspepsia, ileus, abdominal distention (in infants), dysphagia
GU: urine retention, urinary hesitancy, impotence
Skin: decreased sweating, flushing, urticaria, dry skin

Other: thirst, **anaphylaxis**

Interactions
Drug-drug. *Amantadine, antiarrhythmics, anticholinergics, antihistamines, antiparkinsonian drugs, glutethimide, meperidine, muscle relaxants, phenothiazines, tricyclic antidepressants:* increased atropine effects
Antacids, antidiarrheals: decreased atropine absorption
Antimyasthenics: decreased intestinal motility
Cyclopropane: ventricular arrhythmias
Haloperidol: decreased antipsychotic effect
Ketoconazole, levodopa: decreased absorption of these drugs
Metoclopramide: decreased effect of atropine on GI motility
Potassium chloride wax-matrix tablets: increased severity of mucosal lesions
Drug-herb. *Jaborandi tree, pill-bearing spurge:* decreased drug effect
Jimsonweed: changes in cardiovascular function
Squaw vine: reduced metabolic breakdown of drug
Drug-behaviors. *Sun exposure:* increased risk of photophobia

Precautions
Use cautiously in:
• chronic renal, hepatic, pulmonary, or cardiac disease
• intra-abdominal infection, prostatic hypertrophy
• elderly patients
• pregnant or breastfeeding patients
• children.

Patient monitoring
• Watch closely for signs and symptoms of anaphylaxis.
• Monitor heart rate for bradycardia or tachycardia.
• Evaluate fluid intake and output.
• Assess for urine retention or urinary hesitancy.

• Monitor for signs and symptoms of glaucoma.

Patient teaching
• Instruct patient to immediately report allergic response.
◀€ Inform patient that headache, eye pain, and blurred vision may signal glaucoma; encourage him to report these symptoms at once.
• Advise patient to avoid driving and other hazardous activities until he knows how drug affects concentration, alertness, and vision.
• Encourage patient to establish an effective bedtime routine to minimize insomnia.

auranofin
Ridaura

aurothioglucose
Solganal

gold sodium thiomalate
Aurolate

Pharmacologic class: Heavy metal, gold compound
Therapeutic class: Anti-inflammatory
Pregnancy risk category C

Action
Unclear; exerts anti-inflammatory, antiarthritic, and immunoregulatory actions, including stimulation of cell-mediated immunity, suppression of immunoglobulin synthesis and antibody-dependent cytotoxicity, inhibition of neutrophil release from lysosomal enzymes, selective suppression of macrophage function, inhibition of interleukin secretion by T lymphocytes, and inhibition of neovascularization.

Availability
Capsules (Ridaura): 3 mg
Injection (Aurolate): 50 mg/ml in 2-ml
and 10-ml vials for I.M. injection only
Injection (Solganal): 50 mg/ml suspension for I.M. injection (preferably in
upper gluteal muscle)

Indications and dosages
➤ Active early rheumatoid arthritis in
adults and children when disease isn't
adequately controlled by other inflammatory agents or conservative measures (given in conjunction with other
therapy)
Aurothioglucose—
Adults: Initially, 10 mg I.M. in gluteal
muscle once a week; during second
and third weeks, 25 mg I.M.; during
fourth and subsequent weeks, 50 mg
I.M.; then 50 mg I.M. at weekly intervals until patient has received a total
dosage of 0.8 to 1 g. If patient improves
with no signs or symptoms of drug
toxicity, give 50 mg I.M. at 3- to 4-week
intervals indefinitely.
Children ages 6 to 12: One-fourth of
adult dose I.M., depending on body
weight, not to exceed 25 mg/dose
Gold sodium thiomalate—
Adults: Initially, 10 mg I.M. in gluteal
muscle once a week; during second
week, 25 mg I.M.; during third and
subsequent weeks, 25 to 50 mg I.M.
until major clinical improvement or
toxicity occurs or cumulative dose
reaches 1 g. Maintenance dosage is 25
to 50 mg I.M. every other week for 2 to
20 weeks. If patient's clinical status remains stable, give maintenance dosage
of 25 to 50 mg I.M. every 3 or 4 weeks
indefinitely.
Children: Initial test dose of 10 mg
I.M.; then 1 mg/kg, not to exceed
50 mg as single dose. Space doses as
described for adult dosage.
➤ Active classic rheumatoid arthritis
in patients who don't respond sufficiently to or can't tolerate nonsteroidal
anti-inflammatory drugs (NSAIDs),

given in conjunction with nondrug
therapies
Auranofin—
Adults: Initially, 6 mg P.O. daily, given
in single dose or as 3 mg b.i.d. If response isn't adequate after 6 months,
increase to 9 mg P.O. daily, given as
3 mg t.i.d.
Children: Initially, 0.1 mg/kg/day P.O.
Maximum dosage is 0.2 mg/kg/day
P.O. Maintenance dosage is 0.15 mg/
kg/day P.O.

Contraindications
• Hypersensitivity to gold
• Systemic lupus erythematosus
• Renal disease
• Hepatic disease
• Inflammatory bowel disease
• Pregnancy or breastfeeding

Administration
◀€ Give parenteral form I.M. only,
preferably using gluteal site.
• Administer test dose as prescribed,
and monitor patient for reaction.
• Place vial in warm water, and then
shake vigorously to mix drug.
• Have patient lie down for 10 to 20
minutes after injection.
• Keep dimercaprol readily available to
counteract drug toxicity.

Route	Onset	Peak	Duration
P.O.	Unknown	Unknown	Unknown
I.M.	Slow	4-6 hr	Unknown

Adverse reactions
CNS: dizziness, fainting, malaise
CV: syncope, bradycardia
EENT: pharyngitis
GI: nausea, vomiting, diarrhea, dysphagia, abdominal cramps, gastritis,
colitis, glossitis, stomatitis, gingivitis,
metallic taste, anorexia
GU: vaginitis, **acute tubular necrosis,
renal failure, nephrotic syndrome or
glomerulitis with proteinuria and
hematuria**

Hematologic: eosinophilia, anemia, **leukopenia, thrombocytopenia, granulocytopenia**
Hepatic: jaundice, **hepatitis**
Musculoskeletal: joint pain
Respiratory: cough, shortness of breath, dyspnea, tracheal inflammation, **interstitial pneumonitis, fibrosis, gold bronchitis**
Skin: grayish blue skin discoloration, erythema, dermatitis, pruritus, flushing, sweating, **exfoliative dermatitis**
Other: anaphylactic shock

Interactions

Drug-drug. *Antimalarials, cytotoxic drugs (immunosuppressants other than corticosteroids), penicillamine:* increased risk of adverse hematologic and renal effects
Drug-diagnostic tests. *Hematocrit, hemoglobin, platelets, white blood cells:* decreased levels
Liver function tests: altered results
Urine protein: increased level
Drug-behaviors. *Exposure to sun and artificial ultraviolet light:* grayish blue skin discoloration

Precautions

Use cautiously in:
• renal or hepatic disease, marked hypertension, compromised cardiovascular circulation, Sjögren's syndrome, eczema
• history of gold sensitivity.

Patient monitoring

◀€ For 30 minutes after giving dose, monitor patient for signs and symptoms of anaphylaxis.
• Stop therapy and consult prescriber if patient complains of itching, rash, or other skin problems.
• Monitor liver and kidney function test results and complete blood count (especially platelets).

Patient teaching

• Instruct patient to stop taking drug and notify prescriber immediately if he develops itching, rash, or other skin problems.
• Explain that drug may take 3 to 4 months to relieve symptoms.
• Teach patient to report bleeding tendencies or bruising.
• Caution patient to avoid driving and other hazardous activities until he knows how drug affects concentration and alertness.
• Tell patient that he may experience more joint pain for 1 to 2 days after each dose, but that pain usually eases.
• Teach patient to monitor urine output and report significant changes.
• Advise patient to use good oral hygiene; tell him to report metallic taste.
◀€ Teach patient about risks of using drug during pregnancy; advise her to report planned or suspected pregnancy to prescriber.
• Teach patient to minimize GI upset by eating small, frequent servings of foods and drinking plenty of fluids.
• Notify patient that he'll undergo regular blood testing during therapy.

azathioprine
Imuran

azathioprine sodium
Imuran

Pharmacologic class: Purine antagonist
Therapeutic class: Immunosuppressant
Pregnancy risk category D

Action

Prevents proliferation and differentiation of activated B and T cells by interfering with synthesis of purine, deoxyribonucleic acid, and ribonucleic acid

Availability
Injection (azathioprine sodium):
100-mg vial
Tablets (azathioprine): 50 mg

🖊 Indications and dosages
➤ To prevent rejection of kidney transplant
Adults and children: Initially, 3 to 5 mg/kg/day P.O. or I.V. as a single dose. Give on day of transplantation or 1 to 3 days before day of transplantation; then 3 to 5 mg/kg/day I.V. after surgery until patient can tolerate P.O. route. Maintenance dosage is 1 to 3 mg/kg/day P.O.
➤ Rheumatoid arthritis
Adults and children: Initially, 1 mg/kg P.O. in one or two daily doses. Increase dosage in steps at 6 to 8 weeks and thereafter at 4-week intervals; use dosage increments of 0.5 mg/kg/day, to a maximum dosage of 2.5 mg/kg/day. Once patient stabilizes, decrease in increments of 0.5 mg/kg/day to lowest effective dosage.
Dosage adjustment
• Renal disease
• Concurrent allopurinol therapy
• Elderly patients

Off-label uses
• Crohn's disease
• Myasthenia gravis
• Chronic ulcerative colitis

Contraindications
• Hypersensitivity to drug
• Previous treatment with alkylating agents for rheumatoid arthritis
• Pregnancy or breastfeeding

Administration
• For I.V. dose, mix powder with 10 ml of sterile water.
• Use I.V. route only if patient can't tolerate oral dose. Give over 30 to 60 minutes by I.V. push or by infusion in normal saline solution or dextrose 5% in water.
• Give oral doses after meals.

Route	Onset	Peak	Duration
P.O.	6-8 wks	12 wks	Unknown
I.V.	Days-wks	Unknown	Days-wks

Adverse reactions
CNS: malaise
EENT: retinopathy
GI: nausea, vomiting, stomatitis, esophagitis, anorexia, mucositis, diarrhea, **pancreatitis**
Hematologic: thrombocytopenia, leukopenia, pancytopenia, anemia
Hepatic: jaundice, **hepatotoxicity**
Musculoskeletal: muscle wasting, joint and muscle pain
Skin: rash, alopecia
Other: chills, fever, **serum sickness, neoplasms, serious infection**

Interactions
Drug-drug. *Allopurinol:* increased therapeutic and adverse effects of azathioprine
Anticoagulants, cyclosporine: decreased action of these drugs
Atracurium, pancuronium, tubocurarine, vecuronium: reversal of these drugs' actions
Drugs affecting bone marrow and bone marrow cells (such as angiotensin-converting enzyme inhibitors, co-trimoxazole): severe leukopenia
Drug-diagnostic tests. *Alanine aminotransferase, alkaline phosphatase, amylase, aspartate aminotransferase, bilirubin:* increased levels
Albumin, hemoglobin, uric acid: decreased levels
Urine uric acid: decreased level
Drug-herb. *Astragalus, echinacea, melatonin:* interference with immunosuppressant action

Precautions

Use cautiously in:

• chickenpox, herpes zoster, impaired hepatic or renal function, decreased bone marrow reserve

• previous therapy with alkylating agents (cyclophosphamide, chlorambucil, melphalan) for rheumatoid arthritis

• elderly patients

• women of childbearing age.

Patient monitoring

• Monitor complete blood cell count, platelet level, and liver function test results.

• Assess for signs and symptoms of hepatotoxicity (clay-colored stools, pruritus, jaundice, and dark urine).

• Watch for signs and symptoms of infection.

• Monitor for bleeding tendency and hemorrhage.

Patient teaching

• Teach patient that drug lowers resistance to infection. Instruct him to report fever, cough, breathing problems, chills, and other symptoms immediately.

• Instruct patient to report unusual bleeding or bruising.

• Caution patient to avoid activities that may cause injury. Tell him to use soft toothbrush and electric razor to avoid gum and skin injury.

◀€ Teach patient importance of avoiding pregnancy during therapy and for 4 months afterward.

• Tell patient that drug effects may not be obvious for up to 8 weeks in immunosuppression and up to 12 weeks for rheumatoid arthritis relief.

• Advise patient to minimize GI upset by eating small, frequent servings of foods and drinking plenty of fluids.

• Notify patient that he'll undergo regular blood testing during therapy.

azithromycin, azithromycin dihydrate

Zithromax, Zithromax Tri-Pak, Zithromax Z-Pak

Pharmacologic class: Macrolide
Therapeutic class: Anti-infective
Pregnancy risk category B

Action

Bactericidal and bacteriostatic; inhibits protein synthesis after binding with 50S ribosomal subunit of susceptible organisms. Demonstrates cross-resistance to erythromycin-resistant gram-positive strains and resistance to most strains of *Enterococcus faecalis* and methicillin-resistant *Staphylococcus aureus.*

Availability

Capsules: 250 mg, 500 mg
Oral suspension: 100 mg/5 ml in 15-ml bottles; 200 mg/5 ml in 15-ml, 22.5-ml, and 30-ml bottles
Powder for injection: 500 mg in 10-ml vials
Powder for oral suspension: 100 mg/ 5 ml, 200 mg/5 ml, 1,000 mg/packet
Tablets: 250 mg, 500 mg, 600 mg
Tablets (Tri-Pak): three 500-mg tablets
Tablets (Z-Pak): six 250-mg tablets

🕭 Indications and dosages

➤ Mild community-acquired pneumonia, uncomplicated skin and skin-structure infections
Adults: 500 mg P.O. on first day, then 250 mg/day for next 4 days, to a total dosage of 1.5 g
Children ages 6 months and older: 10 mg/kg P.O. (no more than 500 mg/dose) on first day, then 5 mg/kg (no more than 250 mg/dose) for 4 more days

---

➤ Community-acquired pneumonia caused by *Chlamydia pneumoniae, Haemophilus influenzae, Mycoplasma pneumoniae, Streptococcus pneumoniae, Legionella pneumophila, Moraxella catarrhalis,* and *S. aureus*

Adults and adolescents ages 16 and older: 500 mg I.V. daily for at least two doses, then 500 mg P.O. daily for a total of 7 to 10 days

Children ages 6 months to 16 years: 10 mg/kg P.O. as a single dose on first day, then 5 mg/kg P.O. on second through fifth days

➤ Pharyngitis and tonsillitis

Adults: 500 mg P.O. on first day, then 250 mg/day for next 4 days, to a total dosage of 1.5 g

Children ages 2 and older: 12 mg/kg P.O. daily for 5 days; maximum dosage is 500 mg.

➤ Mild to moderate acute exacerbation of chronic obstructive pulmonary disease

Adults: 500 mg P.O. on first day, then 250 mg P.O. daily on second through fifth days

➤ Pelvic inflammatory disease caused by *Chlamydia trachomatis, Neisseria gonorrhoeae,* or *Mycoplasma hominis*

Adults: 500 mg I.V. daily on first and second days, then 250 mg P.O. daily for a total of 7 days. If anaerobes are suspected, give continually with appropriate anti-anaerobic antibiotic, as ordered.

➤ Prevention of bacterial endocarditis in patients allergic to penicillin who are undergoing dental procedures

Adults: 500 mg P.O. 1 hour before procedure

Children: 15 mg/kg P.O. 1 hour before procedure

➤ Nongonococcal urethritis or cervicitis caused by *C. trachomatis,* genital ulcers caused by *Haemophilus ducreyi* (chancroid)

Adults: 1 g P.O. as a single dose

➤ Urethritis and cervicitis caused by *N. gonorrhoeae*

Adults: 2 g P.O. as a single dose

➤ To prevent disseminated *Mycobacterium avium* complex disease in patients with advanced human immunodeficiency virus (HIV)

Adults: 1.2 g P.O. once weekly (given alone or with rifabutin)

➤ Acute otitis media

Children ages 6 months and older: 30 mg/kg as a single dose or 10 mg/kg once daily for 3 days; or 10 mg/kg as a single dose on first day, followed by 5 mg/kg on second through fifth days

Off-label uses

• Uncomplicated gonococcal infections of cervix, urethra, rectum, and pharynx

Contraindications

• Hypersensitivity to drug, erythromycin, or other macrolide anti-infectives

Administration

• Obtain specimen for culture and sensitivity testing before starting therapy.

• Administer tablets and single-dose packets with or without food.

• Give oral suspension 1 hour before meals or 2 hours afterward; with 1-g packet, mix entire contents in 2 oz of water.

◀€ Don't administer as I.V. bolus or I.M. injection.

• For I.V. use, reconstitute 500-mg vial with 4.8 ml of sterile water for injection.

• As appropriate, dilute solution further using normal or half-normal saline solution, dextrose 5% in water, or lactated Ringer's solution.

• Infuse injection over no less than 60 minutes. Infuse 1 mg/ml over 3 hours or 2 mg/2 ml over 1 hour.

• Know that 1,000-mg packet isn't for pediatric use.

Route	Onset	Peak	Duration
P.O.	Rapid	2.5-3.2 hr	24 hr
I.V.	Rapid	End of infusion	24 hr

Adverse reactions

CNS: dizziness, drowsiness, fatigue, headache, vertigo
CV: chest pain, palpitations
GI: nausea, diarrhea, abdominal pain, cholestatic jaundice, dyspepsia, flatulence, melena, **pseudomembranous colitis**
GU: nephritis, vaginitis, candidiasis
Metabolic: hyperglycemia, hyperkalemia
Skin: photosensitivity, rashes, **angioedema**

Interactions

Drug-drug. *Antacids containing aluminum or magnesium:* decreased azithromycin peak blood level
Carbamazepine, cyclosporine, digoxin, dihydroergotamine, ergotamine, hexobarbital, phenytoin, theophylline, triazolam: increased blood levels of these drugs
Pimozide: prolonged QT interval, ventricular tachycardia
Warfarin: increased International Normalized Ratio
Drug-food. *Any food:* decreased absorption of multidose oral suspension
Drug-behaviors. *Sun exposure:* photosensitivity

Precautions

Use cautiously in:
• severe hepatic impairment, severe renal insufficiency, prolonged QT interval
• breastfeeding patients.

Patient monitoring

• Monitor temperature, white blood cell count, and culture and sensitivity results.

• Assess for signs and symptoms of infection.

Patient teaching

• Tell patient he may take tablets with or without food.
• Advise patient to take suspension 1 hour before or 2 hours after meals.
• Remind patient to complete entire course of therapy as ordered, even after symptoms improve

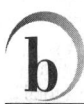

baclofen
Co Baclofen, Lioresal, Lioresal Intrathecal, Liotec✤, Nu-Baclo✤

Pharmacologic class: Skeletal muscle relaxant
Therapeutic class: Antispasmodic
Pregnancy risk category C

Action

Relaxes muscles by acting specifically at spinal end of upper motor neurons

Availability

Intrathecal injection: 10 mg/20 ml (500 mcg/ml), 10 mg/5 ml (2,000 mcg/ml)
Tablets: 10 mg, 20 mg

⚠ Indications and dosages

➤ Reversible spasticity associated with multiple sclerosis or spinal cord lesions
Adults: Initially, 5 mg P.O. t.i.d. May increase by 5 mg q 3 days to a maximum dosage of 80 mg/day.
Children ages 4 and older: 25 to 1,200 mcg/day by intrathecal infusion; (average is 275 mcg/day); dosage deter-

mined by response during screening phase.

➤ Severe spasticity in patients who don't respond to or can't tolerate oral baclofen

Adults: *Screening phase*—Before pump implantation and intrathecal infusion, give test dose to check responsiveness. Administer 1 ml of 50 mcg/ml dilution over 1 minute by barbotage into intrathecal space. Within 4 to 8 hours, muscle spasms should become less severe or frequent and muscle tone should decrease; if patient's response is inadequate, give second test dose of 75 mcg/1.5 ml 24 hours after first dose. If patient is still unresponsive, may give final test dose of 100 mcg/2 ml 24 hours later. Patients unresponsive to 100-mcg dose shouldn't be considered candidates for intrathecal baclofen. Following appropriate responsiveness, adjust dose to twice the screening dose and give over 24 hours. If screening dose efficacy was maintained for 12 hours, don't double the dose. After 24 hours, increase dose slowly as needed and tolerated by 10% to 30% daily. *Maintenance therapy*—During prolonged maintenance therapy, adjust daily dosage by 10% to 40% as needed and tolerated to maintain adequate control of symptoms. Maintenance dosage ranges from 12 mcg to 2,000 mcg daily.

Dosage adjustment
• Renal impairment
• Seizure disorders
• Elderly patients

Off-label uses
• Cerebral palsy
• Tardive dyskinesia
• Trigeminal neuralgia

Contraindications
• Hypersensitivity to drug
• Rheumatic disorders

Administration
• Give oral dose of drug with food or milk.
• Dilute only with sterile, preservative-free sodium chloride for injection.
• Intrathecal infusion should be performed only by those trained in the procedure.

Route	Onset	Peak	Duration
P.O.	Unknown	2-3 hr	Unknown
Intrathecal	0.5-1 hr	4 hr	4-8 hr

Adverse reactions
CNS: dizziness, drowsiness, fatigue, confusion, depression, headache, insomnia, hypotonia, difficulty speaking, **seizures**
CV: edema, hypotension, hypertension, palpitations
EENT: blurred vision, tinnitus, nasal congestion
GI: nausea, vomiting, constipation
GU: urinary frequency, dysuria, impotence
Hepatic: elevated aspartate aminotransferase (AST) and alkaline phosphatase
Metabolic: hyperglycemia
Skin: pruritus, rash, sweating
Other: weight gain, **hypersensitivity reactions**

Interactions
Drug-drug. *CNS depressants:* increased baclofen effect
MAO inhibitors: increased CNS depression, hypotension
Tricyclic antidepressants: hypotonia
Drug-diagnostic tests. *Alkaline phosphatase, AST, glucose:* increased levels
Drug-behaviors. *Alcohol use:* CNS depression

Precautions
Use cautiously in:
• epilepsy
• patients who use spasticity to maintain posture and balance

- elderly patients
- pregnant or breastfeeding patients
- children.

Patient monitoring
- During intrathecal infusion, check pump often for proper functioning and check catheter for patency.
- Monitor patient's response continually to determine appropriate dosage adjustment.
- ◀﹦ Observe closely for signs and symptoms of overdose (drowsiness, light-headedness, dizziness, respiratory depression), especially during initial screening and titration. No specific antidote exists. Immediately remove any solution from pump; if patient has respiratory depression, intubate until drug is eliminated.

Patient teaching
- Advise patient to take oral dose with food or milk.
- Instruct patient to avoid driving and other hazardous activities until he knows how drug affects concentration and alertness.
- Caution patient not to discontinue drug therapy abruptly; doing so may cause hallucinations and rebound spasticity.

balsalazide disodium
Colozal

Pharmacologic class: GI agent
Therapeutic class: Anti-inflammatory
Pregnancy risk category B

Action
Converts to mesalamine in colon and then to 5-aminosalicyclic acid. May decrease inflammation of colonic mucosa by inhibiting production of arachidonic acid metabolites.

Availability
Capsules: 750 mg

⏺ Indications and dosages
➣ Mild to moderate active ulcerative colitis
Adults: 2.25 g (three 750-mg capsules) P.O. t.i.d. for 8 to 12 weeks.

Contraindications
- Hypersensitivity to balsalazide, salicylates, or mesalamine

Administration
- Advise patient to swallow capsules whole, either always with or always without food.

Route	Onset	Peak	Duration
P.O.	Unknown	1-2 hr	Unknown

Adverse reactions
CNS: headache, insomnia, dizziness, anxiety, confusion, agitation, **coma**
EENT: blurred vision, eye irritation, tinnitus, earache, epistaxis, sinusitis, sore throat, nasopharyngitis
GI: nausea, vomiting, diarrhea, constipation, abdominal pain, dyspepsia, anorexia, oral blisters, oral candidiasis, **GI hemorrhage**
GU: urinary tract infection
Musculoskeletal: arthralgia; myalgia; bone, back, neck, or limb pain
Respiratory: cough, upper respiratory tract infection
Skin: erythema
Other: generalized pain

Interactions
Drug-drug. *Oral antibiotics:* interference with balsalazide action

Precautions
Use cautiously in:
- pyloric stenosis
- breastfeeding patients
- children.

Patient monitoring
• Monitor patient for signs and symptoms of hepatotoxicity, such as prolonged abdominal pain and yellow sclera or skin.
• Assess character and frequency of stools.
• Monitor complete blood cell count and liver and kidney function test results.

Patient teaching
• Instruct patient to take drug only as directed.

basiliximab
Simulect

Pharmacologic class: Monoclonal antibody

Therapeutic class: Immunosuppressant

Pregnancy risk category B

Action
Blocks specific interleukin-2 (IL-2) receptor sites on activated T lymphocytes. Specific binding competitively inhibits IL-2–mediated activation and differentiation of lymphocytes responsible for cell-mediated immunity; also impairs immunologic response to antigenic challenges.

Availability
Powder for injection: 10 mg and 20 mg in single-use vials

Indications and dosages
➤ Prevention of acute organ rejection in kidney transplantation
Adults and children weighing 35 kg (77 lb) or more: 20 mg I.V. 2 hours before transplantation surgery; then 20 mg I.V. 4 days after surgery. Withhold second dose if complications,

hypersensitivity reaction, or graft loss occurs.
Children weighing less than 35 kg (77 lb): 10 mg I.V. 2 hours before transplantation surgery; then 10 mg I.V. 4 days after surgery. Withhold second dose if complications, hypersensitivity reaction, or graft loss occurs.

Contraindications
• Hypersensitivity to drug
• Pregnancy or breastfeeding

Administration
◀€ Give by central or peripheral I.V. route only.
• Reconstitute by adding 5 ml of sterile water for injection to vial for bolus injection, or dilute with normal saline solution or dextrose 5% in water to a volume of 50 ml and infuse over 20 to 30 minutes. Use reconstituted vial within 4 hours of preparation (vial contains no preservatives).
• Don't infuse other drugs simultaneously through same I.V. line.
• Know that drug should be used only as part of regimen that includes cyclosporine and corticosteroids.

Route	Onset	Peak	Duration
I.V.	2 hr	Unknown	36 days

Adverse reactions
CNS: headache, insomnia, paresthesia, dizziness, drowsiness, tremor, anxiety, confusion, **coma, seizures**
CV: palpitations, edema, chest pain, electrocardiogram abnormalities, hypotension, hypertension, **prolonged QT interval**
EENT: blurred vision, eye irritation, tinnitus, earache, epistaxis, nasopharyngitis, sinusitis
GI: nausea, vomiting, diarrhea, constipation, abdominal pain, dyspepsia, anorexia, oral blisters, oral candidiasis, **GI hemorrhage**

GU: urinary incontinence, oliguria, intermenstrual bleeding, **renal failure**
Hematologic: anemia, **disseminated intravascular coagulation, hemorrhage, neutropenia, thrombocytopenia**
Metabolic: hypokalemia, hypomagnesemia, hyperglycemia, acidosis, hypoglycemia, hyperkalemia
Musculoskeletal: bone, back, neck, or limb pain
Respiratory: dyspnea, cough, hypoxia, tachypnea, hemoptysis, upper respiratory tract infection, **pleural effusions**
Skin: ecchymosis, pruritus, dermatitis, skin lesions, diaphoresis, night sweats, erythema, hyperpigmentation, urticaria
Other: fever, lymphadenopathy, facial edema, bacterial infection, herpes simplex infection, injection site erythema, **hypersensitivity reaction, sepsis**

Interactions

Drug-drug. *Immunosuppressants:* additive immunosuppression
Drug-diagnostic tests. *ALT, AST, magnesium, calcium, white blood cells:* increased levels
Glucose, potassium: increased or decreased levels
Hemoglobin, neutrophils, platelets: decreased values
Drug-herb. *Astragalus, echinacea, melatonin:* interference with immunosuppressant action

Precautions

Use cautiously in:
• elderly patients
• females of childbearing age.

Patient monitoring

◀≝ Watch for signs and symptoms of hypersensitivity reaction; keep emergency drugs at hand in case these occur.
• Monitor vital signs and observe patient frequently during I.V. infusion.

• Monitor laboratory values and drug blood levels.

Patient teaching

• Teach patient about purpose of therapy. Explain that drug decreases the risk of acute organ rejection.
• Tell patient he may be more susceptible to infection because of drug's immunosuppressant effect.
• Inform patient that he will need lifelong immunosuppressive drug therapy.
• Advise women of childbearing age to use reliable contraception before, during, and for 2 months after therapy.
• As appropriate, review all other significant and life-threatening adverse reactions and interactions, especially those related to the drugs, tests, and herbs mentioned above.

beclomethasone dipropionate
Beclodisk✤, Becloforte✤, Beconase AQ Nasal Spray, QVAR

Pharmacologic class: Corticosteroid
Therapeutic class: Anti-inflammatory
Pregnancy risk category C

Action

Unclear; may decrease inflammation by stabilizing leukocyte lysosomal membrane, decreasing number and activity of inflammatory cells, inhibiting bronchoconstriction (leading to direct smooth muscle relaxation), and reducing airway hyperresponsiveness.

Availability

Inhalation aerosol: 40-mcg metered inhalation in 7.3-g canister; 80-mcg metered inhalation in 7.3-g canister
Inhalation capsules: 100 mcg, 200 mcg
Nasal spray: 0.042% (25-g bottle containing 180 metered inhalations)

⚡ Indications and dosages

➤ Maintenance treatment of asthma as prophylaxis; asthma patients who require systemic steroids for whom adding an inhaled steroid may reduce or eliminate the need for systemic steroids

Adults and children ages 12 and older: When previous therapy was bronchodilator alone, 40 to 80 mcg by oral inhalation (QVAR) b.i.d.; maximum of 320 mcg b.i.d. When previous therapy was inhaled steroid, 40 to 160 mcg by oral inhalation (QVAR) b.i.d.; maximum of 320 mcg b.i.d.

➤ Seasonal or perennial rhinitis

Adults and children ages 12 and older: One or two inhalations (42 to 84 mcg Beconase AQ Nasal Spray) in each nostril b.i.d.

Children ages 6 to 12: One inhalation (42 mcg Beconase AQ Nasal Spray) in each nostril b.i.d.

Contraindications

• Hypersensitivity to drug
• Status asthmaticus

Administration

• Use spacer device to ensure proper delivery of dose and to help prevent candidiasis and hoarseness.
• After inhalation, tell patient to hold his breath for a few seconds before exhaling.
• For greater effectiveness, wait 1 minute between inhalations.
• If patient is also receiving a bronchodilator, administer it at least 15 minutes before beclomethasone.
• Discontinue drug after 3 weeks if symptoms don't improve markedly.

Route	Onset	Peak	Duration
Inhalation (nasal)	5-7 days	3 wk	Unknown
Inhalation (oral)	1-4 wk	Unknown	Unknown

Adverse reactions

CNS: headache
EENT: cataracts; nasal irritation, congestion; epistaxis; perforated nasal septum; anosmia; nasopharyngeal or oropharyngeal fungal infections; hoarseness; throat irritation
GI: esophageal candidiasis
Metabolic: adrenal suppression
Respiratory: cough, wheezing, **bronchospasm**
Skin: urticaria, **angioedema**
Other: Churg-Strauss syndrome, **hypersensitivity reactions**

Interactions

None significant

Precautions

Use cautiously in:
• active untreated infections, diabetes mellitus, glaucoma, underlying immunosuppression
• patients receiving concurrent systemic corticosteroids
• pregnant or breastfeeding patients
• children younger than age 6.

Patient monitoring

• Assess patient's mouth daily for signs of fungal infection.
• Observe patient for proper inhaler use.

Patient teaching

• Instruct patient to hold inhaled drug in airway for several seconds before exhaling and to wait 1 minute between inhalations.
• Advise patient to rinse mouth after using inhaler and to wash and dry inhaler thoroughly to help prevent fungal infections and sore throat.

• Encourage patient to document use of drug and his response in a diary.
• If patient is also using a bronchodilator, teach him to use it at least 15 minutes before beclomethasone.

benazepril hydrochloride
Lotensin

Pharmacologic class: Angiotensin-converting enzyme (ACE) inhibitor
Therapeutic class: Antihypertensive
Pregnancy risk category C (first trimester), *D* (second and third trimesters)

Action

Inhibits conversion of angiotensin I to angiotensin II, vasoconstrictor that stimulates the adrenals and promotes aldosterone secretion, reducing sodium and water reabsorption, ultimately decreasing blood pressure. Decreased angiotensin also causes an increase in potassium levels and fluid loss.

Availability

Tablets: 5 mg, 10 mg, 20 mg, 40 mg

✔ Indications and dosages

➤ Hypertension (used alone or in conjunction with other drugs)
Adults: Initially, 5 to 10 mg/day P.O. as a single dose; increase gradually to a maintenance dosage of 20 to 40 mg/day as a single dose or in two divided doses (start with 5 mg/day in patients receiving diuretics)
Dosage adjustment
• Renal impairment

Off-label uses

• Myocardial infarction
• Nephropathy

Contraindications

• Hypersensitivity to drug

• Angioedema (hereditary or idiopathic)
• Pregnancy (particularly in second and third trimesters)

Administration

◀€ Use extreme caution if patient has family history of angioedema.
• When giving concurrently with diuretics, know that drug may cause excessive hypotension. If possible, stop diuretic therapy 2 to 3 days before starting benazepril.
• Give with or without food.

Route	Onset	Peak	Duration
P.O.	0.5-1 hr	3-4 hr	24 hr

Adverse reactions

CNS: dizziness, drowsiness, fatigue, syncope, light-headedness headache, insomnia
CV: angina pectoris, tachycardia, **hypotension**
EENT: sinusitis
GI: diarrhea, nausea, altered taste, anorexia
GU: proteinuria, impotence, decreased libido, renal failure
Hematologic: agranulocytosis
Metabolic: hyperkalemia
Respiratory: cough, dyspnea, eosinophilic pneumonitis, asthma, bronchitis
Skin: rash, **angioedema**
Other: fever

Interactions

Drug-drug. *Allopurinol:* increased risk of hypersensitivity reaction
Antacids: decreased benazepril absorption
Antihypertensives, diuretics, general anesthetics, nitrates, phenothiazines: excessive hypotension
Cyclosporine, indomethacin, potassium-sparing diuretics, potassium supplements: hyperkalemia

---

Digoxin, lithium: increased lithium blood level, greater risk of lithium toxicity

Nonsteroidal anti-inflammatory drugs: blunting of antihypertensive response

Drug-diagnostic tests. *Alanine aminotransferase, alkaline phosphatase, aspartate aminotransferase, bilirubin, blood urea nitrogen, creatinine, potassium:* increased levels

Antinuclear antibodies: positive result
Sodium: decreased level

Drug-food. *Salt substitutes containing potassium:* hyperkalemia

Drug-herb. *Capsaicin:* cough

Drug-behaviors. *Acute alcohol ingestion:* increased hypotension

Precautions

Use cautiously in:
• renal or hepatic impairment, hypovolemia, hyponatremia, aortic stenosis, hypertrophic cardiomyopathy, cerebrovascular or cardiac insufficiency
• patients receiving concurrent diuretics
• black patients
• elderly patients
• breastfeeding patients
• children.

Patient monitoring

◀᠄ Monitor for signs and symptoms of angioedema, including laryngeal edema and shock.
• Measure blood pressure regularly.
• Monitor complete blood count, electrolyte levels, kidney and liver function test results, and urinary protein level.

Patient teaching

• Instruct patient to record blood pressure at various intervals daily.
• Tell patient to report dizziness, fainting, or light-headedness during initial therapy.
• Advise patient to increase fluid intake during exercise and in hot weather.
• Tell patient to avoid salt substitutes, which may cause hyperkalemia.

benztropine mesylate   b
Apo-Benztropine✤, Bensylate, Cogentin, PMS Benztropine✤

Pharmacologic class: Anticholinergic
Therapeutic class: Antiparkinsonian
Pregnancy risk category C

Action
Blocks cholinergic activity (partially responsible for Parkinson symptoms) in CNS; restores natural balance of neurotransmitters in CNS

Availability
Injection: 1 mg/ml in 2-ml ampules
Tablets: 0.5 mg, 1 mg, 2 mg

🏷 Indications and dosages
➤ Parkinsonism
Adults: Initially, 1 to 2 mg/day P.O. or I.M. at bedtime or in two or four divided doses; dosage range is 0.5 to 6 mg/day.
➤ Acute dystonic reactions
Adults: Initially, 1 to 2 mg I.M. or I.V., then 1 to 2 mg P.O. b.i.d.
➤ Drug-induced extrapyramidal reactions (except tardive dyskinesia)
Adults: 1 to 4 mg P.O. or I.M. once or twice daily.
Dosage adjustment
• Elderly patients

Off-label uses
• Excessive salivation

Contraindications
• Hypersensitivity to drug
• Narrow-angle glaucoma
• Tardive dyskinesia
• Children younger than age 3

Administration
- Know that I.V. route is seldom used.
- Crush tablets if patient has difficulty swallowing.
- Give after meals to prevent GI upset.
- Be aware that entire dose may be given at bedtime (drug has long duration of action).

Route	Onset	Peak	Duration
P.O.	1-2 hr	Unknown	24 hr
I.M., I.V.	15 min	Unknown	24 hr

Adverse reactions
CNS: confusion, depression, dizziness, hallucinations, headache, weakness, toxic psychosis, memory impairment, nervousness, delusions, euphoria, paresthesia, sensation of heaviness in limbs
CV: hypotension, palpitations, tachycardia, **arrhythmias**
EENT: blurred vision, diplopia, mydriasis, closed-angle glaucoma
GI: nausea, constipation, dry mouth, **ileus**
GU: urinary hesitancy or retention, dysuria, difficulty maintaining erection
Musculoskeletal: paratonia, muscle weakness and cramps
Skin: rash, urticaria, decreased sweating, dermatoses

Interactions
Drug-drug. *Antacids, antidiarrheals:* decreased benztropine absorption
Antihistamines, bethanechol, disopyramide, phenothiazines, quinidine, tricyclic antidepressants: additive anticholinergic effects
Drug-herb. *Angel's trumpet, jimsonweed, scopolia:* increased anticholinergic effects
Drug-behaviors. *Alcohol use:* increased sedation

Precautions
Use cautiously in:
- seizure disorders, arrhythmias, tachycardia, hypertension, hypotension, hepatic or renal dysfunction, alcoholism
- elderly patients
- pregnant or breastfeeding patients.

Patient monitoring
- Monitor blood pressure closely, especially in elderly patients.
- Monitor fluid intake and output; check for urinary retention.
- Assess for signs and symptoms of ileus, including constipation and abdominal distention.

Patient teaching
- Advise patient to use caution during activities that require physical or mental alertness, because drug causes sedation.
- Tell patient to avoid increased heat exposure.
- Caution patient against stopping therapy abruptly.

betamethasone
Betnelan✿, Celestone

betamethasone acetate and sodium phosphate
Celestone Soluspan

betamethasone sodium phosphate
Betnesol✿, Celestone Phosphate, Cel-U-Jec, Selestoject

Pharmacologic class: Glucocorticoid (inhalation)
Therapeutic class: Antiasthmatic, anti-inflammatory (steroidal)
Pregnancy risk category C

Action
Stabilizes lysosomal neutrophils and prevents their degranulation, inhibits synthesis of lipoxygenase products and

---

prostaglandins, activates anti-inflammatory genes, and inhibits various cytokines

Availability

Solution for injection: 4 mg/ml of betamethasone sodium phosphate; 3 mg betamethasone sodium phosphate with 3 mg betamethasone acetate/ml
Suspension for injection (acetate, phosphate): 6 mg (total)/ml
Syrup: 0.6 mg/5 ml
Tablets: 0.6 mg
Tablets (effervescent): 0.5 mg
Tablets (extended-release): 1 mg

Indications and dosages

➤ Inflammatory, allergic, hematologic, neoplastic, autoimmune, and respiratory diseases; prevention of organ rejection in patients who've undergone transplantation surgery (given with other immunosuppressants)
Adults: 0.6 to 7.2 mg/day P.O. as a single daily dose or in divided doses; or up to 9 mg I.M. or I.V. of betamethasone sodium phosphate; or 0.5 to 9 mg I.M. of betamethasone sodium phosphate and betamethasone acetate suspension. Typical suspension dosage ranges from one-third to one-half of oral dosage given q 12 hours.
➤ Bursitis or tenosynovitis
Adults: 1 ml of suspension intrabursally
➤ Rheumatoid arthritis or osteoarthritis
Adults: 0.5 to 2 ml of suspension intraarticularly

Off-label uses

• Respiratory distress syndrome

Contraindications

• Hypersensitivity to drug
• Breastfeeding

Administration

• Give as a single daily dose before 9:00 A.M.

• Give oral dose with food or milk.
• Administer I.M. injections deep into gluteal muscle to avoid tissue atrophy.
• Don't give betamethasone acetate I.V.
◀€ To avoid adrenal insufficiency, taper dosage slowly and under close supervision when discontinuing.

Route	Onset	Peak	Duration
P.O.	Unknown	1-2 hr	3-25 days
I.M, I.V. (phosphate)	Rapid	Unknown	Unknown
I.M. (acetate/ phosphate)	1-3 hr	Unknown	1 wk

Adverse reactions

CNS: headache, nervousness, depression, euphoria, psychoses, **increased intracranial pressure**
CV: hypotension, thrombophlebitis, thromboembolism
EENT: cataracts; burning, dryness, and congestion; rebound nasal congestion; sneezing; epistaxis; nasal septum perforation; anosmia; difficulty speaking; oropharyngeal or nasopharyngeal fungal infections
GI: nausea, vomiting, anorexia, dry mouth, esophageal candidiasis, bad taste, peptic ulcers
Metabolic: adrenal insufficiency or suppression, decreased growth, hyperglycemia, cushingoid appearance
Musculoskeletal: muscle wasting, muscle pain, osteoporosis, aseptic joint necrosis
Respiratory: cough, wheezing, **bronchospasm**
Skin: facial edema, rash, contact dermatitis, acne, ecchymosis, hirsutism, petechiae, urticaria, **angioedema**
Other: weight gain or loss, Churg-Strauss syndrome, increased susceptibility to infection, **hypersensitivity reaction**

Interactions

Drug-drug. *Amphotericin B, loop and thiazide diuretics, ticarcillin:* additive hypokalemia

---

Barbiturates, phenytoin, rifampin: stimulation of betamethasone metabolism, causing decreased effects

Digoxin: increased risk of digoxin toxicity

Fluoroquinolones (such as ciprofloxacin, norfloxacin): increased risk of tendon rupture

Hormonal contraceptives: blocking of betamethasone metabolism

Insulin, oral hypoglycemics: increased betamethasone requirement

Live-virus vaccines: decreased antibody response, increased risk of neurologic complications

Nonsteroidal anti-inflammatory drugs: increased risk of adverse GI effects

Drug-diagnostic tests. *Calcium, cholesterol, glucose, potassium:* increased levels

Nitroblue-tetrazolium test for bacterial infection: false-negative result

Drug-herb. *Echinacea:* increased immune-stimulating effects

Ginseng: increased immune-modulating effects

Drug-behaviors. *Alcohol use:* increased risk of gastric irritation and GI ulcers

Precautions

Use cautiously in:
• systemic infections, hypertension, osteoporosis, diabetes mellitus, glaucoma, renal disease, hypothyroidism, cirrhosis, diverticulitis, thromboembolic disorders, seizures, myasthenia gravis, heart failure, ocular herpes simplex, emotional instability
• patients receiving systemic corticosteroids
• pregnant or breastfeeding patients
• children younger than age 6.

Patient monitoring

• Monitor weight daily and report sudden increase, which suggests fluid retention.
• Monitor blood glucose level for hyperglycemia.

• Assess serum electrolyte levels for sodium and potassium imbalances.
• Watch for signs and symptoms of infection (drug may mask these).

Patient teaching

• Advise patient to report signs and symptoms of infection.
• Tell patient to report visual disturbances (long-term drug use may cause cataracts).
• Instruct patient to eat low-sodium, high potassium diet.
• Advise patient to carry medical identification describing drug therapy.
• Inform female patients that drug may cause menstrual irregularities.
• Caution patient not to stop taking drug abruptly.

bethanechol chloride
Duvoid, Myotonachol, PMS-Bethanecol Chloride✸, Urabeth, Urecholine

Pharmacologic class: Cholinergic
Therapeutic class: Urinary and GI tract stimulant
Pregnancy risk category C

Action

Stimulates parasympathetic nervous system and cholinergic receptors, leading to increased muscle tone in bladder (causing contraction) and increased frequency of ureteral peristaltic waves. Also stimulates gastric motility, increases gastric tone, and restores rhythmic GI peristalsis.

Availability

Injection: 5 mg/ml
Tablets: 5 mg, 10 mg, 25 mg, 50 mg

🖊 Indications and dosages

➤ Postpartal and postoperative nonobstructive urinary retention or urinary retention caused by neurogenic bladder

Adults: 10 to 50 mg P.O. three to four times daily. Dosage may be determined by giving 5 or 10 mg hourly until response occurs or a total of 50 mg has been given. Alternatively, 5 mg S.C. three to four times daily. Dosage may be determined by giving 2.5 mg S.C. q 15 to 30 minutes until a response occurs or a total of four doses has been given.

Contraindications

• Hypersensitivity to drug
• Mechanical obstruction of GI or GU tract
• Hyperthyroidism
• Latent or active asthma
• Bradycardia
• Hypotension
• Hypertension
• Atrioventricular conduction defects
• Coronary artery disease
• Vasomotor instability
• Seizure disorders
• Parkinsonism
• Peptic ulcer disease

Administration

• Give on empty stomach to help prevent nausea and vomiting.
• Don't give I.M or I.V. because doing so may cause severe symptoms of cholinergic overstimulation.
• Keep atropine on hand to counteract severe adverse effects.

Route	Onset	Peak	Duration
P.O.	30-90 min	1 hr	6 hr
S.C.	5-15 min	15-30 min	2 hr

Adverse reactions

CNS: headache, malaise
CV: bradycardia, hypotension, **heart block, syncope with cardiac arrest**
EENT: excessive lacrimation, miosis
GI: nausea, vomiting, diarrhea, abdominal discomfort, belching
GU: urinary urgency
Respiratory: increased bronchial secretions, **bronchospasm**
Skin: diaphoresis, flushing
Other: hypothermia

Interactions

Drug-drug. *Anticholinergics:* decreased bethanechol effectiveness
Cholinesterase inhibitors: additive cholinergic effects
Depolarizing neuromuscular blockers: decreased blood pressure
Ganglionic blockers: severe hypotension
Procainamide, quinidine: antagonism of cholinergic effects
Drug-diagnostic tests. *Amylase, hepatic enzymes, lipase:* increased levels
Drug-herb. *Angel's trumpet, jimsonweed, scopolia:* antagonism of cholinergic effects

Precautions

Use cautiously in:
• sensitivity to cholinergics or their effects
• asthma, ulcer disease, cardiovascular disease, seizure disorders, hyperthyroidism
• pregnant or breastfeeding patients
• children.

Patient monitoring

• Monitor blood pressure; hypertensive patients may experience sudden blood pressure drop.
• Monitor vital signs and respirations for 30 to 60 minutes after S.C. injection.
• Stay alert for orthostatic hypotension, a common adverse effect.

Patient teaching
• Tell patient that drug usually is effective within 90 minutes of administration.
• Teach patient to take oral dose on an empty stomach to avoid GI upset.
• Instruct patient to move slowly when sitting up or standing to avoid dizziness or light-headedness from blood pressure decrease.

---

bexarotene
Targretin

Pharmacologic class: Retinoid (second-generation)
Therapeutic class: Antineoplastic
Pregnancy risk category X

Action
Inhibits growth of tumor cells by selectively binding to and activating retinoid X-receptor subtypes. These subtypes regulate cell differentiation, apoptosis, and proliferation.

Availability
Capsules: 75 mg
Topical gel: 1%

⚠ Indications and dosages
➤ Cutaneous T-cell lymphoma in patients unable to tolerate other therapies
Adults: 300 mg/m²/day P.O. as a single dose with a meal; if no response occurs after 8 weeks, increase dosage to 400 mg/m²/day.
➤ Refractory cutaneous lesions in patients with early cutaneous T-cell lymphoma
Adults: Wait 20 minutes after bathing and apply 1% topical gel to affected area every other day for first week; then increase at weekly intervals to one daily application, then three daily applications, and then four daily applications.

Dosage adjustment
• Hepatic insufficiency

Contraindications
• Hypersensitivity to drug or retinoids
• Uncontrolled diabetes mellitus
• Biliary tract disease
• Uncontrolled hyperlipidemia
• Excessive alcohol use
• Pregnancy

Administration
• Give with meals.
• Start therapy on third day of normal menstrual period.

Route	Onset	Peak	Duration
P.O.	Unknown	Unknown	Unknown

Adverse reactions
CNS: headache, insomnia, paresthesia, dizziness, drowsiness, tremor, anxiety, confusion, **coma, seizures**
CV: tachycardia, palpitations, edema, chest pain, electrocardiogram abnormalities, hypotension, hypertension, **prolonged QT interval**
EENT: blurred vision, eye irritation, earache, tinnitus, epistaxis, nasopharyngitis, sinusitis, sore throat
GI: nausea, vomiting, diarrhea, constipation, abdominal pain, dyspepsia, anorexia, oral candidiasis, **GI hemorrhage**
GU: renal impairment, urinary incontinence, oliguria, intermenstrual bleeding, **renal failure**
Hematologic: leukopenia, anemia, lymphadenopathy, **disseminated intravascular coagulation, hemorrhage, neutropenia, thrombocytopenia**
Metabolic: hypokalemia, hypomagnesemia, hyperglycemia, acidosis, hypoglycemia, **hyperkalemia**
Musculoskeletal: bone, back, neck, or limb pain
Respiratory: dyspnea, cough, hypoxia, wheezing, crackles, tachypnea, decreased breath sounds, crepitation,

---

hemoptysis, rhonchi, upper respiratory tract infection, **pleural effusion**
Skin: ecchymosis, dermatitis, diaphoresis, night sweats, erythema, petechiae, hyperpigmentation, urticaria, skin lesions, herpes simplex infection, local exfoliation
Other: weight gain or loss, fever, facial edema, injection site edema, bacterial infection, **hypersensitivity reaction, sepsis**

Interactions
Drug-drug. *CYP450-3A4 inducers (such as phenobarbital, phenytoin, rifampin):* decreased bexarotene blood level
CYP450-3A4 inhibitors (such as erythromycin, gemfibrozil, itraconazole, ketoconazole): increased bexarotene blood level
Insulin, sulfonylureas: enhanced hypoglycemic effect
Products containing diethyltoluamide (DEET): increased DEET toxicity
Vitamin A preparations: increased vitamin A toxicity
Drug-diagnostic tests. *Alanine aminotransferase, amylase, aspartate aminotransferase, bilirubin, cholesterol, creatinine, eosinophils, glucose, lactate dehydrogenase, lipids, platelets:* increased levels
Calcium, hemoglobin, lymphocytes, protein, sodium, white blood cells (WBCs): decreased values
Drug-food. *Any food:* increased drug absorption
Drug-behaviors. *Sun exposure:* increased risk of photosensitivity

Precautions
Use cautiously in:
• renal or hepatic insufficiency
• females of childbearing age.

Patient monitoring
• Monitor blood lipid levels, WBC count with white cell differential, and liver and thyroid function test results

at start of therapy, 2 to 4 weeks after initiation, and then every 8 weeks.

Patient teaching
◀ Advise women of childbearing age to use two reliable contraceptive methods for 1 month before starting therapy, during therapy, and for 1 month after discontinuation.
• Advise patient to limit vitamin A intake to less than 15,000 IU daily.
• Instruct patient to report vision changes.
• Advise male patient to use condoms during sexual intercourse throughout therapy and for 1 month afterward if partner is pregnant or able to become pregnant.
• Instruct patient to minimize exposure to sunlight and wear sunscreen.

bicalutamide
Casodex

Pharmacologic class: Nonsteroidal antiandrogen
Therapeutic class: Antineoplastic
Pregnancy risk category X

Action
Antagonizes effects of androgen at cellular level by binding to androgen receptors on target tissues

Availability
Tablets: 50 mg

Indications and dosages
➤ Metastatic prostate carcinoma
Adults: 50 mg P.O. once daily; must be given with luteinizing hormone-releasing hormone (LHRH) analog

Contraindications
• Hypersensitivity to drug

Administration
• Administer at same time each day.
• Always give in combination with LHRH analog; start both therapies together.

Route	Onset	Peak	Duration
P.O.	Unknown	31 hr	Unknown

Adverse reactions
CNS: headache, weakness, dizziness, depression, hypertonia, paresthesia, lethargy
CV: chest pain, peripheral edema, vasodilation, hypercholesterolemia, hypertension, **thromboembolic disease**
EENT: pharyngitis
GI: nausea, vomiting, diarrhea, constipation, abdominal pain, anorexia, dry mouth, food distaste
GU: urinary tract infection
Musculoskeletal: bone and back pain
Respiratory: dyspnea, cough
Skin: rash, alopecia
Other: weight gain, edema, pain, hot flashes, flulike symptoms

Interactions
Drug-drug. *Warfarin:* increase in bicalutamide effects
Drug-diagnostic tests. *Alanine aminotransferase, alkaline phosphatase, aspartate aminotransferase, bilirubin:* increased levels
Hemoglobin, white blood cells: decreased values

Precautions
Use cautiously in:
• previous hypersensitivity or serious adverse reaction to flutamide or nilutamide
• moderate to severe hepatic impairment
• children.

Patient monitoring
• Monitor prostate-significant antigen levels, complete blood count, and liver and kidney function test results.

• Evaluate prothrombin time and International Normalized Ratio if patient is receiving concurrent warfarin.

Patient teaching
• Teach patient to take drug at same time each day, along with prescribed LHRH analog.
• Tell patient that any drug-related hair loss should reverse once therapy ends.

biperiden
Akineton

Pharmacologic class: Anticholinergic
Therapeutic class: Antiparkinsonian
Pregnancy risk category C

Action
Blocks striatal cholinergic receptors, partially restoring natural balance of neurotransmitters in brain's corpus striatum

Availability
Injection: 5 mg/ml
Tablets: 2 mg

Indications and dosages
➤ Parkinsonism
Adults: Initially, 2 mg P.O. three to four times daily; don't exceed 16 mg/day.
➤ Extrapyramidal reactions
Adults: 2 mg P.O. one to three times daily; or 2 mg I.M. or I.V., repeated as needed q 30 minutes. Don't exceed 8 mg or four doses in 24 hours.

Contraindications
• Hypersensitivity to drug or other anticholinergics
• Narrow-angle glaucoma
• Myasthenia gravis

- GI or GU tract obstruction
- Achalasia
- Paralytic ileus or intestinal atony
- Ulcerative colitis
- Prostatic hypertrophy
- Tardive dyskinesia

Administration

- Give before or after meals, depending on patient's response. If dry mouth occurs, give before meals. When giving with meals, allay thirst with water, mints, or chewing gum.
- For I.V. use, inject drug slowly.
- With parenteral route, patient may experience light-headedness; have him rest in prone position for approximately 20 minutes after injection.

Route	Onset	Peak	Duration
P.O.	1 hr	1-1.5 hr	Unknown
I.V.	Immediate	Unknown	1-8 hr
I.M.	15 min	Unknown	Unknown

Adverse reactions

CNS: confusion, depression, dizziness, hallucinations, headache, sedation, weakness, restlessness, delusions, incoherence, euphoria, tremor, memory loss

CV: hypotension, palpitations, tachycardia, **arrhythmias**

EENT: blurred vision, dry eyes, photophobia, mydriasis, increased intraocular pressure, closed-angle glaucoma, difficulty swallowing

GI: nausea, constipation, abdominal distress, dry mouth, **paralytic ileus**

GU: urinary hesitancy or retention

Skin: rash, urticaria, dermatosis, flushing, decreased sweating

Other: increased body temperature, numbness in fingers, cramping, **heat stroke**

Interactions

Drug-drug. *Antacids, antidiarrheals:* decreased biperiden absorption

Antihistamines, disopyramide, phenothiazines, quinidine, tricyclic antidepressants: additive anticholinergic effects
Bethanechol: antagonistic effects
CNS depressants: increased sedative effect
Haloperidol, phenothiazines: masking of extrapyramidal symptoms, tardive dyskinesia, central anticholinergic syndrome
Drug-herb. *Angel's trumpet, jimsonweed, scopolia:* increased anticholinergic effects
Drug-behaviors. *Alcohol use:* increased CNS depression

Precautions

Use cautiously in:
- enlarged prostate, seizure disorders, arrhythmias, tachycardia, hypotension, hypertension, renal or hepatic dysfunction, chronic illness, alcoholism
- elderly patients
- pregnant or breastfeeding patients.

Patient monitoring

- Monitor vital signs and cardiac status.
- Watch for urinary retention, especially in males.
- Closely monitor patient with pulmonary disease.

Patient teaching

- Advise patient to take drug with food to minimize GI upset.
- Instruct patient to avoid driving and other hazardous activities until he knows how drug affects concentration and alertness.
- Emphasize importance of avoiding alcohol and other CNS depressants.
- Caution patient against heat exposure and exercising in warm weather because drug decreases ability to sweat.
- Instruct patient to have annual eye examinations because drug increases risk of increased intraocular pressure.

bisacodyl

Bisac-Evac, Carter's Little Pills, Correctol, Dacodyl, Deficol, Dulcagen, Dulcolax, Feen-a-Mint, Fleet Laxative, Laxit✤, Reliable Gentle Laxative, Theralax, Women's Gentle Laxative

Pharmacologic class: Stimulant laxative
Therapeutic class: Laxative
Pregnancy risk category B

Action
Unknown; thought to stimulate colonic mucosa, producing parasympathetic reflexes that increase peristalsis and increase water and electrolyte secretion, thereby causing evacuation of the colon

Availability
Enema: 0.33 mg/ml, 10 mg/ml
Powder for rectal solution: 1.5 mg bisacodyl and 2.5 g tannic acid
Suppositories (rectal): 5 mg, 10 mg
Tablets (enteric-coated): 5 mg

🚫 Indications and dosages
➤ Constipation; bowel cleansing for childbirth, surgery, and endoscopic examination
Adults and children ages 12 and older: 5 to 15 mg P.O.; maximum daily dosage is 30 mg/day P.O. or 10 mg P.R.
Children ages 3 to 11: 5 to 10 mg (0.3 mg/kg) P.O. as a single dose or 5 to 10 mg P.R. as a single dose
Children ages 2 and younger: 5 mg P.R. as a single dose

Contraindications
• Hypersensitivity to drug
• Intestinal obstruction
• Gastroenteritis
• Appendicitis

Administration
• Make sure patient swallows tablets whole and doesn't chew them.
• Don't give within 1 hour of dairy products or antacid.
• Know that drug should be used only for short periods.

Route	Onset	Peak	Duration
P.O.	6-12 hr	Variable	Variable
P.R.	15-60 min	Variable	Variable

Adverse reactions
CNS: dizziness, syncope
GI: nausea, vomiting, diarrhea (with high doses), abdominal pain, burning sensation in rectum (with suppositories), laxative dependence, protein-losing enteropathy
Metabolic: alkalosis, hypokalemia, fluid and electrolyte imbalances, tetany
Musculoskeletal: muscle weakness (with excessive use)

Interactions
Drug-drug. *Antacids:* gastric irritation, dyspepsia
Drug-diagnostic tests. *Calcium, magnesium, potassium:* decreased levels
Phosphate, sodium: increased levels
Drug-food. *Dairy products:* gastric irritation

Precautions
Use cautiously in:
• hypersensitivity to tannic acid
• severe cardiovascular disease, anal or rectal fissures
• pregnant or breastfeeding patients.

Patient monitoring
• Assess stools for frequency and consistency.
• Monitor patient for electrolyte imbalances and dehydration.

Patient teaching

• Instruct patient to swallow enteric-coated tablets no sooner than 1 hour before or after ingesting antacids or dairy products. Tell him not to chew tablets.

• Advise patient not to use bisacodyl or other laxatives habitually because this may lead to dependence.

• Suggest other ways to prevent constipation, such as eating more fruits, vegetables, and whole grains to increase dietary bulk and drinking 8 to 10 glasses of water daily.

bismuth subsalicylate

Bismatrol, Bismatrol Extra Strength, Bismed, Pepto-Bismol, Pepto-Bismol Bismuth Maximum Strength, Pink Bismuth, PMS-Bismuth Subsalicylate

Pharmacologic class: Adsorbent
Therapeutic class: Antidiarrheal, antibiotic, antiulcer drug
Pregnancy risk category C

Action

Promotes intestinal adsorption of fluids and electrolytes; decreases synthesis of intestinal prostaglandins. Adsorbent action removes irritant from stomach and soothes irritated bowel lining. Drug also shows antibacterial activity.

Availability

Liquid: 130 mg/15 ml, 262 mg/15 ml, 525 mg/15 ml (maximum strength)
Tablets: 262 mg
Tablets (chewable): 262 mg, 300 mg

Indications and dosages

➣ Adjunctive therapy for mild to moderate diarrhea, nausea, abdominal cramping, heartburn, and indigestion that may accompany diarrheal illnesses

Adults: 2 tablets or 30 ml P.O. (15 ml of maximum strength) q 30 minutes or 2 tablets or 60 ml (30 ml of extra/maximum strength) q 60 minutes as needed. Don't exceed 4.2 g in 24 hours.

Children ages 9 to 12: 1 tablet or 15 ml P.O. (7.5 ml of maximum strength) q 30 to 60 minutes. Don't exceed 2.1 g in 24 hours.

Children ages 6 to 9: 10 ml (5 ml of maximum strength) P.O. q 30 to 60 minutes. Don't exceed 1.4 g in 24 hours.

Children ages 3 to 6: 5 ml (2.5 ml of maximum strength) P.O. q 30 to 60 minutes. Don't exceed 704 mg in 24 hours.

➣ Ulcer disease associated with *Helicobacter pylori* (given with antibiotics)
Adults: 2 tablets or 30 ml P.O. q.i.d. (15 ml of maximum strength)

Off-label uses

• Chronic infantile diarrhea
• Norwalk virus–induced gastroenteritis

Contraindications

• Hypersensitivity to aspirin
• Elderly patients with fecal impaction
• Children or adolescents during or after recovery from chickenpox or flulike illness

Administration

• Know that tablets may be chewed or dissolved in mouth before swallowing.
• Notify prescriber if patient has diarrhea with fever for more than 48 hours.

Route	Onset	Peak	Duration
P.O.	1 hr	Unknown	Unknown

Adverse reactions

EENT: tinnitus, tongue discoloration
GI: nausea, vomiting, diarrhea, constipation, gray-black stools, fecal impaction

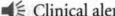

Respiratory: tachypnea
Other: salicylate toxicity

Interactions
Drug-drug. *Aspirin, other salicylates:* salicylate toxicity
Corticosteroids, probenecid (large doses), sulfinpyrazone: decreased bismuth efficacy
Enoxacin: decreased enoxacin bioavailability
Methotrexate: increased risk of bismuth toxicity
Tetracycline: decreased tetracycline absorption
Drug-diagnostic tests. *Radiologic GI tract examination:* test interference

Precautions
Use cautiously in:
• diabetes mellitus, gout
• patients taking concurrent aspirin
• elderly patients
• pregnant or breastfeeding patients
• infants.

Patient monitoring
• Monitor fluid intake and electrolyte levels.
• Monitor frequency and appearance of stools.
• Assess infants and debilitated patients for fecal impaction.

Patient teaching
• Teach patient to chew tablets or dissolve them in mouth before swallowing.
• Inform patient that drug may turn stools gray-black temporarily.

bisoprolol
Monocor✤, Zebeta, Ziac

Pharmacologic class: Beta$_1$-adrenergic blocker
Therapeutic class: Antihypertensive
Pregnancy risk category C

Action
Blocks beta$_1$-adrenergic receptors of sympathetic nervous system in heart and juxtaglomerular apparatus. Decreases myocardial excitability, myocardial oxygen consumption, cardiac output, and renin release from kidneys; lowers blood pressure without affecting beta$_2$-adrenergic (pulmonary, vascular, uterine) receptor sites.

Availability
Tablets: 5 mg, 10 mg

⚕ Indications and dosages
➤ Hypertension (used alone or with other antihypertensives)
Adults: Initially, 2.5 to 5 mg P.O. daily, alone or added to diuretic therapy. Dosages up to 20 mg P.O. daily have been used.
Dosage adjustment
• Renal or hepatic impairment

Contraindications
• Hypersensitivity to drug
• Sinus bradycardia
• Second- or third-degree heart block
• Cardiogenic shock
• Heart failure
• Children (safety and efficacy not established)

Administration
• Give with or without food, but be consistent to minimize variations in absorption.
• Check patient's apical pulse before giving; if it's irregular or below 60 beats/minute, withhold dose and notify prescriber.

Route	Onset	Peak	Duration
P.O.	30-60 min	2 hr	12-15 hr

Adverse reactions
CNS: dizziness, depression, paresthesia, sleep disturbances, hallucinations, memory loss, slurred speech

CV: sinoatrial or atrioventricular (AV) node block, tachycardia, peripheral vascular insufficiency, claudication, hypotension, **second- or third- degree heart block, heart failure, pulmonary edema, cerebrovascular accident, arrhythmias**

EENT: blurred vision, dry eyes, conjunctivitis, tinnitus, rhinitis, pharyngitis

GI: nausea, vomiting, diarrhea, constipation, gastric pain, gastritis, flatulence, anorexia, ischemic colitis, acute pancreatitis, **renal and mesenteric arterial thrombosis**

GU: Peyronie's disease, dysuria, polyuria, nocturia, impotence, decreased libido

Hematologic: eosinophilia, **agranulocytosis, thrombocytopenia**

Hepatic: elevated serum transaminase and alkaline phosphatase, hepatomegaly

Metabolic: hyperglycemia, hypoglycemia, elevated low-density lipoprotein levels

Musculoskeletal: arthralgia, muscle cramps

Respiratory: dyspnea, cough, bronchial obstruction, **bronchospasm**

Skin: rash, purpura, pruritus, dry skin, excessive sweating

Interactions

Drug-drug. *Amphetamines, ephedrine, epinephrine, norepinephrine, phenylephrine, pseudoephedrine:* unopposed alpha-adrenergic stimulation

Antihypertensives, aspirin, bismuth subsalicylate, hormonal contraceptives, magnesium salicylate, nitrates, sulfinpyrazone: increased hypotension

Digoxin: additive bradycardia

Dobutamine, dopamine: decrease in beneficial beta$_1$-adrenergic cardiovascular effects

General anesthetics, I.V. phenytoin, verapamil: additive myocardial depression

Monoamine oxidase (MAO) inhibitors: hypertension when taken within 14 days of bisoprolol

Nonsteroidal anti-inflammatory drugs: decreased antihypertensive effect

Thyroid preparations: decreased bisoprolol efficacy

Drug-diagnostic tests. *Alanine aminotransferase, aspartate aminotransferase, blood urea nitrogen, glucose, potassium, uric acid:* increased levels

Antinuclear antibodies: increased titers

Insulin tolerance tests: test interference

Drug-behaviors. *Acute alcohol ingestion:* additive hypotension

Cocaine use: unopposed alpha-adrenergic stimulation

Precautions

Use cautiously in:
• renal or hepatic impairment, pulmonary disease, asthma, diabetes mellitus, thyrotoxicosis
• elderly patients
• pregnant or breastfeeding patients
• children.

Patient monitoring

• Closely monitor blood glucose levels in diabetic patients.
• Monitor for sudden discontinuation of therapy, which may precipitate angina.
• Assess for signs and symptoms of heart failure, including weight gain.

Patient teaching

• Instruct patient to weigh himself daily at the same time and to report gain of 3 to 4 lb/day.
• Instruct patient to move slowly when sitting up or standing to avoid dizziness or light-headedness from blood pressure decrease.
• Instruct patient to avoid driving and other hazardous activities until he knows how drug affects concentration and alertness.

• Caution patient not to discontinue drug abruptly unless prescriber approves.
• Teach patient to carry medical identification stating that he's taking a beta blocker.

---

bivalirudin
Angiomax

Pharmacologic class: Thrombin inhibitor
Therapeutic class: Anticoagulant
Pregnancy risk category B

Action
Selectively inhibits thrombin by binding to its receptor sites, causing inactivation of coagulation factors V, VIII, and XII, preventing the conversion of fibrinogen to fibrin and the formation of clots

Availability
Powder for injection: 250 mg/vial

🔻 Indications and dosages
➤ Ischemic complications; unstable angina; patients undergoing percutaneous transluminal angioplasty (PCTA)
Adults: 1 mg/kg bolus just before PCTA; then start 4-hour I.V. infusion at 2.5 mg/kg/hour. After 4-hour infusion, may give additional I.V. infusion at 0.2 mg/kg/hour for up to 20 hours as needed, along with aspirin 300 to 325 mg.
Dosage adjustment
• Renal impairment
• Dialysis patients

Contraindications
• Hypersensitivity to drug
• Acute coronary syndrome
• Active major bleeding or unstable angina in patients not undergoing PCTA

Administration
• For I.V. injection and infusion, add 5 ml of sterile water to each 250-mg vial; gently mix until dissolved. Further dilute in 50 ml of dextrose 5% in water or normal saline solution for injection to a final concentration of 5 mg/ml.
• Don't mix with other drugs.
• Don't give by I.M. route.
• Know that drug is intended for use with aspirin.

Route	Onset	Peak	Duration
I.V.	Immediate	Immediate	1-2 hr

Adverse reactions
CNS: headache, anxiety, nervousness, insomnia
CV: hypotension, hypertension, **bradycardia, ventricular fibrillation**
GI: nausea, vomiting, abdominal pain, dyspepsia, **severe spontaneous bleeding**
GU: urinary retention, **severe spontaneous bleeding**
Hematologic: severe spontaneous bleeding
Musculoskeletal: pelvic or back pain
Other: fever, pain at injection site

Interactions
Drug-drug. *Abciximab, anticoagulants (including heparin, low-molecular-weight heparins, and heparinoids), thrombolytics, ticlopidine:* increased risk of bleeding
Glycoprotein IIb/IIIa inhibitors: safety and efficacy of concomitant use not established
Drug-diagnostic tests. *Activated partial thromboplastin time, prothrombin time:* increased
Drug-herb. *Ginkgo biloba:* increased risk of bleeding

Precautions
Use cautiously in:
• renal impairment, severe hepatic dysfunction, bacterial endocarditis, cerebrovascular accident, severe hypertension, heparin-induced thrombocytopenia, thrombosis syndrome
• diseases associated with increased risk of bleeding
• unstable angina in patients not undergoing PCTA
• concurrent use of other platelet aggregation inhibitors
• pregnant or breastfeeding patients
• children.

Patient monitoring
◢€ Monitor blood pressure, hemoglobin, and hematocrit. Be aware that decrease in blood pressure or hematocrit may signal hemorrhagic event.
• Monitor venipuncture site closely for bleeding.

Patient teaching
• Instruct patient to immediately report bleeding, bruising, or tarry stools.
• Tell patient to avoid activities that can cause injury. Advise him to use soft toothbrush and electric razor to avoid gum and skin injury.
• Advise family members to take classes in cardiopulmonary resuscitation.

bleomycin sulfate
Blenoxane

Pharmacologic class: Antitumor antibiotic
Therapeutic class: Antineoplastic
Pregnancy risk category D

Action
Unknown; appears to inhibit DNA synthesis and, to a lesser degree, RNA and protein synthesis. Binds to DNA, causing severing of single DNA strands.

Availability
Injection: 15-unit vials, 30-unit vials

𝌆 Indications and dosages
➤ Hodgkin's lymphoma
Adults: 10 to 20 units/m² I.V., I.M., or S.C. once or twice weekly. After 50% response, maintenance dosage is 1 unit I.M. or I.V. daily or 5 units I.M. or I.V. weekly. Give dosages above 400 units with extreme caution.
➤ Malignant pleural effusion, prevention of recurrent pleural effusions
Adults: 60 units dissolved in 50 to 100 mg of normal saline solution and administered through thoracostomy tube
➤ Squamous cell carcinoma of head, neck, skin, penis, cervix, or vulva; non-Hodgkin's lymphoma; testicular carcinoma
Adults and children ages 12 and older: 10 to 20 units/m² I.V., I.M., or S.C. once or twice weekly. Give dosages above 400 units with extreme caution.
Dosage adjustment
• Renal impairment
• Elderly patients

Off-label uses
• Esophageal carcinoma
• Hemangioma
• AIDS-related Kaposi's sarcoma
• Osteosarcoma
• Verrucous carcinoma
• Warts

Contraindications
• Hypersensitivity to drug
• Pregnancy or breastfeeding

Administration
• Wash hands before and after preparing drug; wear gloves during handling and preparation.
• For I.M. or S.C. use, reconstitute 15-unit vial with 1 to 5 ml and 30-unit

vial with 2 to 10 ml of sterile water for injection, normal saline solution for injection, or bacteriostatic water for injection.

• For I.V. infusion, dissolve contents of 15- or 30-unit vial in 5 or 10 ml, respectively, of normal saline solution for injection.

• For intrapleural use, dissolve 60 units in 50 to 100 ml of normal saline solution for injection, then administer through thoracostomy tube. Clamp tube after instilling drug. During next 4 hours, reposition patient from supine to right and left lateral positions several times. Then unclamp tube and restart suction.

• Premedicate patient with aspirin, as prescribed, to reduce risk of drug fever.

Route	Onset	Peak	Duration
I.V.	Immediate	10-20 min	Unknown
I.M., S.C.	15-20 min	30-60 min	Unknown

Adverse reactions

CNS: disorientation, weakness, aggressive behavior

CV: hypotension, peripheral vasoconstriction

GI: vomiting, diarrhea, anorexia, stomatitis

Hematologic: anemia, **leukopenia, thrombocytopenia**

Hepatic: hepatotoxicity

Metabolic: hyperuricemia

Respiratory: dyspnea, crackles, **pulmonary fibrosis, pneumonitis**

Skin: alopecia, erythema, rash, urticaria, vesicles, striae, hyperpigmentation, mucocutaneous toxicity

Other: fever, chills, weight loss, **anaphylactic reaction**

Interactions

Drug-drug. *Anesthetics:* increased oxygen requirement

Antineoplastics: increased risk of hematologic and pulmonary toxicity

Cardiac glycosides: decreased cardiac glycoside blood level

Cisplatin: decreased bleomycin elimination, increased risk of toxicity

Fosphenytoin, phenytoin: decreased blood levels of these drugs

Vinblastine: increased risk of Raynaud's syndrome

Drug-diagnostic tests. *Uric acid:* increased level

Precautions

Use cautiously in:
• renal or pulmonary impairment
• elderly patients
• women of childbearing age.

Patient monitoring

• Assess baseline pulmonary function status before initiating therapy; monitor throughout therapy.

• Monitor chest X-rays and assess breath sounds to detect signs of pulmonary toxicity.

• Assess oral cavity for sores, ulcers, pain, and bleeding.

• Monitor infusion site for irritation, burning, and signs of infection.

• Evaluate closely for signs and symptoms of drug fever.

Patient teaching

• Advise patient to use reliable method of contraception during therapy.

• Tell patient to avoid activities that can cause injury. Advise him to use soft toothbrush and electric razor to avoid gum and skin injury.

• Teach patient to avoid spicy, hot, or rough foods because they may cause GI upset.

• Inform patient that drug may cause hair loss; reassure him that hair will grow back after treatment ends.

bortezomib
Velcade

Pharmacologic class: Proteasome inhibitor
Therapeutic class: Antineoplastic
Pregnancy risk category D

Action
Inhibits proteasomes (enzyme complexes that regulate protein homeostasis within cell); reversibly inhibits chymotrypsin-like activity at 26S proteasome, leading to activation of signaling cascades, cell-cycle arrest, and apoptosis

Availability
Powder for reconstitution (preservative-free): 3.5 mg (contains 35 mg of mannitol)

Indications and dosages
➤ Multiple myeloma in patients who've undergone at least two previous therapies and demonstrated disease progression during previous therapy
Adults: 1.3 mg/m^2 I.V. twice weekly for 2 weeks (days 1, 4, 8, and 11), followed by 10-day rest period (days 12 to 21). Allow at least 72 hours to elapse between doses. One treatment cycle equals 21 days (3 weeks).

Contraindications
• Hypersensitivity to drug, mannitol, or boron
• Pregnancy

Administration
• Reconstitute drug in vial with 3.5 ml of normal saline for injection.
• Give IV push over 3 to 5 seconds.

Route	Onset	Peak	Duration
I.V.	Unknown	Unknown	Unknown

Adverse reactions
CNS: headache, insomnia, dizziness, anxiety, peripheral neuropathy
CV: tachycardia, hypertension
EENT: throat tightness
GI: nausea, vomiting, diarrhea, abdominal pain, dyspepsia, altered taste
Hematologic: eosinophilia, anemia, **thrombocytopenia, neutropenia**
Metabolic: dehydration, pyrexia
Respiratory: cough, dyspnea, upper respiratory tract infection
Skin: rash, pruritus, urticaria
Other: fever, chills, increased or decreased appetite

Interactions
Drug-drug. *CYP3A4 inducers, including amiodarone, carbamazepine, nevirapine, phenobarbital, phenytoin, rifampin:* possible decreased serum level or efficacy of bortezomib
CYP3A4 inhibitors, including amiodarone, cimetidine, clarithromycin, delavirdine, diltiazem, disulfiram, erythromycin, fluoxetine, fluvoxamine, nefazodone, nevirapine, propoxyphene, quinupristin, verapamil, zafirlukast, zileuton: possible increased serum level or efficacy of bortezomib
Drug-food. *Grapefruit juice:* increased bortezomib blood level, greater risk of toxicity

Precautions
Use cautiously in:
• dehydration, hepatic or renal impairment
• history of syncope
• children.

Patient monitoring
◀€ Monitor vital signs and temperature; especially watch for tachycardia, fever, and hypertension.
• Monitor nutritional and hydration status for changes due to GI adverse effects.

• Monitor complete blood cell count with differential, and watch for signs and symptoms of blood dyscrasias.
• Monitor respiratory status, watching for dyspnea, cough, and other signs and symptoms of upper respiratory tract infection.

Patient teaching

• Teach patient that drug has significant adverse effects. Reassure him he will be closely monitored; advise him to report any significant issues.
• Instruct patient to avoid driving or other hazardous activities until drug's effects on concentration and alertness are known.
• Teach patient to handle GI adverse effects by eating small frequent servings of healthy food and ensuring adequate fluid intake.
• Tell patient to immediately report signs of upper respiratory tract infection.
• Advise patient that drug can cause serious blood dyscrasias; outline signs and symptoms that should be reported right away.

bosentan
Tracleer

Pharmacologic class: Endothelin-receptor antagonist, vasodilator
Therapeutic class: Antihypertensive
Pregnancy risk category X

Action

Binds to and blocks receptor sites for endothelin A and B in endothelium and vascular smooth muscle; this action reduces elevated endothelin levels in patients with pulmonary arterial hypertension. Also inhibits vasoconstriction resulting from endothelin-1 (ET-1).

Availability
Tablets: 62.5 mg, 125 mg

Indications and dosages

➣ To improve exercise ability and slow clinical deterioration in patients with pulmonary arterial hypertension who have World Health Organization class III or class IV symptoms
Adults: Initially, 62.5 mg P.O. b.i.d. for 4 weeks; increase to a maintenance dosage of 125 mg P.O. b.i.d. In patients weighing less than 40 kg (88 lb), initial and maintenance dosages are 62.5 mg b.i.d.
Dosage adjustment
• Moderate to severe hepatic dysfunction
• Hepatic injury in patients with elevated alanine aminotransferase (ALT) or aspartate aminotransferase (AST) levels

Contraindications
• Hypersensitivity to drug
• Severe hepatic impairment
• Patients receiving concurrent cyclosporine or glyburide
• Pregnancy or breastfeeding
• Children younger than age 12 (safety and efficacy not established).

Administration
• Give tablets in morning and evening with or without food.

Route	Onset	Peak	Duration
P.O.	Variable	3-5 hr	Unknown

Adverse reactions
CNS: headache, fatigue
CV: edema, hypotension, palpitations
EENT: nasopharyngitis
GI: dyspepsia
Hematologic: decreased hematocrit and hemoglobin
Hepatic: abnormal liver function, **hepatic injury, hepatotoxicity**
Skin: pruritus, flushing

Interactions
Drug-drug. *Cyclosporine:* decreased cyclosporine blood level, increased bosentan blood level
Glyburide: decreased blood levels of both drugs, increased risk of liver damage
Hormonal contraceptives: decreased bosentan efficacy
Ketoconazole: increased bosentan blood level and effects
Simvastatin: decreased simvastatin effects
Drug-diagnostic tests. *Hematocrit, hemoglobin:* decreased values
Transaminases: increased levels

Precautions
Use cautiously in:
• mitral stenosis
• elderly patients.

Patient monitoring
• Assess serum transaminase levels within first 3 days of therapy and then monthly.
• Evaluate hemoglobin level 1 month after therapy and then every 3 months.
• Assess female patient for pregnancy every month during therapy.

Patient teaching
• Tell patient to take drug with or without food in morning and evening.
• Caution female to avoid pregnancy; discuss reliable contraceptive methods. Instruct her to contact prescriber immediately if she thinks she may be pregnant.
• Inform patient that he'll have complete blood counts and undergo liver function testing regularly during therapy.

botulinum toxin type A
Botox Cosmetic

botulinum toxin type B
Myobloc

Pharmacologic class: Neurotoxin
Therapeutic class: Neuromuscular blocker
Pregnancy risk category C

Action
Blocks neuromuscular transmission by binding to receptor sites on motor nerve terminals and inhibiting acetylcholine release, causing localized muscle denervation. As a result, local muscle paralysis occurs, leading to muscle atrophy and reinnervation if muscle develops new acetylcholine receptors.

Availability
Powder for injection: 100 units/vial

Indications and dosages
Toxin type A
➤ Temporary improvement in appearance of moderate to severe glabellar lines associated with corrugator or procerus muscle activity
Adults: Total of 20 units (0.5-ml solution) injected I.M. as divided doses of 0.1 ml into each of five sites—two in each corrugator muscle and one in the procerus muscle. Injection usually needs to be repeated q 3 to 4 months to maintain effect.
Toxin type B
➤ To relax skeletal muscles and reduce severity of abnormal head position and neck pain associated with cervical dystonia
Adults: 2,500 to 5,000 units I.M. injected locally into affected muscles

Contraindications
- Hypersensitivity to drug
- Active infection at injection site

Administration
Toxin type A
- Reconstitute toxin type A by slowly injecting normal saline solution without preservative into drug vial.
- Rotate vial gently to mix drug; then draw up at least 20 units (0.5-ml solution) and expel air bubbles.
- Remove needle used for reconstituting and attach 30-gauge needle; then inject drug as divided dose of 0.1 ml into each of five sites (two in each corrugator muscle, and one in the procerus muscle).

Toxin type B
- Draw up prescribed dose from preservative-free 3.5-ml single-use vial.
- Divide prescribed dose and inject locally among affected muscles.

Route	Onset	Peak	Duration
I.M.	Mins-hrs	Unknown	3-4 mo

Adverse reactions
CNS: headache, dizziness
CV: hypertension, **arrhythmias, myocardial infarction (MI)**
EENT: blepharoptosis, transient ptosis, sinusitis, pharyngitis
GI: nausea, difficulty swallowing, dyspepsia, tooth disorder
Respiratory: pneumonia, bronchitis, upper respiratory tract infection
Skin: skin tightness, ecchymosis
Other: injection site redness, edema, or pain; flulike symptoms; paralysis of facial muscles; infection; **anaphylaxis**

Interactions
Drug-drug. *Aminoglycosides, anticholinesterase compounds, clindamycin, lincomycin, magnesium sulfate, neuromuscular blockers (such as succinylcholine), polymyxin B, quinidine:* increased risk of adverse effects

Precautions
Use cautiously in:
- cardiovascular disease, peripheral neuropathy, neuromuscular disorders (such as myasthenia gravis)
- inflammation at injection site
- pregnant or breastfeeding patients.

Patient monitoring
- Watch closely for signs of anaphylaxis, particularly after first dose.
- Monitor vital signs and electrocardiogram, watching for signs and symptoms of hypertension, arrhythmias, and MI.
- Assess effect of drug on affected muscles, watching for paralysis.
- Monitor temperature and watch for signs and symptoms of respiratory and eyes, ears, nose and throat (EENT) infections as well as flulike symptoms.

Patient teaching
- Describe desired effect of injection, and advise patient to report paralysis.
- Instruct patient to report signs and symptoms of infections, particularly flulike illness and EENT and respiratory infections.

bretylium tosylate
Bretylate✿, Bretylol

Pharmacologic class: Beta-adrenergic blocker

Therapeutic class: Antiarrhythmic (class III)

Pregnancy risk category C

Action
Unclear; initially may cause norepinephrine release from adrenergic neurons, then may inhibit such release by depressing adrenergic nerve excitability, thus prolonging repolarization. Also thought to increase duration of action

---

potential and refractory period, helping to suppress ventricular tachycardia.

Availability
Injection: 50 mg/ml in 10-ml ampules, vials, and syringes; 2 mg/ml and 4 mg/ml in 250-ml vials
Prefilled syringes: 1 mg/ml, 2 mg/ml, 4 mg/ml
Premixed solution: 500 mg/250 ml, 1,000 mg/250 ml

⚕ Indications and dosages
➣ Immediate, life-threatening ventricular arrhythmias
Adults: 5 mg/kg (undiluted) by I.V. push over 1 minute. May increase to 10 mg/kg if needed, to a total of 30 to 35 mg/kg.
Children: Initially, 5 mg/kg I.V., then 10 mg/kg at 15- to 30-minute intervals; maximum dosage is 30 mg/kg.
➣ Other ventricular arrhythmias
Adults: 5 to 10 mg/kg I.V. infused over more than 8 minutes, repeated q 1 to 2 hours. May repeat q 6 hours for maintenance or continuous I.V. infusion of 1 to 2 mg/minute or 5 to 10 mg/kg undiluted solution I.M. Repeat q 1 to 2 hours as needed.
Children: 2 to 5 mg/kg I.V. q 6 hours; increase dosage as needed.
Dosage adjustment
• Renal impairment

Off-label uses
• Resistant ventricular fibrillation and ventricular tachycardia

Contraindications
• Hypersensitivity to drug
• Pulmonary hypertension
• Aortic stenosis
• Digoxin toxicity

Administration
• Always dilute drug for intermittent or continuous I.V. infusion, unless patient has life-threatening ventricular

fibrillation; in that case, give undiluted as quickly as possible.
• Keep patient supine during administration; observe closely for orthostatic hypotension.
• If given I.M., rotate injection sites. Repeated injections in same site may cause inflammation, fibrosis, and atrophy.

Route	Onset	Peak	Duration
I.V.	Immediate	Immediate	6-24 hr
I.M.	5-40 min	1 hr	6-24 hr

Adverse reactions
CNS: syncope, dizziness, anxiety, confusion, psychosis, vertigo, lightheadedness
CV: transient hypertension, angina, transient arrhythmias, substernal pressure, **bradycardia, increased premature ventricular contractions, severe hypotension**
GI: nausea, vomiting
Respiratory: respiratory depression

Interactions
Drug-drug. *Antihypertensives:* increased hypotension
Digoxin: increased digoxin toxicity
Procainamide, propranolol, quinidine, other antiarrhythmics: increased or decreased antiarrhythmic effects
Sympathomimetics: increased bretylium effect
Drug-herb. *Aloe, buckthorn bark or berry, cascara bark, rhubarb root, senna leaf or fruit:* increased bretylium effect

Precautions
Use cautiously in:
• digoxin-induced arrhythmias, sinus bradycardia, renal impairment
• elderly patients
• pregnant or breastfeeding patients
• children.

Patient monitoring

🔊 Continuously monitor blood pressure and electrocardiogram during administration.

• Assess patient regularly for signs and symptoms of angina.

Patient teaching

• Instruct patient to remain supine during infusion.

bromocriptine mesylate

Alti-Bromocriptine✤, Apo-Bromocriptine✤, Parlodel

Pharmacologic class: Ergot-derivative dopamine agonist
Therapeutic class: Antiparkinsonian
Pregnancy risk category B

Action

Directly stimulates dopamine receptors in hypothalamus, releasing prolactin-inhibitory factors and thereby alleviating akinesia, rigidity, and tremor associated with Parkinson's disease. Also inhibits release of prolactin and specific hormones, thereby restoring testicular or ovarian function and suppressing lactation.

Availability

Capsules: 5 mg
Tablets: 2.5 mg

🕗 Indications and dosages

➤ Parkinson's disease
Adults: Initially, 1.25 mg P.O. b.i.d. with meals; increase by 2.5 mg/day q 14 to 28 days, to a maximum daily dosage of 100 mg.
➤ Acromegaly
Adults: Initially, 1.25 to 2.5 mg/day P.O. h.s. for 3 days; increase up to 1.25 to 2.5 mg/day q 3 to 7 days. Maximum dosage is 100 mg/day.

➤ Hyperprolactinemia
Adults: Initially, 1.25 to 2.5 mg/day P.O.; increase gradually q 3 to 7 days up to 2.5 mg two to three times daily.
➤ Neuroleptic malignant syndrome
Adults: Initially, 5 mg P.O. once daily; increase up to 20 mg/day.

Contraindications

• Hypersensitivity to drug or other ergot derivatives
• Severe peripheral vascular disease
• Uncontrolled hypertension
• Breastfeeding

Administration

• Give with meals or milk.
• If needed, give at bedtime to minimize dizziness and nausea.

Route	Onset	Peak	Duration
P.O.	2 hr	8 hr	24 hr

Adverse reactions

CNS: confusion, headache, dizziness, fatigue, delusions, nervousness, mania, insomnia, nightmares, **seizures, cerebrovascular accident**
CV: hypotension, palpitations, extrasystoles, **arrhythmias, bradycardia, acute myocardial infarction**
EENT: blurred vision, diplopia, burning sensation in eyes, nasal congestion
GI: nausea, vomiting, diarrhea, constipation, abdominal cramps, anorexia, dry mouth, metallic taste, **GI hemorrhage**
GU: urinary incontinence, polyuria, urinary retention, increased urine output
Musculoskeletal: leg cramps
Skin: urticaria, coolness and pallor of fingers and toes, rash on face and arms, alopecia
Other: digital vasospasm (in acromegaly use only)

✤ Canada   🔊 Clinical alert   Reactions in **bold** are life-threatening

Interactions

Drug-drug. *Amitriptyline, estrogens, haloperidol, hormonal contraceptives, imipramine, loxapine, monoamine oxidase inhibitors, phenothiazines, progestins, reserpine:* interference with bromocriptine effects
Erythromycin: increased bromocriptine blood level and greater risk of adverse effects
Levodopa: additive effects of bromocriptine
Risperidone: increased prolactin blood level, interference with bromocriptine effects
Drug-diagnostic tests. *Alanine aminotransferase, alkaline phosphatase, aspartate aminotransferase, blood urea nitrogen, creatine kinase, growth hormone, uric acid:* increased levels
Drug-herb. *Chaste tree fruit:* decrease in bromocriptine effects
Drug-behaviors. *Alcohol use:* disulfiram-like reaction

Precautions

Use cautiously in:
• impaired hepatic or cardiac function, renal disease, hypertension, pituitary tumor
• psychiatric disorders
• pregnant patients
• children younger than age 15.

Patient monitoring

• Monitor blood pressure to detect hypotension.
• When giving drug for hyperprolactinemia, monitor serum prolactin levels.
• With long-term use, monitor respiratory, hepatic, cardiovascular, and renal function.

Patient teaching

• Instruct patient to avoid driving and other hazardous activities until he knows how drug affects concentration and alertness.
• Caution patient not to drink alcohol during therapy.
• Advise patient to have regular dental exams; drug causes dry mouth, possibly resulting in caries and periodontal disorders.
• To minimize constipation, instruct patient to exercise regularly, increase dietary fiber, and drink plenty of fluids (3,000 ml daily).

brompheniramine
Bromfenac, Dimetane, Dimetapp Allergy, Nasahist B, ND-Stat

Pharmacologic class: Histamine antagonist
Therapeutic class: Antihistamine
Pregnancy risk category C

Action

Antagonizes effects of histamine at histamine$_1$-receptor sites; doesn't bind to or inactivate histamine. Also shows anticholinergic, antipruritic, and sedative activity.

Availability

Capsules (liquigels): 4 mg
Elixir: 2 mg/5 ml
Injection: 10 mg/ml
Tablets: 4 mg, 8 mg, 12 mg
Tablets (extended-release): 8 mg, 12 mg

Indications and dosages

➤ Symptomatic relief of allergic symptoms (rhinitis, urticaria) caused by histamine release, severe allergic or hypersensitivity reactions (including anaphylaxis and transfusion reactions)
Adults and children ages 12 and older: 4 to 8 mg P.O. three to four times daily, or 8 to 12 mg extended-release tablets P.O. two or three times daily; maxi-

mum oral dosage is 36 mg/day. Alternatively, 5 to 20 mg I.M., I.V., or S.C. q 6 to 12 hours. Maximum parenteral dosage is 40 mg daily as needed (not to exceed 24 mg/day).

Children ages 6 to 12: 2 mg P.O. q 4 to 6 hours as needed, not to exceed 12 mg/day

Children ages 2 to 6: 1 mg P.O. q 4 to 6 hours as needed, not to exceed 6 mg/day

Contraindications

- Hypersensitivity to drug
- Coronary artery disease
- Angle-closure glaucoma
- Urinary retention
- Pyloroduodenal obstruction
- Peptic ulcer
- Monoamine oxidase (MAO) inhibitor use within past 14 days
- Breastfeeding

Administration

- Give with food if GI upset occurs.
- For I.V. use, give undiluted or diluted with 10 ml of normal saline solution by bolus over 1 minute.
- For continuous I.V. infusion, dilute in dextrose 5% in water or normal saline solution.
- Don't break or crush extended-release tablets.

Route	Onset	Peak	Duration
P.O.	15-60 min	2-5 hr	3-24 hr
I.V.	Rapid	Unknown	8-12 hr
I.M., S.C.	20-30 min	Unknown	8-12 hr

Adverse reactions

CNS: drowsiness, sedation, dizziness, excitation, irritability, syncope, tremor
CV: hypertension, hypotension, palpitations, tachycardia, extrasystole, **arrhythmias, bradycardia**
EENT: blurred vision, nasal stuffiness or dryness, sore throat

GI: nausea, vomiting, constipation, increased or decreased appetite, dry mouth and throat
GU: urinary retention or hesitancy, dysuria, early menses, decreased libido, impotence
Hematologic: hemolytic anemia, hypoplastic anemia, **thrombocytopenia, agranulocytosis, leukopenia, pancytopenia**
Respiratory: thickened bronchial secretions, chest tightness, wheezing
Skin: diaphoresis, urticaria, rash (with parenteral use)
Other: weight gain, local stinging, **anaphylactic shock, hypersensitivity reaction** (with I.V. use)

Interactions

Drug-drug. *CNS depressants (including alcohol, opioids, and sedative-hypnotics):* additive CNS depression
MAO inhibitors: intensified, prolonged anticholinergic effects
Drug-diagnostic tests. *Allergy tests:* false results
Granulocytes, platelets: decreased counts
Drug-behaviors. *Alcohol use:* increased CNS depression

Precautions

Use cautiously in:
- angle-closure glaucoma, liver disease, hyperthyroidism, hypertension, bronchial asthma, prostatic hypertrophy
- elderly patients
- pregnant patients.

Patient monitoring

- Monitor respiratory status.
- Stay alert for urinary retention, urinary frequency, and painful or difficult urination. Discontinue drug if these problems occur.
- With long-term use, monitor complete blood count.
- Monitor elderly patient for dizziness, sedation, and hypotension.

• If patient is taking over-the-counter antihistamines, monitor him closely to avoid potential overdose.

Patient teaching
• Advise patient to take drug with meals if GI upset occurs.
• Instruct patient to avoid driving and other hazardous activities until he knows how drug affects concentration and alertness.
• Instruct patient to tell all prescribers which medications and over-the-counter preparations he's taking.
• Caution patient to avoid alcohol while taking drug.

budesonide
Pulmicort Respules, Pulmicort Turbuhaler, Rhinocort

Pharmacologic class: Corticosteroid (inhalation)
Therapeutic class: Antiasthmatic, steroidal anti-inflammatory
Pregnancy risk category C

Action
Decreases inflammation by inhibiting activity of specific inflammation mediators, such as prostaglandins, leukotrienes, and kinins. Inhibits migration of inflammatory mediators to injury site; reverses dilation and increased vessel permeability of this site. Also decreases plasma exudation and mucus secretions within airway.

Availability
Inhalation powder: 200 mcg/metered inhalation in 200-metered-dose inhaler
Inhalation suspension (Respules): 0.25 mg/2 ml, 0.5 mg/2 ml
Nasal spray: 32 mcg/metered spray (7-g canister)

Indications and dosages
➤ Prophylactic therapy in chronic asthma
Adults previously controlled on bronchodilators alone: One or two inhalations b.i.d. (200 mcg/inhalation)
Adults previously controlled on other inhaled corticosteroids: One or two inhalations b.i.d. (up to four inhalations b.i.d.)
Adults previously controlled on oral corticosteroids: Two to four inhalations b.i.d. (up to four inhalations b.i.d.)
Children ages 6 and older: One inhalation (200 mcg) b.i.d. to a maximum of 400 mcg b.i.d.
Children ages 3 to 6 previously controlled on bronchodilators alone: One to two inhalations b.i.d. (200 mcg/inhalation)
Children ages 3 to 6 previously controlled on other inhaled corticosteroids: One or two inhalations b.i.d.
Children ages 3 to 6 previously controlled on oral corticosteroids: Maximum of two inhalations b.i.d.
Pulmicort Respules—
Children ages 12 months to 8 years previously controlled on bronchodilators alone: 0.25 mg/day as a single dose or in divided doses b.i.d.
Children ages 12 months to 8 years previously controlled on other inhaled corticosteroids: 0.5 mg/day as a single dose or in divided doses of 0.25 mg b.i.d.
Children ages 12 months to 8 years previously controlled on oral corticosteroids: 1 mg/day as a single dose or in divided doses b.i.d. Individualized titration is required.
➤ Seasonal or perennial allergic rhinitis
Adults and children ages 6 and older: Two sprays in each nostril in morning and evening, or four sprays in each nostril in morning. Maintenance

dosage is fewest number of sprays needed to control symptoms.

Dosage adjustment
• Moderate to severe liver disease

Contraindications
• Hypersensitivity to drug
• Status asthmaticus

Administration
• If patient is also using a bronchodilator, give that drug at least 15 minutes before budesonide.
• Know that inhaler use reduces candidiasis incidence.

Route	Onset	Peak	Duration
P.O.	Slow	0.5-10 hr	Unknown
Inhalation (nasal)	Immediate	1-2 wk	Unknown

Adverse reactions
CNS: headache, nervousness, depression, euphoria, psychoses, **increased intracranial pressure**
CV: hypotension, thrombophlebitis, **thromboembolism**
EENT: cataracts, nasal congestion, nasal burning or dryness, epistaxis, perforated nasal septum, anosmia, hoarseness, nasopharyngeal and oropharyngeal fungal infections
GI: nausea, vomiting, peptic ulcers, anorexia, esophageal candidiasis, bad taste, dry mouth
Metabolic: adrenal suppression or insufficiency, hyperglycemia, decreased growth, cushingoid appearance (moon face, buffalo hump)
Musculoskeletal: muscle wasting, muscle pain, osteoporosis, aseptic joint necrosis
Respiratory: cough, wheezing, rebound congestion, **bronchospasm**
Skin: facial edema, rash, petechiae, contact dermatitis, acne, bruising, hirsutism, urticaria
Other: weight gain or loss, Churg-Strauss syndrome, increased suscepti-

bility to infection, **angioedema, hypersensitivity reaction**

Interactions
Drug-drug. *Amphotericin B, mezlocillin, piperacillin, thiazide and loop diuretics, ticarcillin:* additive hypokalemia
Digoxin: increased risk of digoxin toxicity
Erythromycin, indinavir, itraconazole, ketoconazole, ritonavir, saquinavir: increased blood level and effects of budesonide
Fluoroquinolones: increased risk of tendon rupture
Hormonal contraceptives: blockage of budesonide metabolism
Insulin, oral hypoglycemics: increased budesonide requirement
Live-virus vaccines: decreased antibody response to vaccine, increased risk of adverse effects from budesonide
Nonsteroidal anti-inflammatory drugs (including aspirin): increased risk of adverse GI effects
Phenobarbital, phenytoin, rifampin: decreased budesonide efficacy
Somatrem, somatropin: decreased response to budesonide
Drug-food. *Grapefruit juice:* increased blood level and effects of budesonide

Precautions
Use cautiously in:
• renal disease, cirrhosis, heart failure, active untreated infections, systemic infections, hypertension, osteoporosis, diabetes mellitus, glaucoma, underlying immunosuppression, hypothyroidism, diverticulitis, nonspecific ulcerative colitis, recent intestinal anastomoses, thromboembolic disorders, seizures, myasthenia gravis, ocular herpes simplex infection
• patients receiving concurrent systemic corticosteroids
• pregnant or breastfeeding patients
• children younger than age 6.

Patient monitoring

• Monitor respiratory status to evaluate drug efficacy.
• Evaluate liver function test results.
• Periodically observe patient for proper inhaler use.
• Assess oral cavity for signs of infection.

Patient teaching

• Teach patient proper use of inhaler.
• Encourage patient to document medication use and his response in diary.
• Teach patient to report signs and symptoms of fungal infections of the mouth.
• Emphasize importance of rinsing mouth after each treatment and washing and drying inhaler thoroughly after each use.

bumetanide
Bumetanide Injection, Bumex

Pharmacologic class: Loop diuretic
Therapeutic class: Antihypertensive
Pregnancy risk category C

Action

Inhibits the reabsorption of sodium and chloride in the distal renal tubules and ascending limb of the loop of Henle; increases renal excretion of water, sodium, chloride, magnesium, hydrogen, and calcium. Also reduces fluid volume resulting from renal vasodilation.

Availability

Injection: 0.25 mg/ml
Tablets: 0.5 mg, 1 mg, 2 mg

Indications and dosages

➤ Edema caused by heart failure or hepatic or renal disease; adult nocturia

Adults: 0.5 to 2 mg/day P.O. as a single dose; up to two additional doses may be given q 4 to 5 hours (up to 10 mg/day) while patient is awake. Or 0.5 to 1 mg I.V. or I.M. repeated q 2 to 3 hours as needed, up to 10 mg/day.

Dosage adjustment
• Renal impairment
• Elderly patients

Off-label uses

• Drug-related edema

Contraindications

• Hypersensitivity to drug
• Uncorrected electrolyte imbalances
• Hepatic coma
• Anuria and oliguria

Administration

• Know that oral or I.V. route is preferred because I.M. route may cause pain at injection site.
• Dilute drug with dextrose 5% in water, normal saline solution, or lactated Ringer's injection.
• Give I.V. injection slowly over 2 minutes.
• Give P.O. form with food or milk.

Route	Onset	Peak	Duration
P.O.	30-60 min	1 hr	3-6 hr
I.V.	Within min	15-45 min	3-6 hr
I.M.	40 min	1-2 hr	4-6 hr

Adverse reactions

CNS: dizziness, encephalopathy, headache, insomnia, nervousness, vertigo, weakness, paresthesia, confusion, fatigue, hand-flapping tremor
CV: hypotension, electrocardiogram changes, chest pain, thrombophlebitis, **arrhythmias**
EENT: blurred vision, nystagmus, hearing loss, tinnitus
GI: nausea, vomiting, diarrhea, constipation, dyspepsia, dry mouth, anorexia, gastric irritation, acute pancreatitis, jaundice

GU: polyuria, nocturia, glycosuria, oliguria, increased blood urea nitrogen (BUN), premature ejaculation, difficulty maintaining erection, **renal failure**
Metabolic: dehydration, hyperglycemia, hyperuricemia, hypokalemia, hypochloremic alkalosis, hypomagnesemia
Musculoskeletal: arthralgia; muscle cramps, aching, or tenderness
Skin: photosensitivity, hives, rash, pruritus, urticaria, diaphoresis
Other: pain, nipple tenderness

Interactions

Drug-drug. *Aminoglycosides, cisplatin:* increased risk of ototoxicity
Amphotericin B, corticosteroids, mezlocillin, other diuretics, piperacillin, stimulant laxatives: additive hypokalemia
Anticoagulants, thrombolytics: increased bumetanide effects
Antihypertensives, nitrates: additive hypotension
Cardiac glycosides: increased risk of digoxin toxicity
Lithium: decreased lithium excretion, possible lithium toxicity
Neuromuscular blockers: prolonged neuromuscular blockade
Nonsteroidal anti-inflammatory drugs, probenecid: inhibition of diuretic response
Drug-diagnostic tests. *Calcium, magnesium, platelets, potassium, sodium:* decreased levels
Cholesterol, creatinine, glucose, nitrogenous compounds: increased levels
Drug-herb. *Dandelion:* interference with diuretic activity
Licorice: rapid potassium loss
Drug-behaviors. *Acute alcohol ingestion:* additive hypotension

Precautions

Use cautiously in:
• severe liver disease accompanied by cirrhosis or ascites, electrolyte depletion, diabetes mellitus, worsening azotemia
• elderly patients
• pregnant or breastfeeding patients
• children younger than age 18.

Patient monitoring

• Weigh patient at start of therapy, and monitor weight throughout therapy.
• Monitor blood pressure regularly.
• Monitor serum electrolyte, uric acid, urine glucose, and BUN levels.

Patient teaching

• Advise patient to take drug in morning to prevent nocturia, and to take second dose (if required) in late afternoon.
• Instruct patient to move slowly when sitting up or standing to avoid dizziness or light-headedness from blood pressure decrease.
• Caution patient to avoid alcohol because of increased risk of hypotension.
• Teach patient to eat foods high in potassium; provide other dietary counseling as appropriate to prevent or minimize electrolyte imbalances.
• Instruct patient to weigh himself often to help detect fluid retention.

buprenorphine hydrochloride
Buprenex, Subutex

Pharmacologic class: Opioid agonist-antagonist
Therapeutic class: Opioid analgesic
Controlled substance schedule III
Pregnancy risk category C

Action

Unknown; may bind to opiate receptors in CNS, altering perception of and response to painful stimuli while causing generalized CNS depression. Also has partial antagonist properties, which may lead to opioid withdrawal in patients who become physically dependent on drug.

Availability
Injection: 300 mcg (0.3 mg)/ml
Tablets (sublingual): 2 mg, 8 mg

Indications and dosages
➣ Moderate to severe pain
Adults: 0.3 mg I.M. or slow I.V. q 6 hours as needed. Repeat initial dose after 30 to 60 minutes.
Children ages 2 to 12: 2 to 6 mcg (0.002 to 0.006 mg)/kg I.M. or slow I.V. q 4 to 6 hours
➣ Opioid dependence
Adults: 12 to 16 mg/day S.L.
Dosage adjustment
• Elderly patients

Contraindications
• Hypersensitivity to drug
• Elderly patients
• Monoamine oxidase (MAO) inhibitor use within 14 days

Administration
◀€ Use extra caution when giving I.V.; drug may cause respiratory depression (especially initial dose).
• Mix with lactated Ringer's injection, dextrose 5% in water, or normal saline solution.
• When giving I.M., rotate injection sites to prevent induration and abscess.
• If patient is immobilized, reposition him frequently and keep head of bed elevated.

Route	Onset	Peak	Duration
I.V.	Immediate	2 min	6 hr
I.M., S.L.	15 min	1 hr	6 hr

Adverse reactions
CNS: confusion, malaise, hallucinations, dizziness, euphoria, headache, unusual dreams, psychosis, slurred speech, paresthesia, depression, tremor, agitation, **seizures, coma, increased intracranial pressure (ICP)**
CV: hypertension, hypotension, palpitations, tachycardia, Wenckebach block, **bradycardia**
EENT: blurred vision, diplopia, amblyopia, miosis, conjunctivitis, tinnitus
GI: nausea, vomiting, constipation, dry mouth, flatulence, ileus
GU: urinary retention
Respiratory: hypoventilation, dyspnea, cyanosis, apnea, **respiratory depression**
Skin: diaphoresis, clamminess, pruritus
Other: physical or psychological drug dependence, drug tolerance

Interactions
Drug-drug. *Antidepressants, antihistamines, sedative-hypnotics:* additive CNS depression
MAO inhibitors: increased CNS and respiratory depression, increased hypotension
Drug-herb. *Chamomile, hops, kava, skullcap, valerian:* increased CNS depression
Drug-behaviors. *Alcohol use:* increased CNS depression

Precautions
Use cautiously in:
• increased ICP; respiratory impairment; severe renal, hepatic, or pulmonary disease; hepatic coma; hypothyroidism; adrenal insufficiency; undiagnosed abdominal pain; prostatic hypertrophy; systemic lupus erythematosus; gout; kyphoscoliosis; diabetes mellitus; alcoholism; delirium tremens
• elderly patients
• pregnant or breastfeeding patients
• children younger than age 13.

Patient monitoring

• Monitor respiratory status throughout therapy.

Patient teaching

• Instruct patient to move slowly when sitting up or standing to avoid dizziness or light-headedness from blood pressure decrease.

• Tell patient to avoid driving and other hazardous activities until he knows how drug affects concentration and alertness.

• Advise patient to increase daily fluid intake to help prevent or minimize constipation.

---

bupropion hydrochloride
Wellbutrin, Wellbutrin SR, Zyban

Pharmacologic class: Aminoketone
Therapeutic class: Antidepressant, smoking-cessation aid
Pregnancy risk category B

Action

Unknown; believed to decrease neuronal reuptake of dopamine, serotonin, and norepinephrine in CNS. Action as smoking-cessation aid may result from noradrenergic or dopaminergic action.

Availability

Tablets: 75 mg, 100 mg
Tablets (sustained-release): 100 mg, 150 mg, 200 mg

⚕ Indications and dosages

➤ Depression
Adults: Initially, 100 mg P.O. b.i.d. (morning and evening). After 3 days, may increase to 100 mg t.i.d. After 4 weeks, may increase to a maximum dosage of 450 mg/day in divided doses. No single dose should exceed 150 mg. With total daily dosage of 300 mg, wait at least 6 hours between doses; with total daily dosage of 450 mg, wait at least 4 hours between doses. Alternatively, give one 150-mg sustained-release tablet daily; increase to 150-mg sustained-release tablet b.i.d. based on clinical response.

➤ Smoking cessation
Adults: 150-mg sustained-release tablet once daily for 3 days, then 150-mg sustained-release tablet b.i.d. for 7 to 12 weeks. Space doses at least 8 hours apart.

Contraindications

• Hypersensitivity to drug
• Seizures
• Anorexia nervosa
• Monoamine oxidase (MAO) inhibitor use within past 14 days
• Acute alcohol or sedative withdrawal
• Breastfeeding

Administration

• Avoid bedtime doses because they may worsen insomnia.
• Know that drug shouldn't be withdrawn abruptly.

Route	Onset	Peak	Duration
P.O.	Unknown	2 hr	Unknown
P.O. (sustained)	Unknown	3 hr	Unknown

Adverse reactions

CNS: agitation, headache, insomnia, mania, psychoses, depression, dizziness, drowsiness, tremor, anxiety, nervousness, **seizures**
CV: hypertension, hypotension, tachycardia, palpitations, **complete atrioventricular block**
EENT: blurred vision, amblyopia, auditory disturbances, epistaxis, rhinitis, pharyngitis
GI: nausea, vomiting, dyspepsia, abdominal pain, flatulence, mouth ulcers, dry mouth, altered taste, increased or decreased appetite

---

GU: urinary frequency, nocturia, vaginal irritation, testicular swelling
Metabolic: hyperglycemia, hypoglycemia, syndrome of inappropriate antidiuretic hormone secretion, increased libido
Musculoskeletal: arthralgia, myalgia, leg cramps, twitching, neck pain
Respiratory: bronchitis, increased cough, dyspnea
Skin: photosensitivity, dry skin, pruritus, rash, urticaria, diaphoresis, skin temperature changes
Other: weight gain or loss, hot flashes, fever, allergic reaction, flulike symptoms

Interactions
Drug-drug. *Benzodiazepine withdrawal, corticosteroids, other antidepressants, over-the-counter stimulants, phenothiazines, theophylline:* increased risk of seizures
Cimetidine: inhibition of bupropion metabolism
Levodopa, MAO inhibitors: increased risk of adverse reactions
Ritonavir: increased bupropion blood level
Drug-diagnostic tests. *Glucose:* increased level
Drug-behaviors. *Alcohol use or cessation:* increased risk of seizures
Sun exposure: increased risk of photosensitivity

Precautions
Use cautiously in:
• renal or hepatic impairment, unstable cardiovascular status
• elderly patients
• pregnant or breastfeeding patients
• children.

Patient monitoring
• Monitor blood pressure, electrocardiogram, complete blood count, and renal and hepatic function. Monitor tricyclic antidepressant (TCA) blood levels in patients taking TCAs concurrently.
• Assess patient for oral and dental problems.

Patient teaching
• Caution patient not to discontinue drug abruptly.
• Emphasize importance of frequent oral hygiene because dry mouth increases risk of caries and dental problems.
• Teach patient to avoid alcohol because it may increase risk of seizures.
• Advise patient to keep regular appointments for periodic blood testing and hepatic and renal studies.

buspirone hydrochloride
BuSpar

Pharmacologic class: Azaspirodecanedione
Therapeutic class: Anxiolytic
Pregnancy risk category B

Action
Unknown; believed to bind to serotonin and dopamine receptors in brain and increase norepinephrine metabolism; also thought to inhibit neuronal firing and reduce serotonin turnover in cortical, amygdaloid, and septohippocampal tissues.

Availability
Tablets: 5 mg, 7.5 mg, 10 mg, 15 mg, 30 mg

Indications and dosages
➤ Anxiety disorders; short-term relief of anxiety symptoms
Adults: 5 mg P.O. t.i.d.; increase by 5 mg/day q 2 to 3 days as needed (not to exceed 60 mg/day). Common dosage is 20 to 30 mg/day in divided doses.

Off-label uses
- Parkinsonian syndrome
- Symptomatic relief of depression

Contraindications
- Hypersensitivity to drug
- Severe renal or hepatic impairment
- Monoamine oxidase (MAO) inhibitor use within past 14 days

Administration
- Know that full benefit of therapy may take up to 2 weeks.

Route	Onset	Peak	Duration
P.O.	7-10 days	3-4 wk	Unknown

Adverse reactions
CNS: dizziness, drowsiness, nervousness, headache, insomnia, weakness, personality changes, numbness, paresthesia, tremor
CV: chest pain, palpitations, tachycardia, hypertension, hypotension
EENT: blurred vision, conjunctivitis, tinnitus, nasal congestion, sore throat, altered taste or smell
GI: nausea, vomiting, diarrhea, constipation, abdominal pain, dry mouth
GU: dysuria, urinary frequency or hesitancy, menstrual irregularities, menstrual spotting, libido changes
Musculoskeletal: myalgia, poor coordination
Respiratory: chest congestion, hyperventilation, dyspnea
Skin: rash, alopecia, blisters, pruritus, dry skin, easy bruising, edema, flushing, clamminess, excessive sweating
Other: fever

Interactions
Drug-drug. *Erythromycin, itraconazole:* increased buspirone blood level
MAO inhibitors: hypertension
Trazadone: increased risk of adverse hepatic effects
Drug-herb. *Hops, kava, skullcap, valerian:* increased CNS depression

Drug-food. *Grapefruit juice:* increased buspirone blood level and effects
Drug-behaviors. *Alcohol use:* increased CNS depression

Precautions
Use cautiously in:
- patients receiving concurrent anxiolytics or psychotropics
- pregnant or breastfeeding patients
- children.

Patient monitoring
- Monitor mental status closely.
- Assess hepatic and renal function regularly to detect drug toxicity.

Patient teaching
- Instruct patient to take drug with fluids.
- Advise patient not to use drug to manage everyday stress or tension.
- Instruct patient to avoid driving and other hazardous activities until he knows how drug affects concentration and alertness.
- Caution patient to avoid alcohol because it increases CNS depression.
- Emphasize importance of keeping follow-up appointments to check progress.

busulfan
Busulfex, Myleran

Pharmacologic class: Alkylating agent
Therapeutic class: Antineoplastic
Pregnancy risk category D

Action
Unknown; thought to interfere with bacterial cell wall synthesis by cross-linking strands of DNA and disrupting RNA transcription, causing bacterial cell to rupture and die. Overall, exhibits minimal immunosuppressant activity.

Availability
Injection: 6 mg/ml in 10-ml ampules
Tablets: 2 mg

🔵 Indications and dosages
➤ Chronic myelogenous leukemia
Adults: 4 to 8 mg P.O. daily until white blood cell (WBC) count falls to 15,000/mm^3; then discontinue drug until WBC count rises to 50,000/mm^3; then resume as needed. Or 4 to 8 mg P.O. daily until WBC count falls to 10,000 to 20,000/mm^3; then reduce daily dosage as needed to maintain WBC count at this level. (Dosage is highly variable, ranging from 2 to 4 mg/day.)
Children: 0.06 to 0.12 mg/kg/day P.O. or 1.8 to 4.6 mg/m^2/day P.O. Adjust dosage to maintain WBC count at 20,000/mm^3 but never below 10,000/mm^3.
➤ Allogenic hematopoietic stem cell transplantation
Adults: 0.8 mg/kg I.V. q 6 hours for 4 days. Starting 6 hours after 16th dose of busulfan injection, give cyclophosphamide 60 mg/kg/day I.V. over 1 hour for 2 days.

Off-label uses
• Adjunctive therapy in ovarian cancer
• Bone marrow transplantation

Contraindications
• Hypersensitivity to drug
• Patients not definitively diagnosed with chronic myelogenous leukemia
• Pregnancy or breastfeeding

Administration
• Give oral doses on an empty stomach.
• When administering I.V., withdraw dose from ampule using 5-micron filter needle. Remove filter needle and use new needle to add busulfan to diluent.

• Dilute for injection using dextrose 5% in water or normal saline solution.
• Follow facility procedures for safe handling, administration, and disposal of chemotherapeutic drugs.
• Maintain vigorous hydration to reduce risk of renal toxicity.
• Handle patient gently to avoid bruising.

Route	Onset	Peak	Duration
P.O.	1-2 wk	Wks	Up to 1 mo
I.V.	Unknown	Unknown	13 days

Adverse reactions
CNS: anxiety, confusion, depression, dizziness, headache, encephalopathy, weakness, **seizures, cerebral hemorrhage, coma**
CV: chest pain, hypotension, hypertension, tachycardia, thrombosis, atrial fibrillation, electrocardiogram changes, heart block, left-sided heart failure, **pericardial effusion, ventricular extrasystole, arrhythmias, cardiac tamponade, cardiomegaly**
EENT: cataracts, ear disorders, epistaxis, pharyngitis
GI: nausea, vomiting, diarrhea, constipation, abdominal pain, dyspepsia, abdominal enlargement, pancreatitis, hematemesis, dry mouth, stomatitis, anorexia
GU: oliguria, dysuria, hematuria, sterility, gynecomastia
Hematologic: myelosuppression
Hepatic: drug-induced hepatitis, hepatomegaly
Metabolic: hypokalemia, hypomagnesemia, hypophosphatemia, hyperuricemia, hyperglycemia
Musculoskeletal: arthralgia, myalgia, back pain
Respiratory: hyperventilation, dyspnea, **pulmonary fibrosis**
Skin: pruritus, rash, acne, alopecia, erythema nodosum, exfoliative dermatitis, hyperpigmentation

Other: allergic reactions, chills, fever, injection site infection or inflammation

Interactions

Drug-drug. *Anticoagulants, aspirin, nonsteroidal anti-inflammatory drugs:* increased risk of bleeding

Live-virus vaccines: decreased antibody response to vaccine, increased risk of adverse reactions

Myelosuppressives: additive bone marrow depression

Nephrotoxic and ototoxic drugs (such as aminoglycosides, loop diuretics): additive nephrotoxicity and ototoxicity

Thioguanine: increased risk of hepatotoxicity

Drug-diagnostic tests. *Alkaline phosphatase, aspartate aminotransferase, bilirubin, nitrogenous compounds (urea):* increased levels

Hemoglobin, white blood cells (WBCs): decreased values

Precautions

Use cautiously in:
• active infections, decreased bone marrow reserve, chronic debilitating disease, depressed neutrophil and platelet counts, seizure disorders, obesity
• patients receiving concurrent myelosuppressive or radiation therapy
• females of childbearing age.

Patient monitoring

◀️€ Know that diffuse pulmonary fibrosis (busulfan lung) is a rare but potentially life-threatening complication, with symptom onset as late as 10 years after therapy.
• Monitor patient closely for adequate hydration.
• Check for signs and symptoms of local or systemic infections.
• Assess for bleeding and excessive bruising.
• Evaluate oral hygiene regularly.

• Monitor complete blood count, WBC count, and platelet count daily if patient is receiving I.V. busulfan.
• Monitor renal and hepatic function.

Patient teaching

• Inform patient that drug doesn't cure leukemia but may induce remission.
• Advise patient to drink plenty of fluids to avoid dehydration.
• Instruct patient to immediately report inability to eat or drink; prescriber may add another drug to encourage his appetite.
• Inform patient that he's at increased risk for infection. Advise him to avoid contact with people who are obviously sick and to avoid public transportation, if possible.
• Tell patient he's at increased risk for bleeding and bruising.
• Tell patient to avoid activities that can cause injury. Advise him to use soft toothbrush and electric razor to avoid gum and skin injury.
• Inform patient that he'll undergo frequent blood testing to monitor drug effects.

butorphanol tartrate
Stadol, Stadol NS

Pharmacologic class: Agonist-antagonist
Therapeutic class: Opioid analgesic
Controlled substance schedule IV
Pregnancy risk category C

Action

Alters perception of and emotional response to pain by binding with opiate receptors in the brain, causing depression of the CNS. Also exerts antagonistic activity at opioid receptors, reduc-

---

🍁 Canada   ◀️€ Clinical alert   Reactions in **bold** are life-threatening

ing the risk of toxicity, drug dependence, and respiratory depression.

Availability
Injection: 1 mg/ml, 2 mg/ml
Nasal spray: 10 mg/ml

Indications and dosages
➤ Moderate to severe pain
Adults: 1 to 4 mg I.M. q 3 to 4 hours as needed or around the clock, not to exceed 4 mg/dose. Or 0.5 to 2 mg I.V. q 3 to 4 hours as needed or around the clock. With nasal spray, 1 mg (one spray in one nostril) q 3 to 4 hours, repeated in 60 to 90 minutes if pain relief is inadequate.
Dosage adjustment
• Elderly patients

➤ Labor pains
Adults: 1 to 2 mg I.V. or I.M., repeated after 4 hours as needed
➤ Preoperative anesthesia
Adults: 2 mg I.M. 60 to 90 minutes before surgery
➤ Balanced anesthesia
Adults: 2 mg I.V. 60 to 90 minutes before anesthesia induction, or 0.5 to 1 mg I.V. in increments during anesthesia
Dosage adjustment
• Elderly patients

Off-label uses
• Headache
• Symptomatic relief of ureteral colic

Contraindications
• Hypersensitivity to drug

Administration
• Make sure solution is clear and free of particulate matter before giving.
• When using nasal spray, insert tip of the sprayer about ¼″ into nostril, point tip backwards, and administer one spray.
• Be aware that I.V. route is preferred for severe pain.

◀ Know that drug may cause infant respiratory distress in neonate of pregnant patient, especially if administered within 2 hours of delivery.

Route	Onset	Peak	Duration
I.V.	2-3 min	30-60 min	3-4 hr
I.M.	10-15 min	30-60 min	3-4 hr
Intranasal	15 min	1-2 hr	4-5 hr

Adverse reactions
CNS: drowsiness, sedation, dizziness, tremor, irritability, syncope, stimulation
CV: hypertension, hypotension, arrhythmias, palpitations, bradycardia, tachycardia, extrasystole
EENT: blurred vision, nasal stuffiness or dryness, dry or sore throat
GI: nausea, vomiting, constipation, GI tract obstruction, epigastric distress, increased or decreased appetite, dry mouth
GU: urinary retention or hesitancy, dysuria, early menses, decreased libido, impotence
Hematologic: hemolytic anemia, hypoplastic anemia, **thrombocytopenia, agranulocytosis, leukopenia, pancytopenia**
Respiratory: thickened bronchial secretions, chest tightness, wheezing
Skin: urticaria, rash, diaphoresis (with parenteral use)
Other: weight gain, local stinging, **anaphylactic shock, hypersensitivity reaction** (with I.V. use)

Interactions
Drug-drug. *CNS depressants:* additive CNS effects
Drug-behaviors. *Alcohol use:* additive CNS effects

Precautions
Use cautiously in:
• head injury, ventricular dysfunction, coronary insufficiency, respiratory dis-

ease or depression, renal or hepatic dysfunction.

Patient monitoring

• Monitor respiratory status closely, especially after I.V. administration.
• Watch for signs and symptoms of withdrawal in long-term use and in opioid-dependent patients.
• Assess elderly patient closely for sensitivity to opioid analgesic.

Patient teaching

• Teach patient how to use nasal spray properly.
• Emphasize importance of using drug exactly as prescribed.
• Advise patient to avoid driving and other hazardous activities until he knows how drug affects concentration and alertness.
• Caution patient that drug may be habit-forming.

calcitonin (human)
Cibacalcin

calcitonin (salmon)
Calcimar, Caltine, Miacalcin, Miacalcin Nasal Spray, Salmonine

Pharmacologic class: Hormone (calcium-lowering)
Therapeutic class: Hypocalcemic
Pregnancy risk category C

Action

Directly affects bone, kidney, and GI tract. Decreases osteoclastic osteolysis in bone; also reduces mineral release and matrix or collagen breakdown in bone and promotes renal excretion of calcium. In pain relief, acts through prostaglandin inhibition, pain threshold modification, or beta-endorphin stimulation.

Availability

Injection: 0.5 mg/ml (human), 1 mg/ml (human), 200 IU/ml in 2-ml vials (salmon)
Nasal spray: 200 IU/actuation in 2-ml bottles (salmon)

⟩ Indications and dosages

➤ Postmenopausal osteoporosis
Adults: *Calcitonin (salmon)*—100 IU/day I.M. or S.C. or 200 IU/day intranasally
➤ Paget's disease of bone (osteitis deformans)
Adults: *Calcitonin (salmon)*—Initially, 100 IU/day I.M. or S.C.; after titration, maintenance dosage is 50 to 100 IU daily or every other day (three times a week). *Calcitonin (human)*—0.5 mg I.M. or S.C. daily, reduced to 0.25 mg daily
➤ Hypercalcemia
Adults: *Calcitonin (salmon)*—4 IU/kg I.M. or S.C. q 12 hours; after 1 or 2 days, may increase to 8 IU/kg q 12 hours; after 2 more days, may increase further, if needed, to 8 IU q 6 hours

Contraindications

• Hypersensitivity to drug
• Pregnancy or breastfeeding

Administration

◀⟨ Before calcitonin salmon therapy begins, perform skin test, if ordered; don't administer drug if patient has positive reaction.
• Give intranasal dose as one spray in one nostril daily; alternate nostrils every day.
• To minimize adverse effects, give at bedtime.
• Rotate injection sites to decrease inflammatory reactions.

Route	Onset	Peak	Duration
I.M., S.C.	15 min	4 hr	8-24 hr
Intranasal	Rapid	0.5 hr	1 hr

Adverse reactions

CNS: headache, weakness, dizziness, paresthesia

CV: chest pain

EENT: epistaxis, nasal irritation, rhinitis

GI: nausea, vomiting, diarrhea, epigastric pain or discomfort, altered taste

GU: urinary frequency

Musculoskeletal: arthralgia, back pain

Respiratory: dyspnea

Skin: rash

Other: allergic reactions (including facial flushing, swelling, tingling, tenderness in hands, and **anaphylaxis**)

Interactions

Drug-drug. *Previous bisphosphonate therapy (alendronate, etidronate, pamidronate, risedronate):* decreased response to calcitonin

Precautions

Use cautiously in:
• renal insufficiency, pernicious anemia
• children.

Patient monitoring

• Monitor for adverse reactions during first few days of therapy.
• Assess alkaline phosphatase level and 24-hour urinary excretion of hydroxyproline.
• Check urine for casts.

Patient teaching

• Instruct patient to take drug before bedtime to lessen GI upset. Tell him to call prescriber if he can't maintain his usual diet because of GI upset.
• Teach patient to consume a diet rich in calcium and vitamin D.
• Inform patient using nasal spray that runny nose, sneezing, and nasal irritation may occur during first several days as he adjusts to spray.

calcium carbonate

Alka-Mints, Alkets, Amitone, Calcarb 600, Calci-Chew, Calci-Mix, Calcite 500✤, Calcium 600, Calcium Antacid Extra Strength, Calglycine, Caltrate 600, Chooz, Dicarbosil, Equilet, Florical, Mallamint, Nephro-Calci, Nu-Cal✤, Os-Cal, Os-Cal 500, Oysco, Oyst-Cal 500, Oystercal 500, Rolaids Calcium Rich, Tums, Tums Calcium for Life Bone Health, Tums Calcium for Life PMS, Tums E-X, Tums Ultra

calcium chloride

Calciject✤

calcium citrate

Cal-Citrate-225, Cal-Citrate-250, Citracal, Citracal Liquitabs, Citrus Calcium

calcium glubionate

Calcionate, Calciquid, Neo-Calglucon

calcium gluceptate

calcium gluconate

calcium lactate

Cal-Lac

tricalcium phosphate

Posture

Pharmacologic class: Mineral

Therapeutic class: Dietary supplement, electrolyte replacement agent

Pregnancy risk category C (calcium acetate, chloride, glubionate, gluceptate, phosphate), *NR* (calcium carbonate, citrate, gluconate, lactate)

Action
Increases serum calcium level through direct effects on bone, kidney, and GI tract; decreases osteoclastic osteolysis by reducing mineral release and collagen breakdown in bone

Availability
Calcium acetate—
Capsules: 333.5 mg, 364 mg, 667 mg
Gelcaps: 667 mg
Tablets: 364 mg, 667 mg
Calcium carbonate—
Capsules: 1,250 mg
Lozenges: 600 mg
Oral suspension: 1,250 mg
Powder: 6.5 g
Tablets: 650 mg, 1,250 mg, 1,500 mg
Tablets (chewable): 750 mg, 1,000 mg, 1,250 mg
Tablets (gum): 300 mg, 450 mg, 500 mg
Calcium chloride—
Injection: 10% solution
Calcium citrate—
Tablets: 950 mg
Calcium glubionate—
Syrup: 1.8 g/5 ml (contains 115 mg of elemental calcium)
Calcium gluceptate—
Injection: 22% solution
Calcium gluconate—
Injection: 10% solution
Tablets: 500 mg, 650 mg, 975 mg
Calcium lactate—
Tablets: 325 mg, 500 mg, 650 mg
Tricalcium phosphate—
Tablets: 600 mg

ⓘ Indications and dosages
➤ Hypocalcemic emergency
Adults: 7 to 14 mEq I.V. of 10% calcium gluconate solution, 2% to 10% calcium chloride solution, or 22% calcium gluceptate solution
Children: 1 to 7 mEq calcium gluconate I.V.
Infants: Up to 1 mEq calcium gluconate I.V.

➤ Hypocalcemic tetany
Adults: 4.5 to 16 mEq I.V., repeated until tetany is controlled
Children: 0.5 to 0.7 mEq/kg I.V. three to four times daily until tetany is controlled
Neonates: 2.4 mEq/kg I.V. daily in divided doses
➤ Cardiac arrest
Adults: 0.027 to 0.054 mEq/kg calcium chloride I.V., 4.5 to 6.3 mEq calcium gluceptate I.V., or 2.3 to 3.7 mEq calcium gluconate I.V.
Children: 0.27 mEq/kg calcium chloride I.V., repeated in 10 minutes if needed. Check calcium level before giving additional doses.
➤ Magnesium intoxication
Adults: Initially, 7 mEq I.V.; subsequent dosages based on patient response
➤ Exchange transfusions
Adults: 1.35 mEq I.V. with each 100 ml of citrated blood
➤ Hyperphosphatemia
Adults: 1,334 to 2,000 mg calcium acetate P.O. daily, given in divided doses t.i.d. with meals
➤ Dietary supplement
Adults: 500 mg to 2 g P.O. daily

Off-label uses
• Osteoporosis

Contraindications
• Hypersensitivity to drug
• Ventricular fibrillation
• Hypercalcemia and hypophosphatemia
• Cancer
• Renal calculi
• Pregnancy or breastfeeding

Administration
• When infusing I.V., don't exceed rate of 0.5 to 2 ml/minute.
• I.V. route is preferred for children.
• Keep patient supine for 15 minutes after I.V. administration to prevent orthostatic hypotension.

• I.M. administration is never recommended.
• Administer P.O. doses 1 to 1½ hours after meals.

Route	Onset	Peak	Duration
P.O.	Unknown	Unknown	Unknown
I.V.	Immediate	Immediate	0.5-2 hr

Adverse reactions

CNS: headache, weakness, dizziness, syncope, paresthesia
CV: mild blood pressure decrease, vasodilation, **bradycardia, arrhythmias, cardiac arrest** (with rapid I.V. injection)
GI: nausea, vomiting, diarrhea, constipation, epigastric pain or discomfort, altered or chalky taste
GU: urinary frequency, renal calculi
Metabolic: hypercalcemia
Musculoskeletal: joint pain, back pain
Respiratory: dyspnea
Skin: rash
Other: excessive thirst, allergic reactions (including facial flushing, swelling, tingling, tenderness in hands and **anaphylaxis**)

Interactions

Drug-drug. *Atenolol, fluoroquinolones, tetracycline:* decreased bioavailability of these drugs
Calcium channel blockers: decreased calcium effects
Cardiac glycosides: increased risk of digoxin toxicity
Iron salts: decreased iron absorption
Sodium polystyrene sulfonate: metabolic alkalosis
Verapamil: reversal of verapamil effects
Drug-diagnostic tests. *Calcium:* increased level
Drug-food. *Foods containing oxalic acid (such as spinach), phytic acid (such as whole grain cereal), or phosphorus (dairy products):* interference with calcium absorption

Precautions

Use cautiously in:
• renal insufficiency, pernicious anemia, heart disease, sarcoidosis, hyperparathyroidism, hypoparathyroidism, renal calculi
• children.

Patient monitoring

• Monitor calcium levels, especially in elderly patients.

Patient teaching

• Instruct patient to consume plenty of milk and dairy products during therapy.
• Refer patient to dietitian for help in meal planning and preparation.

calcium polycarbophil

Equalactin, FiberCon, Fiber-Lax, FiberNorm, Konsyl, Mitrolan

Pharmacologic class: Bulk-forming agent
Therapeutic class: Laxative
Pregnancy risk category NR

Action

Absorbs water, thereby expanding and increasing bulk and moisture content of stool; increased bulk promotes peristalsis and bowel movement

Availability

Tablets: 500 mg
Tablets (chewable): 500 mg, 1,250 mg

⚕ Indications and dosages

➤ Constipation
Adults and children ages 12 and older: 1 g P.O. q.i.d. as needed; maximum dosage is 6 g daily.
Children ages 7 to 12: 500 mg P.O. one to three times daily as needed; maximum dosage is 3 g daily.

Children ages 3 to 6: 500 mg P.O. b.i.d. as needed; maximum dosage is 1.5 g daily.

➤ Diarrhea, irritable bowel syndrome
Adults and children ages 12 and older: 1 g P.O. q.i.d. as needed; maximum dosage is 6 g daily.
Children ages 7 to 12: 500 mg P.O. one to three times daily as needed; maximum dosage is 3 g in 24-hour period.
Children ages 3 to 6: 500 mg P.O. b.i.d. as needed; maximum dosage is 1.5 g daily.

Contraindications
• GI obstruction
• Difficulty swallowing

Administration
• Give with at least 8 oz of water or other fluid.
• Administer at least 2 hours before or after other drugs.
• Make sure patient maintains adequate fluid intake during therapy.

Route	Onset	Peak	Duration
P.O.	12-24 hr	3 days	Variable

Adverse reactions
CV: chest pain
GI: nausea, vomiting, abdominal pain, flatulence, rectal bleeding, **intestinal obstruction**
Respiratory: difficulty breathing
Other: laxative dependence

Interactions
Drug-drug. *Tetracyclines:* impaired tetracycline absorption
Drug-herb. *Lily of the valley, pheasant's eye, squill:* increased risk of adverse drug reactions

Precautions
Use cautiously in:
• pregnant or breastfeeding patients
• children.

Patient monitoring
• Assess for rectal bleeding or failure to respond to drug
• Monitor fluid intake and output; assess hydration status regularly.

Patient teaching
• Teach patient to take each dose with at least 8 oz of water or other fluid.
• Advise patient to space doses at least 2 hours apart from other drugs.
• Instruct patient to seek immediate medical attention if he experiences chest pain, vomiting, difficulty breathing, or rectal bleeding.
• Advise patient to tell prescriber if he's taking other drugs or if he has abdominal pain, nausea, vomiting, or sudden change in bowel habits lasting 2 weeks or longer.

candesartan cilexetil
Atacand

Pharmacologic class: Angiotensin II receptor antagonist

Therapeutic class: Antihypertensive

Pregnancy risk category C (first trimester), *D* (second and third trimesters)

Action
Blocks aldosterone-producing and vasoconstrictive effects of angiotensin II at various receptor sites, including vascular smooth muscle and adrenal glands

Availability
Tablets: 4 mg, 8 mg, 16 mg, 32 mg

Indications and dosages
➤ Hypertension
Adults: 16 mg P.O. daily. Start at lower dosage if patient is receiving diuretics or is volume depleted. Range is 2 to

32 mg/day as a single dose or divided in two doses.

Dosage adjustment
• Renal impairment

Contraindications
• Hypersensitivity to drug
• Pregnancy or breastfeeding
• Children (safety and efficacy not established)

Administration
• Give with or without food.

◀€ Supervise patient closely if he is receiving concurrent diuretics or is otherwise at risk for intravascular volume depletion.

• Know that diuretic may be added to regimen if drug alone doesn't control blood pressure.

Route	Onset	Peak	Duration
P.O.	2-4 hr	6-8 hr	24 hr

Adverse reactions
CNS: dizziness, syncope, fatigue, headache
CV: hypotension, chest pain, peripheral edema, **mitral or aortic valve stenosis**
EENT: ear congestion or pain, sinus disorders, sore throat, dental pain
GI: nausea, diarrhea, constipation, abdominal pain, dry mouth
GU: albuminuria, **renal failure**
Hepatic: drug-induced hepatitis
Metabolic: hyperkalemia, gout
Musculoskeletal: arthralgia, back pain, muscle weakness
Respiratory: upper respiratory tract infection, cough, bronchitis
Other: fever

Interactions
Drug-drug. *Diuretics, other antihypertensives:* increased risk of hypotension
Lithium: increased lithium blood level
Nonsteroidal anti-inflammatory drugs: decreased antihypertensive effect

Potassium-sparing diuretics, potassium supplements: increased risk of hyperkalemia
Drug-food. *Salt substitutes containing potassium:* increased risk of hyperkalemia

Precautions
Use cautiously in:
• heart failure, renal or hepatic impairment, obstructive biliary disorders
• volume- or salt-depleted patients receiving high doses of diuretics
• black patients
• females of childbearing age
• children younger than age 18.

Patient monitoring
• Monitor electrolyte levels and kidney and liver function test results.
• Assess blood pressure regularly to determine drug efficacy.
• Closely monitor patient with renal dysfunction who is receiving concurrent diuretics.

Patient teaching
• Instruct patient to practice reliable birth control and to contact prescriber if she suspects she's pregnant.
• Teach patient about lifestyle changes that help control blood pressure, such as diet, exercise, stress reduction, smoking cessation, and moderation of alcohol intake.

capecitabine
Xeloda

Pharmacologic class: Fluoropyrimidine, antimetabolite (pyrimidine analog)

Therapeutic class: Antineoplastic
Pregnancy risk category D

Action
Enzymatically converts to 5-fluoro-uracil; injures cells by interfering with DNA synthesis, cell division, RNA processing, and protein synthesis

Availability
Tablets: 150 mg, 500 mg

🕭 Indications and dosages
➤ Metastatic breast cancer resistant to both paclitaxel and chemotherapy regimen that includes anthracycline, or resistant to paclitaxel when further anthracycline therapy isn't indicated; metastatic colorectal cancer when treatment with fluoropyrimidine therapy alone is preferred

Adults: Initially, 2,500 mg/m²/day P.O. in two divided doses for 2 weeks, followed by 1-week rest period; administered in 3-week cycles

Dosage adjustment
• Renal impairment
• Hepatic impairment
• Elderly patients

Contraindications
• Hypersensitivity to drug
• Severe renal impairment
• Pregnancy or breastfeeding

Administration
• Give with water within 30 minutes after a meal.
• If dosage must be decreased because of toxicity, don't increase dosage later.

Route	Onset	Peak	Duration
P.O.	Unknown	1.5-2 hr	Unknown

Adverse reactions
CNS: dizziness, fatigue, headache, insomnia, paresthesia
CV: edema
EENT: eye irritation
GI: nausea, vomiting, diarrhea, constipation, abdominal pain, dyspepsia, anorexia, stomatitis, **intestinal obstruction**

Hematologic: anemia, lymphopenia, **neutropenia, thrombocytopenia**
Hepatic: hyperbilirubinemia
Metabolic: dehydration
Musculoskeletal: myalgia, limb pain
Skin: dermatitis, alopecia, nail disorder, hand and foot syndrome (palmar-plantar erythrodysesthesia)
Other: fever

Interactions
Drug-drug. *Antacids:* increased capecitabine blood level
Leucovorin: increased cytotoxicity
Phenytoin: increased phenytoin blood level
Warfarin: increased risk of bleeding
Drug-diagnostic tests. *Bilirubin:* increased level
Hemoglobin, neutrophils, platelets, white blood cells: decreased counts

Precautions
Use cautiously in:
• renal or hepatic impairment, severe diarrhea, coronary artery disease, intestinal disease, infection, coagulopathy
• children younger than age 18.

Patient monitoring
• Monitor patient for signs and symptoms of toxicity; be prepared to reduce dosage or withhold drug when indicated.
• Carefully assess fluid and electrolyte status if patient has severe diarrhea.
• Monitor weight, complete blood count, International Normalized Ratio, prothrombin time, and kidney and liver function test results.
• Evaluate closely for adverse reactions in patient older than age 80.

Patient teaching
• Instruct patient to immediately report nausea, vomiting, diarrhea, mouth ulcers, swollen joints, temperature above 100.5º F (38º C), or other signs or symptoms of infection.

• Teach patient to take drug with water and within 30 minutes after a meal.
• Tell patient to expect dosage adjustments during therapy.
• Advise patient to use reliable birth control method because drug may harm fetus if she becomes pregnant.
• Caution patient not to breastfeed during therapy.

captopril
Apo-Capto✤, Capoten, Gen-Captopril✤, Novo-Captopril✤, Nu-Capto✤

Pharmacologic class: Angiotensin-converting enzyme (ACE) inhibitor
Therapeutic class: Antihypertensive
*Pregnancy risk category C (*first trimester), *D (*second and third trimesters)

Action
Inhibits conversion of angiotensin I to angiotensin II (a vasoconstrictor); inactivates bradykinin and other vasodilatory prostaglandins. Increases plasma renin levels and reduces aldosterone levels, resulting in systemic vasodilation.

Availability
Tablets: 12.5 mg, 25 mg, 50 mg, 100 mg

⚕ Indications and dosages
➤ Hypertension
Adults: 12.5 to 25 mg P.O. two to three times daily. May be increased up to 150/mg/day at 1- to 2-week intervals; usual dosage is 50 mg t.i.d. If patient is receiving diuretics, start with 6.25 to 12.5 mg P.O. two to three times daily. If blood pressure isn't adequately controlled after 1 to 2 weeks, add diuretic, as prescribed. If further blood pressure decrease is needed, dosage may be

raised to 150 mg P.O. t.i.d. while patient continues on diuretic; maximum dosage is 450 mg/day.
➤ Heart failure
Adults: 25 mg P.O. three times daily; may be increased to 50 to 100 mg P.O. t.i.d. (range is 12.5 to 450 mg/day)
➤ Left ventricular dysfunction after myocardial infarction
Adults: 6.25 mg P.O. as a test dose, followed by 12.5 mg t.i.d.; may increase up to 50 mg t.i.d.
➤ Diabetic nephropathy
Adults: 25 mg P.O. t.i.d.
Dosage adjustment
• Renal impairment

Off-label uses
• Bartter's syndrome
• Hypertension associated with scleroderma
• Management of hypertensive crisis
• Raynaud's syndrome
• Rheumatoid arthritis
• Severe childhood hypertension

Contraindications
• Hypersensitivity to drug or other ACE inhibitors
• Angioedema (hereditary or idiopathic)
• Pregnancy

Administration
• Discontinue other antihypertensives 1 week before starting captopril, if possible.
• Give 1 hour before meals on empty stomach.

Route	Onset	Peak	Duration
P.O.	0.25-1 hr	1-1.5 hr	6-12 hr

Adverse reactions
CNS: headache, dizziness, drowsiness, fatigue, weakness, insomnia
CV: angina pectoris, tachycardia, **hypotension**
EENT: sinusitis

GI: nausea, diarrhea, anorexia, altered taste

GU: proteinuria, impotence, decreased libido, renal failure

Hematologic: anemia, **agranulocytosis, leukopenia, pancytopenia, thrombocytopenia**

Metabolic: hyperkalemia

Respiratory: eosinophilic pneumonitis, cough, asthma, bronchitis, dyspnea

Skin: rash, **angioedema**

Other: fever

Interactions

Drug-drug. *Allopurinol:* increased risk of hypersensitivity reaction

Antacids: decreased captopril absorption

Antihypertensives, general anesthetics that lower blood pressure, nitrates, phenothiazines: additive hypotension

Cyclosporine: hyperkalemia

Digoxin, lithium: increased blood levels of these drugs, increased risk of toxicity

Epoetin alfa: additive hyperkalemia

Indomethacin: reduced antihypertensive effect of captopril

Nonsteroidal anti-inflammatory drugs: decreased antihypertensive response

Potassium-sparing diuretics, potassium supplements: hyperkalemia

Probenecid: decreased elimination and increased blood level of captopril

Drug-diagnostic tests. *Alanine aminotransferase, alkaline phosphatase, aspartate aminotransferase, bilirubin, blood urea nitrogen, creatinine, potassium:* increased levels

Granulocytes, hemoglobin, platelets, red blood cells, sodium, white blood cells: decreased values

Urine acetone: false-positive result

Drug-food. *Any food:* decreased captopril absorption

Salt substitutes containing potassium: hyperkalemia

Drug-herb. *Capsaicin, yohimbine:* cough

Drug-behaviors. *Acute alcohol ingestion:* additive hypotension

Precautions

Use cautiously in:
• renal or hepatic impairment, hypovolemia, hyponatremia, aortic stenosis and hypertrophic cardiomyopathy, cardiac or cerebrovascular insufficiency, systemic lupus erythematous
• family history of angioedema
• black patients with hypertension
• elderly patients
• breastfeeding patients
• children.

Patient monitoring

◀€ Monitor for sudden blood pressure drop within 3 hours of initial dose if patient is receiving concurrent diuretics and on a low-sodium diet.
• Monitor hematologic, kidney, and liver function test results.
• Check for proteinuria monthly and after first 9 months of therapy.

Patient teaching

• Tell patient to take drug 1 hour before meals on empty stomach.
• Advise patient to report fever, rash, sore throat, mouth sores, fast or irregular heartbeat, chest pain, or cough.
• Inform patient that dizziness, fainting, and light-headedness usually disappear once his body adjusts to drug.
• Tell patient his ability to taste may decrease during first 2 to 3 months of therapy.
• Instruct patient not to discontinue drug without prescriber's approval.
• Caution patient to avoid over-the-counter medications unless approved by prescriber.

carbamazepine
Apo-Carbamazepine✿, Atretol,
Carbamaz✿, Carbatrol, Epitol,
Novo-Tegretol, Tegretol-XR

Pharmacologic class: Iminostilbene
derivative
Therapeutic class: Anticonvulsant
Pregnancy risk category D

Action
Unclear; chemically related to tricyclic
antidepressants (TCAs). Anticonvulsant action may result from reduction
in polysynaptic responses and blocking
of post-tetanic potentiation

Availability
Capsules (extended-release): 200 mg,
300 mg
Oral suspension: 100 mg/5 ml
Tablets: 200 mg
Tablets (chewable): 100 mg, 200 mg
Tablets (extended-release): 100 mg,
200 mg, 400 mg

Indications and dosages
➤ Prophylaxis of generalized tonic-
clonic, mixed, and complex-partial
seizures
Adults and children ages 12 and older:
Initially, 200 mg P.O. b.i.d. (tablets) or
100 mg q.i.d. (oral suspension); increase by 200 mg/day q 7 days until
therapeutic blood levels are reached.
Usual maintenance dosage is 600 to
1,200 mg/day in divided doses q 6 to 8
hours; in children ages 12 to 15, don't
exceed 1 g/day. Give extended-release
forms b.i.d.
Children ages 6 to 12: Initially, 100 mg
P.O. b.i.d. (tablets) or 50 mg q.i.d. (oral
suspension); increase by 100 mg/week
until therapeutic levels are reached.
Usual maintenance dosage is 400 to

800 mg/day; don't exceed 1 g/day. Give
extended-release forms b.i.d.
Children younger than age 6: Initially,
10 to 20 mg/kg/day P.O. in two or three
divided doses; may increase by 100 mg/
day at weekly intervals. Usual maintenance dosage is 250 to 350 mg/day;
don't exceed 400 mg/day.
➤ Trigeminal neuralgia
Adults: Initially, 100 mg b.i.d. or 50 mg
q.i.d. (oral suspension). Increase up to
200 mg/day until pain relief occurs;
then give maintenance dosage of 200 to
1,200 mg/day in divided doses. Usual
maintenance range is 400 to 800 mg/
day.

Off-label uses
• Alcohol, cocaine, or benzodiazepine
withdrawal
• Atypical psychoses
• Central diabetes insipidus
• Mood disorders
• Neurogenic pain

Contraindications
• Hypersensitivity to drug or TCAs
• Monoamine oxidase (MAO) in-
hibitor use within past 14 days
• Bone marrow depression
• Pregnancy or breastfeeding

Administration
• Don't give within 14 days of MAO
inhibitor.
• Don't give with grapefruit juice.
• Institute seizure precautions if drug
must be withdrawn suddenly.

Route	Onset	Peak	Duration
P.O.	Up to 1 mo	4-5 hr	6-12 hr
P.O. (extended)	Up to 1 mo	2-12 hr	12 hr

Adverse reactions
CNS: ataxia, drowsiness, fatigue, psychosis, syncope, vertigo, headache,
worsening of seizures

CV: hypertension, hypotension, **arrhythmias, atrioventricular block, aggravation of coronary artery disease, heart failure**

EENT: blurred vision, diplopia, nystagmus, corneal opacities, conjunctivitis, pharyngeal dryness

GI: nausea, vomiting, diarrhea, abdominal pain, stomatitis, glossitis, dry mouth, anorexia

GU: urinary hesitancy, retention, or frequency; albuminuria; glycosuria; impotence

Hematologic: eosinophilia, lymphadenopathy, **agranulocytosis, aplastic anemia, thrombocytopenia, leukopenia**

Hepatic: hepatitis

Metabolic: syndrome of inappropriate antidiuretic hormone secretion

Respiratory: pneumonitis

Skin: photosensitivity, rash, urticaria, diaphoresis, **erythema multiforme, Stevens-Johnson syndrome**

Other: weight gain, chills, fever

Interactions

Drug-drug. *Acetaminophen:* increased risk of acetaminophen-induced hepatotoxicity, decreased acetaminophen efficacy

Anticoagulants, bupropion: increased metabolism of these drugs, leading to decreased efficacy

Barbiturates: decreased barbiturate blood level, increased carbamazepine blood level

Charcoal: decreased carbamazepine absorption

Cimetidine, danazol, diltiazem: increased carbamazepine blood level

Cyclosporine, felbamate, felodipine, haloperidol: decreased blood levels of these drugs

Doxycycline: shortened doxycycline half-life, leading to decreased antimicrobial effect

Hormonal contraceptives: decreased contraceptive efficacy, possibly leading to pregnancy

Hydantoins: increased or decreased hydantoin blood level, decreased carbamazepine blood level

Isoniazid: increased risk of carbamazepine toxicity and isoniazid hepatotoxicity

Lithium: increased risk of CNS toxicity

Macrolide antibiotics (such as clarithromycin, erythromycin), propoxyphene, selective serotonin reuptake inhibitors (such as fluoxetine, fluvoxamine), verapamil: increased carbamazepine blood level, greater risk of toxicity

MAO inhibitors: high fever, hypertension, seizures, and possibly death

Nondepolarizing neuromuscular blockers: shortened carbamazepine duration of action

TCAs: increased carbamazepine blood level and greater risk of toxicity, decreased TCA blood level

Valproic acid: decreased valproic acid blood level with possible loss of seizure control, variable changes in carbamazepine blood level

Drug-diagnostic tests. *Blood urea nitrogen, eosinophils, liver function tests:* increased values

Granulocytes, hemoglobin, platelets, thyroid function tests, white blood cells: decreased values

Drug-food. *Grapefruit juice:* increased drug blood level and effects

Drug-herb. *Plantain (psyllium seed):* inhibited GI absorption of drug

Precautions

Use cautiously in:
• cardiac disease, hepatic disease, increased intraocular pressure, mixed seizure disorders, glaucoma
• elderly males with prostatic hypertrophy
• psychiatric patients.

Patient monitoring

• Assess for history of psychosis; drug may activate symptoms.
• Monitor baseline hematologic, kidney, and liver function test results.

• During dosage adjustments, monitor vital signs and fluid intake and output; stay alert for fluid retention, renal failure, and cardiovascular complications.
• With high doses, monitor complete blood count weekly for first 3 months and then monthly to detect bone marrow depression.

Patient teaching

• Teach patient to take drug with meals to minimize GI upset.
• Instruct patient to avoid driving and other hazardous activities until he knows how drug affects concentration, alertness, and vision.
• Advise patient that coating on extended-release capsules may be visible in stools because it isn't absorbed.
• Tell patient to avoid excessive sun exposure and to wear protective clothing and sunscreen.
• Inform female patient that drug may interfere with hormonal contraception; advise her to use alternative birth-control method.

carbidopa-levodopa
Sinemet, Sinemet CR

Pharmacologic class: Dopamine agonist
Therapeutic class: Antiparkinsonian
Pregnancy risk category C

Action

After conversion to dopamine in CNS, levodopa acts as a neurotransmitter, relieving symptoms of Parkinson's disease. Carbidopa prevents peripheral destruction of levodopa, making more levodopa available to be decarboxylated to dopamine in the brain.

Availability

Tablets: 10 mg carbidopa/100 mg levodopa, 25 mg carbidopa/100 mg levodopa, 25 mg carbidopa/250 mg levodopa
Tablets (extended-release): 25 mg carbidopa/100 mg levodopa, 50 mg carbidopa/200 mg levodopa

⚕️ Indications and dosages

➤ Idiopathic Parkinson's disease, parkinsonism, carbon monoxide or manganese intoxication
Conventional tablets—
Adults not currently receiving levodopa: Initially, 10 mg carbidopa/ 100 mg levodopa P.O. three to four times daily or 25 mg carbidopa/100 mg levodopa t.i.d.; may be increased q 1 to 2 days until desired effect occurs
Adults converting from levodopa alone (less than 1.5 g/day): Initially, 25 mg carbidopa/100 mg levodopa three to four times daily; may be increased q 1 to 2 days until desired effect occurs
Adults converting from levodopa alone (more than 1.5 g/day): Initially, 25 mg carbidopa/250 mg levodopa three to four times daily; may be increased q 1 to 2 days until desired effect occurs
Extended-release tablets—
Adults not currently receiving levodopa: Initially, 50 mg carbidopa/ 200 mg levodopa P.O. b.i.d., with doses spaced at least 6 hours apart
Adults converting from standard carbidopa-levodopa: Initiate therapy with at least 10% more levodopa content/day (may need up to 30% more) given at 4- to 8-hour intervals while awake; wait 3 days between dosage changes. Some patients may need higher dosages and shorter dosing intervals.

Contraindications

• Hypersensitivity to drug or tartrazine
• Angle-closure glaucoma
• Monoamine oxidase (MAO) inhibitor use within past 14 days

- Malignant melanoma
- Breastfeeding

Administration

- Give dose as close as possible to time ordered to ensure stable drug blood level.
- Know that giving extended-release form with food increases drug bioavailability.
- If patient needs general anesthesia, continue drug therapy as appropriate, provided he's allowed to have oral fluids and drugs.

Route	Onset	Peak	Duration
P.O.	Unknown	40-120 min	Unknown

Adverse reactions

CNS: anxiety, dizziness, hallucinations, memory loss, headache, numbness, confusion, insomnia, nightmares, delusions, psychotic changes, depression, dementia

CV: cardiac irregularities, palpitations, orthostatic hypotension

EENT: blurred vision, diplopia, mydriasis, eyelid twitching, tooth grinding (especially at night), difficulty swallowing

GI: nausea, vomiting, diarrhea, constipation, abdominal pain or discomfort, flatulence, excessive salivation, dry mouth, altered or bitter taste, burning sensation of tongue, anorexia, **upper GI hemorrhage** (with history of peptic ulcer)

GU: urinary retention, urinary incontinence, dark urine

Hematologic: hemolytic anemia, **leukopenia**

Hepatic: elevated alanine aminotransferase (ALT), alkaline phosphatase (ALP), aspartate aminotransferase (AST), bilirubin, blood urea nitrogen, low-density lipoprotein, and protein-bound iodine levels; **hepatotoxicity**

Musculoskeletal: muscle twitching, involuntary or spasmodic movements, poor coordination, worsening hand tremor

Respiratory: hyperventilation

Skin: melanoma, flushing, rash

Other: weight changes, hot flashes, abnormally dark sweat, hiccups

Interactions

Drug-drug. *Anticholinergics:* decreased carbidopa-levodopa absorption

Antihypertensives: additive hypotension

Haloperidol, papaverine, phenothiazines, phenytoin, reserpine: reversal of carbidopa-levodopa effects

Inhalation hydrocarbon anesthetics: increased risk of arrhythmias

MAO inhibitors: hypertensive reactions

Methyldopa: altered effectiveness of carbidopa-levodopa, increased risk of adverse CNS reactions

Pyridoxine: antagonism of carbidopa-levodopa effects

Selegiline: increased risk of adverse reactions

Drug-diagnostic tests. *ALP, ALT, AST, bilirubin, lactate dehydrogenase, uric acid:* increased levels

Coombs' test: false-positive result

Granulocytes, hemoglobin, platelets, white blood cells: decreased values

Urine glucose, urine ketones: test interference

Drug-food. *Foods rich in pyridoxine (liver, yeast, cereals):* reversal of carbidopa-levodopa effects

Drug-herb. *Kava:* decreased efficacy of carbidopa-levodopa

Octacosanol: worsening of dyskinesia

Drug-behaviors. *Cocaine use:* increased risk of adverse reactions to carbidopa-levodopa

Precautions

Use cautiously in:
- cerebrovascular, renal, hepatic, or endocrine disease
- history of cardiac, psychiatric, or ulcer disease
- pregnant patients

• children age 18 and under (safety not established).

Patient monitoring
• Monitor patient for orthostatic hypotension.
• Assess patient's need for drug "holiday" if his response to drug decreases.

Patient teaching
◀◥ Inform patient that muscle and eyelid twitching may indicate toxicity; tell him to report these symptoms immediately.
• Instruct patient to swallow extended-release tablets whole without crushing or chewing them.
• Instruct patient to move slowly when sitting up or standing to avoid dizziness or light-headedness caused by blood pressure decrease.
• Tell patient that drug may darken or discolor his urine and sweat.

carbidopa-levodopa-entacapone
Stalevo

Pharmacologic class: Dopamine agonist
Therapeutic class: Antiparkinsonian
Pregnancy risk category C

Availability
Tablets: 12.5 mg carbidopa/50 mg levodopa/200 mg entacapone; 25 mg carbidopa/100 mg levodopa/200 mg entacapone; 37.5 mg carbidopa/150 mg levodopa/200 mg entacapone

Action
After conversion to dopamine in CNS, levodopa acts as a neurotransmitter, relieving symptoms of Parkinson's disease. Carbidopa prevents peripheral destruction of levodopa, making more levodopa available to be decarboxylated to dopamine in the brain. Entacapone increases levodopa blood level by more than 30% and prolongs levodopa's effects.

Indications and dosages
➤ Idiopathic Parkinson's disease, postencephalitic parkinsonism, and symptomatic parkinsonism resulting from carbon monoxide or manganese intoxication (drug-induced extrapyramidal effects)
Adults: Optimal daily dosage determined by careful individual titration. Target carbidopa dosage is 70 mg to 100 mg P.O. daily, not to exceed 200 mg; maximum entacapone dosage is 1,600 mg P.O. daily. Patients should receive no more than eight tablets daily.

Contraindications
• Hypersensitivity to drug
• Malignant melanoma (or history of this disease)
• Monoamine oxidase (MAO) inhibitor use within 14 days
• Narrow-angle glaucoma
• Undiagnosed skin lesions
• Breastfeeding

Administration
• Give with meals if GI upset occurs.
• Don't crush or break tablets.

Route	Onset	Peak	Duration
P.O.	Unknown	2-3 hr	12 hr

Adverse reactions
CNS: involuntary movements, anxiety, dizziness, hallucinations, memory loss, psychiatric problems, increased hand tremor, headache, numbness, weakness, confusion, insomnia, nightmares, delusions, psychotic changes, depression, dementia, bradykinesia
CV: cardiac irregularities, palpitations, orthostatic hypotension, **arrhythmias**

EENT: blurred vision, mydriasis, diplopia, blepharospasm, sialorrhea, trismus

GI: nausea, vomiting, diarrhea, constipation, abdominal pain, dysphagia, burning sensation, flatulence, anorexia, **upper GI hemorrhage**

GU: urinary retention, urinary incontinence, dark urine, elevated blood urea nitrogen

Hematologic: hemolytic anemia, **leukopenia**

Hepatic: hepatotoxicity, elevated alanine aminotransferase (ALT), alkaline phosphatase (ALP), aspartame aminotransferase (AST), bilirubin, and lactate dehydrogenase (LD) levels

Metabolic: elevated protein-bound iodine level

Musculoskeletal: muscle twitching

Respiratory: hiccups, hyperventilation, pulmonary infiltrates

Skin: melanoma, rash

Other: weight changes, darkened sweat, flushing, hot flashes

Interactions

Drug-drug. *Ampicillin, chloramphenicol, cholestyramine, erythromycin, probenecid, rifampin:* interference with biliary excretion, additive increase in entacapone blood level

Anticholinergics: decreased levodopa absorption

Antihypertensives: additive hypotension

Haloperidol, papaverine, phenothiazines, phenytoin, reserpine: reversal of levodopa effects

Inhalation hydrocarbon anesthetics: increased risk of arrhythmias

MAO inhibitors: severe hypertension

Methyldopa: altered levodopa efficacy, increased risk of CNS adverse effects

Pyridoxine: antagonism of beneficial effects of levodopa

Drug-diagnostic tests. *ALP, ALT, AST, LD, bilirubin, uric acid:* increased levels

Coombs' test: false-positive results

Granulocytes, hemoglobin, platelets, white blood cells: decreased values

Urine tests for glucose or ketones: test interference

Drug-food. *Foods high in pyridoxine:* reversal of levodopa effects

Drug-herb. *Kava:* decreased levodopa efficacy

Octacosanol: worsening of dyskinesia

Precautions

Use cautiously in:
• biliary obstruction, renal disease, cerebrovascular disease, endocrine disorders, hepatic impairment, psychiatric disorders
• history of cardiac disease or GI ulcers
• pregnant patients
• children younger than age 18 (safety not established).

Patient monitoring

◀€ Monitor closely for mental changes, especially psychosis and depression. Report suicidal ideation immediately.
• Assess neurologic status closely to evaluate drug efficacy and identify adverse effects.
• Monitor complete blood count with white cell differential; also monitor liver function test results.
• Evaluate vital signs; watch for arrhythmias, orthostatic hypotension, and respiratory problems.
• Assess fluid intake and output; check for urinary problems.

Patient teaching

• Explain to patient or caregiver that drug may cause significant neurologic effects.
• Instruct patient or caregiver to report anxiety, dizziness, hallucinations, memory loss, increased hand tremor, headache, confusion, nightmares, and depression.
• Teach patient or caregiver about recommended home modifications and other safety measures to reduce risk of injury.

• Advise patient to rise slowly and carefully; drug may cause temporary blood pressure drop if he stands up suddenly.

• Instruct patient to avoid hazardous activities until disease is well controlled and he knows how drug affects concentration, alertness, vision, and motor function.

• Teach patient to minimize GI upset by eating small, frequent servings of healthy food and ensuring adequate fluid intake.

• Tell patient that he'll undergo regular blood testing while taking this drug.

carboplatin
Paraplatin, Paraplatin-AQ✤

Pharmacologic class: Alkylating agent
Therapeutic class: Antineoplastic
Pregnancy risk category D

Action
Inhibits DNA synthesis by causing cross-linking of parent DNA strands; interferes with RNA transcription, causing growth imbalance that leads to cell death. Cell-cycle-phase non-specific.

Availability
Injection: 50-mg, 150-mg, and 450-mg vials

⟋ Indications and dosages
➤ Initial treatment of advanced ovarian carcinoma or palliative treatment of ovarian carcinoma unresponsive to other chemotherapeutic modalities (given in combination with other agents)
Adults: Initially, 300 mg/m² I.V. (given with cyclophosphamide) at 4-week intervals. For refractory tumors, 360 mg/m² I.V. as a single dose; may be repeated at 4-week intervals, depending on response. However, single dose shouldn't be repeated until neutrophil count is at least 2,000/mm³ and platelet count at least 100,000/mm³. Subsequent dosages are based on blood counts.

Dosage adjustment
• Renal impairment
• Reduced bone marrow reserve

Off-label uses
• Advanced endometrial cancer
• Advanced or recurrent squamous cell carcinoma of head and neck
• Relapsed and refractory acute leukemia
• Small-cell lung cancer
• Testicular cancer

Contraindications
• Hypersensitivity to drug, cisplatin, or mannitol
• Pregnancy or breastfeeding

Administration
• Premedicate patient with antiemetics, as prescribed.
• Don't use with needles or I.V. sets containing aluminum.
• Make sure patient maintains adequate fluid intake during therapy.
• Be aware that reconstituted solution is stable at room temperature for 8 hours and should be discarded after that time.

Route	Onset	Peak	Duration
I.V.	Rapid	21 days	28 days

Adverse reactions
CNS: weakness, dizziness, confusion, peripheral neuropathy, **cerebrovascular accident**
CV: heart failure, embolism
EENT: visual disturbances, ototoxicity, altered taste
GI: nausea, vomiting, constipation, diarrhea, abdominal pain, stomatitis
GU: gonadal suppression, nephrotoxicity

✤ Canada   ◀€ Clinical alert   Reactions in **bold** are life-threatening

Hematologic: anemia, **leukopenia, thrombocytopenia**
Hepatic: increased blood urea nitrogen (BUN) and creatinine levels, **hepatitis**
Metabolic: hypocalcemia, hypokalemia, hypomagnesemia, hyponatremia
Respiratory: bronchospasm
Skin: alopecia, rash, urticaria, erythema, pruritus
Other: hypersensitivity reactions, **anaphylaxis**

Interactions

Drug-drug. *Aspirin, nonsteroidal anti-inflammatory drugs:* increased risk of bleeding
Live-virus vaccines: decreased antibody response to vaccine, increased risk of adverse reactions
Myelosuppressants: additive bone marrow depression
Nephrotoxic or ototoxic drugs (such as aminoglycosides, loop diuretics): additive nephrotoxicity or ototoxicity
Drug-diagnostic tests. *Alkaline phosphatase (ALP), aspartate aminotransferase (AST), BUN, creatinine:* increased levels
Electrolytes, hematocrit, hemoglobin, neutrophils, platelets, red blood cells, white blood cells: decreased counts

Precautions

Use cautiously in:
• hearing loss, electrolyte imbalances, renal impairment, active infections, diminished bone marrow reserve
• females of childbearing age.

Patient monitoring

• Assess for signs and symptoms of hypersensitivity reactions.
• Monitor complete blood count to help detect drug-induced anemia and other hematologic problems.
• Monitor ALP, AST, and total bilirubin levels.
• Evaluate fluid and electrolyte balance.

Patient teaching

• Instruct patient to report signs and symptoms of allergic response and other adverse reactions, such as breathing problems, mouth sores, rash, itching, and skin redness.
• Advise patient to report unusual bleeding or bruising.
• Caution patient to avoid driving and other hazardous activities until he knows how drug affects concentration and alertness.
• Teach patient to avoid activities that can cause injury; advise him to use soft toothbrush and electric razor to avoid gum and skin injury.
• Instruct patient to drink plenty of fluids to ensure adequate urinary output.
• Provide dietary counseling and refer patient to dietitian as needed if GI adverse effects significantly limit food intake.

carisoprodol
Soma, Vanadom

Pharmacologic class: Carbamate derivative
Therapeutic class: Centrally acting skeletal muscle relaxant
Pregnancy risk category C

Action

Unknown; may modify central perception of pain without modifying pain reflexes; skeletal muscle relaxation may result from sedative properties or from inhibition of activity in descending reticular formation and spinal cord.

Availability

Tablets: 350 mg

Indications and dosages
➤ Adjunctive treatment of muscle spasms associated with acute painful musculoskeletal conditions
Adults: 350 mg P.O. q.i.d.

Contraindications
• Hypersensitivity to drug or meprobamate
• Porphyria or suspected porphyria

Administration
• Give last daily dose at bedtime.
• Administer with food if GI upset occurs.
• If patient can't swallow, mix drug with syrup, chocolate, or jelly.

Route	Onset	Peak	Duration
P.O.	30 min	1-2 hr	4-6 hr

Adverse reactions
CNS: dizziness, drowsiness, agitation, ataxia, depression, headache, insomnia, vertigo, tremor, depression
CV: hypotension, tachycardia
GI: nausea, vomiting, epigastric distress
Hematologic: eosinophilia, **leukopenia**
Respiratory: asthma attacks
Skin: flushing (especially of face), rash, pruritus, **erythema multiforme**
Other: hiccups, fever, psychological drug dependence, **anaphylactic shock**

Interactions
Drug-drug. *Antihistamines, opioids, sedative-hypnotics:* additive CNS depression
Drug-diagnostic tests. *Eosinophils:* increased count
Drug-herb. *Chamomile, hops, kava, skullcap, valerian:* increased CNS depression
Drug-behaviors. *Alcohol use:* increased CNS depression

Precautions
Use cautiously in:
• severe liver or kidney disease

• pregnancy or breastfeeding
• children ages 12 and younger.

Patient monitoring
• When giving to breastfeeding patient, watch for signs of sedation and GI upset in infant.
• Monitor range of motion, stiffness, and discomfort level.

Patient teaching
• Tell patient to avoid over-the-counter drugs and alcohol because they may increase CNS depression.
• Instruct patient to avoid driving and other hazardous activities until he knows how drug affects concentration and alertness.
• Tell patient that psychological drug dependence may occur.

carmustine
BCNU, BiCNU, Gliadel

Pharmacologic class: Alkylating agent
Therapeutic class: Antineoplastic
Pregnancy risk category D

Action
Unknown; thought to interfere with bacterial cell wall synthesis by cross-linking strands of DNA and disrupting RNA transcription, causing bacterial cell to rupture and die. Overall, exhibits minimal immunosuppressant activity.

Availability
Intracavitary wafer implant: 7.7 mg (available in packages of eight wafers)
Powder for injection: 100-mg vials

Indications and dosages
➤ Brain tumor, multiple myeloma, Hodgkin's disease, other lymphomas (used alone or in conjunction with

other treatments, such as surgery or radiation)

Adults and children: 150 to 200 mg/m² I.V. as a single dose q 6 to 8 weeks, or 75 to 100 mg/m²/day for 2 days q 6 weeks, or 40 mg/m²/day for 5 days q 6 weeks. Repeat dose q 6 weeks if platelet count exceeds 100,000/mm³ and white blood cell (WBC) count exceeds 4,000/mm³.

➤ Adjunct to brain surgery

Adults: Up to 61.6 mg (eight wafers) implanted in surgical cavity created during brain tumor resection

Dosage adjustment
• Based on leukocyte and platelet counts

Off-label uses
• Mycosis fungoides

Contraindications
• Hypersensitivity to drug
• Radiation therapy
• Chemotherapy
• Pregnancy or breastfeeding

Administration
• Administer reconstituted I.V. infusion over 1 to 2 hours.
• Know that infusion lasting less than 1 hour causes intense pain and burning at I.V. site.
• Infuse solution in glass containers only; drug is unstable in plastic I.V. bags.
• Know that skin contact with reconstituted drug may cause transient hyperpigmentation. If contact occurs, wash skin thoroughly with soap and water.
• Know that oxidized regenerated cellulose may be placed over wafers to secure them against the surgical cavity surface.
• Irrigate resection cavity after wafer placement; be aware that dura should be closed in watertight fashion.

Route	Onset	Peak	Duration
I.V.	Immediate	15 min	6 wk
Intra-cavitary	Unknown	Unknown	Unknown

Adverse reactions
CNS: ataxia, drowsiness
GI: nausea, vomiting, diarrhea, esophagitis, stomatitis, anorexia
GU: renal failure, nephrotoxicity
Hematologic: anemia, azotemia, **leukopenia, thrombocytopenia, cumulative bone marrow depression, bone marrow dysplasia**
Hepatic: hepatotoxicity
Respiratory: pulmonary fibrosis, pulmonary infiltrates
Skin: alopecia, hyperpigmentation, facial flushing, abnormal bruising
Other: I.V. site pain, **secondary malignancies**

Interactions
Drug-drug. *Anticoagulants, aspirin, nonsteroidal anti-inflammatory drugs:* increased risk of bleeding
Antineoplastics: additive bone marrow depression
Cimetidine: potentiation of bone marrow depression
Digoxin, phenytoin: decreased blood levels of these drugs
Live-virus vaccines: decreased antibody response to vaccines, increased risk of adverse reactions
Drug-diagnostic tests. *Alkaline phosphatase, aspartate aminotransferase, bilirubin, nitrogenous compounds (urea):* increased levels
Hemoglobin, WBCs: decreased values
Drug-behaviors. *Smoking:* increased risk of respiratory toxicity

Precautions
Use cautiously in:
• infection; depressed bone marrow reserve; impaired respiratory, hepatic, or renal function
• females of childbearing age.

Patient monitoring

- Assess baseline kidney and liver function tests.
- Monitor complete blood count for up to 6 weeks after giving dose to detect delayed bone marrow toxicity.

Patient teaching

- Instruct patient to report signs and symptoms of allergic response and other adverse reactions, such as mouth sores and abnormal bruising or bleeding.
- Teach patient to avoid activities that can cause injury; advise him to use soft toothbrush and electric razor to avoid gum and skin injury.
- Advise patient to minimize GI upset by eating small, frequent servings of healthy food and drinking plenty of fluids.
- Instruct patient to monitor urinary output and report significant changes.
- Inform patient that drug may cause hair loss.
- Tell patient that severe flushing may follow I.V. dose but should subside in 2 to 4 hours.
- Advise patient that he'll undergo regular blood testing during therapy.

---

carteolol hydrochloride
Cartrol

Pharmacologic class: Beta-adrenergic blocker (nonselective)

Therapeutic class: Antianginal, antihypertensive

Pregnancy risk category C

Action

Blocks stimulation of cardiac $beta_1$-adrenergic receptor sites and pulmonary $beta_2$-adrenergic receptor sites. Shows intrinsic sympathomimetic activity, resulting in slowing of heart rate, decrease in myocardial excitability, reductions in cardiac output and oxygen consumption, decrease in renin release from kidneys, and reduction in blood pressure.

Availability
Tablets: 2.5 mg, 5 mg

⚠ Indications and dosages
➤ Hypertension

Adults: 2.5 mg P.O. daily, given alone or with diuretic; may be increased up to 10 mg daily. (Dosages above 10 mg may produce no further response or may decrease response.) Maintenance dosage is 2.5 to 5 mg P.O. daily.

Dosage adjustment
- Renal impairment
- Elderly patients

Off-label uses
- Angina pectoris

Contraindications
- Hypersensitivity to beta-adrenergic blockers
- Uncompensated heart failure
- Pulmonary edema
- Cardiogenic shock
- Bradycardia or heart block

Administration
- Give with or without food.
- Don't withdraw drug abruptly; doing so may lead to withdrawal phenomenon (angina exacerbation, myocardial infarction, ventricular arrhythmias, and even death).
- Store at controlled room temperature of 59° to 86° F (15° to 30° C).

Route	Onset	Peak	Duration
P.O.	Variable	1-3 hr	24-48 hr

Adverse reactions
CNS: fatigue, weakness, anxiety, depression, dizziness, insomnia, memory loss, nightmares, paresthesia, hallucinations, disorientation, slurred speech

---

CV: orthostatic hypotension, peripheral vasoconstriction, conduction disturbances, **bradycardia, heart failure**
EENT: blurred vision, dry eyes, tinnitus, nasal congestion or stuffiness, pharyngitis, dry mouth, **laryngospasm**
GI: nausea, vomiting, diarrhea, constipation, abdominal pain, anorexia
GU: impotence, decreased libido, Peyronie's disease, dysuria, polyuria, nocturia, dark urine
Metabolic: hyperglycemia, hypoglycemia
Musculoskeletal: arthralgia, back or leg pain, muscle cramps
Respiratory: wheezing, **bronchospasm, respiratory distress, pulmonary edema**
Skin: pruritus, rash, sweating
Other: drug-induced lupuslike syndrome, **anaphylaxis**

Interactions

Drug-drug. *Adrenergics:* antagonism of carteolol effects
Allergen immunotherapy: increased risk of anaphylaxis
Amphetamines, ephedrine, epinephrine, norepinephrine, phenylephrine, pseudoephedrine: unopposed alpha-adrenergic stimulation, causing excessive hypertension and bradycardia
Antihypertensives, nitrates: additive hypotension
Clonidine: increased hypotension and bradycardia, exaggerated withdrawal phenomenon
Digoxin: additive bradycardia
Dobutamine, dopamine: decrease in beneficial cardiovascular effects
General anesthetics, I.V. phenytoin, verapamil: additive myocardial depression
Insulin, oral hypoglycemics: altered efficacy of these drugs
Monoamine oxidase inhibitors: hypertension
Nonsteroidal anti-inflammatory drugs: decreased antihypertensive effect
Thyroid preparations: decreased carteolol efficacy

Drug-diagnostic tests. *Blood urea nitrogen, lipoproteins, potassium, triglycerides, uric acid:* increased levels
Glucose or insulin tolerance tests: test interference
Drug-behaviors. *Acute alcohol ingestion:* additive hypotension
Cocaine use: unopposed alpha-adrenergic stimulation, causing excessive hypertension and bradycardia
Sun exposure: photophobia

Precautions

Use cautiously in:
• renal or hepatic impairment, pulmonary disease, diabetes mellitus, hypoglycemia, thyrotoxicosis, hypotension, respiratory depression
• elderly patients
• pregnant or breastfeeding patients
• children.

Patient monitoring

• Monitor vital signs (especially blood pressure) and electrocardiogram.
• Evaluate renal function.
• Assess blood glucose levels regularly if patient has diabetes mellitus.

Patient teaching

◀≷ Caution patient not to stop using drug abruptly because doing so may lead to serious reactions.
• Instruct patient to report dizziness, confusion, depression, respiratory problems, or rash.
• Advise patient to move slowly when sitting up or standing to avoid dizziness or light-headedness from sudden blood pressure decrease.
• Caution patient to avoid driving and other hazardous activities until he knows how drug affects concentration and alertness.
• Inform male patient that drug may cause impotence; advise him to discuss this issue with prescriber.

carvedilol
Coreg

Pharmacologic class: Beta-adrenergic blocker (nonselective)
Therapeutic class: Antihypertensive
Pregnancy risk category C

Action
Blocks stimulation of cardiac beta$_1$-adrenergic receptor sites and pulmonary beta$_2$-adrenergic receptor sites. Also shows alpha$_1$-adrenergic blocking action,probably responsible for orthostatic hypotension occurrences.

Availability
Tablets: 3.125 mg, 6.25 mg, 12.5 mg, 25 mg

Indications and dosages
➤ Hypertension
Adults: Initially, 6.25 mg P.O. b.i.d.; may be increased q 7 to 14 days to a maximum dosage of 25 mg b.i.d.
➤ Heart failure caused by ischemia or cardiomyopathy (given with digoxin, diuretics, or angiotensin-converting enzyme inhibitors)
Adults: Initially, 3.125 mg P.O. b.i.d. for 2 weeks; may increase to 6.25 mg b.i.d. Dosage may be doubled q 2 weeks as tolerated, not to exceed 25 mg b.i.d. in patients weighing less than 85 kg (187 lb) or 50 mg b.i.d. in patients weighing more than 85 kg.

Off-label uses
• Angina pectoris
• Idiopathic cardiomyopathy

Contraindications
• Hypersensitivity to drug
• Uncompensated heart failure
• Pulmonary edema
• Cardiogenic shock
• Bradycardia or heart block
• Severe hepatic impairment
• Bronchial asthma
• Bronchospasm

Administration
• Give with food to slow absorption and minimize orthostatic hypotension.
• Be aware that addition of diuretic may cause additive effects and may worsen orthostatic hypotension.
• Know that full antihypertensive effect takes 7 to 14 days.
• Don't withdraw drug abruptly because this may lead to withdrawal phenomenon (angina exacerbation, myocardial infarction, ventricular arrhythmias, and even death).

Route	Onset	Peak	Duration
P.O.	Within 1 hr	1-2 hr	12 hr

Adverse reactions
CNS: dizziness, fatigue, anxiety, depression, insomnia, memory loss, nervousness, nightmares, headache, pain, vertigo
CV: orthostatic hypotension, peripheral vasoconstriction, angina pectoris, chest pain, hypertension, **bradycardia, heart failure, atrioventricular block**
EENT: blurred or abnormal vision, dry eyes, nasal stuffiness, rhinitis, sinusitis, pharyngitis
GI: nausea, diarrhea, constipation
GU: urinary tract infection, hematuria, albuminuria, abnormal renal function, decreased libido, impotence
Hematologic: bleeding, **purpura, thrombocytopenia**
Metabolic: hypovolemia, hypervolemia, hyperglycemia, hypoglycemia, hypertriglyceridemia, hyponatremia, hyperuricemia, hypercholesterolemia, glycosuria, gout
Musculoskeletal: arthralgia, back pain, muscle cramps

C

Respiratory: wheezing, upper respiratory tract infection, dyspnea, bronchitis, **bronchospasm, pulmonary edema**
Skin: pruritus, rash
Other: weight gain, drug-induced lupuslike syndrome, viral infection, **anaphylaxis**

Interactions

Drug-drug. *Antihypertensives:* additive hypotension
Calcium channel blockers, general anesthetics, phenytoin (I.V.): additive myocardial depression
Cimetidine: increased carvedilol toxicity
Clonidine: increased hypotension and bradycardia, exaggerated withdrawal phenomenon
Digoxin: additive bradycardia
Dobutamine, dopamine: decrease in beneficial cardiovascular effects
Insulin, oral hypoglycemics: altered effectiveness of these drugs
Monoamine oxidase inhibitors: hypertension
Nonsteroidal anti-inflammatory drugs: decreased antihypertensive action
Rifampin, thyroid preparations: decreased carvedilol efficacy
Theophyllines: reduced theophylline elimination, antagonistic effect leading to decreased theophylline or carteolol efficacy
Drug-diagnostic tests. *Antinuclear antibodies:* increased titers
Blood urea nitrogen, glucose, lipoproteins, potassium, triglyceride, uric acid: increased levels
Drug-food. *Any food:* delayed drug absorption
Drug-behaviors. *Acute alcohol ingestion:* additive hypotension

Precautions

Use cautiously in:
• renal or hepatic impairment, pulmonary disease, diabetes mellitus, hypoglycemia, thyrotoxicosis, peripheral vascular disease, hypotension, respiratory depression
• elderly patients
• pregnant or breastfeeding patients
• children.

Patient monitoring

• Watch for signs and symptoms of hypersensitivity reaction.
• Assess baseline complete blood count and kidney and liver function test results.
• Monitor vital signs (especially blood pressure), electrocardiogram, and exercise tolerance.
• Measure blood glucose regularly if patient has diabetes mellitus; drug may mask signs and symptoms of hypoglycemia.

Patient teaching

• Instruct patient to take drug exactly as prescribed and with food.
◀€ Caution patient not to stop taking drug abruptly because serious reactions may occur.
• Instruct patient to move slowly when sitting up or standing to avoid dizziness or light-headedness from sudden blood pressure decrease.
• Caution patient to avoid driving and other hazardous activities until he knows how drug affects concentration and alertness.
• Inform male patient that drug may cause impotence; advise him to discuss this issue with prescriber.
• Advise patient to use soft-bristled toothbrush and electric razor to avoid gum and skin injury.

cascara sagrada
Aromatic Cascara Fluidextract,
Cascara, Cascara Sagrada
Fluidextract

Pharmacologic class: Stimulant,
irritant
Therapeutic class: Laxative
Pregnancy risk category C

Action
Exerts laxative action by direct effect
on colonic smooth musculature (stimulation of intramural nerve plexi); as a
result, peristalsis increases and concentration of fluid and ions in colon rises.

Availability
Aromatic fluidextract: 1g/ml
Fluidextract: 1 g/ml
Tablets: 325 mg

⚕ Indications and dosages
➢ Constipation
Adults and children ages 12 and older:
325-mg tablet or 2 to 6 ml of aromatic
fluidextract P.O. at bedtime

Contraindications
• Hypersensitivity to drug
• GI bleeding or obstruction
• Heart failure
• Appendicitis
• Alcoholism
• Breastfeeding

Administration
• Give on empty stomach at bedtime.
• Administer with 8 oz of water or other fluid.

Route	Onset	Peak	Duration
P.O.	30-45 min	6-12 hr	Unknown

Adverse reactions
GI: nausea, vomiting, diarrhea, enteropathy, anorexia
Metabolic: alkalosis, hypocalcemia, hypokalemia, **tetany**

Interactions
Drug-drug. *Antibiotics, digoxin, nitrofurantoin, oral anticoagulants, salicylates, tetracyclines:* decreased absorption of these drugs
Drug-diagnostic tests. *Calcium, potassium:* decreased levels
Glucose: increased level
Drug-herb. *Lily of the valley, pheasant's eye, squill:* increased adverse effects of drug

Precautions
Use cautiously in:
• pregnant patients.

Patient monitoring
• Assess patient for adverse GI and metabolic reactions.
• Monitor serum calcium level.

Patient teaching
• Emphasize importance of taking drug with full glass of water or other fluid.
• Tell patient to consume adequate dietary fiber and to drink plenty of fluids to help reduce the need for laxatives.
• Inform patient that drug may turn urine yellowish brown.

caspofungin acetate
Cancidas

Pharmacologic class: Glucan synthesis
inhibitor
Therapeutic class: Antifungal
Pregnancy risk category C

Action

Inhibits synthesis of beta (1, 3)-D-glucan, an important component of cell wall in *Aspergillus* and other fungal cells; this inhibition leads to cell rupture and death.

Availability

Lyophilized powder for injection: 50 mg and 75 mg in single-use vials

/ Indications and dosages

➤ Invasive aspergillosis in patients refractory to or intolerant of other therapies
Adults: 70 mg I.V. as a single loading dose on first day, followed by 50 mg/day thereafter

Contraindications

• Hypersensitivity to drug

Administration

• Administer by slow I.V. infusion over 1 hour.
• Don't mix with other medications or with diluents containing dextrose.

Route	Onset	Peak	Duration
I.V.	Immediate	9-11 hr	40-50 hr

Adverse reactions

CNS: headache, paresthesia
CV: tachycardia, phlebitis
GI: nausea, vomiting, diarrhea, abdominal pain, anorexia
Hematologic: eosinophilia, anemia
Metabolic: hypokalemia
Musculoskeletal: pain, myalgia
Respiratory: tachypnea
Skin: histamine-mediated symptoms (including rash, facial swelling, pruritus, and warm sensation)

Interactions

Drug-drug. *Cyclosporine:* markedly increased caspofungin blood level
Inducers of drug clearance, mixed inducers-inhibitors (carbamazepine, dexam-ethasone, efavirenz, nelfinavir, nevirapine, phenytoin, rifampin): reduced caspofungin blood level
Tacrolimus: possible altered tacrolimus blood level
Drug-diagnostic tests. *Alkaline phosphatase, eosinophils:* increased levels
Hemoglobin, potassium: decreased levels

Precautions

Use cautiously in:
• hepatic impairment
• bone marrow depression
• renal insufficiency
• pregnant or breastfeeding patients.

Patient monitoring

• Monitor I.V. site carefully for phlebitis or other complications.
• Monitor complete blood cell count and serum electrolyte levels, watching for signs and symptoms of hypokalemia.
• Watch for histamine-mediated signs and symptoms (rash, facial swelling, pruritus, and sensation of warmth).
• Monitor vital signs, especially for tachycardia and tachypnea.
• Monitor nutritional and hydration status.

Patient teaching

• Teach patient signs and symptoms of histamine-mediated symptoms; tell him when to notify prescriber.
• Teach patient to handle GI adverse effects by eating small frequent servings of healthy food and ensuring adequate fluid intake.
• Advise patient that drug can cause problems in vein used for infusion; encourage him to immediately report pain, swelling, or other symptoms.

Proteus mirabilis, and coagulase-negative staphylococci

Adults and children ages 13 to 17:
250 mg P.O. q 8 hours. For severe infections, 500 mg P.O. q 8 hours.
Children: 20 mg/kg/day P.O. in divided doses q 8 hours. For serious infections, 40 mg/kg/day P.O. in divided doses q 8 hours. Maximum dosage is 1g/day.

Dosage adjustment
• Renal insufficiency
• Elderly patients

Contraindications
• Hypersensitivity to cephalosporins or penicillins

Administration
• Obtain specimen for culture and sensitivity testing as necessary before starting therapy.
• Be aware that cross-sensitivity to penicillins may occur.
• Give extended-release tablets with food to enhance absorption.
• Don't give antacids within 2 hours of extended-release form.

Route	Onset	Peak	Duration
P.O.	Rapid	30-60 min	6-12 hr
P.O. (extended)	Unknown	1.5-2.5 hr	12 hr

Adverse reactions
CNS: headache, lethargy, paresthesia, syncope, **seizures**
CV: hypotension, palpitations, chest pain, vasodilation
EENT: hearing loss
GI: nausea, vomiting, diarrhea, abdominal cramps, oral candidiasis, **pseudomembranous colitis**
GU: vaginal candidiasis, **nephrotoxicity**
Hematologic: elevated blood urea nitrogen (BUN), bleeding, lymphocytosis, eosinophilia, hemolytic anemia, **hypoprothrombinemia, neutropenia, thrombocytopenia, agranulocytosis, bone marrow depression**

cefaclor
Apo-Cefaclor✽ Ceclor, Ceclor CD, Ceclor Pulvules, PMS-Cefaclor✽

Pharmacologic class: Second-generation cephalosporin
Therapeutic class: Anti-infective
Pregnancy risk category B

Action
Interferes with bacterial cell wall synthesis, causing cell to rupture and die

Availability
Capsules: 250 mg, 500 mg
Oral suspension: 125 mg/5 ml, 187 mg/5 ml, 250 mg/5 ml, 375 mg/5 ml
Tablets (extended-release): 375 mg, 500 mg

Indications and dosages
➤ Uncomplicated skin infections caused by *Staphylococcus aureus*
Adults and children ages 16 and older: 375 mg P.O. (extended-release tablet) q 12 hours for 7 to 10 days
➤ Pharyngitis and tonsillitis not caused by *Haemophilus influenzae*
Adults and children ages 16 and older: 375 mg P.O. (extended-release tablet) q 12 hours for 10 days
➤ Chronic bronchitis and acute bronchitis not caused by *H. influenzae*
Adults and children ages 16 and older: 500 mg P.O. (extended-release tablet) q 12 hours for 7 days
➤ Otitis media caused by *Staphylococcus pneumoniae, Staphylococcus pyogenes, H. influenzae,* and other staphylococci; lower respiratory tract infections caused by *H. influenzae, S. pyogenes,* and *S. pneumoniae;* pharyngitis and tonsillitis caused by *S. pyogenes;* urinary tract infections caused by *Klebsiella* species, *Escherichia coli,*

Hepatic: hepatic failure, hepatomegaly
Musculoskeletal: arthralgia
Respiratory: dyspnea
Skin: urticaria, maculopapular or erythematous rash
Other: chills, fever, superinfection, **anaphylaxis, serum sickness**

Interactions

Drug-drug. *Aminoglycosides, loop diuretics:* increased risk of nephrotoxicity
Antacids: decreased absorption of cefaclor extended-release tablets
Chloramphenicol: antagonistic effect
Oral anticoagulants: increased anticoagulant effect
Probenecid: decreased excretion and increased blood level of cefaclor
Drug-diagnostic tests. *Alanine aminotransferase, alkaline phosphatase, aspartate aminotransferase, bilirubin, BUN, creatinine, eosinophils, gammaglutamyltransferase, lactate dehydrogenase:* increased levels
Coombs' test, urinary 17-ketosteroids, urine glucose determination with nonenzyme-based tests (Clinitest): false-positive results
Hemoglobin, platelets, white blood cells: decreased values

Precautions

Use cautiously in:
• renal impairment, phenylketonuria
• history of GI disease (especially colitis)
• emaciated patients
• elderly patients
• pregnant or breastfeeding patients
• children.

Patient monitoring

• Assess complete blood count and kidney and liver function test results.
• Monitor for signs and symptoms of superinfection and other serious adverse reactions.

Patient teaching

• Instruct patient to take drug with food or milk to reduce GI upset.
• Teach patient to take drug exactly as prescribed and to complete entire course of therapy even if he feels better.
• Tell patient to report signs and symptoms of allergic response and other adverse reactions, such as rash, easy bruising, bleeding, severe GI problems, or difficulty breathing.
• Teach patient to avoid taking antacids within 2 hours of extended-release cefaclor.

cefadroxil
Duricef, Novo-Cefadroxil✤

Pharmacologic class: First-generation cephalosporin
Therapeutic class: Anti-infective
Pregnancy risk category B

Action

Interferes with bacterial cell wall synthesis, causing cell to rupture and die

Availability

Capsules: 500 mg
Oral suspension: 125 mg/5 ml, 250 mg/5 ml, 500 mg/5 ml
Tablets: 1 g

🖊 Indications and dosages

➤ Pharyngitis and tonsillitis caused by beta-hemolytic streptococci
Adults: 1 g/day P.O. or 500 mg P.O. b.i.d. for 10 days
Children: 30 mg/kg/day P.O. in divided doses q 12 hours for 10 days
➤ Skin infections caused by staphylococci and streptococci
Adults: 1 g/day P.O. or 500 mg P.O. q 12 hours

Children: 30 mg/kg/day P.O. in divided doses q 12 hours

➤ Urinary tract infections (UTIs) caused by *Proteus mirabilis, Escherichia coli,* and *Klebsiella* species

Adults: 1 to 2 g/day P.O. in divided doses q 12 hours

Children: 30 mg/kg/day P.O. in divided doses q 12 hours

Dosage adjustment
• Renal insufficiency
• Elderly patients

Off-label uses
• Bone and joint infections
• Unspecified respiratory infections

Contraindications
• Hypersensitivity to cephalosporins or penicillins

Administration
• Obtain specimen for culture and sensitivity testing as necessary before starting therapy.
• Give with or without food.

Route	Onset	Peak	Duration
P.O.	Rapid	1.5-2 hr	12-24 hr

Adverse reactions
CNS: headache, lethargy, paresthesia, syncope, **seizures**
CV: hypotension, palpitations, chest pain, vasodilation
EENT: hearing loss
GI: nausea, vomiting, diarrhea, cramps, oral candidiasis, **pseudomembranous colitis**
GU: vaginal candidiasis, **nephrotoxicity**
Hematologic: elevated blood urea nitrogen (BUN), bleeding, lymphocytosis, eosinophilia, hemolytic anemia, **hypoprothrombinemia, neutropenia, thrombocytopenia, agranulocytosis, bone marrow depression**
Hepatic: hepatic failure, hepatomegaly
Musculoskeletal: arthralgia

Respiratory: dyspnea
Skin: urticaria, maculopapular or erythematous rash
Other: chills, fever, superinfection, **anaphylaxis**

Interactions
Drug-drug. *Aminoglycosides, loop diuretics:* increased risk of nephrotoxicity
Oral anticoagulants: increased anticoagulant effect
Probenecid: decreased excretion and increased blood level of cefadroxil
Drug-diagnostic tests. *Alanine aminotransferase, alkaline phosphatase, aspartate aminotransferase, bilirubin, BUN, creatinine, eosinophils, gammaglutamyltransferase, lactate dehydrogenase:* increased levels
Coombs' test, urinary 17-ketosteroids, urine glucose determination with nonenzyme-based tests (Clinitest): false-positive results
Hemoglobin, platelets, white blood cells: decreased values

Precautions
Use cautiously in:
• renal impairment, phenylketonuria
• history of GI disease (especially colitis)
• elderly patients
• pregnant or breastfeeding patients
• children.

Patient monitoring
• Assess baseline complete blood count and kidney and liver function test results.
• Monitor for signs and symptoms of superinfection and other serious adverse reactions.
• Be aware that cross-sensitivity to penicillins may occur.

Patient teaching
• Teach patient to take with food or milk if GI upset occurs.

• Instruct patient to take drug exactly as prescribed and to complete entire course of therapy even if he feels better.
• Teach patient to report signs and symptoms of allergic response and other adverse reactions, such as rash, easy bruising, bleeding, severe GI problems, or difficulty breathing.

cefazolin sodium
Ancef, Kefzol

Pharmacologic class: First-generation cephalosporin
Therapeutic class: Anti-infective
Pregnancy risk category B

Action
Interferes with bacterial cell wall synthesis, causing cell to rupture and die

Availability
Powder for injection: 250 mg, 500 mg, 1 g, 5 g, 10 g, 20 g
Premixed containers: 500 mg/50 ml in dextrose 5% in water (D_5W), 1 g/50 ml in D_5W

Indications and dosages
➤ Respiratory tract infections caused by group A beta-hemolytic streptococci, *Klebsiella* species, *Haemophilus influenzae, Staphylococcus aureus,* and *Streptococcus pneumoniae;* skin infections caused by *S. aureus* and beta-hemolytic streptococci; biliary tract infections caused by *Escherichia coli, Klebsiella* species, *Proteus mirabilis,* and *S. aureus;* bone and joint infections caused by *S. aureus;* genital infections caused by *E. coli, Klebsiella* species, *P. mirabilis,* and strains of enterococci; septicemia caused by *E. coli, Klebsiella* species, *P. mirabilis, S. aureus,* and *S. pneumoniae;* endocarditis caused by *S. aureus* or beta-hemolytic streptococci

Adults: For mild infections, 250 to 500 mg q 8 hours I.V. or I.M. For moderate to severe infections, 500 to 1,000 mg I.V. or I.M. q 6 to 8 hours. For life-threatening infections, 1,000 to 1,500 mg I.M. or I.V. q 6 hours to a maximum dosage of 6 g/day.
Children: For mild to moderate infections, 25 to 50 mg/kg/day I.V. or I.M. in divided doses t.i d. or q.i.d. For severe infections, 100 mg/kg/day I.V. or I.M. in divided doses t.i.d. or q.i.d.
➤ Acute uncomplicated urinary tract infections (UTIs) caused by *E. coli, Klebsiella* species, *P. mirabilis,* and strains of *Enterococcus* and *Enterobacter* species
Adults: 1 g I.V. or I.M. q 12 hours
➤ Surgical prophylaxis
Adults: 1g I.V. or I.M. 30 to 60 minutes before surgery, then 0.5 to 1 g I.V. or I.M. q 6 to 8 hours for 24 hours. If surgery exceeds 2 hours, another 0.5- to 1-g dose I.M. or I.V. may be given intraoperatively.
➤ Pneumococcal pneumonia
Adults: 500 mg I.M. or I.V. infusion q 12 hours
Dosage adjustment
• Renal impairment
• Elderly patients

Contraindications
• Hypersensitivity to cephalosporins or penicillins

Administration
• Obtain specimen for culture and sensitivity testing as needed before starting therapy.
• For intermittent I.V. infusion, administer in volume-control set or in separate, secondary I.V. container.
• For direct I.V. injection, dilute reconstituted dose in 5 ml of sterile water for injection and administer slowly over 3 to 5 minutes.

• For I.M. use, reconstitute with sterile water for injection, bacteriostatic water, or normal saline solution for injection; shake well until dissolved.
• Inject I.M. into large muscle mass.

Route	Onset	Peak	Duration
I.V.	Rapid	End of infusion	6-12 hr
I.M.	Rapid	1-2 hr	6-12 hr

Adverse reactions

CNS: headache, lethargy, confusion, hemiparesis, paresthesia, syncope, **seizures**
CV: hypotension, palpitations, chest pain, vasodilation
EENT: hearing loss
GI: nausea, vomiting, diarrhea, abdominal cramps, oral candidiasis, **pseudomembranous colitis**
GU: elevated blood urea nitrogen (BUN), vaginal candidiasis, **nephrotoxicity**
Hematologic: bleeding, lymphocytosis, eosinophilia, hemolytic anemia, **hypoprothrombinemia, neutropenia, thrombocytopenia, agranulocytosis, bone marrow depression**
Hepatic: hepatic failure, hepatomegaly
Musculoskeletal: arthralgia
Respiratory: dyspnea
Skin: urticaria, maculopapular or erythematous rash
Other: chills, fever, superinfection, **anaphylaxis, serum sickness**

Interactions

Drug-drug. *Aminoglycosides, loop diuretics:* increased risk of nephrotoxicity
Chloramphenicol: antagonistic effect
Oral anticoagulants: increased anticoagulant effect
Probenecid: decreased excretion and increased blood level of cefazolin
Drug-diagnostic tests. *Alanine aminotransferase, alkaline phosphatase, aspartate aminotransferase, bilirubin,* *BUN, creatinine, eosinophils, gamma-glutamyltransferase, lactate dehydrogenase:* increased levels
Coombs' test, urinary 17-ketosteroids, urine glucose determination with nonenzyme-based tests (Clinitest): false-positive results
Hemoglobin, platelets, white blood cells: decreased values
Drug-behaviors. *Alcohol use:* acute alcohol intolerance (disulfiram-like reaction) when alcohol is consumed within 72 hours of drug administration

Precautions

Use cautiously in:
• renal impairment, phenylketonuria
• history of GI disease (especially colitis)
• emaciated patients
• elderly patients
• pregnant or breastfeeding patients
• children.

Patient monitoring

◀€ If patient is receiving high doses, monitor for extreme confusion, tonic-clonic seizures, and mild hemiparesis.
• Monitor complete blood count and kidney and liver function test results.
• Watch for signs and symptoms of superinfection and other serious adverse reactions.
• Be aware that cross-sensitivity to penicillins may occur.

Patient teaching

• Tell patient to report reduced urinary output, persistent diarrhea, bruising, or bleeding.
• Instruct patient to take drug exactly as prescribed and to complete full course of therapy even when he feels better.

---

cefdinir
Omnicef

Pharmacologic class: Third-generation cephalosporin
Therapeutic class: Anti-infective
Pregnancy risk category B

Action
Interferes with bacterial cell wall synthesis and division by binding to the cell wall, causing instability and death. Active against gram-negative and gram-positive bacteria but has expanded spectrum of activity against gram-negative bacteria. Overall, exhibits minimal immunosuppressant activity.

Availability
Capsules: 300 mg
Oral suspension: 125 mg/5 ml in 60- and 100-ml bottles

💋 Indications and dosages
➤ Acute bacterial otitis media caused by *Haemophilus influenzae, Streptococcus pneumoniae,* and *Moraxella catarrhalis*
Adults and children ages 13 and older: 300 mg P.O. q 12 hours or 600 mg P.O. q 24 hours for 10 days
Children ages 6 months to 12 years: 7 mg/kg P.O. q 12 hours for 5 to 10 days or 14 mg/kg P.O. q 24 hours for 10 days
➤ Uncomplicated skin and soft-tissue infections caused by *Staphylococcus aureus* and *Streptococcus pyogenes*
Adults and children ages 13 and older: 300 mg P.O. q 12 hours for 10 days; maximum dosage is 600 mg/day.
➤ Acute maxillary sinusitis caused by *H. influenzae, S. pneumoniae,* and *M. catarrhalis*
Adults and children ages 13 and older: 300 mg P.O. q 12 hours or 600 mg P.O.

q 24 hours for 10 days; maximum dosage is 600 mg/day.
Children ages 6 months to 12 years: 7 mg/kg P.O. q 12 hours or 14 mg/kg P.O. q 24 hours for 10 days
➤ Pharyngitis or tonsillitis caused by *S. pyogenes,* chronic bronchitis caused by *H. influenzae, S. pneumoniae,* and *M. catarrhalis*
Adults and children ages 13 and older: 300 mg P.O. q 12 hours for 5 to 10 days or 600 mg P.O. q 24 hours for 10 days; maximum dosage is 600 mg/day.
➤ Community-acquired pneumonia caused by *H. influenzae, Haemophilus parainfluenzae, S. pneumoniae,* and *M. catarrhalis*
Adults and children ages 13 and older: 300 mg P.O. q 12 hours for 10 days; maximum dosage is 600 mg/day.
Dosage adjustment
• Renal impairment

Contraindications
• Hypersensitivity to cephalosporins or penicillins

Administration
• Obtain specimens for culture and sensitivity tests as necessary before starting therapy.
• Give with or without food.
• Administer 2 hours before or after iron supplements or antacids that contain aluminum or magnesium.
• Give capsules, if possible, to diabetic patients (oral suspension contains 2.86 g of sucrose per teaspoon).

Route	Onset	Peak	Duration
P.O.	Rapid	2-4 hr	12-24 hr

Adverse reactions
CNS: headache, lethargy, paresthesia, syncope, **seizures**
CV: hypotension, palpitations, chest pain, vasodilation
EENT: hearing loss

GI: nausea, vomiting, diarrhea, abdominal cramps, oral candidiasis, **pseudomembranous colitis**
GU: vaginal candidiasis, **nephrotoxicity**
Hematologic: bleeding, elevated blood urea nitrogen (BUN), lymphocytosis, eosinophilia, hemolytic anemia, **hypoprothrombinemia, neutropenia, thrombocytopenia, agranulocytosis, bone marrow depression**
Hepatic: hepatic failure, hepatomegaly
Musculoskeletal: arthralgia
Respiratory: dyspnea
Skin: chills, fever, urticaria, maculopapular or erythematous rash
Other: superinfection, **anaphylaxis, serum sickness**

Interactions
Drug-drug. *Aminoglycosides, loop diuretics:* increased risk of nephrotoxicity
Antacids, iron-containing preparations: decreased cefdinir absorption
Oral anticoagulants: increased anticoagulant effect
Probenecid: decreased excretion and increased blood level of cefdinir
Drug-diagnostic tests. *Alanine aminotransferase, alkaline phosphatase, aspartate aminotransferase, bilirubin, BUN, creatinine, eosinophils, gamma-glutamyltransferase, lactate dehydrogenase:* increased levels
Coombs' test, urinary 17-ketosteroids, urine glucose determination with nonenzyme-based tests (Clinitest): false-positive results
Hemoglobin, platelets, white blood cells: decreased values
Drug-herb. *Angelica, anise, arnica, asafetida, bogbean, boldo, celery, chamomile, clove, danshen, fenugreek, feverfew, garlic, ginger, ginkgo, horse chestnut, horseradish, licorice, meadowsweet, onion, ginseng, papain, passionflower, poplar, prickly ash, quassia, red clover, turmeric, wild carrot, wild*

lettuce, willow: increased risk of bleeding

Precautions
Use cautiously in:
• renal impairment, phenylketonuria
• history of GI disease (especially colitis)
• elderly patients
• pregnant or breastfeeding patients
• children.

Patient monitoring
• Monitor complete blood count and kidney and liver function test results.
• Monitor for signs and symptoms of superinfection and other serious adverse reactions.

Patient teaching
• Tell patient he may take drug with or without food.
• Teach patient to report persistent diarrhea (more than four episodes daily) and other adverse effects.
• If patient uses antacids or iron-containing preparations (such as iron supplements), tell him to take them 2 hours before or after drug.
• Inform patient that drug may temporarily discolor stools.

cefditoren pivoxil
Spectracef

Pharmacologic class: Third-generation cephalosporin
Therapeutic class: Anti-infective
Pregnancy risk category B

Action
Interferes with bacterial cell wall synthesis and division by binding to the cell wall, causing instability and death. Active against gram-negative and gram-positive bacteria but has expanded spectrum of activity against gram-

negative bacteria. Overall, exhibits minimal immunosuppressant activity.

Availability

Tablets: 200 mg

⚠ Indications and dosages

➤ Mild to moderate pharyngitis and tonsillitis caused by *Streptococcus pyogenes*

Adults and children ages 12 and older: 200 mg P.O. b.i.d. for 10 days
➤ Mild to moderate uncomplicated skin and soft-tissue infections caused by *S. pyogenes* and *Staphylococcus aureus*

Adults and children ages 12 and older: 200 mg P.O. b.i.d. for 10 days
➤ Mild to moderate chronic bronchitis caused by *Haemophilus influenzae, Haemophilus parainfluenzae, Streptococcus pneumoniae,* and *Moraxella catarrhalis*

Adults and children ages 12 and older: 400 mg P.O. b.i.d. for 10 days
Dosage adjustment
• Renal impairment

Contraindications

• Hypersensitivity to cephalosporins, drug components, penicillins, or milk protein
• Inborn errors of metabolism
• Carnitine deficiency

Administration

• Obtain specimen for culture and sensitivity testing as needed before starting therapy.
• Administer with meals to increase drug's bioavailability.
• Give 2 hours before antacids or other drugs that reduce stomach acid.

Route	Onset	Peak	Duration
P.O.	Unknown	1.5-3 hr	8-10 hr

Adverse reactions

CNS: headache, lethargy, paresthesia, syncope, **seizures**

CV: hypotension, palpitations, chest pain, vasodilation
EENT: hearing loss
GI: nausea, vomiting, diarrhea, abdominal cramps, oral candidiasis, **pseudomembranous colitis**
GU: elevated blood urea nitrogen (BUN), vaginal candidiasis, **nephrotoxicity**
Hematologic: bleeding, lymphocytosis, eosinophilia, hemolytic anemia, **hypoprothrombinemia, neutropenia, thrombocytopenia, agranulocytosis, bone marrow depression**
Hepatic: hepatic failure, **hepatomegaly**
Metabolic: carnitine deficiency
Musculoskeletal: arthralgia
Respiratory: dyspnea
Skin: urticaria, maculopapular or erythematous rash
Other: chills, fever, drug fever, superinfection, **anaphylaxis, serum sickness**

Interactions

Drug-drug. *Aminoglycosides, loop diuretics:* increased risk of nephrotoxicity
Antacids, histamine$_2$-receptor antagonists: decreased cefditoren absorption
Oral anticoagulants: increased anticoagulant effect
Probenecid: decreased excretion and increased blood level of cefditoren
Drug-diagnostic tests. *Alanine aminotransferase, alkaline phosphatase, aspartate aminotransferase, bilirubin, BUN, creatinine, eosinophils, gammaglutamyltransferase, lactate dehydrogenase:* increased levels
Coombs' test, urinary 17-ketosteroids, urine glucose determination with nonenzyme-based tests (Clinitest): false-positive results
Hemoglobin, platelets, white blood cells: decreased values
Drug-food. *Moderate- or high-fat meal:* increased drug bioavailability

Precautions
Use cautiously in:
- renal impairment, phenylketonuria
- history of GI disease (especially colitis)
- emaciated patients
- elderly patients
- pregnant or breastfeeding patients
- children.

Patient monitoring
- Monitor complete blood count and kidney and liver function test results.
- Monitor for signs and symptoms of superinfection and other serious adverse reactions.
- Be aware that cross-sensitivity to penicillins may occur.

Patient teaching
- Teach patient to take drug with food to promote drug absorption.
- Advise patient to take drug exactly as prescribed and to continue to take full amount prescribed even when he feels better.
- Tell patient to avoid taking antacids within 2 hours of drug.
- Instruct patient to report signs and symptoms of allergic response and other adverse reactions, such as rash, easy bruising, bleeding, severe GI problems, or difficulty breathing.
- Tell patient not to take drug with other medications unless prescriber approves.

cefepime hydrochloride
Maxipime

Pharmacologic class: Fourth-generation cephalosporin
Therapeutic class: Anti-infective
Pregnancy risk category B

Action
Interferes with bacterial cell wall synthesis and division by binding to the cell wall, causing instability and death. Active against gram-negative and gram-positive bacteria but has expanded spectrum of activity against gram-negative bacteria. Overall, exhibits minimal immunosuppressant activity.

Availability
Powder for injection: 500-mg vial, 1-g vial, 2-g vial; 1-g and 2-g piggyback bottles; 1 g/15 ml vial

⚕ Indications and dosages
➤ Urinary tract infections (UTIs) caused by *Escherichia coli, Klebsiella pneumoniae,* and *Proteus mirabilis*
Adults: 500 mg to 1g by I.V. infusion or I.M. q 12 hours for 7 to 10 days
➤ Severe UTIs caused by *E. coli* or *K. pneumoniae,* moderate to severe skin infections caused by *Staphylococcus aureus* or *Streptococcus pyogenes*
Adults: 2 g by I.V. infusion q 12 hours for 10 days
➤ Febrile neutropenia
Adults and children ages 2 months to 16 years: 2 g by I.V. infusion q 8 hours for 7 days
➤ Complicated intra-abdominal infections caused by alpha-hemolytic streptococci, *E. coli, K. pneumoniae, Pseudomonas aeruginosa, Enterobacter* species, and *Bacteroides fragilis*
Adults: 2 g by I.V. infusion q 12 hours for 7 to 10 days (given with metronidazole)
➤ Moderate to severe pneumonia caused by *K. pneumoniae, P. aeruginosa, Enterobacter* species, and *Streptococcus pneumoniae*
Adults: 1 to 2 g by I.V. infusion q 12 hours for 10 days
Dosage adjustment
- Renal impairment

Contraindications

• Hypersensitivity to cephalosporins or penicillins

Administration

• Obtain specimen for culture and sensitivity testing as needed before starting therapy.

• Don't mix with ampicillin (at concentrations above 40 mg/ml), metronidazole, aminoglycosides, or aminophylline if ordered concurrently. Give each drug separately.

• For I.V. infusion, use small I.V. needle and large vein.

Route	Onset	Peak	Duration
I.V.	Rapid	End of infusion	12 hr
I.M.	Rapid	1-2 hr	12 hr

Adverse reactions

CNS: headache, lethargy, paresthesia, syncope, **seizures**
CV: phlebitis, hypotension, palpitations, chest pain, vasodilation, **thrombophlebitis**
EENT: hearing loss
GI: nausea, vomiting, diarrhea, abdominal cramps, oral candidiasis, **pseudomembranous colitis**
GU: vaginal candidiasis, **nephrotoxicity**
Hematologic: bleeding, elevated blood urea nitrogen (BUN), lymphocytosis, eosinophilia, hemolytic anemia, **hypoprothrombinemia, neutropenia, thrombocytopenia, agranulocytosis, bone marrow depression**
Hepatic: hepatic failure, hepatomegaly
Musculoskeletal: arthralgia
Respiratory: dyspnea
Skin: urticaria, maculopapular or erythematous rash, redness, swelling, induration
Other: chills, fever, superinfection, pain at I.M. site, phlebitis at I.V. site, **anaphylaxis, serum sickness**

Interactions

Drug-drug. *Aminoglycosides, loop diuretics:* increased risk of nephrotoxicity
Oral anticoagulants: increased anticoagulant effect
Probenecid: decreased excretion and increased blood level of cefepime
Drug-diagnostic tests. *Alanine aminotransferase, alkaline phosphatase, aspartate aminotransferase, bilirubin, BUN, creatinine, eosinophils, gamma-glutamyltransferase, lactate dehydrogenase:* increased levels
Coombs' test, urinary 17-ketosteroids, urine glucose determination with nonenzyme-based tests (Clinitest): false-positive results
Hemoglobin, platelets, white blood cells: decreased values
Drug-herb. *Angelica, anise, arnica, asafetida, bogbean, boldo, celery, chamomile, clove, danshen, fenugreek, feverfew, garlic, ginger, ginkgo, ginseng, horse chestnut, horseradish, licorice, meadowsweet, onion, papain, passionflower, poplar, prickly ash, quassia, red clover, turmeric, wild carrot, wild lettuce, willow:* increased risk of bleeding

Precautions

Use cautiously in:
• renal impairment, phenylketonuria
• history of GI disease
• elderly patients
• pregnant or breastfeeding patients
• children.

Patient monitoring

• Obtain specimen for culture and sensitivity testing as needed before starting therapy.

• Assess baseline complete blood count and kidney and liver function test results.

• Monitor for signs and symptoms of superinfection and other serious adverse reactions.

• Monitor for inflammation at infusion site.

• Be aware that cross-sensitivity to penicillins may occur.

Patient teaching

• Instruct patient to report reduced urinary output, persistent diarrhea, bruising, or bleeding.
• Advise patient not to take herbs without consulting prescriber.

cefixime
Suprax

Pharmacologic class: Third-generation cephalosporin
Therapeutic class: Anti-infective
Pregnancy risk category B

Action

Interferes with bacterial cell wall synthesis and division by binding to the cell wall, causing instability and death. Active against gram-negative and gram-positive bacteria but has expanded spectrum of activity against gram-negative bacteria. Overall, exhibits minimal immunosuppressant activity.

Availability

Oral suspension: 100 mg/5 ml
Tablets: 200 mg, 400 mg

⚕ Indications and dosages

➤ Uncomplicated gonorrhea caused by *Neisseria gonorrhoeae*
Adults and children weighing more than 50 kg (110 lb): 400 mg P.O. daily
➤ Uncomplicated urinary tract infections caused by *Escherichia coli* and *Proteus mirabilis;* otitis media caused by *Haemophilus influenzae, Moraxella catarrhalis,* and *Streptococcus pyogenes;* pharyngitis and tonsillitis caused by *S. pyogenes;* acute bronchitis and acute exacerbation of chronic bronchitis caused by *H. influenzae* and *Streptococcus pneumoniae*

Adults and children older than age 12 or weighing more than 50 kg (110 lb): 400 mg P.O. daily or 200 mg P.O. q 12 hours
Children ages 12 and younger or weighing 50 kg (110 lb) or less: 8 mg/kg P.O. daily or 4 mg/kg P.O. q 12 hours
Dosage adjustment
• Renal impairment

Contraindications

• Hypersensitivity to cephalosporins or penicillins

Administration

• Obtain specimen for culture and sensitivity testing as necessary before starting therapy.

Route	Onset	Peak	Duration
P.O.	Rapid	2-6 hr	24 hr

Adverse reactions

CNS: headache, lethargy, paresthesia, syncope, **seizures**
CV: hypotension, palpitations, chest pain, vasodilation
EENT: hearing loss
GI: nausea, vomiting, diarrhea, abdominal cramps, oral candidiasis, **pseudomembranous colitis**
GU: elevated blood urea nitrogen (BUN), vaginal candidiasis, **nephrotoxicity**
Hematologic: bleeding, lymphocytosis, eosinophilia, hemolytic anemia, **hypoprothrombinemia, neutropenia, thrombocytopenia, agranulocytosis, bone marrow depression**
Hepatic: hepatic failure, hepatomegaly
Musculoskeletal: arthralgia
Respiratory: dyspnea
Skin: urticaria, maculopapular or erythematous rash
Other: chills, fever, superinfection, **anaphylaxis, serum sickness**

Interactions

Drug-drug. *Aminoglycosides, loop diuretics:* increased risk of nephrotoxicity

Oral anticoagulants: increased anticoagulant effect

Probenecid: decreased excretion and increased blood level of cefixime

Drug-diagnostic tests. *Alanine aminotransferase, alkaline phosphatase, aspartate aminotransferase, bilirubin, BUN, creatinine, eosinophils, gammaglutamyltransferase, lactate dehydrogenase:* increased levels

Coombs' test, urinary 17-ketosteroids, urine glucose determination with nonenzyme-based tests (Clinitest): false-positive results

Hemoglobin, platelets, white blood cells: decreased values

Drug-herb. *Angelica, anise, arnica, asafetida, bogbean, boldo, celery, chamomile, clove, danshen, fenugreek, feverfew, garlic, ginger, ginkgo, ginseng, horse chestnut, horseradish, licorice, meadowsweet, onion, papain, passionflower, poplar, prickly ash, quassia, red clover, turmeric, wild carrot, wild lettuce, willow:* increased risk of bleeding

Precautions

Use cautiously in:
• renal impairment, phenylketonuria
• history of GI disease
• elderly patients
• pregnant or breastfeeding patients
• children.

Patient monitoring

• Monitor baseline complete blood count and kidney and liver function test results.
• Monitor for signs of superinfection and other serious adverse reactions.
• Be aware that cross-sensitivity to penicillins may occur.

Patient teaching

• Teach patient to take once-daily doses at same time each day.

• Tell patient to take drug as prescribed and to continue to take full amount prescribed even when he feels better.
• Teach patient to report signs and symptoms of allergic response and other adverse reactions, such as rash, easy bruising, bleeding, severe GI problems, or difficulty breathing.
• Advise patient not to take herbs without consulting prescriber.

cefmetazole sodium
Zefazone

Pharmacologic class: Second-generation cephalosporin
Therapeutic class: Anti-infective
Pregnancy risk category B

Action

Interferes with bacterial cell wall synthesis, causing cell to rupture and die

Availability

Powder for injection: 1 g/50 ml, 2 g/50 ml

🖊 Indications and dosages

➢ Respiratory tract infections, skin infections, urinary tract infections, gynecologic infections, gonorrhea, preoperative prophylaxis

Adults: 2 g I.V. q 6 to 12 hours. For gonorrhea, give 1 g I.M. with or 30 minutes after 1 g probenecid P.O.

Dosage adjustment
• Renal impairment

Contraindications

• Hypersensitivity to cephalosporins or penicillins

Administration

• Obtain specimen for culture and sensitivity testing as necessary before starting therapy.

• Don't give with products containing alcohol.

• Reconstitute powder for injection with sterile water for injection, bacteriostatic water, or normal saline solution for injection. As directed, drug may be diluted further and given as I.V. infusion.

• Administer in volume-control set or separate secondary I.V. container.

• Be aware that cross-sensitivity to penicillins may occur.

Route	Onset	Peak	Duration
I.V.	Unknown	Immediate	Unknown

Adverse reactions

CNS: headache, confusion, hemiparesis, lethargy, paresthesia, syncope, **seizures**

CV: hypotension, palpitations, chest pain, vasodilation

EENT: hearing loss

GI: nausea, vomiting, diarrhea, abdominal cramps, oral candidiasis, **pseudomembranous colitis**

GU: elevated blood urea nitrogen (BUN), vaginal candidiasis, **nephrotoxicity**

Hematologic: bleeding, lymphocytosis, eosinophilia, hemolytic anemia, **hypoprothrombinemia, neutropenia, thrombocytopenia, agranulocytosis, bone marrow depression**

Hepatic: **hepatic failure, hepatomegaly**

Musculoskeletal: arthralgia

Respiratory: dyspnea

Skin: urticaria, maculopapular or erythematous rash

Other: chills, fever, superinfection, **anaphylaxis, serum sickness**

Interactions

Drug-drug. *Oral anticoagulants:* increased risk of bleeding

Probenecid: increased cefmetazole blood level

Drug-diagnostic tests. *Coombs' test, urine glucose determination using Benedict's reagent:* false-positive results

Glucose, hematocrit: decreased levels

Drug-behaviors. *Alcohol use:* disulfiram-like reaction when alcohol is used within 48 to 72 hours of drug

Precautions

Use cautiously in:

• renal impairment, phenylketonuria

• history of GI disease

• elderly patients

• pregnant or breastfeeding patients

• children.

Patient monitoring

◀€ Monitor for extreme confusion, tonic-clonic seizures, and mild hemiparesis when giving high doses.

• Evaluate baseline complete blood count and kidney and liver function test results.

• Monitor for signs of superinfection and other serious adverse reactions.

• Be aware that cross-sensitivity to penicillins may occur.

Patient teaching

• Instruct patient to report reduced urinary output, persistent diarrhea, bruising, and bleeding.

cefonicid sodium
Monocid

Pharmacologic class: Second-generation cephalosporin

Therapeutic class: Anti-infective

Pregnancy risk category B

Action

Interferes with bacterial cell wall synthesis, causing cell to rupture and die

Availability

Powder for injection: 1 g

⚕ Indications and dosages

➢ Respiratory tract infections; skin infections; urinary tract infections; gynecologic infections; severe, life-threatening infections; preoperative prophylaxis

Adults: 0.5 to 1 g I.M. or I.V. q 24 hours; for severe, life-threatening infections, 2 g q 24 hours

Dosage adjustment
• Renal impairment

Contraindications

• Hypersensitivity to cephalosporins or penicillins

Administration

• Obtain specimen for culture and sensitivity testing as necessary before starting therapy.
• For injection, reconstitute powder in single-dose vial with sterile water for injection according to manufacturer's directions; shake well.
• Dilute reconstituted drug for infusion in 50 to 100 ml of compatible solution, such as normal saline solution, dextrose 5% in water (D_5W), dextrose 10% in water, half-normal saline solution, lactated Ringer's injection, D_5W and lactated Ringer's injection, 10% invert sugar in sterile water, or D_5W and 0.15% potassium chloride.
• When piggy-backing with primary I.V. fluids to give as a single dose, reconstitute with 50 to 100 ml of normal saline solution or other fluid listed above.
• For I.V. bolus, give reconstituted solution slowly over 3 to 5 minutes either directly or through tubing if patient is receiving parenteral fluids.
• Inject I.M. deep into large muscle mass; divide 2-g dose in half and inject into separate large muscle masses.

Route	Onset	Peak	Duration
I.V., I.M.	Unknown	Unknown	Unknown

Adverse reactions

CNS: headache, confusion, hemiparesis, lethargy, paresthesia, syncope, **seizures**
CV: hypotension, palpitations, chest pain, vasodilation
EENT: hearing loss
GI: nausea, vomiting, diarrhea, abdominal cramps, oral candidiasis, **pseudomembranous colitis**
GU: elevated blood urea nitrogen (BUN), vaginal candidiasis, **nephrotoxicity**
Hematologic: bleeding, lymphocytosis, eosinophilia, **hemolytic anemia, hypoprothrombinemia, neutropenia, thrombocytopenia, agranulocytosis, bone marrow depression**
Hepatic: hepatic failure, hepatomegaly
Musculoskeletal: arthralgia
Respiratory: dyspnea
Skin: urticaria, maculopapular or erythematous rash
Other: chills, fever, superinfection, **anaphylaxis, serum sickness**

Interactions

Drug-drug. *Aminoglycosides, loop diuretics:* increased risk of nephrotoxicity
Antacids: decreased cefonicid absorption
Chloramphenicol: antagonistic effect
Oral anticoagulants: increased anticoagulant effect
Probenecid: decreased excretion and increased blood level of cefonicid
Drug-diagnostic tests. *Alanine aminotransferase, alkaline phosphatase, aspartate aminotransferase, bilirubin, BUN, creatinine, eosinophils, gamma-glutamyltransferase, lactate dehydrogenase:* increased levels
Coombs' test, urinary 17-ketosteroids, urine glucose determination with nonenzyme-based tests (Clinitest): false-positive results
Hemoglobin, platelets, white blood cells: decreased values

Precautions

Use cautiously in:

- renal impairment, phenylketonuria
- history of GI disease
- elderly patients
- pregnant or breastfeeding patients
- children.

Patient monitoring

◀╪ Monitor for extreme confusion, tonic-clonic seizures, and mild hemiparesis when high doses are used.

- Monitor complete blood count and kidney and liver function test results.
- Assess for signs and symptoms of superinfection and other serious adverse reactions.
- Be aware that cross-sensitivity to penicillins may occur.

Patient teaching

- Advise patient to report reduced urinary output, persistent diarrhea, bruising, or bleeding.

cefoperazone sodium
Cefobid

Pharmacologic class: Third-generation cephalosporin
Therapeutic class: Anti-infective
Pregnancy risk category B

Action

Interferes with bacterial cell wall synthesis and division by binding to the cell wall, causing instability and death. Active against gram-negative and gram-positive bacteria but has expanded spectrum of activity against gram-negative bacteria. Overall, exhibits minimal immunosuppressant activity.

Availability

Powder for injection: 1 g, 2 g, 10 g

Premixed containers: 1 g/50 ml, 2 g/50 ml

🕖 Indications and dosages

➤ Respiratory tract infections caused by *Escherichia coli, Haemophilus influenzae, Enterobacter* species, *Klebsiella* species, *Proteus mirabilis, Staphylococcus aureus, Streptococcus pneumoniae, Streptococcus pyogenes,* and *Pseudomonas aeruginosa;* urinary tract infections caused by *E. coli* and *P. aeruginosa;* uncomplicated gonorrhea caused by *Neisseria gonorrhoeae;* gynecologic infections caused by gram-positive cocci, *Bacteroides* species, *E. coli, Clostridium* species, *Staphylococcus epidermidis,* and *Streptococcus agalactiae;* bacterial septicemia caused by *E. coli, Klebsiella* species, *Serratia marcescens, S. aureus,* and streptococci; skin and soft-tissue infections caused by *P. aeruginosa, S. aureus,* and *S. pyogenes;* intra-abdominal infections caused by gram-negative bacilli, *E. coli,* and *P. aeruginosa*

Adults: 1 to 2 g I.V. or I.M. q 12 hours; maximum dosage is 12 g/day. For severe infections, 6 to 12 g/day I.V. in divided doses two, three, or four times daily.

Dosage adjustment

- Renal impairment
- Hepatic impairment

Contraindications

- Hypersensitivity to cephalosporins or penicillins

Administration

- Obtain specimen for culture and sensitivity testing as necessary before starting therapy.
- Reconstitute powder for injection with at least 2.8 ml diluent per gram of cefoperazone, using a compatible solution, such as dextrose 5% in water (D₅W), D₅W and lactated Ringer's injection, D₅W and normal saline solution, dextrose 10% in water, lactated

---

Ringer's injection, or normal saline solution.

• For intermittent I.V. infusion, further dilute reconstituted drug with 20 to 40 ml of diluent per gram of cefoperazone; give over 15 to 30 minutes.

• For continuous I.V. infusion, dilute to final concentration of 2 to 25 mg/ml.

• For I.M. injection, dilute with bacteriostatic water or sterile water. For concentrations of 250 mg/ml or more, prepare solution using 0.5% lidocaine hydrochloride.

• Administer I.M. injection into large muscle mass.

• Don't mix with aminoglycosides. If both drugs are prescribed, give cefoperazone before aminoglycoside.

Route	Onset	Peak	Duration
I.V.	Rapid	End of infusion	12 hr
I.M.	Rapid	1-2 hr	12 hr

Adverse reactions

CNS: headache, lethargy, paresthesia, syncope, **seizures**
CV: hypotension, palpitations, chest pain, vasodilation
EENT: hearing loss
GI: nausea, vomiting, diarrhea, abdominal cramps, oral candidiasis, **pseudomembranous colitis**
GU: elevated blood urea nitrogen (BUN), vaginal candidiasis, **nephrotoxicity**
Hematologic: bleeding, lymphocytosis, eosinophilia, hemolytic anemia, **hypoprothrombinemia, neutropenia, thrombocytopenia, agranulocytosis, bone marrow depression**
Hepatic: hepatic failure, hepatomegaly
Musculoskeletal: arthralgia
Respiratory: dyspnea
Skin: urticaria, maculopapular or erythematous rash

Other: chills, fever, superinfection, I.M. injection site pain, **anaphylaxis, serum sickness**

Interactions

Drug-drug. *Aminoglycosides, loop diuretics:* increased risk of nephrotoxicity
Oral anticoagulants: increased anticoagulant effect
Probenecid: decreased excretion and increased blood level of cefoperazone
Drug-diagnostic tests. *Alanine aminotransferase, alkaline phosphatase, aspartate aminotransferase, bilirubin, BUN, creatinine, eosinophils, gammaglutamyltransferase, lactate dehydrogenase:* increased levels
Coombs' test, urinary 17-ketosteroids, urine glucose determination with nonenzyme-based tests (Clinitest): false-positive results
Hemoglobin, platelets, white blood cells: decreased values
Drug-herb. *Angelica, anise, arnica, asafetida, bogbean, boldo, celery, chamomile, clove, danshen, fenugreek, feverfew, garlic, ginger, ginkgo, ginseng, horse chestnut, horseradish, licorice, meadowsweet, onion, papain, passionflower, poplar, prickly ash, Quassia, red clover, turmeric, wild carrot, wild lettuce, willow:* increased risk of bleeding

Precautions

Use cautiously in:
• renal impairment, phenylketonuria
• history of GI disease
• elderly patients
• pregnant or breastfeeding patients
• children.

Patient monitoring

• Monitor complete blood count and kidney and liver function test results.
• Monitor for signs and symptoms of superinfection and other serious adverse reactions.
• Be aware that cross-sensitivity to penicillins may occur.

Patient teaching

• Advise patient to report reduced urinary output, persistent diarrhea, bruising, or bleeding.

• Caution patient not to use herbs without consulting prescriber.

cefotaxime sodium
Claforan

Pharmacologic class: Third-generation cephalosporin
Therapeutic class: Anti-infective
Pregnancy risk category B

Action

Interferes with bacterial cell wall synthesis and division by binding to the cell wall, causing instability and death. Active against gram-negative and gram-positive bacteria but has expanded spectrum of activity against gram-negative bacteria. Overall, exhibits minimal immunosuppressant activity.

Availability

Powder for injection: 1 g, 2 g, 10 g
Premixed containers: 1 g/50 ml, 2 g/50 ml

🕭 Indications and dosages

➤ Perioperative prophylaxis
Adults and children weighing more than 50 kg (110 lb): 1 g I.V. or I.M. 30 to 90 minutes before surgery
➤ Preoperative prophylaxis in patients undergoing cesarean delivery
Adults: 1 g I.V. or I.M. as soon as umbilical cord is clamped
➤ Gonococcal urethritis and cervicitis
Adults weighing more than 50 kg (110 lb): 500 mg I.M. as a single dose
➤ Rectal gonorrhea (females)
Adults weighing more than 50 kg (110 lb): 500 mg I.M. as a single dose

➤ Rectal gonorrhea (males)
Adults weighing more than 50 kg (110 lb): 1 g I.M. as a single dose
➤ Disseminated gonorrhea
Adults and children weighing 50 kg (110 lb) or more: 1 g by I.V. infusion q 8 hours
➤ Uncomplicated infections caused by susceptible organisms
Adults and children weighing 50 kg (110 lb) or more: 1 g I.V. or I.M. q 12 hours
Children ages 1 month to 12 years weighing less than 50 kg (110 lb): 50 to 180 mg/kg/day I.V. or I.M. in four to six divided doses
➤ Moderate to severe infections caused by susceptible organisms
Adults and children weighing 50 kg (110 lb) or more: 1 to 2 g I.V. or I.M. q 8 hours
➤ Life-threatening infections caused by susceptible organisms
Adults and children weighing 50 kg (110 lb) or more: 2 g by I.V. infusion q 4 hours; maximum dosage is 12 g/day.
➤ Septicemia and other infections that commonly require antibiotics in higher doses
Adults and children weighing 50 kg (110 lb) or more: 2 g by I.V. infusion q 6 to 8 hours
Dosage adjustment
• Renal impairment

Contraindications

• Hypersensitivity to cephalosporins or penicillins

Administration

• Obtain specimen for culture and sensitivity testing as necessary before starting therapy.
• Reconstitute powder for I.V. injection with at least 10 ml of sterile water; infusion bottles may be reconstituted with 50 or 100 ml of normal saline solution or dextrose 5% in water (D_5W).
• Reconstituted drug may be diluted further for I.V. infusion up to 1,000 ml

with compatible solution, such as normal saline solution, D_5W or dextrose 10% in water, D_5W and normal saline solution, half-normal saline solution, or lactated Ringer's injection.

• For intermittent I.V. infusion, administer 1 or 2 g in 10 ml of sterile water over 3 to 5 minutes; if I.V. line is in place, give over longer period through I.V. tubing.

• Don't mix with diluent that has a pH above 7.5 (such as sodium bicarbonate).

• Inject I.M. deep into large muscle mass; divide 2-g dose in half and give in separate large muscle masses.

Route	Onset	Peak	Duration
I.V.	Rapid	End of infusion	4-12 hr
I.M.	Rapid	0.5 hr	4-12 hr

Adverse reactions

CNS: headache, lethargy, paresthesia, syncope, **seizures**
CV: hypotension, palpitations, chest pain, vasodilation
EENT: hearing loss
GI: nausea, vomiting, diarrhea, abdominal cramps, oral candidiasis, **pseudomembranous colitis**
GU: elevated blood urea nitrogen (BUN), vaginal candidiasis, **nephrotoxicity**
Hematologic: bleeding, lymphocytosis, eosinophilia, hemolytic anemia, **hypoprothrombinemia, neutropenia, thrombocytopenia, agranulocytosis, bone marrow depression**
Hepatic: hepatic failure, hepatomegaly
Musculoskeletal: arthralgia
Respiratory: dyspnea
Skin: urticaria, maculopapular or erythematous rash
Other: chills, fever, superinfection, pain at I.M. injection site, **anaphylaxis, serum sickness**

Interactions

Drug-drug. *Aminoglycosides, loop diuretics:* increased risk of nephrotoxicity
Oral anticoagulants: increased anticoagulant effect
Probenecid: decreased excretion and increased blood level of cefotaxime
Drug-diagnostic tests. *Alanine aminotransferase, alkaline phosphatase, aspartate aminotransferase, bilirubin, BUN, creatinine, eosinophils, gammaglutamyltransferase, lactate dehydrogenase:* increased levels
Coombs' test, urinary 17-ketosteroids, urine glucose determination with nonenzyme-based tests (Clinitest): false-positive results
Hemoglobin, platelets, white blood cells: decreased values
Drug-herb. *Angelica, anise, arnica, asafetida, bogbean, boldo, celery, chamomile, clove, danshen, fenugreek, feverfew, garlic, ginger, ginkgo, ginseng, horse chestnut, horseradish, licorice, meadowsweet, onion, papain, passionflower, poplar, prickly ash, quassia, red clover, turmeric, wild carrot, wild lettuce, willow:* increased risk of bleeding

Precautions

Use cautiously in:
• renal impairment, phenylketonuria
• history of GI disease
• elderly patients
• pregnant or breastfeeding patients
• children.

Patient monitoring

• Monitor complete blood count and kidney and liver function test results.
• Monitor for signs and symptoms of superinfection and other serious adverse reactions.
• Be aware that cross-sensitivity to penicillins may occur.

Patient teaching

• Advise patient to report reduced urinary output, persistent diarrhea, bruising, and bleeding.

cefotetan disodium
Cefotan

Pharmacologic class: Second-generation cephalosporin
Therapeutic class: Anti-infective
Pregnancy risk category B

Action
Interferes with bacterial cell wall synthesis and division by binding to the cell wall, causing instability and death. Active against gram-negative and gram-positive bacteria but has expanded spectrum of activity against gram-negative bacteria. Overall, exhibits minimal immunosuppressant activity.

Availability
Powder for injection: 1 g, 2 g

Indications and dosages
➤ Postcesarean prophylaxis
Adults: 1 to 2 g I.V. as soon as umbilical cord is clamped
➤ Urinary tract infections caused by *Escherichia coli*, *Proteus* species, and *Klebsiella* species
Adults: 0.5 to 2 g I.V. or I.M. q 12 hours, or 1 to 2 g I.V. or I.M. q 24 hours
➤ Skin and soft-tissue infections caused by *E. coli*, *Klebsiella pneumoniae*, *Peptostreptococcus* species, *Staphylococcus aureus*, and *Staphylococcus epidermidis*
Adults: For mild to moderate infections, 1 to 2 g I.V. or I.M. q 12 hours. For severe infections, 2 g I.V. q 12 hours.
➤ Lower respiratory tract infections caused by *E. coli*, *Haemophilus influenzae*, *Klebsiella* species, *Proteus mirabilis*, and *Serratia marcescens*
Adults: For mild to moderate infections, 1 to 2 g I.V. or I.M. q 12 hours.

For severe infections, 2 g I.V. q 12 hours. For life-threatening infections, 3 g I.V. q 12 hours.
Dosage adjustment
• Renal impairment

Contraindications
• Hypersensitivity to cephalosporins or penicillins

Administration
• Obtain specimen for culture and sensitivity testing as necessary before starting therapy.
• For I.V. administration, reconstitute with sterile water.
• For intermittent I.V. infusion, give 1 or 2 g in sterile water over 3 to 5 minutes; if patient has I.V. line in place, give over longer period through I.V. tubing.
• For I.M. injection, reconstitute with sterile water, bacteriostatic water, 0.5% or 1% lidocaine hydrochloride, or normal saline solution.
• Inject I.M. deep into large muscle mass; divide 2-g dose in half and inject into separate large muscle masses.

Route	Onset	Peak	Duration
I.V.	Rapid	End of infusion	12 hr
I.M.	Rapid	1-3 hr	12 hr

Adverse reactions
CNS: headache, confusion, hemiparesis, lethargy, paresthesia, syncope, **seizures**
CV: hypotension, palpitations, chest pain, vasodilation
EENT: hearing loss
GI: nausea, vomiting, diarrhea, abdominal cramps, oral candidiasis, **pseudomembranous colitis**
GU: elevated blood urea nitrogen (BUN), vaginal candidiasis, **nephrotoxicity**
Hematologic: bleeding, lymphocytosis, eosinophilia, hemolytic anemia, **hypoprothrombinemia, neutropenia,**

thrombocytopenia, agranulocytosis, bone marrow depression
Hepatic: hepatic failure, hepatomegaly
Musculoskeletal: arthralgia
Respiratory: dyspnea
Skin: urticaria, maculopapular or erythematous rash
Other: chills, fever, allergic reactions (including superinfection), pain at I.M. injection site, phlebitis at I.V. site, **anaphylaxis, serum sickness**

Interactions
Drug-drug. *Aminoglycosides, loop diuretics:* increased risk of nephrotoxicity
Antacids: decreased absorption
Oral anticoagulants: increased anticoagulant effect
Probenecid: decreased excretion and increased blood level of cefotetan
Drug-diagnostic tests. *Alanine aminotransferase, alkaline phosphatase, aspartate aminotransferase, bilirubin, BUN, creatinine, eosinophils, gamma-glutamyltransferase, lactate dehydrogenase:* increased levels
Coombs' test, urinary 17-ketosteroids, urine glucose determination with nonenzyme-based tests (Clinitest): false-positive results
Hemoglobin, platelets, white blood cells: decreased values
Drug-food. *Moderate- or high-fat meal:* increased drug bioavailability
Drug-behaviors. *Alcohol use:* disulfiram-like reaction when alcohol is consumed within 48 to 72 hours of drug administration

Precautions
Use cautiously in:
• renal impairment, phenylketonuria
• history of GI disease
• elderly patients
• pregnant or breastfeeding patients
• children.

Patient monitoring
◀❧ Monitor for extreme confusion, tonic-clonic seizures, and mild hemiparesis when high doses are used.
• Assess complete blood count and kidney and liver function test results.
• Monitor for signs and symptoms of superinfection and other serious adverse reactions.
• Be aware that cross-sensitivity to penicillins may occur.

Patient teaching
• Instruct patient to report reduced urinary output, persistent diarrhea, bruising, or bleeding.
• Caution patient to avoid alcohol in any form.

cefoxitin sodium
Mefoxin

Pharmacologic class: Second-generation cephalosporin
Therapeutic class: Anti-infective
Pregnancy risk category B

Action
Interferes with bacterial cell wall synthesis and division by binding to the cell wall, causing instability and death. Active against gram-negative and gram-positive bacteria but has expanded spectrum of activity against gram-negative bacteria. Overall, exhibits minimal immunosuppressant activity.

Availability
Powder for injection: 1 g, 2 g
Premixed containers: 1 g/50 ml in dextrose 5% in water (D_5W), 2 g/50 ml in D_5W

Indications and dosages
➤ Respiratory tract infections, skin infections, bone and joint infections,

urinary tract infections, gynecologic infections, septicemia

Adults: For most infections, 1 g I.M. or I.V. q 6 to 8 hours. For severe infections, 1 g I.M. or I.V. q 4 hours or 2 g I.M. or I.V. q 6 to 8 hours. For life-threatening infections, 2 g I.V. q 4 hours or 3 g I.V. q 6 hours.

Children ages 3 months and older: For most infections, 13.3 to 26.7 mg/kg I.M. or I.V. q 4 hours or 20 to 40 mg/kg q 6 hours.

➢ Preoperative prophylaxis

Adults: 1 to 2 g I.V. within 60 minutes of incision, then q 6 hours for up to 24 hours

Dosage adjustment
• Renal failure

Contraindications

• Hypersensitivity to cephalosporins or penicillins

Administration

• Obtain specimens for culture and sensitivity testing as necessary before starting therapy.
• Reconstitute 1-g dose with 10 ml of sterile water; reconstitute 2-g dose with 10 to 20 ml..
• For intermittent I.V. use, give 1- or 2-g dose in 10 ml of sterile water over 3 to 5 minutes; may also give through existing I.V. tubing.
• For continuous I.V. infusion, add compatible solution to I.V. container, such as D_5W, normal saline solution, or D_5W and normal saline solution.
• For I.M. injection, reconstitute each gram with 2 ml of sterile water or 2 ml of 0.5% lidocaine hydrochloride (without epinephrine).
• Inject I.M. deep into large muscle mass; divide 2-g dose in half and inject into separate large muscle masses.
• Know that dry powder and solution may darken, but this doesn't alter drug's effectiveness.

Route	Onset	Peak	Duration
I.V.	Rapid	End of infusion	4-8 hr
I.M.	Rapid	30 min	4-8 hr

Adverse reactions

CNS: headache, lethargy, paresthesia, syncope, **seizures**
CV: hypotension, palpitations, chest pain, vasodilation, thrombophlebitis
EENT: hearing loss
GI: nausea, vomiting, diarrhea, abdominal cramps, oral candidiasis, **pseudomembranous colitis**
GU: elevated blood urea nitrogen (BUN), vaginal candidiasis, **nephrotoxicity**
Hematologic: bleeding, lymphocytosis, eosinophilia, hemolytic anemia, **hypoprothrombinemia, neutropenia, thrombocytopenia, agranulocytosis, bone marrow depression**
Hepatic: hepatic failure, hepatomegaly
Musculoskeletal: arthralgia
Respiratory: dyspnea
Skin: urticaria, maculopapular or erythematous rash
Other: chills, fever, superinfection, pain at I.M. site, **anaphylaxis, serum sickness**

Interactions

Drug-drug. *Aminoglycosides, loop diuretics:* increased risk of nephrotoxicity
Oral anticoagulants: increased anticoagulant effect
Probenecid: decreased excretion and increased blood level of cefoxitin
Drug-diagnostic tests. *Alanine aminotransferase, alkaline phosphatase, aspartate aminotransferase, bilirubin, BUN, creatinine, eosinophils, gamma-glutamyltransferase, lactate dehydrogenase:* increased levels
Coombs' test, urinary 17-ketosteroids, urine glucose determination with nonenzyme-based tests (Clinitest): false-positive results

Hemoglobin, platelets, white blood cells: decreased values

Precautions

Use cautiously in:
• renal impairment, hepatic disease, or biliary obstruction
• history of GI disease
• elderly patients
• children.

Patient monitoring

• Assess complete blood count and kidney and liver function test results.
• Monitor fluid intake and output; report significant decrease in output.
• Monitor for signs and symptoms of superinfection and other serious adverse reactions.
• Be aware that cross-sensitivity to penicillins may occur.

Patient teaching

• Instruct patient to report reduced urinary output, persistent diarrhea, bruising, and bleeding.

cefpodoxime proxetil
Vantin

Pharmacologic class: Third-generation cephalosporin
Therapeutic class: Anti-infective
Pregnancy risk category B

Action

Interferes with bacterial cell wall synthesis and division by binding to the cell wall, causing instability and death. Active against gram-negative and gram-positive bacteria but has expanded spectrum of activity against gram-negative bacteria. Overall, exhibits minimal immunosuppressant activity.

Availability

Oral suspension: 50 mg/5 ml, 100 mg/5 ml
Tablets: 100 mg, 200 mg

Indications and dosages

➤ Acute community-acquired pneumonia due to *Haemophilus influenzae* or *Streptococcus pneumoniae*
Adults and children ages 13 and older: 200 mg P.O. q 12 hours for 14 days
➤ Acute bacterial or chronic bronchitis
Adults and children ages 13 and older: 200 mg P.O. q 12 hours for 10 days
➤ Uncomplicated gonorrhea, rectal gonococcal infection due to *Neisseria gonorrhoeae*
Adults: 200 mg P.O. as a single dose
➤ Uncomplicated urinary tract infections due to *Escherichia coli, Klebsiella pneumoniae, Proteus mirabilis,* and *Staphylococcus saprophyticus*
Adults: 100 mg P.O. q 12 hours for 7 days
➤ Skin and soft-tissue infections due to *Staphylococcus aureus* and *Streptococcus pyogenes*
Adults and children ages 13 and older: 400 mg P.O. q 12 hours for 7 to 14 days
➤ Acute otitis media due to *H. influenzae, Streptococcus pneumoniae,* and *Moraxella catarrhalis*
Children ages 5 months to 12 years: 5 mg/kg P.O. q 12 hours (maximum of 200 mg/dose) or 10 mg/kg q 24 hours (maximum of 400 mg/dose) for 10 days
➤ Tonsillitis and pharyngitis due to *S. pyogenes*
Adults and children ages 13 and older: 100 mg P.O. q 12 hours for 5 to 10 days
Children ages 2 months to 12 years: 5 mg/kg P.O. q 12 hours for 5 to 10 days
Dosage adjustment
• Renal impairment

Contraindications

• Hypersensitivity to cephalosporins or penicillins

Administration

• Obtain specimen for culture and sensitivity testing as necessary before starting therapy.
• Give tablets with food to enhance absorption; oral suspension may be given with or without food.
• Don't give antacids within 2 hours of cefpodoxime.

Route	Onset	Peak	Duration
P.O.	Unknown	2-3 hr	12 hr

Adverse reactions

CNS: headache, lethargy, paresthesia, syncope, **seizures**
CV: hypotension, palpitations, chest pain, vasodilation
EENT: hearing loss
GI: nausea, vomiting, diarrhea, abdominal cramps, oral candidiasis, **pseudomembranous colitis**
GU: elevated blood urea nitrogen (BUN), vaginal candidiasis, **nephrotoxicity**
Hematologic: bleeding, lymphocytosis, eosinophilia, hemolytic anemia, **hypoprothrombinemia, neutropenia, thrombocytopenia, agranulocytosis, bone marrow depression**
Hepatic: hepatic failure, hepatomegaly
Musculoskeletal: arthralgia
Respiratory: dyspnea
Skin: urticaria, maculopapular or erythematous rash
Other: chills, fever, superinfection, **anaphylaxis, serum sickness**

Interactions

Drug-drug. *Aminoglycosides, loop diuretics:* increased risk of nephrotoxicity
Antacids: decreased cefpodoxime absorption
Histamine₂-receptor antagonists: decreased cefpodoxime blood level

Oral anticoagulants: increased anticoagulant effect
Probenecid: decreased excretion and increased blood level of cefpodoxime
Drug-diagnostic tests. *Alanine aminotransferase, alkaline phosphatase, aspartate aminotransferase, bilirubin, BUN, creatinine, eosinophils, gamma-glutamyltransferase, lactate dehydrogenase:* increased levels
Coombs' test, urinary 17-ketosteroids, urine glucose determination with nonenzyme-based tests (Clinitest): false-positive results
Hemoglobin, platelets, white blood cells: decreased values
Drug-herb. *Angelica, anise, arnica, asafetida, bogbean, boldo, celery, chamomile, clove, danshen, fenugreek, feverfew, garlic, ginger, ginkgo, ginseng, horse chestnut, horseradish, licorice, meadowsweet, onion, papain, passionflower, poplar, prickly ash, quassia, red clover, turmeric, wild carrot, wild lettuce, willow:* increased risk of bleeding

Precautions

Use cautiously in:
• renal impairment, phenylketonuria
• history of GI disease
• elderly patients
• pregnant or breastfeeding patients
• children.

Patient monitoring

• Assess complete blood count and kidney and liver function test results.
• Monitor for signs and symptoms of superinfection and other serious adverse reactions.
• Be aware that cross-sensitivity to penicillins may occur.

Patient teaching

• Instruct patient to take drug with food or milk to reduce GI distress and enhance absorption.
• Advise patient to take drug exactly as prescribed and to continue to take full

amount prescribed even when he feels better.

• Teach patient to report signs and symptoms of allergic response and other adverse reactions, such as rash, easy bruising, bleeding, severe GI problems, difficulty breathing, persistent nausea and vomiting, or diarrhea.

• Tell patient not to take antacids within 2 hours of drug.

• If patient is being treated for gonorrhea, instruct him to have partner tested and treated (as needed) and to use barrier contraception to prevent reinfection.

cefprozil
Cefzil

Pharmacologic class: Second-generation cephalosporin
Therapeutic class: Anti-infective
Pregnancy risk category B

Action
Bactericidal; interferes with bacterial cell wall synthesis, causing cell to rupture and die

Availability
Powder for suspension: 125 mg/5 ml, 250 mg/5 ml
Tablets: 250 mg, 500 mg

Indications and dosages
➤ Uncomplicated skin infections due to *Staphylococcus aureus* and *S. pyogenes*
Adults and children ages 13 and older: 250 to 500 mg P.O. q 12 hours or 500 mg P.O. daily for 10 days
➤ Pharyngitis or tonsillitis caused by *Streptococcus pyogenes*
Adults and children ages 13 and older: 500 mg P.O. daily for at least 10 days

➤ Acute bronchitis; acute bacterial chronic bronchitis due to *S. pneumoniae, H. influenzae,* and *M. catarrhalis*
Adults and children ages 13 and older: 500 mg P.O. q 12 hours for 10 days
➤ Acute sinusitis due to *S. pneumoniae, H. influenzae,* and *M. catarrhalis*
Adults and children ages 13 and older: 250 mg P.O. q 12 hours for 10 days; for moderate to severe infections, 500 mg P.O. q 12 hours for 10 days
Children ages 6 months to 12 years: 7.5 mg/kg P.O. q 12 hours for 10 days; for moderate to severe infections, 15 mg/kg P.O. q 12 hours for 10 days
➤ Otitis media due to *Streptococcus pneumoniae, Haemophilus influenzae,* and *Moraxella catarrhalis*
Children ages 6 months to 12 years: 15 mg/kg P.O. q 12 hours for 10 days
Dosage adjustment
• Renal impairment

Contraindications
• Hypersensitivity to cephalosporins or penicillins
• Renal failure
• Pregnancy or breastfeeding

Administration
• Obtain culture and sensitivity test before beginning therapy.
• Give drug with food.

Route	Onset	Peak	Duration
P.O.	Unknown	6-10 hr	24-28 hr

Adverse reactions
CNS: headache, dizziness, drowsiness, hyperactivity, hypotonia, insomnia, confusion, **seizures**
GI: nausea, vomiting, diarrhea, abdominal pain, dyspepsia, **pseudomembranous colitis**
GU: renal dysfunction, vaginal candidiasis, hematuria, increased white blood cells in urine, genital pruritus, **toxic nephropathy**

Hematologic: aplastic anemia, hemolytic anemia, hemorrhage, eosinophilia, **bone marrow depression**
Hepatic: hepatic dysfunction
Skin: erythema multiforme, toxic epidermal necrolysis, **Stevens-Johnson syndrome**
Other: allergic reactions, carnitine deficiency, drug fever, superinfection, **serum sickness–like reaction, anaphylaxis**

Interactions
Drug-drug. *Aminoglycosides:* increased risk of nephrotoxicity
Antacids containing aluminum or magnesium, histamine$_2$-receptor antagonists: increased cefprozil absorption
Oral anticoagulants: increased risk of bleeding
Probenecid: decreased excretion and increased blood level of cefprozil
Drug-diagnostic tests. *Alanine aminotransferase, alkaline phosphatase, aspartate aminotransferase, bilirubin, blood urea nitrogen, creatinine, eosinophils, gamma-glutamyltransferase, lactate dehydrogenase:* increased levels
Blood glucose, Coombs' test, urine glucose determination using Benedict's solution: false-positive results
Platelets, white blood cells: decreased counts
Drug-food. *Moderate- or high-fat meal:* increased drug bioavailability

Precautions
Use cautiously in:
• renal or hepatic impairment
• pregnant or breastfeeding patients
• children.

Patient monitoring
◀€ Monitor for life-threatening reactions, including anaphylaxis, serum sickness–like reaction, Stevens-Johnson syndrome, and pseudomembranous colitis.

• Monitor neurologic status, particularly for signs and symptoms of impending seizures.
• Monitor kidney and liver function test results and intake and output.
• Monitor complete blood cell count with differential; watch for signs and symptoms of blood dyscrasias.
• Monitor temperature; watch for signs and symptoms of superinfection.

Patient teaching
• Advise patient to immediately report rash or bleeding tendency.
• Teach patient signs and symptoms of superinfection, and instruct him to report these right away.
• Instruct patient to report CNS changes.
• Tell patient to take drug with food.

ceftazidime
Ceptaz, Fortaz, Tazicef, Tazidime

Pharmacologic class: Third-generation cephalosporin
Therapeutic class: Anti-infective
Pregnancy risk category B

Action
Interferes with bacterial cell wall synthesis and division by binding to the cell wall, causing instability and death. Active against gram-negative and gram-positive bacteria but has expanded spectrum of activity against gram-negative bacteria. Overall, exhibits minimal immunosuppressant activity.

Availability
Powder for injection: 500 mg, 1 g, 2 g, 6 g, 10 g
Premixed containers: 1 g/50 ml, 2 g/50 ml

⚕️ Indications and dosages

➤ Skin infections; bone and joint infections; urinary tract and gynecologic infections, including gonorrhea; respiratory tract infections; intraabdominal infections; septicemia

Adults and children ages 12 and older: For most infections, 500 mg to 2 g I.V. or I.M. q 8 to 12 hours. For pneumonia and skin infections, 0.5 to 1 g I.V. or I.M. q 8 to 12 hours. For bone and joint infections, 2 g I.V. or I.M. q 12 hours. For severe and life-threatening infections, 2 g I.V. q 8 hours. For complicated urinary tract infections (UTIs), 500 mg q 8 to 12 hours. For uncomplicated UTIs, 250 mg I.M. or I.V. q 12 hours.

Children ages 1 month to 12 years: 30 to 50 mg/kg I.V. q 8 hours

Neonates younger than 4 weeks: 30 mg/kg I.V. q 12 hours

Dosage adjustment
• Renal impairment

Off-label uses
• Febrile neutropenia
• Prophylaxis of perinatal infections

Contraindications
• Hypersensitivity to cephalosporins or penicillins

Administration
• Obtain specimen for culture and sensitivity testing as necessary before starting therapy.
• For I.V. infusion, reconstitute 1- or 2-g dose with 100 ml of sterile water or another compatible fluid, such as normal saline solution or dextrose 5% in water. Follow manufacturer's directions for amount of diluent to use.
• Don't dilute with sodium bicarbonate.
• For I.M. injection, reconstitute with sterile water, bacteriostatic water, or 0.5% or 1% lidocaine hydrochloride.
• Inject I.M. deep into large muscle mass.

Route	Onset	Peak	Duration
I.V.	Rapid	End of infusion	6-12 hr
I.M.	Rapid	1 hr	6-12 hr

Adverse reactions
CNS: headache, confusion, hemiparesis, lethargy, paresthesia, syncope, **seizures**
CV: hypotension, palpitations, chest pain, vasodilation
EENT: hearing loss
GI: nausea, vomiting, diarrhea, abdominal cramps, oral candidiasis, **pseudomembranous colitis**
GU: elevated blood urea nitrogen (BUN), vaginal candidiasis, **nephrotoxicity**
Hematologic: bleeding, lymphocytosis, eosinophilia, hemolytic anemia, **hypoprothrombinemia, neutropenia, thrombocytopenia, agranulocytosis, bone marrow depression**
Hepatic: hepatic failure, hepatomegaly
Musculoskeletal: arthralgia
Respiratory: dyspnea
Skin: urticaria, maculopapular or erythematous rash
Other: chills, fever, superinfection, I.M. site pain, **anaphylaxis, serum sickness**

Interactions
Drug-drug. *Aminoglycosides, loop diuretics:* increased risk of nephrotoxicity
Oral anticoagulants: increased anticoagulant effect
Probenecid: decreased excretion and increased blood level of ceftazidime
Drug-diagnostic tests. *Alanine aminotransferase, alkaline phosphatase, aspartate aminotransferase, bilirubin, BUN, creatinine, eosinophils, gammaglutamyltransferase, lactate dehydrogenase:* increased levels

---

Hemoglobin, platelets, white blood cells: decreased values

Coombs' test, urinary 17-ketosteroids, urine glucose determination using nonenzyme-based tests (Clinitest): false-positive results

Drug-herb. *Angelica, anise, arnica, asafetida, bogbean, boldo, celery, chamomile, clove, danshen, fenugreek, feverfew, garlic, ginger, ginkgo, ginseng, horse chestnut, horseradish, licorice, meadowsweet, onion, papain, passion-flower, poplar, prickly ash, quassia, red clover, turmeric, wild carrot, wild lettuce, willow:* increased risk of bleeding

Precautions

Use cautiously in:
• renal impairment, hepatic disease, biliary obstruction, phenylketonuria
• history of GI disease
• elderly patients
• pregnant or breastfeeding patients
• children.

Patient monitoring

◀€ Monitor for extreme confusion, tonic-clonic seizures, and mild hemiparesis when high doses are used.
• Assess complete blood count and kidney and liver function test results.
• Monitor for signs and symptoms of superinfection and other serious adverse reactions.
• Be aware that cross-sensitivity to penicillins may occur.

Patient teaching

• Instruct patient to report reduced urinary output, persistent diarrhea, bruising, and bleeding.
• Advise patient not to take herbs while receiving this drug.

ceftibuten
Cedax

Pharmacologic class: Third-generation cephalosporin
Therapeutic class: Anti-infective
Pregnancy risk category B

Action

Interferes with bacterial cell wall synthesis and division by binding to the cell wall, causing instability and death. Active against gram-negative and gram-positive bacteria but has expanded spectrum of activity against gram-negative bacteria. Overall, exhibits minimal immunosuppressant activity.

Availability

Capsules: 400 mg
Oral suspension: 90 mg/5 ml, 180 mg/5 ml

Indications and dosages

➤ Acute bacterial exacerbations of chronic bronchitis caused by *Haemophilus influenzae, Moraxella catarrhalis,* and *Streptococcus pneumoniae;* pharyngitis and tonsillitis caused by *Streptococcus pyogenes;* acute bacterial otitis media caused by *H. influenzae, M. catarrhalis,* and *S. pyogenes*
Adults and children ages 12 and older: 400 mg P.O. q 24 hours for 10 days
Children ages 12 and younger: 9 mg/kg P.O. daily for 10 days; maximum dosage shouldn't exceed 400 mg daily.
Dosage adjustment
• Renal impairment

Off-label uses

• Urinary tract infections

Contraindications

• Hypersensitivity to cephalosporins and penicillins

Administration

• Obtain specimen for culture and sensitivity testing as necessary before starting therapy.
• Give oral suspension at least 1 hour before or 2 hours after meal.

Route	Onset	Peak	Duration
P.O.	Rapid	3 hr	24 hr

Adverse reactions

CNS: headache, lethargy, paresthesia, syncope, **seizures**
CV: hypotension, palpitations, chest pain, vasodilation
EENT: hearing loss
GI: nausea, vomiting, diarrhea, abdominal cramps, oral candidiasis, **pseudomembranous colitis**
GU: elevated blood urea nitrogen (BUN), vaginal candidiasis, **nephrotoxicity**
Hematologic: bleeding, lymphocytosis, eosinophilia, hemolytic anemia, **hypoprothrombinemia, neutropenia, thrombocytopenia, agranulocytosis, bone marrow depression**
Hepatic: hepatic failure, hepatomegaly
Musculoskeletal: arthralgia
Respiratory: dyspnea
Skin: urticaria, maculopapular or erythematous rash
Other: chills, fever, superinfection, **anaphylaxis, serum sickness**

Interactions

Drug-drug. *Aminoglycosides, loop diuretics:* increased risk of nephrotoxicity
Oral anticoagulants: increased anticoagulant effect
Probenecid: decreased excretion and increased blood level of ceftibuten
Drug-diagnostic tests. *Alanine aminotransferase, alkaline phosphatase, aspartate aminotransferase, bilirubin, BUN, creatinine, eosinophils, gammaglutamyltransferase, lactate dehydrogenase:* increased levels

Coombs' test, urinary 17-ketosteroids, urine glucose determination with nonenzyme-based tests (Clinitest): false-positive results
Hemoglobin, platelets, white blood cells: decreased values
Drug-herb. *Angelica, anise, arnica, asafetida, bogbean, boldo, celery, chamomile, clove, danshen, fenugreek, feverfew, garlic, ginger, ginkgo, ginseng, horse chestnut, horseradish, licorice, meadowsweet, onion, papain, passionflower, poplar, prickly ash, quassia, red clover, turmeric, wild carrot, wild lettuce, willow:* increased risk of bleeding

Precautions

Use cautiously in:
• renal impairment, hepatic disease, biliary obstruction, phenylketonuria
• history of GI disease
• elderly patients
• pregnant or breastfeeding patients
• children.

Patient monitoring

• Assess complete blood count and kidney and liver function test results.
• Monitor for signs and symptoms of superinfection and other serious adverse reactions.
• Be aware that cross-sensitivity to penicillins may occur.

Patient teaching

• Instruct patient to take oral suspension at least 1 hour before or 2 hours after a meal.
• Instruct patient to take drug exactly as prescribed and to continue to take full amount prescribed even when he feels better.
• Teach patient to report signs and symptoms of allergic response and other adverse reactions, such as rash, easy bruising, bleeding, severe GI problems, difficulty breathing, persistent nausea and vomiting, or diarrhea.

---

ceftizoxime sodium
Cefizox

Pharmacologic class: Third-generation cephalosporin
Therapeutic class: Anti-infective
Pregnancy risk category B

Action
Interferes with bacterial cell wall synthesis and division by binding to the cell wall, causing instability and death. Active against gram-negative and gram-positive bacteria but has expanded spectrum of activity against gram-negative bacteria. Overall, exhibits minimal immunosuppressant activity.

Availability
Powder for injection: 500 mg, 1 g, 2 g, 10 g
Premixed containers: 1 g/50 ml, 2 g/50 ml

Indications and dosages
➢ Skin infections, bone and joint infections, urinary tract and gynecologic infections (including gonorrhea), respiratory tract infections, intra-abdominal infections, septicemia
Adults: For mild or moderate infections, 1g I.V. or I.M. q 8 to 12 hours. For uncomplicated urinary tract infections, 500 mg I.V. or I.M. q 12 hours. For severe infections, 2 g I.V. q 8 to 12 hours. For life-threatening infections, 4 g I.V. q 8 hours.
Children age 6 months and older: 50 mg/kg I.M. or I.V. q 6 to 8 hours
Dosage adjustment
• Renal impairment

Contraindications
• Hypersensitivity to cephalosporins or penicillins

Administration
• Obtain specimen for culture and sensitivity testing as necessary before starting therapy.
• Reconstitute powder with sterile water; follow manufacturer's guidelines for amount of diluent to use.
• For intermittent or continuous I.V. administration, dilute reconstituted drug in compatible solutions, such as normal saline solution, dextrose 5% in water (D_5W), dextrose 10% in water, D_5W and normal saline solution, half-normal saline solution, Ringer's injection, lactated Ringer's injection, or D_5W in lactated Ringer's injection (only when reconstituted with 4% bicarbonate injection).
• For administration in piggyback vials, reconstitute with 50 to 100 ml of any compatible I.V. solution listed above.
• Divide high I.M. doses equally and administer in two separate sites. Inject deep into large muscle mass.

Route	Onset	Peak	Duration
I.V.	Rapid	End of infusion	6-12 hr
I.M.	Rapid	0.5-1.5 hr	6-12 hr

Adverse reactions
CNS: headache, confusion, hemiparesis, lethargy, paresthesia, syncope, **seizures**
CV: hypotension, palpitations, chest pain, vasodilation
EENT: hearing loss
GI: nausea, vomiting, diarrhea, abdominal cramps, oral candidiasis, **pseudomembranous colitis**
GU: elevated blood urea nitrogen (BUN), vaginal candidiasis, **nephrotoxicity**
Hematologic: bleeding, lymphocytosis, eosinophilia, hemolytic anemia, **hypoprothrombinemia, neutropenia, thrombocytopenia, agranulocytosis, bone marrow depression**

Hepatic: hepatic failure, hepatomegaly
Musculoskeletal: arthralgia
Respiratory: dyspnea
Skin: urticaria, maculopapular or erythematous rash
Other: chills, fever, superinfection, pain at I.M. injection site, **anaphylaxis, serum sickness**

Interactions
Drug-drug. *Aminoglycosides, loop diuretics:* increased risk of nephrotoxicity
Oral anticoagulants: increased anticoagulant effect
Probenecid: decreased excretion and increased blood level of ceftizoxime
Drug-diagnostic tests. *Alanine aminotransferase, alkaline phosphatase, aspartate aminotransferase, bilirubin, BUN, creatinine, eosinophils, gamma-glutamyltransferase, lactate dehydrogenase:* increased levels
Coombs' test, urinary 17-ketosteroids, urine glucose determination with nonenzyme-based tests (Clinitest): false-positive results
Hemoglobin, platelets, white blood cells: decreased values
Drug-herb. *Angelica, anise, arnica, asafetida, bogbean, boldo, celery, chamomile, clove, danshen, fenugreek, feverfew, garlic, ginger, ginkgo, ginseng, horse chestnut, horseradish, licorice, meadowsweet, onion, papain, passionflower, poplar, prickly ash, quassia, red clover, turmeric, wild carrot, wild lettuce, willow:* increased risk of bleeding.

Precautions
Use cautiously in:
• renal impairment, hepatic disease, biliary obstruction, phenylketonuria
• history of GI disease
• elderly patients
• pregnant or breastfeeding patients
• children.

Patient monitoring
◀≋ Monitor for extreme confusion, tonic-clonic seizures, and mild hemiparesis when high doses are used.
• Assess complete blood count and kidney and liver function test results.
• Monitor for signs and symptoms of superinfection and other serious adverse reactions.
• Be aware that cross-sensitivity to penicillins may occur.

Patient teaching
• Advise patient to report reduced urinary output, persistent diarrhea, bruising, and bleeding.

ceftriaxone sodium
Rocephin

Pharmacologic class: Third-generation cephalosporin
Therapeutic class: Anti-infective
Pregnancy risk category B

Action
Interferes with bacterial cell wall synthesis and division by binding to the cell wall, causing instability and death. Active against gram-negative and gram-positive bacteria but has expanded spectrum of activity against gram-negative bacteria. Overall, exhibits minimal immunosuppressant activity.

Availability
Powder for injection: 250 mg, 500 mg, 1 g, 2 g
Premixed containers: 1 g/50 ml, 2 g/50 ml

⚕ Indications and dosages
➤ Infections of respiratory system, bones, joints, and skin and septicemia caused by susceptible organisms

---

Adults: 1 to 2 g/day I.M. or I.V. or in equally divided doses q 12 hours; maximum daily dosage is 4 g.

➤ Uncomplicated gonorrhea

Adults: 250 mg I.M. as a single dose

➤ Surgical prophylaxis

Adults: 1 g I.V. as a single dose 30 minutes to 2 hours before start of surgical procedure

➤ Meningitis

Adults: 1 g to 2 g I.V. q 12 hours for 10 to 14 days

Children: Initially, 100 mg/kg/day I.M. or I.V. (not to exceed 4 g). Then 100 mg/kg/day I.M. or I.V. once daily or in equally divided doses q 12 hours (not to exceed 4 g) for 7 to 14 days.

Off-label uses

- Disseminated gonorrhea
- Endocarditis
- Epididymitis
- Gonorrhea-associated meningitis
- Lyme disease
- *Neisseria meningitides* carriers
- Pelvic inflammatory disease

Contraindications

- Hypersensitivity to cephalosporins or penicillins

Administration

- Obtain specimen for culture and sensitivity testing as necessary before starting therapy.
- Know that drug for I.V. injection is compatible with sterile water, normal saline solution, dextrose 5% in water (D_5W), D_5W and normal saline solution, and half-normal saline solution.
- After reconstitution, dilute further to desired concentration for intermittent I.V. infusion.
- For I.M. use, reconstitute powder for injection with compatible solution by adding 0.9 ml of diluent to 250-mg vial, 1.8 ml to 500-mg vial, 3.6 ml to 1-g vial, or 7.2 ml to 2-g vial to yield concentration averaging 250 mg/ml.

- Divide high I.M. doses equally and administer in two separate sites. Inject deep into large muscle mass.

Route	Onset	Peak	Duration
I.V.	Rapid	End of infusion	12-24 hr
I.M.	Rapid	1-2 hr	12-24 hr

Adverse reactions

CNS: headache, confusion, hemiparesis, lethargy, paresthesia, syncope, **seizures**

CV: hypotension, palpitations, chest pain, vasodilation

EENT: hearing loss

GI: nausea, vomiting, diarrhea, abdominal cramps, oral candidiasis, **pseudomembranous colitis**

GU: elevated blood urea nitrogen (BUN), vaginal candidiasis, **nephrotoxicity**

Hematologic: bleeding, lymphocytosis, eosinophilia, hemolytic anemia, **hypoprothrombinemia, neutropenia, thrombocytopenia, agranulocytosis, bone marrow depression**

Hepatic: **hepatic failure, hepatomegaly**

Musculoskeletal: arthralgia

Respiratory: dyspnea

Skin: urticaria, maculopapular or erythematous rash

Other: chills, fever, superinfection, pain at I.M. injection site, **anaphylaxis, serum sickness**

Interactions

Drug-drug. *Aminoglycosides, loop diuretics:* increased risk of nephrotoxicity
Oral anticoagulants: increased anticoagulant effect
Probenecid: decreased excretion and increased blood level of ceftriaxone

Drug-diagnostic tests. *Alanine aminotransferase, alkaline phosphatase, aspartate aminotransferase, bilirubin, BUN, creatinine, eosinophils, gamma-glutamyltransferase, lactate dehydrogenase:* increased levels

Coombs' test, urinary 17-ketosteroids, urine glucose determination with nonenzyme-based tests (Clinitest): false-positive results
Hemoglobin, platelets, white blood cells: decreased values
Drug-herb. *Angelica, anise, arnica, asafetida, bogbean, boldo, celery, chamomile, clove, danshen, fenugreek, feverfew, garlic, ginger, ginkgo, ginseng, horse chestnut, horseradish, licorice, meadowsweet, onion, papain, passion-flower, poplar, prickly ash, quassia, red clover, turmeric, wild carrot, wild lettuce, willow:* increased risk of bleeding.

Precautions
Use cautiously in:
• renal impairment, hepatic disease, biliary obstruction, phenylketonuria
• history of GI disease
• elderly patients
• pregnant or breastfeeding patients.

Patient monitoring
◀◣ Monitor for extreme confusion, tonic-clonic seizures, and mild hemiparesis when high doses are used.
• Monitor coagulation studies.
• Assess complete blood count and kidney and liver function test results.
• Monitor for signs and symptoms of superinfection and other serious adverse reactions.
• Be aware that cross-sensitivity to penicillins may occur.

Patient teaching
• Instruct patient to report reduced urinary output, persistent diarrhea, bruising, or bleeding.
• Advise patient not to use herbs.

cefuroxime axetil
Ceftin

cefuroxime sodium
Kefurox, Zinacef

Pharmacologic class: Second-generation cephalosporin
Therapeutic class: Anti-infective
Pregnancy risk category B

Action
Interferes with bacterial cell wall synthesis and division by binding to the cell wall, causing instability and death. Active against gram-negative and gram-positive bacteria but has expanded spectrum of activity against gram-negative bacteria. Overall, exhibits minimal immunosuppressant activity.

Availability
Oral suspension: 125 mg/5 ml
Powder for injection: 750 mg, 1.5 g, 7.5 g
Premixed containers: 750 mg/50 ml, 1.5 g/50 ml
Tablets: 125 mg, 250 mg, 500 mg

ⓘ Indications and dosages
➤ Moderate to severe infections, including those of the urinary tract, respiratory tract, skin, bone, and joints, gynecologic infections, and septicemia
Adults and children ages 12 and older: 750 mg to 1.5 g I.M. or I.V. q 8 hours for 5 to 10 days or 250 to 500 mg P.O. q 12 hours
Children ages 3 months to 12 years: 50 to 100 mg/kg/day I.V. or I.M. in divided doses q 6 to 8 hours
➤ Gonorrhea
Adults: 750 mg to 1.5 g I.M. or I.V. as a single dose, or 1.5 g I.M. (750 mg in two separate sites) given with 1 g probenecid P.O.

➤ Bacterial meningitis

Adults and children ages 12 and older:
Up to 3 g I.V. or I.M. q 8 hours

Children ages 3 months to 12 years:
200 to 240 mg/kg I.V. daily in divided doses q 6 to 8 hours

➤ Otitis media

Children ages 3 months to 12 years:
15 mg/kg P.O. q 12 hours (oral suspension) for 10 days, or 250 mg (tablets) P.O. q 12 hours for 10 days

➤ Pharyngitis and tonsillitis

Adults and children ages 13 and older:
250 mg P.O. b.i.d. for 10 days

Children ages 3 months to 12 years:
125 mg P.O. q 12 hours for 10 days, or 20 mg/kg/day P.O. in two divided doses for 10 days as oral suspension (maximum 500 mg/day)

Dosage adjustment
• Renal impairment

Contraindications

• Hypersensitivity to cephalosporins or penicillins
• Carnitine deficiency

Administration

• Reconstitute drug in vial with sterile water for injection.
• Give by direct I.V. injection over 3 to 5 minutes into a large vein or flowing I.V. line.
• For intermittent I.V. infusion, reconstitute drug with 100 ml of dextrose 5% in water or normal saline solution and administer over 15 minutes to 1 hour.
• Inject I.M. doses deep into large muscle mass.
• Give oral form with food

Route	Onset	Peak	Duration
P.O.	Unknown	2 hr	8-12 hr
I.V., I.M.	Rapid	End of infusion	6-12 hr

Adverse reactions

CNS: headache, hyperactivity, hypertonia, **seizures**

GI: nausea, vomiting, diarrhea, abdominal pain, dyspepsia, **pseudomembranous colitis**

GU: renal dysfunction, vaginal candidiasis, hematuria, increased urinary white blood cells, **toxic nephropathy**

Hematologic: hemolytic anemia, **aplastic anemia, hemorrhage**

Hepatic: hepatic dysfunction

Metabolic: hyperglycemia

Skin: erythema multiforme, toxic epidermal necrolysis, **Stevens-Johnson syndrome**

Other: allergic reaction, drug fever, superinfection, **anaphylaxis**

Interactions

Drug-drug. *Antacids containing aluminum or magnesium, histamine$_2$-receptor antagonists:* increased cefuroxime absorption

Oral anticoagulants: increased risk of bleeding

Probenecid: decreased excretion and increased blood level of cefuroxime

Drug-diagnostic tests. *Benedict's solution test, blood glucose, Coombs' test:* false-positive results

Glucose, hematocrit: decreased levels

Drug-food. *Moderate- or high-fat meal:* increased drug bioavailability

Precautions

Use cautiously in:
• renal or hepatic impairment
• pregnant or breastfeeding patients
• children.

Patient monitoring

• Monitor for life-threatening effects, including anaphylaxis, serum sickness–like reaction, Stevens-Johnson syndrome, and pseudomembranous colitis.
• Monitor neurologic status, particularly for signs of impending seizures.

• Monitor kidney and liver function test results and intake and output.
• Monitor complete blood cell count with differential; watch for signs and symptoms of blood dyscrasias.
• Monitor temperature; watch for signs and symptoms of superinfection.

Patient teaching
• Advise patient to immediately report rash or bleeding tendency.
• Teach patient signs and symptoms of superinfection; instruct him to report these right away.
• Instruct patient to report CNS changes.
• Tell patient to take drug every 12 hours as prescribed, with food.

celecoxib
Celebrex

Pharmacologic class: Nonsteroidal cyclooxygenase-2 (COX-2) inhibitor, anti-inflammatory drug (NSAID)
Therapeutic class: Antirheumatic
Pregnancy risk category C

Action
Exhibits anti-inflammatory, analgesic, and antipyretic action due to inhibition of the enzyme COX-2

Availability
Capsules: 100 mg, 200 mg

Indications and dosages
➤ Osteoarthritis
Adults: 200 mg/day P.O. as a single dose or 100 mg P.O. b.i.d.
➤ Rheumatoid arthritis
Adults: 100 to 200 mg P.O. b.i.d.
➤ Adjunctive treatment to decrease the number of adenomatous colorectal polyps in familial adenomatous polyposis
Adults: 400 mg P.O. b.i.d.

Dosage adjustment
• Hepatic impairment
• Patients weighing less than 50 kg (110 lb)

Contraindications
• Hypersensitivity to drug, sulfonamides, or other NSAIDs
• Severe hepatic impairment
• History of asthma or urticaria
• Advanced renal disease
• Late pregnancy
• Breastfeeding

Administration
• Give with food or milk.

Route	Onset	Peak	Duration
P.O.	Unknown	3 hr	Unknown

Adverse reactions
CNS: dizziness, drowsiness, headache, insomnia, fatigue
CV: peripheral edema
EENT: ophthalmic effects, tinnitus, pharyngitis, rhinitis, sinusitis
GI: nausea, diarrhea, constipation, abdominal pain, dyspepsia, flatulence, dry mouth, **GI bleeding**
GU: menorrhagia
Hematologic: decreased hemoglobin or hematocrit, eosinophilia, epistaxis, bruising, **neutropenia, leukopenia, pancytopenia, thrombocytopenia, agranulocytosis, granulocytopenia, aplastic anemia, bone marrow depression**
Hepatic: hepatotoxicity
Metabolic: hyperchloremia, hypophosphatemia
Musculoskeletal: back pain, leg cramps
Respiratory: upper respiratory tract infection
Skin: rash
Other: anaphylactic reaction

Interactions
Drug-drug. *Angiotensin-converting enzyme inhibitors, furosemide, thiazides:* reduced celecoxib efficacy

Antacids containing aluminum and magnesium: decreased celecoxib blood level

Aspirin (regular doses): increased risk of GI bleeding and GI ulcers

Fluconazole: increased celecoxib blood level

Lithium: increased lithium blood level

Warfarin: increased risk of bleeding

Drug-diagnostic tests. *Alanine aminotransferase, aspartate aminotransferase, blood urea nitrogen:* increased levels

Drug-herb. *Dong quai, feverfew, garlic, ginger, horse chestnut, red clover:* increased risk of bleeding

White willow: increased risk of GI ulcers

Drug-behaviors. *Long-term alcohol use, smoking:* GI irritation and bleeding

Precautions
Use cautiously in:
• renal insufficiency, hypertension
• history of asthma, renal disease, hepatic dysfunction, heart failure
• patients on long-term NSAID therapy
• elderly patients
• pregnant patients
• children younger than age 18 (safety not established).

Patient monitoring
• Monitor complete blood count, electrolyte levels, creatinine clearance, and occult fecal blood test and liver function test results every 6 to 12 months.

Patient teaching
◀€ Advise patient to immediately report bloody stools, blood in vomit, or signs or symptoms of liver damage (nausea, fatigue, lethargy, pruritus, yellowing of eyes or skin, tenderness on upper right side of abdomen, or flulike symptoms).

• Instruct patient to take drug with food or milk.

• Teach patient to avoid aspirin and other NSAIDs (such as ibuprofen and naproxen) during therapy.

c

cephalexin hydrochloride
Keftab

cephalexin monohydrate
Apo-Cephalex✤, Biocef, Keflex, Novo-Lexin✤, Nu-Cephalex✤, PMS-Cephalexin✤

Pharmacologic class: First-generation cephalosporin
Therapeutic class: Anti-infective
Pregnancy risk category B

Action
Bactericidal; inhibits bacterial cell wall synthesis, causing osmotic instability and cell death

Availability
Capsules: 250 mg, 500 mg
Oral suspension: 100 mg/ml, 125 mg/ 5 ml, 250 mg/5 ml
Tablets: 250 mg, 500 mg

ⓘ Indications and dosages
➤ Respiratory tract infections caused by *Streptococcus pneumoniae* and group A beta-hemolytic streptococci; skin and skin-structure infections caused by staphylococci and streptococci; bone infections caused by staphylococci or *Proteus mirabilis;* genitourinary infections caused by *Escherichia coli, P. mirabilis,* and *Klebsiella* species; *Haemophilus influenzae,* staphylococci, streptococci, and *Moraxella catarrhalis* infections
Adults: 1 to 4 g P.O. daily in divided doses (usually 250 mg P.O. q 6 hours). For uncomplicated cystitis, skin and

---

✤ Canada   ◀€ Clinical alert   Reactions in **bold** are life-threatening

soft-tissue infections, and streptococcal pharyngitis, 500 mg P.O. q 12 hours.
Children: 25 to 50 mg/kg/day P.O. in divided doses

➤ Otitis media caused by *S. pneumoniae*
Children: 75 to 100 mg/kg/day P.O. in four divided doses

Dosage adjustment
• Renal impairment

Contraindications
• Hypersensitivity to cephalosporins or penicillin

Administration
• Give with or without food.
• Refrigerate oral suspension.

Route	Onset	Peak	Duration
P.O.	Rapid	1 hr	6-12 hr

Adverse reactions
CNS: fever, headache, lethargy, paresthesia, **seizures**
CV: edema, hypotension, vasodilation, palpitations, chest pain, syncope
EENT: hearing loss
GI: nausea, vomiting, diarrhea, abdominal cramps, oral candidiasis, **pseudomembranous colitis**
GU: elevated blood urea nitrogen (BUN), vaginal candidiasis, **nephrotoxicity**
Hematologic: lymphocytosis, eosinophilia, **hemolytic anemia, neutropenia, thrombocytopenia, bleeding, agranulocytosis, myelosuppression**
Musculoskeletal: joint pain
Respiratory: dyspnea
Skin: rash, maculopapular and erythematous urticaria, induration, sterile abscesses
Other: superinfections, chills, pain, allergic reaction, serum sickness, **anaphylaxis**

Interactions
Drug-drug. *Aminoglycosides, loop diuretics:* increased risk of nephrotoxicity

Chloramphenicol: antagonistic effect
Probenecid: increased cephalexin blood level

Drug-diagnostic tests. *Coombs' test:* false-positive result (especially in neonates whose mothers received drug before delivery)
Alanine aminotransferase, alkaline phosphatase, aspartate aminotransferase, bilirubin, BUN, creatinine, eosinophils, lactate dehydrogenase, lymphocytes,: increased values
Granulocytes, neutrophils, white blood cells: decreased counts

Precautions
Use cautiously in:
• renal impairment, phenylketonuria
• history of GI disease
• debilitated or emaciated patients
• elderly patients
• pregnant or breastfeeding patients.

Patient monitoring
• Assess for signs and symptoms of serious adverse reactions, including hypersensitivity, severe diarrhea, and bleeding.
• Monitor liver and renal function test results and complete blood cell count during long-term therapy.

Patient teaching
◀€ Instruct patient to stop taking drug and contact prescriber immediately if he develops a rash or breathing difficulties.
• Tell patient to take drug with full glass of water.
• Teach patient to report severe diarrhea.

cephradine
Velosef

Pharmacologic class: First-generation cephalosporin
Therapeutic class: Anti-infective
Pregnancy risk category B

Action
Bactericidal; inhibits bacterial cell wall synthesis, causing osmotic instability and cell death

Availability
Capsules: 250 mg, 500 mg
Oral suspension: 125 mg/5 ml, 250 mg/5 ml

⊘ Indications and dosages
➤ Respiratory, skin, and other infections (including otitis media and urinary tract infections)
Adults: 250 to 1,000 mg P.O. q 6 to 12 hours
Children older than age 9 months: 25 to 50 mg/kg/day P.O. q 6 hours in divided doses
Dosage adjustment
• Renal impairment

Contraindications
• Hypersensitivity to cephalosporins or penicillin
• Breastfeeding

Administration
• Give drug with food if it causes gastric upset.

Route	Onset	Peak	Duration
P.O.	Rapid	1-2 hr	6-12 hr

Adverse reactions
CNS: headache, lethargy, paresthesia, syncope, **seizures**

CV: phlebitis, thrombophlebitis, hypotension, vasodilation, palpitations, chest pain
EENT: hearing loss
GI: nausea, vomiting, constipation, abdominal cramps, oral candidiasis, **pseudomembranous colitis**
GU: elevated blood urea nitrogen (BUN), vaginal candidiasis, **nephrotoxicity**
Hematologic: anemia, bleeding, eosinophilia, leukopenia, bone marrow depression, lymphocytosis, hypoprothrombinemia, **neutropenia, thrombocytopenia, agranulocytosis**
Hepatic: transient rise in hepatic enzyme levels, **hepatomegaly**
Musculoskeletal: joint pain
Respiratory: dyspnea
Skin: rash, maculopapular and erythematous urticaria, induration, sterile abscesses, yellowing of skin and sclera
Other: chills; fever; edema; allergic reactions, including superinfections, serum sickness, and **anaphylaxis**

Interactions
Drug-drug. *Aminoglycosides, loop diuretics:* increased risk of nephrotoxicity
Probenecid: increased cephradine blood level

Drug-diagnostic tests. *Alanine aminotransferase, alkaline phosphatase, aspartate aminotransferase, bilirubin, BUN, creatinine, eosinophils, lactate dehydrogenase, lymphocytes:* increased levels
Coombs' test: false-positive result (especially in neonates whose mothers received drug before delivery)
Granulocytes, neutrophils, white blood cells: decreased counts

Precautions
Use cautiously in:
• renal impairment, phenylketonuria
• history of GI disease
• debilitated or emaciated patients
• elderly patients
• pregnant or breastfeeding patients.

Patient monitoring

• Assess for signs and symptoms of serious adverse reactions, including hypersensitivity, jaundice, and bleeding.
• Monitor hepatic and renal function test results.

Patient teaching

• Tell patient to take drug with full glass of water.
◀€ Instruct patient to immediately report severe diarrhea, abdominal pain, or vomiting.
◀€ Teach patient to stop taking drug and contact prescriber immediately if rash occurs.

cetirizine hydrochloride
Reactine✦, Zyrtec

Pharmacologic class: Histamine₁-receptor antagonist (peripherally selective)

Therapeutic class: Allergy, cold, and cough agent; antihistamine

Pregnancy risk category B

Action
Antagonizes histamine's effects at histamine₁-receptor sites, preventing allergic response. Also has mild bronchodilation effects and blocks histamine-induced bronchoconstriction in asthma.

Availability
Syrup: 5 mg/5 ml
Tablets: 5 mg, 10 mg

🅿 Indications and dosages
➢ Allergic symptoms caused by histamine release, including allergic rhinitis and chronic urticaria
Adults and children older than age 6: 5 to 10 mg P.O. daily
Children ages 2 to 5: 2.5 mg to 5 mg P.O. daily

Dosage adjustment
• Renal impairment
• Hepatic impairment

Off-label uses
• Bronchial asthma

Contraindications
• Hypersensitivity to drug or hydroxyzine
• Acute asthma attacks
• Narrow-angle glaucoma
• Pyloroduodenal obstruction
• Breastfeeding

Administration
• Give with or without food.
• Administer at same time each day.

Route	Onset	Peak	Duration
P.O.	30 min	1-4 hr	24 hr

Adverse reactions
CNS: dizziness, drowsiness, fatigue
CV: palpitations, edema
EENT: pharyngitis
GI: nausea, vomiting, abdominal distress, dry mouth
Musculoskeletal: myalgia, joint pain
Respiratory: bronchospasm
Skin: photosensitivity, rash, angioedema
Other: fever

Interactions
Drug-drug. *CNS depressants:* additive CNS effects
Theophylline: decreased cetirizine clearance
Drug-diagnostic tests. *Allergy skin testing:* false-negative results
Drug-behaviors. *Alcohol use:* additive CNS effects
Sun exposure: photosensitivity

Precautions
Use cautiously in:
• renal impairment, significant hepatic dysfunction
• elderly patients

✦ Canada   ◀€ Clinical alert   Reactions in **bold** are life-threatening

- pregnant patients
- children younger than age 2 (safety not established).

Patient monitoring
- Monitor creatinine levels in patients with renal dysfunction.
- Assess hepatic enzyme levels in patients with hepatic disease.

Patient teaching
- Tell patient to take with full glass of water.
- Inform patient that drug may impair alertness and that alcohol may exaggerate this effect.
- Advise patient to avoid driving and other hazardous activities until he knows how drug affects concentration and alertness.

cetrorelix acetate
Cetrotide

Pharmacologic class: Gonadotropin-releasing hormone (GnRH) antagonist
Therapeutic class: Infertility drug
Pregnancy risk category X

Action
Binds to membrane receptors on pituitary cells, disrupting natural GnRH; resulting antagonistic activity causes increased production and release of luteinizing hormone (LH) and follicle-stimulating hormone

Availability
Powder for injection: 0.25 mg, 3 mg

Indications and dosages
➤ Inhibition of premature LH surges in women undergoing controlled ovarian stimulation
Adults: *Single-dose regimen*—3 mg S.C. once daily, given when estradiol level indicates appropriate stimulation response (usually on day 7). If patient hasn't received human chorionic gonadotropin (hCG) within 4 days after injection, give cetrorelix 0.25 mg S.C. once daily until day of hCG administration. *Multidose regimen*—0.25 mg S.C. given on stimulation day 5 or 6 and continued daily until day of hCG administration.

Contraindications
- Hypersensitivity to drug
- Latex allergy
- Pregnancy or breastfeeding

Administration
- Preferably, inject into lower abdomen around navel; rotate sites as necessary.
- Know that drug may be self-administered by patient after thorough instruction.

Route	Onset	Peak	Duration
S.C.	1-2 hr	1-2 hr	≥4 days

Adverse reactions
CNS: headache
GI: nausea
GU: ovarian hyperstimulation syndrome
Other: pain or infection at injection site (redness, bruising, itching, or swelling), **fetal death**

Interactions
Drug-diagnostic tests. *Alanine aminotransferase (ALT), alkaline phosphatase (ALP), aspartate aminotransferase (AST), gamma-glutamyltransferase (GGT):* increased levels

Precautions
None

Patient monitoring
- Assess for pregnancy before starting therapy; if patient's pregnant, don't give drug.

• Monitor ALP, ALT, AST, and GGT levels.
• Assess patient's ability to self-administer drug.

Patient teaching
• Before allowing self-administration, teach patient how to prepare and administer S.C. injection; observe return demonstration.
• Instruct patient to immediately report vaginal bleeding or abdominal discomfort.

cevimeline hydrochloride
Evoxac

Pharmacologic class: Muscarinic, cholinergic agonist
Therapeutic class: Miscellaneous mouth and throat agent
Pregnancy risk category C

Action
Binds with and activates muscarinic receptors of the parasympathetic nerves, causing increased secretion of salivary and sweat glands. Also increases smooth-muscle tone in GI and urinary tracts.

Availability
Tablets: 30 mg

Indications and dosages
➤ Dry mouth in patients with Sjögren's syndrome
Adults: 30 mg P.O. t.i.d.

Contraindications
• Hypersensitivity to drug
• Narrow-angle glaucoma
• Uncontrolled asthma
• Acute iritis

Administration
• Give with water; ensure adequate fluid intake during therapy.

Route	Onset	Peak	Duration
P.O.	Unknown	1.5-2 hr	Unknown

Adverse reactions
CNS: headache, migraine, dizziness, fatigue, insomnia, rigors, anxiety, tremor, vertigo, depression, hypoesthesia, hyporeflexia, hypertonia
CV: peripheral edema, chest pain
EENT: conjunctivitis, abnormal vision, xerophthalmia, eye pain, earache, epistaxis, sinusitis, rhinitis, pharyngitis, sialadenitis, salivary gland pain, salivary gland enlargement, toothache
GI: nausea, vomiting, diarrhea, constipation, dyspepsia, abdominal pain, gastroesophageal reflux, flatulence, ulcerative stomatitis, dry mouth, increased salivation, anorexia
GU: urinary tract infection, cystitis, vaginitis
Hematologic: anemia
Musculoskeletal: back pain, joint pain, skeletal pain, myalgia, leg cramps
Respiratory: upper respiratory tract infection, coughing, bronchitis, pneumonia
Skin: erythematous or other rash, pruritus, diaphoresis, skin disorder
Other: hot flashes, hiccups, injury, pain, fever, flulike symptoms, fungal infection, edema, allergic reaction, abscess

Interactions
Drug-drug. *CYP2D6, CYP3A3, or CYP3A4 inhibitors:* inhibition of cevimeline metabolism
Parasympathomimetic drugs: additive effects

Precautions
Use cautiously in:
• cholelithiasis, cardiovascular disease, chronic bronchitis, chronic obstructive pulmonary disease

• history of nephrolithiasis.

Patient monitoring
• Monitor patient for signs and symptoms of toxicity (headache, visual disturbances, respiratory distress, GI cramps, nausea, vomiting, diarrhea, atrioventricular block, tachycardia, bradycardia, hypotension, shock, mental confusion, arrhythmias, tremor, and excessive sweating, salivation, or lacrimation).
• Assess fluid intake and output to detect dehydration early.

Patient teaching
◀≶ Tell patient to immediately report eye pain or vision changes.
• Teach patient to avoid driving and other hazardous activities until he knows how drug affects vision, concentration, and alertness.
• Inform patient that drug may make him sweat more and cause dehydration. Advise him to drink one glass of water every hour when awake.

---

chloral hydrate
Aquachloral Supprettes, Novo-Chloralhydrate✦, PMS-Chloral Hydrate✦

Pharmacologic class: CNS agent
Therapeutic class: Sedative-hypnotic
Controlled substance schedule IV
Pregnancy risk category C

Action
Unknown; thought to produce CNS depression by converting into its metabolite, trichloroethanol

Availability
Capsules: 250 mg, 500 mg
Suppositories: 324 mg, 500 mg, 648 mg
Syrup: 250 mg/ml, 500 mg/ml

Indications and dosages
➤ Nighttime sedation
Adults: 500 mg to 1 g 15 to 30 minutes before bedtime, not to exceed 2 g
Children: 50 mg/kg/day P.O., up to a maximum dosage of 1 g as a single dose or in divided doses
➤ Sedation
Adults: 250 mg P.O. or P.R. t.i.d. after meals
Children: 25 mg/kg/day P.O. or P.R., to a maximum daily dosage of 500 mg; may be given as a single dose or in divided doses

Contraindications
• Hypersensitivity to drug or tartrazine
• Coma, CNS depression, esophagitis, ulcer disease
• Pregnancy or breastfeeding

Administration
• Know that drug may take 45 to 60 minutes to achieve adequate preprocedural sedation in children.
◀≶ When giving to children for preprocedural sedation, be aware that drug may cause unpredictable or paradoxical effects.

Route	Onset	Peak	Duration
P.O.	30 min	1 hr	4-8 hr
P.R.	0.5-1 hr	Unknown	4-8 hr

Adverse reactions
CNS: dizziness, drowsiness, nightmares, ataxia, paradoxical stimulation, hangover, delirium, light-headedness, hallucinations, confusion
GI: nausea, vomiting, diarrhea, flatulence
Hematologic: eosinophilia, **leukopenia**
Skin: hypersensitivity reactions
Other: physical and psychological drug dependence

✦ Canada   ◀≶ Clinical alert   Reactions in **bold** are life-threatening

Interactions
Drug-drug. *CNS depressants (including antidepressants, antihistamines, narcotics, and other sedative-hypnotics):* excessive CNS depression
Furosemide: diaphoresis, flushing, variable blood pressure, nausea, uneasiness
Oral anticoagulants: increased risk of bleeding
Phenytoin: decreased phenytoin blood level
Drug-diagnostic tests. *Eosinophils:* increased count
Urinary 17-hydroxycorticosteroids: interference with test interpretation
White blood cells: decreased count
Drug-behaviors. *Alcohol use:* excessive CNS and respiratory depression

Precautions
Use cautiously in:
• hepatic dysfunction, severe renal impairment
• elderly patients.

Patient monitoring
• Monitor respiratory status, including oxygen saturation (using pulse oximetry), especially in children.
• Assess creatinine levels in patients with chronic renal disease.
• Monitor hepatic enzyme levels in patients with chronic hepatic disease.
• After giving to child, turn down lights in room and minimize other stimulation.

Patient teaching
• Instruct patient to avoid driving and other hazardous activities until he knows how drug affects concentration and alertness.
• Caution patient not to drink alcohol during therapy.
• When administering to a child, instruct parents to minimize stimulation to decrease risk of paradoxical reactions.

chlorambucil
Leukeran

Pharmacologic class: Alkylating agent, nitrogen mustard

Therapeutic class: Antineoplastic, immunosuppressant

Pregnancy risk category D

Action
Interacts with cellular DNA to produce cytotoxic cross-linkage; cell-cycle-phase nonspecific

Availability
Tablets: 2 mg

💊 Indications and dosages
➤ Chronic lymphocytic leukemia, malignant lymphoma
Adults: Initially, 0.1 to 0.2 mg/kg/day P.O. for 3 to 6 weeks as a single dose or in divided doses. Maintenance dosage is based on blood counts; shouldn't exceed 0.1 mg/kg/day.

Off-label uses
• Idiopathic membranous nephropathy
• Meningoencephalitis associated with Behçet's disease
• Rheumatoid arthritis

Contraindications
• Hypersensitivity to drug or other alkylating agents
• Pregnancy or breastfeeding

Administration
• Ask the patient about history of seizures or head trauma before starting therapy.
• After full-course radiation or chemotherapy, wait 4 weeks before giving full doses because of bone marrow vulnerability.

Route	Onset	Peak	Duration
P.O.	Unknown	1 hr	Unknown

Adverse reactions

CNS: peripheral neuropathy, tremor, confusion, agitation, ataxia, flaccid paresis, **seizures**

GI: nausea, vomiting, diarrhea

GU: sterile cystitis, amenorrhea, sterility, decreased sperm count

Hematologic: anemia, **leukopenia, thrombocytopenia, neutropenia, bone marrow depression**

Hepatic: jaundice, **hepatotoxicity**

Metabolic: hyperuricemia

Musculoskeletal: muscle twitching

Respiratory: interstitial pneumonitis, **pulmonary fibrosis**

Skin: rash, keratitis, erythema multiforme, **epidermal necrolysis**

Other: drug fever, allergic reactions, **Stevens-Johnson syndrome, secondary malignancies**

Interactions

Drug-drug. *Anticoagulants, aspirin:* increased risk of bleeding

Immunosuppressants, myelosuppressants (such as antineoplastics): additive bone marrow depression

Live-virus vaccines: decreased antibody response to vaccine, increased risk of adverse reactions

Drug-diagnostic tests. *Alanine aminotransferase, alkaline phosphatase, aspartate aminotransferase, uric acid:* increased levels (may reflect hepatotoxicity)

Granulocytes, hemoglobin, neutrophils, platelets, red blood cells, white blood cells (WBCs): decreased counts

Drug-herb. *Astragalus, echinacea, melatonin:* interference with immunosuppressant action

Precautions

Use cautiously in:

• hematopoietic depression, infection, other chronic debilitating diseases

• elderly patients

• females of childbearing age

• children (safety and efficacy not established).

Patient monitoring

◀≶ Monitor complete blood count with white cell differential and platelet count weekly.

• Monitor WBC count every 3 to 4 days.

• Assess liver function test results.

Patient teaching

• Teach patient to immediately report unusual bleeding or bruising, fever, nausea, vomiting, rash, chills, sore throat, cough, shortness of breath, seizures, amenorrhea, unusual lumps or masses, flank or stomach pain, joint pain, lip or mouth sores, or yellowing of skin or sclera.

• Tell patient to take drug with full glass of water.

• Inform patient that drug may increase his risk for infection. Advise him to wash hands frequently, wear a mask in public places, and avoid people with infections.

• Instruct patient to contact prescriber before receiving vaccines.

• Advise female patients to use reliable contraception.

chloramphenicol

AK-Chlor, Chloromycetin Ophthalmic, Chloroptic, Chloroptic S.O.P., Chlorsig, Novochlorocap✽, Pentamycetin✽, Sopamycetin

Pharmacologic class: Dichloroacetic acid derivative

Therapeutic class: Anti-infective

Pregnancy risk category NR

Action
Bacteriostatic action by binding with 50S subunit of ribosome and inhibiting protein synthesis

Availability
Injection: 1-g vial
Ointment (ophthalmic): 10 mg/g
Powder for solution (ophthalmic): 25 mg/vial
Solution (ophthalmic): 5 mg/ml

⚕ Indications and dosages
➤ Serious infections when less potentially dangerous drugs are ineffective or contraindicated
Adults: 50 to 100 mg/kg/day I.V. in divided doses q 6 hours, to a maximum dosage of 4 g/day
Children: 50 to 75 mg/kg/day I.V. in divided doses q 6 hours
➤ Bacteremia or meningitis
Children: 50 to 100 mg/kg/day I.V. in divided doses q 6 hours
➤ Ocular infections when less potentially dangerous drugs are ineffective or contraindicated
Adults and children: Instill two drops of ophthalmic solution in each eye q.i.d.; apply small amount of ophthalmic ointment to conjunctival sac at bedtime as supplement to solution. (Solution and ointment may be used together or alone.)
Dosage adjustment
• Hepatic impairment
• Renal impairment

Off-label uses
• Unspecified acne

Contraindications
• Hypersensitivity to drug
• Severe renal or hepatic impairment
• Prophylaxis for bacterial infections
• Acute porphyria

Administration
• Dilute parenteral dose with aqueous solution (for example, water for injection or dextrose 5% in water injection) to at least 100 mg/ml.
• Give parenteral form by I.V. infusion over at least 2 minutes.
• Don't give I.M.
• Be aware that drug should be used only when safer anti-infectives are ineffective or contraindicated.

Route	Onset	Peak	Duration
I.V.	Immediate	1-2 hr	8 hr
Ophthalmic	Unknown	Unknown	Unknown

Adverse reactions
CNS: confusion, delirium, depression, headache, peripheral neuropathy
EENT: optic neuritis, vision loss
GI: nausea, vomiting, diarrhea, abdominal pain, glossitis, colitis, pruritus ani, dry mouth
Hematologic: reticulocytopenia, **aplastic anemia, bone marrow depression, granulocytopenia, hypoplastic anemia, leukopenia, thrombocytopenia**
Skin: angioedema, rash, itching, urticaria, contact dermatitis
Other: fever, **anaphylaxis, gray syndrome in neonates**

Interactions
Drug-drug. *Aminoglycosides, penicillins:* decreased activity of these drugs
Barbiturates: increased barbiturate level, decreased chloramphenicol blood level
Hepatic enzyme inducers: decreased chloramphenicol blood level
Hydantoins: increased hydantoin blood level
Iron salts: increased iron level
Myelosuppressants, drugs that cause blood dyscrasias: increased bone marrow depression
Vitamin B_{12}: antagonism of hematopoietic response
Warfarin: enhanced warfarin action
Drug-diagnostic tests. *Alanine aminotransferase, aspartate aminotransferase,*

hemoglobin, platelets, red blood cells, white blood cells: altered values

Precautions
Use cautiously in:
• hepatic disease, renal disease, bone marrow depression
• pregnant or breastfeeding patients
• infants and children.

Patient monitoring
◀€ Monitor patient for signs and symptoms of aplastic anemia, which may occur weeks or months after therapy ends.
• Monitor complete blood cell count closely.
• Assess hepatic enzyme levels in patients with hepatic disease.
• Monitor creatinine levels in patients with renal insufficiency or failure.

Patient teaching
◀€ Instruct patient to report bleeding or bruising, even if therapy ended several weeks or months earlier.
• Teach patient to report rash or itching.
• Caution patient to avoid pregnancy during therapy. If she's using hormonal contraceptives, advise her to use additional birth control method; drug may make these contraceptives ineffective.

chlordiazepoxide hydrochloride
Apo-Chlordiazepoxide✤, Librium, Mitran, Novo-Poxide, Reposans-10

Pharmacologic class: Benzodiazepine
Therapeutic class: Anxiolytic, sedative-hypnotic
Controlled substance schedule IV
Pregnancy risk category D

Action
Unknown; may potentiate effects of gamma-aminobutyric acid (an inhibitory neurotransmitter) and depress CNS at limbic and subcortical levels of brain. Anxiolytic effect occurs at doses well below those that cause sedation or ataxia.

Availability
Capsules: 5 mg, 10 mg, 25 mg
Injection: 100-mg ampules

🖋 Indications and dosages
➤ Mild to moderate anxiety
Adults: 5 to 10 mg P.O. three to four times daily
➤ Severe anxiety
Adults: Initially, 50 to 100 mg I.M. or I.V.; then 25 to 50 mg P.O. three to four times daily as needed
➤ Preoperative apprehension or anxiety
Adults: 5 to 10 mg P.O. for several days before surgery or 50 to 100 mg I.M. 1 hour before surgery
➤ Acute alcohol withdrawal
Adults: Initially, 50 to 100 mg P.O., I.V., or I.M.; repeat dose as needed up to 300 mg/day.
Dosage adjustment
• Renal impairment
• Age 65 or older

Contraindications
• Hypersensitivity to drug, benzodiazepines, or tartrazine
• CNS depression
• Uncontrolled severe pain
• Porphyria
• Pregnancy or breastfeeding
• Children younger than age 6

Administration
• Dilute I.V. preparation with 5 ml of normal saline solution. Administer dose over at least 1 minute.
• When giving I.M., use 2 ml of special I.M. diluent.

✤ Canada   ◀€ Clinical alert   Reactions in **bold** are life-threatening

• Don't use I.M. diluent for I.V. preparation.

• After I.V. or I.M. administration, observe patient closely; enforce bedrest for several hours.

Route	Onset	Peak	Duration
P.O.	Rapid	0.5-4 hr	Up to 24 hr
I.V.	1-5 min	Unknown	0.25-1 hr
I.M.	15-30 min	Unknown	Unknown

Adverse reactions

CNS: dizziness, drowsiness, hangover, headache, depression, paradoxical stimulation

EENT: blurred vision

GI: nausea, vomiting, constipation, diarrhea

Hematologic: agranulocytosis

Hepatic: jaundice

Skin: rash

Other: physical or psychological drug dependence, drug tolerance, pain at I.M. site

Interactions

Drug-drug. *Antidepressants, antihistamines, opioids:* additive CNS depression

Barbiturates, rifampin: decreased chlordiazepoxide efficacy

Cimetidine, disulfiram, fluoxetine, hormonal contraceptives, isoniazid, ketoconazole, metoprolol, propoxyphene, propranolol, valproic acid: enhanced chlordiazepoxide effect

Levodopa: decreased levodopa efficacy

Drug-diagnostic tests. *Alanine aminotransferase, aspartate aminotransferase, bilirubin:* increased levels

Granulocytes: decreased count

Metyrapone test: decreased response

Radioactive iodine uptake test (^{123}I or ^{131}I): decreased uptake

Urine 17-ketogenic steroids, urine 17-ketosteroids: altered test results

Drug-herb. *Chamomile, hops, kava, skullcap, valerian:* increased CNS depression

Drug-behaviors. *Alcohol use:* increased CNS depression

Precautions

Use cautiously in:

• hepatic dysfunction, severe renal impairment

• debilitated or elderly patients.

Patient monitoring

• Monitor complete blood count and hepatic enzyme levels in prolonged therapy.

• Monitor renal and hepatic studies.

• Assess patient for apnea, bradycardia, and hypotension.

Patient teaching

• Instruct patient to avoid driving and other hazardous activities until he knows how drug affects concentration and alertness.

• Advise patient to avoid alcohol during therapy.

• Tell patient not to stop taking drug abruptly after several weeks or more of continuous use; instruct him to consult prescriber regarding dosage-tapering schedule.

• Caution female patient not to take drug if she's pregnant or might become pregnant during therapy. Advise her to use reliable contraception.

chloroquine hydrochloride
Aralen HCl

chloroquine phosphate
Aralen

Pharmacologic class: 4-amino-
quinolone derivative
Therapeutic class: Antimalarial,
amebicide
Pregnancy risk category C

Action
Unknown; antimalarial action may occur through inhibition of protein synthesis and alteration of DNA in susceptible parasites

Availability
Injection (hydrochloride): 50 mg/ml
(40-mg base)
Tablets (phosphate): 250 mg (150-mg
base), 500 mg (300-mg base)

Indications and dosages
➣ Uncomplicated acute malarial attacks
Adults: Initially, 1 g (600-mg base)
P.O., then an additional 500 mg (300-
mg base) P.O. 6 hours later and a single
dose of 500 mg (300-mg base) P.O. on
second and third days. Or initially, 160-
to 200-mg base I.M., repeated in 6
hours (800-mg base maximum dosage
during first 24 hours); continue for 3
days until total dosage of 1.5-g base has
been given. Switch to oral therapy as
soon as possible.
Children: Initially, 10 mg (base)/kg
P.O., then 5 mg (base)/kg 6 hours, 24
hours, and 36 hours later; don't exceed
recommended adult dosage. Or initially, 5 mg (base)/kg I.M. repeated 6
hours later, 18 hours after second dose,
and then 24 hours after third dose;

don't exceed recommended adult
dosage.
➣ Malaria prophylaxis
Adults: 500 mg (300-mg base) P.O.
weekly 1 to 2 weeks before visiting endemic area and continued for 4 weeks
after leaving area. If therapy starts after
malaria exposure, initial dosage is 600-
mg base P.O. in two divided doses 6
hours apart.
Children: 5 mg (base)/kg P.O. weekly
for 1 to 2 weeks before visiting endemic area and continued for 4 weeks after
leaving area, to a maximum dosage
of 300 mg weekly. If treatment starts
after exposure, 10 mg (base)/kg P.O. in
two divided doses 6 hours apart and
continued for 8 weeks after leaving
area.
➣ Extraintestinal amebiasis
Adults: Initially, 1 g (600-mg base) P.O.
chloroquine phosphate daily for 2
days, then 500 mg (300-mg base) daily
for 2 to 3 weeks. When oral therapy
isn't tolerated, give 160- to 200-mg
base I.M. daily for 10 to 12 days; switch
to oral therapy as soon as possible.
Children: 10 mg (base)/kg P.O. once
daily for 2 to 3 weeks, to a maximum
dosage of 300 mg (base) daily

Off-label uses
• Lupus erythematosus
• Rheumatoid arthritis

Contraindications
• Hypersensitivity to drug
• Retinal and visual field changes
• Porphyria

Administration
• Administer parenteral form I.M.
only.
• For obese patients, determine
weight-based dosages from lean body
weight (drug is stored in body tissues
and eliminated slowly).

Route	Onset	Peak	Duration
P.O.	Unknown	1-3 hr	Unknown
I.M.	Unknown	30 min	Unknown

Adverse reactions

CNS: mild and transient headache, psychic stimulation, dizziness, neuropathy, **seizures**

CV: hypotension, electrocardiogram changes

EENT: blurred vision, difficulty focusing, reversible corneal changes, irreversible retinal damage leading to vision loss, scotomas, ototoxicity, tinnitus, nerve deafness, vertigo

GI: nausea, vomiting, diarrhea, abdominal pain, stomatitis, anorexia

Hematologic: agranulocytosis, aplastic anemia, hemolytic anemia, thrombocytopenia

Skin: lichen planus eruptions, skin and mucosal pigmentation changes, pruritus, pleomorphic skin eruptions

Interactions

Drug-drug. *Aluminum and magnesium salts, kaolin:* decreased GI absorption of chloroquine

Cimetidine: decreased hepatic metabolism of chloroquine

Drug-diagnostic tests. *Granulocytes, hemoglobin, platelets:* decreased values

Drug-behaviors. *Sun exposure:* exacerbation of drug-induced dermatoses

Precautions

Use cautiously in:
• severe GI, neurologic, or blood disorders; hepatic impairment; glucose-6-phosphate dehydrogenase deficiency; neurologic disease; eczema
• alcoholism
• pregnant patients
• children.

Patient monitoring

• Monitor hepatic enzyme levels in patients with hepatic disease.

• Assess creatinine levels in patients with renal insufficiency or failure.

• With long-term therapy (as for lupus or rheumatoid arthritis), be aware that desired effects may not occur for up to 6 months.

• Be aware that drug is secreted in breast milk but not in sufficient amounts to prevent malaria in infant.

Patient teaching

• Teach patient to take drug with food at evenly spaced intervals.

◀€ Instruct patient to immediately report blurred vision or hearing changes.

• In areas where malaria is endemic, advise pregnant patient to check with prescriber about taking drug.

• Inform patient on long-term therapy that beneficial effects may take up to 6 months.

chlorothiazide
Diurigen, Diuril

Pharmacologic class: Thiazide
Therapeutic class: Diuretic, antihypertensive
Pregnancy risk category B

Action

Increases sodium and water excretion and inhibits sodium reabsorption in distal tubule, promoting excretion of chloride, potassium, magnesium, and bicarbonate.

Availability

Oral suspension: 250 mg/5 ml
Powder for injection: 500 mg
Tablets: 250 mg, 500 mg

⧸ Indications and dosages

➤ Edema associated with heart failure, renal dysfunction, cirrhosis, corticosteroid therapy, and estrogen therapy

Adults: 0.5 to 1 g P.O. daily (or I.V. for emergency use or for patients unable to receive oral form) as a single dose or in two divided doses

Children ages 3 to 6 months: 10 to 20 mg/kg P.O. daily as a single dose or in two divided doses

➣ Mild to moderate hypertension
Adults: 0.5 to 1 g P.O. daily as a single dose or in divided doses; adjust dosage to blood pressure response. (Rarely, patients may require up to 2 g/day in divided doses.)

Children: 10 to 20 mg/kg P.O. daily as a single dose or in two divided doses, not to exceed 375 mg/day (2.5 to 7.5 ml or ½ to 1½ tsp of oral suspension) in infants up to age 2, or 1 g/day in children ages 2 to 12. Infants younger than 6 months may require up to 30 mg/kg/day in two divided doses. I.V. use isn't recommended.

Contraindications
• Hypersensitivity to drug, other thiazides, benzodiazepines, sulfonamides, or tartrazine
• Anuria
• Gout
• Systemic lupus erythematosus
• Glucose tolerance abnormalities
• Hyperparathyroidism
• Bipolar disorder
• Breastfeeding

Administration
• Know that drug is not safe for I.M. or S.C. use.
• Be aware that drug may be ineffective in patients with renal insufficiency.

Route	Onset	Peak	Duration
P.O.	2 hr	4 hr	6-12 hr
I.V.	15 min	30 min	Unknown

Adverse reactions
CNS: dizziness, drowsiness, lethargy, weakness, encephalopathy, headache, insomnia, nervousness, vertigo, weakness, paresthesia, confusion, fatigue, asterixis

CV: hypotension, electrocardiogram changes, chest pain, hypovolemia, arrhythmias, thrombophlebitis

EENT: nystagmus

GI: nausea, vomiting, abdominal cramps, pancreatitis, anorexia

GU: polyuria, nocturia, impotence, loss of libido

Hematologic: blood dyscrasias

Hepatic: jaundice, **hepatitis**

Metabolic: dehydration, hypovolemia, hyperglycemia, hypokalemia, hypocalcemia, hypochloremic alkalosis, hypomagnesemia, hyponatremia, hypophosphatemia, hyperuricemia, hyperlipidemia, gout attack

Musculoskeletal: muscle cramps or spasms

Skin: photosensitivity, rash, urticaria, flushing

Other: fever, weight loss, hypersensitivity reactions

Interactions
Drug-drug. *Allopurinol:* increased risk of hypersensitivity reaction
Amphotericin B, corticosteroids, mezlocillin, piperacillin, ticarcillin: additive hypokalemia
Antihypertensives, barbiturates, nitrates, opiates: increased hypotension
Cholestyramine, colestipol: increased chlorothiazide absorption
Digoxin: increased risk of hypokalemia
Lithium: decreased lithium excretion, lithium toxicity
Nonsteroidal anti-inflammatory drugs: decreased chlorothiazide efficacy

Drug-diagnostic tests. *Bilirubin, serum and urine glucose (in diabetic patients), calcium, creatinine, uric acid:* increased levels
Cholesterol, low-density lipoproteins, triglycerides: decreased levels
Magnesium, potassium, protein-bound iodine, sodium: decreased levels
Urine calcium: decreased level

Drug-herb. *Ginkgo:* decreased antihypertensive effect
Licorice, stimulant laxative herbs (aloe, cascara sagrada, senna): increased risk of hypokalemia
Drug-behaviors. *Acute alcohol ingestion:* additive hypotension
Sun exposure: increased risk of photosensitivity

Precautions

Use cautiously in:
• renal or severe hepatic impairment
• pregnant patients.

Patient monitoring

• Monitor blood pressure.
• Assess electrolyte, bilirubin, creatinine, uric acid, magnesium, cholesterol, low-density lipoprotein, and triglyceride levels.
• Monitor urine calcium levels.
• Evaluate blood and urine glucose levels in patients with diabetes.

Patient teaching

• Advise patient to take drug in morning to avoid interrupting sleep with nighttime trips to bathroom.
◀≣ Instruct patient to immediately report yellow discoloration of eyes or skin, nausea, vomiting, diarrhea, fatigue, or lethargy.
• Advise patient not to stop taking drug abruptly; advise him to discuss dosage-tapering schedule with prescriber.
• Caution patient to use alcohol cautiously, if at all.
• Inform patient that drug makes him prone to dehydration. Tell him to stay indoors in hot weather and to increase fluid intake if he sweats more than usual.

chlorpheniramine maleate

Aller-Chlor, Allergy Chlo-Amine, Chlorate, Chlor-Trimeton, Chlor-Trimeton Allergy 4 Hour, Chlor-Trimeton Allergy 8 Hour, Chlor-Trimeton Allergy 12 Hour, Chlor-Tripolon♣, Novo-Pheniram♣, PediaCare Allergy Formula, Phenetron, Teldrin, Telachlor

Pharmacologic class: Propylamine (nonselective)

Therapeutic class: Antihistamine; allergy, cold, and cough remedy

Pregnancy risk category B

Action

Antagonizes effects of histamine at histamine$_2$-receptor sites, preventing histamine-mediated responses

Availability

Capsules (sustained-release): 8 mg, 12 mg
Syrup: 1 mg/5 ml, 2 mg/5 ml, 2.5 mg/5 ml
Tablets: 4 mg, 8 mg, 12 mg
Tablets (chewable): 2 mg
Tablets (timed-release): 8 mg, 12 mg

⑦ Indications and dosages

➤ Allergy symptoms caused by histamine release (as from nasal allergies and allergic dermatoses); management of hypersensitivity reactions (including anaphylaxis and transfusion reactions)
Adults: 4 mg q 4 to 6 hours P.O. or 8 to 12 mg of sustained-release form q 8 to 12 hours; maximum dosage is 24 mg/day
Children ages 6 to 12: 2 mg P.O. q 4 to 6 hours daily; maximum dosage is 12 mg/day
Dosage adjustment
• Glaucoma

- Gastric ulcer
- Hyperthyroidism
- Heart disease

Contraindications
- Hypersensitivity to drug
- Acute asthma attacks
- Narrow-angle glaucoma
- Stenosing peptic ulcer
- Symptomatic prostatic hypertrophy
- Breastfeeding

Administration
- Don't crush or break timed-release tablets or sustained-release capsules.
- Discontinue drug 4 days before allergy skin tests; drug may cause false-negative reactions.

Route	Onset	Peak	Duration
P.O.	15-30 min	1-2 hr	4-12 hr
P.O. (sustained)	Unknown	Unknown	Unknown

Adverse reactions
CNS: dizziness, drowsiness, excitation (in children), sedation, disturbed coordination, fatigue, confusion, restlessness, nervousness, tremor, headache, hysteria, tingling sensation, heaviness and weakness in hands
CV: palpitations, bradycardia, tachycardia, extrasystoles, hypotension, **arrhythmias**
EENT: blurred vision, diplopia, vertigo, tinnitus, acute labyrinthitis, nasal congestion, dry nose, dry throat, sore throat
GI: nausea, vomiting, diarrhea, constipation, GI obstruction, epigastric distress, anorexia, dry mouth
GU: urinary retention, urinary hesitancy, dysuria, early menses, decreased libido, impotence
Hematologic: hemolytic anemia, hypoplastic anemia, thrombocytopenia, leukopenia, agranulocytosis, pancytopenia
Respiratory: thickened bronchial secretions, chest tightness, wheezing

Skin: urticaria, rash, photosensitivity, diaphoresis
Other: chills, increased appetite, weight gain, **anaphylactic shock**

Interactions
Drug-drug. *CNS depressants (such as opioids, sedative-hypnotics):* additive CNS depression
Anticholinergics, anticholinergic-like drugs (such as some antidepressants, atropine, haloperidol, phenothiazines, quinidine, disopyramide): additive anticholinergic effects
Monoamine oxidase inhibitors: intensified, prolonged anticholinergic effects
Drug-diagnostic tests. *Allergy skin tests:* false-negative reactions
Drug-behaviors. *Alcohol use:* additive CNS depression
Sun exposure: photosensitivity

Precautions
Use cautiously in:
- hepatic or renal disease, narrow-angle glaucoma
- elderly patients
- pregnant patients (safety not established).

Patient monitoring
- Assess for urinary retention and frequency.
- Monitor respiratory status throughout therapy.

Patient teaching
- Advise patient to take drug with full glass of water.
- Tell patient not to crush timed-release tablets or sustained-release capsules; instruct him to swallow them whole.
- Instruct patient to avoid driving and other hazardous activities until he knows how drug affects concentration and alertness.
- Advise parents to give dose to children in evening because morning doses may cause inattention in school.

chlorpromazine hydrochloride

Chlorpromanyl✤, Largactil✤,
Novo-Chlorpromazine✤, Thorazine,
Thorazine Spansule, Thor-Prom

Pharmacologic class: Phenothiazine
Therapeutic class: Antipsychotic,
anxiolytic, antiemetic
Pregnancy risk category C

Action

Unknown; may block postsynaptic
dopamine receptors in brain and depress areas involved in wakefulness and
emesis. Also possesses anticholinergic,
antihistaminic, and adrenergic-
blocking properties.

Availability

Capsules (sustained-release): 30 mg,
75 mg, 150 mg, 200 mg, 300 mg
Injection: 25 mg/ml
Oral concentrate: 30 mg/ml, 40 mg/ml,
100 mg/ml
Suppositories: 25 mg, 100 mg
Syrup: 10 mg/5 ml, 25 mg/5 ml,
100 mg/5 ml
Tablets: 10 mg, 25 mg, 50 mg, 100 mg,
200 mg

⑦ Indications and dosages

➤ Acute schizophrenia or mania
Adults: *For hospitalized patients*—Initially, 25 mg I.M; if necessary, give an
additional 25 to 50 mg in 1 hour. Increase gradually, as needed, for several
days (up to 400 mg q 4 to 6 hours in
exceptionally severe cases) until symptoms are controlled; then give 500 mg
P.O. daily. In less acutely disturbed patients, 25 mg P.O. t.i.d., increased gradually until effective dosage is reached
(usually 400 mg P.O. daily). *For acutely
disturbed outpatients*—Initially, 10 mg
P.O. three or four times daily or 25 mg

P.O. two or three times daily. In more
severe cases, 25 mg P.O. t.i.d.; after 1 or
2 days, increase daily dosage by 20 to
50 mg at semiweekly intervals until effective dosage is reached.
Children ages 6 months to 12 years:
0.55 mg/kg P.O. (15 mg/m²) q 4 to 6
hours as needed, or 0.55 mg/kg I.M.
(15 mg/m²) q 6 to 8 hours (not to exceed 40 mg/day in children ages 6
months to 5 years, or 75 mg/day in
children ages 6 to 12), or 1 mg/kg P.R.
q 6 to 8 hours p.r.n.
➤ Nausea and vomiting
Adults: 10 to 25 mg P.O. q 4 to 6 hours,
increased if necessary; or 25 mg I.M. If
no hypertension occurs, give 25 to
50 mg I.M. q 3 to 4 hours as needed
until vomiting stops; then switch to
oral dosing or one 100-mg suppository
q 6 to 8 hours p.r.n.
➤ Nausea and vomiting during surgery
Adults: 12.5 mg I.M., repeated in 30
minutes p.r.n. if no hypotension occurs, or 2 mg I.V. at 2-minute intervals
(not to exceed 25 mg)
Children ages 6 months to 12 years:
0.275 mg/kg I.M.; may repeat in 30
minutes as needed
➤ Preoperative sedation
Adults: 25 to 50 mg P.O. 2 to 3 hours
before surgery, or 12.5 to 25 mg I.M. 1
to 2 hours before surgery
Children ages 6 months to 12 years:
0.55 mg/kg P.O. (15 mg/m²) 2 to 3
hours before surgery, or 0.55 mg/kg
I.M. 1 to 2 hours before surgery
➤ Intractable hiccups
Adults: 25 to 50 mg P.O. three to four
times daily. If symptoms continue for 2
to 3 days, give 25 to 50 mg I.M.; if
symptoms still persist, give 25 to 50 mg
by slow I.V. infusion with patient flat in
bed.
➤ Acute intermittent porphyria
Adults: 25 to 50 mg P.O. three to four
times daily. Drug usually is discontinued after several weeks, but some patients require maintenance doses. Or

25 mg I.M. t.i.d. until patient can tolerate oral doses.

➢ Tetanus

Adults: 25 to 50 mg P.O. three to four times daily (given with barbiturates, as prescribed); total dosage and frequency determined by patient response.

Children ages 6 months to 12 years: 0.55 mg/kg I.M. or 0.55 mg/kg I.V. q 6 to 8 hours

Dosage adjustment

• Age over 60

Off-label uses

• Anxiety disorders
• Migraine
• Phencyclidine (PCP) psychosis

Contraindications

• Hypersensitivity to drug, other phenothiazines, sulfites (injection), benzyl alcohol (sustained-release capsules)
• Narrow-angle glaucoma
• Bone marrow depression
• Severe hepatic or cardiovascular disease

Administration

◀€ Know that I.V. infusion is recommended only for severe hiccups.
• When giving by I.V. infusion for intractable hiccups, dilute in 500 to 1,000 ml of normal saline solution and infuse slowly.
• For direct I.V. injection during surgery, dilute to 1 mg/ml, using normal saline solution.
• For direct I.V. injection for tetanus, dilute to at least 1 mg/ml and administer at a rate of 1 mg/minute.
• When giving I.M., use Z-track injection method to minimize tissue irritation.
• Don't inject S.C.
• Know that in preoperative use, drug increases risk of neuromuscular excitation and hypotension when followed by barbiturate anesthetics.

Route	Onset	Peak	Duration
P.O.	30-60 min	Unknown	4-6 hr
P.O. (sustained)	30-60 min	Unknown	10-12 hr
I.V.	Rapid	Unknown	Unknown
I.M.	Unknown	Unknown	4-8 hr
P.R.	1-2 hr	Unknown	3-4 hr

Adverse reactions

CNS: sedation, extrapyramidal reactions, tardive dyskinesia, drowsiness, pseudoparkinsonism, **neuroleptic malignant syndrome, seizures**

CV: tachycardia, hypotension (especially with I.M. or I.V. use)

EENT: blurred vision, dry eyes, lens opacities, nasal congestion

GI: constipation, ileus, anorexia, dry mouth

GU: urinary retention, menstrual irregularities, galactorrhea, gynecomastia, inhibited ejaculation, priapism

Hematologic: eosinophilia, **agranulocytosis, leukopenia, hemolytic anemia, aplastic anemia, thrombocytopenia**

Hepatic: jaundice, **hepatitis**

Skin: rash, photosensitivity, pigmentation changes, sterile abscess

Other: allergic reactions, hyperthermia, pain at injection site

Interactions

Drug-drug. *Activated charcoal:* decreased chlorpromazine absorption
Adsorbent antidiarrheals, antacids: decreased chlorpromazine absorption
Antidepressants, antihistamines, general anesthetics, monoamine oxidase inhibitors, opioids, sedative-hypnotics: additive CNS depression
Antihistamines, disopyramide, quinidine, tricyclic antidepressants: increased anticholinergic effects
Antihypertensives: additive hypotension
Barbiturates: increased metabolism and decreased efficacy of chlorpromazine

Bromocriptine: decreased bromocriptine efficacy

Epinephrine: antagonism of peripheral vasoconstriction, epinephrine reversal

Guanethidine: inhibition of antihypertensive effects

Lithium: disorientation, loss of consciousness, extrapyramidal symptoms

Meperidine: excessive sedation and hypotension

Norepinephrine: reduced pressor effect, elimination of bradycardia

Phenytoin: altered phenytoin blood level, lowered seizure threshold

Pimozide: increased risk of potentially serious CV reactions

Propranolol: increased blood levels of both drugs

Tricyclic antidepressants (TCAs): increased TCA blood levels and effects

Valproic acid: decreased elimination and increased effects of valproic acid

Drug-diagnostic tests. *Alanine aminotransferase, alkaline phosphatase, aspartate aminotransferase, bilirubin:* increased levels

Granulocytes, hematocrit, hemoglobin, leukocytes, platelets: decreased values

Pregnancy tests: false-positive or false-negative results

Urine bilirubin: false-positive results

Drug-herb. *Angel's trumpet, jimsonweed, scopolia:* increased anticholinergic effects

Chamomile, hops, kava, skullcap, valerian: increased CNS depression

St. John's wort: photosensitivity

Yohimbe: increased risk of toxicity

Drug-behaviors. *Alcohol use:* increased CNS depression

Sun exposure: increased risk of photosensitivity

Precautions

Use cautiously in:
• diabetes mellitus, respiratory disease, prostatic hypertrophy, CNS tumors, epilepsy, intestinal obstruction
• elderly patients

• pregnant or breastfeeding patients
• children.

Patient monitoring

• Monitor blood pressure closely during I.V. infusion.
• Evaluate patient for signs and symptoms of neuroleptic malignant syndrome (hyperpyrexia, muscle rigidity, altered mental status, irregular pulse or blood pressure, tachycardia, diaphoresis, and arrhythmias). Stop drug immediately if these occur.
• Assess for extrapyramidal symptoms.

Patient teaching

• Instruct patient not to crush sustained-release capsules.
• Teach patient to take capsules or tablets with full glass of water, with or without food.
• Tell patient to mix oral concentrate in juice, soda, applesauce, or pudding.
• Instruct patient to avoid driving and other hazardous activities until he knows how drug affects concentration and alertness.

chlorpropamide
Apo-Chlorpropamide✚, Chloronase✚, Diabinese, Novo-Propamide✚

Pharmacologic class: Sulfonylurea
Therapeutic class: Hypoglycemic
Pregnancy risk category C

Action

Unknown; thought to reduce blood glucose level primarily by stimulating secretion of endogenous insulin from pancreatic beta cells

Availability

Tablets: 100 mg, 250 mg

Indications and dosages

➤ To lower glucose level in patients with non-insulin-dependent diabetes mellitus

Adults: 250 mg P.O. daily with breakfast

➤ Insulin to oral hypoglycemic therapy

Adults: For patient on 40 units of insulin or less, stop insulin and start chlorpropamide at 250 mg P.O. daily. If patient is receiving more than 40 units, start chlorpropamide at 250 mg P.O. daily with insulin dosage reduced 50%; further insulin decreases depend on patient response.

Dosage adjustment
• Renal impairment
• Debilitated patients
• Elderly patients

Off-label uses
• Diabetes insipidus

Contraindications
• Hypersensitivity to drug
• Diabetic ketoacidosis
• Type 1 diabetes mellitus

Administration
• Give before meals for best results.
• If drug causes gastric upset, give with food.
• To prevent hypoglycemia, adjust dosage during times of stress, illness, or decreased caloric intake.

Route	Onset	Peak	Duration
P.O.	1 hr	2-4 hr	24 hr

Adverse reactions
CNS: paresthesia, fatigue, dizziness, vertigo, malaise, headache
CV: increased risk of CV mortality
EENT: tinnitus
GI: nausea, heartburn, epigastric distress
GU: tea-colored urine

Hematologic: leukopenia, thrombocytopenia, aplastic anemia, agranulocytosis, hemolytic anemia
Hepatic: cholestatic jaundice
Metabolic: dilutional hyponatremia, **prolonged hypoglycemia**
Skin: rash, pruritus, erythema, urticaria
Other: hypersensitivity reaction, disulfiram-like reaction

Interactions
Drug-drug. *Anabolic steroids, chloramphenicol, clofibrate, guanethidine, monoamine oxidase inhibitors, salicylates, sulfonamides:* increased hypoglycemia
Beta-adrenergic blockers: prolonged hypoglycemia
Corticosteroids, glucagons, rifampin, thiazide diuretics: decreased hypoglycemic response
Hydantoins: increased hydantoin blood level
Oral anticoagulants: increased hypoglycemic activity
Drug-diagnostic tests. *Alanine aminotransferase, alkaline phosphatase, aspartate aminotransferase, bilirubin, blood urea nitrogen (BUN), cholesterol, creatinine, lactate dehydrogenase:* increased levels
Glucose, granulocytes, hemoglobin, platelets, sodium, white blood cells: decreased values
Drug-herb. *Bitter melon, burdock, dandelion, eucalyptus, ginkgo, marshmallow:* increased hypoglycemic activity
Drug-behaviors. *Alcohol use:* altered glycemic control (most commonly, leading to hypoglycemia), disulfiram-like reaction

Precautions
Use cautiously in:
• insulin hypersensitivity, hepatic or renal impairment, severe infection, trauma, major surgery
• elderly patients
• pregnant or breastfeeding patients.

Patient monitoring

• Assess electrolyte levels before starting therapy.

◀◤ Watch for signs and symptoms of jaundice.

• Monitor patient for fluid and electrolyte imbalances.

• Check blood pressure frequently.

• Monitor urine for ketones and glucose.

Patient teaching

• If patient takes drug once daily, instruct him to take it before breakfast. If he takes it more than once a day, teach him to take it before meals.

◀◤ Teach patient to recognize signs and symptoms of hypoglycemia (such as shaking, irritability, inability to think clearly, and flushed skin). Tell him to keep orange juice or other high-energy food available at all times to raise blood glucose level quickly. Instruct him to report hypoglycemia promptly.

◀◤ Advise patient to immediately report yellowing of eyes or skin.

• Teach patient how to test urine or blood for glucose; stress the need for regular testing.

◀◤ If patient is switching from insulin, instruct him to test his urine three times a day for glucose and ketones and to immediately report positive results.

• Emphasize importance of following recommendations regarding diet, exercise, and weight loss (if needed) to help control diabetes.

• Tell patient to consult prescriber before breastfeeding; drug may cause low blood glucose level in infant.

• Caution patient not to take over-the-counter weight-loss, cough, cold, or allergy preparations without consulting prescriber.

chlorthalidone

Apo-Chlorthalidone✤, Hygroton, Novo-Thalidone✤, Thalitone, Uridon✤

Pharmacologic class: Thiazide-like diuretic

Therapeutic class: Diuretic, antihypertensive

Pregnancy risk category B

Action

Unknown; enhances excretion of sodium, chloride, other electrolytes, and water by interfering with the transport of sodium ions across renal tubular epithelium. Also may dilate arterioles.

Availability

Tablets: 15 mg, 25 mg, 50 mg, 100 mg

💊 Indications and dosages

➤ Edema associated with heart failure, renal dysfunction, cirrhosis, corticosteroid therapy, and estrogen therapy

Adults: 50 to 100 mg/day P.O. (30 to 60 mg Thalitone) or 100 mg every other day P.O. (60 mg Thalitone), up to 200 mg/day (120 mg Thalitone)

➤ Management of mild to moderate hypertension

Adults: 25 mg/day P.O. (15 mg Thalitone). Based on patient response, may increase to 50 mg/day P.O. (30 to 50 mg Thalitone), then up to 100 mg/day P.O. (except Thalitone).

Contraindications

• Hypersensitivity to drug, other thiazides, sulfonamides, or tartrazine

• Renal decompensation

Administration

• Know that dosages above 25 mg/day are likely to increase potassium excretion without further increasing sodium excretion or decreasing blood pressure.

Route	Onset	Peak	Duration
P.O.	2 hr	4 hr	48-72 hr

Adverse reactions

CNS: dizziness, drowsiness, lethargy, weakness, fatigue, encephalopathy, headache, insomnia, nervousness, vertigo, asterixis, paresthesia, confusion, nystagmus

CV: hypotension, electrocardiogram changes, chest pain, volume depletion, arrhythmias, thrombophlebitis

GI: nausea, vomiting, cramping, anorexia, **pancreatitis**

GU: polyuria, nocturia, impotence, loss of libido

Hematologic: blood dyscrasias

Metabolic: gout attack, dehydration, hyperglycemia, hypokalemia, hypocalcemia, hypochloremic alkalosis, hypomagnesemia, hyponatremia, hypophosphatemia, hypovolemia, hyperuricemia, hyperlipidemia

Musculoskeletal: muscle cramps, muscle spasm

Skin: flushing, photosensitivity, hives, rash, exfoliative dermatitis, **toxic epidermal necrolysis**

Other: fever, weight loss, hypersensitivity reactions

Interactions

Drug-drug. *Allopurinol:* increased risk of hypersensitivity reaction

Amphotericin B, corticosteroids, mezlocillin, piperacillin, ticarcillin: additive hypokalemia

Antihypertensives, barbiturates, nitrates, opiates: increased hypotension

Cholestyramine, colestipol: decreased chlorthalidone blood level

Digoxin: increased risk of hypokalemia

Lithium: increased risk of lithium toxicity

Nonsteroidal anti-inflammatory drugs: decreased diuretic effect

Drug-diagnostic tests. *Bilirubin, calcium, creatinine, uric acid:* increased levels

Calcium: decreased urine level

Glucose (in diabetic patients): increased blood and urine levels

Magnesium, potassium, protein-bound iodine, sodium: decreased levels

Drug-herb. *Ginkgo:* decreased antihypertensive effects

Licorice, stimulant laxative herbs (aloe, cascara sagrada, senna): increased risk of potassium depletion

Drug-behaviors. *Acute alcohol ingestion:* additive hypotension

Sun exposure: increased risk of photosensitivity

Precautions

Use cautiously in:
• renal or severe hepatic impairment or disease, glucose tolerance abnormalities, gout, systemic lupus erythematosus, hyperparathyroidism, bipolar disorder
• elderly patients
• pregnant or breastfeeding patients.

Patient monitoring

• Closely monitor patient with renal insufficiency.
• Assess for signs and symptoms of hematologic disorders.
• Monitor complete blood count with white cell differential and serum uric acid and electrolyte levels.
• Monitor patient for hypersensitivity reactions, especially dermatitis.
• Assess for fluid and electrolyte imbalances.

Patient teaching

• Instruct patient to consume low-sodium diet containing plenty of potassium-rich foods and beverages, such as bananas, green leafy vegetables, and citrus juice.
• Caution patient to avoid driving and other hazardous activities until he

knows whether drug makes him dizzy or affects concentration and alertness.
• Teach patient with diabetes to check urine or blood glucose level frequently.

chlorzoxazone
EZE-DS, Paraflex, Parafon Forte DSC, Relaxazone, Remular, Remular-S, Strifon Forte DSC

Pharmacologic class: Autonomic nervous system agent
Therapeutic class: Skeletal muscle relaxant (centrally acting)
Pregnancy risk category C

Action
Unknown; thought to act primarily at spinal cord and subcortical level of brain to inhibit multisynaptic reflex arcs responsible for skeletal muscle activity.

Availability
Caplets: 250 mg, 500 mg
Tablets: 250 mg, 500 mg

Indications and dosages
➤ Adjunct to rest and physical therapy in treatment of muscle spasms associated with acute, painful musculoskeletal conditions
Adults: 250 to 750 mg P.O. three to four times daily

Contraindications
• Hypersensitivity to drug
• Hepatic impairment

Administration
• If desired, crush tablets and mix with food or water.
• Don't withdraw drug abruptly.

Route	Onset	Peak	Duration
P.O.	30-60 min	1-2 hr	3-4 hr

Adverse reactions
CNS: dizziness, drowsiness, light-headedness, malaise, headache, over-stimulation, tremor
GI: nausea, vomiting, constipation, diarrhea, heartburn, abdominal distress, anorexia
GU: orange or purplish-red urine
Hepatic: hepatic dysfunction
Skin: angioedema, allergic dermatitis, urticaria, erythema, pruritus, petechiae, ecchymosis
Other: allergic reactions

Interactions
Drug-drug. *CNS depressants (including antihistamines, antidepressants, opioids, sedative-hypnotics):* increased risk of CNS depression
Drug-diagnostic tests. *Alanine aminotransferase, alkaline phosphatase, bilirubin:* increased levels
Drug-herb. *Chamomile, hops, kava, skullcap, valerian:* increased CNS depression
Drug-behaviors. *Alcohol use:* increased sedation

Precautions
Use cautiously in:
• underlying cardiovascular disease, renal impairment
• children (safety not established).

Patient monitoring
◀€ Stay alert for signs and symptoms of hepatic disease. Withhold drug and notify prescriber right away if these occur.
• Monitor hepatic enzyme and electrolyte levels.

Patient teaching
• Caution patient not to consume alcohol during therapy.
• Instruct patient to avoid driving and other hazardous activities until he knows how drug affects concentration and alertness.

🔊 Instruct patient to promptly report yellowing of eyes or skin.
• Tell patient that drug may turn his urine red or orange.

cholestyramine
LoCHOLEST, LoCHOLEST Light, Novo-Cholamine✤, Novo-Cholamine Light✤, Prevalite, Questran, Questran Light

Pharmacologic class: Bile acid sequestrant
Therapeutic class: Lipid-lowering agent
Pregnancy risk category C

Action
Combines with bile acid in GI tract, forming an insoluble complex excreted in feces; complex regulates and increases cholesterol synthesis, causing serum cholesterol and low-density lipoprotein levels to decrease

Availability
Powder for suspension with aspartame (strawberry flavor [LoCHOLEST], unflavored [Prevalite, Questran Light]): 4 g cholestyramine/packet or scoop
Powder for suspension (strawberry flavor [LoCHOLEST], unflavored [Questran, generic]): 4 g cholestyramine/packet or scoop

⚱ Indications and dosages
➣ Primary hypercholesterolemia and pruritus caused by biliary obstruction; primary hyperlipidemia
Adults: Initially, 4 g P.O. once or twice daily; may increase as needed and tolerated, up to 24 g/day in six divided doses

Off-label uses
• Anti-infective–induced pseudomembranous colitis
• Adjunct in infantile diarrhea
• Digoxin toxicity

Contraindications
• Hypersensitivity to drug, its components, or other bile-acid sequestering resins
• Complete biliary obstruction
• Phenylketonuria (products containing aspartame)

Administration
• Mix powder with soup, cereal, pulpy fruit, juice, milk, or water.
• Administer 1 hour before or 4 to 6 hours after other drugs.

Route	Onset	Peak	Duration
P.O.	24-48 hr	1-3 wk	2-4 wk

Adverse reactions
CNS: headache, anxiety, vertigo, dizziness, insomnia, fatigue, syncope
EENT: tinnitus, tongue irritation
GI: nausea, vomiting, constipation, abdominal discomfort, fecal impaction, flatulence, hemorrhoids, perianal irritation, steatorrhea
GU: hematuria, dysuria, diuresis, burnt odor to urine
Hematologic: anemia, ecchymosis, increased prothrombin time
Hepatic: abnormal hepatic function
Metabolic: vitamin A, D, and K deficiencies; hyperchloremic acidosis
Musculoskeletal: joint pain, arthritis, back pain, muscle pain
Respiratory: wheezing, asthma
Skin: hypersensitivity reaction (irritation, rash, urticaria)

Interactions
Drug-drug. *Acetaminophen, amiodarone, clindamycin, clofibrate, corticosteroids, digoxin, diuretics, fat-soluble vitamins (A, D, E, and K), gemfibrozil, glipizide, imipramine, methotrexate,*

methyldopa, mycophenolate, niacin, nonsteroidal anti-inflammatory drugs, penicillin, phenytoin, phosphates, propranolol, tetracyclines, tolbutamide, thyroid preparations, ursodiol, warfarin: decreased absorption and effects of these drugs

Drug-diagnostic tests. *Alkaline phosphatase:* increased level
Hemoglobin: decreased value

Precautions
Use cautiously in:
• history of constipation or abnormal intestinal function
• pregnant patients
• children.

Patient monitoring
• Monitor complete blood count with white cell differential and liver function test results.
• If bleeding or bruising occurs, monitor prothrombin time; drug may reduce vitamin K absorption.
• Watch for constipation, especially in patients with coronary artery disease; take appropriate steps to prevent this problem.

Patient teaching
◄€ Instruct patient to immediately report yellowing of skin or eyes, bruising, or easy bleeding.
• Tell patient to take drug 1 hour before or 4 to 6 hours after other drugs.
• Teach patient about role of diet in controlling cholesterol level and preventing constipation.
• Instruct patient to avoid inhaling or ingesting raw powder; it must be mixed with food, juice, or milk before consuming.

choline salicylate
Arthropan, Teejel✦

Pharmacologic class: Nonsteroidal anti-inflammatory drug (NSAID)
Therapeutic class: Nonopioid analgesic, antipyretic, antiplatelet agent
Pregnancy risk category C (first and second trimesters), ***D*** (third trimester)

Action
Anti-inflammatory and analgesic actions result from inhibition of prostaglandin production; antipyretic action, from peripheral vasodilation; and antiplatelet action, from inhibition of synthesis of thromboxane A_2 (a potent vasoconstrictor and inducer of platelet aggregation)

Availability
Oral solution: 870 mg/5 ml

⬤ Indications and dosages
➤ Inflammatory disorders, including rheumatoid arthritis and osteoarthritis
Adults and children older than age 12: For rheumatoid arthritis, initially 870 mg P.O. up to q.i.d.
➤ Pain relief, fever reduction
Adults and children older than age 12: 870 mg P.O. q 3 to 4 hours, up to six times daily

Contraindications
• Hypersensitivity to salicylates
• Bleeding conditions
• Chickenpox
• Influenza
• Pregnancy (third trimester)
• Fever and dehydration in children

Administration
• Give with food or mix with fruit juice.
• Avoid giving to patients with gastric ulcers.

• Be aware that 435 mg of choline salicylate is equivalent to 325 mg of aspirin.

Route	Onset	Peak	Duration
P.O.	5-30 min	1-3 hr	3-6 hr

Adverse reactions

CNS: stimulation, drowsiness, dizziness, confusion, headache, flushing, hallucinations, depression, **seizures, coma**
CV: rapid pulse
EENT: hearing loss, tinnitus, **laryngeal edema**
GI: nausea, vomiting, dyspepsia, epigastric distress, heartburn, abdominal pain, anorexia, **GI bleeding**
Hematologic: prolonged bleeding time, prothrombin time, and activated partial thromboplastin time; shortened red blood cell life span; **leukopenia, agranulocytosis, thrombocytopenia, hemolytic anemia**
Hepatic: hepatotoxicity, hepatitis
Metabolic: hypoglycemia, hyponatremia, hypokalemia
Respiratory: wheezing, hyperpnea, **pulmonary edema**
Skin: angioedema, rash, urticaria, ecchymosis
Other: mild salicylism, **Reye's syndrome, anaphylaxis**

Interactions

Drug-drug. *Activated charcoal:* decreased choline salicylate absorption
Angiotensin-converting enzyme inhibitors: decreased antihypertensive effect
Antacid, urine alkalinizers: decreased choline salicylate efficacy
Anticoagulants: increased risk of bleeding
Beta-adrenergic blockers, probenecid, spironolactone, sulfinpyrazone, sulfonylureas: decreased effects of these drugs
Carbonic anhydrase inhibitors: salicylism

Cefamandole, clopidogrel, eptifibatide, plicamycin, thrombolytics, ticlopidine, tirofiban: increased bleeding
Corticosteroids: increased choline salicylate excretion, decreased blood level
Insulin, oral hypoglycemics, penicillin, phenytoin, valproic acid: increased effects of these drugs
Methotrexate: decreased excretion and increased blood level of methotrexate, possibly causing toxicity
Nizatidine: increased choline salicylate blood level
Vancomycin: increased risk of ototoxicity
Drug-diagnostic tests. *Alanine aminotransferase, alkaline phosphatase, amylase, aspartate aminotransferase, coagulation studies, $PacO_2$, uric acid:* increased levels
Cholesterol, potassium, protein-bound iodine: decreased levels
Pregnancy tests, protirelin-induced thyroid stimulating hormone, radionuclide thyroid imaging, serum uric acid, urine catecholamines, urine glucose, urine hydroxyindoleacetic acid determination, urine ketone determination by ferric chloride method, urine vanillylmandelic acid: test interference
Urine protein: increased level
Drug-food. *Urine-acidifying foods:* increased choline salicylate blood level
Drug-herb. *Anise, arnica, chamomile, clove, fenugreek, feverfew, garlic, ginger, ginkgo, ginseng, horse chestnut, kelpware, licorice:* increased risk of bleeding
Drug-behaviors. *Alcohol use:* increased risk of GI bleeding

Precautions

Use cautiously in:
• renal disease or impairment, anemia, hepatic disorders, Hodgkin's disease, gastritis, asthma, nasal polyps, hypoprothrombinemia, vitamin K deficiency
• elderly patients
• pregnant or breastfeeding patients
• children.

Patient monitoring

- Closely monitor patients receiving anticoagulants or corticosteroids concurrently.
- Monitor complete blood count with white cell differential and liver function test results.

Patient teaching

- Teach patient to take drug with food.
- Tell patient to mix solution with 30 ml of fruit juice.
- ◀╪ Instruct patient to immediately report yellowing of eyes or skin.
- ◀╪ Tell patient to contact prescriber right away if he experiences stomach pain, blood in stool or vomit, or ringing in ears.
- Inform patient that this drug contains aspirin.
- Stress that anyone with chickenpox or who has received chickenpox vaccine in past 6 months shouldn't take drug.

choriogonadotropin alfa
Ovidrel

Pharmacologic class: Gonadotropin
Therapeutic class: Ovulation stimulant
Pregnancy risk category X

Action

Stimulates late follicular maturation and resumption of oocyte meiosis; initiates rupture of preovulatory ovarian follicle

Availability

Powder for injection: 285-mcg vial

⊘ Indications and dosages

➤ Final follicular maturation in infertile women undergoing assisted reproductive technology and ovulation induction

Adults: 250 mcg S.C. 1 day after last dose of follicle-stimulating agent

Contraindications

- Hypersensitivity to drug
- Uncontrolled thyroid or adrenal dysfunction
- Abnormal uterine bleeding
- Ovarian cysts
- Sex hormone–dependent tumors of reproductive tract
- Pregnancy

Administration

- Obtain pregnancy test before starting therapy; drug may cause birth defects when given during pregnancy.
- Be aware that drug is intended for single S.C. injection.
- Reconstitute with 1 ml of sterile water for injection.

Route	Onset	Peak	Duration
S.C.	Unknown	12-24 hr	Unknown

Adverse reactions

CNS: dizziness, headache, malaise, paresthesia
CV: heart murmur, **arterial thromboembolism, arrhythmias**
EENT: pharyngitis
GI: nausea, vomiting, diarrhea, abdominal pain, flatulence
GU: dysuria, urinary tract infection, urinary incontinence, albuminuria, ovarian hyperstimulation syndrome, spontaneous abortion, congenital abnormalities in infants, premature labor, postpartum fever, cervical lesion, leukorrhea, breast pain, intermenstrual bleeding, uterine disorders, vaginitis, genital candidiasis, genital herpes, vaginal discomfort, **ectopic pregnancy, cervical cancer, vaginal hemorrhage**
Hematologic: leukocytosis
Metabolic: hyperglycemia
Musculoskeletal: back pain

Respiratory: upper respiratory tract infection

Skin: rash, pruritus

Other: hiccups; fever; hot flashes; body pain; bruising, inflammation, and pain at injection site

Interactions

Drug-diagnostic tests. *Glucose:* increased level

Precautions

Use cautiously in:
• thromboembolic disease, diabetes mellitus
• breastfeeding patients.

Patient monitoring

• Assess for signs and symptoms of thromboembolic disease.
• Monitor blood glucose level in patients with diabetes.

Patient teaching

◀§ Inform patient that drug may cause potentially fatal ovarian hyperstimulation syndrome (especially during first cycle of therapy). Tell her to immediately report nausea, vomiting, diarrhea, decreased urination, abdominal or pelvic pain, or swelling in hands or legs.
• Advise patient that drug increases risk of multiple births, which may pose a risk to patient and unborn fetuses.
• Teach patient and her partner how to inject S.C. medication at home.

cidofovir
Vistide

Pharmacologic class: Purine nucleotide cytosine analog

Therapeutic class: Antiviral

Pregnancy risk category C

Action

Exerts antiviral effect by interfering with DNS synthesis and inhibiting viral replication

Availability

Solution for injection: 75 mg/ml in 5-ml, single-use vial

⟋ Indications and dosages

➤ CMV retinitis in AIDS patients

Adults: 5 mg/kg I.V. infused over 1 hour q week for 2 continuous weeks (given with oral probenecid); then 5 mg/kg I.V. once q 2 weeks as maintenance dose (given with oral probenecid)

Dosage adjustment
• Renal impairment

Contraindications

• Hypersensitivity to drug, probenecid, or other sulfa-containing agents
• Creatinine level above 1.5 mg/dl, calculated creatinine clearance of 55 ml/minute or less, or urine protein level of 100 mg/dl or more
• Concurrent use of nephrotoxic drugs

Administration

◀§ Be aware that drug carries a high risk of nephrotoxicity. Follow administration instructions carefully, including preinfusion and postinfusion hydration with I.V. normal saline solution.
• Premedicate with probenecid 2 g P.O. as prescribed 3 hours before starting cidofovir infusion.
• Mix I.V. dose in 100 ml of normal saline solution.
• Before starting infusion, give 1 L of normal saline solution over 1 to 2 hours.
• Give 1 L of normal saline solution during or immediately after infusion (unless contraindicated).
• Administer probenecid 1 g 2 hours and 8 hours after infusion ends, as ordered.

• If drug contacts skin, flush thoroughly with water.

Route	Onset	Peak	Duration
I.V.	Rapid	End of infusion	Unknown

Adverse reactions

CNS: headache, asthenia, **seizures, coma**
EENT: decreased intraocular pressure
GI: nausea, vomiting, diarrhea, anorexia, oral candidiasis
GU: proteinuria, increased creatinine level, **nephrotoxicity**
Hematologic: neutropenia
Hepatic: hepatomegaly
Metabolic: metabolic acidosis
Musculoskeletal: muscle contractions
Respiratory: dyspnea, increased cough
Skin: rash, alopecia
Other: pain, fever, chills, infection, pain at injection site

Interactions

Drug-drug. *Nephrotoxic drugs:* increased risk of nephrotoxicity
Drug-diagnostic tests. *Alanine aminotransferase, alkaline phosphatase, aspartate aminotransferase, blood urea nitrogen, creatinine, lactate dehydrogenase:* increased levels
Bicarbonate, creatinine clearance, hemoglobin, neutrophils, platelets: decreased values

Precautions

Use cautiously in:
• mild renal impairment
• elderly patients
• pregnant or breastfeeding patients
• children younger than age 12 (safety and efficacy not established).

Patient monitoring

• Assess white blood cell count and creatinine and urine protein levels within 48 hours of each dose.
• Closely monitor intraocular pressure and visual acuity.

• Monitor hepatic enzyme levels in patients with hepatic disease.

Patient teaching

◀╫ Teach patient to immediately report postinfusion fever, vision changes, nausea, vomiting, rash, or urinary output changes.
• Emphasize importance of taking probenecid with each dose, as prescribed.
• Instruct patient to have regular eye examinations.
• Advise female patients of childbearing age to use effective contraception during and for 1 month after therapy.
• Instruct male patients to use barrier contraception during and for 3 months after therapy.

cilostazol
Pletal

Pharmacologic class: Quinolone derivative
Therapeutic class: Antiplatelet agent
Pregnancy risk category C

Action

Unclear; thought to inhibit phosphodiesterase III by increasing cyclic adenosine monophosphate in platelets and blood vessels, causing vasodilation

Availability

Tablets: 50 mg, 100 mg

⟋ Indications and dosages
➢ Intermittent claudication
Adults: 100 mg P.O. b.i.d. at least 30 minutes before or 2 hours after breakfast and dinner
Dosage adjustment
• Concurrent use of erythromycin, ketoconazole, or omeprazole

Contraindications

- Hypersensitivity to drug
- Heart failure

Administration

- Give with water 30 minutes before or 2 hours after patient consumes food or milk.
- Don't give with grapefruit juice.
- Be aware that although response may appear within 2 to 3 weeks, patient should continue therapy for up to 12 weeks or as prescribed.

Route	Onset	Peak	Duration
P.O.	Gradual	4-6 hr	Unknown

Adverse reactions

CNS: dizziness, headache, vertigo
CV: tachycardia
GI: abdominal pain, abnormal stools, dyspepsia, flatulence
EENT: rhinitis, pharyngitis
Musculoskeletal: back pain, myalgia
Respiratory: increased cough
Other: infection

Interactions

Drug-drug. *Diltiazem, erythromycin, macrolides, omeprazole, CYP3A4 and CYP2C19 inhibitors:* increased cilostazol blood level
Drug-food. *Grapefruit juice, high-fat meals:* increased cilostazol blood level
Drug-behaviors. *Smoking:* decreased exposure to cilostazol

Precautions

Use cautiously in:
- cardiovascular disorders
- patients receiving other antiplatelet agents concurrently
- pregnant or breastfeeding patients
- children (safety and efficacy not established).

Patient monitoring

- Monitor cardiovascular status.
- Closely monitor patients receiving other antiplatelet drugs.

Patient teaching

- Instruct patient to take drug with full glass of water, 30 minutes before or 2 hours after food or milk.
- Tell patient not to drink grapefruit juice during therapy.
- Advise patient to report nausea, vomiting, or abdominal pain.
- Instruct patient not to smoke because smoking interferes with drug effects.

cimetidine

Apo-Cimetidine✦, Gen-Cimetidine✦, Novo-Cimetine✦, Nu-Cimet✦, Peptol✦, Tagamet, Tagamet HB, Tagamet HB 200 Suspension

Pharmacologic class: Histamine$_2$-receptor antagonist
Therapeutic class: Antiulcer drug
Pregnancy risk category B

Action

Inhibits action of histamine at histamine$_2$-receptor sites (located primarily in gastric parietal cells), resulting in inhibition of gastric acid secretion

Availability

Oral liquid: 200 mg/5 ml, 300 mg/5 ml
Solution for injection: 300 mg/2-ml vials, 300 mg/50 ml premixed in normal saline solution
Tablets: 100 mg, 200 mg, 300 mg, 400 mg, 600 mg, 800 mg

Indications and dosages

➤ Active duodenal ulcer (short-term therapy)
Adults and children older than age 16: 800 mg P.O. at bedtime, or 300 mg P.O. q.i.d. with meals and at bedtime, or 400 mg P.O. b.i.d.; maintenance dosage is 400 mg P.O. at bedtime.

➤ Active benign gastric ulcer (short-term therapy)

Adults and children older than age 16: 800 mg P.O. at bedtime or 300 mg P.O. q.i.d. with meals and at bedtime

➤ Gastric hypersecretory conditions (such as Zollinger-Ellison syndrome), intractable ulcers

Adults and children older than age 16: 300 mg P.O. q.i.d with meals and at bedtime; in hospitalized patients, 300 mg I.M. or I.V. q 6 hours

➤ Erosive gastroesophageal reflux disease

Adults and children older than age 16: 1,600 mg P.O. daily in divided doses (800 mg b.i.d. or 400 mg q.i.d.) for 12 weeks

➤ Prevention of stress-induced upper GI bleeding in critically ill patients

Adults and children older than age 16: 50 mg/hour as continuous I.V. infusion

➤ Heartburn, acid indigestion

Adults and children older than age 16: 200 mg (2 tablets of over-the-counter product only) P.O. with water as directed, up to twice daily. Give maximum dosage for no longer than 2 weeks continuously, unless directed by prescriber.

Dosage adjustment
• Renal impairment

Off-label uses
• Acetaminophen overdose
• Adjunctive therapy in burns
• Barrett's esophagus
• Renal carcinoma
• Anaphylaxis

Contraindications
• Hypersensitivity to drug
• Intolerance to alcohol (oral forms)

Administration
• Give I.M. dose undiluted.
• Dilute I.V. dose in normal saline solution or other compatible solution.
• Administer I.V. dose over at least 5

minutes; may give intermittently over 15 to 20 minutes.
• Give continuous I.V. infusion at a rate of 37.5 mg/hour.
• When giving drug to prevent stress ulcers, administer by continuous I.V. infusion at a rate of 50 mg/hour.

Route	Onset	Peak	Duration
P.O.	30 min	45-90 min	4-5 hr
I.V., I.M.	10 min	30 min	4-5 hr

Adverse reactions
CNS: confusion, dizziness, drowsiness, hallucinations, agitation, psychosis, depression, anxiety, headache
GI: diarrhea
GU: reversible impotence, gynecomastia
Hepatic: elevated transaminase levels
Other: pain at I.M. site

Interactions
Drug-drug. *Calcium channel blockers, carbamazepine, chloroquine, lidocaine, metformin, metronidazole, moricizine, pentoxifylline, phenytoin, propafenone, quinidine, quinine, some benzodiazepines, some beta blockers (chlordiazepoxide, diazepam, midazolam), sulfonylureas, tacrine, theophylline, triamterene, tricyclic antidepressants, valproic acid, warfarin:* decreased metabolism of these drugs, possible toxicity
Drug-diagnostic tests. *Creatinine, transaminases:* increased levels
Parathyroid hormone: decreased level
Prolactin (after I.V. bolus of cimetidine): increased level
Skin tests using allergenic extracts: false-negative results (drug should be discontinued 24 hours before testing)
Drug-food. *Caffeine-containing foods and beverages (such as coffee, chocolate):* increased drug blood level, increased risk of toxicity
Drug-herb. *Pennyroyal:* change in rate at which herb's toxic metabolite forms
Yerba maté: decreased yerba maté

clearance, possible toxicity
Drug-behaviors. *Alcohol use:* increased blood alcohol level

Precautions
Use cautiously in:
• renal impairment
• elderly patients
• pregnant or breastfeeding patients.

Patient monitoring
• Monitor creatinine levels in patients with renal insufficiency or failure.
• Assess elderly or chronically ill patients for confusion (which usually resolves once therapy ends).

Patient teaching
• Inform patient that gastric ulcer may take up to 2 months to heal. Advise him not to discontinue therapy, even if he feels better, without first contacting prescriber. Ulcer may recur if therapy ends too soon.
• Advise patient not to take over-the-counter cimetidine for more than 2 weeks continuously, except with prescriber's advice and supervision.

---

ciprofloxacin
Cipro, CiproHC Otic, Cipro I.V.

Pharmacologic class: Fluoroquinolone
Therapeutic class: Anti-infective
Pregnancy risk category C

Action
Inhibits bacterial DNA synthesis by inhibiting DNA gyrase in susceptible gram-negative and gram-positive aerobic and anaerobic organisms

Availability
Injection: 200 mg/20 ml, 400 mg/40 ml, 200 mg/100 ml premixed in dextrose 5% in water (D_5W), 400 mg/200 ml

premixed in D_5W, 1,200 mg/120-ml bulk package
Oral suspension: 5 g/100 ml (5%), 10 g/100 ml (10%)
Tablets: 250 mg, 500 mg, 750 mg

Indications and dosages
➤ Acute sinusitis
Adults: 500 mg P.O. q 12 hours or 400 mg I.V. for 10 days
➤ Prostatitis
Adults: 500 mg P.O. q 12 hours or 400 mg I.V. for 28 days
➤ Intra-abdominal infections
Adults: 500 mg P.O. q 12 hours or 400 mg I.V. for 7 to 14 days
➤ Febrile neutropenic patients
Adults: 400 mg I.V. q 8 hours
➤ Gonorrhea
Adults: 250 mg P.O. as a single dose
➤ Infectious diarrhea
Adults: 500 mg P.O. q 12 hours for 5 to 7 days
➤ Inhalation anthrax (postexposure)
Adults: 500 mg P.O. q 12 hours for 60 days or 400 mg I.V. q 12 hours for 60 days
Children: 15 mg/kg P.O. q 12 hours for 60 days (not to exceed 500 mg/dose) or 10 mg/kg I.V. q 12 hours for 60 days. Maximum dosage shouldn't exceed 400 mg/dose.
➤ Lower respiratory tract, skin and skin-structure, bone, and joint infections
Adults: 500 mg to 750 mg P.O. q 12 hours or 400 mg I.V. q 8 hours for 7 to 14 days. Severe bone and joint infections may necessitate up to 6 weeks of therapy.
➤ Nosocomial pneumonia
Adults: 400 mg I.V. q 8 hours
➤ Typhoid fever
Adults: 500 mg P.O. q 12 hours for 10 days
➤ Urinary tract infections
Adults: 250 to 500 mg P.O. q 12 hours, or 200 to 400 mg I.V. q 12 hours for 3

---

days in acute uncomplicated infection or for 7 to 14 days in mild to severe complicated infection
Dosage adjustment
• Renal impairment or insufficiency

Off-label uses
• Chancroid
• Cystic fibrosis
• Pseudomembranous anti-infective–associated colitis

Contraindications
• Hypersensitivity to drug or other fluoroquinolones

Administration
• Infuse I.V. dose over at least 1 hour; use pump to ensure 1-hour duration.
• Be aware that oral suspension isn't suitable for use in nasogastric tube.

Route	Onset	Peak	Duration
P.O.	Rapid	1-2 hr	12 hr
I.V.	Rapid	End of infusion	12 hr

Adverse reactions
CNS: agitation, headache, restlessness, confusion, delirium, myoclonus, toxic psychosis
CV: orthostatic hypotension, vasculitis
EENT: nystagmus, anosmia
GI: nausea, vomiting, diarrhea, constipation, abdominal pain or discomfort, dyspepsia, dysphagia, flatulence, altered taste, **pseudomembranous colitis, pancreatitis**
GU: albuminuria, candiduria, renal calculi
Hematologic: methemoglobinemia, prolonged prothrombin time, **agranulocytosis, hemolytic anemia**
Hepatic: jaundice, elevated hepatic enzyme levels, **hepatic necrosis**
Metabolic: elevated cholesterol level, hypertriglyceridemia, hyperglycemia, hyperkalemia
Musculoskeletal: myalgia, tendinitis, tendon rupture

Skin: rash, erythema multiforme, exfoliative dermatitis, **toxic epidermal necrolysis**
Other: exacerbation of myasthenia gravis, hypersensitivity reactions including **anaphylaxis** and **Stevens-Johnson syndrome**

Interactions
Drug-drug. *Antacids, bismuth subsalicylate, iron salts, sucralfate, zinc salts:* decreased ciprofloxacin absorption
Cyclosporine: transient creatinine increase
Hormonal contraceptives: reduced contraceptive efficacy
Oral anticoagulants: increased anticoagulant effects
Phenytoin: increased or decreased phenytoin blood level
Probenecid: decreased renal elimination of ciprofloxacin, causing increased blood level
Theophylline: increased theophylline blood level, increased risk of toxicity
Drug-diagnostic tests. *Alanine aminotransferase, alkaline phosphatase, aspartate aminotransferase, bilirubin, glucose, lactate dehydrogenase, potassium, triglycerides:* increased levels
Drug-food. *Caffeine:* interference with caffeine clearance
Concurrent tube feedings: impaired drug absorption (because of metal cations)
Milk, yogurt (when consumed alone with ciprofloxacin): decreased drug absorption
Drug-herb. *Fennel:* decreased drug absorption

Precautions
Use cautiously in:
• cirrhosis, renal impairment, underlying CNS disease
• elderly patients
• pregnant or breastfeeding patients
• children younger than age 18.

Patient monitoring

• In patients with renal insufficiency, assess creatinine level before giving dose and at least once a week during prolonged therapy. Monitor drug blood level closely.

• Watch for signs and symptoms of serious adverse reactions, including GI problems, jaundice, and hypersensitivity reactions.

Patient teaching

• Teach patient to take drug 2 hours after a meal.

• Instruct patient to swallow microcapsules in oral suspension whole without chewing.

• Advise patient not to take drug with dairy products alone or with caffeinated beverages.

• Instruct patient to drink 8 oz of water every hour when awake to ensure proper hydration.

• Advise patients taking hormonal contraceptives to use supplemental birth control method, such as condoms; drug reduces contraceptive efficacy.

• Inform breastfeeding patient that drug is excreted in breast milk and can affect infant's bone growth. Advise her to consult prescriber before taking.

cisatracurium besylate
Nimbex

Pharmacologic class: Neuromuscular blocker

Therapeutic class: Skeletal muscle relaxant

Pregnancy risk category B

Action

Competively binds to cholinergic receptors on motor endplate, antagonizing the action of acetylcholine and blocking neuromuscular transmission

Availability

Injection: 2 mg/ml, 10 mg/ml

Indications and dosages

➤ Adjunct to general anesthesia; skeletal muscle relaxation during mechanical ventilation

Adults: Initially, 0.15 mg/kg I.V., then maintain on dosage of 0.03 mg/kg I.V. q 40 to 50 minutes; or initially, 0.2 mg/kg I.V., then maintain on dosage of 0.03 mg/kg I.V. q 50 to 60 minutes. Or initially, a maintenance I.V. infusion of 3 mcg/kg/minute, titrating to 1 to 2 mcg/kg/minute p.r.n.

Children ages 2 to 12: 0.1 mg/kg I.V. over 5 to 10 seconds; then give maintenance infusion at 3 mcg/kg/ minute, titrating to 1 to 2 mcg/kg/ minute p.r.n.

Contraindications

• Hypersensitivity to drug

Administration

◀ Don't give unless mechanical ventilation support and emergency equipment are available.

• Initial dose may be given as I.V. bolus, followed by continuous infusion at prescribed rate.

Route	Onset	Peak	Duration
I.V.	1-2 min	2-5 min	25-44 min

Adverse reactions

CV: hypotension, flushing, **bradycardia**

Respiratory: bronchospasm, **prolonged apnea**

Skin: rash

Interactions

Drug-drug. *Aminoglycosides, bacitracin, clindamycin, colistimethate sodium, colistin, lincomycin, lithium, local anesthetics, magnesium salts, polymyxins, procainamide, quinidine, tetracyclines:* enhanced neuromuscular blockade

Carbamazepine, phenytoin: shortened duration of neuromuscular blockade
Enflurane or isoflurane given with nitrous oxide or oxygen: prolonged duration of cisatracurium action
Succinylcholine: faster onset of maximal neuromuscular blockade
Drug-herb. *St. John's wort:* increased risk of cardiovascular collapse, delayed emergence from anesthesia

Precautions

Use cautiously in:
• neuromuscular disease, peripheral neuropathy
• concurrent anticonvulsant therapy
• pregnant or breastfeeding patients.

Patient monitoring

• Monitor vital signs and electrocardiogram; stay alert for respiratory depression, bradycardia, and hypotension.
• Use peripheral nerve stimulator to monitor degree of neuromuscular blockade during administration. Continue to use nerve stimulator to monitor recovery from neuromuscular blockade after drug therapy is stopped.

Patient teaching

• Be aware that patient's hearing is intact during neuromuscular blockade; continue to provide explanations and reassurance during therapy.

---

cisplatin
Platinol, Platinol-AQ

Pharmacologic class: Alkylating agent, platinum coordination complex
Therapeutic class: Antineoplastic
Pregnancy risk category D

Action

Inhibits DNA synthesis by causing intrastrand and interstrand cross-linking of DNA

Availability

Injection: 1 mg/ml in 50-mg and 100-mg vials

🖊 Indications and dosages

➤ Metastatic testicular tumors
Adults: 20 mg/m² I.V. daily for 5 days/cycle, repeated q 3 to 4 weeks
➤ Metastatic ovarian cancer
Adults: 75 to 100 mg/m² I.V. repeated q 4 weeks in combination with cyclophosphamide, or 100 mg/m² q 4 weeks as a single agent
➤ Advanced bladder cancer
Adults: 50 to 70 mg/m² I.V. q 3 to 4 weeks as a single agent; dosage varies depending on whether patient has undergone radiation or chemotherapy.

Off-label uses

• Cervical carcinoma

Contraindications

• Hypersensitivity to drug or other platinum-containing compounds
• Impaired renal function
• Hearing impairment
• Bone marrow depression
• Pregnancy or breastfeeding

Administration

• Prepare drug with equipment that doesn't contain aluminum.
• Give 2 L of I.V. fluids, as prescribed, 8 to 12 hours before drug infusion to help prevent toxicity.
• Infuse over 6 to 8 hours to minimize toxicity, or over 30 minutes in well-hydrated patients with good renal function.
• Follow facility policy for handling and disposal of antineoplastics.
• If solution contacts skin, wash immediately and thoroughly with soap and

---

water; if solution contacts mucosa, flush with water immediately.

• Protect drug from light.

Route	Onset	Peak	Duration
I.V.	Unknown	18-23 days	39 days

Adverse reactions

CNS: malaise, weakness, **seizures**

EENT: ototoxicity, tinnitus

GI: severe nausea, vomiting, diarrhea

GU: nephrotoxicity, sterility

Hematologic: anemia, **leukopenia, thrombocytopenia**

Hepatic: hepatotoxicity

Metabolic: hypocalcemia, hypokalemia, hypomagnesemia, hyperuricemia

Skin: alopecia

Other: phlebitis at I.V. site, **anaphylactic reactions**

Interactions

Drug-drug. *Amphotericin B, loop diuretics:* increased risk of hypokalemia and hypomagnesemia

Antineoplastics: additive bone marrow depression

Live-virus vaccines: decreased antibody response to vaccine, increased risk of adverse reactions

Nephrotoxic drugs (such as aminoglycosides): additive nephrotoxicity

Ototoxic drugs (such as loop diuretics): additive ototoxicity

Phenytoin: reduced phenytoin blood level

Drug-diagnostic tests. *Aspartate aminotransferase, bilirubin, blood urea nitrogen, creatinine, uric acid:* increased levels

Calcium, magnesium, phosphate, potassium, sodium: decreased levels

Coombs' test: positive result

Precautions

Use cautiously in:

• renal impairment, active infection, myelosuppression, chronic debilitating illness, heart failure, electrolyte abnormalities

• females of childbearing age.

Patient monitoring

• Monitor neurologic status, hepatic enzyme and uric acid levels, and audiogram results.

• Before starting therapy and before each subsequent dose, assess complete blood count with white cell differential and renal function test results.

• Monitor urine output closely.

Patient teaching

• Teach patient to drink 8 oz of water every hour while awake.

• Advise patient to report bleeding, bruising, hearing loss, yellowing of skin or eyes, decreased urine production, or suspected infection.

• Tell patient that drug may cause hair loss.

• Instruct female patients to use reliable contraception; drug can harm fetus.

citalopram hydrobromide
Celexa

Pharmacologic class: Selective serotonin reuptake inhibitor

Therapeutic class: Antidepressant

Pregnancy risk category C

Action

Unclear; thought to potentiate serotonergic activity in CNS by inhibiting neuronal uptake of serotonin

Availability

Oral solution: 10 mg/5 ml

Tablets: 10 mg, 20 mg, 40 mg

⏀ Indications and dosages

➤ Depression (often used in conjunction with psychotherapy)

244 citalopram hydrobromide

Adults: Initially, 20 mg P.O. once daily; may increase by 20 mg/day at weekly intervals, up to 60 mg/day. Usual dosage is 40 mg/day.

Dosage adjustment
• Hepatic impairment
• Elderly patients

Off-label uses
• Alcoholism
• Panic disorder
• Premenstrual dysphoria
• Social phobia

Contraindications
• Hypersensitivity to drug
• Monoamine oxidase (MAO) inhibitor use within 14 days

Administration
◀€ Don't give within 14 days of MAO inhibitor use; life-threatening interactions may occur.

Route	Onset	Peak	Duration
P.O.	1-4 wk	Unknown	Unknown

Adverse reactions
CNS: apathy, confusion, drowsiness, insomnia, migraine, weakness, agitation, amnesia, anxiety, dizziness, fatigue, impaired concentration, deepening of depression, tremor, paresthesia, **suicide attempt**
CV: orthostatic hypotension, tachycardia
EENT: abnormal visual accommodation
GI: nausea, vomiting, diarrhea, abdominal pain, dyspepsia, flatulence, increased saliva, altered taste, dry mouth, anorexia
GU: polyuria, amenorrhea, dysmenorrhea, ejaculation delay, impotence, decreased libido
Musculoskeletal: joint pain, myalgia
Respiratory: cough
Skin: rash, pruritus, diaphoresis, photosensitivity

Other: fever, yawning, increased appetite, weight changes

Interactions
Drug-drug. *Carbamazepine:* decreased citalopram blood level
Centrally acting drugs (such as antihistamines, opioids, sedative-hypnotics): additive CNS effects
5-hydroxytryptamine$_1$ receptor agonists (such as sumatriptan, zolmitriptan): increased risk of adverse reactions
Erythromycin, itraconazole, ketoconazole, omeprazole: increased citalopram blood level
Lithium: potentiation of serotonergic effects
MAO inhibitors: life-threatening reactions
Tricyclic antidepressants (TCAs): altered TCA pharmacokinetics
Drug-herb. *St. John's wort, S-adenosylmethionine (SAM-e):* increased risk of serotonergic reactions, including serotonin syndrome
Drug-behaviors. *Alcohol use:* additive CNS depression
Sun exposure: photosensitivity

Precautions
Use cautiously in:
• severe renal impairment, hepatic impairment, conditions likely to cause altered metabolism or hemodynamic responses
• history of mania or seizure disorder
• elderly patients
• pregnant patients
• children (safety not established).

Patient monitoring
• If patient is receiving lithium concurrently, watch closely for potentiation of serotonergic effects.
• Assess for signs and symptoms of drug efficacy.

Patient teaching
• Instruct patient to take drug with full glass of water at same time every day.

✦ Canada   ◀€ Clinical alert   Reactions in **bold** are life-threatening

- Advise patient to avoid alcohol during therapy.
- Instruct patient to move slowly when sitting up or standing to avoid dizziness or light-headedness caused by sudden blood pressure decrease.
- Tell patient it may take several weeks before he starts to feel better.

◀≶ Advise patient to immediately report suicidal thoughts or extreme depression.

- Inform patient that he may experience inadequate filling of penile erectile tissue; advise him to consult prescriber if he experiences adverse sexual effects.

clarithromycin
Biaxin, Biaxin XL

Pharmacologic class: Macrolide
Therapeutic class: Anti-infective, antiulcer drug
Pregnancy risk category B

Action
Reversibly binds to 50S ribosomal subunit of susceptible bacterial organisms, thereby blocking protein synthesis; bactericidal or bacteriostatic

Availability
Granules for oral suspension: 125 mg/5 ml, 250 mg/5 ml
Tablets: 250 mg, 500 mg
Tablets (extended-release): 500 mg

⃕ Indications and dosages
➤ Pharyngitis, tonsillitis
Adults: 250 mg P.O. q 12 hours for 10 days
➤ Acute maxillary sinusitis
Adults: 500 mg P.O. q 12 hours for 14 days or two 500-mg extended-release tablets q 24 hours for 14 days

➤ Chronic bronchitis
Adults: 500 mg P.O. for 7 to 14 days or two 500-mg extended-release tablets q 24 hours for 7 days
➤ Community-acquired pneumonia caused by *Streptococcus pneumoniae*, *Mycoplasma pneumoniae*, and *Chlamydia pneumoniae*; acute exacerbation of chronic bronchitis caused by *S. pneumoniae* and *Moraxella catarrhalis*
Adults: 250 mg P.O. q 12 hours for 7 to 14 days or two 500-mg extended-release tablets q 24 hours for 7 days
➤ Community-acquired pneumonia caused by *H. influenzae*
Adults: 250 mg P.O. for 7 days or two 500-mg extended-release tablets q 24 hours for 7 days
➤ Community-acquired pneumonia caused by *H. parainfluenzae* or *M. catarrhalis*
Adults: Two 500-mg extended-release tablets q 24 hours for 7 days
➤ Uncomplicated skin and skin-structure infections
Adults: 250 mg P.O. q 12 hours for 7 to 14 days
Dosage adjustment
- Renal impairment
- Hepatic impairment

Off-label uses
- *Borrelia burgdorferi* infection

Contraindications
- Hypersensitivity to drug, erythromycin, or other macrolide anti-infectives
- Concurrent use of pimozide, astemizole, or cisapride
- Cardiac disease

Administration
- Obtain culture and sensitivity testing before starting therapy.
- Take with or without food.
- Discard oral suspension 14 days after mixing.
- Don't refrigerate drug.

Route	Onset	Peak	Duration
P.O.	Unknown	2 hr	12 hr
P.O. (extended)	Unknown	4 hr	24 hr

Adverse reactions

CNS: headache

CV: ventricular arrhythmias

GI: nausea, diarrhea, abdominal pain or discomfort, dyspepsia, abnormal taste

GU: elevated blood urea nitrogen (BUN)

Hematologic: increased prothrombin time, decreased white blood cell (WBC) count

Metabolic: elevated alkaline phosphatase level

Interactions

Drug-drug. *Carbamazepine, digoxin, theophylline:* increased blood levels of these drugs, greater risk of toxicity

Digoxin: increased digoxin blood level, leading to digoxin toxicity

HMG-CoA reductase inhibitors (such as lovastatin, simvastatin): rhabdomyolysis

Pimozide: increased risk of arrhythmias

Zidovudine: increased or decreased zidovudine peak blood level

Drug-diagnostic tests. *Alkaline phosphatase, BUN, prothrombin time:* increased values

WBCs: decreased count

Precautions

Use cautiously in:
• severe hepatic or renal impairment.
• pregnant or breastfeeding patients.

Patient monitoring

• Monitor hepatic enzyme and creatinine levels during long-term therapy.
• Assess cardiovascular status.

Patient teaching

• Advise patient to take with full glass of water, either with food or on an empty stomach.
• Tell patients using hormonal contraceptives to use supplemental birth-control method to avoid pregnancy.

clindamycin hydrochloride
Cleocin, Dalacin C

clindamycin palmitate hydrochloride
Cleocin Pediatric, Dalacin C Flavored Granules✤

clindamycin phosphate
Cleocin Phosphate, Cleocin T, Clinda-Derm, Clindets, C/T/S, Dalacin C Phosphate✤, Dalacin T✤

Pharmacologic class: Lincosamide
Therapeutic class: Anti-infective
Pregnancy risk category B

Action

Inhibits protein synthesis in susceptible bacteria at level of 50S ribosome, thereby inhibiting peptide bond formation and causing cell death; bactericidal or bacteriostatic

Availability

Capsules: 75 mg, 150 mg, 300 mg
Granules for oral suspension: 75 mg/5 ml
Injection: 150 mg base/ml
Topical: 1% gel, lotion, single-use applicators, solution, suspension
Vaginal cream: 2% cream
Vaginal suppositories (ovules): 100 mg

⚠ Indications and dosages
➤ Severe infections caused by sensitive organisms (such as *Bacteroides*

fragilis, *Clostridium perfringens, Fusobacterium,* pneumococci, staphylococci, and streptococci)

Adults: 300 to 450 mg P.O. q 6 hours, or (for other than *C. perfringens*) 1.2 to 2.7 g/day I.M. or I.V. in two to four equally divided doses

Children: 16 to 20 mg/kg/day P.O. (hydrochloride) in three to four equally divided doses, or 13 to 25 mg/kg/day P.O. (palmitate hydrochloride) in three to four equally divided doses

➤ Acute pelvic inflammatory disease

Adults: 900 mg I.V. q 8 hours (given with gentamicin)

➤ Acne vulgaris

Adults and children older than age 12: Apply a thin film of topical gel, lotion, or solution to affected area b.i.d.

Off-label uses

• Bacterial vaginosis (phosphate)
• *Chlamydia trachomatis* infection in females
• CNS toxoplasmosis in AIDS patients (given with pyrimethamine)
• *Pneumocystis jiroveci* (formerly *Pneumocystis carinii*) pneumonia (given with primaquine)
• Rosacea (lotion)

Contraindications

• Hypersensitivity to drug or lincomycin

Administration

• Give oral doses with full glass of water, with or without food.
• Administer I.V. dose every 6 hours, as ordered.
• Don't give as I.V. bolus.
• Dilute I.V. solution to a concentration of 18 mg/ml using normal saline solution, dextrose 5% in water, or lactated Ringer's solution. Infuse no faster than 30 mg/minute.
• Don't administer I.M. dosages above 600 mg.

• Inject I.M. doses deep into large muscle mass to prevent induration and sterile abscess.

Route	Onset	Peak	Duration
P.O.	Rapid	45 min	6-8 hr
I.V.	Rapid	End of infusion	6-8 hr
I.M.	Rapid	1-3 hr	6-8 hr
Topical, vaginal	Unknown	Unknown	Unknown

Adverse reactions

GI: nausea, vomiting, diarrhea, abdominal pain, esophagitis, bitter taste (I.V. use only), **pseudomembranous colitis**

Hematologic: neutropenia, leukopenia, **agranulocytosis, thrombocytopenia purpura**

Hepatic: jaundice, hepatic function changes

Skin: maculopapular rash, generalized morbiliform-like rash

Other: phlebitis at I.V. site, induration and sterile abscess (with I.M. use), **anaphylaxis**

Interactions

Drug-drug. *Erythromycin:* antagonistic effect

Kaolin/pectin: decreased GI absorption of clindamycin

Hormonal contraceptives: decreased contraceptive efficacy

Neuromuscular blockers: enhanced neuromuscular blockade

Drug-diagnostic tests. *Alanine aminotransferase, alkaline phosphatase, aspartate aminotransferase, bilirubin, creatine kinase:* increased levels

Platelets, white blood cells: transient decrease in levels

Precautions

Use cautiously in:
• renal or hepatic impairment
• known alcohol intolerance

- pregnant patients
- neonates.

Patient monitoring
- Monitor creatinine level closely in patients with renal insufficiency.
- Monitor hepatic enzyme levels in patients with known hepatic disease.
- Assess for signs and symptoms of hypersensitivity reactions.

Patient teaching
- Tell patient to take drug with food if it causes stomach upset.
- 🔊 Teach patient to contact prescriber immediately if he experiences diarrhea during or after treatment.
- Tell patient that I.V. use may cause bitter taste; reassure him that this effect will resolve on its own.
- Caution patient not to rely on condoms or a diaphragm for contraception for 72 hours after using vaginal preparation; drug may weaken latex products and cause breakage.
- Instruct patient taking hormonal contraceptives to use supplemental birth control method, such as condoms (unless she's using vaginal preparation); drug may reduce hormonal contraceptive efficacy.

clomiphene citrate
Clomid, Milophene, Serophene

Pharmacologic class: Chlorotrianisene derivative
Therapeutic class: Fertility drug, ovulation stimulant
Pregnancy risk category X

Action
Binds with estrogen receptors in cytoplasm, increasing secretion of follicle-stimulating hormone, luteinizing hormone, and gonadotropin in hypothalamus and pituitary gland

Availability
Tablets: 50 mg

💊 Indications and dosages
➤ Ovarian failure
Adults: 50 mg/day P.O. for 5 days starting any time in patients who've had no recent uterine bleeding; or 50 mg/day P.O. starting on fifth day of menstrual cycle. If ovulation doesn't occur, increase to 100 mg/day P.O. for 5 days. Start second course of therapy as early as 30 days after first; if patient doesn't respond to second course, no further doses are recommended.

Off-label uses
- Male sterility (controversial)

Contraindications
- Hepatic disease
- Organic intracranial lesions
- Uncontrolled thyroid or adrenal dysfunction
- Ovarian cyst
- Pregnancy

Administration
- Obtain pregnancy test before therapy begins.
- Be aware that patient should undergo pelvic and eye examinations before starting therapy.

Route	Onset	Peak	Duration
P.O.	5-8 days	Unknown	6 wk

Adverse reactions
CNS: nervousness, insomnia, dizziness, light-headedness
CV: vasomotor flushing
EENT: visual disturbances
GI: nausea; vomiting; abdominal discomfort, distention, and bloating
GU: breast tenderness, uterine bleeding, ovarian enlargement, multiple pregnancies, birth defects in resulting pregnancies, **ovarian hyperstimulation syndrome**

Interactions
None significant

Precautions
None

Patient monitoring
• Monitor patient for bleeding and other adverse reactions.

Patient teaching
◄€ Instruct patient to immediately report signs and symptoms of ovarian hyperstimulation syndrome, including nausea, vomiting, diarrhea, abdominal or pelvic pain, and swelling in hands or legs.

• Tell patient that drug increases risk of multiple births, which heightens maternal risk.

• Advise patient not to take drug if she is or may become pregnant.

• As appropriate, review all significant and life-threatening adverse reactions.

clomipramine hydrochloride
Anafranil, Apo-Clomipramine✤, Gen-Clomipramine✤, Novo-Clopamine✤

Pharmacologic class: Tricyclic antidepressant (TCA)

Therapeutic class: Antiobsessional agent, antidepressant

Pregnancy risk category C

Action
Unknown; may influence obsessive-compulsive behavior by selectively inhibiting norepinephrine and serotonin reuptake at presynaptic neuron; also possesses moderate anticholinergic properties.

Availability
Capsules: 25 mg, 50 mg, 75 mg

Indications and dosages
➣ Obsessive-compulsive disorder
Adults: Initially, 25 mg/day P.O., increased over 2 weeks to 100 mg/day given in divided doses. May be increased further over several weeks, up to 250 mg/day given in divided doses.
Elderly patients: Initially, 20 to 30 mg/day P.O.; may be increased p.r.n.
Children ages 10 to 17: Initially, 25 mg/day P.O., increased over 2 weeks to 3 mg/kg/day or 100 mg/day (whichever is smaller) given in divided doses. May be increased further to 3 mg/kg/day or 200 mg/day (whichever is smaller) given in divided doses.

Off-label uses
• Panic disorder

Contraindications
• Hypersensitivity to drug or other TCAs
• Recent myocardial infarction (MI)
• Concurrent monoamine oxidase (MAO) inhibitor or clonidine use

Administration
• Don't give with grapefruit juice.
• Once stabilizing dosage is reached, entire daily dose may be given at bedtime.

Route	Onset	Peak	Duration
P.O.	Unknown	2-6 hr	Unknown

Adverse reactions
CNS: lethargy, sedation, weakness, aggressive behavior, extrapyramidal reactions, poor concentration, feeling of unreality, delusions, anxiety, restlessness, panic, asthenia, insomnia, **seizures**
CV: electrocardiogram changes, orthostatic hypotension, hypertension, syncope, tachycardia, palpitations, **ar-**

rhythmias, MI, precipitation of heart block

EENT: blurred vision, dry eyes, vestibular disorder, nasal congestion, laryngitis

GI: nausea, vomiting, constipation, abdominal cramps, eructation, paralytic ileus, epigastric distress, flatulence, dysphagia, abnormal taste, increased salivation, stomatitis, parotid gland swelling, black tongue, dry mouth

GU: urinary retention, urinary hesitancy, urinary tract dilation, male sexual dysfunction, testicular swelling, impotence, gynecomastia, breast enlargement, menstrual irregularities, galactorrhea, libido changes

Hematologic: eosinophilia, purpura, anemia, **bone marrow depression, agranulocytosis, thrombocytopenia, leukopenia**

Metabolic: hyperthermia, hypothermia, elevated blood glucose and prolactin levels, syndrome of inappropriate antidiuretic hormone secretion

Musculoskeletal: muscle weakness

Skin: sweating, dry skin, photosensitivity, rash, pruritus, vasculitis, petechiae, flushing

Other: chills, edema, increased appetite, weight gain

Interactions

Drug-drug. *Adrenergics, anticholinergics:* additive adrenergic or anticholinergic effects

Cimetidine, hormonal contraceptives, phenothiazines, selective serotonin reuptake inhibitors: increased TCA effects, greater risk of toxicity

Clonidine: hypertensive crisis

CNS depressants (including antihistamines, opioid analgesics, sedative-hypnotics): additive CNS depression

Disulfiram: transient delirium

Guanethidine: interference with antihypertensive response

MAO inhibitors: severe or life-threatening adverse reactions

Sparfloxacin: increased risk of adverse cardiovascular reactions

Drug-food. *Grapefruit juice:* increased clomipramine blood level and effects

Drug-herb. *Chamomile, hops, kava, skullcap, valerian:* increased CNS depression

St. John's wort, S-adenosylmethionine (SAM-e): increased serotonergic effects, possibly causing serotonin syndrome

Drug-behaviors. *Alcohol use:* additive CNS depression

Nicotine use: increased metabolism and decreased efficacy of clomipramine

Sun exposure: photosensitivity

Precautions

Use cautiously in:
• glaucoma, hyperthyroidism, prostatic hypertrophy, preexisting cardiovascular disease
• elderly patients
• pregnant or breastfeeding patients
• children younger than age 10 (safety not established).

Patient monitoring

• Monitor patient for cardiovascular, CNS, and hematologic adverse reactions.

• Assess for suicidal ideation; if necessary, institute suicide precautions.

Patient teaching

◀€ Teach patient to immediately report suicidal thoughts or severe depression.

• Instruct patient not to drink grapefruit juice during therapy.

• Teach patient to avoid driving and other hazardous activities until he knows how drug affects concentration and alertness.

• Instruct patient to avoid alcohol because it increases drowsiness.

• Tell patient to move slowly when sitting up or standing to avoid dizziness or light-headedness caused by sudden blood pressure decrease.

• Caution patient not to stop taking drug abruptly because this may cause nausea, headache, or malaise.

clonazepam

Apo-Clonazepam✤, Clonapam✤, Gen-Clonazepam✤, Klonopin, Rivotril✤, Syn-Clonazepam

Pharmacologic class: Benzodiazepine
Therapeutic class: Anticonvulsant
Controlled substance schedule IV
Pregnancy risk category D

Action

Unknown; may enhance activity of gamma-aminobutyric acid, an inhibitory neurotransmitter in CNS

Availability

Tablets: 0.5 mg, 1 mg, 2 mg

🖉 Indications and dosages

➤ Absence seizures (Lennox-Gastaut syndrome), akinetic and myoclonic seizures

Adults: Initially, 1.5 mg/day P.O. in three divided doses; may increase by 0.5 to 1 mg q 3 days until seizures are adequately controlled or drug intolerance occurs. Maximum dosage is 20 mg/day.

Infants and children ages 10 and younger or weighing 30 kg (66 lb) or less: Initially, 0.01 to 0.03 mg/kg/day P.O. Give total dosage (not to exceed 0.05 mg/kg/day) in two to three equally divided doses; increase by no more than 0.25 to 0.5 mg q 3 days until dosage of 0.1 to 0.2 mg/kg/day is reached, seizures are adequately controlled, or drug intolerance occurs.

Off-label uses

• Acute manic episodes of bipolar disorder

• Multifocal tic disorders
• Neuralgias
• Parkinsonian dysarthria
• Periodic leg movements during sleep
• Adjunctive treatment of schizophrenia

Contraindications

• Hypersensitivity to drug or other benzodiazepines
• Severe hepatic disease
• Acute narrow-angle glaucoma
• Untreated open-angle glaucoma

Administration

• Be aware that overdose may cause fatal respiratory depression or cardiovascular collapse.

Route	Onset	Peak	Duration
P.O.	20-60 min	1-2 hr	6-12 hr

Adverse reactions

CNS: ataxia, fatigue, behavioral changes, depression, dizziness, nervousness, reduced intellectual ability, drowsiness
CV: palpitations
EENT: abnormal eye movements, blurred vision, diplopia, nystagmus, sinusitis, rhinitis, pharyngitis
GI: constipation, diarrhea, hypersalivation
GU: dysuria, nocturia, urinary retention, dysmenorrhea, delayed ejaculation, impotence
Hematologic: anemia, eosinophilia, **leukopenia, thrombocytopenia**
Hepatic: hepatitis
Musculoskeletal: myalgia
Respiratory: increased respiratory secretions, upper respiratory tract infection, coughing, bronchitis, **respiratory depression**
Other: appetite changes, fever, physical or psychological drug dependence, drug tolerance, allergic reaction

---

Interactions

Drug-drug. *Antidepressants, antihistamines, opioids, other benzodiazepines:* additive CNS depression
Barbiturates, rifampin: increased metabolism and decreased efficacy of clonazepam
Cimetidine, disulfiram, fluoxetine, hormonal contraceptives, isoniazid, ketoconazole, metoprolol, propoxyphene, propranolol, valproic acid: decreased clonazepam metabolism
Phenytoin: decreased clonazepam blood level

Drug-diagnostic tests. *Liver function tests, eosinophils:* increased values
Platelets, white blood cells: decreased counts

Drug-herb. *Chamomile, hops, kava, skullcap, valerian:* increased CNS depression

Drug-behaviors. *Alcohol use:* increased CNS depression

Precautions

Use cautiously in:
• renal impairment, chronic respiratory disease, open-angle glaucoma
• history of porphyria
• pregnant or breastfeeding patients
• children.

Patient monitoring

• Monitor patient for respiratory depression; assess respiratory rate and quality, oxygen saturation (using pulse oximetry), and mental status.
• Monitor liver function and hematologic test results.

Patient teaching

🔊 Instruct patient to immediately report easy bleeding or bruising or yellowing of skin or eyes.
• Teach patient to avoid driving and other hazardous activities until he knows how drug affects concentration and alertness.
• Caution patient not to stop taking drug abruptly; advise him to consult

prescriber for dosage-tapering schedule if he wishes to discontinue drug.

clonidine
Catapres-TTS

clonidine hydrochloride
Apo-Clonidine✤, Catapres, Dixarit✤, Duraclon, Nu-Clonidine✤

Pharmacologic class: Centrally acting sympatholytic
Therapeutic class: Antihypertensive
Pregnancy risk category C

Action

Stimulates alpha-adrenergic receptors in CNS, decreasing sympathetic outflow and inhibiting vasoconstriction. Prevents transmission of pain impulses to CNS by stimulating alpha-adrenergic receptors in spinal cord.

Availability

Solution for epidural injection: 100 mcg/ml in 10-ml vials, 500 mcg/ml in 10-ml vials
Tablets: 25 mcg (0.025 mg), 100 mcg (0.1 mg), 200 mcg (0.2 mg), 300 mcg (0.3 mg)
Transdermal systems: 2.5 mg total released as 0.1 mg/24 hours (TTS 1), 5 mg total released as 0.2 mg/24 hours (TTS 2), 7.5 mg total released as 0.3 mg/24 hours (TTS 3)

💊 Indications and dosages

➤ Mild to moderate hypertension
Adults: 0.1 mg P.O. b.i.d. (in morning and at bedtime) alone or with other antihypertensives; increase in increments of 0.1 mg/day q week until desired response occurs. Or, one transdermal system applied once q 7 days to hairless area of intact skin on upper outer arm or chest.

➤ Severe pain in cancer patients unresponsive to opioids alone

Adults: Initially, 30 mcg/hour by continuous epidural infusion, titrated upward or downward depending on patient response

Dosage adjustment
• Renal impairment

Off-label uses
• Acute alcohol withdrawal
• Akathisia
• Diarrhea
• Prolonged surgical anesthesia

Contraindications
• Hypersensitivity to drug
• Hypersensitivity to components of adhesive layer (transdermal form)
• Infection at epidural injection site
• Bleeding problems (epidural use)
• Concurrent anticoagulant therapy

Administration
• To minimize sedative effects, give largest portion of maintenance P.O. dose at bedtime.

Route	Onset	Peak	Duration
P.O.	30-60 min	2-4 hr	8-12 hr
Epidural	Rapid	19 min	Variable
Transdermal	Slow	2-3 days	7 days

Adverse reactions
CNS: drowsiness, depression, dizziness, nervousness, nightmares
CV: hypotension (especially with epidural use), palpitations, bradycardia
GI: nausea, vomiting, constipation, dry mouth
GU: urinary retention, impotence, nocturia
Metabolic: sodium retention
Skin: rash, sweating, pruritus, dermatitis
Other: weight gain, withdrawal phenomenon

Interactions
Drug-drug. *Amphetamines, beta-adrenergic blockers, monoamine oxidase inhibitors, prazosin, tricyclic antidepressants:* decreased antihypertensive effect
Antihypertensives, nitrates: additive hypotension
Beta-adrenergic blockers: increased withdrawal phenomenon
CNS depressants (including antihistamines, opioids, sedative-hypnotics): additive sedation
Epidurally administered local anesthetics: prolongation of clonidine effects
Levodopa: decreased levodopa efficacy
Myocardial depressants (including beta-adrenergic blockers): additive bradycardia
Verapamil: increased risk of adverse cardiovascular reactions
Drug-herb. *Capsicum:* reduced antihypertensive effects
Drug-behaviors. *Alcohol use:* increased sedation

Precautions
Use cautiously in:
• renal insufficiency, serious cardiac or cerebrovascular disease
• elderly patients
• pregnant or breastfeeding patients.

Patient monitoring
• Monitor patient for signs and symptoms of adverse cardiovascular reactions.
• Frequently assess vital signs, especially blood pressure and pulse.
• Monitor patient for drug tolerance and efficacy.

Patient teaching
• Instruct patient to move slowly when sitting up or standing to avoid dizziness or light-headedness caused by sudden blood pressure decrease.
• Tell patient not to stop taking drug abruptly.

clopidogrel bisulfate
Plavix

Pharmacologic class: Platelet aggregation inhibitor
Therapeutic class: Antiplatelet drug
Pregnancy risk category B

Action
Inhibits platelet aggregation by blocking the binding of adenosine diphosphate to platelets, preventing thrombus from forming

Availability
Tablets: 75 mg

🖊 Indications and dosages
➤ To reduce atherosclerotic events in patients who have had a recent myocardial infarction (MI) or cerebrovascular accident and in those with established peripheral arterial disease or acute coronary syndrome
Adults: 75 mg/day P.O.
➤ Acute coronary syndrome (unstable angina or non-Q-wave MI)
Adults: 300 mg P.O. as a loading dose, then 75 mg/day P.O.

Contraindications
• Hypersensitivity to drug
• Active pathologic bleeding

Administration
• Give with or without food.
• Know that drug may need to be discontinued 5 days before surgery.

Route	Onset	Peak	Duration
P.O.	Variable	60 min	3-4 hr

Adverse reactions
CNS: depression, dizziness, fatigue, headache
CV: chest pain, hypertension
EENT: epistaxis, rhinitis

GI: diarrhea, abdominal pain, dyspepsia, gastritis, **GI bleeding**
Hematologic: bleeding, neutropenia, thrombotic thrombocytopenic purpura
Metabolic: hypercholesterolemia, gout
Musculoskeletal: joint pain, back pain
Respiratory: cough, dyspnea, bronchitis, upper respiratory tract infection, **bronchospasm**
Skin: pruritus, rash, angioedema
Other: hypersensitivity reactions, **anaphylactic reactions**

Interactions
Drug-drug. *Abciximab, aspirin, eptifibatide, heparin, heparinoids, nonsteroidal anti-inflammatory drugs (NSAIDs), thrombolytics, ticlopidine, tirofiban, warfarin:* increased risk of bleeding
Fluvastatin, many NSAIDs, phenytoin, tamoxifen, tolbutamide, torsemide: interference with metabolism of these drugs
Drug-diagnostic tests. *Bilirubin, hepatic enzymes, nonprotein nitrogen, total cholesterol, uric acid:* increased levels
Platelets: decreased count
Drug-herb. *Anise, arnica, chamomile, clove, fenugreek, feverfew, garlic, ginger, ginkgo, ginseng:* increased risk of bleeding

Precautions
Use cautiously in:
• severe hepatic impairment, GI bleeding, ulcer disease
• increased risk of bleeding
• pregnant or breastfeeding patients
• children.

Patient monitoring
• Monitor hemoglobin and hematocrit periodically.
• Monitor patient for unusual bleeding or bruising; drug significantly increases risk of bleeding.

• Assess for occult GI blood loss if patient is receiving naproxen concurrently with clopidogrel.

Patient teaching

• Advise patient to immediately report unusual or acute chest pain, respiratory difficulty, rash, unresolved bleeding, diarrhea, GI distress, nosebleed, or acute headache.

• Instruct patient to tell all health care providers that he's taking clopidogrel, especially if surgery is scheduled or new drugs are prescribed.

• Tell patient that drug may cause headache and dizziness; advise him to avoid driving and other hazardous activities until he knows how drug affects concentration and alertness.

• Teach patient to minimize adverse GI effects by eating small, frequent meals or chewing gum.

clorazepate dipotassium
Apo-Clorazepate✤, Gen-XENE, Novo-Clopate✤, Tranxene, Tranxene-SD, Tranxene-SD Half Strength, Tranxene-T

Pharmacologic class: Benzodiazepine
Therapeutic class: Anticonvulsant, anxiolytic
Controlled substance schedule IV
Pregnancy risk category D

Action

Unknown; thought to potentiate effects of gamma-aminobutyric acid (GABA) and other neurotransmitters, thus promoting inhibitory neurotransmission and causing CNS depression. Suppresses seizures by raising seizure threshold and promoting presynaptic inhibition.

Availability

Capsules: 3.75 mg, 7.5 mg, 15 mg
Tablets: 3.75 mg, 7.5 mg, 11.25 mg, 15 mg, 22.5 mg

Indications and dosages

➤ Anxiety
Adults: 7.5 to 15 mg P.O. two to four times daily

➤ Adjunctive therapy in partial seizure disorder
Adults and children older than age 12: Initially, 7.5 mg P.O. t.i.d.; increase by no more than 7.5 mg/week. Don't exceed 90 mg/day.
Children ages 9 to 12: Initially, 7.5 mg P.O. b.i.d; increase by no more than 7.5 mg/week. Don't exceed 60 mg/day.

➤ Management of alcohol withdrawal
Adults: 30 mg P.O. initially, followed by 15 mg P.O. two to four times daily on first day. On second day, give 45 to 90 mg P.O. in divided doses, then decrease gradually over subsequent days to 7.5 mg to 15 mg P.O. daily.

Dosage adjustment
• Elderly or debilitated patients

Contraindications

• Benzodiazepine hypersensitivity
• Acute narrow-angle glaucoma
• Psychosis
• Concurrent ketoconazole or itraconazole therapy
• Children younger than age 9

Administration

• If GI upset occurs, give with food.
• When discontinuing therapy after long-term use, taper dosage gradually over 4 to 8 weeks to avoid withdrawal symptoms.
• Take suicide precautions if patient is depressed or anxious.

Route	Onset	Peak	Duration
P.O.	Rapid	1-2 hr	Days

✤ Canada   ◀€ Clinical alert   Reactions in **bold** are life-threatening

Adverse reactions

CNS: dizziness, drowsiness, lethargy, sedation, depression, fatigue, nervousness, confusion, irritability, headache, slurred speech, difficulty articulating words, stupor, rigidity, tremor, poor coordination

CV: hypertension, hypotension, palpitations

EENT: blurred or double vision

GI: dry mouth

Hematologic: neutropenia

Hepatic: jaundice

Skin: rash, diaphoresis

Other: weight gain or loss, drug dependence or tolerance

Interactions

Drug-drug. *Antacids:* altered clorazepate absorption rate

Antidepressants, antihistamines, opioids: additive CNS depression

Barbiturates, monoamine oxidase inhibitors, other antidepressants, phenothiazines: potentiation of clorazepate effects

Cimetidine, disulfiram, fluoxetine, hormonal contraceptives, isoniazid, itraconazole, ketoconazole, metoprolol, propoxyphene, propranolol, valproic acid: decreased clorazepate metabolism, leading to enhanced drug action or markedly increased CNS effects

Levodopa: decreased antiparkinsonian effect

Probenecid: rapid onset or prolonged action of clorazepate

Rifampin: increased metabolism and decreased efficacy of clorazepate

Theophylline: decreased sedative effect of clorazepate

Drug-diagnostic tests. *Alanine aminotransferase, alkaline phosphatase, aspartate aminotransferase:* increased levels

Drug-herb. *Chamomile, hops, kava, skullcap, valerian:* increased CNS depression

Drug-behaviors. *Alcohol use:* increased CNS depression

Precautions

Use cautiously in:
- depression or suicidal ideation
- psychotic reaction
- elderly patients
- females of childbearing age
- pregnant or breastfeeding patients.

Patient monitoring

- Monitor blood counts and liver function test results during long-term therapy; drug may cause neutropenia and jaundice.
- Evaluate patient for depression and drug dependence or tolerance.
- Assess for pregnancy before initiating therapy.

Patient teaching

- Instruct patient to avoid driving and other hazardous activities until he knows how drug affects concentration and alertness.
- Teach patient to avoid alcohol and other CNS depressants.
- Caution patient not to stop therapy abruptly because withdrawal symptoms may occur.

clozapine
Clozaril

Pharmacologic class: Dibenzodiazepine derivative

Therapeutic class: Antipsychotic agent

Pregnancy risk category B

Action

Unclear; thought to interfere with dopamine binding in limbic system of CNS, with high affinity for dopamine$_4$ receptors. May antagonize adrenergic, cholinergic, histaminergic, and serotonergic receptors.

Availability

Tablets: 25 mg, 100 mg

Indications and dosages

> Schizophrenia in patients unresponsive to other therapies

Adults: 12.5 mg P.O. daily or b.i.d.; increase daily in 25- to 50-mg increments, as tolerated, to target dosage of 300 to 450 mg/day by end of second week. Make subsequent dosage increases once or twice weekly in increments of 100 mg or less, to a maximum dosage of 900 mg/day P.O. in divided doses.

Dosage adjustment
- Renal impairment
- Elderly patients

Contraindications
- Hypersensitivity to drug
- Uncontrolled seizures
- Severe CNS depression or coma
- Concurrent use of drugs that cause agranulocytosis or bone marrow depression

Administration
◄£ Obtain white blood cell (WBC) count before initiating therapy. Don't give drug if WBC count is below 3,500/mm³.
- When discontinuing drug, taper dosage gradually over 1 to 2 weeks.

Route	Onset	Peak	Duration
P.O.	Unknown	2.5 hr	4-12 hr

Adverse reactions
CNS: sedation, drowsiness, dizziness, vertigo, headache, tremor, insomnia, disturbed sleep, nightmares, agitation, lethargy, fatigue, weakness, confusion, anxiety, parkinsonism, slurred speech, depression, restlessness, extrapyramidal reactions, tardive dyskinesia, akathisia, syncope, **neuroleptic malignant syndrome, autonomic disturbances, seizures**
CV: hypotension, tachycardia, electrocardiogram (ECG) changes, chest pain, myocarditis

EENT: blurred vision, dry eyes, nasal congestion, sinusitis
GI: nausea, vomiting, constipation, dyspepsia, salivation, dry mouth, anorexia
GU: urinary retention, urinary incontinence, urinary frequency and urgency, inhibited ejaculation
Musculoskeletal: rigidity, back and muscle pain, muscle spasms
Hematologic: agranulocytosis, leukopenia, hemolytic anemia, aplastic anemia, thrombocytopenia, neutropenia, eosinophilia
Hepatic: abnormal liver function test results
Respiratory: dyspnea
Skin: rash, sweating
Other: weight gain, fever

Interactions
Drug-drug. *Anticholinergics, antihypertensives, digoxin, warfarin:* increased effects of these drugs
Cimetidine, erythromycin: increased therapeutic and toxic effects of clozapine
Epinephrine: increased hypotension
Fluoxetine, fluvoxamine, paroxetine, sertraline: increased clozapine blood level
Phenytoin, rifampin: decreased clozapine blood level
Psychoactive drugs: additive psychoactive effect
Drug-diagnostic tests. *Granulocytes, hematocrit, hemoglobin, platelets, white blood cells:* decreased values
Liver function tests: abnormal values
Pregnancy test: false-positive result
Drug-food. *Caffeine:* increased clozapine blood level
Drug-herb. *Angel's trumpet, jimsonweed, scopolia:* increased anticholinergic effects
Nutmeg: decreased clozapine efficacy
St. John's wort: decreased clozapine blood level
Drug-behaviors. *Alcohol use:* increased CNS depression

Smoking: decreased clozapine blood level

Precautions
Use cautiously in:
- hypersensitivity to phenothiazines
- cardiac, hepatic, or renal impairment; CNS tumors; diabetes mellitus; seizures; prostatic hypertrophy; intestinal obstruction; paralytic ileus; narrow-angle glaucoma
- elderly patients
- pregnant or breastfeeding patients
- children.

Patient monitoring
◀᠄ Monitor WBC count weekly for first 6 months of therapy; if it's normal, WBC testing can be reduced to every other week. Notify prescriber immediately if WBC count decreases or agranulocytosis occurs.
- Monitor ECG and liver function test results.
- If drug must be withdrawn abruptly, monitor patient for psychosis and cholinergic rebound (headache, nausea, vomiting, diarrhea).
- Continue to monitor WBC count weekly for 4 weeks after therapy ends.

Patient teaching
- Teach patient about significant risk of agranulocytosis; tell him he'll need to undergo weekly blood testing to check for this blood disorder. Mention that clozapine tablets are available only through special program designed to ensure required blood monitoring.
- Advise patient to immediately report new onset of lethargy, weakness, fever, sore throat, malaise, mucous membrane ulcers, flulike symptoms, or other signs and symptoms of infection.

coagulation factor VIIa (recombinant)
NovoSeven

Pharmacologic class: Coagulation factor VIIa
Therapeutic class: Antihemophilic
Pregnancy risk category C

Action
Promotes hemostasis by activating intrinsic pathway of coagulation cascade

Availability
Lyophilized powder for injection: 1.2 mg/vial, 4.8 mg/vial

🖊 Indications and dosages
➤ Bleeding episodes in patients with hemophilia A or B who have inhibitors to factor VIII or IX
Adults: 90 mcg/kg I.V. bolus q 2 hours until hemostasis occurs or therapy is deemed inadequate

Contraindications
- Hypersensitivity to drug or mouse, hamster, or bovine products

Administration
◀᠄ Give by I.V. bolus only.
- Reconstitute only with specified volume of sterile water for injection.
◀᠄ Don't mix with infusion solutions.
- Administer within 3 hours after reconstituting.

Route	Onset	Peak	Duration
I.V.	Unknown	Unknown	Unknown

Adverse reactions
CNS: headache
CV: hypertension, hypotension, bradycardia
GU: abnormal renal function

Hematologic: purpura, **hemorrhage, hemarthrosis, disseminated intravascular coagulation, coagulation disorders, decreased fibrinogen plasma, thrombosis**
Musculoskeletal: arthrosis
Skin: pruritus, rash
Other: fever, edema, pain, redness or reaction at injection site, hypersensitivity reaction

Interactions
Drug-drug. *Activated prothrombin complex concentrates or prothrombin complex concentrates:* risk of potential interaction, but not evaluated

Precautions
Use cautiously in:
• pregnant or breastfeeding patients
• children.

Patient monitoring
• Monitor for signs and symptoms of coagulation activation or thrombosis.
• Be aware that laboratory coagulation parameters may be used as an adjunct to clinical evaluation of hemostasis to monitor drug efficacy and treatment schedule. However, these parameters have shown no direct correlation with achieving hemostasis.

Patient teaching
• Instruct patient to report swelling, pain, burning, or itching at infusion site.
• Tell patient to inform prescriber if she's pregnant or intends to become pregnant.

codeine phosphate
Paveral✤

codeine sulfate

Pharmacologic class: Opioid agonist
Therapeutic class: Opioid analgesic
Controlled substance schedule II
Pregnancy risk category C

Action
Binds to opiate receptors in CNS, altering perception of painful stimuli. Causes generalized CNS depression, decreases cough reflex, and reduces GI motility.

Availability
Injection (phosphate): 30 mg/ml, 60 mg/ml
Oral solution (phosphate): 10 mg/5 ml, 15 mg/5 ml
Tablets (sulfate): 15 mg, 30 mg, 60 mg; 30 mg, 60 mg (soluble)

💊 Indications and dosages
➤ Pain
Adults: 15 to 60 mg P.O. or 15 to 60 mg (phosphate) I.M., I.V., or S.C. q 4 to 6 hours. Usual daily dosage is 30 mg; maximum daily dosage is 360 mg.
Children ages 1 and older: 0.5 mg/kg or 15 mg/m^2 P.O., I.M., or S.C. q 4 to 6 hours
➤ Cough
Adults: 10 to 20 mg P.O. q 4 to 6 hours as needed; don't exceed 120 mg/day.
Children ages 6 to 12: 5 to 10 mg P.O. q 4 to 6 hours as needed; don't exceed 60 mg/day.
Children ages 2 to 6: 2.5 to 5 mg P.O. q 4 to 6 hours as needed; don't exceed 30 mg/day.
Dosage adjustment
• Elderly or debilitated patients

Contraindications

- Hypersensitivity to narcotics
- Respiratory disease
- Labor and delivery of premature neonate
- Premature neonates

Administration

- If GI upset occurs, give with food.
- Titrate dosage for appropriate analgesic effect.
- When changing administration route, be aware that oral dose is two-thirds as effective as parenteral dose.
- Don't give I.V. to children.
- If overdose occurs, give naloxone I.V. as prescribed; repeat administration as needed (up to manufacturer's recommended maximum dosage) to reverse toxic effects.
- Don't mix with other solutions; drug isn't compatible with other drugs.

Route	Onset	Peak	Duration
P.O.	30-45 min	60-120 min	4 hr
I.M.	10-30 min	30-60 min	4 hr
S.C.	10-30 min	Unknown	4 hr

Adverse reactions

CNS: confusion, sedation, malaise, agitation, euphoria, floating feeling, headache, hallucinations, unusual dreams, apathy, mood changes
CV: hypotension, bradycardia, peripheral vasodilation, reduced peripheral resistance
EENT: blurred or double vision, miosis, reddened sclera
GI: nausea, vomiting, constipation, decreased gastric motility
GU: urinary retention, urinary tract spasms, urinary urgency
Respiratory: respiratory depression, suppressed cough reflex
Skin: flushing, sweating
Other: physical or psychological drug dependence, drug tolerance

Interactions

Drug-drug. *Antidepressants, antihistamines, sedative-hypnotics:* additive CNS depression
Nalbuphine, pentazocine: decreased analgesic effect
Opioid partial agonists (buprenorphine, butorphanol, nalbuphine, pentazocine): precipitation of opioid withdrawal in physically dependent patients
Drug-herb. *Chamomile, hops, kava, skullcap, valerian:* increased CNS depression
Drug-behaviors. *Alcohol use:* increased CNS depression

Precautions

Use cautiously in:
- severe renal, hepatic, or pulmonary disease
- adrenal insufficiency, head trauma, hypothyroidism, increased intracranial pressure, prostatic hypertrophy, undiagnosed abdominal pain, alcoholism
- elderly patients
- pregnant or breastfeeding patients.

Patient monitoring

- Monitor vital signs and CNS status.
- Assess pain level and efficacy of pain relief.
- Evaluate patient for adverse reactions.
- Stay alert for overdose signs and symptoms, such as CNS and respiratory depression, GI cramping, and constipation.
- Assess other drugs that patient is taking for possible additive or adverse interactions.
- Monitor patient for signs and symptoms of drug dependence or tolerance.

Patient teaching

- With oral use, teach patient to minimize adverse GI effects by taking doses with food or milk.
- Tell patient to notify prescriber if he experiences shortness of breath or difficulty breathing or if nausea, vomit-

ing, or constipation become pronounced.

• Advise patient to avoid driving and other hazardous activities until he knows how drug affects concentration, alertness, vision, coordination, and physical dexterity.

• Instruct patient to move slowly when sitting up or standing to avoid dizziness or light-headedness from sudden blood pressure decrease.

colchicine

Pharmacologic class: Colchicum alkaloid
Therapeutic class: Antigout drug
Pregnancy risk category C

Action

Unclear; antigout action may occur through white blood cell (WBC) migration and reduced lactic acid production by WBCs. This action in turn decreases uric acid deposition, kinetin formation, and phagocytosis, leading to reduction of inflammatory response.

Availability

Injection: 0.5 mg/ml
Tablets: 0.5 mg, 0.6 mg

Indications and dosages

➤ Acute gouty arthritis
Adults: Initially, 0.6 to 1.2 mg P.O.; then 0.6 to 1.2 mg P.O. q 1 to 2 hours or until relief is achieved, adverse GI reactions occur, or patient has received total cumulative dosage of 8 mg. Or 2 mg I.V., followed by 0.5 mg I.V. q 6 hours as needed, not to exceed 4 mg daily.
➤ Prophylaxis for recurrent gouty arthritis
Adults: In patients who have one yearly attack or less, 0.6 mg P.O. daily 3

days per week. In patients who have more than one yearly attack, 0.6 mg P.O. daily; in severe cases, 1 to 1.8 mg P.O. daily.

Dosage adjustment
• Mild hepatic or renal impairment

Off-label uses

• Hepatic cirrhosis
• Chronic progressive multiple sclerosis
• Pyoderma gangrenosum associated with Crohn's disease
• Psoriasis
• Dermatitis herpetiformis

Contraindications

• Hypersensitivity to drug
• Blood dyscrasias
• Serious GI, renal, hepatic, or cardiac disorders

Administration

• Initiate therapy at first sign of acute gout attack.
• Don't administer I.M. or S.C. because of local irritation.
• For I.V. injection, give by slow I.V. push over 2 to 5 minutes.
• Know that GI symptoms may be troublesome in patients with peptic ulcer or irritable bowel.

Route	Onset	Peak	Duration
P.O.	12 hr	24-72 hr	Unknown

Adverse reactions

CNS: peripheral neuritis, neuropathy
GI: nausea, vomiting, diarrhea, abdominal pain
GU: anuria, hematuria, reversible azoospermia, renal damage
Hematologic: purpura, **agranulocytosis, aplastic anemia, thrombocytopenia**
Metabolic: vitamin B_{12} malabsorption
Musculoskeletal: myopathy
Skin: dermatosis, alopecia
Other: hypersensitivity reactions

Interactions
Drug-drug. *Vitamin B$_{12}$:* reversible vitamin malabsorption
Drug-diagnostic tests. *Alkaline phosphatase, aspartate aminotransferase:* increased levels
Hematocrit, hemoglobin, platelets: decreased values
Urine hemoglobin, urinary red blood cells: false-positive results

Precautions
Use cautiously in:
• renal impairment
• elderly or debilitated patients
• pregnant or breastfeeding patients
• children (safety not established).

Patient monitoring
◀€ Monitor patient for signs and symptoms of toxicity (nausea, vomiting, abdominal pain, bloody diarrhea, burning sensations, muscle weakness, oliguria, hematuria, ascending paralysis, delirium, and seizures). Discontinue drug if these occur.
• Be aware that patient may need opioids to control drug-induced diarrhea (especially if receiving maximum dosage).
• Monitor complete blood count and renal function test results regularly.

Patient teaching
• Instruct patient to report rash, sore throat, fever, unusual bleeding, bruising, tiredness, weakness, numbness, or tingling.
• Tell patient to immediately report muscle tremors, weakness, fatigue, bruising, bleeding, yellowing of eyes or skin, pale stools, dark urine, severe vomiting, watery or bloody diarrhea, or abdominal pain.
• Teach patient to increase fluid intake to prevent renal calculi, unless prescriber advises him to restrict fluids.

colesevelam hydrochloride
Welchol

Pharmacologic class: Bile acid sequestrant
Therapeutic class: Antihyperlipidemic
Pregnancy risk category B

Action
Binds bile acids in GI tract and forms insoluble complex, causing bile acid excretion in feces and impeding reabsorption. As a result, cholesterol and low-density lipoprotein (LDL) levels decrease.

Availability
Tablets: 625 mg

⏀ Indications and dosages
➢ Adjunct to diet and exercise to reduce LDL cholesterol in patients with primary hypercholesterolemia
Adults: Three tablets P.O. b.i.d., or six tablets P.O. once daily; maximum daily dosage is 4,375 mg.

Contraindications
• Hypersensitivity to drug
• Bowel obstruction
• Vitamin K deficiency

Administration
• Give with meals and fluids.
• Ensure that patient swallows tablets whole without crushing or chewing them.
• Store tablets at room temperature.

Route	Onset	Peak	Duration
P.O.	Unknown	2 wk	Unknown

Adverse reactions
CNS: headache, anxiety, vertigo, dizziness, insomnia, fatigue, syncope
EENT: tinnitus

GI: nausea, vomiting, diarrhea, constipation, abdominal discomfort, flatulence, fecal impaction, loose stools, fatty stools, rectal or hemorrhoidal bleeding, other GI bleeding
GU: increased libido
Hematologic: anemia, bleeding tendencies
Metabolic: malabsorption of vitamins A, D, E, and K
Musculoskeletal: back, muscle, or joint pain
Skin: bruising

Interactions
Drug-drug. *Fat-soluble vitamins (A, D, E, and K):* decreased vitamin absorption

Precautions
Use cautiously in:
• serum triglyceride level above 300 mg/dl
• children (safety and efficacy not established).

Patient monitoring
• Monitor lipid levels before initiating therapy and periodically thereafter.

Patient teaching
• Teach patient to take drug with meals as directed.
• Tell patient to report persistent GI upset, back or muscle pain or weakness, or respiratory difficulties.
• If drug causes constipation, instruct patient to increase exercise, drink plenty of fluids, consume more fruits and fiber, or take a stool softener.
• As appropriate, review all significant adverse reactions and interactions, especially those related to the drug mentioned above.

colestipol hydrochloride
Colestid

Pharmacologic class: Bile acid sequestrant
Therapeutic class: Antihyperlipidemic
Pregnancy risk category NR

Action
Combines with bile acids in the intestines to form insoluble complex that's excreted through feces. Liver then synthesizes and increases the production of cholesterol, resulting in reduction in low density-lipoprotein level.

Availability
Flavored granules for suspension (orange flavor with aspartame): 5 g/packet or scoop
Granules for suspension (unflavored): 5 g/packet or scoop
Tablets: 1 g

🖊 Indications and dosages
➤ Primary hypercholesterolemia
Adults: *Granules*—5 g P.O. once or twice daily; may increase q 1 to 2 months up to 30 g/day P.O. taken in one or two divided doses. *Tablets*—2 g once or twice daily; may increase q 1 to 2 months up to 16 g/day taken in one or two divided doses.

Off-label uses
• Digoxin toxicity

Contraindications
• Hypersensitivity to drug

Administration
• Mix granules with at least 90 ml of liquid, and stir until completely mixed.
• Give tablets with large amount of water.
• Administer other drugs 1 hour before or 4 hours after colestipol.

Route	Onset	Peak	Duration
P.O.	24-48 hr	1 mo	1 mo

Adverse reactions
CNS: dizziness, headache, vertigo, anxiety, syncope, fatigue
CV: chest pain
EENT: tongue irritation
GI: nausea, vomiting, constipation, abdominal discomfort, fecal impaction, flatulence, fatty stools, hemorrhoids, perianal irritation
Metabolic: hyperchloremic acidosis
Musculoskeletal: osteoporosis, backache, muscle and joint pain, arthritis
Skin: irritation, rashes
Other: deficiency of vitamins A, D, E, and K and folic acid

Interactions
Drug-drug. *Amiodarone, corticosteroids, digoxin, diuretics, fat-soluble vitamins (A, D, E, K), folic acid, gemfibrozil, imipramine, methotrexate, mycophenolate, nonsteroidal antiinflammatory drugs, penicillin G, phosphates, propranolol, tetracyclines, thyroid preparations, ursodiol:* decreased absorption of these drugs (when given orally)
Drug-diagnostic tests. *Alanine aminotransferase, alkaline phosphatase, aspartate aminotransferase, phosphorus:* increased levels
Prothrombin time: prolonged

Precautions
Use cautiously in
• history of constipation
• breastfeeding patients
• children (safety and efficacy not established).

Patient monitoring
• Monitor lipid levels frequently during first few months of therapy and periodically thereafter.
• Evaluate patient for signs and symptoms of abnormal bleeding.

• Be aware that prolonged use may increase bleeding tendency (from hypoprothrombinemia resulting from vitamin K deficiency). As prescribed and needed, give oral or parenteral vitamin K to reverse this effect.

Patient teaching
• Teach patient to take granules with 3 to 4 oz of water, fruit juice, soup with high fluid content, cereal, or pulpy fruits (crushed).
• Tell patient to swallow tablets whole, one at a time and not to crush, cut, or chew them.
• Inform patient that drug may interfere with absorption of many other drugs. Advise him to take other drugs 1 hour before or 4 hours after colestipol.

cortisone acetate
Cortone Acetate

Pharmacologic class: Glucocorticoid
Therapeutic class: Adrenocorticoid
Pregnancy risk category C

Action
Unclear; reduces inflammation, possibly by suppressing cell-mediated immune reactions; decreasing leukocyte, monocyte, and eosinophil levels; reducing binding of immunoglobulins to cell surface receptors; and inhibiting interleukin synthesis. Also stabilizes lysosomal membranes, curbs migration of polymorphonuclear leukocytes, interrupts phagocytosis, and diminishes antibody formation in infected and injured tissues. Interferes with histamine synthesis, fibroblast development, and capillary permeability.

Availability
Injection: 50 mg/ml
Tablets: 5 mg, 10 mg, 25 mg

Indications and dosages

➤ Asthma; adrenal insufficiency; chronic inflammatory, allergic, hematologic, neoplastic, and autoimmune disorders; prevention of organ rejection in organ transplant recipients (given with other immunosuppressants)

Adults: 25 to 300 mg P.O. daily, or 20 to 300 mg I.M. daily or on alternate days. Individualize dosage based on disease and patient response.

Dosage adjustment
- Renal impairment
- Elderly patients

Contraindications
- Hypersensitivity to drug
- Systemic fungal infections

Administration
- To help prevent peptic ulcer, give large doses between meals with antacids.
- If possible, administer in morning before 9 A.M. (Exogenous corticosteroids suppress adrenocortical activity the least when given at time of maximal activity.)

Route	Onset	Peak	Duration
P.O.	Rapid	2 hr	1.25-1.5 days
I.M.	24-48 hr	Variable	Variable

Adverse reactions
CNS: depression, euphoria, psychosis, vertigo, headache, **increased intracranial pressure, seizures**
CV: hypertension, thrombophlebitis, **thromboembolism**
EENT: cataracts, glaucoma, increased intraocular pressure, exophthalmos
GI: nausea, abdominal distention, **pancreatitis, peptic ulcers, ulcerative esophagitis**
GU: menstrual irregularities

Hepatic: elevated alanine aminotransferase, alkaline phosphatase, and aspartate aminotransferase levels
Metabolic: sodium retention, fluid retention, potassium loss, hypokalemic acidosis, carbohydrate intolerance, negative nitrogen balance, hyperglycemia, cushingoid appearance (moon face, buffalo hump)
Musculoskeletal: muscle wasting, osteoporosis, aseptic joint necrosis, muscle pain or weakness, vertebral compression fractures, steroid myopathy, tendon rupture, decreased growth (in children)
Skin: decreased wound healing, bruising, fragile skin, hirsutism, petechiae, urticaria, facial erythema, diaphoresis
Other: weight gain or loss, facial edema, increased susceptibility to infection, hypersensitivity reactions

Interactions
Drug-drug. *Anticoagulants:* increased or decreased anticoagulant blood level
Barbiturates, phenytoin, rifampin: decreased cortisone effects
Digoxin: increased risk of digitalis toxicity
Estrogens, hormonal contraceptives: increased cortisone effects
Fluoroquinolones: increased risk of tendon rupture
Itraconazole, ketoconazole: increased cortisone blood level
Live-virus vaccines: decreased antibody response to vaccine, increased risk of adverse reactions
Somatrem, somatropin: inhibition of growth-promoting effect
Thiazide and loop diuretics: additive hypokalemia
Drug-diagnostic tests. *Calcium, potassium:* decreased levels
Cholesterol, glucose: increased levels
Nitroblue-tetrazolium test: false-negative results
Drug-herb. *Echinacea:* increased immune-stimulating effects

c

Ginseng: increased immune-modulating response

Precautions
Use cautiously in:
• renal insufficiency, cirrhosis, diabetes mellitus, diverticulitis, nonspecific ulcerative colitis, recent intestinal anastomoses, peptic ulcer (active or latent), heart failure, hypertension, thromboembolic disorders, hypoprothrombinemia, hypothyroidism, myasthenia gravis, glaucoma, ocular herpes simplex, osteoporosis, seizures, underlying immunosuppression, systemic infections, active untreated infections
• emotional instability or psychotic tendencies
• pregnant or breastfeeding patients
• children.

Patient monitoring
• Monitor patient closely for signs and symptoms of infection; be aware that drug may mask these.
• Watch for weight gain, edema, and signs and symptoms of hypokalemia.
• Measure blood pressure regularly to detect hypertension.
◀‌≶ When discontinuing drug after long-term therapy, taper dosage gradually; abrupt withdrawal may be fatal.
• With long-term therapy, evaluate patient for negative nitrogen balance (drug may cause protein catabolism). Also check vital signs and evaluate laboratory findings (including 2-hour postprandial blood glucose level, potassium level, and chest X-ray) at regular intervals.
• Monitor upper GI X-rays in patients with suspected peptic ulcer disease or significant dyspepsia or gastric distress.

Patient teaching
• Advise patient to take drug with meal or snack.
• Teach patient to take single daily dose or alternate-day doses in morning before 9 A.M. Instruct him to take multiple doses at evenly spaced intervals throughout day.
• Instruct patient to carry identification stating that he's on long-term steroid therapy.
• Tell patient to report unusual weight gain, leg or foot swelling, muscle weakness, puffy face, cold, or infection.
◀‌≶ Caution patient never to stop therapy abruptly; doing so can cause life-threatening adrenal insufficiency.
◀‌≶ Tell patient to contact prescriber immediately if signs or symptoms of adrenal insufficiency follow dosage reduction or drug discontinuation.
• Inform patient that he'll require continued supervision after discontinuing drug because his disease or disorder may suddenly reappear.

cromolyn sodium
Crolom, Gastrocrom, Intal, Nalcrom✿, Nasalcrom

Pharmacologic class: Chromone derivative

Therapeutic class: Mast cell stabilizer, antiasthmatic, ophthalmic decongestant

Pregnancy risk category B

Action
Inhibits release of histamine and reacting substances of anaphylaxis from mast cells, stabilizing the membrane and reducing allergic response and inflammatory reaction

Availability
Aerosol spray for inhalation: 800 mcg/spray in 8.1-g container (112 sprays) or 14.2-g container (200 sprays)
Nasal solution: 40 mg/ml (5.2 mg/spray) in 13-ml container (100 sprays) or 26-ml container (200 sprays)
Ophthalmic solution: 4%
Oral solution: 100 mg/5 ml

Solution for nebulization: 10 mg/ml

⑩ Indications and dosages

➤ Prevention of exercise-induced bronchospasm; adjunct in prevention of allergic disorders, including rhinitis and asthma

Adults and children ages 5 and older: One aerosol spray in each nostril (5.2 mg/spray) q.i.d., or two metered-dose sprays using inhaler at regular intervals or shortly before exposure to triggering event

Children ages 2 to 5: 20 mg q.i.d. via nebulization at regular intervals or no more than 1 hour before exposure to triggering event

➤ Mastocytosis

Adults and children ages 13 and older: 200 mg P.O. q.i.d.

Children ages 2 to 12: 100 mg P.O. q.i.d.

➤ Vernal keratoconjunctivitis, vernal conjunctivitis, and vernal keratitis

Adults and children ages 4 and older: One to two drops of ophthalmic solution in each eye four to six times daily at regular intervals

Off-label uses

- Proctitis
- Ulcerative colitis
- Urticaria

Contraindications

- Hypersensitivity to drug
- Status asthmaticus

Administration

- Administer oral form 30 minutes before meals and at bedtime.
- Before giving by inhalation, shake canister gently.
- Don't immerse canister in water.
- Have patient clear nasal passages by blowing nose before using nasal spray.
- Don't expose solutions to direct sunlight.

Route	Onset	Peak	Duration
P.O., inhalation, nasal, ophthalmic	<1 wk	2-4 wk	Unknown

Adverse reactions

CNS: headache, drowsiness, dizziness

EENT: nasal irritation, sneezing, epistaxis, postnasal drip (with nasal solution); stinging, lacrimation (with ophthalmic solution)

GI: nausea, diarrhea, stomachache, altered taste, swollen parotid glands

GU: difficult or painful urination, urinary frequency

Musculoskeletal: myopathy

Respiratory: wheezing, cough, **bronchospasm**

Skin: erythema, rash, urticaria, angioedema

Other: substantial burning, serum sickness, allergic reactions including **anaphylaxis**

Interactions

None significant

Precautions

Use cautiously in:
- renal or hepatic impairment, acute bronchospasm attacks
- pregnant or breastfeeding patients
- children younger than age 5.

Patient monitoring

- Monitor pulmonary function periodically.
- Evaluate patient for signs and symptoms of overdose, including bronchospasm and difficult or painful urination.

Patient teaching

Nebulizer

- Instruct patient to prepare nebulizer according to package instructions, to clear as much mucus as possible before use, and to rinse mouth after each use to prevent opportunistic infections and reduce unpleasant aftertaste.

Nasal form

• Teach patient to instill nasal spray as directed.

• Tell patient that drug may cause unpleasant taste, but that rinsing mouth and performing frequent oral care may help. Also inform him that drug may cause headache.

• Advise patient to report increased sneezing; nasal burning, stinging, or irritation; sore throat; hoarseness; or nosebleed.

Oral form

• Tell patient to take oral form 30 minutes before meals.

Ophthalmic form

• Instruct patient to wash hands before using.

• Teach patient how to instill drops: He should tilt his head back and look up, place drops inside lower eyelid, close his eye, and then roll eyeball in all directions. Tell him not to blink for about 30 seconds, and then to apply gentle pressure to inner corner of eye for 30 seconds.

• Caution patient not to let applicator tip touch eye or any other surface.

• Tell patient that drug may cause temporary stinging of eye or blurred vision.

• Advise patient not to wear contact lenses during therapy.

cyclobenzaprine hydrochloride
Apo-Cyclobenzaprine✤, Flexeril, Novo-Cycloprine✤

Pharmacologic class: Autonomic nervous system drug
Therapeutic class: Skeletal muscle relaxant (centrally acting)
Pregnancy risk category B

Action
Unclear; thought to act primarily at brain stem (and to a lesser extent at spinal cord level) to relieve skeletal muscle spasm of local origin without altering muscle function.

Availability
Tablets: 5 mg, 10 mg

💊 Indications and dosages
➤ Adjunct to physical therapy to relieve muscle spasms
Adults: 5 mg P.O. t.i.d.; may increase to 10 mg P.O. t.i.d. as needed

Contraindications
• Hypersensitivity to drug
• Acute recovery phase after myocardial infarction (MI)
• Heart failure
• Arrhythmias
• Hyperthyroidism
• Monoamine oxidase (MAO) inhibitor use within past 14 days

Administration
◀€ Don't give within 14 days of MAO therapy; drug interaction may cause hypertensive crisis and severe seizures.

• Know that drug shouldn't be used for more than 3 weeks.

• Be aware that drug may not be first-line agent for elderly patients because of its anticholinergic effects.

Route	Onset	Peak	Duration
P.O.	1 hr	4-6 hr	12-24 hr

Adverse reactions
CNS: dizziness, drowsiness, confusion, fatigue, headache, nervousness, decreased mental acuity, irritability, weakness, insomnia, depression, disorientation, delusions, peripheral neuropathy, Bell's palsy, electroencephalogram changes, extrapyramidal symptoms, **cerebrovascular accident**

CV: vasodilation, tachycardia, syncope, chest pain, hypotension, **MI, heart block**

EENT: blurred vision

GI: nausea, constipation, dyspepsia, swollen parotid glands, mouth inflammation, tongue discoloration, dry mouth, unpleasant taste, **paralytic ileus**

GU: galactorrhea, urinary retention, urinary frequency, gynecomastia, testicular swelling, libido changes, impotence

Hematologic: purpura, eosinophilia, **bone marrow depression, leukopenia, thrombocytopenia**

Metabolic: hyperglycemia, hypoglycemia, syndrome of inappropriate diuretic hormone secretion

Musculoskeletal: muscle ache, abnormal gait

Respiratory: dyspnea

Skin: photosensitization, alopecia, angioedema

Other: weight gain or loss, edema

Interactions

Drug-drug. *Anticholinergics, anticholinergic-like drugs (including antihistamines, antidepressants, disopyramide, haloperidol, phenothiazines):* additive anticholinergic effects

Antihistamines, CNS depressants, opioids, sedative-hypnotics: additive CNS depression

Guanadrel, guanethidine: reduction or blockage of these drugs' actions

MAO inhibitors: hyperpyretic crisis, seizures, death

Drug-herb. *Chamomile, hops, kava, skullcap, valerian:* increased CNS depression

Drug-behaviors. *Alcohol use:* increased CNS depression

Precautions

Use cautiously in:

• cardiovascular disease, closed-angle glaucoma, hepatic impairment, increased intraocular pressure, urinary retention

• elderly patients

• pregnant or breastfeeding patients

• children younger than age 15.

Patient monitoring

• Assess for adverse CNS effects, such as drowsiness, dizziness, and decreased mental acuity.

• Monitor patient for signs and symptom of drug interactions, especially when giving with CNS depressants.

Patient teaching

• Caution patient to avoid driving and other hazardous activities until he knows how drug affects concentration, alertness, and vision.

• Tell patient that drug may cause dry mouth.

• Advise patient not to use alcohol, sedatives, pain medications, over-the-counter preparations, or herbs without consulting prescriber.

cyclophosphamide
Cytoxan, Neosar, Procytox❧

Pharmacologic class: Alkylating agent, nitrogen mustard

Therapeutic class: Antineoplastic

Pregnancy risk category D

Action

Unknown; thought to prevent cell division by cross-linking DNA strands and interfering with growth of susceptible cancer cells

Availability

Powder for injection: 100 mg, 200 mg, 500 mg, 1 g, 2 g

Tablets: 25 mg, 50 mg

Indications and dosages

➤ Hodgkin's disease, malignant lymphoma, multiple myeloma, leukemia, advanced mycosis fungoides, neuroblastoma, ovarian cancer, breast cancer, certain other tumors

Adults and children: 40 to 50 mg/kg I.V. in divided doses over 2 to 5 days, or 10 to 15 mg/kg I.V. q 10 days, or 3 to 5 mg/kg I.V. twice weekly. Initial and maintenance P.O. dosages range from 1 to 5 mg/kg/day. When drug is given with other antineoplastics, dosage decrease may be required.

➤ Nephrotic syndrome in children (proven by biopsy)

Children: 2.5 to 3 mg/kg/day P.O. for 60 to 90 days

Off-label uses

• Severe rheumatologic conditions
• Selected cases of severe progressive rheumatoid arthritis and systemic lupus erythematosus

Contraindications

• Hypersensitivity to drug
• Severe bone marrow depression
• Pregnancy or breastfeeding

Administration

• Verify that patient isn't pregnant before administering.
• Don't cut or crush tablets; Administer tablets on empty stomach; if drug causes severe GI upset, give with food.
• Reconstitute I.V. solution with compatible fluid, such as 5% dextrose injection, 5% dextrose and normal saline solution for injection, 5% dextrose and Ringer's injection, lactated Ringer's injection, or half-normal saline solution for injection.
• Use solution prepared with bacteriostatic water for injection within 24 hours if stored at room temperature or within 6 days if refrigerated.
• To minimize bladder toxicity, increase patient's fluid intake during therapy and for 1 to 2 days afterward; most adults require fluid intake of at least 2 L/day.

Route	Onset	Peak	Duration
P.O., I.V.	7 days	7-15 days	21 days

Adverse reactions

CV: cardiotoxicity
GI: nausea, vomiting, diarrhea, abdominal pain or discomfort, stomatitis, oral mucosal ulcers, anorexia, **hemorrhagic colitis**
GU: urinary bladder fibrosis, hematuria, acute hemorrhagic cystitis, renal tubular necrosis, hemorrhagic ureteral inflammation, amenorrhea, decreased sperm count, sterility
Hematologic: anemia, **leukopenia, thrombocytopenia, bone marrow depression, neutropenia**
Hepatic: jaundice
Metabolic: hyperuricemia
Respiratory: interstitial pulmonary fibrosis
Skin: changes in nails and pigmentation, alopecia
Other: poor wound healing, infections, allergic reactions including **anaphylaxis, secondary cancer**

Interactions

Drug-drug. *Allopurinol, thiazide diuretics:* increased risk of leukopenia
Digoxin: decreased digoxin blood level
Cardiotoxic drugs (cytarabine, daunorubicin, doxorubicin): additive cardiotoxicity
Chloramphenicol: prolonged cyclophosphamide half-life
Phenobarbital: increased risk of cyclophosphamide toxicity
Quinolones: decreased antimicrobial effect
Succinylcholine: prolonged neuromuscular blockade
Warfarin: increased anticoagulant effect
Drug-diagnostic tests. *Hemoglobin, platelets, pseudocholinesterase, red blood*

cells (RBCs), white blood cells: decreased values
Uric acid: increased level

Precautions

Use cautiously in:
• renal or hepatic impairment, adrenalectomy, bone marrow depression, other chronic debilitating illnesses
• females of childbearing age
• breastfeeding patients.

Patient monitoring

• Assess infusion site for signs of extravasation.
• Monitor hematologic profile to determine degree of hematopoietic suppression; be aware that leukopenia is an expected effect and is used to help determine dosage.
• Monitor urine regularly for RBCs, which may precede hemorrhagic cystitis.

Patient teaching

• Tell patient to take tablets on empty stomach; if GI upset occurs, instruct him to take them with food.
• Teach patient to report unusual bleeding or bruising, fever, chills, sore throat, cough, shortness of breath, seizures, lack of menstrual flow, unusual lumps or masses, flank or stomach pain, joint pain, mouth or lip sores, or yellowing of skin or eyes.
• Instruct patient to drink 2 to 3 L of fluids daily (unless prescriber has told him to restrict fluids).
• Tell patient that drug may cause hair loss, but that hair usually grows back after treatment ends.
• Advise female patient to use barrier contraception during therapy and for 1 month afterward.

cyclosporine
Gengraf, Neoral, Sandimmune

Pharmacologic class: Polypeptide antibiotic
Therapeutic class: Immunosuppressant
Pregnancy risk category C

Action

Unclear; thought to act by specific, reversible inhibition of immunocompetent lymphocytes in G_0-G_1 phase of cell cycle. Preferentially inhibits T lymphocytes; also inhibits lymphokine production.

Availability

Capsules: 25 mg, 100 mg
Injection: 50 mg/ml
Oral solution: 100 mg/ml

Indications and dosages

➤ Psoriasis
Adults: *Neoral only*—1.25 mg/kg P.O. b.i.d. for 4 weeks. Based on patient response, may increase by 0.5 mg/kg/day once q 2 weeks, to a maximum dosage of 4 mg/kg/day.
➤ Severe active rheumatoid arthritis
Adults: *Neoral only*—1.25 mg/kg P.O. b.i.d. May adjust dosage by 0.5 to 0.75 mg/kg/day after 8 weeks and again after 12 weeks, to a maximum dosage of 4 mg/kg/day. If no response occurs after 16 weeks, discontinue therapy. *Gengraf only*—2.5 mg/kg daily given b.i.d.; after 8 weeks, may increase to a maximum dosage of 4 mg/kg/day.
➤ To prevent organ rejection in kidney, liver, or heart transplantation
Adults and children: *Sandimmune only*—Initially, 15 mg/kg P.O. 4 to 12 hours before transplantation; then daily for 1 to 2 weeks postoperatively. Reduce dosage by 5% weekly to a maintenance level of 5 to 10 mg/kg/day. Or 5

to 6 mg/kg I.V. 4 to 12 hours before transplantation as a continuous infusion.

Off-label uses
- Aplastic anemia
- Atopic dermatitis

Contraindications
- Hypersensitivity to drug
- Rheumatoid arthritis, psoriasis, abnormal renal function, uncontrolled hypertension, or cancer (Neoral only)

Administration
- Administer I.V. dose over 2 to 6 hours.
- Mix Neoral solution with orange juice or apple juice to improve its taste.
- Dilute Sandimmune oral solution with milk, chocolate milk, or orange juice. Be aware that grapefruit and grapefruit juice affect drug metabolism.
- Switch to P.O. dosage as tolerance allows in postoperative patients.
- Be aware that Sandimmune and Neoral aren't bioequivalent; don't use interchangeably.

Route	Onset	Peak	Duration
P.O.	Unknown	1.5-3.5 hr	Unknown
I.V.	Rapid	1-2 hr	Unknown

Adverse reactions
CNS: tremor, headache, confusion, paresthesia, insomnia, anxiety, depression, lethargy, weakness
CV: hypertension, chest pain, **myocardial infarction**
EENT: visual disturbances, hearing loss, tinnitus, rhinitis, gum hyperplasia
GI: nausea, vomiting, diarrhea, constipation, abdominal discomfort, gastritis, upper GI bleeding, peptic ulcer, mouth sores, difficulty swallowing, anorexia, **pancreatitis**

GU: gynecomastia, hematuria, **nephrotoxicity, renal dysfunction, glomerular capillary thrombosis**
Hematologic: anemia, **leukopenia, thrombocytopenia**
Metabolic: increased low-density lipoprotein (LDL) level, hyperglycemia, hypomagnesemia, hyperkalemia, hyperuricemia, metabolic acidosis
Musculoskeletal: muscle and joint pain
Respiratory: cough, dyspnea, *Pneumocystis jiroveci* **pneumonia** (formerly *Pneumocystis carinii*), **bronchospasm**
Skin: acne, hirsutism, brittle fingernails, hair breakage, night sweats
Other: flulike symptoms, edema, fever, weight loss, hiccups, **anaphylaxis**

Interactions
Drug-drug. *Acyclovir, aminoglycosides, amphotericin B, cimetidine, diclofenac, gentamicin, ketoconazole, melphalan, naproxen, ranitidine, sulindac, sulfamethoxazole, tacrolimus, tobramycin, trimethoprim, vancomycin:* increased risk of nephrotoxicity
Allopurinol, amiodarone, bromocriptine, clarithromycin, colchicine, danazol, diltiazem, erythromycin, fluconazole, imipenem and cilastatin, itraconazole, ketoconazole, methylprednisolone, nicardipine, prednisolone, quinupristin/dalfopristin, verapamil: increased cyclosporine blood level
Azathioprine, corticosteroids, cyclophosphamide: increased immunosuppression
Carbamazepine, isoniazid, nafcillin, octretide, orlistat, phenobarbital, phenytoin, rifabutin, rifampin, ticlopidine: decreased cyclosporine blood level
Digoxin: decreased digoxin clearance
Live-virus vaccines: decreased antibody response to vaccine
Lovastatin: decreased lovastatin clearance, increased risk of myopathy and rhabdomyolysis

Potassium-sparing diuretics: increased risk of hyperkalemia

Drug-diagnostic tests. *Alanine aminotransferase, aspartate aminotransferase, bilirubin, blood urea nitrogen, creatinine, glucose, LDLs:* increased levels
Hemoglobin, platelets, white blood cells: decreased values

Drug-food. *Grapefruit, grapefruit juice:* decreased metabolism and increased blood level of cyclosporine
High-fat diet: decreased drug absorption (Neoral)

Drug-herb. *Alfalfa sprouts, astragalus, echinacea, licorice:* interference with immunosuppressive action
St. John's wort: reduced cyclosporine blood level, possibly leading to organ rejection

Precautions

Use cautiously in:
• hepatic impairment, renal dysfunction, active infection, hypertension
• pregnant or breastfeeding patients
• children.

Patient monitoring

• Observe patient for first 30 to 60 minutes of infusion; monitor frequently thereafter.
• Monitor cyclosporine blood level, electrolyte levels, and liver and kidney function test results.
• Assess for signs and symptoms of hyperkalemia if patient is receiving potassium-sparing diuretic concurrently.

Patient teaching

• Teach patient to dilute Neoral oral solution with orange or apple juice (preferably at room temperature) to improve its flavor.
• Teach patient to use glass container when taking oral solution, not to let solution stand before drinking, to stir solution well and drink all at once, and to rinse glass with same liquid and then drink again to ensure that he takes entire dose.

• Tell patient taking Neoral to avoid high-fat meals, grapefruit, and grapefruit juice.
• Advise patient to dilute Sandimmune oral solution with milk, chocolate milk, or orange juice to improve its flavor.
• Inform patient that he's at increased risk for infection; teach him to avoid crowds and exposure to illness.
• Inform patient that he will need repeated laboratory tests during therapy.

cyproheptadine hydrochloride
Periactin, PMS-Cyproheptadine✽

Pharmacologic class: Piperidine (nonselective)
Therapeutic class: Antihistamine
Pregnancy risk category B

Action

Antagonizes effects of histamine at histamine$_1$-receptor sites, preventing histamine-mediated responses. Also blocks effects of serotonin, causing increased appetite.

Availability

Syrup: 2 mg/5 ml
Tablets: 4 mg

🖊 Indications and dosages

➤ Allergy symptoms caused by histamine release (including seasonal and perennial allergic rhinitis), chronic urticaria, angioedema, dermographism, cold urticaria, adjunctive therapy for anaphylactic reactions
Adults: Initially, 4 mg P.O. q 8 hours; maintenance dosage is 4 to 20 mg/day in three divided doses, to a maximum dosage of 0.5 mg/kg/day.
Children ages 7 to 14: 2 to 4 mg P.O. q 12 hours. Don't exceed 16 mg/day.

Children ages 2 to 6: 2 mg P.O. q 12 hours. Don't exceed 12 mg/day.

Off-label uses
• Vascular cluster headaches

Contraindications
• Hypersensitivity to drug
• Alcohol intolerance (syrup only)
• Bladder neck obstruction
• Narrow-angle glaucoma
• Ulcer disease
• Symptomatic prostatic hypertrophy
• Monoamine oxidase (MAO) inhibitor use within past 14 days
• Elderly patients
• Pregnancy (third trimester) and breastfeeding

Administration
• Give with food or milk to decrease GI upset.

Route	Onset	Peak	Duration
P.O.	15-60 min	1-2 hr	8 hr

Adverse reactions
CNS: drowsiness, dizziness, excitation (especially in children), fatigue, sedation, hallucinations, disorientation, tremor
CV: arrhythmias, palpitations, hypotension
EENT: blurred vision, dry stuffy nose, dry throat
GI: constipation, dry mouth
GU: urinary retention, urinary frequency, ejaculatory inhibition, early menses
Respiratory: thickened bronchial secretions
Skin: rash, photosensitivity
Other: weight gain

Interactions
Drug-drug. *CNS depressants (including opioid analgesics, sedative-hypnotics):* increased CNS depression

MAO inhibitors: intensified, prolonged anticholinergic effects
Drug-diagnostic tests. *Allergy skin tests:* false-negative reactions
Drug-behaviors. *Alcohol use:* increased CNS depression

Precautions
Use cautiously in:
• hepatic impairment
• elderly patients
• pregnant patients (safety not established)
• breastfeeding patients.

Patient monitoring
• Monitor patient for excess anticholinergic effects.
• Assess for excessive CNS depression.
• Discontinue drug 4 days before diagnostic skin testing.

Patient teaching
• Advise patient to take drug with food to minimize GI upset.
• Teach patient not to use other CNS depressants, sleep aids, or alcohol during therapy.
• Instruct patient to avoid driving and other hazardous activities until he knows how drug affects concentration and alertness.

cytarabine
Cytosar✦, Cytosar-U, DepoCyt

Pharmacologic class: Antimetabolite, pyrimidine analog
Therapeutic class: Antineoplastic
Pregnancy risk category D

Action
Unclear; cytotoxic effect may stem from inhibition of DNA polymerase by active metabolite.

Availability

Injection (conventional form): 20 mg
Liposome injection for intrathecal use (sustained-release): 50 ml/5-ml vial
Powder for injection (conventional form): 100 mg, 500 mg, 1g, 2 g

🖊 Indications and dosages

➤ To induce remission of acute non-lymphocytic leukemia
Adults: Injection (conventional form)—100 mg/m²/day by continuous I.V. infusion on days 1 through 7, or 100 mg/m² I.V. q 12 hours on days 1 through 7, given with other antineoplastics
➤ Meningeal leukemia
Adults: Injection (conventional form)—5 to 75 mg/m²/day intrathecally for 4 days or once q 4 days. Most common dosage is 30 mg/m² q 4 days until cerebrospinal fluid is normal.
➤ Lymphomatous meningitis
Adults: Liposome injection—50 mg intrathecally q 14 days for two doses (at first and third weeks); then q 14 days for three doses (at fifth, seventh, and ninth weeks), with one additional dose at 13th week; then q 28 days for four doses

Contraindications

• Hypersensitivity to drug

Administration

• Be aware that conventional and liposomal forms can be administered inthrathecally.
◀🔊 Don't use intrathecal route for formulations containing benzyl alcohol.
• When giving conventional form intrathecally, reconstitute with autologous spinal fluid or preservative-free normal saline solution for injection; use immediately.
• If patient is receiving liposomal cytarabine concurrently with dexamethasone, provide appropriate care to ease symptoms of chemical arachnoiditis.

Route	Onset	Peak	Duration
I.V.	Unknown	Unknown	Unknown
Intrathecal	Rapid	5 hr	14-28 hr

Adverse reactions

CNS: malaise, dizziness, headache, neuritis, **neurotoxicity, chemical arachnoiditis**
CV: thrombophlebitis, chest pain
EENT: conjunctivitis
GI: nausea, vomiting, diarrhea, abdominal pain, anal ulcers, esophagitis, esophageal ulcers, oral ulcers (in 5 to 10 days), anorexia, **bowel necrosis**
GU: urinary retention, renal dysfunction
Hematologic: reticulocytopenia, megaloblastosis, anemia, **leukopenia, thrombocytopenia**
Hepatic: hepatic dysfunction
Metabolic: hyperuricemia
Musculoskeletal: muscle ache, bone pain
Respiratory: pneumonia, shortness of breath
Skin: rash, pruritus, freckling, skin ulcers, urticaria, alopecia
Other: flulike symptoms, edema, infection, fever, cellulitis at injection site, **anaphylaxis**

Interactions

Drug-drug. *Digoxin:* decreased digoxin blood level
Fluorocytosine: decreased fluorocytosine blood level
Gentamicin: decreased gentamicin effect
Drug-diagnostic tests. *Megaloblasts, uric acid:* increased levels
Hemoglobin, platelets, red blood cells, reticulocytes, white blood cells: decreased values

Precautions

Use cautiously in:
• renal or hepatic disease, active infection, decreased bone marrow reserve, other chronic illnesses

---

- females of childbearing age
- pregnant or breastfeeding patients
- children.

Patient monitoring
- Observe for signs and symptoms of cytarabine syndrome (malaise, fever, muscle ache, bone pain, occasional chest pain, maculopapular rash, and conjunctivitis).
- When giving liposomal form, assess for signs and symptoms of chemical arachnoiditis, such as neck rigidity and pain, nausea, vomiting, headache, fever, and back pain.
- Monitor liver function test results, complete blood count with differential, platelet count, blood urea nitrogen, and serum creatinine and uric acid levels.

Patient teaching
- Tell patient to contact prescriber immediately if he develops signs or symptoms of cytarabine syndrome (fever, muscle ache, bone pain, chest pain, rash, eye infection, or fatigue) or chemical arachnoiditis (neck rigidity or pain, nausea, vomiting, headache, fever, or back pain).
- Advise patient to increase fluid intake to promote uric acid excretion.

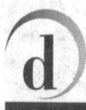

dacarbazine
DTIC✤, DTIC-Dome

Pharmacologic class: Alkylating drug, triazene

Therapeutic class: Antineoplastic
Pregnancy risk category C

Action
Unclear; thought to inhibit DNA synthesis by acting as purine analog. Also causes alkylation and may interact with sulfhydryl groups.

Availability
Injection: 100-mg and 200-mg vials

ⓘ Indications and dosages
➤ Hodgkin's disease
Adults: 150 mg/m^2 I.V. daily for 5 days in combination with other drugs, repeated q 4 weeks. Or 375 mg/m^2 I.V. on first day of combination therapy, repeated q 15 days.
➤ Metastatic malignant melanoma
Adults: 2 to 4.5 mg/kg I.V. daily for 10 days, repeated q 4 weeks. Or 250 mg/m^2 I.V. daily for 5 days, repeated q 3 weeks.

Off-label uses
- Malignant pheochromocytoma
- Metastatic malignant melanoma

Contraindications
- Hypersensitivity to drug

Administration
◀ Administer by I.V. infusion only.
- Take steps to prevent extravasation, which may cause tissue damage and severe pain.
- Reconstitute with sterile water for injection according to manufacturer's directions.
- Further dilute reconstituted drug with 5% dextrose or 5% sodium chloride solutions.

Route	Onset	Peak	Duration
I.V.	Unknown	Unknown	Unknown

Adverse reactions
CNS: malaise, paresthesia
GI: nausea, vomiting, dyspepsia, anorexia

Hematologic: anemia, **leukopenia, thrombocytopenia, bone marrow depression**
Musculoskeletal: myalgia
Skin: dermatitis, erythematous or urticarial rash, alopecia, flushing, photosensitivity
Others: flulike symptoms, fever, **hypersensitivity reactions** including **anaphylaxis**

Interactions
Drug-diagnostic tests. *Platelets, red blood cells, white blood cells:* decreased counts
Drug-behaviors. *Sun exposure:* photosensitivity reaction

Precautions
Use cautiously in:
• hepatic dysfunction, impaired bone marrow function
• pregnant or breastfeeding patients.

Patient monitoring
• Frequently monitor complete blood count with white cell differential and platelet count; hematopoietic depression is most common toxicity.
• Assess infusion site closely for extravasation.

Patient teaching
• Instruct patient to immediately report pain, burning, or swelling at infusion site; numbness in arms or legs; gait changes; respiratory distress; difficulty breathing; rash; easy bruising; or bleeding.
• Teach patient to minimize adverse GI effects by eating small, frequent servings of healthy food and drinking plenty of fluids.
• Tell patient he'll undergo regular blood testing during therapy.

daclizumab
Zenapax

Pharmacologic class: Immunomodulator, humanized immunoglobulin G_1 monoclonal antibody

Therapeutic class: Immunosuppressant

Pregnancy risk category C

d

Action
Binds to alpha subunit of high-affinity interleuken-2 (IL2) receptor complex, inhibiting IL2 binding and preventing critical pathway in cellular immune response against allografts. Also impedes immunologic response to antigenic challenges.

Availability
Injection: 25 mg/5 ml

⚡ Indications and dosages
➤ Prevention of acute organ rejection in kidney transplants (given as part of immunosuppressive combination therapy)
Adults: 1 mg/kg by I.V. infusion, usually for five doses. First dose is given no more than 24 hours before transplantation; remaining doses ar given at 14-day intervals.

Contraindications
• Hypersensitivity to drug

Administration
• Don't give by direct injection.
• Mix calculated dose with 50 ml of sterile normal saline solution.
• Deliver through peripheral or central vein over 15 minutes.
• Don't add or infuse other drugs through same I.V. line.
• Administer diluted drug within 4 hours of preparation if stored at room temperature or within 24 hours if re-

frigerated. Discard prepared solution after 24 hours.

• Protect undiluted solution from direct light.

Route	Onset	Peak	Duration
I.V.	Rapid	After 5th dose	120 days

Adverse reactions

CNS: headache, tremor, dizziness, prickly sensations, insomnia, fatigue, weakness, depression, anxiety
CV: tachycardia, chest pain, hypotension, hypertension, **thrombosis**
EENT: blurred vision, rhinitis, pharyngitis
GI: nausea, vomiting, constipation, diarrhea, abdominal pain, abdominal distention, epigastric pain, heartburn, dyspepsia, gastritis, hemorrhoids, flatulence
GU: oliguria, kidney enlargement, urinary tract bleeding, dysuria, urinary retention, renal insufficiency, **renal tubular necrosis**
Hematologic: bleeding
Metabolic: diabetes mellitus, dehydration, fluid overload
Musculoskeletal: myalgia; joint, back, and leg pain
Respiratory: dyspnea, cough, hypoxia, crackles, crepitus, rhonchi, atelectasis, congestion, abnormal or decreased breath sounds, hemoptysis, upper respiratory tract infection, **pleural effusion**
Skin: acne, wound infection, impaired wound healing
Other: lymphocele (cystic mass), pain, edema at injection site, peripheral edema, cellulitis, cytomegalovirus infection, shivering, fever

Interactions

None significant

Precautions

Use cautiously in:
• elderly patients
• pregnant or breastfeeding patients
• children.

Patient monitoring

• Monitor patient closely; drug increases risk of infectious complications and secondary cancers.
• Assess cardiovascular, respiratory, and renal function during infusion and periodically between infusions.
• Monitor blood glucose level, especially in patients receiving high-dose corticosteroids concurrently with daclizumab.

Patient teaching

• Explain that drug's purpose is to prevent transplant rejection.
◀€ Instruct patient to immediately report difficulty breathing or swallowing, tightness in jaw or throat, chest pain, or pain at infusion site.
• Tell patient to report changes in urinary pattern, unusual bleeding or bruising, rash, fever, and other adverse effects.
• Inform patient that drug increases risk of infection; advise him to avoid crowds and exposure to illness.

dactinomycin
(actinomycin D, ACT)
Cosmegen

Pharmacologic class: Anti-infective
Therapeutic class: Antineoplastic
Pregnancy risk category D

Action

Inhibits RNA synthesis, resulting in cell death; cell-cycle-phase nonspecific.

Availability
Lyophilized powder for injection: 500-mcg vial

Indications and dosages
➤ Wilms' tumor, childhood rhabdomyosarcoma, Ewing's sarcoma
Children: Maximum dosage is 15 mcg/kg/day I.V. for 5 days, or 500 mcg/day or 2.5 mg/m² in equally divided doses over 7-day period (given with other chemotherapeutic drugs). Regimen may be repeated in 3 weeks if toxicity signs and symptoms have disappeared.
➤ Metastatic nonseminomatous testicular carcinoma
Adults: 1,000 mcg/m² I.V. on first day as part of combination regimen with cyclophosphamide, bleomycin, vinblastine, and cisplatin
➤ Gestational trophoblastic neoplasia
Adults: 12 mcg/kg/day I.V. for 5 days as a single drug. Or 500 mcg I.V. on first and second days as part of combination regimen with etoposide, methotrexate, folinic acid, vincristine.
Dosage adjustment
• Obesity
• Edema

Contraindications
• Hypersensitivity to drug
• Chickenpox
• Herpes zoster
• Infants younger than age 12 months

Administration
◀︎ Know that drug is highly toxic, so prepare and administer with care. Don't inhale dust or vapors or let drug contact skin or mucous membranes. If contact occurs, irrigate with copious amounts of water.
• Reconstitute powder by adding 1.1 ml of sterile water for injection (free of preservatives). Add reconstituted solution directly to infusion solution of 5% dextrose injection or sodium chloride injection or to tubing of running I.V. infusion.

• Be aware that dosages are almost always expressed in micrograms rather than milligrams.
◀︎ Remember that drug is an extremely corrosive vesicant. Take care to avoid extravasation because severe tissue damage will result. If extravasation occurs, discontinue drug immediately and apply cold compresses to area.
• Premedicate with antiemetic, as prescribed, because drug usually causes severe nausea and vomiting for up to 24 hours.
• Know that toxic reactions are common and may limit amount of drug that can be given.

Route	Onset	Peak	Duration
I.V.	Unknown	Unknown	Unknown

Adverse reactions
CNS: malaise, fatigue, lethargy
EENT: lip inflammation and cracking, pharyngitis
GI: nausea, vomiting, diarrhea, dyspepsia, abdominal pain, proctitis, difficulty swallowing, esophagitis, dry mouth, stomatitis, anorexia
Hematologic: anemia, petechiae, **leukocytosis, thrombocytopenia, bleeding, leukopenia, pancytopenia, agranulocytosis, aplastic anemia, reticulocytopenia**
Hepatic: abnormal liver function test results, **hepatotoxicity**
Metabolic: hypocalcemia
Musculoskeletal: joint pain, growth retardation (in children)
Respiratory: pneumonitis
Skin: skin eruptions, acne, erythema, increased pigmentation, diaphoresis, alopecia
Other: phlebitis and soft-tissue damage at injection site, fever, infection, edema

Interactions
Drug-drug. *Myelosuppressants:* additive toxicity

Drug-diagnostic tests. *Antibacterial drug assays:* test interference
Calcium, granulocytes, hemoglobin, platelets, red blood cells, white blood cells: decreased values

Precautions

Use cautiously in:
• renal or hepatic disease
• bone marrow depression in patients undergoing radiation therapy
• pregnant or breastfeeding patients.

Patient monitoring

• Monitor patient for severe nausea and vomiting.
• Watch infusion site closely for irritation and signs of extravasation.
• Monitor daily platelet count and complete blood count with white cell differential; be prepared to withhold drug if any of these values drops significantly.
• Check liver and renal function test results frequently.

Patient teaching

• Tell patient that he'll be premedicated to help minimize nausea and vomiting (common drug effects).
• Inform patient that drug may cause fatigue, appetite loss, and diarrhea; teach him to report these symptoms if they persist.
• Teach patient to report pain or swelling at I.V. site.
• Teach patient to minimize adverse GI effects by eating small, frequent servings of healthy food and drinking plenty of fluids.
• Inform patient that drug makes him more susceptible to infection, so he should avoid crowds and exposure to illness.
• Tell patient that drug may cause hair loss but that hair usually grows back after therapy.
• Notify patient that he'll undergo regular blood testing during therapy.

dalteparin sodium
Fragmin

Pharmacologic class: Low-molecular-weight heparin
Therapeutic class: Anticoagulant
Pregnancy risk category B

Action

Inhibits thrombus and clot formation by blocking factor Xa and thrombin

Availability

Solution for injection (prefilled syringes): 2,500 antifactor Xa IU/0.2 ml; 5,000 antifactor Xa IU/0.2 ml; 7,500 antifactor Xa IU/0.3 ml; 10,000 antifactor Xa IU/1 ml

⬤ Indications and dosages

➤ To prevent deep-vein thrombosis and pulmonary embolism in patients undergoing surgery that increases the risk of these complications (abdominal surgery, hip replacement)
Adults: *Abdominal surgery*—2,500 IU S.C. 1 to 2 hours before surgery; then once daily for 5 to 10 days. For high-risk patient, 5,000 IU S.C. on evening before surgery; then once daily for 5 to 10 days. For cancer patient, 2,500 IU S.C. 1 to 2 hours before surgery; repeat dose 12 hours later, then give 5,000 IU S.C. daily for 5 to 10 days. *Hip replacement surgery*—5,000 IU S.C. 10 to 14 hours before surgery; repeat dose 4 to 8 hours after surgery, then give 5,000 IU daily for 5 to 10 days.
➤ To prevent ischemic complications in patients with unstable angina and non-Q-wave myocardial infarction
Adults: 120 IU/kg (not to exceed 10,000 IU) S.C. q 12 hours (concurrently with aspirin P.O.) for 5 to 8 days

---

Off-label uses
• Systemic anticoagulation

Contraindications
• Hypersensitivity to drug, heparin, pork products, sulfites, or benzyl alcohol
• Active major bleeding
• Thrombocytopenia

Administration
◀€ Administer S.C. only; don't administer by I.M. or I.V. route.
• To minimize bruising at injection site, massage site with ice cube before giving injection.
• Administer by S.C. injection with patient sitting or lying down. Inject in U-shaped area around navel, upper outer side of thigh, or upper outer quadrangle of buttock; rotate injection sites daily.
• Don't use interchangeably with heparin or other low-molecular-weight heparins.

Route	Onset	Peak	Duration
S.C.	20-60 min	3-5 hr	12 hr

Adverse reactions
Hematologic: anemia, ecchymosis, bleeding, **thrombocytopenia, hemorrhage**
Hepatic: transaminase elevations
Skin: rash, urticaria
Other: pain, irritation, and hematoma at injection site; fever; edema

Interactions
Drug-drug. *Antiplatelet drugs (aspirin, clopidogrel, dipyridamole, ticlopidine), thrombolytics, warfarin:* increased risk of bleeding
Drug-diagnostic tests. *Alanine aminotransferase, aspartate aminotransferase:* increased levels
Platelets: decreased count
Drug-herb. *Anise, arnica, chamomile, clove, feverfew, garlic, ginger, ginkgo, ginseng:* increased risk of bleeding

Precautions
Use cautiously in:
• bacterial endocarditis, bleeding disorders, hemorrhagic stroke, severe uncontrolled hypertension, GI ulcer, severe renal or hepatic insufficiency, hypertensive or diabetic retinopathy
• spinal or epidural anesthesia
• history of thrombocytopenia from heparin use, history of congenital or acquired bleeding disorder
• recent CNS or ophthalmologic surgery or recent GI disease
• pregnant or breastfeeding patients
• children (safety not established).

Patient monitoring
◀€ Monitor patient for increased risk of bleeding if he is also receiving other drugs that affect platelet function.
• Check complete blood count and platelet count.
• Monitor stools for occult blood.

Patient teaching
• Tell patient that drug may cause him to bleed easily; to avoid injury, advise him to brush his teeth with soft toothbrush, use electric razor, and avoid scissors and sharp knives.
◀€ Advise patient to immediately report bleeding, bruising, dizziness, light-headedness, itching, rash, fever, swelling, or difficulty breathing.

danazol
Cyclomen✲, Danocrine

Pharmacologic class: Androgen (synthetic)
Therapeutic class: Sex hormone
Pregnancy risk category X

Action
Suppresses pituitary-ovarian axis, probably through a combination of de-

pressed hypothalamic-pituitary response to reduced estrogen production, altered sex hormone metabolism, and interaction with sex hormone receptors

Availability
Capsules: 50 mg, 100 mg, 200 mg

Indications and dosages

➤ Moderate endometriosis amenable to hormonal management
Adults and adolescents: 400 mg P.O. b.i.d for up to 9 months. In milder cases, 100 to 200 mg P.O. b.i.d. initially, with dosage adjustments based on patient response.
➤ Fibrocystic breast disease
Adults and adolescents: 100 to 200 mg P.O. b.i.d. for 2 to 6 months
➤ Hereditary angioedema
Adults and adolescents: 200 mg P.O. two to three times daily. If possible, decrease dosage by 50% or less q 1 to 3 months; if acute angioedema attack occurs, increase dosage up to 200 mg/day.

Off-label uses
• Menorrhagia
• Precocious puberty

Contraindications
• Hypersensitivity to drug
• Abnormal genital bleeding
• Porphyria
• Severe hepatic, renal, or cardiac disease
• Pregnancy or breastfeeding

Administration
• Verify that patient isn't pregnant before initiating therapy; start therapy during menstruation.
• Don't give to female of childbearing age unless she's willing and able to use barrier contraception during therapy.

Route	Onset	Peak	Duration
P.O. (endo-metriosis)	Unknown	6-8 wk	60-90 days
P.O. (fibro-cyst.)	1 mo	2-6 mo	1 yr
P.O. (angio-edema)	Unknown	1-3 mo	Unknown

Adverse reactions
CNS: headache, tremor, emotional lability, irritability, nervousness, anxiety, depression, sleep disorders, epilepsy exacerbation, **benign intracranial hypertension**
CV: increased blood pressure, palpitations, tachycardia, **thrombotic events, myocardial infarction**
EENT: cataracts, blurred vision, **papilledema**
GI: nausea, vomiting, constipation, indigestion, gastroenteritis, anorexia, **pancreatitis**
GU: hematuria; amenorrhea; menstrual cycle disturbances (spotting, altered cycle); anovulation; vaginal dryness; changes in breast size; clitoral enlargement; testicular atrophy; abnormalities in semen volume, viscosity, mobility, and sperm count; decreased libido
Hematologic: reversible erythrocytosis, eosinophilia, leukocytosis, splenic peliosis, polycythemia, thrombocytosis, **leukopenia, thrombocytopenia**
Hepatic: elevated hepatic enzyme levels, cholestatic jaundice, **peliosis hepatitis, hepatic adenoma, malignant hepatic tumor**
Metabolic: increased insulin requirement (in diabetic patients)
Musculoskeletal: muscle cramps, spasms, pain, or fasciculations; joint pain and swelling; joint "lock-up"; pain in back, neck, or limbs; carpal tunnel syndrome
Respiratory: nasal congestion
Skin: acne, hirsutism, oily skin, rash, photosensitivity, yellowing of skin and sclera, pigmentation changes, seborrhea, sweating

Other: weight gain, edema, deepening of voice, **Stevens-Johnson syndrome**

Interactions
Drug-drug. *Carbamazepine:* increased carbamazepine blood level
Cyclosporine, tacrolimus: increased blood levels of these drugs, increased risk of nephrotoxicity
Insulin, oral hypoglycemics: increased blood glucose level and insulin resistance, necessitating adjustment of insulin and oral hypoglycemic dosages
Warfarin: prolonged prothrombin time
Drug-diagnostic tests. *Creatine phosphokinase, glucagon, glucose, hepatic enzymes, low-density lipoproteins, plasma proteins, sex hormone-binding globulins:* increased levels
Glucose tolerance, thyroid function: altered test results
High-density lipoproteins: decreased level

Precautions
Use cautiously in:
• coronary artery disease, conditions aggravated by edema
• hepatic disease
• children.

Patient monitoring
◀≋ Assess for early indications of benign intracranial hypertension, such as headache, nausea, vomiting, and visual disturbances. Screen for papilledema; if present, refer patient to neurologist immediately.
• Watch for hepatic problems; long-term use is linked to peliosis hepatitis and hepatic tumors, which may be silent until complicated by acute, life-threatening intra-abdominal hemorrhage.
• Monitor patient for thromboembolism and thrombophlebitis.
• Check hepatic and renal function test results regularly.

Patient teaching
• Advise female of childbearing age to use barrier contraception because drug causes fetal abnormalities.
• Inform female patient that drug frequently causes amenorrhea after 6 to 8 weeks of therapy.
• Instruct patient to notify prescriber if she notices masculinizing effects, such as facial hair or deepening of voice.
• Tell male patient that drug may cause sperm reduction during therapy.
• Teach patient to report signs and symptoms of fluid retention (swelling of ankles, feet, or hands; difficulty breathing; sudden weight gain), change in urine or stool color, or yellowing of eyes and skin.

d

dantrolene sodium
Dantrium, Dantrium Intravenous

Pharmacologic class: Hydantoin derivative
Therapeutic class: Skeletal muscle relaxant (direct-acting)
Pregnancy risk category C

Action
Relaxes skeletal muscle by affecting contractile response at a site beyond myoneural junction. Dissociates excitation-contraction coupling in skeletal muscle, probably by interfering with calcium release from sarcoplasmic reticulum.

Availability
Capsules: 25 mg, 50 mg, 100 mg
Powder for injection: 20 mg/vial

⟐ Indications and dosages
➤ Chronic spasticity resulting from upper motor neuron disorders, such as multiple sclerosis, cerebral palsy, or spinal cord injury

---

Adults: Initially, 25 mg P.O. daily, increased gradually in 25-mg increments, if needed, up to 100 mg two or three times daily, to a maximum dosage of 400 mg P.O. daily. Maintain dosage level for 4 to 7 days to gauge patient response.

Children: Initially, 0.5 mg/kg P.O. b.i.d., increased to 0.5 mg/kg P.O. three or four times daily. Then increase by 0.5 mg/kg P.O. daily, as needed, to 3 mg/kg two or three times daily. Maximum dosage is 100 mg q.i.d.

➤ Malignant hyperthermic crisis
Adults and children: Initially, 1 mg/kg by I.V. push, repeated as needed up to a cumulative dosage of 10 mg/kg/day

➤ To prevent or minimize malignant hyperthermia in patients who require surgery
Adults and children: 4 to 8 mg/kg P.O. daily in three or four divided doses for 1 to 2 days before surgery; give last dose 3 to 4 hours before surgery. Or 2.5 mg/kg I.V. infused over 1 hour before anesthetics are administered.

➤ To prevent recurrence of malignant hyperthermic crisis
Adults: 4 to 8 mg/kg daily P.O. in four divided doses for up to 3 days after initial hyperthermic crisis

Off-label uses
• Heat stroke
• Neuroleptic malignant syndrome

Contraindications
• Active hepatic disease (oral form)
• Patients who use spasticity to maintain posture or balance (oral form)
• Breastfeeding

Administration
• For I.V. use, add 60 ml of sterile water for injection to each vial; shake until solution is clear. Protect from direct light and use within 6 hours.
• Give therapeutic or emergency dose by rapid I.V. push; administer follow-up dose over 2 to 3 minutes.

• Prevent extravasation when giving I.V.; drug has high pH and causes tissue irritation.

Route	Onset	Peak	Duration
P.O.	Slow	Unknown	6-12 hr
I.V.	Rapid	Unknown	Unknown

Adverse reactions
CNS: dizziness, drowsiness, fatigue, malaise, weakness, confusion, depression, insomnia, nervousness, headache, light-headedness, speech disturbances, **seizures**
CV: tachycardia, blood pressure fluctuations, phlebitis, **heart failure**
EENT: double vision, excessive tearing
GI: nausea; vomiting; diarrhea; constipation; abdominal cramps; GI reflux, bleeding, and irritation; hematemesis; difficulty swallowing; altered taste; anorexia
GU: urinary frequency, painful or difficult urination, hematuria, crystalluria, urinary incontinence, nocturia, prostatitis
Hematologic: aplastic anemia, leukopenia, lymphocytic lymphoma, thrombocytopenia
Hepatic: hepatitis
Musculoskeletal: myalgia, backache
Respiratory: suffocating sensation, respiratory depression, **pleural effusion with pericarditis**
Skin: rash, urticaria, pruritus, eczema-like eruptions, sweating, photosensitivity, abnormal hair growth
Other: chills, fever, edema

Interactions
Drug-drug. *CNS depressants:* increased CNS depression
Estrogen: increased risk of hepatotoxicity
Verapamil (I.V.): cardiovascular collapse (when given with I.V. dantrolene)
Drug-diagnostic tests. *Alanine aminotransferase, alkaline phosphatase, aspar-*

tate aminotransferase, bilirubin, blood urea nitrogen: increased values
Drug-behaviors. *Alcohol use:* increased CNS depression
Sun exposure: phototoxicity

Precautions
Use cautiously in:
• cardiac, hepatic, renal, or respiratory dysfunction or impairment
• women (especially pregnant women)
• patients older than age 35
• children younger than age 5.

Patient monitoring
• Obtain baseline liver function test results; monitor periodically during therapy.
• With long-term oral therapy, monitor patient for signs and symptoms of hepatotoxicity; be prepared to discontinue drug if these occur.
• Assess for muscle weakness, poor coordination, and reduced reflexes before and during therapy; drug may weaken muscles and impair ambulation.

Patient teaching
◀€ Instruct patient on prolonged oral therapy to immediately report weakness, malaise, fatigue, nausea, rash, itching, severe diarrhea, bloody or black tarry stools, or yellowing of skin or eyes.
• Inform patient that drug may cause drowsiness, dizziness, or light-headedness.
• Teach patient to avoid driving and other hazardous activities until he knows how drug affects his concentration and alertness.

dapsone (DDS)
Avlosulfon✦, Dapsone

Pharmacologic class: Synthetic sulfone
Therapeutic class: Antileprotic, antimalarial
Pregnancy risk category C

d

Action
Unknown; bactericidal and bacteriostatic against *Mycobacterium leprae*. Action in dermatitis herpetiformis not established.

Availability
Tablets: 25 mg, 100 mg

⬤ Indications and dosages
➤ Leprosy
Adults: 100 mg/day P.O. (given with one or more antileprotics) for 6 to 12 months depending on disease course
Children ages 10 to 14 years: 50 mg daily for 6 to 12 months depending on disease course
Children under age 10: As appropriate
➤ Dermatitis herpetiformis
Adults: Initially, 50 mg/day P.O., increased as needed to a maximum dosage of 300 mg/day, then reduced to a minimum maintenance level as soon as possible
Dosage adjustment
• Children

Off-label uses
• Inflammatory bowel disorders
• Malaria prophylaxis
• *Pneumocystis jiroveci* (formerly *Pneumocystis carinii*) pneumonia
• Rheumatic and connective tissue disorders

Contraindications
• Hypersensitivity to drug or its derivatives

Administration
• Give with meals if GI upset occurs.

Route	Onset	Peak	Duration
P.O.	Unknown	4-8 hr	Unknown

Adverse reactions
CNS: headache, vertigo, insomnia, paresthesia, peripheral neuropathy, psychosis
CV: tachycardia
EENT: blurred vision, retinal and optic nerve damage, tinnitus
GI: nausea, vomiting, abdominal pain, anorexia, **pancreatitis**
GU: albuminuria, male infertility, **nephrotic syndrome, renal papillary necrosis**
Hematologic: elevated reticulocyte and methemoglobin values, **hemolytic anemia, agranulocytosis, aplastic anemia, hypoalbuminemia**
Respiratory: pulmonary eosinophilia
Skin: photosensitivity, exfoliative dermatitis, **lupus erythematosus**
Other: fever, hypersensitivity reaction, infectious mononucleosis–like syndrome, **sulfone syndrome**

Interactions
Drug-drug. *Activated charcoal:* decreased dapsone absorption
Didanosine: therapeutic failure of dapsone
Folic acid antagonists (such as methotrexate): increased risk of adverse reactions from dapsone
Para-aminobenzoic acid: antagonistic effect
Probenecid: reduced urinary excretion of dapsone metabolites
Rifampin: increased hepatic metabolism of dapsone, causing reduced blood level
Trimethoprim: increased blood levels of both drugs
Drug-diagnostic tests. *Albumin, granulocytes, hemoglobin:* decreased values
Methemoglobin, reticulocytes: increased values

Drug-behaviors. *Sun exposure:* photosensitivity

Precautions
Use cautiously in:
• renal or hepatic impairment, cardiopulmonary disease, refractory anemia, glucose-6-phosphate dehydrogenase deficiency
• pregnant or breastfeeding patients.

Patient monitoring
◀€ Monitor patient for sulfone syndrome, a potentially fatal reaction that causes fever, malaise, jaundice with hepatic necrosis, exfoliative dermatitis, lymphadenopathy, methemoglobinemia, and hemolytic anemia.
• Evaluate complete blood count weekly for first month of therapy, monthly for next 6 months, and then every 6 months. Discontinue drug if tests show decreased white blood cell or platelet count or reduction in hematopoiesis.
• Monitor liver function test results.

Patient teaching
◀€ Instruct patient to immediately report persistent sore throat, fever, chills, malaise, fatigue, swollen lymph nodes, yellowing of skin or eyes, or easy bruising or bleeding.
• Caution patient to avoid driving and other hazardous activities until he knows whether drug affects vision or balance.
• Tell patient that drug is intended for long-term use.
• Teach patient to minimize GI upset by eating small, frequent servings of healthy food and drinking plenty of fluids.

darbepoetin alfa
Aranesp

Pharmacologic class: Recombinant human erythropoietin
Therapeutic class: Hematopoietic
Pregnancy risk category C

Action
Stimulates erythropoiesis in bone marrow, increasing red blood cell production

Availability
Albumin solution for injection: 25 mcg/ml, 40 mcg/ml, 60 mcg/ml, 100 mcg/ml, 200 mcg/ml, 300 mcg/ml, 500 mcg/ml
Polysorbate solution for injection: 25 mcg/ml, 40 mcg/ml, 60 mcg/ml, 100 mcg/ml, 200 mcg/ml

Indications and dosages
➤ Anemia caused by chronic renal failure
Adults: Initially, 0.45 mcg/kg I.V. or S.C. as a single dose once weekly. Titrate dosage to maintain target hemoglobin concentration no higher than 12 g/dl. Adjust dosage no more often than once monthly.
➤ Chemotherapy-induced anemia
Adults: 2.25 mcg/kg I.V. or S.C. q week. Titrate dosage to maintain target hemoglobin concentration no higher than 12 g/dl.
Dosage adjustment
• Conversion from epoetin therapy

Contraindications
• Hypersensitivity to drug
• Uncontrolled hypertension

Administration
• Give by S.C. or I.V. injection only.
• Don't dilute or give with other drug solutions.

◀€ Don't shake; vigorous shaking may denature drug, making it biologically inactive.
• Discard unused portion; drug contains no preservative.

Route	Onset	Peak	Duration
I.V., S.C.	2-6 wk	Unknown	Unknown

d

Adverse reactions
CNS: dizziness, headache, fatigue, weakness, **seizures,** transient ischemic attack, **cerebrovascular accident**
CV: hypertension, hypotension, chest pain, peripheral edema, **arrhythmias, heart failure, cardiac arrest, myocardial infarction, vascular access thrombosis**
GI: nausea, vomiting, diarrhea, constipation, abdominal pain
Metabolic: fluid overload
Musculoskeletal: myalgia; joint, back, and limb pain
Respiratory: cough, upper respiratory tract infection, dyspnea, bronchitis
Skin: pruritus
Other: fever, flulike symptoms, infection, pain at injection site

Interactions
None significant

Precautions
Use cautiously in:
• anemia, thalassemia, porphyria, seizures
• underlying hematologic disease, including hemolytic and sickle cell anemia
• pregnant or breastfeeding patients
• children.

Patient monitoring
• Assess hemoglobin concentration before starting therapy; monitor weekly during therapy.
• Observe closely for serious CNS and cardiovascular adverse reactions.
• Be aware that supplemental iron is recommended for patients with serum

ferritin level below 100 mcg/ml or serum transferrin saturation less than 20%.

Patient teaching

• Teach patient to report chest pain or other pain, muscle tremors, weakness, and cough or other respiratory symptoms.

• If patient will self-administer drug, tell him to follow exact directions for injection and needle disposal.

• Instruct patient to avoid driving and other hazardous activities until he knows how drug affects concentration and alertness.

• Teach patient to minimize GI upset by eating small, frequent servings of healthy food and drinking plenty of fluids.

• Tell patient he'll undergo frequent blood testing during therapy to determine correct dosage.

daunorubicin citrate liposome
DaunoXome

Pharmacologic class: Anthracycline glycoside

Therapeutic class: Anti-infective antineoplastic

Pregnancy risk category D

Action

Exerts antineoplastic activity by inhibiting DNA synthesis and DNA-dependent RNA synthesis through intercalation. Formulation increases selectivity of daunorubicin for solid tumors; may increase permeability of tumor neovasculature to some particles in drug's size range.

Availability

Injection: 2 mg/ml

Indications and dosages

➤ First-line cytotoxic therapy for advanced Kaposi's sarcoma associated with human immunodeficiency virus (HIV)

Adults: 40 mg/m² I.V. over 1 hour. Repeat q 2 weeks until evidence of disease progression or other complications occur.

Dosage adjustment
• Renal impairment
• Hepatic impairment

Contraindications

• Hypersensitivity to drug

Administration

• Follow facility policy for preparing and handling antineoplastics.

• Dilute 1:1 with 5% dextrose injection.

• Don't use in-line filter for I.V. infusion.

• If prescribed, premedicate with allopurinol to help prevent hyperuricemia.

• Take steps to prevent extravasation.

• Protect solution from light.

Route	Onset	Peak	Duration
I.V.	Unknown	Unknown	Unknown

Adverse reactions

CNS: headache, fatigue, malaise, confusion, depression, dizziness, drowsiness, emotional lability, anxiety, hallucinations, syncope, tremors, rigors, insomnia, neuropathy, amnesia, hyperactivity, abnormal thinking, meningitis, **seizures**

CV: hypertension, chest pain, palpitations

EENT: abnormal vision, conjunctivitis, eye pain, deafness, earache, tinnitus, rhinitis, sinusitis, dental caries

GI: nausea, vomiting, diarrhea, constipation, abdominal pain, dyspepsia, gastritis, enlarged spleen, melena, fecal incontinence, hemorrhoids, tenesmus, difficulty swallowing, bleeding gums, dry mouth, mouth inflammation, altered taste, **GI hemorrhage**

GU: dysuria, nocturia, polyuria

Hematologic: thrombocytopenia, neutropenia

Hepatic: hepatomegaly

Metabolic: hyperuricemia, dehydration

Musculoskeletal: joint pain, myalgia, muscle rigidity, back pain, abnormal gait

Respiratory: dyspnea, cough, hemoptysis, increased sputum, **pulmonary infiltrations**

Skin: pruritus, dry skin, seborrhea, folliculitis, alopecia, sweating

Other: lymphadenopathy, opportunistic infections, fever, hot flashes, hiccups, thirst, infusion site inflammation, edema, allergic reactions

Interactions

Drug-diagnostic tests. *Granulocytes:* decreased count
Uric acid: increased level

Precautions

Use cautiously in:

• renal or hepatic impairment, bone marrow depression, cardiac disease, gout, infections

• pregnant or breastfeeding patients.

Patient monitoring

• Assess cardiac, renal, and hepatic function before each course of treatment.

• Evaluate complete blood count and white cell differential before each dose; withhold dose if granulocyte count is below 750 cells/mm³.

• Monitor serum uric acid level.

Patient teaching

◀€ Instruct patient to immediately report swelling, pain, burning, or redness at infusion site as well as persistent nausea, vomiting, diarrhea, chest pain, arm or leg swelling, difficulty breath-

ing, palpitations, rapid heartbeat, yellowing of skin or eyes, abdominal pain, or bloody stools.

• Inform patient that drug will make him more susceptible to infection; advise him to avoid crowds and exposure to illness.

• Teach patient to minimize GI upset by eating small, frequent servings of healthy foods, drinking plenty of fluids, and chewing gum.

daunorubicin hydrochloride
Cerubidine

Pharmacologic class: Anthracycline glycoside

Therapeutic class: Anti-infective antineoplastic

Pregnancy risk category D

Action

Antimitotic and cytotoxic. Forms complexes with DNA by intercalation between base pairs. Inhibits topoisomerase II activity by stabilizing topoisomerase II complex; causes breaks in single- and double-stranded DNA. May also inhibit polymerase activity, influence regulation of gene expression, and cause free radical damage to DNA.

Availability

Injection: 5 mg/ml
Lyophilized powder for injection: 21.4 mg, 53.5 mg

⒜ Indications and dosages

➤ Acute nonlymphocytic leukemia

Adults over age 60: 30 mg/m² /day I.V. on days1, 2, and 3 of first course and on days 1 and 2 of subsequent courses, given with cytarabine I.V. infusion (7 days for first course, 5 days for subsequent courses)

Adults younger than age 60: 45 mg/m²/day I.V. on days 1, 2, and 3 of first course and on days 1 and 2 of subsequent courses, given with cytarabine I.V. infusion (7 days for first course, 5 days for subsequent courses)

➤ Acute lymphocytic leukemia

Adults: 45 mg/m²/day I.V. on days 1, 2, and 3; vincristine I.V. on days 1, 8, and 15; prednisone P.O. on days 1 through 22, then tapered between days 22 and 29; then asparaginase I.V. on days 22 to 32

Children ages 2 and older: 25 mg/m²/day I.V. on first day every week; may be given in combination with vincristine I.V. on first day every week and prednisone P.O. daily

Dosage adjustment
• Renal impairment
• Hepatic impairment

Contraindications
• Hypersensitivity to drug

Administration
• Follow facility policy for preparing and handling antineoplastics.
• If prescribed, premedicate with allopurinol to help prevent hyperuricemia.
◀≶ Give by I.V. route only.
• Reconstitute vial contents with 4 ml of sterile water for injection to produce 5 mg/ml solution.
• Don't mix with other drugs or heparin.
• Withdraw desired dosage into syringe containing 10 to 15 ml of normal saline solution; then inject into tubing or sidearm of compatible, rapidly flowing I.V. solution
◀≶ Take care to prevent extravasation; drug causes severe local tissue necrosis. If extravasation occurs, stop infusion immediately; following facility policy, intervene to avoid severe tissue necrol-

ysis, severe cellulitis, thrombophlebitis, and painful induration.

Route	Onset	Peak	Duration
I.V.	Unknown	Unknown	Unknown

Adverse reactions
CV: cardiotoxicity
GI: acute nausea, vomiting, GI mucosal inflammation
GU: urine discoloration
Hematologic: bone marrow depression
Metabolic: hyperuricemia
Skin: rash, contact dermatitis, urticaria, reversible alopecia

Interactions
Drug-drug. *Other antineoplastic, hepatotoxic, and myelosuppressive drugs:* increased risk of toxicity
Drug diagnostic tests. *Granulocytes:* decreased count
Uric acid: increased level

Precautions
Use cautiously in:
• renal or hepatic impairment, bone marrow depression, cardiac disease, gout, infections
• elderly patients
• pregnant or breastfeeding patients.

Patient monitoring
◀≶ Observe I.V. site closely for extravasation.
• Monitor cardiac, renal, and hepatic function before each course of treatment.
• Evaluate complete blood count and white cell differential before each dose; withhold dose if granulocyte count is below 750 cells/mm³.
• Monitor serum uric acid level.

Patient teaching
◀≶ Instruct patient to immediately report swelling, pain, burning, or redness at infusion site, as well as persistent nausea, vomiting, diarrhea, bloody

stools, abdominal or chest pain, swollen arm or leg, difficulty breathing, palpitations, rapid heartbeat, or yellowing of skin or eyes.
• Inform patient that drug makes him more susceptible to infection; tell him to avoid crowds and exposure to illness.
• Teach patient to minimize GI upset by eating small, frequent servings of healthy food, drinking plenty of fluids, and chewing gum.
• Tell patient that drug may redden his urine.
• As appropriate, review all other significant and life-threatening adverse reactions and interactions, especially those related to drugs and tests mentioned above.

delavirdine mesylate
Rescriptor

Pharmacologic class: Nonnucleoside reverse transcriptase inhibitor
Therapeutic class: Antiretroviral
Pregnancy risk category C

Action
Binds to reverse transcriptase enzyme, blocking RNA-dependent and DNA-dependent DNA polymerase synthesis

Availability
Tablets: 100 mg, 200 mg

Indications and dosages
➤ Human immunodeficiency virus (HIV)–1 infection
Adults: 400 mg P.O. t.i.d., given with at least two other antiretrovirals

Contraindications
• Hypersensitivity to drug
• Concurrent use of terfenadine, ergot derivatives, pimozide, alprazolam, midazolam, or triazolam

Administration
• If patient can't swallow tablets, dissolve 100-mg tablets in water by adding four tablets to at least 3 oz of water; let stand for a few minutes and then stir until completely dissolved. Have patient swallow entire mixture immediately; add small amount of water to glass and then have him swallow this mixture as well to ensure that he consumes entire dose.
• Give 200-mg tablets intact; don't dissolve in water.
• If patient has achlorhydria, give drug with acidic beverage, such as orange juice.

Route	Onset	Peak	Duration
P.O.	Unknown	1 hr	Unknown

Adverse reactions
CNS: confusion, disorientation, dizziness, drowsiness, agitation, amnesia, changes in dreams, hallucinations, hyperesthesia, poor concentration, mania, nervousness, restlessness, paranoia, paresthesia, tremor, migraine, neuropathy, paralysis, **seizures**
CV: abnormal heart rate and rhythm, peripheral vascular disorder, peripheral edema, hypertension, orthostatic hypotension, cardiac insufficiency, cardiomyopathy
EENT: blurred or double vision, nystagmus, conjunctivitis, dry eyes, ear pain, otitis media, tinnitus, epistaxis, rhinitis, tooth abscess, toothache, gingivitis, gum hemorrhage, increased saliva
GI: nausea, diarrhea, constipation, abdominal pain or cramps, dyspepsia, enteritis, abdominal distention, bloody stools, colitis, diverticulitis, gastroenteritis, gastroesophageal reflux, mouth and tongue irritation and ulcers, difficulty swallowing, **GI bleeding, pancreatitis**
GU: renal calculi, kidney pain, chromaturia, hematuria, nocturia, polyuria, proteinuria, urinary tract infection, gy-

d

necomastia, impotence, epididymitis, hemospermia, testicular pain, vaginal candidiasis, amenorrhea, irregular uterine bleeding

Hematologic: purpura, spleen disorders, increased prothrombin time, eosinophilia, **granulocytosis, disseminated intravascular coagulation, leukopenia, neutropenia, pancytopenia, hemolytic anemia**

Hepatic: bilirubinemia, elevated alanine aminotransferase (ALT) and aspartate aminotransferase (AST) levels, **hepatotoxicity, hepatic failure, hepatomegaly**

Metabolic: hyperkalemia; hypomagnesemia; hyperglycemia; hypoglycemia; acidosis; hypertriglyceridemia; hyperuricemia; hypocalcemia; hyponatremia; elevated lipase, gamma glutamyl transpeptidase, alkaline phosphatase, and creatinine levels

Musculoskeletal: joint pain, arthritis, bone disorders, myalgia, muscle cramps, muscle weakness, bone pain, bone disorders, tendon disorders, tenosynovitis, rhabdomyolysis, neck pain and rigidity, limb pain, tetany

Respiratory: lung congestion, dyspnea, pneumonia

Skin: pallor, bruising, yellowing of skin and sclera, angioedema, dermal leukocytoblastic vasculitis, dermatitis, skin dryness and discoloration, erythema, folliculitis, herpes zoster or herpes simplex infection, petechiae, petechial rash, pruritic rash, seborrhea, alopecia, skin nodules, urticaria. sebaceous cyst, epidermal cyst, erythema multiforme

Others: weight gain or loss, fever, lymphadenopathy, adenopathy, increased thirst, hiccups, facial edema, bacterial infection, pain, abscess, *Mycobacterium tuberculosis* infection, body fat redistribution, hypersensitivity reaction, **sepsis, Stevens-Johnson syndrome**

Interactions

Drug-drug. *Antacids, histamine₂-receptor antagonists:* reduced delavirdine absorption

Bepridil, clarithromycin, estrogen, hormonal contraceptives, indinavir, lopinavir-ritonavir, saquinavir, sildenafil, warfarin: increased blood levels of these drugs

Carbamazepine, phenobarbital, phenytoin, rifabutin, rifampin: loss of virologic response, resistance to delavirdine

Dexamethasone: decreased delavirdine blood level

Didanosine: decreased blood levels of both drugs

Drug-diagnostic tests. *ALT, AST, bilirubin, partial thromboplastin time:* increased values

Granulocytes, hemoglobin, neutrophils, platelets, red blood cells, white blood cells: decreased values

Drug-herb. *St. John's wort:* loss of virologic response or resistance to delavirdine

Precautions

Use cautiously in:
• hepatic impairment
• pregnant or breastfeeding patients.

Patient monitoring

• Monitor liver function test results frequently when giving drug concurrently with saquinavir.
• Check electrolyte and uric acid levels regularly.
• Monitor patient for serious hepatic, cardiovascular, and CNS problems and hypersensitivity reactions.

Patient teaching

• Tell patient he can take drug with or without food.
• If patient can't swallow tablets, teach him how to dissolve 100-mg tablets in water.
◀╟ Tell patient to discontinue drug and consult prescriber immediately if he develops severe rash accompanied

by fever, blistering, oral lesions, conjunctivitis, swelling, or muscle aches.
• Inform patient that drug doesn't cure HIV or reduce its transmission.
• Inform patient that rash is a major adverse effect, usually occurring 1 to 3 weeks after therapy starts and resolving in 3 to 14 days.

demeclocycline hydrochloride
Declomycin

Pharmacologic class: Tetracycline
Therapeutic class: Antibiotic
Pregnancy risk category D

Action
Binds with bacterial cell and inhibits reproduction and protein synthesis

Availability
Tablets: 150 mg, 300 mg

Indications and dosages
➤ Infections caused by rickettsiae, *Mycoplasma pneumoniae, Borrelia recurrentis, Haemophilus ducreyi, Yersinia pestis, Francisella tularensis, Bartonella bacilliformis, Bacteroides* species, *Vibrio cholerae, Campylobacter fetus, Brucella* species, *Escherichia coli, Enterobacter aerogenes, Shigella* species, *Acinetobacter, Haemophilus influenzae, Klebsiella* species, *Streptococcus pneumoniae, Staphylococcus aureus;* organisms causing psittacosis, ornithosis, lymphogranuloma venereum, and granuloma inguinale. When penicillin is contraindicated, infections caused by *Neisseria gonorrhoeae, Treponema pallidum, Treponema pertenue, Listeria monocytogenes, Clostridium* species; *Bacillus anthracis, Fusobacterium fusiforme, Actinomyces israelii, Neisseria meningitides.* Also, adjunct to amebicides in

acute intestinal amebiasis, treatment of severe acne and nongonococcal urethritis, and trachoma and inclusion conjunctivitis caused by *Chlamydia trachomatis.*
Adults: 150 mg P.O. q.i.d. or 300 mg P.O. b.i.d. For gonococcal infections, initially 600 mg P.O., followed by 300 mg q 12 hours for 4 days, to a maximum dosage of 3 g.
Children older than age 8: 3 to 6 mg/ lb/day (6 to 12 mg/kg/day) P.O. in two to four divided doses

Off-label uses
• Syndrome of inappropriate antidiuretic hormone secretion (limited use)

Contraindications
• Hypersensitivity to tetracyclines
• Children younger than age 8

Administration
• Give with full glass of water 1 hour before or 2 hours after meals.
• If patient is receiving antacids, give at least 2 hours after demeclocycline.

Route	Onset	Peak	Duration
P.O.	Variable	3-4 hr	18-20 hr

Adverse reactions
CNS: dizziness, light-headedness, headache, vertigo, pseudotumor cerebri
EENT: blurred vision, tinnitus, discolored and poorly calcified permanent teeth (when used during dental development period in children), discolored and poorly calcified primary teeth of fetus (when used by pregnant patient)
GI: nausea, vomiting, diarrhea, tongue inflammation, difficulty swallowing, anorexia, enterocolitis, **pancreatitis, esophageal ulcers**
GU: nephrogenic diabetes insipidus, increased blood urea nitrogen, **acute renal failure**
Hematologic: leukocytosis, eosinophilia, **hemolytic anemia, thrombocyto-**

---

penia, **neutropenia, leukopenia**
Hepatic: increased hepatic enzyme levels, **liver failure, hepatitis**
Skin: phototoxicity, rash, urticaria, changes in skin and mucous membrane pigmentation, exfoliative dermatitis, erythema multiforme
Other: superinfection, **Stevens-Johnson syndrome**

Interactions

Drug-drug. *Aluminum, antacids, calcium, iron preparations, magnesium:* decreased demeclocycline absorption
Hormonal contraceptives: decreased contraceptive efficacy
Methoxyflurane: increased risk of nephrotoxicity
Penicillin: decreased demeclocycline activity
Drug-food. *Any food (especially dairy products):* decreased drug absorption

Precautions

Use cautiously in:
• marked renal impairment
• significant exposure to sun or ultraviolet light
• pregnant patients.

Patient monitoring

• Monitor patient for serious GI, hepatic, and skin reactions.
• Monitor hepatic enzyme levels, complete blood count, and white cell differential.

Patient teaching

• Tell patient to take drug on empty stomach with a full glass of water at least 1 hour before or 2 hours after meals.
• Advise patient to avoid dairy products, laxatives, and iron preparations.
• Instruct patient to report unusual bleeding or bruising.
• Instruct patient to avoid driving and other hazardous activities until he knows if drug causes dizziness.

• Teach patient to minimize GI upset by eating small, frequent servings of healthy food and drinking plenty of fluids.

denileukin diftitox
Ontak

Pharmacologic class: Biological response modifier
Therapeutic class: Antineoplastic
Pregnancy risk category C

Action

Recombinant DNA-derived cytotoxic protein; interacts with interleukin-2 (IL-2) receptors on cell surface and inhibits cellular protein synthesis, causing cell death

Availability

Frozen solution for injection: 150 mcg/ml

⏴ Indications and dosages

➢ Persistent or recurrent cutaneous T-cell lymphoma that expresses CD25 component of IL-2 receptor
Adults: 9 or 18 mcg/kg/day I.V. infused over 15 minutes for 5 consecutive days q 21 days

Contraindications

• Hypersensitivity to drug, its components, diphtheria toxin, or IL-2

Administration

◀⟨ Administer by I.V. infusion only; don't give by I.V. bolus.
• Infuse over at least 15 minutes.
• During infusion, observe closely for signs and symptoms of hypersensitivity reaction.
• Gently swirl vial to mix, but avoid vigorous agitation.
• Don't mix with other drugs.
• Don't deliver through in-line filter.

Route	Onset	Peak	Duration
I.V.	Variable	Variable	Variable

Adverse reactions

CNS: dizziness, paresthesia, nervousness, confusion, insomnia, syncope, headache

CV: vascular leak syndrome (with extravasation), hypotension, hypertension, vasodilation, tachycardia, chest pain, **thrombosis, arrhythmias**

EENT: rhinitis, pharyngitis, laryngeal spasm

GI: nausea, vomiting, diarrhea, constipation, flatulence, dyspepsia, difficulty swallowing, anorexia

GU: hematuria, albuminuria, pyuria, urine creatinine elevation

Hematologic: anemia, **thrombocytopenia, leukopenia**

Musculoskeletal: myalgia, back or joint pain

Metabolic: hypoalbuminemia, hypocalcemia, hypokalemia, dehydration

Respiratory: dyspnea, cough, lung disorder

Skin: rash, pruritus, sweating

Other: weight loss, edema, flulike symptoms, injection site reaction, **hypersensitivity reactions** including **anaphylaxis**

Interactions

Drug-drug. *Live-virus vaccines:* decreased antibody reaction

Drug-diagnostic tests. *Albumin, calcium, potassium:* decreased levels

Precautions

Use cautiously in:
• cardiovascular disease
• elderly patients
• pregnant and breastfeeding patients
• children (safety and efficacy not established).

Patient monitoring

• Monitor patient closely during first infusion and for 24 hours afterward.

• Evaluate patient for vascular leak syndrome (marked by at least two of the following: edema, hypotension, hypoalbuminemia).

• Monitor complete blood count, blood chemistry panel, renal and hepatic function, and albumin level. Repeat all tests weekly during therapy.

Patient teaching

◀€ Instruct patient to immediately report chest pain; difficulty breathing; chills; throat tightness, redness, swelling, or pain; or burning at infusion site.

• Instruct patient to avoid driving and other hazardous activities until he knows how drug affects concentration and alertness.

• Inform patient that drug makes him more susceptible to infection; advise him to avoid crowds and exposure to illness.

desipramine hydrochloride
Norpramin

Pharmacologic class: Tricyclic antidepressant

Therapeutic class: Antidepressant

Pregnancy risk category NR

Action

Inhibits reuptake of norepinephrine or serotonin at presynaptic neuron

Availability

Tablets: 10 mg, 25 mg, 50 mg, 75 mg, 100 mg, 150 mg

🖋 Indications and dosages

➤ Depression

Adults: Initially, 100 to 200 mg/day P.O; increase gradually if needed to a maximum dosage of 300 mg/day.

Adolescents and elderly adults: 25 to 100 mg/day P.O. as a single dose or in divided doses; increase gradually if needed to a maximum dosage of 150 mg/day.

Off-label uses
- Arthritic pain
- Cancer pain
- Diabetic neuropathy
- Peripheral neuropathy
- Tic douloureux

Contraindications
- Hypersensitivity to drug
- Recovery phase of myocardial infarction (MI)
- Monoamine oxidase (MAO) inhibitor use within past 14 days

Administration
- Before giving, measure sitting and supine blood pressure to assess for orthostasis.
- Discontinue drug 2 days before surgery.
- Give full dose at bedtime to avoid daytime drowsiness.

Route	Onset	Peak	Duration
P.O.	Unknown	4-6 hr	Unknown

Adverse reactions
CNS: sedation, weakness, anxiety, restlessness, insomnia, delusions, confusion, agitation, hallucinations, disorientation, extrapyramidal reactions, electroencephalogram changes, **neuroleptic malignant syndrome, seizures**
CV: hypotension, hypertension, tachycardia, palpitations, **arrhythmias, MI, heart block**
EENT: blurred vision, dry eyes, laryngitis
GI: nausea, vomiting, constipation, abdominal cramps, epigastric distress, difficulty swallowing, parotid gland swelling, peculiar taste, mouth inflammation, dry mouth, black tongue
GU: urinary retention, delayed voiding, urinary tract dilation, testicular swelling, impotence, male sexual dysfunction, gynecomastia, menstrual irregularities, galactorrhea, increased or decreased libido
Hematologic: purpura, eosinophilia, **bone marrow depression, agranulocytosis, thrombocytopenia**
Metabolic: blood glucose elevation, syndrome of inappropriate antidiuretic hormone secretion
Musculoskeletal: muscle weakness
Skin: dry skin, photosensitivity, rash, pruritus, petechiae, flushing, sweating
Other: weight gain, edema, hypothermia, flushing, withdrawal symptoms on abrupt cessation (dizziness, nausea, vomiting, headache, malaise, sleep disturbances, hyperthermia, irritability, worsening of depression), **sudden death (in children)**

Interactions
Drug-drug. *Adrenergics, anticholinergics:* additive adrenergic or anticholinergic effects
Cimetidine, phenothiazines, quinidine, selective serotonin reuptake inhibitors: increased desipramine effects, possible toxicity
Clonidine: hypertensive crisis
CNS depressants (antihistamines, opioid analgesics, sedative-hypnotics): additive CNS depression
MAO inhibitors: hyperpyretic crisis, severe seizures, death
Sparfloxacin: increased risk of adverse cardiovascular reactions
Drug-diagnostic tests. *Glucose:* increased or decreased level
Drug-food. *Grapefruit juice:* increased drug blood level and effects
Drug-herb. *Chamomile, hops, kava, skullcap, valerian:* increased CNS depression
S-adenosylmethionine (SAM-e), St. John's wort: adverse serotonergic effects, including serotonin syndrome
Drug-behaviors. *Alcohol use:* increased response to alcohol
Smoking: increased metabolism and decreased efficacy of desipramine

Precautions

Use cautiously in:

- cardiovascular disorders, glaucoma, thyroid disorders
- urinary retention
- children younger than age 12.

Patient monitoring

- Assess for suicidal tendencies before starting therapy.
- Monitor blood glucose level, complete blood count, and white cell differential during therapy.
- Watch for severe CNS, cardiovascular, and hematologic adverse reactions.

Patient teaching

- Tell patient to take full dose at bedtime to avoid daytime drowsiness.
- Inform patient that desired therapeutic effect may take 2 to 3 weeks.
- Caution patient that drug may cause physical or psychological dependence.
- Instruct patient to avoid driving and other hazardous activities until he knows how drug affects alertness, vision, and coordination.

desloratadine
Clarinex, Clarinex Reditabs

Pharmacologic class: Peripherally selective piperidine, selective histamine$_1$-receptor antagonist
Therapeutic class: Antihistamine (nonsedating, second generation)
Pregnancy risk category C

Action

Suppresses the release of histamine at peripheral histamine$_1$-receptor sites

Availability

Tablets: 5 mg

Indications and dosages

➤ Seasonal and perennial allergic rhinitis; chronic idiopathic urticaria and allergies caused by indoor and outdoor allergens

Adults and children ages 12 and older: 5 mg/day P.O.

Dosage adjustment
- Hepatic impairment
- Renal impairment

Contraindications

- Hypersensitivity to drug, its components, or loratadine

Administration

- Give with or without food.

Route	Onset	Peak	Duration
P.O.	1 hr	3 hr	24 hr

Adverse reactions

CNS: dizziness, drowsiness, fatigue, headache
CV: tachycardia, palpitations
EENT: pharyngitis, dry throat
GI: nausea, dyspepsia, dry mouth
GU: dysmenorrhea
Hepatic: elevated hepatic enzyme and bilirubin levels
Musculoskeletal: myalgia
Other: flulike symptoms, hypersensitivity reaction

Interactions

Drug-diagnostic tests. *Bilirubin, hepatic enzymes:* increased values
Skin tests: interference with positive reaction to dermal reactivity indicators

Precautions

Use cautiously in:
- renal or hepatic impairment
- elderly patients
- pregnant or breastfeeding patients
- children younger than age 12 (safety and efficacy not established).

Patient monitoring
• Monitor hepatic and renal function test results.

Patient teaching
• Tell patient he may take drug with or without food.
• Teach patient to report rapid heartbeat, shortness of breath, rash, persistent flulike symptoms, or muscle ache.
• Caution patient to avoid driving and other hazardous activities until he knows how drug affects concentration and alertness.

desmopressin acetate
(1-deamino-8-D-arginine vasopressin)
DDAVP, Desmospray, Minirin, Stimate

Pharmacologic class: Posterior pituitary hormone

Therapeutic class: Antidiuretic hormone

Pregnancy risk category B

Action
Enhances water reabsorption by increasing permeability of renal collecting ducts to adenosine monophosphate and water, thereby reducing urinary output. Also increases factor VIII (antihemophilic factor) activity.

Availability
Injection: 4 mcg/ml in single-dose 1-ml ampules and multidose 10-ml vials
Intranasal solution: 0.1 mg/ml, 1.5 mg/ml
Tablets: 0.1 mg, 0.2 mg

🖊 Indications and dosages
➤ Diabetes insipidus
Adults and children older than age 12: 0.05 mg P.O. b.i.d; adjust dosage based on patient response. Or 0.1 to 0.4 ml (10 to 40 mcg) daily intranasally as a single dose or in two or three divided doses. Or 0.5 ml (2 mcg) to 1 ml (4 mcg) daily I.V. or S.C., usually in two divided doses.
Children ages 3 months to 12 years: 0.05 to 0.3 ml/day intranasally in one or two divided doses
➤ Hemophilia A, von Willebrand's disease
Adults and children: 0.3 mcg/kg I.V. infused over 15 to 30 minutes; may repeat dose if needed. Or 300 mcg intranasally of solution containing 1.5 mcg/ml; for patients weighing less than 50 kg (110 lb), total dosage of 150 mcg (one spray of solution containing 1.5 mg/ml into a single nostril) is usually sufficient. If needed to maintain hemostasis during surgery, give intranasal dose 2 hours before surgery or give I.V. dose 30 minutes before surgery.
➤ Primary nocturnal enuresis
Children ages 6 and older: Initially, 20 mcg intranasally at bedtime; maximum dosage is 40 mcg/day.

Off-label uses
• Chronic autonomic failure (such as nocturnal polyuria, overnight weight loss, morning orthostatic hypotension)

Contraindications
• Hypersensitivity to drug
• Hemophilia A with factor VIII levels less than or equal to 5%
• Von Willebrand's disease
• Impaired level of consciousness (intranasal form)

Administration
• Adjust morning and evening dosages as appropriate to minimize frequent urination and risk of water intoxication.
🔊 When giving to child with diabetes insipidus, carefully restrict fluid intake to prevent hyponatremia and water intoxication.

Route	Onset	Peak	Duration
P.O.	1 hr	1-5 hr	8-12 hr
I.V.	15-30 min	Unknown	4-12 hr
Intranasal	1 hr	1-1.5 hr	8-12 hr

Adverse reactions
CNS: headache, dizziness, insomnia
CV: slight blood pressure increase, chest pain, palpitations
EENT: rhinitis, epistaxis, sore throat
GI: nausea, abdominal pain
GU: vulvar pain
Respiratory: cough
Other: local erythema, flushing, swelling or burning after injection

Interactions
Drug-drug. *Carbamazepine, chlorpropamide, pressor drugs:* potentiation of desmopressin effects

Precautions
Use cautiously in:
• coronary artery disease, hypertensive cardiovascular disease, fluid and electrolyte imbalances
• breastfeeding patients.

Patient monitoring
• Monitor urine volume and specific gravity, plasma and urine osmolality, and electrolyte levels in patients with diabetes insipidus.
• Monitor factor VIII antigen levels, activated partial thromboplastin time, and bleeding time in patients with hemophilia.
◀◁ When giving to child with diabetes insipidus, carefully monitor fluid intake and output.

Patient teaching
• Instruct patient to take drug exactly as prescribed and not to interchange strengths or delivery systems.
• Teach patient how to use prescribed delivery system if taking drug by other than oral route.

• Instruct patient with diabetes insipidus to avoid overhydration and to weigh himself daily. Tell him to report weight gain or swelling of arms or legs. If he's using nasal spray, teach him to inspect nasal membranes regularly and to report increased nasal congestion or swelling.
• Caution elderly patients not to increase fluid intake beyond that sufficient to satisfy thirst.
• As appropriate, review all significant adverse reactions and interactions, especially those related to drugs mentioned above.

d

dexamethasone
Alti-Dexamethasone✦, Decadron, Dexameth, Dexamethosone Intensol, Dexone, Hexadrol

dexamethasone acetate
Cortastat LA, Dalalone D.P.

dexamethasone sodium phosphate
Cortastat, Dalalone, Decadron Phosphate

Pharmacologic class: Glucocorticoid
Therapeutic class: Anti-inflammatory
Pregnancy risk category C

Action
Unclear; reduces inflammation by suppressing migration of polymorphonuclear leukocytes, reversing increased capillary permeability, and stabilizing leukocyte lysosomal membranes. Also suppresses immune response, stimulates bone marrow, and influences protein, fat, and carbohydrate metabolism.

Availability

Elixir: 0.5 mg/5 ml
Oral solution: 0.5 mg/5 ml, 1 mg/ml
Solution for injection (sodium phosphate): 4 mg/ml, 10 mg/ml, 20 mg/ml, 24 mg/ml
Suspension for injection (acetate): 8 mg/ml, 16 mg/ml
Tablets: 0.25 mg, 0.5 mg, 0.75 mg, 1 mg, 1.5 mg, 2 mg, 4 mg, 6 mg

⃠ Indications and dosages

➤ Allergic and inflammatory conditions

Adults: 0.75 to 9 mg/day (dexamethasone) P.O. as a single dose or in divided doses; in severe cases, much higher dosages may be needed. Or 8 to 16 mg (acetate) I.M. q 1 to 3 weeks. Dosage requirements vary and must be individualized based on disease and patient response.

➤ Cerebral edema

Adults: Initially, 10 mg (sodium phosphate) I.V., followed by 4 mg I.M. q 6 hours. Then reduce dosage gradually over 5 to 7 days.

➤ Suppression test for Cushing's syndrome

Adults: 1 mg P.O. at 11 P.M. or 0.5 mg P.O. q 6 hours for 48 hours (with urine collection testing, as ordered)

Off-label uses

• Acute altitude sickness
• Bacterial meningitis
• Bronchopulmonary dysplasia in preterm infants
• Hirsutism
• Suppression test (for detection, diagnosis, or management of depression)

Contraindications

• Hypersensitivity to drug, alcohol, bisulfites, EDTA, creatinine, polysorbate 80, or methylparaben
• Systemic fungal infections

Administration

• Give P.O. dose with food or milk.

• When giving I.M., inject deep into gluteal muscle and rotate sites as needed.

Route	Onset	Peak	Duration
P.O.	Unknown	1-2 hr	2.75 days
I.V.	1 hr	1 hr	Variable
I.M. (acetate)	Unknown	8 hr	6 days
I.M. (sodium phosphate)	1 hr	1 hr	6 days

Adverse reactions

CNS: headache, malaise, vertigo, psychiatric disturbances, **increased intracranial pressure, seizures**

CV: hypotension, thrombophlebitis, **myocardial rupture after recent myocardial infarction, thromboembolism**

EENT: cataracts

GI: nausea, vomiting, abdominal distention, dry mouth, anorexia, **peptic ulcer, bowel perforation, pancreatitis, ulcerative esophagitis**

Metabolic: adrenal insufficiency, hyperglycemia, cushingoid appearance (moon face, buffalo hump), decreased growth (in children), latent diabetes mellitus, reduced carbohydrate tolerance, sodium and fluid retention, hypokalemic alkalosis, negative nitrogen balance, **adrenal suppression**

Musculoskeletal: muscle wasting, muscle pain, osteoporosis, aseptic joint necrosis, tendon rupture, long bone fractures

Skin: diaphoresis, angioedema, erythema, rash, pruritus, urticaria, contact dermatitis, acne, decreased wound healing, bruising, skin fragility, petechiae

Other: facial edema, weight gain or loss, increased susceptibility to infection, hypersensitivity reactions

Interactions

Drug-drug. *Barbiturates, phenytoin, rifampin:* decreased dexamethasone effect

Digoxin: increased risk of digoxin toxicity

Ephedrine: increased dexamethasone clearance

Estrogen, hormonal contraceptives: blocking of dexamethasone metabolism

Fluoroquinolones: increased risk of tendon rupture

Itraconazole, ketoconazole: increased dexamethasone blood level and effects

Live-virus vaccines: decreased antibody response to vaccine, increased risk of adverse reactions

Loop and thiazide diuretics: additive hypokalemia

Somatrem, somatropin: decreased response to these drugs

Drug-diagnostic tests. *Calcium, potassium:* decreased levels

Cholesterol, glucose: increased levels

Nitroblue-tetrazolium test: false-negative results

Drug-herb. *Echinacea:* increased immune-stimulating effect

Ginseng: potentiation of immune-modulating response

Drug-behaviors. *Alcohol use:* increased risk of gastric irritation and GI ulcers

Precautions

Use cautiously in:
• renal insufficiency, cirrhosis, diabetes mellitus, diverticulitis, GI disease, cardiovascular disease, hypoprothrombinemia, hypothyroidism, myasthenia gravis, glaucoma, osteoporosis, infections, underlying immunosuppression, psychotic tendencies
• pregnant or breastfeeding patients
• children.

Patient monitoring

• Monitor blood glucose level closely in diabetic patients receiving drug orally.

• Monitor hemoglobin and potassium levels.

• Assess for occult blood loss.

◀€ With long-term therapy, never discontinue abruptly; taper dosage gradually.

Patient teaching

◀€ Instruct patient to immediately report sudden weight gain, swelling of face or limbs, excessive nervousness or sleep disturbances, excessive body hair growth, vision changes, difficulty breathing, muscle weakness, stool color changes, or persistent abdominal pain.

• Teach patient to take oral medication with or after meals.

• Tell patient to report vision changes.

• Inform patient that drug makes him more susceptible to infection; advise him to avoid crowds and exposure to illness.

◀€ Instruct patient not to stop drug abruptly.

dexmedetomidine hydrochloride
Precedex

Pharmacologic class: Alpha$_2$-adrenoceptor agonist

Therapeutic class: Nonbarbiturate sedative-hypnotic

Pregnancy risk category C

Action

Produces sedation through alpha$_1$ and alpha$_2$ stimulation

Availability

Injection: 100 mcg/ml

⚕ Indications and dosages

➢ Sedation of intubated and mechanically ventilated patients

Adults: 1 mcg/kg I.V. as a loading dose given over 10 minutes, then 0.2 to 0.7 mcg/kg/hour. Don't infuse longer than 24 hours.
Dosage adjustment
• Hepatic or renal impairment
• Elderly patients

Contraindications
• Hypersensitivity to drug
• Complete heart block

Administration
◄€ Use controlled infusion device; calculate infusion rate according to patient's weight and desired sedation level.
• To prepare infusion, add 2 ml of drug to 48 ml of normal saline solution, for a total volume of 50 ml.
• Don't infuse through same I.V. line with plasma or blood.
• Administer only in continually monitored setting.

Route	Onset	Peak	Duration
I.V.	Unknown	Unknown	Unknown

Adverse reactions
CV: bradycardia, hypotension, hypertension, **atrial fibrillation, myocardial infarction**
GI: nausea
GU: oliguria
Hematologic: leukocytosis, anemia
Respiratory: hypoxia, **pulmonary edema, pleural effusion**
Other: thirst

Interactions
Drug-drug. *Antipsychotics, inhalation anesthetics, opioids, sedative-hypnotics, skeletal muscle relaxants:* increased CNS depression
Drug-behaviors. *Alcohol use:* increased CNS depression

Precautions
Use cautiously in:
• renal or hepatic impairment, respiratory depression, arrhythmias
• elderly patients
• pregnant or breastfeeding patients
• children.

Patient monitoring
• Assess renal and hepatic function before starting therapy.
• Monitor for hypertension when giving loading dose.
• Monitor cardiovascular status continuously.
• Evaluate infusion site for burning and irritation.

Patient teaching
• Advise patient not to get up or walk without assistance while sedated.
• Tell patient he'll be closely supervised during period of sedation and on arousal.

dexmethylphenidate hydrochloride
Focalin

Pharmacologic class: Methylphenidate derivative
Therapeutic class: CNS stimulant
Controlled substance schedule II
Pregnancy risk category C

Action
Thought to block norepinephrine and dopamine reuptake, increasing the concentration of these neurotransmitters in the extraneuronal space

Availability
Tablets: 2.5 mg, 5 mg, 10 mg

Indications and dosages

> Attention deficit hyperactivity disorder

Adults and children over age 6: In patients not receiving methylphenidate concurrently, 2.5 mg P.O. b.i.d. at least 4 hours apart without regard to meals; increase as needed in 2.5- to 5-mg increments to a maximum of 10 mg b.i.d. (Individualize dosage according to patient needs and response.) In patients receiving methylphenidate concurrently, start with half of methylphenidate dosage; maximum dosage is 10 mg P.O. b.i.d.

Contraindications

- Hypersensitivity to drug
- Glaucoma
- Anxiety
- Family history or diagnosis of Tourette syndrome
- Monoamine oxidase (MAO) inhibitor use within 14 days
- Children younger than age 6

Administration

- Administer at same time each day.
- Don't give within 14 days of MAO inhibitor therapy.

Route	Onset	Peak	Duration
P.O.	Variable	1-1.5 hr	Unknown

Adverse reactions

CNS: nervousness, insomnia, dizziness, headache, dyskinesia, chorea, drowsiness, Tourette syndrome, toxic psychosis

CV: increased or decreased pulse rate and blood pressure, tachycardia, angina, palpitations, arrhythmias

EENT: blurred vision, visual accommodation problems

GI: nausea, abdominal pain

Hematologic: anemia, **leukopenia, thrombocytopenia**

Hepatic: abnormal hepatic function, **hepatic coma**

Skin: rash, alopecia

Other: fever, decreased appetite, weight loss, psychological drug dependence, drug tolerance

Interactions

Drug-drug. *Anticoagulants, phenobarbital, phenytoin, primidone, selective serotonin reuptake inhibitors, tricyclic antidepressants:* inhibited metabolism and additive effects of these drugs

Antihypertensives, pressor agents (dopamine, epinephrine): decreased efficacy of these drugs

MAO inhibitors: severe hypertensive crisis

Precautions

Use cautiously in:
- hypertension, depression, seizures, cardiovascular disorders, psychosis, drug abuse
- pregnant or breastfeeding patients
- children under age 6 (safety and efficacy not established).

Patient monitoring

◀€ Monitor blood pressure closely, especially in patients receiving antihypertensives concurrently.
- Evaluate cardiac status; report palpitations and other signs and symptoms of arrhythmias.
- During prolonged therapy, regularly monitor complete blood count with white cell differential and platelet count.

Patient teaching

- Advise patient or parents that drug should be taken at same time each day.
- Tell patient or parents that drug usually is discontinued if symptoms don't improve within 1 month.
- Instruct parents to monitor child's height and weight; drug may suppress growth.

dextran, high-molecular-weight (dextran 70, dextran 75)

Gendex 75, Gentran 70, Gentran 75, Macrodex

dextran, low-molecular-weight (dextran 40)

Gentran 40, Rheomacrodex

Pharmacologic class: Polysaccharide

Therapeutic class: Plasma volume expander

Pregnancy risk category C

Action

Expands plasma volume through colloidal osmotic effects during hypovolemic shock; pulls fluid from interstitial space, moving it into intravascular space

Availability

Injection: 6% dextran 70 in dextrose 5% in water (D_5W) or normal saline solution; 6% dextran 75 in D_5W or normal saline solution; 10% dextran 40 in D_5W or normal saline solution

Indications and dosages

➣ Plasma volume expansion

Adults: Dosage and infusion rate based on amount of fluid lost and hemoconcentration. Usual initial dosage of dextran 70 or 75 is 500 ml of 6% solution I.V., not to exceed 20 ml/kg during first 24 hours. Usual initial dosage of dextran 40 is 500 ml of 10% solution I.V., not to exceed 20 ml/kg during first 24 hours; beyond 24 hours, total daily dosage not to exceed 10 ml/kg and therapy not to exceed 5 days.

Children: Dosage based on weight or body surface area, not to exceed 20 ml/kg I.V. daily.

Contraindications

• Hypersensitivity to drug
• Pulmonary edema, cardiac decompensation, and severe heart failure
• Thrombocytopenia
• Renal disease with severe oliguria or anuria
• Hypovolemic conditions

Administration

• Give by I.V. infusion only.
• In normovolemic patients, infuse no faster than 4 ml/minute.

Route	Onset	Peak	Duration
I.V.	Immediate	Immediate	Unknown

Adverse reactions

CV: thrombophlebitis, hypotension, **cardiac arrest**

GI: nausea, vomiting

GU: increased urine viscosity, **osmotic nephrosis, renal failure**

Hematologic: decreased hematocrit, reduced platelet function, **prolonged bleeding time, decreased coagulation times**

Hepatic: elevated alanine aminotransferase (ALT) and aspartate aminotransferase (AST) levels

Metabolic: hyponatremia

Respiratory: wheezing, dyspnea, **bronchospasm, pulmonary edema**

Skin: urticaria, rash, flushing, pruritus, angioedema

Other: chills, infection at injection site, **anaphylaxis**

Interactions

Drug-drug. *Abciximab, aspirin, heparin, thrombolytics, warfarin:* increased bleeding

Drug-diagnostic tests. *ALT, AST:* increased levels

Bilirubin, glucose, hematocrit, hemoglobin, total protein, urine protein: falsely increased levels

Bleeding time: prolonged

Blood typing and cross-matching, Rh typing: test interference

Precautions
Use cautiously in:
• active hemorrhage, diabetes mellitus, chronic liver disease, abdominal conditions
• pregnant or breastfeeding patients.

Patient monitoring
◀≣ Observe patient closely for signs and symptoms of anaphylaxis during first 30 minutes of infusion.
• Know that bleeding time may be prolonged temporarily in patients receiving more than 1,000 ml of drug.
• Monitor amount and pattern of fluid intake and output.
• Assess patient's vital signs frequently. Suspect circulatory overload if patient has increased heart and respiratory rates, shortness of breath, and wheezing.
• Evaluate for dehydration after infusion.

Patient teaching
• Instruct patient to immediately report signs of bleeding, such as easy bruising, blood in urine, or dark tarry stools.

dextroamphetamine sulfate
Dexedrine, Dexedrine Spansule, DextroStat

Pharmacologic class: Amphetamine
Therapeutic class: Sympathomimetic amine, CNS stimulant
Controlled substance schedule II
Pregnancy risk category C

Action
Produces CNS and respiratory stimulation by promoting release of norepinephrine from nerve terminals

Availability
Capsules (sustained-release): 5 mg, 10 mg, 15 mg
Tablets: 5 mg, 10 mg

⚕ Indications and dosages
➤ Attention-deficit hyperactivity disorder
Adults: 5 to 60 mg P.O. daily in divided doses
Children ages 6 and older: 5 mg P.O. once or twice daily, increased by 5 mg at weekly intervals
Children ages 3 to 5: 2.5 mg P.O. daily, increased by 2.5 mg at weekly intervals
➤ Narcolepsy
Adults: 5 to 60 mg P.O. daily as a single dose or in divided doses
Children ages 12 and older: 10 mg P.O. daily, increased by 10 mg at weekly intervals until desired response occurs or adult dosage is reached
Children ages 6 to 11: 5 mg P.O. daily, increased by 5 mg at weekly intervals until desired response occurs or adult dosage is reached

Contraindications
• Hypersensitivity to drug or tartrazine
• Glaucoma
• Psychotic disorders
• Pregnancy or breastfeeding

Administration
• Ensure that patient swallows the sustained-release capsule whole and that he does not chew or crush it.
• Give last daily dose at least 6 hours before patient's bedtime.

Route	Onset	Peak	Duration
P.O.	1-2 hr	Unknown	2-10 hr
P.O. (sustained)	Unknown	Unknown	Up to 24 hr

Adverse reactions

CNS: hyperactivity, insomnia, restlessness, tremor, depression, dizziness, headache, irritability
CV: palpitations, tachycardia, hypertension, hypotension, **arrhythmias**
GI: nausea, vomiting, constipation, diarrhea, abdominal cramps, dry mouth, metallic taste
GU: impotence, increased libido
Skin: urticaria
Other: decreased appetite, physical or psychological drug dependence

Interactions

Drug-drug. *Acetazolamide, sodium bicarbonate:* urine alkalinization, which increases dextroamphetamine effects
Adrenergic blockers: additive effects
Ammonium chloride, ascorbic acid (large doses): urine acidification, which decreases dextroamphetamine effects
Beta-adrenergic blockers, tricyclic antidepressants: increased risk of adverse cardiovascular effects
Guanethidine: reversal of hypotensive effect
Monoamine oxidase inhibitors: hypertensive crisis
Phenothiazines: decreased dextroamphetamine effects
Selective serotonin reuptake inhibitors: increased risk of serotonin syndrome
Drug-diagnostic tests. *Plasma corticosteroids:* increased levels
Drug-food. *Caffeine:* increased stimulant effect
Drug-herb. *Caffeine-containing herbs, ephedra:* increased stimulant effect

Precautions

Use cautiously in:
• cardiovascular disease, hypertension, diabetes mellitus
• history of substance abuse
• elderly patients.

Patient monitoring

• Interrupt therapy or reduce dosage periodically to assess drug efficacy in patients with behavior disorders.
• Monitor blood and urine glucose levels carefully in diabetic patients; drug may alter regular insulin requirements.

Patient teaching

• Tell patient to swallow sustained-release capsules whole with liquid and not to chew or crush them.
• Advise patient to take drug early in day to avoid insomnia.
• Instruct patient to avoid driving and other hazardous activities until he knows how drug affects him.
• Advise patient not to stop therapy abruptly but to taper dosage gradually.

dextromethorphan hydrobromide

Balminil DM♣, Benylin Adult Formula Cough Syrup, Benylin Pediatric, Broncho-Grippol-DM♣, Calmylin #1♣, Children's Hold, Creo-Terpin, Delsym, DexAlone, DM Syrup, Drixoral Cough and Congestion Liquid Caps, Hold, Koffex-DM♣, Mediquell, Neo-DM♣, Ornex DM, Pertussin Cough Suppressant, Pertussin CS, Pertussin ES, Robidex, Robitussin Cough Calmers, Robitussin Maximum Strength Cough Suppressant, Robitussin Pediatric Cough and Cold, Sedatuss♣, Sucrets Cough Control Formula, Vicks Pediatric Formula 44D

Pharmacologic class: Levorphanol derivative
Therapeutic class: Antitussive (nonnarcotic)
Pregnancy risk category C

Action

Depresses cough reflex through direct effect on cough center in medulla; although related to opioids structurally, lacks analgesic and addictive properties

Availability

Gelcaps: 30 mg
Liquid: 3.5 mg/5 ml, 7.5 mg/5 ml, 15 mg/5 ml
Lozenges: 5 mg, 7.5 mg
Oral suspension (extended-release): 30 mg/5 ml
Syrup: 7.5 mg/5 ml, 10 mg/15 ml

Indications and dosages

➤ Cough caused by minor viral upper respiratory tract infections or inhaled irritants
Adults and children over age 12: 10 to 20 mg P.O. q 4 hours, or 30 mg P.O. q 6 to 8 hours, or 60 mg of extended-release form P.O. b.i.d. (not to exceed 120 mg/day)
Children ages 6 to 12: 5 to 10 mg P.O. q 4 hours, or 15 mg P.O. q 6 to 8 hours, or 30 mg of extended-release form P.O. q 12 hours (not to exceed 60 mg/day)
Children ages 2 to 6: 2.5 to 5 mg P.O. q 4 hours, or 7.5 mg q 6 to 8 hours, or 15 mg of extended-release form P.O. q 12 hours (not to exceed 30 mg/day)
Dosage adjustment
• Elderly patients

Contraindications

• Hypersensitivity to drug
• Chronic productive cough
• Monoamine oxidase (MAO) inhibitor use within past 14 days

Administration

• Don't give lozenges to children younger than age 6.
• Make sure patient swallows extended-release tablet whole and doesn't crush or chew it.

Route	Onset	Peak	Duration
P.O.	15-30 min	Unknown	3-6 hr
P.O. (extended)	Unknown	Unknown	9-12 hr

Adverse reactions

CNS: dizziness and sedation
GI: nausea, vomiting, stomach pain

Interactions

Drug-drug. *Amiodarone, fluoxetine, quinidine:* increased dextromethorphan blood level, greater risk of adverse reactions
Antidepressants, antihistamines, opioids, sedative-hypnotics: additive CNS depression
MAO inhibitors, sibutramine: serotonin syndrome (nausea, confusion, blood pressure changes)
Drug-behaviors. *Alcohol use:* additive CNS depression

Precautions

Use cautiously in:
• diabetes mellitus (with sucrose-containing products)
• pregnant or breastfeeding patients
• children younger than age 2 (safety not established).

Patient monitoring

• Monitor cough frequency and type; assess sputum characteristics.
• Assess hydration status; increase patient's fluid input to help moisten secretions.

Patient teaching

• Teach patient to avoid irritants, such as smoking, dust, and fumes. Suggest use of humidifier to filter air pollutants.
• Inform patient that treatment aims to decrease coughing frequency and intensity without completely eliminating protective cough reflex.

• Instruct patient to contact health care provider if cough lasts more than 7 days.

---

dextrose (d-glucose)
B-D Glucose, Glutose, Insta-Glucose

Pharmacologic class: Monosaccharide
Therapeutic class: Carbohydrate caloric nutritional supplement
Pregnancy risk category C

Action
Prevents protein and nitrogen loss; promotes glycogen deposition and the accumulation of ketones (acts as osmotic diuretic)

Availability
Injection: 2.5%, 5%, 10%, 20%, 25%, 30%, 40%, 50%, 60%, 70%
Oral gel: 40%
Tablets (chewable): 5 g

🖊 Indications and dosages
➤ Insulin-dependent hypoglycemia
Adults and children: Initially, 10 to 20 g P.O., repeated in 10 to 20 minutes if needed based on blood glucose level; or 20 to 50 ml by I.V. infusion or injection of 50% solution given at 3 ml/minute. Maintenance dosage is 10% to 15% solution given by continuous I.V. infusion until blood glucose level reaches therapeutic range.
Infants and neonates: 2 ml/kg of 10% to 25% solution given by slow I.V. infusion until blood glucose level reaches therapeutic range
➤ Calorie replacement
Adults and children: 2.5%, 5%, or 10% solution given through peripheral I.V. line, with dosage tailored to patient's need for fluid or calories; or 10% to 70% solution given through large central vein, if needed (typically mixed with amino acids or other solution)

Off-label uses
• Varicose veins
• Insulin-secreting islet-cell adenoma

Contraindications
• Hypersensitivity to drug
• Hyperglycemia and diabetic coma
• Hemorrhage
• Heart failure

Administration
• Use aseptic technique when preparing solution; bacteria thrive in high-glucose environments.
◀€ Infuse concentrations above 10% through central vein.
• Don't infuse concentrated solution rapidly because doing so may cause hyperglycemia and fluid shifts.
◀€ Never stop infusion abruptly.

Route	Onset	Peak	Duration
P.O.	10-20 min	40 min	Unknown
I.V.	2-3 min	Unknown	Unknown

Adverse reactions
CNS: confusion, loss of consciousness
CV: phlebitis, hypertension, **venous thrombosis, heart failure**
GU: glycosuria, osmotic diuresis
Metabolic: hyperglycemia, hypervolemia, hypovolemia, electrolyte imbalances, **hyperosmolar coma**
Respiratory: pulmonary edema
Skin: flushing, urticaria
Other: chills, fever, dehydration, injection site reaction, infection

Interactions
Drug-drug. *Corticosteroids, corticotropin:* increased risk of fluid and electrolyte imbalances
Drug-diagnostic tests. *Glucose:* increased level

Precautions

Use cautiously in:
• renal, cardiac, or hepatic impairment; diabetes mellitus.

Patient monitoring

◀€ Monitor infusion site frequently to prevent irritation, tissue sloughing, necrosis, and phlebitis.
• Check blood glucose level at regular intervals.
• Monitor fluid intake and output.
• Weigh patient regularly.
• Assess patient for confusion.

Patient teaching

• Teach patient to recognize signs and symptoms of hypoglycemia and hyperglycemia.
• Provide instructions on glucose self-monitoring.

diazepam

Apo-Diazepam✦, Diastat, Diazemuls✦, Diazepam Intensol, Dizac, Novo-Dipam✦, PMS-Diazepam✦, Valium, Vivol✦

Pharmacologic class: Benzodiazepine
Therapeutic class: Anxiolytic, anticonvulsant, sedative-hypnotic, skeletal muscle relaxant (centrally acting)
Controlled substance schedule IV
Pregnancy risk category D

Action

Produces anxiolytic effect and CNS depression by stimulating gamma-aminobutyric acid (GABA) receptors; relaxes skeletal muscles of the spine by inhibiting polysynaptic afferent pathways; controls seizures by enhancing presynaptic inhibition

Availability

Capsules (extended-release): 15 mg
Injection: 5 mg/ml
Oral solution: 5 mg/ml, 5 mg/5 ml
Rectal gel delivery system: 2.5 mg, 10 mg, 15 mg, 20 mg
Sterile emulsion for injection: 5 mg/ml
Tablets: 2 mg, 5 mg, 10 mg

🕗 Indications and dosages

➤ Anxiety
Adults: 2 to 10 mg P.O. two to four times daily
Children age 6 months and older: 1 to 2.5 mg P.O. three to four times daily; may be increased gradually as needed
➤ Before cardioversion
Adults: 5 to 15 mg I.V. 5 to 10 minutes before cardioversion
➤ Before endoscopy
Adults: 2.5 to 20 mg I.V. or 5 to 10 mg I.M. 30 minutes before endoscopy
➤ Status epilepticus, seizure activity
Adults and children age 12 and older: 5 to 10 mg I.V., repeated as necessary q 10 to 15 minutes to a maximum dosage of 30 mg; may repeat regimen if needed in 2 to 4 hours. Or 0.2 mg/kg P.R.; may repeat 4 to 12 hours later.
Children ages 6 to 11: 0.3 mg/kg P.R.; may repeat 4 to 12 hours later
Children ages 3 to 5: 1 mg I.M. or I.V. q 2 to 5 minutes, to a maximum dosage of 10 mg; repeat q 2 to 4 hours.
Children ages 1 month to 3 years: 0.2 to 0.5 mg I.M. or I.V. q 2 to 5 minutes, to a maximum dosage of 5 mg
➤ Skeletal muscle relaxation
Adults: 2 to 10 mg P.O. three to four times daily or 15 to 30 mg P.O. extended-release once daily. Or 5 to 10 mg I.M. or I.V.; may repeat in 2 to 4 hours.
Elderly or debilitated patients: Initially, 2 to 2.5 mg P.O. once or twice daily or 2 to 5 mg I.M. or I.V.; may repeat in 2 to 4 hours.
Children: 1 to 2.5 mg P.O. three to four times daily

d

➤ Tetanus
Children age 5 and older: 5 to 10 mg
I.M. or I.V. q 3 to 4 hours
Children over 1 month to 5 years: 1 to
2 mg I.M. or I.V. q 3 to 4 hours
➤ Alcohol withdrawal
Adults: Initially, 10 mg P.O. three to
four times during first 24 hours, decreased to 5 mg P.O. three to four times
daily. Or initially, 10 mg I.M. or I.V.;
then 5 to 10 mg I.M. or I.V. in 3 to 4
hours, as needed.

Off-label uses

• Panic attacks
• Adjunct to general anesthesia

Contraindications

• Hypersensitivity to drug, other ben-
zodiazepines, alcohol, or tartrazine
• Coma or CNS depression
• Narrow-angle glaucoma
• Pregnancy or breastfeeding

Administration

◀€ Give I.V. infusion slowly into large
vein, taking at least 1 minute for each
5 mg for adults or 3 minutes for each
0.25 mg/kg for children.
• Know that I.V. route is preferred over
I.M. route because of slow or erratic
I.M. absorption.
• Don't mix with other drugs or solutions in syringe or container.
• Inject I.M. dose deeply and slowly
into large muscle mass.
• Ensure patient swallows extended-
release form whole without chewing or
crushing it.
• If desired, mix oral solution with liquid or soft food.

Route	Onset	Peak	Duration
P.O.	30-60 min	1-2 hr	Up to 24 hr
I.V.	1-5 min	15-30 min	15-60 min
I.M.	Within 20 min	0.5-1.5 hr	Unknown
P.R.	Unknown	1-2 hr	4-12 hr

Adverse reactions

CNS: dizziness, drowsiness, lethargy,
depression, light-headedness, disorientation, anger, manic or hypomanic
episodes, restlessness, paresthesia,
headache, slurred speech, dysarthria,
stupor, tremor, dystonia, vivid dreams,
extrapyramidal reactions, mild paradoxical excitation
CV: bradycardia, tachycardia, hypertension, hypotension, palpitations, **cardiovascular collapse**
EENT: blurred vision, diplopia, nystagmus, nasal congestion, difficulty swallowing
GI: nausea, vomiting, diarrhea, constipation, gastric disorders, increased salivation
GU: urinary retention or incontinence,
menstrual irregularities, gynecomastia,
libido changes
Hematologic: blood dyscrasias (including eosinophilia, **leukopenia,
agranulocytosis,** and **thrombocytopenia**)
Hepatic: elevated alanine aminotransferase (ALT), alkaline phosphatase
(ALP), aspartate aminotransferase
(AST), and lactate dehydrogenase levels; hepatic dysfunction
Musculoskeletal: muscle rigidity, muscular disturbances
Respiratory: respiratory depression
Skin: dermatitis, rash, pruritus, urticaria, diaphoresis
Other: weight gain or loss, decreased
appetite, edema, hiccups, fever, physical or psychological drug dependence
or tolerance

Interactions

Drug-diagnostic tests. *ALP, ALT, AST,
liver function tests:* increased values
Neutrophils: decreased count
Drug-drug. *Antidepressants, antihista-
mines, barbiturates, opioids:* additive
CNS depression
*Cimetidine, disulfiram, fluoxetine, hor-
monal contraceptives, isoniazid, keto-*

conazole, metoprolol, propoxyphene, propranolol, valproic acid: decreased metabolism and enhanced action of diazepam
Digoxin: increased digoxin blood level, possible toxicity
Levodopa: decreased levodopa efficacy
Rifampin: increased metabolism and decreased efficacy of diazepam
Theophylline: decreased sedative effects of diazepam
Drug-herb. *Chamomile, hops, kava, skullcap, valerian:* increased CNS depression
Drug-behaviors. *Alcohol use:* increased CNS depression

Precautions
Use cautiously in:
• hepatic dysfunction, severe renal impairment
• elderly patients
• children.

Patient monitoring
• Supervise ambulation, especially in elderly patients.
• Monitor complete blood count and kidney and liver function test results.
• Avoid sudden withdrawal. Taper dosage gradually to termination.

Patient teaching
• Instruct patient to avoid driving and other hazardous activities until he knows how drug affects concentration and alertness.
• Teach patient to move slowly when sitting up or standing to avoid dizziness or light-headedness. Advise him to dangle legs briefly before getting out of bed.

diazoxide
Hyperstat IV

Pharmacologic class: Vasodilator
Therapeutic class: Antihypertensive (nondiuretic), antihypoglycemic
Pregnancy risk category C

Action
Unclear; relaxes peripheral arterioles of smooth muscle cells and reduces peripheral vascular resistance as a result of vasodilation

Availability
Capsules: 50 mg
Injection: 15 mg/ml in 20-ml ampules

Indications and dosages
➤ Hypertensive crisis
Adults and children: 1 to 3 mg/kg I.V. bolus, to a maximum dosage of 150 mg q 5 to 15 minutes until adequate response occurs; repeat as needed every 4 hours or more
➤ Hypoglycemia secondary to hyperinsulinism
Adults and children: 3 to 8 mg/kg P.O. daily in two to three divided doses q 8 to 12 hours

Off-label uses
• Pregnancy-induced hypertension
• Obesity

Contraindications
• Hypersensitivity to drug, thiazides, or sulfonamides
• Compensatory hypertension
• Pheochromocytoma

Administration
• Keep patient recumbent during I.V. administration and for at least 30 minutes afterward.

• I.V. infusion can be given at a constant rate (7.5 to 30 mg/minute) until adequate response occurs.

Route	Onset	Peak	Duration
I.V.	1 min	2-5 min	2-12 hr

Adverse reactions

CNS: headache, light-headedness, dizziness, weakness, euphoria, **seizures, paralysis, cerebral ischemia**
CV: electrocardiogram (ECG) changes, orthostatic hypotension, angina pectoris, **myocardial ischemia, myocardial infarction, arrhythmias, shock, supraventricular tachycardia**
EENT: optic nerve damage
GI: nausea, vomiting, diarrhea, constipation, abdominal discomfort, dry mouth
GU: increased blood urea nitrogen, breast tenderness
Metabolic: hyperglycemia, hyperuricemia, fluid and electrolyte imbalances, sodium and water retention
Skin: inflammation and pain from extravasation, diaphoresis, flushing
Other: sensation of warmth

Interactions

Drug-drug. *Antihypertensives (such as beta-adrenergic blockers, hydralazine, methyldopa, minoxidil, nitrates, prazosin, reserpine):* additive hypotension
Hydantoins: decreased hydantoin level
Sulfonylureas: hyperglycemia
Thiazide diuretics: increased diazoxide effects
Drug-diagnostic tests. *Glucose, uric acid:* increased levels
Eosinophils, hematocrit, hemoglobin, platelets, white blood cells: decreased values

Precautions

Use cautiously in:
• fluid and electrolyte imbalances, impaired renal, hepatic, cerebral, or cardiac circulation

• pregnant or breastfeeding patients
• children.

Patient monitoring

• Measure blood pressure every 5 minutes for first 15 to 30 minutes of infusion or until patient is stabilized.
• Monitor ECG and pulse continuously during and after infusion; be aware that tachycardia may immediately follow I.V. infusion.
• Assess fluid status; promptly report intake and output changes. If fluid retention occurs, give diuretic, as prescribed.
• Inspect I.V. site regularly for infiltration or extravasation.
• Observe closely for signs and symptoms of heart failure.
• Monitor diabetic patient for loss of glycemic control.

Patient teaching

• Instruct patient to report chest pain, dizziness, and severe headache.
• Teach patient to weigh himself daily and report significant gains.

diclofenac potassium
Cataflam, Novo-Difenac-K✦, Novo-Difenac-SR✦

diclofenac sodium
Voltaren, Voltaren SR

Pharmacologic class: Cyclooxygenase inhibitor, nonsteroidal anti-inflammatory drug (NSAID)

Therapeutic class: Nonopioid analgesic, antiarthritic

Pregnancy risk category B (third trimester: *D*)

Action

Unknown; thought to block activity of cyclooxygenase, thereby inhibiting inflammatory responses of vasodilation and swelling and blocking transmission of painful stimuli

Availability
Tablets (delayed-release): 25 mg, 50 mg, 75 mg
Tablets (extended-release): 100 mg
Tablets (immediate-release): 50 mg, 75 mg

⚠ Indications and dosages
➤ Analgesia, dysmenorrhea
Adults: Initially, 100 mg P.O., then 50 mg t.i.d. as needed
➤ Rheumatoid arthritis
Adults: Initially, 50 mg P.O. three to four times daily; after initial response, reduce to lowest dosage that controls symptoms. Usual maintenance dosage is 25 mg t.i.d.
➤ Osteoarthritis
Adults: Initially, 50 mg P.O. two to three times daily; after initial response, reduce to lowest dosage that controls symptoms.
➤ Ankylosing spondylitis
Adults: 25 mg P.O. four to five times daily; after initial response, reduce to lowest dosage that controls symptoms.
Dosage adjustment
• Renal impairment
• Elderly patients

Off-label uses
• Post-radial keratotomy symptoms
• Dental pain

Contraindications
• Hypersensitivity to drug or its components, other NSAIDs, or aspirin
• Active GI bleeding or ulcer disease

Administration
• Make sure patient swallows extended-release or enteric-coated form whole without chewing or crushing it.
• Give on empty stomach 1 hour before or after a meal.

• If drug causes GI upset, give with milk or meals.

Route	Onset	Peak	Duration
P.O.	30 min	Unknown	8 hr

Adverse reactions
CNS: dizziness, drowsiness, headache
CV: hypertension
EENT: tinnitus
GI: diarrhea, abdominal pain, dyspepsia, heartburn, **GI bleeding**
GU: dysuria, frequent urination, hematuria, nephritis, proteinuria, **acute renal failure**
Hematologic: prolonged bleeding time
Hepatic: hepatotoxicity
Skin: eczema, photosensitivity, rash, contact dermatitis, dry skin, exfoliation
Other: allergic reactions (including edema), **anaphylaxis**

Interactions
Drug-drug. *Anticoagulants, antiplatelet agents, cephalosporins, plicamycin, thrombolytics:* increased risk of bleeding
Antihypertensives, diuretics: decreased efficacy of these drugs
Antineoplastics: increased risk of hematologic adverse reactions
Colchicine, corticosteroids, NSAIDs: additive adverse GI effects
Cyclosporine, probenecid: increased risk of diclofenac toxicity
Digoxin, lithium, methotrexate, phenytoin, theophylline: increased levels and greater risk of toxicity of these drugs
Potassium-sparing diuretics: increased risk of hyperkalemia
Drug-diagnostic tests. *Alanine aminotransferase, alkaline phosphatase, aspartate aminotransferase, blood urea nitrogen, creatinine, electrolytes, lactate dehydrogenase, urine uric acid:* increased values
Hematocrit, hemoglobin, platelets, serum uric acid, urine electrolytes, white blood cells: decreased values

---

Drug-herb. *Anise, arnica, chamomile, clove, dong quai, fenugreek, feverfew, garlic, ginger, ginkgo, ginseng, and others:* increased risk of bleeding

Drug-behaviors. *Alcohol use:* increased risk of adverse GI effects

Precautions

Use cautiously in:
• severe cardiovascular, renal, or hepatic disease
• bleeding tendency
• history of porphyria or ulcer disease
• concurrent anticoagulant use
• elderly patients
• pregnant or breastfeeding patients
• children.

Patient monitoring

• Monitor hepatic and renal function.
• Observe for and report signs and symptoms of bleeding.
• Assess for hypertension.
• Monitor sodium and potassium levels in patients receiving potassium-sparing diuretics.
• Weigh patient to detect fluid retention; report gain of more than 2 lb in 24 hours.

Patient teaching

• Instruct patient to take drug on empty stomach 1 hour before or after a meal.
• Advise patient not to lie down for 15 to 30 minutes after taking drug to minimize esophageal irritation.
• Instruct patient to stop taking drug and contact prescriber if he experiences ringing or buzzing in ears, dizziness, GI discomfort, or bleeding.
• Caution patient not to take over-the-counter analgesics during diclofenac therapy.

dicloxacillin sodium

Dycill, Dynapen, Pathocil

Pharmacologic class: Penicillinase-resistant penicillin
Therapeutic class: Anti-infective
Pregnancy risk category B

Action

Inhibits cell wall synthesis during bacterial cell division and multiplication; resists penicillinase enzymes produced by bacteria

Availability

Capsules: 125 mg, 250 mg, 500 mg
Oral solution: 62.5 mg/5 ml

🖊 Indications and dosages

➣ Systemic infections caused by penicillinase-producing staphylococci
Adults and children weighing 40 kg (88 lb) or more: 125 to 250 mg P.O. q 6 hours; more severe infection may require higher dosage
Children weighing less than 40 kg (88 lb): 12.5 to 25 mg/kg P.O. daily in divided doses q 6 hours, depending on severity of infection

Contraindications

• Hypersensitivity to drug or other penicillins
• Allergy to cephalosporins

Administration

• Give on empty stomach at least 1 hour before or 2 hours after meals.
• Administer with water only; don't give with acidic juices or carbonated beverages, which may inactivate drug effects.

Route	Onset	Peak	Duration
P.O.	Unknown	2 hr	6 hr

Adverse reactions

CNS: lethargy, hallucinations, anxiety, confusion, agitation, depression, fatigue, dizziness, **seizures**

CV: vein irritation, thrombophlebitis, **heart failure**

GI: nausea, vomiting, diarrhea, bloody diarrhea, abdominal pain, gastritis, enterocolitis, oral and rectal candidiasis, stomatitis, glossitis, sore mouth, **pseudomembranous colitis**

GU: nephropathy, vaginitis, **interstitial nephritis**

Hematologic: eosinophilia, anemia, neutropenia, hemolytic anemia, **agranulocytosis, leukopenia, thrombocytopenic purpura, thrombocytopenia**

Hepatic: hepatitis

Respiratory: wheezing

Skin: rash, urticaria

Other: overgrowth of nonsusceptible organisms, superinfection, fever, hypersensitivity reactions, serum sickness, **anaphylaxis**

Interactions

Drug-drug. *Aminoglycosides:* decreased levels

Chloramphenicol, tetracycline: decreased efficacy of both drugs

Hormonal contraceptives: decreased contraceptive efficacy

Drug-diagnostic tests. *Conjugated estrone or estriol-glucuronide (in pregnant women), estradiol, granulocytes, hemoglobin, platelets, total conjugated estriol, white blood cells:* decreased levels

Coombs' test, urine glucose: false-positive results

Eosinophils: increased count

Drug-food. *Any food:* interference with absorption and efficacy of drug

Carbonated beverages, juices: drug inactivation

Precautions

Use cautiously in:
• severe renal insufficiency, infectious mononucleosis
• pregnant or breastfeeding patients.

Patient monitoring

• In long-term therapy, monitor renal, hepatic, and hematopoietic functions and evaluate blood cultures weekly.

Patient teaching

• Advise patient to notify prescriber if nausea, diarrhea, or other GI adverse effects occur.

d

dicyclomine

Bentyl, Bentylol✤, Formulex✤, Spasmoban

Pharmacologic class: Anticholinergic
Therapeutic class: Antispasmodic
Pregnancy risk category B

Action

May exert a direct effect on GI smooth muscle by inhibiting acetylcholine at receptor sites, reducing GI tract motility and tone

Availability

Capsules: 10 mg, 20 mg
Solution for injection: 10 mg/ml
Syrup: 10 mg/5 ml
Tablets: 10 mg, 20 mg

Indications and dosages

➣ Irritable bowel syndrome in patients unresponsive to usual interventions

Adults: 20 mg P.O. or I.M. q.i.d.; may increase up to 160 mg/day

Contraindications

• Hypersensitivity to drug
• GI or genitourinary tract obstruction
• Severe ulcerative colitis
• Unstable cardiovascular status
• Glaucoma
• Myasthenia gravis
• Breastfeeding
• Infants less than 6 months old

✤ Canada   ◀€ Clinical alert   Reactions in **bold** are life-threatening

Administration

• Give 30 to 60 minutes before meals; give bedtime dose at least 2 hours after last meal.

◀╠ Don't give drug by I.V. route.

• Be aware that drug shouldn't be given I.M. for more than 2 days.

Route	Onset	Peak	Duration
P.O., I.M.	Unknown	Unknown	Unknown

Adverse reactions

CNS: confusion, drowsiness, light-headedness (with I.M. use), psychosis

CV: palpitations, tachycardia

EENT: blurred vision, increased intraocular pressure

GI: nausea, vomiting, constipation, heartburn, decreased salivation, dry mouth, **paralytic ileus**

GU: urinary hesitancy or retention, impotence, decreased lactation

Skin: decreased sweating

Other: pain and redness at I.M. site, allergic reactions including **anaphylaxis**

Interactions

Drug-drug. *Adsorbent antidiarrheals, antacids:* decreased dicyclomine absorption

Cyclopropane anesthetics: increased risk of cardiovascular adverse reactions

Oral drugs: altered absorption of these drugs

Potassium (oral): increased GI mucosal lesions

Other anticholinergics (including antihistamines, disopyramide, quinidine): additive anticholinergic effects

Drug-diagnostic tests. *Gastric acid secretion test:* antagonism of pentagastrin and histamine (testing agents)

Precautions

Use cautiously in:

• hepatic or renal impairment, autonomic neuropathy, cardiovascular disease, prostatic hypertrophy

• elderly patients

• pregnant patients (safety not established).

Patient monitoring

• Be alert for an anaphylactic reaction.

• Monitor vital signs and fluid intake and output; ask patient about palpitations.

• Assess for confusion and light-headedness (after I.M. injection).

• Evaluate patient's vision, particularly for blurred vision and other signs and symptoms of increasing intraocular pressure.

• Assess bowel pattern, particularly for signs and symptoms of paralytic ileus.

Patient teaching

• Instruct patient to take drug 30 to 60 minutes before meals and to take bedtime dose at least 2 hours after last meal.

• Advise patient not to take antacids or adsorbent antidiarrheals within 2 hours of dicyclomine.

• Urge patient to promptly report abdominal pain, decreased urinary output, or absence of bowel movements.

• Instruct patient to avoid driving or other hazardous activities until he knows how drug affects concentration, vision, and alertness.

• Teach patient to minimize GI upset by eating small, frequent servings of healthy food and drinking plenty of fluids.

didanosine
(ddI, 2,3-dideoxyinosine)
Videx, Videx EC

Pharmacologic class: Nucleoside reverse transcriptase inhibitor

Therapeutic class: Antiretroviral, antiviral

Pregnancy risk category B

Action
Inhibits replication of human immunodeficiency virus (HIV) by preventing replication of DNA polymerase, an enzyme crucial to DNA and RNA formation

Availability
Capsules (delayed-release): 125 mg, 200 mg, 250 mg, 400 mg
Powder for oral solution (buffered): 100 mg/packet, 167 mg/packet, 250 mg/packet
Powder for oral solution (pediatric): 2 g in 4-oz glass bottle, 4 g in 8-oz glass bottle
Tablets (buffered, chewable): 25 mg, 50 mg, 100 mg, 150 mg, 200 mg

💊 Indications and dosages
➤ HIV infection (given with other antiretrovirals)
Adults weighing 60 kg (132 lb) or more: 200 mg P.O. (tablets) q 12 hours, 400 mg P.O. (capsules) once daily, or 250 mg P.O. (buffered powder) q 12 hours
Adults weighing less than 60 kg (132 lb): 125 mg P.O. (tablets) q 12 hours, 250 mg P.O. (capsules) once daily; or 167 mg P.O. (buffered powder) q 12 hours
Children: 90 to 120 mg/m² P.O. q 12 hours
Dosage adjustment
• Renal impairment

Contraindications
• Hypersensitivity to drug

Administration
• Give on empty stomach 30 minutes before or 2 hours after a meal.
• Don't administer with fruit juice.
• Know that pharmacist must prepare pediatric powder for oral solution by diluting with water and antacid to a concentration of 10 mg/ml.

Route	Onset	Peak	Duration
P.O.	Unknown	0.5-1 hr	Unknown

Adverse reactions
CNS: dizziness, anxiety, abnormal thinking, hypoesthesia, agitation, confusion, hypertonia, asthenia, peripheral neuropathy, **seizures**, **coma**
CV: pseudoaneurysm, peripheral coldness, palpitations, incomplete atrioventricular (AV) block, nodal arrhythmias, thrombophlebitis, hypotension, bradycardia, weak pulse, **ventricular tachycardia**, **complete AV block**, **embolism**
EENT: diplopia, abnormal vision, ocular hypotony, iritis, retinal detachment
GI: nausea, vomiting, diarrhea, abdominal enlargement, dyspepsia, ileus, GI reflux, hematemesis, dysphagia, dry mouth, **pancreatitis**
GU: urinary retention, frequency, or incontinence; dysuria; renal dysfunction; cystalgia; prostatitis; **nephrotoxicity**
Hematologic: leukocytosis, anemia, **thrombocytopenia**, **bleeding**, **neutropenia**
Hepatic: **hepatomegaly with steatosis**
Metabolic: hyperkalemia, diabetes mellitus, **lactic acidosis**
Musculoskeletal: muscle contractions
Respiratory: pneumonia, crackles, bronchitis, pleurisy, rhonchi, dyspnea, wheezing, **pleural effusion**, **pulmonary edema**, **pulmonary embolism**, **bronchospasm**
Skin: diaphoresis, pallor, rash, urticaria, pruritus, bullous eruption, petechiae, cellulitis, abscess
Other: edema, development of human antichimeric antibodies

Interactions
Drug-drug. *Amprenavir, delavirdine, indinavir, ritonavir, saquinavir:* altered didanosine pharmacokinetics
Antacids, other drugs that increase gastric pH: increased risk of didanosine toxicity

---

Co-trimoxazole, pentamidine: increased risk of pancreatic toxicity
Dapsone, fluoroquinolones, ketoconazole: decreased blood levels of these drugs
Itraconazole: decreased itraconazole blood level
Drug-diagnostic tests. *Alanine aminotransferase, alkaline phosphatase, aspartate aminotransferase, bilirubin, uric acid:* increased levels
Granulocytes, hemoglobin, platelets, white blood cells: decreased values
Drug-food. *Any food:* decreased rate and extent of drug absorption

Precautions
Use cautiously in:
• renal or hepatic impairment, peripheral neuropathy, phenylketonuria, hyperuricemia
• elderly patients
• pregnant or breastfeeding patients
• children.

Patient monitoring
◀͟ Monitor for signs and symptoms of pancreatitis; report these to prescriber immediately.
• Assess carefully for signs and symptoms of lactic acidosis, such as dizziness, light-headedness, and bradycardia.
• Monitor for signs and symptoms of peripheral neuropathy.
• In patients with renal impairment, watch for drug toxicity and hypermagnesemia (suggested by muscle weakness and confusion).

Patient teaching
• Teach patient to take drug on empty stomach and to chew tablets without crushing or breaking them.
• Advise patient using buffered powder to mix with water, not juice, and to let powder dissolve for several minutes before taking.

◀͟ Instruct patient to immediately report abdominal pain, nausea, or vomiting.

diflunisal
Dolobid

Pharmacologic class: Nonsteroidal anti-inflammatory drug
Therapeutic class: Nonopioid analgesic, anti-inflammatory
Pregnancy risk category C

Action
Unknown; thought to act by inhibiting prostaglandin synthesis

Availability
Tablets: 250 mg, 500 mg

⏀ Indications and dosages
➤ Osteoarthritis, rheumatoid arthritis
Adults: 500 to 1,000 mg P.O. daily in two divided doses, usually q 12 hr, up to a maximum dosage of 1,500 mg/day
➤ Mild to moderate pain
Adults: 1 g P.O., followed by 500 mg q 8 to 12 hours; or 500 mg P.O., followed by 250 mg q 8 to 12 hours (depending on severity of pain and patient's age, weight, or response)
Dosage adjustment
• Elderly patients

Contraindications
• Hypersensitivity to drug
• Acute asthmatic attacks
• Bleeding disorders
• Vitamin K deficiency
• Children younger than age 12

Administration
• Give tablets whole with food or milk.

Route	Onset	Peak	Duration
P.O.	1 hr	2-3 hr	8-12 hr

Adverse reactions

CNS: dizziness, insomnia, drowsiness, headache, fatigue

EENT: tinnitus

GI: nausea, vomiting, diarrhea, constipation, flatulence, stomatitis

GU: renal impairment, hematuria, **interstitial nephritis**

Skin: rash, pruritus, sweating, erythema multiforme

Other: Stevens-Johnson syndrome

Interactions

Drug-drug. *Acetaminophen, hydrochlorothiazide, indomethacin:* increased levels of these drugs

Antacids, aspirin: decreased diflunisal blood level

Anticoagulants, thrombolytics: enhanced anticoagulant effect

Cyclosporine: increased risk of nephrotoxicity

Methotrexate: increased risk of methotrexate toxicity

Precautions

Use cautiously in:
• renal impairment, compromised cardiac function, hypertension, peptic ulcer
• elderly patients.

Patient monitoring

• Monitor fluid intake and output for signs of renal impairment; assess for dysuria and hematuria.

◀€ Watch for signs and symptoms of erythema multiforme (sore throat, fever, rash, cough, iris lesions, mouth sores); report early signs before condition can progress to Stevens-Johnson syndrome.

• Assess nutritional and hydration status.

• Monitor neurologic status.

Patient teaching

• Instruct patient to swallow tablets whole with food or milk.

• If patient needs antacids, advise him not to take them within 2 hours of diflusinal.

• Instruct patient to avoid driving and other hazardous activities until he knows how drug affects concentration, balance, hearing, and alertness.

• Teach patient to minimize GI upset by eating small, frequent servings of healthy food and ensuring adequate fluid intake.

◀€ Advise patient to promptly report rash or other signs of erythema multiforme.

d

digoxin
Digitek, Lanoxicaps, Lanoxin, Novo-Digoxin✦

Pharmacologic class: Cardiac glycoside
Therapeutic class: Inotropic, antiarrhythmic
Pregnancy risk category C

Action

Increases the force and velocity of myocardial contraction and prolongs the refractory period of atrioventricular (AV) node due to an increase in calcium entering myocardial cells; slows conduction through sinoatrial and AV nodes and produces antiarrhythmic effect.

Availability

Capsules: 0.05 mg, 0.1 mg, 0.2 mg
Elixir (pediatric): 0.05 mg/ml
Injection: 0.05 mg/ml, 0.1 mg/ml, 0.25 mg/ml
Tablets: 0.125 mg, 0.25 mg, 0.5 mg

🖊 Indications and dosages

➢ Heart failure, tachyarrhythmias, atrial fibrillation and flutter, paroxysmal atrial tachycardia

---

Adults: For rapid digitalizing, 0.6 to 1 mg I.V. over 24 hours, with 50% of total dosage given initially and additional fractions given at 4- to 8-hour intervals; or digitalizing dose of 0.75 to 1.25 mg P.O. over 24 hours, with 50% of total dosage given initially and additional fractions given at 4- to 8-hour intervals. Maintenance dosage is 0.063 to 0.5 mg/day (tablets) or 0.35 to 0.5 mg/day (gelatin capsules), depending on lean body weight, renal function, and drug blood level.

Children older than age 10: For rapid digitalizing, 8 to 12 mcg/kg I.V. over 24 hours, with 50% of total dosage given initially and additional fractions given at 4- to 8-hour intervals; or digitalizing dose of 10 to 15 mcg/kg P.O. over 24 hours, with 50% of total dosage given initially and additional fractions given at 6- to 8-hour intervals. Maintenance dosage is 25% to 35% of loading dose, given daily as a single dose (determined by renal function).

Children ages 5 to 10: For rapid digitalizing, 15 to 30 mcg/kg I.V. over 24 hours, with 50% of total dosage given initially and additional fractions given at 4- to 8-hour intervals; or digitalizing dose of 20 to 35 mcg/kg P.O. over 24 hours, with 50% of total dosage given initially and additional fractions given at 6- to 8-hour intervals. Maintenance dosage is 25% to 35% of loading dose, given daily in two divided doses (determined by renal function).

Children ages 2 to 5: For rapid digitalizing, 25 to 35 mcg/kg I.V. over 24 hours, with 50% of total dosage given initially and additional fractions given at 4- to 8-hour intervals; or digitalizing dose of 30 to 40 mcg/kg P.O. over 24 hours, with 50% of total dosage given initially and additional fractions given at 6- to 8-hour intervals. Maintenance dosage is 25% to 35% of loading dose, given daily in two divided doses (determined by renal function).

Children ages 1 to 2: For rapid digitalizing, 30 to 50 mcg/kg I.V. over 24 hours, with 50% of total dosage given initially and additional fractions given at 4- to 8-hour intervals; or digitalizing dose of 35 to 60 mcg/kg P.O. over 24 hours, with 50% of total dosage given initially and additional fractions given at 6- to 8-hour intervals. Maintenance dosage is 25% to 35% of loading dose, given daily in two divided doses (determined by renal function).

Infants (full-term): For rapid digitalizing, 20 to 30 mcg/kg I.V. over 24 hours, with 50% of total dosage given initially and additional fractions given at 4- to 8-hour intervals; or digitalizing dose of 25 to 35 mcg/kg P.O. over 24 hours, with 50% of total dosage given initially and additional fractions given at 6- to 8-hour intervals. Maintenance dosage is 25% to 35% of loading dose, given daily in two divided doses (determined by renal function).

Infants (premature): For rapid digitalizing, 15 to 25 mcg/kg I.V. over 24 hours, with 50% of total dosage given initially and additional fractions given at 4- to 8-hour intervals; or digitalizing dose of 20 to 30 mcg/kg P.O. over 24 hours, with 50% of total dosage given initially and additional fractions given at 6- to 8-hour intervals. Maintenance dosage is 20% to 30% of loading dose, given daily in two divided doses (determined by renal function).

Dosage adjustment
- Renal impairment
- Hyperthyroidism
- Elderly patients

Off-label uses
- Supraventricular tachyarrhythmias
- Intrauterine tachyarrhythmias

Contraindications
- Hypersensitivity to drug
- Uncontrolled ventricular arrhythmias, AV block

• Idiopathic hypertrophic subaortic stenosis
• Constrictive pericarditis

Administration

• Measure apical pulse for 1 full minute before administering drug. If rate is below 60 beats/minute, withhold dose, notify prescriber, and check drug blood level for toxicity.
• Administer I.V. drug undiluted, or dilute with sterile water for injection, normal saline solution, or dextrose 5% in water as directed.
• Know that for rapid effect, initial digitalizing dose generally is given in several divided doses over 12 to 24 hours.
• Be aware that dosages used for atrial arrhythmias generally are higher than those used for inotropic effect.

Route	Onset	Peak	Duration
P.O.	0.5-2 hr	2-6 hr	2-4 days
I.V.	5-30 min	1-5 hr	2-4 days

Adverse reactions

CNS: fatigue, headache, asthenia
CV: bradycardia, electrocardiogram (ECG) changes, **arrhythmias**
EENT: blurred vision, yellow vision
GI: nausea, vomiting, diarrhea
GU: gynecomastia
Hematologic: thrombocytopenia
Other: decreased appetite

Interactions

Drug-drug. *Amiodarone, cyclosporine, diclofenac, diltiazem, propafenone, quinidine, quinine, verapamil:* increased digoxin blood level, possibly leading to toxicity
Amphotericin B, corticosteroids, mezlocillin, piperacillin, thiazide and loop diuretics, ticarcillin: hypokalemia, increased risk of digoxin toxicity
Antacids, cholestyramine, colestipol, kaolin and pectin: decreased digoxin absorption

Beta-adrenergic blockers, other antiarrhythmics (including disopyramide, quinidine): additive bradycardia
Laxatives (excessive use): hypokalemia, increased risk of digoxin toxicity
Spironolactone: reduced digoxin clearance, increased risk of digoxin toxicity
Thyroid hormones: decreased digoxin efficacy
Drug-diagnostic tests. *Creatine kinase:* increased level
Drug-food. *High-fiber meal:* decreased digoxin absorption
Drug-herb. *Coca seed, coffee seed, cola seed, guarana seed, horsetail, licorice, yerba maté:* increased risk of hypokalemia
Ephedra (ma huang): arrhythmias
Hawthorn: adverse cardiovascular effects
Indian snakeroot: bradycardia
Licorice, natural stimulants (such as aloe): increased risk of hypokalemia and digoxin toxicity
Psyllium: decreased digoxin absorption
St. John's wort: decreased blood level and effects of digoxin

Precautions

Use cautiously in:
• renal or hepatic impairment, electrolyte imbalances, myocardial infarction, thyroid disorders
• obesity
• elderly patients
• pregnant or breastfeeding patients.

Patient monitoring

• Assess apical pulse regularly for 1 full minute; if pulse rate is less than 60 beats/minute, withhold next dose and notify prescriber.
◀ Monitor for signs and symptoms of drug toxicity (such as nausea, vomiting, visual disturbances, arrhythmias, and altered mental status). Be aware that therapeutic digoxin levels range from 0.5 to 2 ng/ml.

• Monitor ECG and blood levels of digoxin, potassium, magnesium, calcium, and creatinine.

Patient teaching

• Advise patient to check pulse rate regularly and to notify prescriber and withhold dose if pulse rate is below 60 or above 110 beats/minute.
• Instruct patient not to take over-the-counter drugs without prescriber's approval.
• Teach patient to recognize and report signs and symptoms of digoxin toxicity.
• Stress importance of follow-up testing as directed by prescriber.

digoxin immune FAB (ovine)
Digibind, DigiFab

Pharmacologic class: Digoxin-specific antigen-binding fragment

Therapeutic class: Cardiac glycoside antidote

Pregnancy risk category C

Action
Binds with free digoxin intravascularly and in extracellular fluid; resulting complex is excreted by kidneys. As digoxin blood level falls, new digoxin from tissues enters serum and is excreted.

Availability
Injection: 38 mg/vial (binds 0.5 mg digoxin)

🕜 Indications and dosages
➤ Digoxin toxicity when amount of drug ingested is known

Adults and children: I.V. dosage individualized based on amount of digoxin

to be eliminated and calculated as follows: Amount of drug ingested (mg) times 0.8, divided by 0.5 and rounded to next whole vial. Average adult dosage is six vials (228 mg).

➤ Digoxin toxicity when amount of drug ingested is unknown

Adults and children: Twenty vials (760 mg) usually are adequate to treat life-threatening digoxin ingestion; alternatively, may give 10 vials followed by an additional 10 vials if needed.

Contraindications
• Hypersensitivity to drug, papain, or sheep products
• Mild digoxin toxicity

Administration
• Perform allergy skin test before administering, if time permits.
• Reconstitute vial with 4 ml of sterile water for injection.
• Give I.V. infusion over 30 minutes or as bolus injection if cardiac arrest is imminent.
🔊 Keep resuscitation equipment at hand during administration.

Route	Onset	Peak	Duration
I.V.	15-30 min	Unknown	8-12 hr

Adverse reactions
CV: increased ventricular rate, low cardiac output, atrial fibrillation
Metabolic: hypokalemia
Respiratory: impaired respiratory function, tachypnea
Skin: erythema
Other: facial swelling, hypersensitivity reactions, **anaphylaxis**

Interactions
Drug-drug. *Any drug in syringe or solution:* possible incompatibility
Drug-diagnostic tests. *Immune digoxin assay:* test interference
Potassium: decreased level

Precautions

Use cautiously in:
• cardiovascular disease, renal impairment
• elderly patients
• pregnant or breastfeeding patients
• children.

Patient monitoring

• Assess baseline vital signs; monitor frequently during administration.
• Monitor electrocardiogram during administration.
• Monitor digoxin and potassium blood levels before, during, and after therapy.
• Monitor cardiac status closely.

Patient teaching

• Explain purpose of therapy and what to expect.

---

dihydroergotamine mesylate

D.H.E. 45, Dihydroergotamine-Sandoz✚, Migranal

Pharmacologic class: Alpha-adrenergic blocker

Therapeutic class: Vasoconstrictor, vascular headache suppressant

Pregnancy risk category X

Action

Stimulates alpha-adrenergic receptors, causing intracranial and peripheral vasoconstriction; also activates 5-hydroxytryptamine-1D ($5\text{-}HT_{1D}$) receptors to inhibit release of proinflammatory neuropeptides

Availability

Injection: 1 mg/ml
Nasal spray: 4 mg/ml in ampule with applicator

✪ Indications and dosages

➢ Vascular headaches, including migraine and cluster headaches
Adults: 1 mg I.M. or S.C.; may repeat in 1 hour to a total dosage of 3 mg (not to exceed 3 mg/day or 6 mg/week). Or 1 mg I.V.; may repeat in 1 hour (not to exceed 2 mg/day or 6 mg/week). Or one spray (0.5 mg) in each nostril, repeated after 15 minutes to a total dosage of 2 mg (not to exceed 3 mg/24 hours or 4 mg/week).

Off-label uses

• Intracranial hypertension
• Prevention of orthostatic hypotension
• Deep-vein thrombosis, pulmonary embolism

Contraindications

• Hypersensitivity to drug
• Concurrent use of potent CYP450-3A4 inhibitors
• Peripheral vascular disease
• Cardiovascular disease, hypertension
• Severe renal or hepatic disease
• Pregnancy or breastfeeding

Administration

• Give at first sign of migraine or as soon as possible after symptom onset.

Route	Onset	Peak	Duration
I.V.	<5 min	15 min-2 hr	8 hr
I.M., S.C.	15-30 min	15 min-2 hr	8 hr
Nasal	Within 30 min	Unknown	Unknown

Adverse reactions

CNS: dizziness, fatigue
CV: angina pectoris, intermittent claudication, sinus tachycardia, sinus bradycardia, **myocardial infarction**
EENT: rhinitis, throat irritation
GI: nausea, vomiting, diarrhea, abdominal pain, altered taste

---

Musculoskeletal: stiffness or weakness of arms, legs, neck, or shoulders; muscle pain

Other: numbness or tingling in fingers or toes, polydipsia

Interactions

Drug-drug. *Almotriptan, frovatriptan, naratriptan, rizatriptan, sumatriptan, zolmitriptan:* prolonged vasoconstriction

Beta-adrenergic blockers, CYP450-3A4 inhibitors (such as macrolides, protease inhibitors), hormonal contraceptives, vasoconstrictors: increased risk of peripheral vasoconstriction

Nitrates: antagonism of antianginal effects

Vasoconstrictors: additive effects

Drug-behaviors. *Smoking:* increased risk of peripheral vasoconstriction

Precautions

Use cautiously in:
• peripheral vascular disease, diabetes mellitus)
• children younger than age 6.

Patient monitoring

• Monitor cardiac status, especially when giving large doses.
• Assess for and report numbness and tingling of fingers and toes, arm or leg weakness, muscle pain, and intermittent claudication.

Patient teaching

• Advise patient to take drug at first sign of migraine.
• Instruct patient to lie down in quiet, darkened room for several hours after taking dose.
◀ Tell patient to immediately report chest pain, nausea, vomiting, change in heartbeat, numbness, tingling, or pain or weakness in arms or legs.

diltiazem hydrochloride
Apo-Diltiaz✦, Apo-Diltiazem✦, Cardizem, Cartia XT, Dilacor-XR, Diltia XT, Gen-Diltiazem✦, Novo-Diltiazem✦, Nu-Diltiaz✦, Syn-Diltiazem, Tiazac

Pharmacologic class: Calcium channel blocker

Therapeutic class: Antianginal, antiarrhythmic (class IV), antihypertensive

Pregnancy risk category C

Action

Inhibits calcium from entering myocardial and vascular smooth muscle cells, thereby depressing mechanical contraction of myocardial and smooth muscle while also depressing impulse formation and conduction velocity, reducing systolic and diastolic pressures

Availability

Capsules (extended-release, sustained-release): 60 mg, 90 mg, 120 mg, 180 mg, 240 mg, 300 mg, 360 mg, 420 mg
Injection: 5 mg/ml in 10-ml vials, 25-mg ready-to-use syringes, 100-mg Monovial
Tablets: 30 mg, 60 mg, 90 mg, 120 mg

🖊 Indications and dosages

➤ Angina pectoris and vasospastic (Prinzmetal's) angina; hypertension; supraventricular tachyarrhythmias; atrial flutter; atrial or fibrillation

Adults: 30 to 90 mg P.O. three to four times daily (tablets); or 60 to 120 mg b.i.d. (sustained-release capsules); or 180 to 240 mg once daily (extended-release capsules), adjusted after 14 days as needed, up to a total daily dosage of 360 mg. Or 0.25 mg/kg by I.V. bolus over 2 minutes; if response is inadequate, may give 0.35 mg/kg over 15 minutes; may follow with continuous I.V. infusion at 10 mg/ hour (at a range 5 to 15 mg/hour) for up to 24 hours.

Dosage adjustment
• Severe hepatic or renal impairment
• Elderly patients

Off-label uses
• Unstable angina, coronary artery bypass graft, myocardial infarction (MI)
• Tardive dyskinesia
• Migraine
• Hyperthyroidism
• Raynaud's phenomenon

Contraindications
• Hypersensitivity to drug
• Atrial and atrioventricular arrhythmias
• Recent MI or pulmonary congestion

Administration
• When giving I.V., dilute in dextrose 5% in water or normal saline solution.
• Give I.V. bolus dose over 2 minutes; a second bolus may be given after 15 minutes.
• Administer continuous I.V. infusion at 5 to 15 mg/hour.
• Don't crush tablets or sustained-release capsules; they must be swallowed whole.
• Withhold dose if systolic blood pressure falls below 90 mm Hg, diastolic pressure is below 60 mm Hg, or apical pulse is slower than 60 beats/minute.

Route	Onset	Peak	Duration
P.O.	30 min	2-3 hr	6-8 hr
P.O. (sustained)	Unknown	Unknown	12 hr
P.O. (extended)	Unknown	14 hr	Up to 24 hr
I.V.	2-5 min	2-4 hr	Unknown

Adverse reactions
CNS: headache, abnormal dreams, anxiety, confusion, dizziness, drowsiness, nervousness, psychiatric disturbances, asthenia, paresthesia, syncope, tremor
CV: peripheral edema, bradycardia, chest pain, hypotension, palpitations, tachycardia, **arrhythmias, heart failure**
EENT: blurred vision, tinnitus, epistaxis, gingival hyperplasia
GI: nausea, vomiting, diarrhea, constipation, dyspepsia, dry mouth, bad taste
GU: urinary frequency, dysuria, nocturia, polyuria, gynecomastia, sexual dysfunction
Hematologic: anemia, **leukopenia, thrombocytopenia**
Hepatic: abnormal liver function test results
Metabolic: hyperglycemia
Musculoskeletal: joint stiffness, muscle cramps
Respiratory: cough, dyspnea
Skin: rash, dermatitis, erythema multiforme, flushing, diaphoresis, photosensitivity, pruritus, urticaria
Other: weight gain, decreased appetite, **Stevens-Johnson syndrome**

Interactions
Drug-drug. *Beta-adrenergic blockers, digoxin, disopyramide, phenytoin:* bradycardia, conduction defects, heart failure
Carbamazepine, cyclosporine, quinidine: decreased diltiazem metabolism, increased risk of toxicity
Cimetidine, ranitidine: increased blood level and effects of diltiazem
Fentanyl, nitrates, other antihypertensives, quinidine: additive hypotension
HMG-CoA reductase inhibitors, imipramine, sirolimus, tacrolimus: increased blood levels of these drugs
Lithium: decreased lithium level, reduced antimanic control

d

Nonsteroidal anti-inflammatory drugs: decreased antihypertensive effects of diltiazem
Theophylline: increased theophylline effects
Drug-diagnostic tests. *Hepatic enzymes:* increased levels
Drug-food. *Grapefruit juice:* increased blood level and effects of diltiazem
Drug-behaviors. *Acute alcohol ingestion:* additive hypotension

Precautions

Use cautiously in:
• severe hepatic or renal impairment, heart failure
• history of serious ventricular arrhythmias
• elderly patients
• pregnant or breastfeeding patients
• children (safety not established).

Patient monitoring

• Check blood pressure and electrocardiogram before initiating therapy, and monitor closely during dosage adjustment period. Withhold dose if systolic pressure is below 90 mm Hg.
• Monitor for signs and symptoms of heart failure.
• Supervise patient during ambulation.

Patient teaching

• Advise patient to change position slowly to minimize light-headedness and dizziness.
• Instruct patient to avoid driving and other hazardous activities until he knows how drug affects concentration and alertness.

dimenhydrinate

Apo-Dimenhydrinate✦, Calm X, Dimetabs, Dinate, Dramamine, Dramanate✦, Gravol✦, Hydrate, PMS-Dimenhydrinate✦, Travamine✦ Triptone Caplets

Pharmacologic class: Anticholinergic
Therapeutic class: Antiemetic, antivertigo agent
Pregnancy risk category B

Action

Prevents nausea and vomiting by inhibiting vestibular stimulation of chemoreceptor trigger zone and inhibiting stimulation of vomiting center in brain

Availability

Capsules: 50 mg
Capsules (extended-release): 25 mg
Elixir: 12.5 mg/5 ml, 15 mg/5 ml
Injection: 50 mg/ml
Liquid: 12.5 mg/4 ml
Suppositories: 50 mg, 100 mg
Tablets: 50 mg
Tablets (chewable): 50 mg

Indications and dosages

➤ Prevention and treatment of nausea, vomiting, dizziness, and vertigo
Adults and children age 12 and older: 50 to 100 mg P.O. q 4 hours (not to exceed 400 mg/day), or 50 to 100 mg P.R. q 6 to 8 hours, or 50 mg I.M. or I.V. q 4 hours p.r.n.
Children ages 6 to 12: 25 to 50 mg P.O. q 6 to 8 hours (not to exceed 150 mg/day), or 25 to 50 mg P.R. q 8 to 12 hours, or 1.25 mg/kg I.M. (37.5 mg/m^2) q 6 hours p.r.n.
Children ages 2 to 6: 12.5 to 25 mg P.O. q 6 to 8 hours (not to exceed 75 mg/day)

Contraindications
• Hypersensitivity to drug or tartrazine
• Alcohol intolerance

Administration
• Give each 50-mg I.V. dose over 2 minutes.
• For I.V. administration, dilute with dextrose 5% in water or normal saline solution.
◀€ Don't administer by I.V. route to premature or low-birth-weight infants; solution contains benzyl alcohol, which can cause fatal "gasping" syndrome.

Route	Onset	Peak	Duration
P.O.	15-60 min	1-2 hr	3-6 hr
I.V.	Rapid	Unknown	3-6 hr
I.M.	20-30 min	1-2 hr	3-6 hr
P.R.	30-45 min	Unknown	6-12 hr

Adverse reactions
CNS: drowsiness, dizziness, headache, paradoxical stimulation (in children)
CV: hypotension, palpitations
EENT: blurred vision, tinnitus
GI: diarrhea, constipation, dry mouth
GU: dysuria, urinary frequency
Skin: photosensitivity
Other: pain at I.M. site, decreased appetite

Interactions
Drug-drug. *Disopyramide, quinidine, tricyclic antidepressants:* increased anticholinergic effects
Monoamine oxidase inhibitors: intensified and prolonged anticholinergic effects
Other CNS depressants (such as antihistamines, opioids, sedative-hypnotics): additive CNS depression
Ototoxic drugs (such as aminoglycosides, ethacrynic acid): masking of signs or symptoms of ototoxicity
Drug-diagnostic tests. *Allergy skin tests:* false-negative results

Drug-behaviors. *Alcohol use:* increased CNS depression

Precautions
Use cautiously in:
• narrow-angle glaucoma, seizure disorders, prostatic hypertrophy.

Patient monitoring
• Assess for lethargy and drowsiness.
• Monitor for dizziness, nausea, and vomiting (possible indicators of drug toxicity).

Patient teaching
• To prevent motion sickness, advise patient to take drug 30 minutes before traveling and to repeat dose before meals and at bedtime.
• Instruct patient to avoid driving and other hazardous activities until he knows how drug affects concentration and alertness.
• Caution patient to avoid alcohol and sedative-hypnotics during therapy.

dinoprostone
(prostaglandin E₂, PGE₂)
Cervidil Vaginal Insert, Prepidil Endocervical Gel, Prostin E2 Vaginal Suppository

Pharmacologic class: Oxytocic, prostaglandin
Therapeutic class: Abortifacient, cervical ripening agent
Pregnancy risk category C

Action
Initiates strong contractions of uterine smooth muscle by stimulating myometrium and initiating cervical softening, effacement, and dilation (ripening); also stimulates GI tract smooth muscle

Availability

Endocervical gel: 0.5 mg in 3-g gel vehicle in prefilled syringe with catheters
Vaginal insert: 10 mg
Vaginal suppositories: 20 mg

🖊 Indications and dosages

➤ Cervical ripening
Adults: 0.5 mg endocervical gel vaginally; if response is poor, may repeat in 6 hours (not to exceed 1.5 mg in 24 hours). Or one 10-mg vaginal insert.
➤ To induce abortion
Adults: One 20-mg vaginal suppository; repeat q 3 to 5 hours (not to exceed total dosage of 240 mg or duration of 48 hours)

Off-label uses

• Drug-induced GI bleeding

Contraindications

• Hypersensitivity to prostaglandins or additives in gel or suppository
• Active genital herpes infection
• Acute pelvic inflammatory disease

Administration

• Keep patient prone for 10 minutes after administration to prevent drug expulsion and enhance absorption.
• Store suppositories in freezer; bring to room temperature before using.

Route	Onset	Peak	Duration
Cervical ripening (gel)	Rapid	30-45 min	Unknown
Cervical ripening (insert)	Rapid	Unknown	12 hr
Abortion (suppository)	10 min	Unknown	2-3 hr

Adverse reactions

CNS: headache, drowsiness, syncope
CV: hypotension, hypertension
GI: nausea, vomiting, diarrhea
GU: urinary tract infection, uterine hyperstimulation, vaginal or uterine pain, uterine contractile abnormalities, warm vaginal sensation, **uterine rupture**
Musculoskeletal: back pain
Respiratory: cough, dyspnea, wheezing
Other: allergic reactions including chills, fever, and **anaphylaxis**

Interactions

Drug-drug. *Other oxytocics:* increased effects

Precautions

Use cautiously in:
• pulmonary, cardiac, renal, or hepatic disease; asthma; hypotension; adrenal disorders; diabetes mellitus; epilepsy; glaucoma
• multiparity

Patient monitoring

◀≶ Monitor uterine contractions and observe for excessive vaginal bleeding and cramping; record pad count.
• Monitor vital signs and assess for drug-induced fever. Report significant blood pressure and pulse changes.
• Assess for wheezing, chest pain, and dyspnea.
• Evaluate for GI upset; to minimize, give antiemetic before therapy.

Patient teaching

• Advise patient to stay in prone position for 10 minutes after administration.
• Instruct patient to report fever, bleeding, or abdominal cramps.
• Teach patient to avoid douches, tampons, sexual intercourse, and tub baths for at least 2 weeks after receiving drug

diphenhydramine hydrochloride

Allerdryl✦, AllerMax, Banophen, Benadryl, Benadryl Allergy, Benadryl Dye-Free Allergy, Compoz, Compoz Nighttime Sleep Aid, Diphen AF, Diphen Cough, Diphenhist, Genahist, Hyrexin, Maximum Strength Nytol, Maximum Strength Sleepinal, Midol PM, Nervine Nighttime Sleep Aid, Nytol, Siladryl, Sleep-Eze D, Sominex, Twilite, Unisom Nighttime Sleep-Aid

Pharmacologic class: Ethanolamine derivative, nonselective histamine$_1$-receptor antagonist

Therapeutic class: Antihistamine, antitussive, antiemetic, antivertigo agent, antidyskinetic

Pregnancy risk category B

Action

Interferes with histamine effects at histamine$_1$-receptor sites; prevents but doesn't reverse histamine-mediated response. Also exerts significant CNS depressant and anticholinergic activity.

Availability

Capsules: 25 mg, 50 mg
Elixir: 12.5 mg/5 ml
Injection: 10 mg/ml, 50 mg/ml
Syrup: 12.5 mg/5 ml
Tablets: 25 mg, 50 mg
Tablets (chewable): 25 mg

⊘ Indications and dosages

➤ Allergy symptoms caused by histamine release (including anaphylaxis, seasonal and perennial allergic rhinitis, allergic dermatoses); nausea; vertigo
Adults and children over age 12: 25 to 50 mg P.O. q 4 to 6 hours or 10 to 50 mg I.V. or I.M. q 2 to 3 hours as need-ed. (Some patients may need up to 100 mg.) Don't exceed 400 mg/day.
Children ages 6 to 12: 12.5 to 25 mg P.O. q 4 to 6 hours or 1.25 mg/kg (37.5 mg/m^2) I.M. or I.V. q.i.d.; don't exceed 150 mg/day.
Children ages 2 to 5: 6.25 mg P.O. q 4 to 6 hours; don't exceed 37.5 mg/day.
➤ Cough
Adults: 25 mg P.O. q 4 hours p.r.n., not to exceed 150 mg/day
Children ages 6 to 12: 12.5 mg P.O. q 4 hours; don't exceed 75 mg/day.
Children ages 2 to 5: 6.25 mg P.O. q 4 hours; don't exceed 37.5 mg/24 hours.
➤ Dyskinesia, Parkinson's disease
Adults: Initially, 25 mg P.O. t.i.d.; may be increased to a maximum of 50 mg q.i.d.
➤ Mild nighttime sedation
Adults: 50 mg P.O. 20 to 30 minutes before bedtime
Dosage adjustment
• Elderly patients

Off-label uses

• Drug-induced extrapyramidal reactions

Contraindications

• Hypersensitivity to drug
• Alcohol intolerance
• Acute asthma attacks
• Breastfeeding

Administration

• For motion sickness, administer 30 minutes before activity.
• Give oral doses with food or milk to minimize adverse GI effects.
• For I.V. use, check compatibility before mixing with other drugs.
• Inject I.M. dose deep into large muscle mass; rotate sites.
• Discontinue drug 4 days before skin testing to avoid misleading results.

Route	Onset	Peak	Duration
P.O.	15-60 min	1-4 hr	4-8 hr
I.V.	Rapid	Unknown	4-8 hr
I.M.	20-30 min	1-4 hr	4-8 hr

Adverse reactions

CNS: drowsiness, dizziness, headache, paradoxical stimulation (especially in children)
CV: hypotension, palpitations
EENT: blurred vision, tinnitus
GI: diarrhea, constipation, dry mouth
GU: dysuria, urinary frequency or retention
Skin: photosensitivity
Other: decreased appetite, pain at I.M. site

Interactions

Drug-drug. *Antihistamines, opioids, sedative-hypnotics:* additive CNS depression
Disopyramide, quinidine, tricyclic antidepressants: increased anticholinergic effects
Monoamine oxidase inhibitors: intensified and prolonged anticholinergic effects
Drug-diagnostic tests. *Skin allergy tests:* false-negative results
Hemoglobin, platelets: decreased values
Drug-herb. *Angel's trumpet, jimson weed, scopolia:* increased anticholinergic effects
Chamomile, hops, kava, skullcap, valerian: increased CNS depression
Drug-behaviors. *Alcohol use:* increased CNS depression

Precautions

Use cautiously in:
• severe hepatic disease, narrow-angle glaucoma, seizure disorders, prostatic hypertrophy
• elderly patients
• pregnant patients (safety not established).

Patient monitoring

• Monitor cardiovascular status, especially in patients with cardiovascular disease.
• Supervise patient during ambulation; use side rails as necessary.

Patient teaching

• Advise patient to take drug with food if it causes GI upset.
• Caution patient to avoid driving and other hazardous activities until he knows how drug affects concentration and alertness.

diphenoxylate hydrochloride and atropine sulfate
Logen, Lomanate, Lomotil, Lonox

Pharmacologic class: Anticholinergic, meperidine congener
Therapeutic class: Antidiarrheal
Controlled substance schedule V
Pregnancy risk category C

Action

Slows gastric motility by decreasing peristalsis of gastric mucosa. (Small amounts of atropine added to reduce abuse potential.)

Availability

Liquid: 2.5 mg diphenoxylate and 0.025 mg atropine/5 ml
Tablets: 2.5 mg diphenoxylate and 0.025 mg atropine

🚫 Indications and dosages

➤ Diarrhea
Adults: Initially, 5 mg P.O. three to four times daily, then 5 mg/day as needed (not to exceed 20 mg/day). Decrease dosage when desired response occurs.

Children: Initially, 0.3 to 0.4 mg/kg P.O. (liquid only) daily in four divided doses. Decrease dosage when desired response occurs.

Dosage adjustment
• Respiratory disease
• Elderly patients

Contraindications
• Hypersensitivity to drug
• Alcohol intolerance
• Severe liver disease
• Narrow-angle glaucoma
• Children younger than age 2

Administration
• Withhold drug if patient has severe fluid or electrolyte imbalance.
• Administer with food if GI upset occurs.

Route	Onset	Peak	Duration
P.O.	45-60 min	2 hr	3-4 hr

Adverse reactions
CNS: dizziness, confusion, drowsiness, headache, insomnia, nervousness
CV: tachycardia
EENT: blurred vision, dry eyes
GI: nausea, vomiting, constipation, epigastric distress, ileus, dry mouth
GU: urinary retention
Skin: flushing

Interactions
Drug-drug. *CNS depressants (including antihistamines, sedative-hypnotics, opioids):* increased CNS depression
Anticholinergic-like drugs (including tricyclic antidepressants, disopyramide): increased anticholinergic effects
Monoamine oxidase inhibitors: hypertensive crisis
Drug-diagnostic tests. *Amylase:* increased level
Drug-herb. *Angel's trumpet, jimson weed, scopolia:* increased anticholinergic effects
Drug-behaviors. *Alcohol use:* increased CNS depression

Precautions
Use cautiously in:
• inflammatory bowel disease, prostatic hypertrophy
• elderly patients
• pregnant or breastfeeding patients
• children (safety not established in children under age 12; drug shouldn't be given to children younger than age 2).

d

Patient monitoring
◀ Assess for and report abdominal distention and signs or symptoms of decreased peristalsis.
• Watch for signs and symptoms of dehydration.
• Assess frequency and consistency of bowel movements.

Patient teaching
• Instruct patient to report persistent diarrhea.
• Advise patient to avoid driving and other hazardous activities until he knows how drug affects concentration and alertness.
• Caution patient that prolonged use may lead to dependence.

dipyridamole
Apo-Dipyridamole FC✦, Apo-Dipyridamole SC✦, Dipridacot, Novo-Dipiradol✦, Persantine, Persantine IV

Pharmacologic class: Platelet adhesion inhibitor

Therapeutic class: Antiplatelet agent, diagnostic agent (coronary vasodilator)

Pregnancy risk category B

Action
Unclear; may reduce platelet aggregation by inhibiting phosphodiesterase,

adenosine uptake, or formation of thromboxane A_2. Produces vasodilation, increasing coronary blood flow.

Availability
Injection: 10 mg/2 ml
Tablets: 25 mg, 50 mg, 75 mg, 100 mg

Indications and dosages
➤ To prevent thromboembolism in patients with prosthetic heart valves (given with warfarin)
Adults: 75 to 100 mg P.O. q.i.d.
➤ Alternative to exercise in thallium myocardial perfusion imaging
Adults: 0.57 mg/kg I.V. infused over 4 minutes (0.142 mg/kg/minute). Maximum I.V. dosage is 60 mg.

Off-label uses
• Prevention of myocardial reinfarction (given with aspirin)
• Thrombotic thrombocytopenia purpura

Contraindications
• Hypersensitivity to drug
• Hypotension

Administration
• Dilute I.V. solution with dextrose 5% in water or normal or half-normal saline solution, as directed.
• Give single I.V dose over 4 minutes.
• When used as diagnostic agent, administer within 5 minutes of thallium injection.
• Give oral form with a full glass of water at least 1 hour before or 2 hours after meals. If gastric distress occurs, give with food.

Route	Onset	Peak	Duration
P.O.	Unknown	Unknown	Unknown
I.V.	Unknown	6.5 min	30 min

Adverse reactions
CNS: dizziness, headache, syncope; transient cerebral ischemia or weakness (with I.V. use)
CV: hypotension, **arrhythmias, myocardial infarction** (all with I.V. use)
GI: nausea, vomiting diarrhea, dyspepsia
Hematologic: increased bleeding time
Respiratory: bronchospasm (with I.V. use)
Skin: rash, flushing (with I.V. use)

Interactions
Drug-drug. *Anticoagulants, cefamandole, cefoperazone, cefotetan, thrombolytics, nonsteroidal anti-inflammatory drugs, plicamycin, sulfinpyrazone, valproic acid:* increased risk of bleeding
Aspirin: increased effects on platelet aggregation
Theophylline: negation of dipyridamole's effects during thallium imaging
Drug-behaviors. *Alcohol use:* increased risk of hypotension

Precautions
Use cautiously in:
• hypotension, platelet defects
• pregnant or breastfeeding patients (safety not established)
• children younger than age 12 (safety not established).

Patient monitoring
• Monitor for therapeutic efficacy, including improved exercise tolerance and decreased need for nitrates.
• Assess platelet and coagulation studies regularly.
• Monitor electrocardiogram and vital signs, especially blood pressure.

Patient teaching
• Advise patient to take drug 1 hour before or 2 hours after meals for best absorption.

2005 Nursing Spectrum Drug Handbook
Photogallery of common tablets and capsules

This special section helps you identify unlabeled drugs that patients bring from home. It can also serve as a visual aid for patients who can't recall the names of the drugs they're taking. Drugs are shown alphabetically by generic name; corresponding trade names also appear. Dosage forms appear in increasing order of strength.

alendronate sodium	**Fosamax**			
	5 mg	10 mg	35 mg	70 mg

alprazolam	**Xanax**		
	0.25 mg	0.5 mg	1 mg
	2 mg		

alprazolam	**Xanax XR**			
	0.5 mg	1 mg	2 mg	3 mg

amitriptyline hydrochloride	**Elavil**		
	10 mg	25 mg	50 mg
	75 mg	100 mg	150 mg

amlodipine besylate	**Norvasc**		
	2.5 mg	5 mg	10 mg

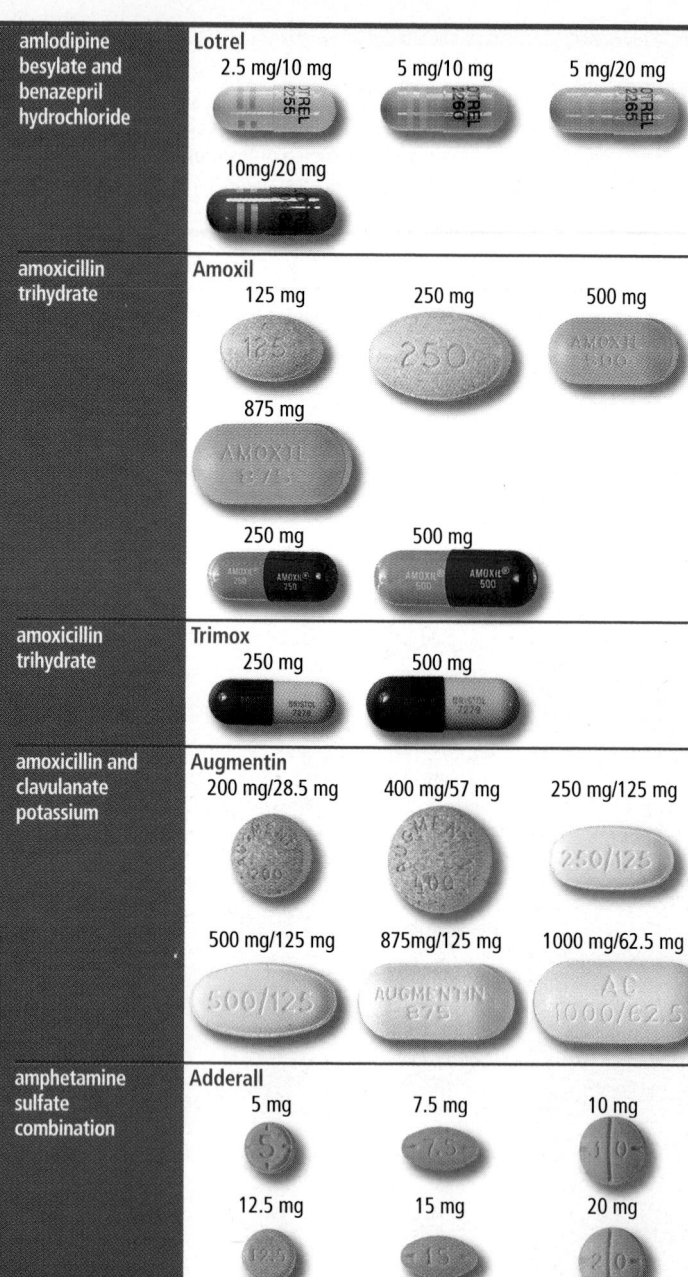

amlodipine besylate and benazepril hydrochloride	**Lotrel**
	2.5 mg/10 mg 5 mg/10 mg 5 mg/20 mg
	10mg/20 mg

amoxicillin trihydrate	**Amoxil**
	125 mg 250 mg 500 mg
	875 mg
	250 mg 500 mg

| amoxicillin trihydrate | **Trimox** |
| | 250 mg 500 mg |

amoxicillin and clavulanate potassium	**Augmentin**
	200 mg/28.5 mg 400 mg/57 mg 250 mg/125 mg
	500 mg/125 mg 875mg/125 mg 1000 mg/62.5 mg

amphetamine sulfate combination	**Adderall**
	5 mg 7.5 mg 10 mg
	12.5 mg 15 mg 20 mg

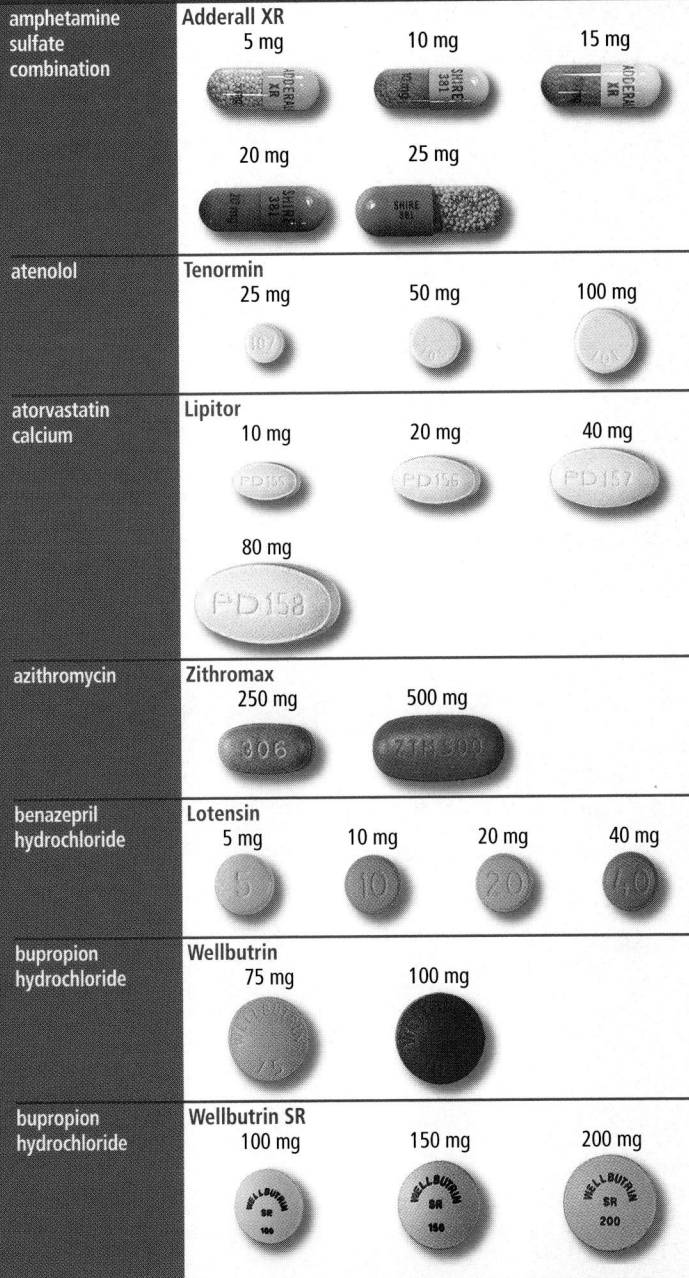

amphetamine sulfate combination	**Adderall XR**
atenolol	**Tenormin**
atorvastatin calcium	**Lipitor**
azithromycin	**Zithromax**
benazepril hydrochloride	**Lotensin**
bupropion hydrochloride	**Wellbutrin**
bupropion hydrochloride	**Wellbutrin SR**

Adderall XR
5 mg   10 mg   15 mg   20 mg   25 mg

Tenormin
25 mg   50 mg   100 mg

Lipitor
10 mg   20 mg   40 mg   80 mg

Zithromax
250 mg   500 mg

Lotensin
5 mg   10 mg   20 mg   40 mg

Wellbutrin
75 mg   100 mg

Wellbutrin SR
100 mg   150 mg   200 mg

bupropion hydrochloride	**Wellbutrin XL**
	150 mg, 300 mg

carvedilol	**Coreg**
	3.125 mg, 6.25 mg, 12.5 mg, 25 mg

cefprozil	**Cefzil**
	250 mg, 500 mg

celecoxib	**Celebrex**
	100 mg, 200 mg, 400 mg

cephalexin monohydrate	**Keflex**
	250 mg, 500 mg

cetirizine hydrochloride	**Zyrtec**
	5 mg, 10 mg

ciprofloxacin hydrochloride	**Cipro**
	100 mg, 250 mg, 500 mg, 750 mg

ciprofloxacin and ciprofloxacin hydrochloride	**Cipro XR**
	500 mg

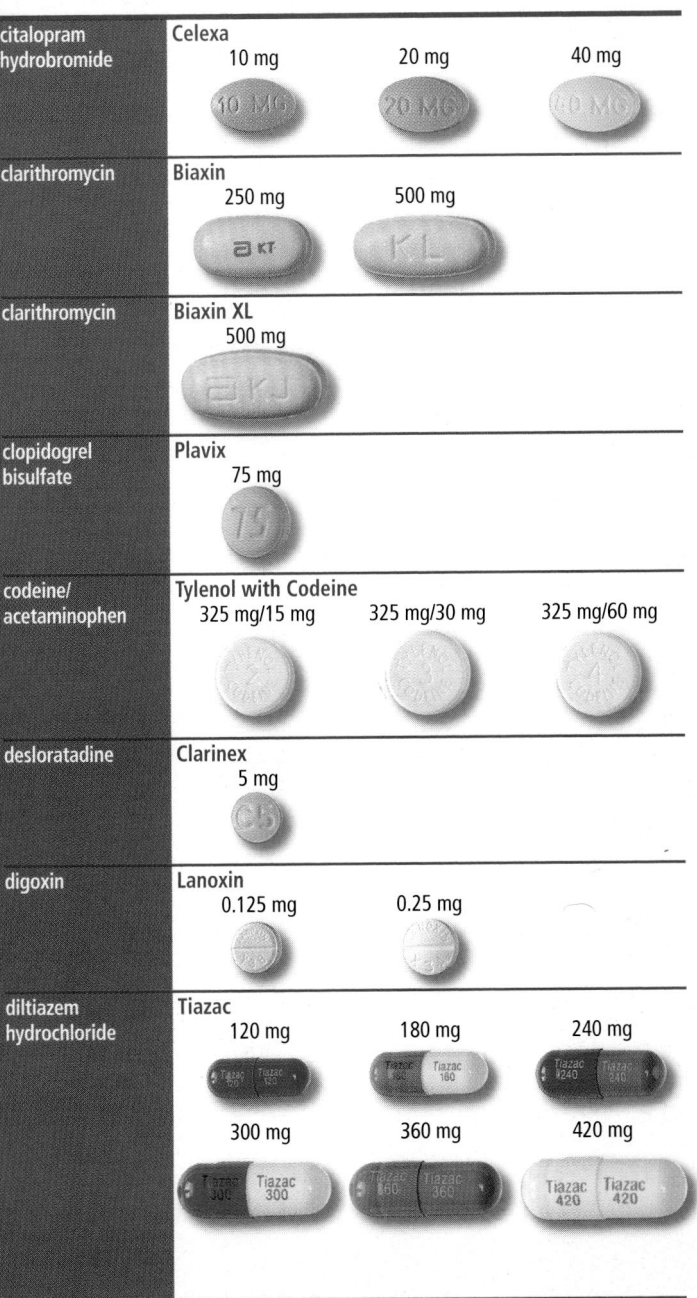

citalopram hydrobromide	**Celexa**		
	10 mg	20 mg	40 mg

clarithromycin	**Biaxin**	
	250 mg	500 mg

clarithromycin	**Biaxin XL**
	500 mg

clopidogrel bisulfate	**Plavix**
	75 mg

codeine/ acetaminophen	**Tylenol with Codeine**		
	325 mg/15 mg	325 mg/30 mg	325 mg/60 mg

desloratadine	**Clarinex**
	5 mg

digoxin	**Lanoxin**	
	0.125 mg	0.25 mg

diltiazem hydrochloride	**Tiazac**		
	120 mg	180 mg	240 mg
	300 mg	360 mg	420 mg

divalproex sodium	**Depakote** 125 mg	250 mg	500 mg
	125 mg		
divalproex sodium	**Depakote ER** 250 mg	500 mg	
esomeprazole magnesium	**Nexium** 20 mg	40 mg	
estrogens, conjugated	**Premarin** 0.3 mg	0.625 mg	0.9 mg
	1.25 mg	2.5 mg	
fenofibrate	**Tricor** 54 mg	160 mg	
fexofenadine hydrochloride	**Allegra** 30 mg	60 mg	180 mg
fexofenadine hydrochloride and pseudoephedrine hydrochloride	**Allegra-D** 60 mg/120 mg		

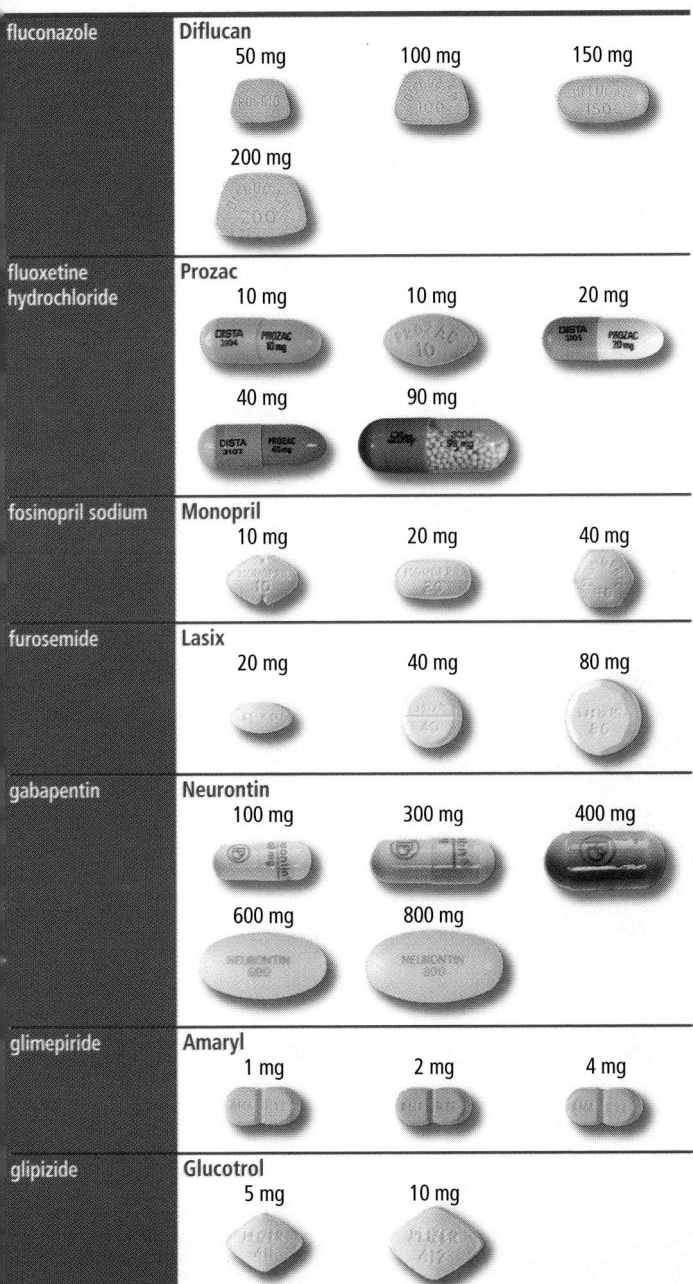

fluconazole	**Diflucan**
fluoxetine hydrochloride	**Prozac**
fosinopril sodium	**Monopril**
furosemide	**Lasix**
gabapentin	**Neurontin**
glimepiride	**Amaryl**
glipizide	**Glucotrol**

glipizide	**Glucotrol XL**		
	2.5 mg	5 mg	10 mg

glyburide and metformin hydrochloride	**Glucovance**		
	1.25 mg/250 mg	2.5 mg/500 mg	5 mg/500 mg

hydrochlorothiazide	**HydroDIURIL**	
	25 mg	50 mg

hydrocodone bitartrate and acetaminophen	**Lortab**		
	2.5 mg/500 mg	5 mg/500 mg	7.5 mg/500 mg
	10 mg/500 mg		

ibuprofen	**Motrin**		
	400 mg	600 mg	800 mg

irbesartan	**Avapro**		
	75 mg	150 mg	300 mg

lansoprazole	**Prevacid**	
	15 mg	30 mg

levofloxacin	**Levaquin**		
	250 mg	500 mg	750 mg

levothyroxine sodium	**Levoxyl**		
	25 mcg	50 mcg	75 mcg
	88 mcg	100 mcg	112 mcg
	125 mcg	137 mcg	150 mcg
	175 mcg	200 mcg	300 mcg

levothyroxine sodium	**Synthroid**		
	25 mcg	50 mcg	75 mcg
	88 mcg	100 mcg	112 mcg
	125 mcg	137 mcg	150 mcg
	175 mcg	200 mcg	300 mcg

lisinopril	**Prinivil**		
	2.5 mg	5 mg	10 mg
	20 mg	40 mg	

lisinopril	**Zestril**		
	2.5 mg	5 mg	10 mg
	20 mg	30 mg	40 mg

lisinopril and hydrochlorothiazide	**Zestoretic** 10 mg/12.5 mg	20 mg/12.5 mg	20 mg/25 mg
loratadine	**Claritin** 10 mg		
lorazepam	**Ativan** 0.5 mg	1 mg	2 mg
losartan potassium	**Cozaar** 25 mg	50 mg	100 mg
losartan potassium and hydrochlorothiazide	**Hyzaar** 50 mg/12.5 mg	100 mg/25 mg	
metformin hydrochloride	**Glucophage** 500 mg	850 mg	1,000 mg
metformin hydrochloride	**Glucophage XR** 500 mg	750 mg	
methylphenidate hydrochloride	**Concerta** 18 mg	27 mg	36 mg
	54 mg		

metoprolol succinate	**Toprol-XL**		
	25 mg	50 mg	100 mg
	200 mg		

mirtazapine	**Remeron**		
	15 mg	30 mg	45 mg

montelukast sodium	**Singulair**		
	4 mg	5 mg	10 mg

nitrofurantoin macrocrystals	**Macrodantin**		
	25 mg	50 mg	100 mg

nitrofurantoin monohydrate	**Macrobid**		
	100 mg		

olanzapine	**Zyprexa**		
	2.5 mg	5 mg	7.5 mg
	10 mg	15 mg	20 mg

omeprazole	**Prilosec**		
	10 mg	20 mg	40 mg

oxybutynin chloride	**Ditropan**		
	5 mg		

oxybutynin chloride	**Ditropan XL**		
	5 mg	10 mg	15 mg

oxycodone hydrochloride	**OxyContin**			
	10 mg	20 mg	40 mg	80 mg

pantoprazole sodium	**Protonix**
	40 mg

paroxetine hydrochloride	**Paxil**			
	10 mg	20 mg	30 mg	40 mg

paroxetine hydrochloride	**Paxil CR**		
	12.5 mg	25 mg	37.5 mg

penicillin V potassium	**Veetids**	
	250 mg	500 mg

phenytoin sodium (extended)	**Dilantin**	
	30 mg	100 mg

pioglitazone hydrochloride	**Actos**		
	15 mg	30 mg	45 mg

pravastatin sodium	**Pravachol**		
	10 mg	20 mg	40 mg
	80 mg		

propoxyphene napsylate and acetaminophen	Darvocet-N 50 50 mg	Darvocet-N 100 100 mg	

quetiapine fumarate	**Seroquel** 25 mg	100 mg	200 mg
	300 mg		

quinapril hydrochloride	**Accupril** 5 mg	10 mg	20 mg
	40 mg		

rabeprazole sodium	**Aciphex** 20 mg		

raloxifene hydrochloride	**Evista** 60 mg		

ramipril	**Altace** 1.25 mg	2.5 mg	5 mg
	10 mg		

risedronate sodium	**Actonel** 5 mg	30 mg	35 mg

risperidone	Risperdal		
	0.25 mg	0.5 mg	1 mg
	2 mg	3 mg	4 mg

rofecoxib	Vioxx		
	12.5 mg	25 mg	50 mg

rosiglitazone maleate	Avandia		
	2 mg	4 mg	8 mg

sertraline hydrochloride	Zoloft		
	25 mg	50 mg	100 mg

sildenafil citrate	Viagra		
	25 mg	50 mg	100 mg

simvastatin	Zocor		
	5 mg	10 mg	20 mg
	40 mg	80 mg	

sumatriptan succinate	Imitrex		
	25 mg	50 mg	100 mg

tamsulosin hydrochloride	**Flomax** 0.4 mg

| tolterodine tartrate | **Detrol** 1 mg | 2 mg |

| tolterodine tartrate | **Detrol LA** 2 mg | 4 mg |

| topiramate | **Topamax** 25 mg | 100 mg | 200 mg |

| topiramate | **Topamax Sprinkle** 15 mg | 25 mg |

| tramadol hydrochloride | **Ultram** 50 mg |

| tramadol hydrochloride and acetaminophen | **Ultracet** 37.5 mg/325 mg |

| triamterene and hydrochlorothiazide | **Maxzide** 37.5 mg/25 mg | 75 mg/50 mg |

| valacyclovir hydrochloride | **Valtrex** 500 mg | 1,000 mg |

| valdecoxib | **Bextra** 10 mg | 20 mg |

valsartan	**Diovan**		
	80 mg	160 mg	320 mg

valsartan and hydrochlorothiazide	**Diovan HCT**		
	80 mg/12.5 mg	160 mg/12.5 mg	160 mg/25 mg

venlafaxine hydrochloride	**Effexor**		
	25 mg	37.5 mg	50 mg
	75 mg	100 mg	

venlafaxine hydrochloride	**Effexor XR**		
	37.5 mg	75 mg	150 mg

warfarin sodium	**Coumadin**		
	1 mg	2 mg	2.5 mg
	3 mg	4 mg	5 mg
	6 mg	7.5 mg	10 mg

zolpidem tartrate	**Ambien**	
	5 mg	10 mg

dirithromycin
Dynabac

Pharmacologic class: Macrolide
Therapeutic class: Anti-infective
Pregnancy risk category C

Action
Binds to 50S ribosomal subunit of susceptible bacteria, inhibiting protein synthesis

Availability
Tablets: 250 mg

Indications and dosages
➤ Acute and chronic bronchitis or other respiratory infections caused by *Moraxella catarrhalis, Streptococcus pneumoniae,* or *Haemophilus influenzae;* secondary bacterial infection of acute bronchitis caused by *M. catarrhalis* or *S. pneumoniae;* uncomplicated skin infections caused by *Staphylococcus aureus*

Adults and children age 12 and older: 500 mg P.O. daily for 5 to 7 days
➤ Community-acquired pneumonia caused by *Legionella pneumophila, Mycoplasma pneumoniae,* or *S. pneumoniae*

Adults and children age 12 and older: 500 mg P.O. daily for 14 days
➤ Pharyngitis or tonsillitis caused by *Streptococcus pyogenes*

Adults and children age 12 and older: 500 mg P.O. daily for 10 days

Contraindications
• Hypersensitivity to drug or other macrolides
• Hypotension

Administration
• Obtain specimen for culture and sensitivity testing as necessary before starting therapy.
• Give with food or within 1 hour of a meal.
• Make sure patient swallows tablets whole without cutting, crushing, or chewing them.

Route	Onset	Peak	Duration
P.O.	Unknown	4 hr	Unknown

Adverse reactions
CNS: headache, dizziness, vertigo, asthenia, insomnia
GI: nausea, diarrhea, vomiting, abdominal pain, dyspepsia, flatulence
Metabolic: hyperkalemia
Respiratory: increased cough, dyspnea
Other: nonspecific pain

Interactions
Drug-drug. *Antacids, histamine$_2$-receptor antagonists:* increased absorption of dirithromycin
Digoxin: increased digoxin blood level
Drug-diagnostic tests. *Alanine aminotransferase, alkaline phosphatase, aspartate aminotransferase, bilirubin, creatine kinase, eosinophils, gamma-glutamyltransferase, lactate dehydrogenase, neutrophils, platelets, potassium:* increased levels
Drug-food. *Any food:* increased absorption of dirithromycin

Precautions
Use cautiously in:
• renal or hepatic impairment, colitis
• pregnant or breastfeeding patients.

Patient monitoring
• Monitor for signs and symptoms of superinfection.

Patient teaching
• Instruct patient to take tablets whole, within 1 hour of a meal.

◀€ Tell patient to report signs and symptoms of worsening infection, superinfection (such as loose, foul-smelling stools, vaginal itching, sudden fever, cough), or pseudomembranous enterocolitis (such as severe diarrhea or vomiting).

disopyramide
Rythmodan✦, Rythmodan-LA✦

disopyramide phosphate
Norpace, Norpace CR

Pharmacologic class: Pyridine derivative

Therapeutic class: Ventricular and supraventricular antiarrhythmic (class IA), antitachyarrhythmic

Pregnancy risk category C

Action
Slows diastolic depolarization rate, reduces upstroke velocity, and prolongs duration of action potential and refractory period. Also decreases disparity in refractoriness between infarcted and adjacent normally perfused myocardium.

Availability
Capsules: 100 mg, 150 mg
Capsules (extended-release): 100 mg, 150 mg
Tablets (extended-release): 150 mg

⟋ Indications and dosages
➤ Ventricular tachycardia and other ventricular arrhythmias not severe enough to require cardioversion
Adults weighing more than 50 kg (110 lb): Initially, 200 to 300 mg P.O. as a loading dose, then 150 mg P.O. q 6 hours (conventional capsules) or 300 mg P.O. q 12 hours (extended-release forms)

Adults weighing 50 kg (110 lb) or less: 100 mg P.O. q 6 hours (conventional capsules) or 200 mg P.O. q 12 hours (extended-release capsules)
Children ages 12 to 18: 6 to 15 mg/kg P.O. daily in four divided doses given q 6 hours
Children ages 4 to 11: 10 to 15 mg/kg P.O. daily in four divided doses given q 6 hours
Children ages 1 to 3: 10 to 20 mg/kg P.O. daily in four divided doses given q 6 hours
Children younger than age 1: 10 to 30 mg/kg P.O. daily in four divided doses given q 6 hours
Dosage adjustment
• Renal or hepatic insufficiency
• Acute myocardial infarction

Off-label uses
• Paroxysmal supraventricular tachycardia

Contraindications
• Hypersensitivity to drug
• Cardiogenic shock
• Second- or third-degree heart block
• Sick sinus syndrome

Administration
• Start therapy 6 to 12 hours after last quinidine dose or 3 to 6 hours after last procainamide dose.
◀€ Know that patients with atrial flutter or fibrillation should receive digitalis before beginning disopyramide therapy to ensure that drug doesn't increase ventricular rate.

Route	Onset	Peak	Duration
P.O.	0.5-3.5 hr	2.5 hr	1.5-8.5 hr
P.O. (extended)	0.5-3.5 hr	4.9 hr	12 hr
I.V.	Unknown	Unknown	Unknown

Adverse reactions
CNS: dizziness, agitation, depression,

---

fatigue, headache, nervousness, acute psychosis, syncope

CV: chest pain, orthostatic hypotension, **heart failure, heart block, arrhythmias**

EENT: blurred vision, narrow-angle glaucoma, dry eyes, dry nose

GI: nausea, vomiting, diarrhea, constipation, abdominal pain, bloating, flatulence, dry mouth

GU: urinary hesitancy or retention, impotence

Hematologic: anemia, decreased hemoglobin and hematocrit, **thrombocytopenia, agranulocytosis**

Hepatic: jaundice

Metabolic: hypoglycemia, hypokalemia

Musculoskeletal: muscle weakness, myalgia

Respiratory: dyspnea

Skin: rash, pruritus, dermatoses

Other: edema, decreased appetite, weight gain

Interactions

Drug-drug. *Antiarrhythmics:* increased QRS complex or QT interval

Anticholinergics: increased risk of adverse effects

Erythromycin: increased disopyramide blood level

Phenytoin: increased disopyramide metabolism and blood level

Rifampin: decreased disopyramide blood level

Drug-diagnostic tests. *Blood urea nitrogen, creatinine, hepatic enzymes, lipids:* increased levels

Glucose, hematocrit, hemoglobin: decreased levels

Drug-herb. *Aloe, buckthorn bark or berry, cascara sagrada bark, senna pod or leaf:* increased drug action

Jimsonweed: adverse cardiovascular effects

Precautions

Use cautiously in:

• heart failure, left ventricular dysfunction, hepatic or renal insufficiency,

prostate enlargement, myasthenia gravis, glaucoma, diabetes mellitus, conduction abnormalities

• pregnant or breastfeeding patients

• children.

Patient monitoring

• Check apical pulse before administering. Withhold dose if pulse rate is below 60 or above 120 beats/minute.

• Monitor electrocardiogram for complete heart block.

• Assess for signs and symptoms of heart failure.

• Evaluate for signs and symptoms of fluid retention, such as rapid weight gain.

• Monitor electrolyte levels regularly, checking especially for hypokalemia.

Patient teaching

• Teach patient to weigh himself daily and report weekly gain of more than 2 lb (1 kg).

• Instruct patient to watch for and report ankle swelling.

• Advise patient to move slowly when sitting up or standing to avoid dizziness or light-headedness from sudden blood pressure decrease.

• Instruct patient to avoid driving and other hazardous activities until he knows how drug affects concentration and alertness.

dobutamine hydrochloride
Dobutrex

Pharmacologic class: Sympathomimetic, adrenergic

Therapeutic class: Inotropic

Pregnancy risk category B

Action

Stimulates beta$_1$-adrenergic receptors of heart, causing a positive inotropic effect, which increases myocardial contractility and stroke volume; reduces peripheral vascular resistance, decreases ventricular filling pressure, and promotes atrioventricular conduction.

Availability
Injection: 12.5 mg/ml in 20-ml vial

⚠ Indications and dosages
➤ Short-term treatment of cardiac decompensation caused by depressed contractility (such as during refractory heart failure) and as adjunct in cardiac surgery
Adults: 2.5 to 10 mcg/kg/minute I.V. as a continuous infusion, adjusted to hemodynamic response
Dosage adjustment
• Elderly patients

Off-label uses
• Adjunct in myocardial infarction (MI) and septic shock
• Diagnostic aid in coronary artery disease
• Echocardiography stress test, ventriculography, computed tomography

Contraindications
• Hypersensitivity to drug
• Idiopathic hypertrophic subaortic stenosis

Administration
• Use infusion pump or microdrip I.V. infusion set.
• Dilute with dextrose 5% in water or normal saline solution to at least 50 ml of solution. Know that drug is incompatible with alkaline solutions, such as sodium bicarbonate injection.

Route	Onset	Peak	Duration
I.V.	1-2 min	10 min	Brief

Adverse reactions
CNS: headache
CV: hypertension, hypotension, tachycardia, premature ventricular contrac-

tions, angina, palpitations, nonspecific chest pain, phlebitis
GI: nausea, vomiting
Metabolic: hypokalemia
Respiratory: dyspnea, **asthma attacks**
Skin: extravasation with tissue necrosis
Other: hypersensitivity reaction, **anaphylaxis**

Interactions
Drug-drug. *Beta-adrenergic blockers:* increased alpha-adrenergic effects
Bretylium: potentiation of vasopressor activity
Cyclopropane, halothane: serious arrhythmias
Guanethidine: decreased hypotensive effects
Thyroid hormone: increased cardiovascular effects
Tricyclic antidepressants: potentiation of cardiovascular and vasopressor effects
Drug-herb. *Rue:* increased inotropic potential

Precautions
Use cautiously in:
• hypertension, MI, atrial fibrillation, hypovolemia
• pregnant or breastfeeding patients
• children.

Patient monitoring
• As needed, correct hypovolemia before initiating therapy by giving volume expanders, as prescribed.
• Monitor electrocardiogram and blood pressure continuously during administration.
• Monitor fluid intake and output.
◀€ Assess electrolyte levels; stay especially alert for hypokalemia.

Patient teaching
• Instruct patient to report anginal pain, headache, leg cramps, and shortness of breath.
• Explain need for close observation and monitoring.

• Mix solution thoroughly and infuse over 1 hour, using a polyethylene-lined infusion set.

docetaxel
Taxotere

Pharmacologic class: Miotic inhibitor
Therapeutic class: Antineoplastic
Pregnancy risk category D

Action
Inhibits cellular mitosis by disrupting microtubular network

Availability
Injection concentrate: 20 mg, 80 mg

Indications and dosages
➤ Metastatic breast cancer unresponsive to previous regimens
Adults: 60 to 100 mg/m^2 I.V. over 1 hour q 3 weeks
➤ Metastatic non-small-cell lung cancer
Adults: 75 mg/m^2 I.V. over 1 hour q 3 weeks
Dosage adjustment
• Febrile neutropenia

Contraindications
• Hypersensitivity to drug or polysorbate 80
• Hepatic impairment
• Neutrophil count below 1,500 cells/mm^3

Administration
• Don't allow drug concentrate to come in contact with plasticized polyvinyl chloride equipment or devices.
• Dilute with accompanying diluent solution, and rotate vial gently to mix. Once foam has largely dissipated, withdraw prescribed amount of drug and mix in glass or polypropylene bottle or in plastic bag with 250 ml of normal saline solution or dextrose 5% in water.

Route	Onset	Peak	Duration
I.V.	Rapid	Unknown	7 days

Adverse reactions
CNS: fatigue, asthenia, neurosensory deficits, peripheral neuropathy
CV: peripheral edema, **cardiac tamponade, pericardial effusion**
GI: nausea, vomiting, diarrhea, stomatitis, ascites
Hematologic: anemia, **thrombocytopenia, leukopenia**
Musculoskeletal: myalgia, joint pain
Respiratory: bronchospasm, **pulmonary edema**
Skin: alopecia, rash, dermatitis, desquamation, erythema, nail disorders
Other: edema, hypersensitivity reactions including **anaphylaxis**

Interactions
Drug-drug. *Antineoplastics:* additive bone marrow depression
Cyclosporine, erythromycin, ketoconazole, troleandomycin: significant change in docetaxel effects
Live vaccines: increased risk of infection

Precautions
Use cautiously in:
• females of childbearing age
• pregnant or breastfeeding patients.

Patient monitoring
◀ᔕ Watch for signs and symptoms of anaphylaxis or other hypersensitivity reactions, especially with first two doses.
• Monitor vital signs and fluid intake and output; watch for signs and symptoms of fluid overload and bronchospasm.

• Monitor complete blood count, and assess for signs and symptoms of blood dyscrasias.
• Observe I.V. site frequently for extravasation.
• Assess neurologic status to detect neurosensory deficits and peripheral neuropathy.

Patient teaching
• Instruct patient to weigh himself daily and to immediately report sudden weight gain or difficulty breathing.
• Teach patient signs and symptoms of blood dyscrasias to report, and tell him that he'll have frequent blood tests to monitor these effects.
• Inform patient that hair loss is common with docetaxel use but that hair will grow back after therapy ends.
• Advise female patient of childbearing age to use an effective contraceptive method during therapy and to notify prescriber if she suspects pregnancy.

docusate calcium
DC Softgels, Pro-Cal-Sof, Stool Softener DC, Sulfolax, Surfak Liquigels

docusate sodium
Colace, Diocto, D.O.S. Softgels, D-S-S, Genasoft Plus Softgels, Modane Soft, Regulax SS, Silace

Pharmacologic class: Emollient
Therapeutic class: Stool softener, surfactant
Pregnancy risk category C

Action
Increases absorption of liquid into stool, resulting in softening of fecal mass; also promotes electrolyte and water secretion into colon

Availability
docusate calcium
Capsules: 50 mg, 240 mg
docusate sodium
Capsules: 50 mg, 100 mg
Capsules (soft gel): 100 mg
Liquid: 150 mg/15 ml
Syrup: 50 mg/15 ml, 60 mg/15 ml
Tablets: 100 mg

Indications and dosages
➢ Stool softener
Adults and children older than age 12: 240 mg (docusate calcium) or 50 to 200 mg (docusate sodium) P.O. daily until bowel movements are normal
Children ages 6 to 12: 40 to 120 mg (docusate sodium) P.O. daily
Children ages 3 to 6: 20 to 60 mg (docusate sodium) P.O. daily

Contraindications
• Hypersensitivity to drug
• Abdominal pain, nausea, or vomiting
• Intestinal obstruction

Administration
• Give tablets and capsules with full glass of water.
• Give liquid solution with milk or fruit juice.
• Be aware that excessive or long-term use may lead to laxative dependence.

Route	Onset	Peak	Duration
P.O.	24-48 hr (up to 5 days)	Unknown	Unknown

Adverse reactions
EENT: throat irritation, bitter taste
GI: nausea, diarrhea, mild cramps
Skin: rash
Other: decreased appetite, laxative dependence

Interactions
Drug-drug. *Mineral oil:* increased mineral oil absorption, causing toxicity

Precautions
Use cautiously in:
• pregnant or breastfeeding patients.

Patient monitoring
• If diarrhea occurs, withhold drug and notify prescriber.
• Know that therapeutic efficacy usually becomes apparent 1 to 3 days after first dose.

Patient teaching
• Instruct patient to drink sufficient fluids with each dose and to increase fluid intake during the day.
• Advise patient to prevent constipation by increasing fluids and consuming more dietary fiber (as in fruits and bran).
• Inform patient that excessive or prolonged used may lead to laxative dependence.

dofetilide
Tikosyn

Pharmacologic class: Methanesulfonamide derivative

Therapeutic class: Antiarrhythmic (class III)

Pregnancy risk category C

Action
Selectively blocks potassium channels, prolonging ventricular refractory period and action potential; has no effect on sodium channels

Availability
Capsules: 125 mcg, 250 mcg, 500 mcg

ⓘ Indications and dosages
➤ To convert atrial fibrillation and atrial flutter to normal sinus rhythm; maintenace of normal sinus rhythm

Adults: 500 mcg P.O. b.i.d. if creatinine clearance exceeds 60 ml/minute
Dosage adjustment
• Renal impairment

Off-label uses
• Ventricular arrhythmias

Contraindications
• Hypersensitivity to drug
• Arrhythmias
• Severe renal impairment
• Pregnancy or breastfeeding

Administration
◀€ Be aware that therapy must be initiated in setting that allows continuous electrocardiogram (ECG) monitoring by trained personnel for at least 3 days; such monitoring must be repeated with dosage changes.
• Know that patients with atrial fibrillation require anticoagulation before and during therapy.
• Know that dosage must be individualized according to creatinine clearance and QTc interval (or QT interval if heart rate is below 60 beats/minute), as determined before first dose.
• Be aware that patient shouldn't be discharged for at least 12 hours after conversion to normal sinus rhythm.

Route	Onset	Peak	Duration
P.O.	Unknown	2-3 hr	Unknown

Adverse reactions
CNS: headache, dizziness, insomnia, anxiety, migraine, asthenia, paresthesia, syncope, cerebral ischemia, **cerebrovascular accident**
CV: chest pain, angina, hypertension, palpitations, bradycardia, cerebral ischemia, peripheral edema, **atrial or ventricular fibrillation, ventricular tachycardia, cardiac arrest, myocardial infarction, torsades de pointes, AV block, bundle-branch block**

GI: nausea, diarrhea, abdominal pain
GU: urinary tract infection
Hepatic: hepatic damage
Musculoskeletal: back pain, joint pain, facial paralysis
Respiratory: respiratory tract infection, dyspnea, increased cough
Skin: rash, diaphoresis, angioedema
Other: flulike symptoms

Interactions
Drug-drug. *Amiloride, cimetidine, diltiazem, ketoconazole, macrolides, metformin, nefazodone, norfloxacin, protease inhibitors, quinine, selective serotonin reuptake inhibitors (SSRIs), sulfamethoxazole, triamterene, trimethoprim, verapamil, zafirlukast:* increased dofetilide blood level
CYP450-3A4 inhibitors (such as amiodarone, azole antifungals, cannabinoids, diltiazem, macrolides, nefazodone, norfloxacin, protease inhibitors, quinine, SSRIs, zafirlukast): increased blood level of and systemic exposure to dofetilide
Drug-food. *Grapefruit juice:* decreased metabolism and increased blood level of dofetilide

Precautions
Use cautiously in:
• renal or hepatic impairment, ventricular arrhythmias
• pregnant patients
• children under age 18.

Patient monitoring
• Monitor ECG regularly during first 3 months of therapy, then periodically.
• Monitor electrolyte levels, QTc interval, renal function, and creatinine clearance.
• Assess patient for signs and symptoms of electrolyte imbalances, such as nausea, vomiting, diaphoresis, and diarrhea.

Patient teaching
• Explain reason for initial monitoring and follow-up.
◀€ Instruct patient to immediately report prolonged vomiting, diarrhea, or excessive sweating.

dolasetron mesylate
Anzemet

Pharmacologic class: Selective serotonin subtype 3 (5-HT$_3$) receptor antagonist
Therapeutic class: Antiemetic
Pregnancy risk category B

Action
Blocks serotonin activation at receptor sites in vagal nerve terminals and in chemoreceptor trigger zone in CNS, decreasing the vomiting reflex

Availability
Injection: 12.5 mg/0.625-ml ampules, 20 mg/ml in 5-ml vials
Tablets: 50 mg, 100 mg

🖊 Indications and dosages
➤ Chemotherapy-induced nausea and vomiting
Adults: 100 mg P.O. 1 hour before chemotherapy or 1.8 mg/kg I.V. 30 minutes before chemotherapy
Children ages 2 to 16: 1.8 mg/kg P.O. within 1 hour before chemotherapy or 1.8 mg/kg I.V. (not to exceed 100 mg) 30 minutes before chemotherapy
➤ Prevention or treatment of postoperative nausea and vomiting
Adults: 100 mg P.O. within 2 hours before surgery or 12.5 mg I.V. 15 minutes before cessation of anesthesia (for prevention) or as soon as nausea or vomiting begins (for treatment)
Children ages 2 to 16: 1.2 mg/kg P.O. (up to 100 mg/dose) within 2 hours

---

before surgery or 0.35 mg/kg I.V. (up to 12.5 mg) 15 minutes before cessation of anesthesia (for prevention) or as soon as nausea or vomiting begins (for treatment)

Contraindications
• Hypersensitivity to drug
• Arrhythmias

Administration
• Give oral dose at least 1 hour before chemotherapy for best results.
• To prevent postoperative nausea, give oral dose within 2 hours before surgery.
• If patient has difficulty swallowing tablet, injection solution may be mixed with apple or apple-grape juice and given orally.
• For I.V. use, dilute in normal saline solution, dextrose 5% in water, or lactated Ringer's solution, as ordered. Don't mix with other drugs.
• Flush I.V. line before and after infusion.

Route	Onset	Peak	Duration
P.O.	Unknown	1-2 hr	Up to 24 hr
I.V.	Unknown	15-30 min	Up to 24 hr

Adverse reactions
CNS: headache (increased in cancer patients), dizziness, fatigue, syncope
CV: bradycardia, electrocardiogram (ECG) changes, hypertension, hypotension, tachycardia
GI: diarrhea, constipation, dyspepsia, abdominal pain
GU: oliguria, urinary retention
Skin: pruritus, rash
Other: chills, fever, decreased appetite

Interactions
Drug-drug. *Antiarrhythmics, anthracycline (high cumulative doses), diuretics:* increased risk of conduction abnormalities

Drugs that affect hepatic microsomal enzymes: altered dolasetron blood level
Drug-diagnostic tests. *Alanine aminotransferase, aspartate aminotransferase:* increased levels

Precautions
Use cautiously in:
• patients with risk factors for prolonged cardiac conduction intervals
• pregnant or breastfeeding patients (safety not established).

Patient monitoring
• Monitor closely for excessive diuresis.
◀ Watch for ECG changes, including prolonged PR interval and widened QRS complex, especially in patients receiving antiarrhythmics concurrently.

Patient teaching
• Instruct patient to take drug 1 to 2 hours before chemotherapy.
• Inform patient that drug commonly causes headache.

donepezil hydrochloride
Aricept

Pharmacologic class: Acetylcholinesterase inhibitor
Therapeutic class: Anti-Alzheimer's agent
Pregnancy risk category C

Action
Reversibly inhibits hydrolysis of acetylcholinesterase in CNS, resulting in increased acetylcholine level and temporary cognitive improvement in patients with Alzheimer's disease

Availability
Tablets: 5 mg, 10 mg

⚠️ Indications and dosages

➤ Alzheimer's disease

Adults: Initially, 5 mg P.O. daily at bedtime. After 4 to 6 weeks, dosage may be increased to 10 mg.

Contraindications

• Hypersensitivity to drug
• Pregnancy or breastfeeding

Administration

• For best response, give at bedtime.
• Know that drug may be given with or without food.

Route	Onset	Peak	Duration
P.O.	Unknown	3-4 hr	Unknown

Adverse reactions

CNS: headache, insomnia, dizziness, fatigue, depression, tremor, irritability, paresthesia, aggression, vertigo, restlessness, nervousness, abnormal dreams, aphasia, **seizures**
CV: chest pain, bradycardia, hypertension, hypotension, vasodilation, **atrial fibrillation**
EENT: cataracts, blurred vision, eye irritation, sore throat, toothache
GI: nausea, vomiting, diarrhea, bloating, epigastric pain, GI bleeding, fecal incontinence
GU: urinary frequency, increased libido
Hepatic: hepatotoxicity
Metabolic: dehydration
Musculoskeletal: muscle cramps, arthritis, bone fracture
Respiratory: dyspnea, bronchitis
Skin: pruritus, urticaria, bruising, diaphoresis, rash, flushing
Other: weight loss, hot flashes, decreased appetite, influenza

Interactions

Drug-drug. *Anticholinergics:* reduced donepezil effects
Anticholinesterases, cholinomimetics: synergistic effects

Carbamazepine, dexamethasone, phenobarbitol, phenytoin, rifampin: accelerated donepezil elimination
Nonsteroidal anti-inflammatory drugs (NSAIDs): increased risk of GI bleeding
Drug-herb. *Jaborandi tree, pill-bearing spurge:* increased risk of drug toxicity

Precautions

Use cautiously in:
• cardiovascular disease, chronic obstructive pulmonary disease (COPD)
• history of ulcers, sick sinus syndrome, or GI bleeding
• concurrent NSAID use.

Patient monitoring

• Closely monitor patients with history of asthma or COPD for increased bronchoconstriction.
• Assess cardiovascular status; drug may cause bradycardia from increased vagal tone.
• Monitor closely for signs and symptoms of GI ulcers and bleeding, especially if patient is using NSAIDs concurrently.

Patient teaching

• Advise patient to take drug at bedtime.
• Inform patient that slowing of heart rate may lead to fainting episodes.
◀❦ Instruct patient to immediately report signs or symptoms of GI ulcers, such as "coffee ground" vomitus, black tarry stools, and abdominal pain.

dopamine hydrochloride
Intropin, Revimine❦

Pharmacologic class: Catecholamine, adrenergic

Therapeutic class: Inotropic, vasopressor

Pregnancy risk category C

Action
Causes norepinephrine release (mainly on dopaminergic receptors), which leads to vasodilation of renal and mesenteric arteries; also exerts inotropic effects on heart, which results in increased heart rate, blood flow, myocardial contractility, and stroke volume

Availability
Injection for dilution: 40 mg/ml, 80 mg/ml, 160 mg/ml
Premixed injection: 0.8 mg/ml, 1.6 mg/ml, 3.2 mg/ml in 250 ml and 500 ml of dextrose 5% in water

⚠ Indications and dosages
➤ To treat shock and hemodynamic imbalance unresponsive to fluid replacement; hypotension
Adults and children: Give 1 to 5 mcg/kg/minute by I.V. infusion. Titrate dosage to desired hemodynamic or renal response; may increase infusion by 1 to 4 mcg/kg/minute at 10- to 30-minute intervals.

Off-label uses
• Chronic obstructive pulmonary disease
• Heart failure

Contraindications
• Hypersensitivity to drug or bisulfites
• Tachyarrhythmias, ventricular fibrillation
• Pheochromocytoma
• Hypovolemia

Administration
• Give I.V. infusion using metered pump or other device that controls flow.
• Add 200 to 400 mg of drug to 250 to 500 ml of normal saline solution, 5% dextrose injection, 5% dextrose and half-normal saline solution, or 5% dextrose in lactated Ringer's solution.
• Infuse into large (preferably central) vein to avoid extravasation.

Route	Onset	Peak	Duration
I.V.	1-2 min	Unknown	<10 min

Adverse reactions
CNS: headache
CV: hypotension, angina, electrocardiogram changes, palpitations, tachycardia, vasoconstriction, **arrhythmias**
EENT: mydriasis
GI: nausea, vomiting
GU: elevated urine catecholamine level
Metabolic: azotemia, hyperglycemia
Respiratory: dyspnea, asthma attacks
Skin: piloerection, necrosis
Other: irritation at injection site, **anaphylactic reactions**

Interactions
Drug-drug. *Alpha-adrenergic blockers, beta-adrenergic blockers:* antagonism of dopamine effects
Ergot alkaloids: extreme blood pressure increase
Guanethidine: decreased cardiostimulatory effects
Inhalation anesthetics: increased risk of hypertension, arrhythmias
Monoamine oxidase (MAO) inhibitors: hypertensive crisis
Oxytocics: severe, persistent hypotension
Phenytoin: seizures, severe hypotension, bradycardia
Tricyclic antidepressants: decreased pressor response
Drug-diagnostic tests. *Glucose, nitrogenous compounds:* increased levels

Precautions
Use cautiously in:
• hypovolemia, myocardial infarction, occlusive vascular disease, diabetic endarteritis, atrial embolism
• concurrent MAO inhibitor use
• pregnant or breastfeeding patients
• children.

Patient monitoring

• Monitor blood pressure, pulse, urinary output, and pulmonary artery wedge pressure during infusion.
• Inspect I.V. site regularly for irritation and extravasation.
• Monitor color and temperature of extremities.

◀€ Never stop infusion abruptly because this may cause severe hypotension. Instead, taper dosage gradually.

Patient teaching

• Explain the need for close observation during infusion.
• Instruct patient to report adverse reactions and I.V. site discomfort.

---

dornase alfa
Pulmozyme

Pharmacologic class: Recombinant human deoxyribonuclease 1

Therapeutic class: Cystic fibrosis agent, mucolytic enzyme, respiratory inhalant

Pregnancy risk category B

Action

Selectively cleaves to DNA in sputum, decreasing the viscosity of pulmonary secretions in patients with cystic fibrosis

Availability

Inhalation solution: 2.5-mg ampule (1 mg/ml)

⚕ Indications and dosages

➤ Moderate to severe respiratory tract infections in patients with cystic fibrosis

Adults and children over age 5: One ampule (2.5 mg) inhaled once daily

Contraindications

• Hypersensitivity to drug, its components, or products derived from Chinese hamster ovary cells
• Status asthmaticus
• Respiratory tract infection

Administration

• Don't shake or dilute drug.
• Use only with approved nebulizer.
• Discard cloudy or discolored solution.

Route	Onset	Peak	Duration
Inhalation	3-7 days	9 days	Unknown

Adverse reactions

CV: chest pain
EENT: conjunctivitis, rhinitis, pharyngitis, hemoptysis, voice changes
Respiratory: dyspnea, increased sputum, wheezing
Skin: rash, urticaria, pruritus
Other: hypersensitivity reactions

Precautions

Use cautiously in:
• nonasthmatic bronchial disease, asthma controlled by bronchodilators
• pregnant or breastfeeding patients.

Patient monitoring

• Assess patient periodically; report improvement in dyspnea and sputum clearance.
• Monitor for signs and symptoms of hypersensitivity reaction.

Patient teaching

• Teach patient proper use of nebulizer.
• Instruct patient to report rash, hives, and itching.

---

doxacurium chloride
Nuromax

Pharmacologic class: Neuromuscular blocker (nondepolarizing)

Therapeutic class: Muscle relaxant, adjunct to anesthesia

Pregnancy risk category C

Action
Competes with the neurotransmitter acetylcholine for receptor sites at motor end plates of skeletal muscles, inhibiting impulse transmission, thereby causing relaxation

Availability
Injection: 1 mg/ml

Indications and dosages
➤ To sustain neuromuscular blockade during prolong procedures

Adults: Initially, 0.05 mg/kg I.V.; for maintenance, 0.005 to 0.01 mg/kg to prolong neuromuscular blockade for an average of 30 to 45 minutes

➤ Adjunct to general anesthesia to relax skeletal muscles during surgery

Adults: 0.05 mg/kg rapid I.V.; produces adequate neuromuscular blockade for endotracheal intubation in 5 minutes when used as part of thiopental-narcotic induction technique. Adequate neuromuscular blockade at this dosage lasts an average of 100 minutes.

Children over age 2: Initially, 0.03 mg/kg I.V. with halothane anesthesia; produces effective neuromuscular blockade in 7 minutes, with duration of 30 minutes. Or 0.05 mg/kg produces neuromuscular blockade in 4 minutes, with duration of 45 minutes.

Dosage adjustment
• Hepatic impairment
• Renal impairment

Contraindications
• Hypersensitivity to drug
• Neonates

Administration
◀℈ Be aware that drug contains benzyl alcohol, which has been linked to fatal complications in neonates.

• Know that children require higher dosages than adults (on a mg/kg basis) to achieve same level of blockade.

• Dilute each 1 mg with 10 ml of dextrose 5% in water, normal saline solution, lactated Ringer's solution, or dextrose 5% in lactated Ringer's solution to yield a concentration of 0.1 mg/ml.

• Give by I.V. push over 5 to 10 seconds.

• Always give concurrently with sedative, amnesiac, or analgesic, as prescribed.

• Store undiluted at room temperature.

Route	Onset	Peak	Duration
I.V.	Variable	Variable	Variable

Adverse reactions
Musculoskeletal: prolonged muscle weakness

Respiratory: dyspnea, **respiratory depression or insufficiency, apnea**

Interactions
Drug-drug. *Acetylcholinesterase inhibitors:* inhibition of muscle relaxation and reversal of neuromuscular blockade

Aminoglycosides, beta-adrenergic blockers, enflurane, halothane, isoflurane, lithium, procainamide, trimethaphan, verapamil: increased muscle relaxation

Carbamazepine, phenytoin, theophylline: resistance to or reversal of neuromuscular blockade; possibly prolonged time to maximum blockade or shortened blockade duration

Clindamycin, lithium, magnesium salts, opioids, polymyxin antibiotics (colistin, polymyxin B sulfate), procainamide,

quinine, thiazide and loop diuretics: increased neuromuscular blockade
Corticosteroids: prolonged weakness
Edrophonium, neostigmine, pyridostigmine: reversal of neuromuscular blockade, inhibition of doxacurium effect
Succinylcholine: quicker onset and increased depth of muscle relaxation

Precautions
Use cautiously in:
• renal or hepatic impairment, severe electrolyte imbalances, metastatic cancer, myasthenia gravis
• elderly patients.

Patient monitoring
• Evaluate for adequate neuromuscular blockade.
• Assess vital signs; monitor closely for hypoxia and hypercapnia.
◀€ Monitor for respiratory depression, which may occur up to 48 hours after administration.
◀€ Keep lifesaving equipment in immediate area; drug may cause profound, prolonged paralysis leading to respiratory insufficiency, apnea, fatal bronchospasm, ventricular fibrillation, or acute myocardial infarction (MI).
• Keep suction equipment available to control secretions and saliva.
• Support ventilation until patient has recovered fully from neuromuscular blockade.

Patient teaching
• Inform patient that he may experience mild to moderate discomfort in neck, upper back, and abdominal muscles when he first starts walking around after drug administration.
• Explain importance of coughing, deep breathing, and incentive spirometry after recovery.

doxapram hydrochloride
Dopram

Pharmacologic class: CNS and respiratory stimulant
Therapeutic class: Analeptic
Pregnancy risk category B

Action
Activates peripheral carotid, aortic, and other chemoreceptors to stimulate respiration; also increases tidal volume and respiratory rate by directly stimulating respiratory center in medulla oblongata

Availability
Injection: 20 mg/ml

⃫ Indications and dosages
➤ Respiratory depression after anesthesia
Adults and adolescents: 5 mg/minute by I.V. infusion until desired response is achieved; then reduce to 1 to 3 mg/minute, to a maximum cumulative dosage of 4 mg/kg (or 300 mg); or 0.5 to 1 mg/kg I.V. injection, repeated q 5 minutes, if needed, to a maximum total dose of 1.5 mg/kg
➤ Chronic pulmonary disease related to acute hypercapnia
Adults: 1 to 2 mg/minute by I.V. infusion, using a concentration of 2 mg/ml, to a maximum of 3 mg/minute; infusion not to exceed 2 hours
➤ Drug-induced CNS depression
Adults: Initially, 2 mg/kg I.V., repeated in 5 minutes and then q 1 to 2 hours until patient awakens, to a maximum daily dosage of 3 g. For infusion, priming dose of 2 mg/kg I.V.; if no response occurs, continue for 1 to 2 hours as needed; if some response occurs, give I.V. infusion of 250 mg in 250 ml of saline solution or dextrose 5% in water

---

at 1 to 3 mg/minute until patient awakens. Don't infuse longer than 2 hours or give more than 3 g/day.

Off-label uses

• Laryngospasm secondary to postoperative tracheal extubation

Contraindications

• Hypersensitivity to drug
• Cardiovascular disorders
• Cerebrovascular accident
• Head injury, seizures
• Respiratory failure or restrictive respiratory disease
• Neonates

Administration

• Ensure adequate airway and oxygenation before giving drug.
• Give slowly to avoid hemolysis.

Route	Onset	Peak	Duration
I.V.	20-40 sec	1-2 min	5-12 min

Adverse reactions

CNS: weakness, dysarthria, dysphonia, dizziness, drowsiness, headache, loss of consciousness, disorientation, hyperactivity, paresthesia, **seizures**
CV: hypotension, bradycardia, chest pain or tightness, heart rate changes, thrombophlebitis (with I.V. use), **atrioventricular block, arrhythmias, cardiac arrest**
EENT: lacrimation, diplopia, miosis, conjunctival hyperemia, sneezing, **laryngospasm**
GI: nausea, vomiting, diarrhea, abdominal cramps, increased salivation, dysphagia
GU: urinary frequency or incontinence, albuminuria
Musculoskeletal: muscle cramps, fasciculations
Respiratory: dyspnea, increased secretions, **respiratory muscle paralysis, central respiratory paralysis, bronchospasm, respiratory depression, respiratory arrest**
Skin: rash, diaphoresis, flushing
Other: anaphylaxis

Interactions

Drug-drug. *General anesthetics:* increased risk of self-limiting arrhythmias
Monoamine oxidase inhibitors, sympathomimetics: potentiation of adverse cardiovascular effects
Skeletal muscle relaxants: masking of residual effects of muscle relaxant
Drug-diagnostic tests. *Blood urea nitrogen:* increased level
Erythrocytes, hematocrit, hemoglobin, red blood cells, white blood cells: decreased values

Precautions

Use cautiously in:
• bronchial asthma, arrhythmias, increased intracranial pressure, hyperthyroidism, pheochromocytoma, metabolic disorders
• pregnant or breastfeeding patients.

Patient monitoring

• Assess blood pressure, pulse, deep tendon reflexes, airway, and arterial blood gas values before initiating therapy and frequently during infusion.
• Monitor I.V. site frequently for irritation or thrombophlebitis.
◀€ Discontinue infusion immediately if hypotension or dyspnea suddenly develops.

Patient teaching

• Teach patient about purpose of drug.
• Instruct patient to report adverse reactions promptly.

doxazosin mesylate
Cardura

Pharmacologic class: Sympatholytic, peripherally acting antiadrenergic
Therapeutic class: Antihypertensive
Pregnancy risk category C

Action
Blocks alpha$_1$-adrenergic receptors, promoting vasodilation; also reduces urethral resistance, relieving obstruction and improving urine flow and symptoms of benign prostatic hypertrophy (BPH)

Availability
Tablets: 1 mg, 2 mg, 4 mg, 8 mg

⚕ Indications and dosages
➤ Hypertension
Adults: 1 mg P.O. once daily; may increase dosage gradually q 2 weeks, up to 2 to 16 mg daily
➤ BPH
Adults: 1 mg P.O. once daily; may increase dosage gradually, up to 8 mg daily

Off-label uses
- Pheochromocytoma
- Syndrome X

Contraindications
- Hypersensitivity to drug or quinazoline derivatives

Administration
- Give initial dose at bedtime to minimize orthostatic hypotension and syncope.
- Know that incidence of orthostatic hypotension increases greatly when daily dosage exceeds 4 mg; usually occurs within 6 hours of administration.

Route	Onset	Peak	Duration
P.O.	1-2 hr	2-6 hr	24 hr

Adverse reactions
CNS: dizziness, vertigo, headache, depression, drowsiness, fatigue, nervousness, weakness, asthenia
CV: orthostatic hypotension, chest pain, palpitations, tachycardia, **arrhythmias**
EENT: abnormal or blurred vision, conjunctivitis, epistaxis, rhinitis, pharyngitis
GI: nausea, vomiting, diarrhea, constipation, abdominal discomfort, flatulence, dry mouth
GU: decreased libido, sexual dysfunction
Respiratory: dyspnea
Musculoskeletal: joint pain, arthritis, gout, myalgia
Skin: flushing, rash, pruritus
Other: edema

Interactions
Drug-drug. *Clonidine:* decreased antihypertensive effect of clonidine
Nitrates, other antihypertensives: additive hypotension
Drug-diagnostic tests. *Neutrophils, white blood cells:* decreased counts
Drug-herb. *Butcher's broom:* decreased doxazosin effects
Drug-behaviors. *Alcohol use:* additive hypotension

Precautions
Use cautiously in:
- renal or hepatic impairment, heart failure
- elderly patients
- pregnant or breastfeeding patients
- children (safety not established).

Patient monitoring
- Monitor blood pressure with patient both lying down and standing every 2 to 6 hours after initial dose or dosage

---

increase (when orthostatic hypotension is most likely to occur).

Patient teaching
• Instruct patient not to drive or engage in other potentially hazardous activities for 12 to 24 hours after first dose.
• Teach patient to move slowly when sitting up or standing to avoid dizziness or light-headedness from sudden blood pressure decrease.
• Advise patient to report episodes of dizziness or palpitations.

doxepin hydrochloride
Apo-Doxepin✤, Novo-Doxepin✤, Sinequan

Pharmacologic class: Tricyclic antidepressant
Therapeutic class: Antidepressant, anxiolytic
Pregnancy risk category C

Action
Unknown; may prevent reuptake of norepinephrine, serotonin, or both at presynaptic neurons, increasing levels of these neurotransmitters in CNS

Availability
Capsules: 10 mg, 25 mg, 50 mg, 75 mg, 100 mg, 150 mg
Oral concentrate: 10 mg/ml

🔾 Indications and dosages
➤ Endogenous depression (in conjunction with psychotherapy); anxiety
Adults: Initially, 25 mg P.O. t.i.d.; increased as needed up to 150 mg daily in outpatients and 300 mg daily in inpatients. (Some patients may require only 25 to 50 mg daily.) Once stabilized, patient may receive entire daily dose at bedtime.

Elderly adults: Initially, 25 to 50 mg P.O. daily; may be increased as needed

Off-label uses
• Adjunct in peptic ulcer disease

Contraindications
• Hypersensitivity to drug or bisulfites
• Untreated narrow-angle glaucoma
• Recent myocardial infarction (MI)
• Monoamine oxidase (MAO) inhibitor use within past 14 days
• Pregnancy or breastfeeding

Administration
• If desired, mix capsule contents with food.
• Dilute oral concentrate with 120 ml of water, milk, or juice; be aware that drug is incompatible with carbonated beverages.
• Know that drug may be given at bedtime to prevent daytime sleepiness.
◀◧ Don't give within 14 days of MAO inhibitor; drug interaction may cause cardiovascular instability.
◀◧ Avoid concurrent use of other CNS depressants because inadvertent overdose may occur.

Route	Onset	Peak	Duration
P.O.	Unknown	2 hr	Unknown

Adverse reactions
CNS: fatigue, sedation, agitation, confusion, hallucinations, drowsiness, dizziness, extrapyramidal reactions, poor concentration, syncope, **seizures, cerebrovascular accident (CVA)**
CV: hypotension, orthostatic hypotension, hypertension, electrocardiogram changes, tachycardia, palpitations, **arrhythmias, MI, heart block**
EENT: blurred vision, increased intraocular pressure, lacrimation, tinnitus, nasal congestion
GI: nausea, constipation, dry mouth, **paralytic ileus**
GU: urinary retention, delayed voiding, urinary tract dilation, gynecomas-

tia, galactorrhea, menstrual irregularities, testicular swelling, libido changes

Hematologic: purpura, **blood dyscrasias, bone marrow depression, eosinophilia, agranulocytosis, thrombocytopenia, leukopenia**

Hepatic: elevated hepatic enzyme levels, bilirubinemia, **hepatitis**

Metabolic: hypoglycemia, hyperglycemia

Skin: photosensitivity, rash, urticaria, pruritus, diaphoresis, flushing, vasculitis, petechiae, alopecia

Other: increased appetite, weight gain or loss, hyperthermia, chills, edema, drug-induced fever, hypersensitivity reactions

Interactions

Drug-drug. *Barbiturates, CNS depressants (including antihistamines, clonidine, opioids, sedative-hypnotics):* additive CNS depression

Carbamazepine, class IC antiarrhythmics (flecainide, propafenone), other antidepressants, other CYP450-2D6 inhibitors (amiodarone, cimetidine, quinidine, ritonavir), phenothiazines: increased doxepin blood level and effects

Clonidine: hypertensive crisis

Guanethidine: antagonism of antihypertensive effects

Levodopa: delayed or decreased levodopa absorption, hypertension

MAO inhibitors: tachycardia, seizures, potentially fatal reactions

Rifamycin: decreased doxepin effects

Selective serotonin reuptake inhibitors (SSRIs): increased risk of toxicity

Sparfloxacin: increased risk of adverse cardiovascular effects

Drug-diagnostic tests. *Alkaline phosphatase, bilirubin:* increased levels

Glucose: increased or decreased level

Liver function tests: altered results

Drug-herb. *Angel's trumpet, jimsonweed, scopolia:* increased anticholinergic effects

Chamomile, hops, kava, skullcap, valerian: increased CNS depression

Evening primrose oil: additive or synergistic effects

S-adenosylmethionine (SAM-e), St. John's wort, yohimbe: serotonin syndrome

Drug-behaviors. *Alcohol use:* increased CNS depression

Smoking: increased drug metabolism and altered effects

Sun exposure: increased risk of photosensitivity reactions

Precautions

Use cautiously in:
• cardiovascular disease, prostatic enlargement, seizures
• elderly patients.

Patient monitoring

• Evaluate efficacy of concurrent antihypertensives.
• Record mood changes; watch for suicidal tendencies.
• Assess bowel elimination pattern; increase fluids and administer stool softeners as ordered to ease constipation.
• Monitor fluid intake and output; report changes in voiding pattern.
• Monitor liver function test results and glucose level.

Patient teaching

• Advise patient on long-term therapy not to stop taking drug abruptly because this may lead to nausea, headache, and malaise.
• Instruct patient to avoid driving and other hazardous activities until he knows how drug affects concentration and alertness.
• Instruct patient to move slowly when sitting up or standing to avoid dizziness or light-headedness from sudden blood pressure decrease.
• Explain that drowsiness and dizziness usually subside after several weeks.

doxorubicin hydrochloride
Adriamycin PFS, Adriamycin RDF, Rubex

Pharmacologic class: Anthracycline
Therapeutic class: Antibiotic antineoplastic
Pregnancy risk category D

Action
Unclear; thought to inhibit DNA and RNA synthesis by forming complex with DNA; also has immunosuppressive activity. Cell-cycle–S-phase specific.

Availability
Injection (preservative-free): 2 mg/ml
Powder for injection: 10 mg, 20 mg, 50 mg, 100 mg, 150 mg

Indications and dosages
➤ Solid tumors, including bladder, breast, lung, stomach, and thyroid cancers; malignant lymphomas including Hodgkin's disease; acute leukemia; Wilms' tumor; neuroblastoma
Adults: 60 to 75 mg/m² I.V. as a single dose on 21-day cycles, or 30 mg/m² I.V. as a single daily dose on first to third days of 4-week cycle, or 20 mg/m² I.V. once weekly. Maximum cumulative dosage is 550 mg/m².
Dosage adjustment
• Bone marrow depression
• Impaired cardiac or hepatic function

Off-label uses
• Endometrial carcinoma and islet cell carcinoma
• Chronic lymphocytic leukemia
• Multiple myeloma

Contraindications
• Hypersensitivity to drug
• Severe bone marrow depression

• Previous treatment with maximum cumulative doses of doxorubicin or other anthracyclines or anthracenes

Administration
• Follow facility policy for handling and preparation of antineoplastics.
◀€ Don't dilute solution with bacteriostatic diluent. Don't mix with other drugs.
• Dilute as directed with normal saline solution to a final concentration of 2 mg/ml.
• Administer slowly over 3 to 5 minutes into tubing of free-flowing I.V. infusion of normal saline solution or dextrose 5% in water.
• Deliver into large vein using butterfly needle. Avoid veins over joints or extremities with compromised venous or lymphatic drainage.
◀€ Avoid rapid infusion because this may increase risk of acute infusion-related reactions (back pain, chest tightness, flushing).
◀€ If extravasation occurs, stop infusion immediately, apply ice, and notify prescriber.

Route	Onset	Peak	Duration
I.V.	Rapid	2 hr	24-36 days

Adverse reactions
CNS: asthenia, paresthesia, headache, drowsiness, dizziness, depression, insomnia, anxiety, malaise, emotional lability, fatigue
CV: chest pain, hypotension, tachycardia, peripheral edema, **cardiomyopathy, heart failure, arrhythmias, pericardial effusion**
GI: nausea, vomiting, diarrhea, constipation, enlarged abdomen, abdominal pain, dyspepsia, oral candidiasis, moniliasis, stomatitis, glossitis, esophagitis, dysphagia, abnormal taste
GU: albuminuria, hyperuricuria, red urine

Hematologic: anemia, **leukopenia, thrombocytopenia, neutropenia, bone marrow depression**
Hepatic: increased alkaline phosphatase and bilirubin levels
Metabolic: hyperglycemia, hypocalcemia
Musculoskeletal: myalgia, back pain
Respiratory: dyspnea, increased cough, pneumonia
Skin: exfoliative dermatitis, diaphoresis, alopecia, palmar-plantar erythrodysesthesia, rash, dry skin, pruritus, skin discoloration
Other: infection, chills, fever, herpes zoster, injection site reactions, allergic reactions, **acute infusion-associated reactions, anaphylaxis**

Interactions

Drug-drug. *Antineoplastics:* additive bone marrow depression
Cyclophosphamide: increased risk of hemorrhagic cystitis, increased cardiotoxicity
Cyclosporine: profound and prolonged hematologic toxicity, increased risk of coma and seizures
Dactinomycin (in children): increased risk of pneumonitis
Live-virus vaccines: decreased antibody response to vaccine, increased risk of adverse reactions
Mercaptopurine: hepatitis
Paclitaxel (if given first): reduced doxorubicin clearance, increased incidence and severity of neutropenia and stomatitis
Phenobarbital: increased clearance and decreased effects of doxorubicin
Phenytoin: decreased phenytoin blood level
Progesterone: increased incidence and severity of neutropenia and thrombocytopenia
Streptozocin: increased doxorubicin half-life
Verapamil: increased doxorubicin blood level

Drug-diagnostic tests. *Bilirubin, glucose, prothrombin time, serum and urine uric acid:* increased levels
Calcium, hemoglobin, neutrophils, platelets, white blood cells (WBCs): decreased values

Precautions

Use cautiously in:
• cardiac disease, hepatic impairment, depressed bone marrow reserve, CNS metastases, brain tumor, malignant melanoma, renal carcinoma
• elderly patients
• females of childbearing age
• pregnant or breastfeeding patients
• children.

Patient monitoring

◀Ɛ Watch for acute life-threatening arrhythmias, which may occur during or within a few hours after administration.

◀Ɛ Monitor for cardiomyopathy and subsequent heart failure with chronic overdose (more common in children).

• Stay alert for erythematous streaking along vein next to injection site, which may indicate too-rapid infusion.

• Watch for nausea and vomiting; administer antiemetics as needed.

• Check for superinfection or hemorrhage from persistent bone marrow depression (but expect WBC counts as low as 1,000/mm³ during therapy).

• Monitor complete blood count; hepatic profile; coagulation tests; glucose, uric acid, and calcium blood levels; and ejection fraction.

Patient teaching

• Caution patient to avoid people with colds, flu, or other contagious illnesses.
• Explain that drug may cause complete but reversible hair loss.
• Inform patient that drug may turn urine red for 1 or 2 days.

---

doxorubicin hydrochloride liposomal
Caelyx✦, Doxil

Pharmacologic class: Anthracycline
Therapeutic class: Antibiotic anti-neoplastic
Pregnancy risk category D

Action
Unclear; thought to inhibit DNA and RNA synthesis by forming complex with DNA; also has immunosuppressive activity. Liposomal encapsulation increases uptake by tumors, prolongs drug action, and may decrease toxicity. Cell-cycle–S-phase specific.

Availability
Liposomal dispersion for injection: 20 mg/10 ml in 10-ml vials

⊘ Indications and dosages
➤ First-line therapy for AIDS-related Kaposi's sarcoma i
Adults: 20 mg/m² I.V. over 30 minutes once q 3 weeks
➤ Metastatic ovarian carcinoma in patients with disease that resists paclitaxel- and platinum-based chemotherapy
Adults: Initially, 50 mg/m² I.V. at a rate of 1 mg/minute q 4 weeks for at least four courses. If no adverse reactions appear, increase infusion rate to complete over 1 hour.
Dosage adjustment
• Hepatic impairment

Contraindications
• Hypersensitivity to drug
• Malignant melanoma
• CNS metastases
• Bone marrow depression
• Cardiac disease

Administration
• Follow facility policy for handling and preparation of antineoplastics.
• Dilute dose (up to 90 mg) in 250 ml of dextrose 5% in water. Don't use any other diluent.
◀€ Don't dilute solution with bacteriostatic diluent. Don't mix with other drugs.
• Don't use in-line filter.
• Administer slowly by I.V. infusion; don't give as I.V. bolus.
◀€ Avoid rapid infusion because this may increase risk of infusion-related reactions (back pain, chest tightness, flushing).
• Don't give I.M. or S.C.
◀€ If extravasation occurs, stop infusion immediately, apply ice, and notify prescriber.
• Know that drug is a translucent red dispersion, not a clear solution.

Route	Onset	Peak	Duration
I.V.	10 days	14 days	21-24 days

Adverse reactions
CNS: asthenia, paresthesia, headache, drowsiness, dizziness, depression, insomnia, anxiety, malaise, emotional lability, fatigue
CV: chest pain, hypotension, tachycardia, peripheral edema, **cardiomyopathy, heart failure, arrhythmias, pericardial effusion**
GI: nausea, vomiting, diarrhea, constipation, abdominal pain, enlarged abdomen, dyspepsia, moniliasis, stomatitis, glossitis, oral candidiasis, esophagitis, dysphagia, altered taste
GU: albuminuria, red urine
Hematologic: anemia, **leukopenia, thrombocytopenia, neutropenia, bone marrow depression**
Hepatic: jaundice, elevated alkaline phosphatase and bilirubin levels
Metabolic: hypocalcemia, hyperglycemia
Musculoskeletal: myalgia, back pain

Respiratory: dyspnea, increased cough, pneumonia

Skin: exfoliative dermatitis, diaphoresis, alopecia, palmar-plantar erythrodysesthesia, rash, dry skin, pruritus, skin discoloration

Other: fever, chills, infection, herpes zoster, injection site reactions, allergic reactions, **infusion reaction, anaphylaxis**

Interactions

Drug-drug. *Antineoplastics:* additive bone marrow depression

Cyclophosphamide: increased risk of hemorrhagic cystitis

Cyclosporine: profound, prolonged hematologic toxicity, increased risk of coma and seizures, increased cardiotoxicity

Dactinomycin (in children): increased risk of pneumonitis

Live-virus vaccines: decreased antibody response to vaccine, increased risk of adverse reactions

Mercaptopurine: hepatitis

Paclitaxel (if administered first): reduced doxorubicin clearance, increased incidence and severity of neutropenia and stomatitis

Phenobarbital: increased clearance and decreased effects of doxorubicin

Phenytoin: decreased phenytoin blood level

Progesterone: increased risk and severity of neutropenia and thrombocytopenia

Streptozocin: prolonged doxorubicin half-life

Verapamil: increased doxorubicin blood level

Drug-diagnostic tests. *Bilirubin, glucose, prothrombin time, serum and urine uric acid:* increased values

Calcium, hemoglobin, neutrophils, platelets, white blood cells: decreased values

Precautions

Use cautiously in:
• cardiac disease, hepatic impairment, depressed bone marrow reserve, CNS metastases, brain tumor, malignant melanoma, renal carcinoma
• elderly patients
• females of childbearing age
• pregnant or breastfeeding patients
• children.

Patient monitoring

◀€ Observe closely for anaphylaxis and bleeding problems.

◀€ Monitor for acute life-threatening arrhythmias, which may occur during or within a few hours of administration.

◀€ Assess for cardiomyopathy and subsequent heart failure with chronic overdose (more common in children).

• Assess for and report liver engorgement and yellowing of skin or eyes.

• Check bilirubin, glucose, and calcium levels; coagulation tests; uric acid levels; hepatic profile; and complete blood count.

• Watch for nausea and vomiting; give antiemetics, as needed and prescribed.

• Assess for constipation and give fluids and stool softeners, as prescribed.

Patient teaching

• Instruct patient to immediately report shortness of breath, peripheral edema, chest pain, or palpitations.

• Advise patient to avoid people with colds, flu, or other contagious illnesses.

• As appropriate, review all significant life-threatening adverse reactions and interactions, especially those drugs and tests mentioned above.

doxycycline
Periostat, Vibramycin

doxycycline calcium
Vibramycin

doxycycline hyclate
Apo-Doxy✿, Doryx, Doxy 100, Doxy-Caps, Doxychel Hyclate, Doxycin✿, Periostat, Vibramycin, Vibra-Tabs

doxycycline monohydrate
Monodox, Vibramycin

Pharmacologic class: Tetracycline
Therapeutic class: Anti-infective
Pregnancy risk category D

Action
Unclear; thought to inhibit bacterial protein synthesis at 30S and 50S ribosomal submit and alters cytoplasmic membrane of susceptible organisms

Availability
Capsules: 20 mg, 50 mg, 100 mg
Capsules (coated pellets): 75 mg, 100 mg
Powder for injection: 100 mg, 200 mg
Powder for oral suspension: 25 mg/5 ml
Syrup: 50 mg
Tablets: 20 mg, 50 mg, 75 mg, 100 mg

Indications and dosages
➤ Infections caused by unusual organisms, including *Mycoplasma, Chlamydia, Rickettsia,* and *Borrelia burgdorferi*
Adults and children weighing more than 45 kg (99 lb): 100 mg P.O. q 12 hours on first day, then 100 to 200 mg P.O. once daily; or 50 to 100 mg P.O. q 12 hours; or 200 mg I.V. once daily; or 100 mg I.V. q 12 hours on first day, then 100 to 200 mg I.V. once daily; or 50 to 100 mg I.V. q 12 hours

Children weighing 45 kg (99 lb) or less: 2.2 mg/kg P.O. q 12 hours on first day, then 2.2 to 4.4 mg/kg/day P.O. once daily; or 1.1 to 2.2 mg/kg P.O. q 12 hours; or 4.4 mg/kg I.V. once daily; or 2.2 mg/kg I.V. q 12 hours on first day, then 2.2 to 4.4 mg/kg I.V. once daily; or 1.1 to 2.2 mg/kg I.V. q 12 hours

➤ Gonorrhea in penicillin-allergic patients
Adults and children weighing more than 45 kg (99 lb): 100 mg P.O. q 12 hours for 7 days; or 300 mg P.O. initially, followed by another 300 mg P.O. 1 hour later

➤ Lyme disease
Adults and children weighing more than 45 kg (99 lb): 100 mg P.O. b.i.d. for 10 to 30 days

➤ Periodontitis
Adults and children weighing more than 45 kg (99 lb): 20 mg P.O. b.i.d. for up to 9 months

➤ Anthrax
Adults and children weighing more than 45 kg (99 lb): 100 mg P.O. b.i.d. for 60 days; or 100 mg I.V. q 12 hours, changing to oral route when appropriate, for 60 days
Children weighing 45 kg (99 lb) or less: 2.2 mg/kg P.O. b.i.d. for 60 days; or 100 mg I.V. q 12 hours, changing to oral route when appropriate, for 60 days

➤ Prevention of malaria caused by *Plasmodium falciparum* in short-term travelers (less than 4 months) to areas with strains resistant to chloroquine or pyrimethamine and sulfadoxine
Adults: 100 mg/day P.O. starting 1 to 2 days before travel begins and continuing during travel and for 4 weeks afterward
Children: 2 mg/kg/day P.O., up to adult dosage of 100 mg/day, starting 1 to 2 days before travel begins and continuing during travel and for 4 weeks afterward

d

Off-label uses

- Traveller's diarrhea
- Pleural effusion

Contraindications

- Hypersensitivity to drug or bisulfites
- Pregnancy or breastfeeding (except in anthrax treatment)
- Children younger than age 8 (except in anthrax treatment)

Administration

- Obtain specimen for culture and sensitivity testing, as ordered, before first dose.
- ◀€ Don't give in conjunction with methoxyflurane anesthetic; severe or fatal kidney damage may result.
- Reconstitute powder for injection with dextrose 5% in water, normal saline solution, lactated Ringer's solution, or dextrose 5% in lactated Ringer's solution.
- Don't infuse solution with concentrations of more than 1 mg/ml.
- Know that 100-mg dose should be infused over at least 1 hour.
- Complete infusion within 12 hours of dilution, unless diluted with lactated Ringer's solution or dextrose 5% in lactated Ringer's solution; in this case, complete infusion within 6 hours.
- Don't give during last half of pregnancy or to children under age 8; drug may cause tooth discoloration and malformation and bone growth retardation.

Route	Onset	Peak	Duration
P.O.	1-2 hr	1.5-4 hr	12 hr
I.V.	Rapid	End of infusion	12 hr

Adverse reactions

CNS: benign intracranial hypertension (pseudotumor cerebri), paresthesia
CV: thrombophlebitis, phlebitis, pericarditis
EENT: vestibular reactions, black hairy tongue, glossitis, hoarseness, oral candidiasis, tooth enamel defects, pharyngitis
GI: nausea, vomiting, diarrhea, esophagitis, epigastric distress, enterocolitis, anogenital lesions or inflammation, **pancreatitis**
GU: dark yellow or brown urine, elevated blood urea nitrogen (BUN), vaginal candidiasis
Hematologic: eosinophilia, hemolytic anemia, **neutropenia, thrombocytopenia**
Hepatic: elevated aspartate aminotransferase (AST), alanine aminotransferase (ALT), alkaline phosphatase (ALP), bilirubin, and amylase levels; **hepatotoxicity**
Musculoskeletal: bone growth retardation (in children younger than age 8)
Skin: photosensitivity, maculopapular or erythematous rash, hyperpigmentation, urticaria
Other: increased appetite, phlebitis at I.V. site, hypersensitivity reactions, superinfection, **anaphylaxis**

Interactions

Drug-drug. *Adsorbent antidiarrheals; antacids; calcium, iron, and magnesium preparations:* decreased doxycycline absorption
Barbiturates, carbamazepine, hormonal contraceptives containing estrogen, phenytoin, rifamycin: decreased doxycycline efficacy
Cholestyramine, colestipol: decreased oral absorption of doxycycline
Methoxyflurane: increased nephrotoxicity
Penicillin: decreased penicillin activity
Sucralfate: prevention of doxycycline absorption from GI tract
Warfarin: enhanced warfarin effects
Drug-diagnostic tests. *ALP, ALT, amylase, AST, bilirubin, BUN:* increased levels
Hemoglobin, neutrophils, platelets, white blood cells: decreased values
Urine catecholamines: false elevation

Drug-food. *Calcium-containing foods, dairy products:* decreased drug absorption

Drug-behaviors: *Alcohol use:* decreased anti-infective effect
Sun exposure: increased risk of photosensitivity

Precautions

Use cautiously in:
• renal disease, hepatic impairment, nephrogenic diabetes insipidus, cachexia.

Patient monitoring

• Evaluate I.V. site regularly; apply cool compresses as needed.
• Monitor hepatic profile, complete blood count, and BUN and creatinine levels.
• Assess for hypercoagulability in patients taking warfarin concurrently.
• Monitor for digoxin toxicity in patients taking digoxin concurrently.

Patient teaching

• Advise patient to take with 8 oz of water to ensure passage into stomach.
• Tell patient to take on empty stomach at least 1 hour before meals or 2 hours afterwards.
• Instruct patient to take drug at least 1 hour before bedtime to prevent esophagitis.
◀ Tell patient to immediately report painful swallowing.
• Stress importance of good oral hygiene.

dronabinol
Marinol

Pharmacologic class: Cannabinoid
Therapeutic class: Antiemetic
Controlled substance schedule IV
Pregnancy risk category B

Action

Unknown; may exert antiemetic effect by inhibiting vomiting control mechanism in medulla oblongata

Availability

Capsules: 2.5 mg, 5 mg, 10 mg

d

🚫 Indications and dosages

➤ Prevention of nausea and vomiting caused by chemotherapy

Adults and children: Initially, 5 mg/m² P.O. 1 to 3 hours before chemotherapy. Repeat dose q 2 to 4 hours after chemotherapy up to four to six doses per day. If 5-mg/m² dose is ineffective and patient has no significant adverse reactions, dosage may be increased in increments of 2.5 mg/m² to a maximum dosage of 15 mg/m².

➤ Appetite stimulant

Adults and children: Initially, 2.5 mg P.O. b.i.d. May reduce dosage to 2.5 mg/day given as a single evening or bedtime dose. Maximum dosage is 10 mg P.O. b.i.d.

Contraindications

• Hypersensitivity to cannabinoids or sesame oil
• Breastfeeding

Administration

• When used as an appetite stimulant, give before lunch and dinner.

Route	Onset	Peak	Duration
P.O.	30-60 min	2-4 hr	4-6 hr

Adverse reactions

CNS: drowsiness, anxiety, impaired coordination, irritability, depression, headache, hallucinations, memory loss, paresthesia, ataxia, paranoia, disorientation, nightmares, speech difficulties, syncope, **suicidal ideation**
CV: tachycardia, hypotension, hypertension
EENT: visual disturbances, tinnitus

GI: dry mouth
Skin: facial flushing, diaphoresis

Interactions
Drug-drug. *Anticholinegics, antihistamines, tricyclic antidepressants:* increased tachycardia and hypertension
CNS depressants: increased CNS depression
Ritonavir: increased dronabinol blood level and risk of toxicity
Drug-behaviors. *Alcohol use:* increased CNS depression

Precautions
Use cautiously in:
• hypertension, heart disease, bipolar disorder, schizophrenia, drug abuse
• pregnant patients.

Patient monitoring
• Monitor vital signs for hypotension and tachycardia.
• Check for adverse CNS reactions and report significant depression, paranoid reaction, or emotional lability.
• Monitor nutritional status and hydration.

Patient teaching
• Instruct patient to take drug only as prescribed and needed, emphasizing its significant adverse CNS and cardiovascular effects.
• Advise patient (and significant others) to immediately report depression, suicidal thoughts, paranoid reactions, and other serious CNS reactions.
• Instruct patient to avoid driving or other hazardous activities until he knows how drug affects concentration and alertness.

droperidol
Inapsine

Pharmacologic class: Butyrophenone
Therapeutic class: General anesthetic, antiemetic
Pregnancy risk category C

Action
Produces marked sedation by directly blocking subcortical receptors; produces antiemetic effect by blocking CNS receptors in chemoreceptor trigger zone

Availability
Injection: 2.5 mg/ml in 1-ml, 2-ml, and 5-ml ampules and in 2-ml, 5-ml, and 10-ml vials

Indications and dosages
➤ Adjunct for general anesthesia induction
Adults and children older than age 12: 0.22 to 0.275 mg/kg I.M. or I.V., given with anesthetic
Children ages 2 to 12: 0.088 to 0.165 mg/kg I.M. or I.V., given with anesthetic
➤ Anesthetic premedication
Adults and children older than age 12: 2.5 to 10 mg I.M. 30 to 60 minutes before induction of anesthesia
Children ages 2 to 12: 0.088 to 0.165 mg/kg I.M. or I.V. 30 to 60 minutes before induction of anesthesia
➤ For use without a general anesthetic in diagnostic procedures
Adults and children older than age 12: 2.5 to 10 mg I.M. 30 to 60 minutes before procedure; may give additional doses of 1.25 to 2.5 mg
➤ Adjunct to regional anesthesia when additional sedation is needed
Adults: 2.5 to 5 mg I.M. or slow I.V.

Dosage adjustment
• Elderly patients

Off-label uses
• Hyperemesis gravidarum

Contraindications
• Hypersensitivity to drug
• Narrow-angle glaucoma
• Bone marrow depression
• CNS depression
• Severe cardiac or renal disease

Administration
• Know that drug needn't be diluted for I.V. or I.M. use.
• Inject I.M. into large muscle.
• Store at room temperature protected from sunlight.

Route	Onset	Peak	Duration
I.V., I.M.	3-10 min	30 min	2-4 hr

Adverse reactions
CNS: weakness, dysarthria, dysphonia, dizziness, extrapyramidal reactions, headache, loss of consciousness, depression, tremor, irritability, paresthesia, aggression, vertigo, ataxia, **seizures**
CV: chest pain, hypertension, hypotension, vasodilation, **arrhythmias, atrial fibrillation**
EENT: cataracts, blurred vision, eye irritation, sore throat, toothache
GI: nausea, vomiting, diarrhea, abdominal cramps, bloating, epigastric pain, fecal incontinence, increased salivation, dysphagia, **GI bleeding**
GU: urinary frequency, increased libido
Metabolic: dehydration
Musculoskeletal: muscle cramps, arthritis, bone fractures
Respiratory: bronchitis, dyspnea
Skin: bruising, rash, urticaria, diaphoresis, pruritus, flushing
Other: weight loss, hot flashes, influenza, chills, facial sweating

Interactions
Drug-drug. *Antihypertensives, nitrates:* additive hypertension
CNS depressants (including antidepressants, antihistamines, opioids): additive CNS depression
Drug-herb. *Chamomile, hops, kava, skullcap, valerian:* increased CNS depression
Drug-behaviors. *Alcohol use:* additive CNS depression

Precautions
Use cautiously in:
• diabetes mellitus, respiratory insufficiency, prostatic hypertrophy, CNS tumors, intestinal obstruction
• elderly patients
• pregnant or breastfeeding patients
• children younger than age 2.

Patient monitoring
• Monitor QT interval; report prolongation.
• Watch for torsades de pointes.
• Assess vital signs frequently. Stay alert for orthostatic hypotension and tachycardia. Keep I.V. fluids and vasopressors on hand for treatment of pronounced hypotension.
◄€ Don't place hypotensive patient in Trendelenburg position because this may deepen anesthesia, precipitating respiratory arrest.
• Avoid abrupt position changes.
• Observe for signs and symptoms of respiratory compromise when drug is used concurrently with narcotics.
• Monitor for and report extrapyramidal symptoms, such as restlessness, tremor, and facial tics.
• Observe patient for signs of worsening depression.

Patient teaching
• Advise patient not to drink alcohol or take CNS depressants for 24 hours after receiving drug.

• Inform patient that drug may cause extreme drowsiness for several days after administration.

• Caution patient not to participate in activities requiring mental alertness.

• Instruct patient to change positions slowly.

• Tell patient to report abdominal discomfort.

• As appropriate, review all significant life-threatening adverse reactions and interactions, especially those drugs, herbs, and behaviors mentioned above.

drotrecogin alfa (activated)
Xigris

Pharmacologic class: Activated protein C (recombinant)
Therapeutic class: Antisepsis drug
Pregnancy risk category C

Action
Antisepsis action unknown; may produce indirect profibrinolytic activity by hindering plasminogen activator inhibitor-1 and limiting generation of activated thrombin-activatable-fibrinolysis-inhibitor. Produces anti-inflammatory effect by inhibiting human tumor necrosis factor production and suppressing thrombin-induced inflammatory responses.

Availability
Powder for injection (lyophilized): 5 mg, 20 mg

⚠ Indications and dosages
➤ Severe sepsis in adults to reduce mortality
Adults: 24 mcg/kg/hour I.V. for a total duration of 96 hours

Contraindications
• Hypersensitivity to drug

• Intracranial neoplasm or lesion or evidence of cerebral herniation
• Hemorrhagic stroke
• High risk for bleeding
• Patients undergoing bone marrow therapy

Administration
• Mix with normal saline solution, lactated Ringer's solution, or dextrose 5% in water.

• Prepare immediately before use. Hang infusion bag within 3 hours of reconstitution; complete infusion within 12 hours after preparation.

• Administer only through infusion pump.

• Don't infuse with any other drug.

• Give entire regimen over 96 hours.

• Discontinue drug 2 hours before invasive procedures.

• Be aware that once hemostasis occurs, drug may be resumed immediately after uncomplicated invasive procedures or 12 hours after major invasive procedures (such as surgery).

Route	Onset	Peak	Duration
I.V.	Rapid	Unknown	Unknown

Adverse reactions
CNS: intracranial hemorrhage
GI: GI, intra-abdominal, or retroperitoneal bleeding
GU: GU tract bleeding
Hematologic: decreased hematocrit, prolonged activated partial thromboplastin time (APTT), **bleeding**
Skin: bruising
Other: skin and soft-tissue bleeding, **intrathoracic bleeding**

Interactions
Drug-drug. *Anticoagulants, aspirin, glycoprotein IIb/IIIa inhibitors, indomethacin, phenylbutazone, thrombolytics:* increased risk of bleeding
Drug-diagnostic tests. *APTT, prothrombin time (PT):* prolonged

Precautions

Use cautiously in:

• intracranial arteriovenous malformation, chronic severe hepatic disease, recent GI bleeding

• concurrent use of heparin, thrombolytics, oral anticoagulants, or aspirin

• pregnant patients

• children (safety and efficacy not established).

Patient monitoring

◀❧ Know that no antidote exists. Monitor closely for signs and symptoms of hemorrhage; stop infusion if clinically significant bleeding occurs.

• Monitor PT and complete blood count (especially platelet count).

• Realize that drug may variably prolong APTT and thus doesn't reliably indicate coagulopathy.

Patient teaching

• Advise patient to inform prescribers about all over-the-counter preparations and herbal or alternative remedies he's using.

---

dutasteride
Avodart

Pharmacologic class: Synthetic 4-azasteroid compound

Therapeutic class: 5-alpha-reductase inhibitor, sex hormone

Pregnancy risk category X

Action

Inhibits the steroid 5-alpha-reductase, an intracellular enzyme present in the liver, skin, and prostate. Conversion of testosterone to 5-alpha-dihydrotestosterone (DHT) depends on this enzyme, and DHT appears to be the principal androgen responsible for stimulation of prostatic growth.

Availability

Capsules: 0.5 mg

⏀ Indications and dosages

➢ Benign prostatic hypertrophy

Adults: 0.5 mg P.O. daily

d

Contraindications

• Hypersensitivity to drug, its components, other 5-alpha-reductase inhibitors, xanthines (such as coffee, theobromine), or ethylenediamine

• Women

• Children

Administration

◀❧ Wear gloves when handling and administering; drug may be absorbed through skin.

• Don't handle if you're pregnant or plan to become pregnant.

• Don't open or crush capsule.

• Give without regard to food.

Route	Onset	Peak	Duration
P.O.	Rapid	2-3 hr	Unknown

Adverse reactions

GI: dyspepsia

GU: decreased libido, decreased ejaculatory volume, impotence, gynecomastia, decreased prostate-specific antigen (PSA) level

Metabolic: thyroid-stimulating hormone (TSH) elevation

Interactions

Drug-drug. *Cimetidine, ciprofloxacin, diltiazem, ketoconazole, other drugs metabolized by CYP450-3A4 pathway, ritonavir, verapamil:* increased dutasteride blood level

Drug-diagnostic tests. *PSA:* decreased level

TSH: increased level

Precautions

Use cautiously in:

• hepatic impairment

• elderly patients.

Patient monitoring
• Monitor fluid intake and output; assess for ease of starting urine stream and for urinary urgency or frequency.
• Check baseline PSA level; reevaluate at 3 to 6 months.

Patient teaching
• Teach patient to take drug with full glass of water without crushing or opening capsule.
• Instruct patient not to take capsule if it's cracked or leaking.
• Inform patient that drug decreases testosterone production in prostate.
• Advise patient not to donate blood for at least 6 months after discontinuing drug.
• Inform patient that drug may decrease ejaculatory volume.
• Explain that sexual side effects eventually will subside.
• Tell patient to report dysuria and urinary urgency.

dyphylline
(dihydroxypropyl theophylline)
Dilor, Dyflex-200, Dylline, Lufyllin

Pharmacologic class: Xanthine, theophylline derivative
Therapeutic class: Bronchodilator
Pregnancy risk category C

Action
Produces bronchodilation by relaxing bronchial smooth muscles; also shows peripheral vasodilatory and other smooth muscle–relaxant activity

Availability
Elixir: 33.3 mg/5 ml, 53.3 mg/5 ml
Injection: 250 mg/ml
Tablets: 200 mg, 400 mg

⏀ Indications and dosages
➤ Prevention or relief of bronchospasm caused by acute or chronic bronchial asthma, chronic bronchitis, or emphysema
Adults: Up to 15 mg/kg P.O. q 6 hours; or 250 to 500 mg I.M. q 6 hours, as needed, not to exceed 15 mg/kg q 6 hours

Contraindications
• Hypersensitivity to xanthines (such as coffee, theobromine) or ethylenediamine
• Active peptic ulcer
• Seizure disorder
• Rectal or colonic irritation

Administration
• Give oral dose with 8 oz of water 1 hour before or 2 hours after a meal.
• Administer I.M. injection slowly into a large muscle.
◀⟨ Don't give by I.V. route.

Route	Onset	Peak	Duration
P.O.	1 hr	6 hr	Unknown
I.M.	30-45 min	6 hr	Unknown

Adverse reactions
CNS: dizziness, nervousness, restlessness, headache, insomnia, abnormal behavior, mutism, **seizures**
CV: palpitations, extrasystole, **sinus tachycardia, arrhythmias, marked hypotension, circulatory failure**
GI: nausea, vomiting, diarrhea, epigastric pain, hematemesis
GU: urinary retention (in men with prostatic enlargement), diuresis, increased excretion of renal tubular cells and red blood cells, proteinuria
Metabolic: hyperglycemia, syndrome of inappropriate antidiuretic hormone secretion
Musculoskeletal: muscle twitching
Respiratory: tachypnea, **respiratory arrest**

Skin: urticaria, rash, flushing
Other: increased appetite, hypersensitivity reactions

Interactions

Drug-drug. *Adrenergics, barbiturates, ketoconazole, nicotine (in cigarettes, gum, transdermal patches), phenytoin, rifampin:* increased metabolism and decreased efficacy of dyphylline
Allopurinol (large doses), beta-adrenergic blockers, cimetidine, clarithromycin, corticosteroids, disulfiram, erythromycin, fluvoxamine, hormonal contraceptives, influenza vaccine, interferons, mexiletine, thiabendazole: decreased dyphylline metabolism, possibly leading to toxicity
Carbamazepine, isoniazid, loop diuretics: increased or decreased dyphylline blood level
Lithium: decreased lithium efficacy
Oral anticoagulants: enhanced anticoagulant effect
Drug-diagnostic tests. *Serum uric acid:* false elevation
Drug-food. *Xanthine-containing foods and beverages (including caffeine):* increased drug blood level, increased risk of adverse cardiovascular and CNS reactions
Drug-herb. *Ephedra:* increased stimulant effects
St. John's wort: decreased drug blood level and efficacy

Precautions

Use cautiously in:
• cardiac or circulatory impairment, chronic obstructive pulmonary disease, renal or hepatic disease, hyperthyroidism, diabetes mellitus, glaucoma, peptic ulcer, hypertension, alcoholism
• elderly patients
• pregnant or breastfeeding patients
• neonates, infants, and young children (safety and efficacy not established).

Patient monitoring

• Monitor baseline and periodic pulmonary function tests.
• Monitor heart rate and blood pressure; report extreme tachycardia and hypotension.
• Assess for abdominal discomfort; if necessary, give drug after meals to relieve stomach upset.
• Watch closely for toxicity in patients with heart failure or hepatic impairment and in elderly patients and infants.
• Assess drug blood level regularly.

Patient teaching

• Instruct patient to take drug at same times each day.
• Tell patient to avoid foods cooked over charcoal; also caution him not to smoke or use nicotine products.

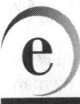

edetate calcium disodium (calcium EDTA)
Calcium Disodium Versenate

Pharmacologic class: Heavy metal antagonist
Therapeutic class: Antidote
Pregnancy risk category B

Action

Chelates with many metals (particularly calcium) to form stable, soluble complexes that are excreted in urine, resulting in reduced calcium blood level

Availability

Injection: 200 mg/ml

⚠ Indications and dosages

➤ Acute lead encephalopathy
Adults and children: 1 to 1.5 g/m^2/day I.V. or I.M. in divided doses at 8- to 12-hour intervals for 5 days. Start second course after at least two drug-free days.
➤ Lead poisoning without encephalopathy
Children: 1 g/m^2/day I.V. or I.M. in divided doses for 5 days

Contraindications

• Hypersensitivity to drug
• Renal disease
• Active or healed tubercular lesions
• Intracranial lesions
• History of seizures

Administration

◀♪ Don't confuse drug with edetate disodium, used to treat hypercalcemia.
• Be aware that I.M. route is preferred.
• Dilute I.V. dose with 250 to 500 ml of normal saline solution or dextrose 5% in water.
◀♪ Know that rapid infusion may be lethal; infuse at rate suggested by manufacturer.
• As desired, add procaine hydrochloride to minimize pain at injection site.
• Force fluids as tolerated, unless patient has elevated intracranial pressure.

Route	Onset	Peak	Duration
I.V., I.M.	1 hr	24-48 hr	Unknown

Adverse reactions

CNS: headache, paresthesia, circumoral paresthesia, tremor, malaise
CV: hypotension, thrombophlebitis, **arrhythmias**
GI: nausea, vomiting, diarrhea
GU: nocturia, dysuria, polyuria, proteinuria, renal insufficiency, hematuria, glycosuria, large epithelial cells in urine, **renal tubular necrosis, renal failure**
Hematologic: anemia, **transient bone marrow depression**

Hepatic: elevated hepatic enzyme levels
Metabolic: electrolyte imbalances
Musculoskeletal: myalgia, joint pain
Skin: erythema, exfoliative dermatitis, rash, flushing, diaphoresis
Other: increased appetite, excessive thirst, hypersensitivity reactions (such as sneezing, nasal congestion, lacrimation)

Interactions

Drug-drug. *Insulin:* interference with insulin's action
Drug-diagnostic tests. *Alanine aminotransferase, aspartate aminotransferase, calcium:* increased levels
Hemoglobin: decreased value

Precautions

Use cautiously in:
• cardiac disease, heart failure
• breastfeeding patients.

Patient monitoring

• Monitor infusion closely to ensure slow rate.
• Assess neurologic status frequently.
• Watch for and report febrile reactions, which may occur 4 to 8 hours after administration.
• Assess fluid intake and output; report changes.
• Know that toxicity may develop rapidly. Stop therapy if urine output decreases or anuria develops.
• Monitor hepatic profile, electrocardiogram, and blood urea nitrogen, creatinine, calcium, phosphate, and electrolyte levels daily.
◀♪ Discontinue drug at first sign of renal toxicity.

Patient teaching

• Teach patient to notify prescriber if he hasn't urinated in 12 hours.
• Instruct patient to report fever.

• Alternate I.V. sites daily to decrease risk of thrombophlebitis.

Route	Onset	Peak	Duration
I.V.	Unknown	Unknown	Unknown

edetate disodium (disodium EDTA)
Endrate

Pharmacologic class: Chelating agent
Therapeutic class: Antidote, potassium-removing resin, heavy metal antagonist
Pregnancy risk category C

Action
Chelates with many metals (particularly calcium) to form stable, soluble complexes that are excreted in urine, resulting in reduced calcium blood level

Availability
Injection: 150 mg/ml

Indications and dosages
➤ Hypercalcemic emergency
Adults: 50 mg/kg/day by slow I.V. infusion over at least 3 hours, up to a maximum of 3 g/day

Off-label uses
• Cardiac glycoside–induced arrhythmias and corneal calcium deposits
• Hypercalcemic emergencies in children

Contraindications
• Hypersensitivity to drug
• Renal disease
• Active or healed tubercular lesions
• Intracranial lesions
• History of seizures

Administration
◀≶ Don't confuse drug with edetate calcium disodium, used as lead poisoning antidote.
• Dilute with normal saline solution or dextrose 5% in water.
• Don't infuse rapidly.

Adverse reactions
CNS: headache, circumoral paresthesia, numbness
CV: orthostatic hypotension, thrombophlebitis
GI: nausea, vomiting, diarrhea
GU: nocturia, dysuria, polyuria, proteinuria, hyperuricemia, renal insufficiency, **renal tubular necrosis, renal failure**
Hematologic: anemia
Metabolic: electrolyte imbalances, **severe hypocalcemia**
Skin: rash, exfoliative dermatitis, erythema, diaphoresis, flushing
Other: pain at infusion site, fever

Interactions
Drug-diagnostic tests. *Calcium, potassium:* decreased levels

Precautions
Use cautiously in:
• cardiac disease, heart failure, hypokalemia
• breastfeeding patients.

Patient monitoring
• Keep patient in bed bed for 15 minutes after infusion to avoid orthostatic hypotension.
◀≶ Know that drug may cause profound hypocalcemia, leading to tetany, seizures, arrhythmias, and respiratory arrest. Keep I.V. calcium readily available.
• Monitor blood pressure closely.
• Monitor electrocardiogram, blood urea nitrogen, and creatinine levels frequently.
• Measure calcium blood level after each dose.

Patient teaching

• Instruct patient to move slowly when sitting up or standing to avoid dizziness or light-headedness from sudden blood pressure decrease.

• Tell patient to report adverse reactions, which may occur 4 to 8 hours after administration.

edrophonium chloride
Enlon, Reversol, Tensilon

Pharmacologic class: Anticholinesterase

Therapeutic class: Diagnostic drug, muscle stimulant, antidote

Pregnancy risk category C

Action

Reversibly inhibits cholinesterase, blocking acetylcholine from its release sites in parasympathetic and somatic efferent nerves and increasing acetylcholine concentration in synapses

Availability

Injection: 10 mg/ml in 1-ml ampules and in 10-ml and 15-ml vials

Indications and dosages

➤ Diagnostic aid in myasthenia gravis (Tensilon test)
Adults: 1 to 2 mg I.V. over 15 to 30 seconds; if no response occurs within 45 seconds, give 8 mg. Alternatively, 10 mg I.M.

Children weighing more than 34 kg (75 lb): 2 mg I.V.; if no response occurs within 45 seconds, give 1 mg q 45 seconds, to a maximum of 10 mg. Alternatively, 5 mg I.M.

Children weighing 34 kg (75 lb) or less: 1 mg I.V.; if no response occurs within 45 seconds, give 1 mg q 45 seconds, to a maximum of 5 mg. Alternatively, 2 mg I.M.

➤ To differentiate myasthenic crisis from cholinergic crisis
Adults: 1 mg I.V.; if no response occurs in 1 minute, repeat dose once. Increased muscle strength confirms myasthenic crisis; weakness or no increase in muscle strength confirms cholinergic crisis.

➤ Antidote for curare to reverse nondepolarizing neuromuscular blocking action
Adults: 10 mg I.V. given over 30 to 45 seconds; repeat dose q 5 to 10 minutes p.r.n. to a maximum of 40 mg.

Contraindications

• Hypersensitivity to drug
• Mechanical GI or urinary tract obstruction
• Peritonitis
• Sulfite sensitivity
• Breastfeeding

Administration

• Withdraw anticholinesterase drugs (cholinergics) at least 8 hours before test.

◀≤ Keep atropine (edrophonium antidote) readily available.

◀≤ Drug may cause respiratory distress, so have advanced life-saving equipment on hand during administration.

• Administer only when continuous electrocardiogram (ECG) monitoring is available.

• Know that drug may be given undiluted.

• Be aware that maximum concentration is 10 mg/ml.

• Frequently assess muscle strength when drug is used for diagnostic or differentiating indications.

Route	Onset	Peak	Duration
I.V.	<1 min	Unknown	5-20 min
I.M.	2-10 min	Unknown	10-40 min

Adverse reactions
CNS: asthenia, dysarthria, dysphonia, dizziness, drowsiness, headache, syncope, loss of consciousness, **seizures**
CV: hypotension, thrombophlebitis (with I.V. use), **atrioventricular (AV) block, cardiac arrest, bradycardia**
EENT: lacrimation, diplopia, miosis, conjunctival hyperemia
GI: nausea, vomiting, diarrhea, abdominal cramps, increased salivation, dysphagia
GU: urinary frequency or incontinence
Musculoskeletal: muscle cramps, fasciculations
Respiratory: laryngospasm, increased secretions, respiratory depression, dyspnea, **respiratory muscle paralysis, central respiratory paralysis, respiratory arrest, bronchospasm**
Skin: rash, diaphoresis, flushing
Other: anaphylaxis

Interactions
Drug-drug. *Aminoglycosides:* prolonged or enhanced muscle weakness
Cholinergics: increased cholinergic effects that mimic myasthenia weakness
Corticosteroids, magnesium, procainamide, quinidine: antagonism of cholinergic effects
Depolarizing neuromuscular blockers: increased neuromuscular blockade, prolonged respiratory depression
Local and general anesthetics: antagonism of cholinergic effects
Drug-diagnostic tests. *Urine cannabinoid test:* false-positive result
Drug-food. *High-fat meals:* decreased drug absorption
Drug-herb. *Jaborandi, pill-bearing spurge:* additive effects

Precautions
Use cautiously in:
• bronchial asthma, peptic ulcer, bradycardia, arrhythmias, vagotonia, recent coronary occlusion, hyperthyroidism, epilepsy
• pregnant patients.

Patient monitoring
• Monitor closely for cholinergic crisis (skeletal muscle fasciculations and increased muscle weakness, especially in respiratory muscles) after 2-mg dose when giving drug as test for myasthenia gravis. If cholinergic crisis occurs, discontinue drug and give atropine I.V. as prescribed.
• Assess for bradycardia, hypotension, and cardiac arrest.
• Monitor I.V. site closely.
• Observe for nausea and vomiting; give antiemetics, as prescribed.

Patient teaching
• Inform patient that increased muscle strength is a positive response to drug.
• Instruct patient to avoid driving and other hazardous activities until he knows how drug affects concentration and alertness.
• Advise patient to report vision changes.

efavirenz
Sustiva

Pharmacologic class: Nonnucleoside reverse transcriptase inhibitor
Therapeutic class: Antiretroviral
Pregnancy risk category C

Action
Inhibits human immunodeficiency virus (HIV) reverse transcriptase (required for transcription of HIV-1 RNA to DNA), leading to viral cell death

Availability
Capsules: 50 mg, 100 mg, 200 mg
Tablets: 600 mg

Indications and dosages
➤ HIV infection
Adults and children older than age 3

and weighing more than 40 kg (88 lb):
600 mg P.O. once daily (given with one
or more other antiretrovirals)
**Children weighing 32.5 to 40 kg (71.5
to 88 lb):** 400 mg P.O. once daily
**Children weighing 25 to 32.5 kg
(55 to 71.5 lb):** 350 mg P.O. once daily
**Children weighing 20 to 25 kg
(44 to 55 lb):** 300 mg P.O. once daily
**Children weighing 15 to 20 kg
(33 to 44 lb):** 250 mg P.O. once daily
**Children weighing 10 to 15 kg
(22 to 33 lb):** 200 mg P.O. once daily

Contraindications

• Hypersensitivity to drug
• Concurrent use of astemizole, midazolam, triazolam, or ergot derivatives

Administration

• Give on empty stomach.
• Store at room temperature protected
from light.

Route	Onset	Peak	Duration
P.O.	Rapid	3-5 hr	24 hr

Adverse reactions

CNS: abnormal dreams, hypoesthesia,
depression, dizziness, drowsiness, fatigue, headache, poor concentration,
insomnia, nervousness, anxiety, CNS
depression, **suicidal ideation**
CV: arrhythmias
GI: nausea, diarrhea, flatulence, abdominal pain, dyspepsia
GU: hematuria, renal calculi
Hepatic: elevated aspartate aminotransferase (AST) and alanine aminotransferase (ALT) levels, **hepatotoxicity**
Metabolic: elevated cholesterol, triglyceride, and gamma-glutamyltransferase
(GGT) levels
Respiratory: respiratory depression
Skin: rash, diaphoresis, pruritus, erythema multiforme, **toxic epidermal
necrolysis**

Other: increased appetite, **Stevens-
Johnson syndrome**

Interactions

Drug-drug. *Clarithromycin, indinavir:*
reduced blood levels of these drugs
*CNS depressants (including antidepres-
sants, antihistamines, opioids):* increased CNS depression
*CYP450 inducers (including phenobar-
bital, rifabutin, rifampin):* increased
clearance and decreased blood level of
efavirenz
*Ergot alkaloids, estrogen, midazolam,
ritonavir, triazolam:* increased blood
levels of these drugs, greater risk of
serious adverse reactions (including
arrhythmias, CNS and respiratory
depression, and hepatotoxicity)
Hormonal contraceptives: increased
ethinyl estradiol blood level
Saquinavir: decreased saquinavir blood
level
Warfarin: increased or decreased warfarin effects
Drug-diagnostic tests. *ALT, AST, GGT,
total cholesterol, triglycerides:* increased
levels
Urine cannabinoid test: false-positive
result
Drug-food. *High-fat meals:* increased
drug absorption
Drug-herb. *St. John's wort:* decreased
efavirenz blood level and efficacy, drug
resistance
Drug-behaviors. *Alcohol use:* increased
CNS depression

Precautions

Use cautiously in:
• hypercholesterolemia, hepatic impairment (including hepatitis B or C or
concurrent use of hepatotoxic drugs),
mental illness, or substance abuse
• pregnant or breastfeeding patients
(use in pregnancy only if other options
have been exhausted)
• children.

Patient monitoring

• Monitor hepatic and lipid profile.

• Closely monitor patients with hepatic failure.

• Be aware that drug may cause hypercholesterolemia.

• Monitor dietary intake.

• Be aware that amount of HIV in blood may increase if patient stops therapy even briefly.

Patient teaching

• Instruct patient to take drug with full glass of water, preferably at bedtime to improve tolerance of CNS effects. Also tell him to avoid taking drug with high-fat meals.

• Inform patient that drug must be taken in combination with other antiretrovirals.

• Teach patient that drug doesn't cure HIV or AIDS and that he can still transmit virus to others during therapy.

• Tell patient to report suicidal thoughts and other psychiatric symptoms.

• Instruct patient to avoid driving and other hazardous activities until he knows how drug affects concentration and alertness.

• Tell female patient to immediately inform prescriber if she becomes pregnant.

eletriptan hydrobromide
Relpax

Pharmacologic class: 5-hydroxytryptamine-1 (5-HT$_1$) receptor agonist
Therapeutic class: Antimigraine agent
Pregnancy risk category C

Action

Binds with vascular 5-HT$_1$ receptors; this effect is thought to cause vasoconstriction of cranial arteries, thereby relieving migraine

Availability

Tablets: 20 mg, 40 mg

Indications and dosages

➤ Migraine with or without aura
Adults: Initially, 20 to 40 mg P.O.; may repeat in 2 hours if headache returns after initial improvement. Maximum dosage is 80 mg/day.

Contraindications

• Hypersensitivity to drug

• Severe hepatic disease, ischemic bowel disease

• Cerebrovascular syndromes

• Basilar and hemiplegic migraine

• Uncontrolled hypertension, ischemic heart disease

• Concurrent use of ergotamine-containing drugs

Administration

• Give first dose as soon as migraine symptoms develop.

• Be aware that for patients with coronary artery disease, first dose should be given under close supervision.

• If headache improves but then recurs, give second dose at least 2 hours after first.

Route	Onset	Peak	Duration
P.O.	2 hr	2-3 hr	Unknown

Adverse reactions

CNS: dizziness, insomnia, drowsiness, headache, fatigue, anxiety, paresthesia, asthenia, cerebrovascular ischemia
CV: chest pain, palpitations, hypertension, cardiovascular ischemia
GI: nausea, vomiting, diarrhea, dry mouth
Musculoskeletal: muscle weakness
Respiratory: chest tightness or pressure
Skin: flushing
Other: hot or cold sensation

Interactions
Drug-drug. *Antihistamines, ergotamine, ergot derivatives:* increased vasospastic effects
CYP450-3A4 inhibitors (such as clarithromycin, ketoconazole, propranolol): increased eletriptan blood level
MAO inhibitors: increased eletriptan effects

Precautions
Use cautiously in:
• hepatic or renal impairment, diabetes, hypercholesterolemia, cardiac disorders
• elderly patients
• pregnant or breastfeeding patients
• children.

Patient monitoring
• Monitor vital signs and assess for chest pain, tightness, or pressure.

Patient teaching
• Instruct patient to take first dose as soon as migraine symptoms occur. If headache improves but then recurs, advise him to take second dose at least 2 hours after first.
• Advise patient to avoid driving and other hazardous activities until drug no longer affects concentration and alertness.
• Caution patient to report chest pain, pressure, or tightness.
• Inform patient that drug won't prevent migraines and isn't effective against other headache types.

emtricitabine
Emtriva

Pharmacologic class: Nucleoside reverse transcriptase inhibitor
Therapeutic class: Antiretroviral
Pregnancy risk category B

Action
Inhibits activity of human immunodeficiency virus (HIV)-1 reverse transcriptase by competing with natural substrate and by its incorporation into nascent viral DNA, which causes termination of chain

Availability
Capsules: 200 mg

⬤ Indications and dosages
➤ HIV-1 infection (in combination with other antiretrovirals)
Adults: 200 mg P.O. once daily
Dosage adjustment
• Renal impairment

Contraindications
• Hypersensitivity to drug

Administration
• Don't give drug at same time as other antiretrovirals.
• Give with or without food.

Route	Onset	Peak	Duration
P.O.	Rapid	1-2 hr	Unknown

Adverse reactions
CNS: headache, abnormal dreams, depression, dizziness, insomnia, peripheral neuritis or neuropathy, paresthesia
EENT: rhinitis
GI: nausea, vomiting, diarrhea, abdominal pain, dyspepsia
Hematologic: decreased neutrophil count
Hepatic: elevated bilirubin and liver function test results
Metabolic: increased or decreased glucose level, elevated triglyceride and creatine kinase levels, cushingoid appearance (buffalo hump, moon face)
Musculoskeletal: joint pain, myalgia
Respiratory: increased cough
Skin: rash, skin discoloration
Other: body fat redistribution

Interactions
Drug-drug. *Tenofovir disoproxil fumarate:* increased emtricitabine effect

Drug-diagnostic tests. *Alanine aminotransferase, amylase, aspartate aminotransferase, bilirubin, creatine kinase, lipase, triglycerides:* increased levels
Glucose: increased or decreased levels
Neutrophils: decreased count

Precautions
Use cautiously in:
• renal impairment
• obese patients
• elderly patients
• children.

Patient monitoring
• Assess neurologic status, checking especially for depression, peripheral neuropathy, and paresthesia.
• Monitor neutrophil count, lipid panel, liver function test results, and blood glucose levels.
• Monitor nutritional and hydration status in light of GI adverse effects and underlying disease.
• Watch for cushingoid appearance and body fat redistribution.

Patient teaching
• Instruct patient to not take drug at same time as other antiretrovirals.
• Advise patient to notify prescriber of adverse CNS reactions and to use good judgment about driving and other hazardous activities.
• Caution patient that drug may cause depression and instruct him to notify prescriber if he develops symptoms.
• Inform patient that drug may cause body fat redistribution, skin discoloration, and rash.

enalapril maleate
Vasotec

enalaprilat
Vasotec IV

Pharmacologic class: Angiotensin-converting enzyme (ACE) inhibitor

Therapeutic class: Antihypertensive

Pregnancy risk category C (second and third trimesters: *D*)

Action
Inhibits conversion of angiotensin I to angiotensin II, a potent vasoconstrictor; inactivates bradykinin and prostaglandins. Also increases plasma renin and potassium levels and reduces aldosterone levels, resulting in systemic vasodilation.

Availability
Injection: 1.25 mg/ml
Tablets: 2.5 mg, 5 mg, 10 mg, 20 mg

Indications and dosages
➤ Hypertension
Adults: Initially, 5 mg P.O. once daily, increased after 1 to 2 weeks as needed to a maintenance dosage of 10 to 40 mg P.O. daily as a single dose or in two divided doses. Or 1.25 mg I.V. q 6 hours.
Children: 0.08 mg/kg P.O. once daily; may be increased, based on blood pressure response, up to 5 mg daily; maximum dosage is 0.58 mg/kg/dose.
➤ Heart failure
Adults: Initially, 2.5 mg P.O. once or twice daily, increased after 1 to 2 weeks as needed to a maintenance dosage of 5 to 40 mg P.O. daily as a single dose or in two divided doses
➤ Asymptomatic left ventricular dysfunction
Adults: Initially, 2.5 mg P.O. once or

twice daily, increased after 1 to 2 weeks as needed to a maximum of 20 mg/day in divided doses

Dosage adjustment
• Renal impairment

Off-label uses
• Diabetic nephropathy
• Hypertensive emergency

Contraindications
• Hypersensitivity to drug or other ACE inhibitors
• Angioedema
• Pregnancy

Administration
• Give oral doses with food or beverage.
• Administer I.V. dose either undiluted or diluted in 50 ml of dextrose 5% in water, normal saline solution, dextrose 5% in normal saline solution, or dextrose 5% in lactated Ringer's solution.
• Give I.V. dose by push or piggyback over 5 minutes.
• Store at room temperature protected from heat and light.

Route	Onset	Peak	Duration
P.O.	1 hr	4-6 hr	24 hr
I.V.	15 min	3-4 hr	6 hr

Adverse reactions
CNS: dizziness, fatigue, headache, insomnia, drowsiness, vertigo, asthenia, paresthesia, ataxia, confusion, depression, nervousness, **cerebrovascular accident**
CV: orthostatic hypotension, palpitations, angina pectoris, tachycardia, peripheral edema, **arrhythmias, cardiac arrest**
EENT: sinusitis
GI: nausea, vomiting, constipation, dyspepsia, abdominal pain, altered taste, dry mouth, **pancreatitis**

GU: proteinuria, elevated creatinine level, oliguria, urinary tract infection, impotence, decreased libido
Hematologic: agranulocytosis, bone marrow depression
Hepatic: elevated hepatic enzyme levels, hyperbilirubinemia, **hepatitis**
Metabolic: hyperkalemia, hyponatremia
Respiratory: cough, eosinophilic pneumonitis, upper respiratory tract infection, asthma, bronchitis, dyspnea
Skin: rash, alopecia, photosensitivity, diaphoresis, exfoliative dermatitis, erythema multiforme, angioedema
Other: fever, increased appetite

Interactions
Drug-drug. *Allopurinol:* increased risk of hypersensitivity reaction
Antacids: decreased enalapril absorption
Cyclosporine, indomethacin, potassium-sparing diuretics, potassium supplements: hyperkalemia
Digoxin, lithium: increased blood levels of these drugs, possibly causing toxicity
Diuretics, nitrates, other antihypertensives, phenothiazines: additive hypotension
Nonsteroidal anti-inflammatory drugs: decreased antihypertensive response
Rifampin: decreased enalapril efficacy
Drug-diagnostic tests. *Alanine aminotransferase, alkaline phosphatase, aspartate aminotransferase, bilirubin, blood urea nitrogen (BUN), creatinine, potassium:* increased levels
Antinuclear antibodies: positive titer
Sodium: decreased level
Drug-food. *Salt substitutes containing potassium:* hyperkalemia
Drug-herb. *Capsaicin:* increased incidence of cough
Drug-behaviors. *Acute alcohol ingestion:* additive hypotension
Sun exposure: photosensitivity reaction

Precautions
Use cautiously in:
• renal or hepatic impairment, hypovolemia, hyponatremia, aortic stenosis, hypertrophic cardiomyopathy, cerebrovascular or cardiac insufficiency
• black patients with hypertension
• concurrent diuretic use
• elderly patients
• breastfeeding patients
• children.

Patient monitoring
◀€ Assess for rapid blood pressure decline leading to cardiovascular collapse, especially when giving with diuretics.
◀€ Monitor patients with renal insufficiency or renal artery stenosis for worsening renal function.
• Monitor fluid intake and output, daily weight, and vital signs.
• Supervise patient during ambulation until effects of drug are known.
• Monitor liver function test results and BUN, creatinine, and electrolyte levels.

Patient teaching
• Inform patient that full effect of drug may not be evident for several weeks.
• Tell patient to report persistent dry cough with nasal congestion.
• Teach patient to report swelling of face, eye area, tongue, lips, hands, or feet.
• Instruct patient to move slowly when sitting up or standing to avoid dizziness or light-headedness from sudden blood pressure decrease.

enoxacin
Penetrex

Pharmacologic class: Fluoroquinolone
Therapeutic class: Anti-infective
Pregnancy risk category C

Action
Inhibits bacterial DNA synthesis primarily by inhibiting gyrase, an enzyme involved in DNA replication, transcription, and repair; bactericidal

Availability
Tablets: 200 mg, 400 mg

🕖 Indications and dosages
➤ Complicated urinary tract infections (UTIs)
Adults: 400 mg P.O. q 12 hours for 14 days
➤ Uncomplicated UTIs
Adults: 200 mg P.O. q 12 hours for 7 days
➤ Gonorrhea
Adults: 400 mg P.O. as a single dose
Dosage adjustment
• Renal impairment

Off-label uses
• Chancroid
• Adjunct in transurethral prostatic resection

Contraindications
• Hypersensitivity to fluoroquinolones or quinolones
• Pregnancy
• Children younger than age 18

Administration
• Withhold tube feedings for 1 hour before and after giving drug.
• Protect drug from excessive heat, moisture, and direct sunlight.

Route	Onset	Peak	Duration
P.O.	Unknown	1-3 hr	Unknown

Adverse reactions
CNS: toxic psychosis, tremor, nervousness, anxiety, agitation, myoclonus, depersonalization, hypertonia, **seizures, increased intracranial pressure**
CV: prolonged QT interval, vasodilation, **arrhythmias**

GI: bloody stools, gastritis, stomatitis, **pseudomembranous colitis**

GU: vaginal moniliasis, urinary incontinence, **renal failure**

Metabolic: hyperkalemia

Skin: photosensitivity, rash, urticaria, diaphoresis, mycotic infection, erythema multiforme

Other: superinfection, decreased appetite, hypersensitivity reactions including **anaphylaxis, Stevens-Johnson syndrome**

Interactions

Drug-drug. *Antacids, bismuth subsalicylate, iron salts, sucralfate, zinc salts:* decreased enoxacin absorption

Antineoplastics: decreased enoxacin blood level

Cimetidine, probenecid: decreased elimination of enoxacin

Cyclosporine: increased cyclosporine blood level

Digoxin: increased digoxin blood level, leading to toxicity

Nonsteroidal anti-inflammatory drugs: increased risk of CNS stimulation and seizures

Theophylline: increased theophylline blood level, leading to toxicity

Warfarin: decreased clearance and increased effects of warfarin

Drug-diagnostic tests. *Potassium:* increased level

Drug-food. *Caffeine:* increased caffeine effects

Concurrent tube feedings: impaired drug absorption

Drug-herb. *Dong quai, St. John's wort:* photosensitivity

Precautions

Use cautiously in:
• underlying CNS disease, renal impairment, cirrhosis, myasthenia gravis
• elderly patients
• breastfeeding patients.

Patient monitoring

• Monitor electrocardiogram; report prolonged QT interval.

• Watch for seizures because drug may lower seizure threshhold.

• Stay alert for digoxin toxicity in patients taking digoxin concurrently.

• Check blood culture and sensitivity test results.

• Monitor creatinine clearance as well as blood urea nitrogen, creatinine, and electrolyte levels.

• Watch for and report rash.

Patient teaching

• Tell patient to take drug on empty stomach with full glass of water.

• Instruct patient to complete entire course of therapy, even if he feels better.

• Instruct patient not to take drug with antacids.

enoxaparin sodium
Lovenox

Pharmacologic class: Low-molecular-weight heparin

Therapeutic class: Anticoagulant

Pregnancy risk category B

Action

Inhibits thrombus and clot formation by blocking factor Xa and factor IIa, which accelerates the formation of antithrombin III-thrombin complex (a coagulation inhibitor). This action deactivates thrombin and prevents conversion of fibrinogen to fibrin.

Availability

Solution for injection: 30 mg/0.3 ml, 40 mg/0.4 ml, 60 mg/0.6 ml, 80 mg/0.8 ml, 100 mg/1 ml (all in prefilled syringes); 300 mg/3 ml (in multidose vials)

Indications and dosages

➤ Prevention of pulmonary embolism and deep vein thrombosis (DVT) after abdominal surgery

Adults: 40 mg S.C. 2 hours before surgery, repeated 24 hours after initial dose (provided hemostasisis is established) and continued once daily for 7 to 10 days until risk of DVT has diminished

➤ Prevention of pulmonary embolism and DVT after hip or knee replacement surgery

Adults: 30 mg S.C. 12 to 24 hours after surgery (provided hemostasisis is established), repeated q 12 hours for 7 to 10 days until risk of DVT has diminished. Alternatively, hip replacement patient may receive 40 mg S.C. 12 hours before surgery and once daily for 3 weeks.

➤ Prevention of ischemic complications of unstable angina or non-Q-wave myocardial infarction

Adults: 1 mg/kg S.C. q 12 hours given with aspirin 100 to 325 mg P.O. once daily until patient is clinically stable

➤ Inpatients with acute DVT with or without pulmonary embolism (PE) (given with warfarin sodium)

Adults: 1 mg/kg S.C. q 12 hours or 1.5 mg/kg S.C. once daily for 5 to 7 days until therapeutic effect is established. Warfarin therapy usually begins within 72 hours of enoxaparin injection.

➤ Outpatients with acute DVT without PE (given with warfarin sodium)

Adults: 1 mg/kg S.C. q 12 hours for 5 to 7 days until therapeutic effect is established. Warfarin therapy usually begins within 72 hours of enoxaparin injection.

Dosage adjustment

• Patients weighing less than 45 kg (99 lb) and with creatinine clearance below 30 ml/minute

Off-label uses

• Prevention of clots associated with hemodialysis
• Prevention of thrombosis during pregnancy

Contraindications

• Hypersensitivity to drug, pork products, sulfites, or benzyl alcohol
• Thrombocytopenia

Administration

• Use tuberculin syringe with multidose vials to ensure accurate dose.
• Don't expel air bubble from syringe before giving drug.
• Inject deep S.C. with patient in supine position; alternate left and right anterolateral and posterolateral abdominal wall sites.
• Don't rub injection site.
◀€ Don't give by I.M. or I.V. route.

Route	Onset	Peak	Duration
S.C.	Unknown	3-5 hr	24 hr

Adverse reactions

CNS: dizziness, headache, insomnia, confusion, **cerebrovascular accident**
CV: edema, chest pain, **atrial fibrillation, heart failure**
GI: nausea, vomiting, constipation
GU: urinary retention
Hematologic: bleeding, anemia, **thrombocytopenia, hemorrhage**
Hepatic: reversible hepatic enzyme elevation
Metabolic: hyperkalemia
Skin: bruising, pruritus, rash, urticaria
Other: fever; pain, irritation, or erythema at injection site

Interactions

Drug-drug. *Warfarin, other drugs that affect platelet function (including abciximab, aspirin, clopidogrel, dextran, dipyridamole, eftifibatide, nonsteroidal anti-inflammatory drugs [NSAIDs], some penicillins, ticlopidine, and tirofiban):* increased risk of bleeding

Drug-diagnostic tests. *Alanine aminotransferase, aspartate aminotransferase:* increased levels
Hemoglobin, platelets: decreased levels
Drug-herb. *Anise, arnica, chamomile, clove, feverfew, garlic, ginger, ginkgo, ginseng:* increased risk of bleeding

Precautions

Use cautiously in:
• severe hepatic or renal disease, retinopathy (hypertensive or diabetic), uncontrolled hypertension, hemorrhagic stroke, bacterial endocarditis, GI bleeding or other bleeding disorders
• recent history of ulcer disease, history of congenital or acquired bleeding disorder or of thrombocytopenia related to heparin use
• recent CNS surgery
• pregnant or breastfeeding patients
• children.

Patient monitoring

• Monitor complete blood count and platelet counts, and watch for signs of bleeding or bruising.
• Monitor fluid intake and output; watch for fluid retention and edema.

Patient teaching

• If patient will self-administer drug, teach proper injection technique.
• Instruct patient to report unusual bleeding or bruising, rash, or hives.
• Teach patient safety measures to avoid bruising or bleeding.
• Advise patient to weigh himself regularly and to report sudden increases.
• Inform patient that many over-the-counter drugs (such as aspirin and NSAIDs) and herbal remedies increase anticoagulant effect of enoxaparin. Instruct him to avoid these products unless prescriber approves them.

entacapone
Comtan

Pharmacologic class: Catechol-O-methyltransferase (COMT) inhibitor
Therapeutic class: Antidyskinetic
Pregnancy risk category C

Action

Inhibits COMT, the primary enzyme involved in metabolizing levodopa, thereby increasing levodopa blood levels and duration of action and lessening symptoms of Parkinson's disease

Availability

Tablets: 200 mg

Indications and dosages

➤ Adjunctive treatment of idiopathic Parkinson's disease in patients experiencing "wearing off" of carbidopa-levodopa's effects
Adults and children: 200 mg P.O. with each carbidopa-levodopa dose, up to a maximum of eight times/day

Contraindications

• Hypersensitivity to drug
• Pregnancy or breastfeeding

Administration

• Give drug at same time as carbidopa-levodopa; remind patient to swallow it whole.
• Avoid abrupt discontinuation.

Route	Onset	Peak	Duration
P.O.	Variable	1 hr	Unknown

Adverse reactions

CNS: disorientation, memory loss, agitation, delusions, paranoia, euphoria, light-headedness, dizziness, depression, drowsiness, paresthesia, heaviness of limbs, numbness of fingers, dyskinesia, hyperkinesia, hallucinations

CV: tachycardia, orthostatic hypotension, hypertension
GI: nausea, vomiting, epigastric pain, flatulence
GU: urine discoloration
Respiratory: upper respiratory tract infection, dyspnea, sinus congestion
Other: fever

Interactions
Drug-drug. *Ampicillin, chloramphenicol, cholestyramine, erythromycin, probenecid, rifampin:* decreased excretion of entacapone
Bitolterol, dobutamine, dopamine, epinephrine, isoetherine, methyldopa, norephinephrine: increased heart rate, increased risk of arrhythmias, excessive blood pressure changes
MAO inhibitors: increased risk of toxicity
Drug-behaviors. *Alcohol use:* increased risk of adverse effects

Precautions
Use cautiously in:
• hepatic or renal dysfunction, hypertension, heart disease.

Patient monitoring
• Monitor vital signs, watching especially for orthostatic hypotension.
• Evaluate neurologic status closely; check for hallucinations and new onset or exacerbation of dyskinesia.
• Assess respiratory status; watch particularly for dyspnea, fever, and other signs and symptoms of upper respiratory tract infection.
• Monitor nutritional and hydration status if patient experiences vomiting.

Patient teaching
• Instruct patient to swallow tablet whole and to take it at same time as carbidopa-levodopa.
• Caution patient (and caregiver as appropriate) to institute safety measures at home to prevent injury related to disease or drug's adverse CNS effects.

• Teach patient to move slowly when sitting up or standing to avoid dizziness or light-headedness from sudden blood pressure decrease.

ephedrine

ephedrine sulfate
Pretz-D, Vick's Vatronol

Pharmacologic class: Sympathomimetic

Therapeutic class: Bronchodilator, vasopressor, nasal decongestant

Pregnancy risk category C

Action
Stimulates beta$_2$-adrenergic receptors, relaxing bronchial smooth muscle and relieving bronchospasm. Also stimulates alpha- and beta-adrenergic receptors and promotes norepinephrine release from sympathetic neurons, which increases blood pressure and cardiac output.

Availability
Capsules: 25 mg, 50 mg
Injection: 25 mg/ml, 30 mg/ml, 50 mg/ml
Nasal spray: 0.25%

⚠ Indications and dosages
➤ Hypotension
Adults: 25 mg P.O. one to four times daily, or 25 to 50 mg I.M. or S.C., or 10 to 25 mg I.V. p.r.n. Maximum dosage is 150 mg daily
Children: 3 mg/kg or 25 to 100 mg/m^2 S.C. or I.V. daily in four to six divided doses
➤ Bronchodilation, nasal decongestion
Adults and children older than age 12: 12.5 to 50 mg P.O. q 3 to 4 hours p.r.n; maximum dosage is 150 mg daily. Two

or three sprays in each nostril q 4 hours as a nasal decongestant.

Children ages 6 to 12: 6.25 to 12.5 mg P.O. q 4 hours; maximum dosage is 75 mg daily. One or two sprays in each nostril q 4 hours as a nasal decongestant.

Children older than age 2: 2 to 3 mg/kg or 100 mg/m^2 P.O. daily in four to six divided doses. One or two sprays in each nostril q 4 hours as a nasal decongestant.

Contraindications

• Hypersensitivity to drug
• Severe coronary artery disease
• Angina pectoris
• Narrow-angle glaucoma
• Monoamine oxidase (MAO) inhibitor use within past 14 days

Administration

• Give by direct I.V. injection slowly; monitor response and repeat dose as needed.
• Give I.M. or S.C. doses as prescribed; monitor response and repeat dose as needed.

Route	Onset	Peak	Duration
P.O.	15-60 min	Unknown	3-5 hr
I.V.	5 min	Unknown	1 hr
I.M., S.C.	10-20 min	Unknown	0.5-1 hr

Adverse reactions

CNS: insomnia, nervousness, dizziness, headache, euphoria, confusion, delirium, tremor, **cerebral hemorrhage**
CV: palpitations, tachycardia, hypertension, precordial pain, **arrhythmias**
EENT: dry nose or throat
GI: nausea, vomiting, epigastric pain, flatulence
GU: urinary retention, painful urination
Musculoskeletal: muscle weakness
Skin: diaphoresis

Interactions

Drug-drug. *Acetazolamide:* increased ephedrine blood level
Alpha-adrenergic blockers: unopposed beta-adrenergic effects, resulting in hypotension
Antihypertensives: decreased antihypertensive effects
Beta-adrenergic blockers: unopposed alpha-adrenergic effects, resulting in hypertension
Cardiac glycosides, general anesthetics: increased risk of ventricular arrhythmias
Ergot alkaloids: enhanced vasoconstrictor and pressor effects
Guanadrel, guanethidine: potentiation of pressor response
MAO inhibitors, tricyclic antidepressants: severe hypertension
Methyldopa, reserpine: inhibition of ephedrine's effects

Precautions

Use cautiously in:
• hypertension, heart disease, hepatic or renal dysfunction, hyperthyroidism, diabetes, prostatic hypertrophy
• elderly patients
• breastfeeding patients.

Patient monitoring

◀€ Monitor vital signs and electrocardiogram, particularly for tachycardia, arrhythmia, or hypertension.
• Assess cardiovascular status closely; ask patient about precordial pain.
• Monitor neurologic status, particularly for signs and symptoms of cerebral hemorrhage.
• Measure fluid intake and output, and watch for urinary retention.

Patient teaching

• Explain to patient that oral form of drug can cause insomnia; encourage him to take it at least 2 hours before bedtime.
• Inform patient that drug may cause abnormal heartbeats; assure him that

he'll be closely monitored, and instruct him to report any chest pain.

◀€ Urge patient to report severe headache or significant CNS changes right away.

• Instruct patient to avoid driving and other hazardous activities until he knows how drug affects concentration and alertness.

• Tell patient to report painful urination or urinary retention.

epinephrine
Bronkaid Mist, Bronkaid Mistometer✿, Primatene Mist

epinephrine bitartrate
AsthmaHaler Mist, Bronkaid Mist, Primatene Mist

epinephrine hydrochloride
Adrenalin Chloride, EpiPen, EpiPen Jr., Glaucon, Nephron, Sus-Phrine, Vaponefrin

Pharmacologic class: Sympathomimetic (direct acting)
Therapeutic class: Bronchodilator
Pregnancy risk category C

Action
Stimulates alpha- and beta-adrenergic receptors, resulting in relaxation of cardiac and bronchial smooth muscle and dilation of skeletal muscle vessels

Availability
Aerosol inhaler: 160 mcg, 200 mcg, 220 mcg, 250 mcg
Auto-injector for I.M. injection: 1:2,000 (0.5 mg/ml)
Injection: 0.01 mg/ml, 0.1 mg/ml, 0.5 mg/ml, 1 mg/ml, 5 mg/ml parenteral suspension
Nebulizer inhaler: 1%, 1.25%, 2.25%

Ophthalmic drops: 0.5%, 1%, 2%
Solution: 1:200,000

💉 Indications and dosages
➤ Bronchodilation, hypersensitivity reaction, anaphylaxis
Adults: 0.1 to 0.5 ml of 1:1,000 solution S.C. or I.M., repeated q 10 to 15 minutes p.r.n. Or 0.1 to 0.25 ml of 1:10,000 solution I.V. slowly over 5 to 10 minutes; may repeat q 5 to 15 minutes p.r.n. or follow with a continuous infusion of 1 mcg/minute, increased to 4 mcg/minute p.r.n. For emergency treatment, EpiPen delivers 0.3 mg I.M. of 1:1,000 epinephrine. EpiPen Jr. may be more appropriate for patients weighing less than 30 kg (66 lb).
Children: For emergency treatment, EpiPen Jr. delivers 0.15 mg I.M. of 1:2,000 epinephrine
➤ Acute asthma attack
Adults and children ages 4 and older: 160 to 250 mcg metered aerosol (equivalent to one inhalation); repeat once if needed after 1 minute. Subsequent doses shouldn't be given for at least 3 hours. Or one to three deep inhalations of 1% solution with handheld nebulizer, repeated q 3 hours p.r.n.
➤ To restore cardiac rhythm in cardiac arrest
Adults: 0.5 to 1 mg I.V., repeated q 3 to 5 minutes, if needed; if no response, may give 3 to 5 mg I.V. q 3 to 5 minutes
➤ Chronic simple glaucoma
Adults: One drop in affected eye once or twice daily; adjust dosage to meet patient's needs.
➤ To prolong local anesthetic effects
Adults and children: 1:200,000 concentration with local anesthetic

Contraindications
• Hypersensitivity to drug, its components, or sulfites
• Narrow-angle glaucoma
• Cardiac disease
• Cerebral arteriosclerosis

- Labor
- Breastfeeding

Administration

- To treat anaphylaxis, use I.M. route rather than S.C. route when possible.
🔊 Inject EpiPen and EpiPen Jr. only into anterolateral aspect of thigh. Don't inject into buttocks or give I.V.
- Use Epi-Pen Jr. for patients weighing less than 30 kg (66 lb).

Route	Onset	Peak	Duration
I.V.	Immediate	5 min	Short
I.M.	Variable	Unknown	1-4 hr
S.C.	5-15 min	0.5 hr	1-4 hr
Inhalation	1-5 min	Unknown	1-3 hr

Adverse reactions

CNS: nervousness, anxiety, tremor, vertigo, headache, disorientation, agitation, drowsiness, fear, dizziness, asthenia, **cerebral hemorrhage, cerebrovascular accident (CVA)**
CV: palpitations, widened pulse pressure, hypertension, tachycardia, angina, electrocardiogram changes, **ventricular fibrillation, shock**
GI: nausea, vomiting
GU: decreased urinary output, urinary retention, painful urination
Respiratory: dyspnea, **pulmonary edema**
Skin: urticaria, pallor, diaphoresis, necrosis
Other: hemorrhage at injection site

Interactions

Drug-drug. *Alpha-adrenergic blockers:* hypotension from unopposed beta-adrenergic effects
Antihistamines, thyroid hormone, tricyclic antidepressants: severe sympathomimetic effects
Beta-adrenergic blockers (such as propranolol): vasodilation and reflex tachycardia

Cardiac glycosides, general anesthetics: increased risk of ventricular arrhythmias
Diuretics: decreased vascular response
Doxapram, mazindol, methylphenidate: enhanced CNS stimulation or pressor effects
Ergot alkaloids: decreased vasoconstriction
Guanadrel, guanethidine: enhanced pressor effects of epinephrine
Levodopa: increased risk of arrhythmias
Levothyroxine: potentiation of epinephrine effects
MAO inhibitors: increased risk of hypertensive crisis
Drug-diagnostic tests. *Glucose:* transient elevation
Lactic acid: elevated level with prolonged use

Precautions

Use cautiously in:
- hypertension, hyperthyroidism, diabetes, prostatic hypertrophy
- elderly patients
- pregnant patients
- children.

Patient monitoring

🔊 Monitor vital signs, electrocardiogram, and cardiovascular status; watch for ventricular fibrillation, tachycardia, arrhythmias, and signs of shock. Ask patient about anginal pain.
- Assess drug's effect on underlying problem (such as anaphylaxis or asthma attack), and repeat doses as needed.
🔊 Monitor neurologic status, particularly for decreased level of consciousness and other signs and symptoms of cerebral hemorrhage or CVA.
- Monitor fluid intake and output, watching for urinary retention or decreased urinary output.
- Inspect injection site for hemorrhage or skin necrosis.

Patient teaching

• Teach patient who uses auto-injector how to use syringe correctly, when to inject drug, and when to repeat doses.
• Teach patient who uses hand-held nebulizer correct use of equipment and drug, and explain indications for both initial dose and repeat doses.
• Caution patient that drug may cause serious adverse effects, and explain which symptoms he should report.
• If patient will self-administer drug outside of health care setting, explain need for prompt evaluation by a health care provider to ensure that underlying disorder has been corrected.

epirubicin hydrochloride
Ellence, Pharmorubicin RDF

Pharmacologic class: Anthracycline
Therapeutic class: Antibiotic antineoplastic
Pregnancy risk category D

Action
Unknown; thought to act by forming a complex with DNA by intercalation between base pairs, causing inhibition of DNA, RNA, and protein synthesis and resulting in cytocidal activity. Also disrupts DNA replication and transcription.

Availability
Injection: 2 mg/ml, 50 mg/25 ml, 200 mg/dl

⚕ Indications and dosages
➤ Adjunct therapy in patients with axillary-node tumor involvement after resection of primary breast cancer
Adults: 100 to 120 mg/m² by I.V. infusion over 3 to 5 minutes on first day of each cycle or divided equally in two doses on first and eighth days of each cycle; cycle repeated q 3 to 4 weeks for six cycles in conjunction with cyclophosphamide and fluorouracil. Dosage adjustments after first cycle are based on toxicity. For patient with a platelet count less than 50,000/mm³, absolute neutrophil count (ANC) below 250/mm³, neutropenic fever, or grade 3 or 4 nonhematologic toxicity, reduce first day's dose in subsequent cycles to 75% and delay subsequent cycles until platelet count is at least 100,000/mm³, ANC is at least 1,500/mm³, and nonhematologic toxicity recovers to grade 1 or better.

Off-label uses
• Cancer of bladder, lung, nasopharynx, endometrium, and ovaries

Contraindications
• Hypersensitivity to drug
• Baseline neutrophil count below 1,500/mm³
• Myocardial insufficiency
• Severe hepatic dysfunction

Administration
• Follow facility policy for administration of carcinogenic drugs.
◀€ Avoid extravasation; if patient complains of burning or stinging, switch infusion to a different vein.
• Administer premixed solution over 3 to 5 minutes into tubing of free-flowing I.V. line containing dextrose 5% in water or normal saline solution.
• If patient develops facial flushing or red streak in vein being infused, slow infusion rate.

Route	Onset	Peak	Duration
I.V.	Unknown	Unknown	Unknown

Adverse reactions
CNS: lethargy
CV: **cardiomyopathy, heart failure**

EENT: conjunctivitis, keratitis
GI: nausea, vomiting, diarrhea, mucositis
GU: amenorrhea, reddish urine
Hematologic: anemia, **leukopenia, neutropenia, thrombocytopenia**
Skin: alopecia; rash; pruritus; darkening of soles, palms, or nails
Other: infection, fever, increased appetite, hot flashes, tissue necrosis

Interactions

Drug-drug. *Calcium channel blockers:* increased risk of heart failure
Cimetidine: increased epirubicin blood levels
Cytotoxic drugs: additive toxicity
Live-virus vaccines: increased risk of infection
Trastuzumab: increased risk of cardiac dysfunction
Drug-diagnostic tests. *Hemoglobin, neutrophils, platelets, white blood cells:* decreased values

Precautions

Use cautiously in:
• heart disease, liver disease
• previous or recent radiation therapy.

Patient monitoring

◀€ Monitor vital signs, left ventricular ejection fraction, and cardiovascular status carefully; watch for signs and symptoms of cardiomyopathy and heart failure.
• Assess nutritional status and hydration in light of GI adverse effects.
• Monitor complete blood count with white cell differential; watch for signs and symptoms of blood dyscrasias.
• Check temperature; watch for fever and other signs of infection.

Patient teaching

• Inform patient that drug can cause tissue damage at injection site. Tell him to report pain, burning, or swelling.

◀€ Instruct patient to immediately report sudden weight gain, swelling, or shortness of breath.
• Tell patient to notify prescriber of unusual bruising or bleeding, fever, or signs and symptoms of infection.
• Explain that drug will probably cause hair loss but that hair should regrow within a few months after therapy.
• Advise female patients that drug may cause premature menopause or permanent cessation of menses.

eplerenone
Inspra

Pharmacologic class: Aldosterone receptor blocker
Therapeutic class: Antihypertensive
Pregnancy risk category B

Action

Binds to aldosterone receptors, blocking the action of aldosterone, which normally causes sodium and water reabsorption; as a result, more sodium and water are excreted, lowering blood volume and blood pressure

Availability

Tablets: 25 mg, 50 mg, 100 mg

🕖 Indications and dosages

➤ Hypertension (alone or in combination with other antihypertensives)
Adults: 50 mg/day P.O. as a single dose; if necessary, may increase to 50 mg P.O. b.i.d. after a 4-week trial period
➤ Heart failure, postmyocardial infarction (MI)
Adults: Initially, 25 mg P.O. once daily; after 1 month, may increase to maximum dosage of 50 mg P.O. once daily

---

Contraindications

- Hypersensitivity to drug
- Hyperkalemia
- Type 2 diabetes mellitus with micro-albuminuria
- Severe renal impairment
- Breastfeeding

Administration

- Give drug with or without food.

Route	Onset	Peak	Duration
P.O.	Slow	1.5 hr	Unknown

Adverse reactions

CNS: headache, dizziness, fatigue
CV: angina, **MI**
GI: diarrhea, abdominal pin
GU: vaginal bleeding, albuminuria, changes in sexual function, gynecomastia and breast pain (in men)
Metabolic: hypercholesterolemia, **hyperkalemia**
Respiratory: cough
Other: flulike symptoms

Interactions

Drug-drug. *Angiotensin-converting enzyme inhibitors:* increased risk of hyperkalemia
CYP450-3A4 inhibitors: serious toxic effects
Lithium: increased risk of toxicity
Nonsteroidal anti-inflammatory drugs: decreased hypertensive effect of eplerenone

Precautions

Use cautiously in:
- hepatic impairment
- pregnant patients.

Patient monitoring

- Monitor electrolyte levels, and watch for signs of hyperkalemia.
- Check vital signs and ask patient about chest pain.
- Monitor lipid panel.
- Assess for new onset of persistent dry cough or flulike symptoms.

Patient teaching

- ◀〰 Advise patient to immediately report chest pain, flulike symptoms, or persistent dry cough.
- Instruct patient to avoid driving and other hazardous activities until he knows how drug affects concentration and alertness.
- Inform patient that drug may affect sexual function; encourage him to discuss these issues with prescriber.

e

---

epoetin alfa
Epogen, Eprex ✤, Procrit

Pharmacologic class: Recombinant human erythropoietin
Therapeutic class: Biological response modifier
Pregnancy risk category C

Action

Binds to erythropoietin, stimulating mitotic activity of erythroid progenitor cells in bone marrow and inducing release of reticulocytes from bone marrow into bloodstream, where they become mature red blood cells

Availability

Injection: 2,000 units/ml, 3,000 units/ml, 4,000 units/ml, 10,000 units/ml; 10,000 units/ml and 20,000 units/ml in multidose vials

⏺ Indications and dosages

➤ Anemia associated with chronic renal failure
Adults: Initially, 50 to 100 units/kg I.V. or S.C. three times weekly; may be increased after 8 weeks if hematocrit is still below target range
➤ Anemia caused by zidovudine therapy in patients with human immunodeficiency virus infection

---

Adults: 100 units/kg I.V. or S.C. three times weekly for 8 weeks or until adequate hematocrit level is reached. If desired response isn't reached after 8 weeks, dosage may be increased by 50 to 100 units/kg I.V. or S.C. three times weekly; after 4 to 8 weeks, dosage may be further increased as prescribed, up to a maximum dosage of 300 units/kg I.V. or S.C. three times weekly.

➤ Anemia caused by cancer chemotherapy

Adults: 150 units/kg S.C. three times weekly for 8 weeks or until the adequate hematocrit level is reached. If desired response isn't reached after 8 weeks, dosage may be increased up to a maximum of 300 units/kg S.C. three times weekly.

➤ To reduce need for blood transfusion in surgical patients

Adults: 300 units/kg S.C. daily for 10 days before surgery, on day of surgery, and for 4 days after surgery; or 600 units/kg S.C. once a week starting 3 weeks before surgery, then an additional dose on day of surgery

➤ Anemia in children with chronic renal failure on dialysis

Children ages 1 month to 16 years: 50 units/kg I.V. or S.C. three times weekly; maintenance dosage is individualized to maintain hematocrit within target range.

Contraindications

• Hypersensitivity to drug, human albumin, or products derived from mammal cells
• Uncontrolled hypertension
• Breastfeeding

Administration

• For I.V. use, give by direct I.V. injection, and follow with saline flush.
• If patient is on hemodialysis, administer drug into venous return line of dialysis tubing after patient has completed dialysis session.

• Know that supplemental iron may be needed to support erythropoiesis and avoid depletion of iron stores.

🔊 Avoid using multidose vials in premature infants because of benzyl alcohol content.

Route	Onset	Peak	Duration
I.V.	Immediate	Immediate	Unknown
S.C.	Unknown	5-24 hr	Unknown

Adverse reactions

CNS: headache, paresthesia, fatigue, dizziness, asthenia, **seizures**
CV: hypertension, edema, increased clotting of arteriovenous grafts
GI: nausea, vomiting, diarrhea
Metabolic: hyperuricemia, hyperkalemia, hyperphosphatemia
Musculoskeletal: joint pain
Respiratory: cough, dyspnea
Skin: rash, urticaria
Other: fever, injection site pain

Interactions

Drug-diagnostic tests. *Blood urea nitrogen, creatinine, phosphate, potassium, uric acid:* increased levels

Precautions

Use cautiously in:
• renal insufficiency
• pregnant patients.

Patient monitoring

• Monitor vital signs and cardiovascular status, especially for hypertension and edema.
• Assess arteriovenous graft for patency (drug may increase clotting at graft).
• Monitor electrolyte and uric acid levels; watch closely for hyperuricemia, hyperkalemia, and hyperphosphatemia.
• Check temperature for fever.
• Monitor neurologic status for signs of impending seizures.
• Evaluate nutritional status and hydration in light of GI adverse effects.

Patient teaching

🔈 Instruct patient to monitor weight and blood pressure regularly and to immediately report hypertension, sudden weight gain, or swelling.

• Instruct patient to avoid driving and other hazardous activities until he knows how drug affects concentration, motor skills, and alertness.

• Teach patient to minimize GI upset by eating small, frequent servings of healthy food and drinking plenty of fluids.

eprosartan mesylate
Teveten

Pharmacologic class: Angiotensin II receptor antagonist

Therapeutic class: Antihypertensive

Pregnancy risk category C (second and third trimesters: *D*)

Action
Blocks aldosterone-producing and vasoconstricting effects of angiotensin II at various receptor sites in vascular smooth muscles, adrenal glands, and other tissues, decreasing vascular resistance

Availability
Tablets: 400 mg, 600 mg

🚺 Indications and dosages
➤ Hypertension
Adults: 600 mg P.O. once daily or in divided doses b.i.d.

Contraindications
• Hypersensitivity to drug
• Hypotension
• Pregnancy or breastfeeding

Administration
• Give initial dose in supervised medical setting, and monitor blood pressure for 2 hours after administration.

• Be prepared to treat transient hypotension by placing patient in supine position and giving I.V. normal saline infusion as needed.

Route	Onset	Peak	Duration
P.O.	Unknown	6 hr	24 hr

Adverse reactions
CNS: dizziness, fatigue, headache, syncope

CV: hypotension, chest pain, peripheral edema

EENT: sinus disorders, dental pain

GI: nausea, diarrhea, abdominal pain, constipation, dry mouth

GU: albuminuria, **renal failure**

Hepatic: drug-induced hepatitis

Metabolic: hyperkalemia, gout

Musculoskeletal: joint pain, back pain, muscle weakness

Respiratory: upper respiratory tract infection, cough, bronchitis

Skin: angioedema

Other: fever, facial edema

Interactions
Drug-drug. *Antihypertensives, diuretics:* increased risk of hypotension
Nonsteroidal anti-inflammatory drugs: decreased antihypertensive effects of eprosartan
Potassium-sparing diuretics, potassium supplements: increased risk of hyperkalemia

Drug-diagnostic tests. *Albumin:* elevated level

Drug-food. *Salt substitutes containing potassium:* increased risk of hyperkalemia

Drug-herb. *Ma huang:* antagonism of eprosartan's action

Drug-behaviors. *Alcohol use:* increased CNS depression

Precautions

Use cautiously in:

- heart failure, renal or hepatic impairment, obstructive biliary disorders, volume or sodium depletion
- concurrent high-dose diuretic therapy
- black patients
- females of childbearing age
- children younger than age18 (safety not established).

Patient monitoring

- Monitor vital signs, particularly for hypotension after administration.
- Check for signs and symptoms of angioedema.
- Assess cardiovascular status, especially for chest pain, syncope, and edema.
- Monitor liver and kidney function test results, watching for drug-induced hepatitis or renal failure.
- Assess respiratory status, watching for dry, persistent cough and signs or symptoms of respiratory infections.
- Monitor electrolyte levels, and watch for signs and symptoms of hyperkalemia.

Patient teaching

- Instruct patient to take drug at same time each day, with or without food.
- Inform patient that drug may cause angioedema. Instruct him to immediately report facial or lip swelling, fever, or sore throat.
- Instruct patient to immediately report chest pain, fainting, decreased urine output, or swelling.
- Caution female patient to contact prescriber right away if she suspects she may be pregnant.

eptifibatide
Integrilin

Pharmacologic class: Platelet aggregation inhibitor

Therapeutic class: Antiplatelet agent
Pregnancy risk category B

Action

Decreases platelet aggregation by binding to platelet receptor glycoprotein, preventing the binding of fibrinogen to active and resting platelets

Availability

Injection: 10-ml vial (2 mg/ml), 100-ml vial (0.75 mg/ml)

Indications and dosages

➤ Acute coronary syndrome (unstable angina or non-Q-wave myocardial infarction)

Adults: 180 mcg/kg I.V. (to a maximum of 22.6 mg) given over 1 to 2 minutes, followed by a continuous infusion of 2 mcg/kg/minute (to a maximum of 15 mg/hour) for up to 72 hours. May reduce infusion rate to 0.5 mcg/kg/minute during percutaneous coronary intervention (PCI); then continue infusion for 20 to 24 hours after procedure.

➤ Prevention of thrombosis related to PCI

Adults: 180 mcg/kg (to a maximum of 22.6 mg) I.V. bolus immediately before PCI, then a continuous infusion of 2 mcg/kg/minute (to a maximum of 15 mg/hour), followed by a second 180-mcg/kg bolus 10 minutes after first bolus. Continue infusion until discharge or for up to 24 hours.

Dosage adjustment

- Renal impairment

Contraindications
- Hypersensitivity to drug
- Severe hypertension
- Recent cerebrovascular accident
- Recent surgery
- Bleeding disorders
- Renal dialysis or creatinine level of at least 4 mg/dl

Administration
- Withdraw bolus dose from 10-ml vial into syringe, and give by I.V. push over 1 to 2 minutes .
- Follow I.V. push with continuous I.V. infusion administered undiluted from a 100-ml vial spiked with an infusion set connected to the infusion control device.
- Don't administer through same I.V. line as furosemide.

Route	Onset	Peak	Duration
I.V.	Immediate	Immediate	4-6 hr

Adverse reactions
CNS: headache, dizziness, asthenia, syncope
CV: hypotension
GI: nausea, diarrhea, constipation
GU: hematuria
Hematologic: bleeding, thrombocytopenia
Skin: flushing
Other: bleeding at femoral artery access site

Interactions
Drug-drug. *Clopidogrel, dipyridamole, nonsteroidal anti-inflammatory drugs, oral anticoagulants, thrombolytics, ticlopidine:* increased risk of bleeding
Other platelet aggregation inhibitors: serious bleeding
Drug-diagnostic tests. *Platelets:* decreased count
Drug-herb. *Most commonly used herbs:* increased anticoagulant effect of eptifibatide

Precautions
Use cautiously in:
- renal insufficiency
- elderly patients
- pregnant or breastfeeding patients.

Patient monitoring
- Monitor vital signs and assess cardiovascular status, especially for syncope and hypotension.
- Monitor coagulation studies, complete blood count, and platelet count; watch for signs of abnormal bleeding or bruising and hematuria.
- Check carefully for bleeding at all sites of invasive procedures, particularly femoral access site.

Patient teaching
- Inform patient that drug causes serious adverse effects but can help prevent more chest pain or a heart attack. Reassure him that he'll be closely monitored during therapy.
- ◀ Instruct patient to report fainting or abnormal bruising or bleeding immediately.
- Teach patient safety measures to avoid bruising or bleeding.

ergonovine maleate
Ergotrate, Ergotrate Maleate✤

Pharmacologic class: Amine ergot alkaloid
Therapeutic class: Oxytocic
Pregnancy risk category NR

Action
Directly stimulates uterine muscle to increase strength, duration, and frequency of uterine contractions and decreases bleeding

Availability
Injection: 0.2 mg/ml
Tablets: 0.2 mg

🚫 Indications and dosages
➣ Prevention or treatment of post-partum and postabortion hemorrhage
Adults: 0.2 mg I.M.; may repeat q 2 to 4 hours for no more than five doses. Or 0.2 mg I.V. in emergencies over at least 1 minute. After initial I.M. or I.V. administration, drug may be given orally in doses of 0.2 to 0.4 mg q 6 to 12 hours for 2 to 7 days.

Contraindications
• Hypersensitivity to drug
• Labor induction
• Threatened spontaneous abortion

Administration
• Be aware that I.V. use is for emergencies only and that drug may be given undiluted or diluted in 5 ml of normal saline for injection over at least 1 minute.

Route	Onset	Peak	Duration
I.V.	Immediate	45 min	Unknown
I.M.	2-5 min	3 hr	Unknown

Adverse reactions
CNS: dizziness, headache, confusion, coma
CV: hypertension, angina, chest pain, **shock, arrhythmias**
EENT: tinnitus
GI: nausea, vomiting, diarrhea
Other: ergotism, cold and numb extremities, **allergic reaction**

Interactions
Drug-drug. *Cardiac glycosides, sympathomimetic amines:* increased vasoconstriction
Triptans: prolonged vasospastic reactions
Drug-behaviors. *Smoking:* increased vasoconstriction

Precautions
Use cautiously in:
• hepatic or renal impairment, hypertension, heart disease, vascular disease, sepsis
• breastfeeding patients.

Patient monitoring
◀€ Monitor vital signs, especially for hypertension (which may be severe) and shock secondary to allergic response.
• Assess neurologic status closely; check for headache, loss of consciousness, or coma.
• Monitor circulatory status for numb, cold extremities, which may lead to gangrene of fingers and toes.

Patient teaching
◀€ Caution patient that drug causes serious adverse effects. Instruct him to immediately report headache, chest pain, seizures, and numbness and coldness of arms and legs.
• Reassure patient that he'll be closely monitored.

---

ergotamine tartrate
Ergomar✦, Ergostat, Gynergen✦

Pharmacologic class: Alpha-adrenergic blocker

Therapeutic class: Vascular headache suppressant

Pregnancy risk category X

Action
Produces vasoconstriction of peripheral and cranial blood vessels by stimulating alpha-adrenergic and serotoninergic receptors

Availability
Tablets: 1 mg
Tablets (sublingual): 2 mg

Indications and dosages

➤ Vascular headaches (including migraine and cluster headaches)
Adults: Initially, 1 to 2 mg P.O. or S.L., repeated q 30 minutes until attack subsides or a total of 6 mg has been given. Alternatively, 1 to 2 mg P.O. daily at bedtime for 10 to 14 days to terminate series of cluster headaches. Drug shouldn't be used more than twice weekly, with at least 5 days between courses.

Contraindications

- Serious infections
- Cardiovascular or peripheral vascular disease
- Severe renal or hepatic disease
- Pregnancy or breastfeeding

Administration

- Give first tablet as soon as vascular headache symptoms occur.
- Repeat doses every 30 minutes as needed, but don't give more than three tablets in 24-hour period.

Route	Onset	Peak	Duration
P.O.	1-2 hr	1-5 hr	Unknown
S.L.	Unknown	Unknown	Unknown

Adverse reactions

CNS: dizziness, fatigue
CV: angina pectoris, peripheral vasospasm, intermittent claudication, sinus bradycardia or tachycardia, **myocardial infarction (MI)**
EENT: rhinitis
GI: nausea, vomiting, diarrhea, abdominal pain, altered taste
Musculoskeletal: muscle pain; leg weakness; stiff neck, shoulders, or extremities
Other: excessive thirst

Interactions

Drug-drug. *Almotriptan, frovatriptan, naratriptan, rizatriptan, sumatriptan,*

zolmitriptan: prolonged vasoconstriction
Beta-adrenergic blockers, hormonal contraceptives, macrolides, vasoconstrictors: increased risk of peripheral vasoconstriction
Nitrates: antagonism of antianginal effects
Vasoconstrictors: additive effects
Drug-behaviors. *Heavy smoking:* increased risk of peripheral vasoconstriction

Precautions

Use cautiously in:
- illnesses associated with peripheral vascular disease, such as diabetes mellitus
- children younger than age 6 (safety not established).

Patient monitoring

- Monitor vital signs, especially for tachycardia or bradycardia.
- Assess cardiovascular status closely. Watch for intermittent claudication and signs and symptoms of MI.
- Monitor neurologic status, particularly for numbness and tingling in arms and legs.

Patient teaching

- Instruct patient to take first tablet as soon as symptoms appear and to repeat doses every 30 minutes as needed; emphasize that he should take no more than three tablets in 24 hours or five tablets in 7 days.
- Advise patient to avoid driving and other hazardous activities until he knows how drug affects concentration, alertness, and strength.

ertapenem sodium
Invanz

Pharmacologic class: Carbapenem
Therapeutic class: Anti-infective
Pregnancy risk category B

Action
Inhibits cell wall synthesis in bacteria, causing cell death

Availability
Powder for infusion (lyophilized): 1 g/vial

Indications and dosages
➣ Community-acquired pneumonia caused by *Streptococcus pneumoniae, Haemophilus influenzae,* or *Moraxella catarrhalis;* skin infections caused by *Staphylococcus aureus, Streptococcus pyogenes, Escherichia coli,* and *Peptostreptococcus* species; complicated genitourinary (GU) infections caused by *E. coli* and *Klebsiella pneumoniae;* complicated intra-abdominal infections caused by *E. coli, Clostridium clostridioforme, Eubacterium lentum, Peptostreptococcus* species, *Bacteroides fragilis, B. thetaiotaomicron,* or *B. uniformis;* acute pelvic infections caused by *Streptococcus agalactiae, E. coli, B. fragilis, Peptostreptococcus* species, or *Prevotella bivia*
Adults: 1 g I.M. or I.V. daily. Length of treatment varies with type of infection: community-acquired pneumonia, 10 to 14 days; skin and skin structures, 7 to 14 days; GU, 10 to 14 days; intra-abdominal, 5 to 14 days; acute pelvic, 3 to 10 days.
Dosage adjustment
• Renal impairment

Contraindications
• Hypersensitivity to drug
• Allergy to lidocaine

Administration
• Reconstitute for I.V. use by adding to vial 10 ml of sterile or bacteriostatic water or normal saline for injection.
• Further dilute reconstituted drug in 50 ml of normal saline solution. Infuse over 30 minutes; don't mix with other drugs.
• Reconstitute for I.M. use by adding 3.2 ml of 1% lidocaine to vial and shaking well.
• Give I.M. dose deep into large muscle mass, such as gluteus maximus or lateral thigh.

Route	Onset	Peak	Duration
I.V.	Rapid	30 min	Unknown
I.M.	10 min	2.3 hr	Unknown

Adverse reactions
CNS: headache, dizziness, asthenia, fatigue, insomnia, altered mental status, anxiety, **seizures**
CV: edema, hypotension, hypertension, chest pain, phlebitis, thrombophlebitis, **arrhythmias, heart failure**
EENT: pharyngitis
GI: nausea, vomiting, diarrhea, constipation, abdominal pain, dyspepsia, gastroesophageal reflux disease, **pseudomembranous colitis**
GU: vaginitis
Hepatic: hepatotoxicity
Respiratory: crackles, cough, dyspnea, wheezing, **respiratory distress**
Skin: rash, erythema multiforme, **Steven Johnson syndrome, toxic epidermal necrolysis**
Other: fever, pain, and inflammation at I.V. site

Interactions
Drug-drug. *Probenecid:* increased blood level and half-life of ertapenem

Precautions
Use cautiously in:
• seizure disorder

- pregnant or breastfeeding patients
- children.

Patient monitoring
- Monitor vital signs, electrocardiogram, and cardiovascular status closely. Stay alert for arrhythmias, edema, blood pressure changes, and signs and symptoms of heart failure.
- Assess neurologic status, and watch for signs of impending seizures.
- Monitor bowel pattern, watching for signs of pseudomembranous colitis.
- Inspect injection site for signs of thrombophlebitis and tissue necrosis.
- Watch for indications of erythema multiforme (sore throat, rash, cough, iris lesions, mouth sores, fever). Report early signs before condition progresses to Stevens-Johnson syndrome.
- Be alert for respiratory distress, abnormal breath sounds, and dyspnea.

Patient teaching
- Tell patient to notify nurse right away if drug causes pain or swelling at injection site.
- Advise patient that drug can be toxic to many organ systems. Encourage him to report significant adverse effects right away.
- Reassure patient that he'll be closely monitored.

erythromycin
Apo-Erythro✤, Apo-Erythro-EC, Diomycin✤, E-Base, E-Mycin, Erybid✤, ERYC, Ery-Tab, Erythromid✤, PCE✤

erythromycin estolate
Ilosone, Novo-rythro✤

erythromycin ethylsuccinate
Apo-Erythro-ES✤, E.E.S., EryPed

erythromycin gluceptate
Ilotycin Glucceptate

erythromycin lactobionate
Erythrocin

erythromycin stearate
Erythrocot, My-E

erythromycin (topical)
Akne-Mycin, A/T/S, Emgel, Erycette, Erygel, EryMax, Ery-Sol, ETS, Sans-Acne✤, Staticin, Theramycin Z, T-Stat

Pharmacologic class: Macrolide
Therapeutic class: Anti-infective
Pregnancy risk category B

Action
Binds with 50S subunit of susceptible bacterial ribosomes, thereby suppressing protein synthesis in bacterial cells and causing cell death

Availability
erythromycin base
Capsules (delayed-release): 250 mg
Tablets (enteric-coated): 250 mg, 333 mg
Tablets (film-coated): 500 mg

Tablets (with polymer-coated particles):
333 mg, 500 mg
erythromycin estolate
Capsules: 250 mg
Oral suspension (cherry flavor):
250 mg/5 ml
Oral suspension (orange flavor):
125 mg/5 ml
Tablets: 500 mg
erythromycin ethylsuccinate
Drops: 100 mg/2.5 ml
Oral suspension (cherry, fruit flavors):
200 mg/5 ml
*Oral suspension (banana, orange
flavors):* 400 mg/5 ml
Tablets: 400 mg
Tablets (chewable): 200 mg
erythromycin gluceptate
Powder for injection: 500 mg, 1 g
erythromycin lactobionate
Powder for injection: 500 mg, 1 g
erythromycin stearate
Tablets (film-coated): 250 mg
erythromycin (topical)
Gel: 2%
Ointment: 2%
Solution: 2%

Indications and dosages
➤ Pelvic inflammatory disease
Adults: 500 mg (base) I.V. q 6 hours
for 3 days, then 250 mg (base, estolate,
or stearate) or 400 mg (ethylsuccinate)
q 6 hours for 7 days
➤ Syphilis
Adults: 500 mg (base, estolate, or
stearate) P.O. q.i.d. for 14 days
➤ Most upper and lower respiratory
tract infections, otitis media, skin infections, legionnaires' disease
Adults: 250 mg P.O. q 6 hours, or 333
mg P.O. q 8 hours, or 500 mg P.O. q 12
hours (base, estolate, or stearate); or
400 mg P.O. q 6 hours or 800 mg P.O. q
12 hours (ethylsuccinate); or 250 to
500 mg I.V. (up to 1 g) q 6 hours (gluceptate or lactobionate)
Children: 30 to 50 mg/kg/day (base,
estolate, ethylsuccinate, or lactobionate) I.V. or P.O., in divided doses q 6

hours for I.V. and q 6 to 8 hours for
P.O. Maximum dosage is 2 g/day for
base or estolate, 3.2 g/day for ethylsuc-
cinate, and 4 g/day for lactobionate.
➤ Intestinal amebiasis
Adults: 250 mg (base, estolate, or
stearate) or 400 mg (ethylsuccinate)
P.O. q 6 hours for 10 to 14 days
Children: 30 to 50 mg/kg/day (base,
estolate, ethylsuccinate, or stearate)
P.O. in divided doses over 10 to 14 days
➤ Conjunctivitis of the newborn
Neonates: 50 mg/kg/day (ethylsucci-
nate or estolate) P.O. in four divided
doses for at least 14 days
➤ Pertussis
Children: 40 to 50 mg/kg/day (estolate
preferred) P.O. in four divided doses
for 14 days
➤ Pneumonia of infancy
Infants: 50 mg/kg/day (ethylsuccinate
or estolate) P.O. in four divided doses
for at least 3 weeks
➤ Acne
Adults and children older than age 12:
2% ointment, gel, or solution applied
topically b.i.d.
Dosage adjustment
• Hepatic impairment

Off-label uses
• Chancroid

Contraindications
• Hypersensitivity to drug or tartrazine
• Hepatic impairment (with estolate)
• Pregnancy (with estolate)

Administration
• Give ethylsuccinate and delayed-
release products without regard to
meals.
• Give erythromycin base or stearate 1
hour before or 2 hours after meals for
optimal absorption.
• Follow label directions to reconstitute drug for I.V. use, then infuse each
250 mg in at least 100 ml of normal
saline solution over 1 hour.

Route	Onset	Peak	Duration
P.O.	1 hr	1-4 hr	6-12 hr
I.V.	Rapid	End of infusion	6-12 hr

Adverse reactions
CV: torsades de pointes, **arrythmias**
EENT: ototoxicity
GI: nausea, vomiting, diarrhea, abdominal pain or cramps
Hepatic: hepatic dysfunction, **hepatitis**
Skin: rash
Other: increased appetite, allergic reactions, superinfection, phlebitis at I.V. site

Interactions
Drug-drug. *Alfentanil, alprazolam, bromocriptine, buspirone, carbamazepine, clozapine, cyclosporine, diazepam, disopyramide, ergot alkaloids, felodipine, methylprednisolone, midazolam, tacrolimus, theophylline, triazolam, vinblastine, warfarin:* increased blood levels and risk of toxicity of these drugs
Clindamycin, lincomycin: antagonism of erythromycin's effects
Digoxin: increased digoxin blood level
HMG-CoA reductase inhibitors: increased risk of myopathy and rhabdomyolysis
Hormonal contraceptives: decreased contraceptive efficacy
Pimozide, sparfloxacin: increased risk of serious arrhythmias
Rifabutin, rifampin: decreased effects of erythromycin, increased risk of adverse GI reactions
Theophylline: increased theophylline blood level, decreased erythromycin blood level
Drug-diagnostic tests. *Alanine aminotransferase, alkaline phosphatase, aspartate aminotransferase, bilirubin:* increased levels
Urine catecholamines: false elevations

Precautions
Use cautiously in:
• hepatic disease.

Patient monitoring
• Check temperature and watch for signs and symptoms of superinfection.
• Monitor liver function test results. Watch for signs and symptoms of hepatoxicity.
• Assess patient's hearing for signs of ototoxicity.

Patient teaching
• Instruct patient to take drug with 8 oz of water 1 hour before or 2 hours after meals.
• If drug causes GI upset, encourage patient to take it with food.
• Caution patient not to swallow chewable tablets whole and not to chew or crush enteric-coated tablets.
• Advise patient to immediately report signs and symptoms of infection.
• Tell patient he'll undergo blood tests to monitor liver function.

escitalopram
Lexapro

Pharmacologic class: Selective serotonin reuptake inhibitor
Therapeutic class: Antidepressant
Pregnancy risk category C

Action
Prevents reuptake of the neurotransmitter serotonin by CNS neurons, making more serotonin available in brain and thereby relieving depression

Availability
Oral solution: 5 mg/5 ml
Tablets: 10 mg, 20 mg

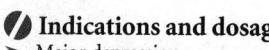 Indications and dosages
➤ Major depression

Adults: Initially, 10 mg P.O. daily as a single dose; after at least 1 week, may increase to 20 mg P.O. daily
Elderly adults and patients with hepatic impairment: Maximum dosage of 10 mg P.O. daily as a single dose

Off-label uses
• Anxiety with depression

Contraindications
• Hypersensitivity to drug
• Monoamine oxidase (MAO) inhibitor use within past 14 days

Administration
• Give drug with or without food.

Route	Onset	Peak	Duration
P.O.	Slow	3.5-6.5 hr	Unknown

Adverse reactions
CNS: drowsiness, dizziness, insomnia, fatigue
EENT: rhinitis, sinusitis
GI: nausea, vomiting, diarrhea, constipation, dyspepsia, abdominal pain, dry mouth
GU: ejaculatory disorders, impotence, anorgasmia (in females), decreased libido
Other: flulike symptoms, increased appetite, serotonin syndrome

Interactions
Drug-drug. *Carbamazepine, lithium:* decreased effects of escitalopram
Citalopram: increased risk of serious toxic effects
MAO inhibitors: increased escitalopram blood level and risk of toxicity
Triptans: weakness, hyperreflexia, incoordination
Drug-herb. *Ginkgo, St. John's wort:* increased risk of adverse effects
Drug-behaviors. *Alcohol use:* increased motor impairment

Precautions
Use cautiously in:
• renal or hepatic impairment, suicidal tendency
• elderly patients
• pregnant or breastfeeding patients.

Patient monitoring
• Assess patient's mood carefully, watching for signs of increased depression or suicidal ideation.
• Monitor patient's prescription refills to help detect drug hoarding or overuse.
• Check nutritional and hydration status in light of GI adverse effects.

Patient teaching
• Inform patient that full drug effect may take up to 4 weeks. Caution him not to overuse drug.
• Advise patient (and significant others as appropriate) to contact prescriber immediately if depression worsens or suicidal thoughts develop.
• Instruct patient to avoid driving and other hazardous activities until he knows how drug affects concentration and alertness.
• Teach patient to minimize GI upset by eating small, frequent servings of healthy food and drinking plenty of fluids.

esmolol hydrochloride
Brevibloc

Pharmacologic class: Beta-adrenergic blocker (cardioselective)

Therapeutic class: Antiarrhythmic, antihypertensive

Pregnancy risk category C

Action
Blocks stimulation of beta-adrenergic receptors (primarily beta$_1$ receptors), reducing atrioventricular conduction

---

and cardiac output, decreasing blood pressure

Availability
Injection: 10 mg/ml, 250 mg/ml

⚠ Indications and dosages
➤ Supraventricular tachycardia
Adults: Initially, a loading dose of 500 mcg/kg/minute by I.V. infusion over 1 minute, followed by a maintenance infusion of 50 mcg/kg/minute over 4 minutes. If desired response isn't achieved after 5 minutes, repeat loading dose and follow with a maintenance infusion of 100 mcg/kg/minute for 4 minutes. Sequence is repeated as needed, with a maintenance dosage increased in increments of 50 mcg/kg/minute, up to a maximum maintenance infusion of 200 mcg/kg/minute for 48 hours.
➤ Perioperative and postoperative tachycardia or hypertension
Adults: Initially, 80 mg (1 mg/kg) by I.V. bolus over 30 seconds; then 150 mcg/kg/minute by I.V. infusion, up to a maximum of 300 mcg/kg/minute

Off-label uses
• Acute myocardial ischemia

Contraindications
• Hypersensitivity to drug
• Heart failure
• Cardiogenic shock

Administration
• Dilute 250-mg/ml dose in a compatible I.V. solution to a concentration of 10 mg/ml and administer by infusion control device.
• Know that maximum I.V. solution concentration is 10 mg/ml.
• Because large fluid volumes may be needed to infuse drug, use caution when excessive fluid could be harmful.

Route	Onset	Peak	Duration
I.V.	Immediate	30 min	30 min after infusion

Adverse reactions
CNS: anxiety, depression, dizziness, drowsiness, headache, agitation, fatigue, confusion, speech disorders, asthenia
CV: edema, peripheral ischemia, chest pain, **bradycardia**, hypotension
GI: nausea, vomiting, heartburn, altered taste
GU: urinary retention
Respiratory: wheezing, dyspnea
Skin: flushing, pallor, erythema
Other: fever, chills, midscapular pain, inflammation or induration at infusion site

Interactions
Drug-drug. *Alpha$_1$-adrenergic blockers:* exaggerated antihypertensive effect
Catecholamines, reserpine: increased bradycardia and hypotension
Digoxin: increased digoxin blood level
Morphine: increased esmolol blood level
Succinylcholine: prolonged neuromuscular blockade
Drug-herb. *Ma huang, St. John's wort, yohimbe:* decreased antihypertensive effect

Precautions
Use cautiously in:
• renal impairment, diabetes, bronchospasm, cardiac disease, cerebrovascular insufficiency, peripheral vascular disease, hyperthyroidism, myasthenic conditions
• pregnant or breastfeeding patients.

Patient monitoring
• Monitor vital signs and electrocardiogram, particularly for hypotension.
• Assess neurologic status, and institute safety measures as needed.

- Monitor fluid intake and output, watching for urinary retention.
- Check I.V. site regularly.

Patient teaching
- Explain to patient that drug is an emergency measure to control blood pressure, arrhythmias, or heart rate.
- Ensure patient he'll be closely monitored throughout drug therapy.
- Tell patient to report pain or redness at I.V. site.

esomeprazole magnesium
Nexium

Pharmacologic class: Proton pump inhibitor
Therapeutic class: Antiulcer agent
Pregnancy risk category C

Action
Reduces gastric acid production by inhibiting proton pump enzyme system in gastric parietal cells, preventing final transport of hydrogen ions into gastric lumen

Availability
Capsules (delayed-release): 20 mg, 40 mg

⏀ Indications and dosages
➤ Gastroesophageal reflux disease (GERD)
Adults: 20 to 40 mg P.O. once daily for 4 to 8 weeks
➤ Symptomatic GERD
Adults: 20 mg P.O. once daily for 4 to 8 weeks p.r.n.;
➤ Prevention of erosive esophagitis
Adults: 20 mg P.O. once daily
➤ Duodenal ulcer associated with *Helicobacter pylori* infection (triple therapy)
Adults: 40 mg P.O. once daily for 10 days, given in combination with amox-

icillin 1,000 mg b.i.d. for 10 days and with clarithromycin 500 mg b.i.d. for 10 days

Contraindications
- Hypersensitivity to drug
- Breastfeeding

Administration
- Give drug 1 hour before or 2 hours after a meal.
- Know that contents of capsules may be mixed with applesauce.
- Don't crush capsules or pellets.

Route	Onset	Peak	Duration
P.O.	Rapid	1.6 hr	24 hr

Adverse reactions
CNS: headache, dizziness, asthenia, vertigo, insomnia, apathy, anxiety, paresthesia, abnormal dreams
EENT: sinusitis, epistaxis
GI: nausea, vomiting, diarrhea, constipation, abdominal pain, flatulence, dry mouth
Respiratory: upper respiratory tract infection, cough
Skin: rash, inflammation, urticaria, pruritus, alopecia, dry skin

Interactions
Drug-drug. *Digoxin, ketoconazole, iron salts:* altered absorption and effects of these drugs
Drug-diagnostic tests. *Alanine aminotransferase, alkaline phosphatase, aspartate aminotransferase, bilirubin, creatinine, uric acid:* increased levels
Hemoglobin, platelets, potassium, sodium, thyroxine, white blood cells: altered levels

Precautions
Use cautiously in:
- severe hepatic impairment
- pregnant patients
- children younger than age18 (safety not established).

Patient monitoring

• Monitor neurologic status, especially for dizziness, headache, paresthesia, and asthenia.
• Watch for signs and symptoms of EENT and respiratory infections.
• Assess nutritional and hydration status in light of GI adverse effects.
• Check for rash and other signs of hypersensitivity.
• Monitor liver function test results if patient is on long-term therapy.

Patient teaching

• Instruct patient to take drug 1 hour before or 2 hours after a meal.
• If patient has trouble swallowing capsule, teach him to open it, sprinkle pellets into soft food such as applesauce, and take right away.
• Advise patient to report rash or other signs of hypersensitivity.
• Instruct patient to avoid driving and other hazardous activities until he knows how drug affects concentration and alertness.
• Teach patient to minimize GI upset by eating small, frequent servings of healthy food and drinking plenty of fluids.
• As appropriate, review all significant adverse reactions and interactions, especially the drugs and tests mentioned above.

estradiol
Estrace, Gynodiol

estradiol cypionate
depGynogen, Depo-Estradiol, Depogen, Dura-Estrin, E-Cypionate, Estragyn LA 5, Estro-Cyp, Estrofem, Estro-L.A.

estradiol transdermal system
Alora, Climara, Esclim, Estraderm, FemPatch, Vivelle

estradiol valerate
Clinagen LA 40, Delestrogen, Dioval XX, Duragen-20, Estra-L 40, Estro-Span, Femogex✤, Gynogen L.A. 20, Menaval, Valergen-20

Pharmacologic class: Estrogen
Therapeutic class: Hormone
Pregnancy risk category X

Action

Stimulates DNA and RNA synthesis, promoting development of female sex organs, including secondary sex characteristics in women; also increases cervical secretion and improves uterine tonicity.

Availability

Injection (cypionate in oil): 5 mg/ml
Injection (valerate in oil): 10 mg/ml, 20 mg/ml, 40 mg/ml
Tablets: 0.5 mg, 1 mg, 1.5 mg, 2 mg
Transdermal system: 25 mcg/24-hour release rate, 37.5 mcg/24-hour release rate, 50 mcg/24-hr release rate, 75 mcg/24-hour release rate, 100 mcg/ 24-hour release rate

Vaginal cream: 100 mcg/g
Vaginal ring: 2 mg released over 90 days
Vaginal tablets: 25 mcg

💋 Indications and dosages

➤ Symptoms of menopause, atrophic vaginitis, female hypogonadism, ovarian failure, and osteoporosis
Adults: 0.5 to 2 mg (estradiol) P.O. daily or cyclically. Or 1 to 5 mg (cypionate) or 10 to 20 mg (valerate) I.M. monthly. Or 50- or 100-mcg/24-hour transdermal patch applied twice weekly (Alora, Estraderm) or weekly (Climara). Or 25-mcg/24-hour patch applied q 7 days (FemPatch) or 37.5- to 100-mcg transdermal patch applied twice weekly (Vivelle). Or 2 to 4 g (0.2 to 0.4 mg) vaginal cream (estradiol) daily for 1 to 2 weeks, then decreased to 1 to 2 g/day for 1 to 2 weeks, then a maintenance dose of 1 g one to three times weekly for 3 weeks, then off for 1 week; cycle repeated once vaginal mucosa has been restored. Or 2-mg vaginal ring q 3 months or 25-mcg vaginal tablet once daily for 2 weeks, then twice weekly.
➤ Postmenopausal breast cancer
Adults: 10 mg P.O. t.i.d. (estradiol)
➤ Prostate cancer
Adults: 1 to 2 mg P.O. t.i.d. (estradiol) or 30 mg I.M. q 1 to 2 weeks (valerate)

Contraindications

• Hypersensitivity to drug
• Thromboembolic disease
• Vaginal bleeding
• Pregnancy or breastfeeding

Administration

• Inject I.M. dose deep into large muscle mass and rotate injection sites.
• If switching from oral estrogen to transdermal, apply patch 1 week after withdrawal of oral therapy.

Route	Onset	Peak	Duration
P.O.	Slow	Days	Unknown
I.M.	Unknown	Unknown	Unknown
Trans-dermal	Unknown	Unknown	3-4 days (Estraderm) 7 days (Climara)
Vaginal ring	Unknown	Unknown	90 days
Vaginal tablet	Unknown	Unknown	3-4 days

Adverse reactions

CNS: headache, dizziness, lethargy, depression
CV: edema, hypertension, **myocardial infarction (MI), thromboembolism**
EENT: contact lens intolerance, worsening of myopia or astigmatism
GI: nausea, vomiting
GU: amenorrhea, dysmenorrhea, breakthrough bleeding, cervical erosions, decreased libido, vaginal candidiasis, impotence, testicular atrophy, gynecomastia, breast pain or tenderness
Hepatic: jaundice
Metabolic: hypercalcemia, sodium and water retention, hyperglycemia
Musculoskeletal: leg cramps
Skin: oily skin, acne, pigmentation changes, urticaria
Other: weight loss or gain, increased appetite

Interactions

Drug-drug. *Insulin, oral hypoglycemics, warfarin:* altered dosage requirements for these drugs
Drug-diagnostic tests. *Antithrombin III, folate, low-density lipoproteins, pyridoxine, total cholesterol, urine pregnanediol:* decreased levels
Cortisol; factors VII, VIII, IX, and X; glucose; high-density lipoproteins; phospholipids; prolactin; prothrombin; sodium; triglycerides: increased levels
Metyrapone test: false decrease
Thyroid function tests: false interpretation

Drug-behaviors. *Smoking:* increased risk of adverse CV reactions

Precautions
Use cautiously in:
• cardiovascular, hepatic, and renal disease.

Patient monitoring
◀€ Monitor vital signs and cardiovascular status, especially for hypertension, edema, thromboembolism, or MI.
• Assess vision.
• In diabetic patients, monitor blood glucose levels and watch for signs and symptoms of hyperglycemia.

Patient teaching
• Instruct patient to place transdermal patches on clean, dry skin areas and to replace patches as instructed on product label.
• Teach proper technique for use of vaginal tablets, rings, and creams, as appropriate.
• Inform patient that drug may cause loss of libido (in women) or impotence (in men). Encourage patient to discuss these issues with prescriber.
• Advise patient that drug may worsen nearsightedness or astigmatism and make contact lenses uncomfortable.

estrogens, conjugated
C.E.S.♣, Congest♣, Premarin, Premarin Intravenous

Pharmacologic class: Estrogen
Therapeutic class: Replacement hormone, antineoplastic, antiosteoporotic
Pregnancy risk category X

Action
Bind to nuclear receptors in responsive tissues (such as female genital organs, breasts, and pituitary gland), enhancing DNA, RNA, and protein synthesis. In androgen-dependent prostate cancer, estrogens compete for androgen receptor sites, inhibiting androgens. Also decreases pituitary release of follicle-stimulating hormone and luteinizing hormone.

Availability
Powder for injection: 25 mg/5 ml
Tablets: 0.3 mg, 0.625 mg, 0.9 mg, 1.25 mg, 2.5 mg
Vaginal cream: 0.625 mg/g

🖋 Indications and dosages
➤ Ovariectomy, primary ovarian failure
Adults: 1.25 mg P.O. daily or in cycles of 3 weeks on and 1 week off
➤ Osteoporosis and menopausal symptoms
Adults: 0.3 to 1.25 mg P.O. daily or in cycles of 3 weeks on and 1 week off
➤ Female hypogonadism
Adults: 0.3 to 0.625 mg P.O. daily, given cyclically 3 weeks on and 1 week off
➤ Inoperable breast cancer in men and postmenopausal women
Adults: 10 mg P.O. t.i.d. for 3 months or more
➤ Inoperable prostate carcinoma
Adults: 1.25 to 2.5 mg P.O. t.i.d.
➤ Uterine bleeding caused by hormonal imbalance
Adults: 25 mg I.M. or I.V., repeated in 6 to 12 hours if necessary
➤ Atrophic vaginitis
Adults: 0.5 to 2 g (vaginal cream) intravaginally daily in cycles of 3 weeks on and 1 week off

Contraindications
• Hypersensitivity to drug
• Thromboembolic disease (current or previous)
• Undiagnosed vaginal bleeding
• Breast or reproductive system cancer (except in metastatic disease)

- Estrogen-dependent neoplasms
- Pregnancy

Administration

- Know that drug is compatible with dextrose 5% in water and normal saline solution.
- Give oral doses in cycles of 3 weeks on, 1 week off.

Route	Onset	Peak	Duration
P.O., I.M.	Unknown	Unknown	6-12 hr
I.V.	Rapid	Unknown	6-12 hr
Intravaginal	Unknown	Unknown	Unknown

Adverse reactions

CNS: headache, dizziness, lethargy, depression, asthenia, paresthesia, syncope, **cerebrovascular accident (CVA), seizures**

CV: hypertension, chest pain, **myocardial infarction (MI), thromboembolism**

EENT: contact lens intolerance, worsening of myopia or astigmatism, otitis media, sinusitis, rhinitis, pharyngitis

GI: nausea, vomiting, diarrhea, abdominal cramps, bloating, enlarged abdomen, dyspepsia, flatulence, gastritis, gastroenteritis, hemorrhoids, colitis, gallbladder disease, cholestatic jaundice, anorexia, **pancreatitis**

GU: urinary incontinence, dysuria, amenorrhea, dysmenorrhea, endometrial hyperplasia, vaginal candidiasis, urinary tract infection, leukorrhea, vaginal hemorrhage, genital eruptions, gynecomastia, breast tenderness, breast enlargement or secretion, reduced libido, impotence, testicular atrophy, **increased risk of breast cancer, endometrial cancer, hemolytic uremic syndrome**

Hepatic: hepatic adenoma

Metabolic: hyperglycemia, hypercalcemia, sodium and water retention, reduced carbohydrate tolerance

Musculoskeletal: leg cramps, back pain, skeletal pain

Respiratory: upper respiratory tract infection, bronchitis, **pulmonary embolism**

Skin: acne, oily skin, changes in pigmentation, urticaria, pruritus, erythema nodosum or multiforme, hemorrhagic eruption, skin hypertrophy, hirsutism, alopecia

Other: edema, weight changes, increased appetite, hypersensitivity reaction

Interactions

Drug-drug. *Corticosteroids:* enhanced corticosteroid effects

CYP450 inducers (such as barbiturates, rifampin): decreased estrogen efficacy

Hypoglycemics, warfarin: altered requirement for these drugs

Phenytoin: loss of seizure control

Tamoxifen: interference with tamoxifen effects

Tricyclic antidepressants: reduced antidepressant effects

Drug-diagnostic tests. *Antithrombin III, folate, low-density lipoproteins, pyridoxine, total cholesterol, urine pregnanediol:* decreased values

Cortisol; factors VII, VIII, IX, and X; glucose; high-density lipoproteins; phospholipids; prolactin; prothrombin; sodium; triglycerides: increased values

Metyrapone test: false decrease

Thyroid function tests: false interpretation

Drug-food. *Caffeine:* increased caffeine blood level

Drug-herb. *Black cohosh:* increased risk of adverse reactions

Red clover: interference with estrogen effects

Saw palmetto: antiestrogenic effects

St. John's wort: decreased drug blood level and effects

Drug-behaviors. *Smoking:* increased risk of adverse cardiovascular reactions

---

Precautions
Use cautiously in:
• cardiovascular disease, severe hepatic or renal disease, asthma, bone disease, migraine, seizures, breast disease
• family history of breast or genital tract cancer
• breastfeeding.

Patient monitoring
• Monitor liver function test results and assess abdomen for liver enlargement.
• Evaluate patient for breast tenderness and swelling; as needed, administer analgesics and apply cool compresses.
• Monitor fluid intake and output; weigh patient daily.
◀€ Know that drug increases risk of thromboembolism, CVA, and MI.
• Check serum phosphatase levels in patients with prostate cancer.
• Monitor calcium, glucose, and folic acid levels and liver function test results.
• Evaluate bone density annually.

Patient teaching
• Teach patient to recognize and report signs and symptoms of thrombophlebitis and thromboembolism.
• Tell patient to report breakthrough vaginal bleeding.
• Recommend that patient have routine breast examinations.
• Mention that contact lens intolerance may occur; instruct patient to report vision changes.
• As appropriate, review all other significant and life-threatening adverse reactions and interactions, especially those related to the drugs, tests, foods, herbs, and behaviors mentioned above.

estrogens, esterified
Estratab, Estratest, Estratest H.S., Menest

Pharmacologic class: Estrogen
Therapeutic class: Replacement hormone, antineoplastic, antiosteoporotic
Pregnancy risk category X

Action
Bind to nuclear receptors in responsive tissues (such as female genital organs, breasts, and pituitary gland), enhancing DNA, RNA, and protein synthesis. In androgen-dependent prostate cancer, estrogens compete for androgen receptor sites, inhibiting androgens. Also decreases pituitary release of follicle-stimulating hormone and luteinizing hormone.

Availability
Tablets: 0.3 mg, 0.625 mg, 1.25 mg, 2.5 mg

🖊 Indications and dosages
➤ Moderate to severe vasomotor symptoms or atrophic vaginitis
Adults: 0.3 to 1.25 mg P.O. daily, adjusted to lowest effective dosage; usually given in cycles of 3 weeks on, 1 week off
➤ Female hypogonadism
Adults: 2.5 to 7.5 mg P.O. daily in divided doses for 20 days, followed by rest period of 10 days. If no bleeding occurs, repeat same dosing schedule. If bleeding occurs before end of rest period, start 20-day estrogen-progestin cycle, with progestin P.O. given during last 5 days of estrogen therapy.
➤ Inoperable prostate cancer
Adults: 1.25 to 2.5 mg P.O. t.i.d. In long-term therapy, gauge efficacy by symptomatic response and serum phosphatase level.

> Selected breast cancers (inoperable, progressing)

Adults: 10 mg P.O. t.i.d. for at least 3 months in selected men and post-menopausal women

> Prevention of osteoporosis

Adults: Initially, 0.3 mg P.O. daily, increased as needed to a maximum dosage of 1.25 mg/day

Contraindications

• Hypersensitivity to drug
• Thromboembolic disease (current or previous)
• Undiagnosed vaginal bleeding
• Breast and reproductive cancers (except in metastatic disease)
• Estrogen-dependent neoplasms
• Pregnancy

Administration

• Administer with food or fluids.
• Give cyclically as prescribed, except when used palliatively for cancer treatment.

Route	Onset	Peak	Duration
P.O.	Slow	Days	Unknown

Adverse reactions

CNS: headache, dizziness, lethargy, depression, asthenia, paresthesia, syncope, **increased risk of cerebrovascular accident (CVA)**, **seizures**

CV: hypertension, chest pain, **myocardial infarction (MI)**, **thromboembolism**, **pulmonary embolism**

EENT: contact lens intolerance, worsening of myopia or astigmatism, otitis media, sinusitis, rhinitis, pharyngitis

GI: nausea, vomiting, diarrhea, dyspepsia, flatulence, gastritis, gastroenteritis, enlarged abdomen, hemorrhoids, colitis, gallbladder disease, anorexia, **pancreatitis**

GU: urinary incontinence, dysuria, amenorrhea, dysmenorrhea, endometrial hyperplasia, urinary tract infection, leukorrhea, vaginal discomfort or pain, vaginal hemorrhage, genital eruptions, gynecomastia, breast tenderness, breast enlargement or secretion, reduced libido, impotence, testicular atrophy, **increased risk of breast cancer**, **endometrial cancer**, **hemolytic uremic syndrome**

Hepatic: cholestatic jaundice, hepatic adenoma

Metabolic: hyperglycemia, hypercalcemia, sodium and fluid retention, reduced carbohydrate tolerance

Musculoskeletal: leg cramps, back pain, skeletal pain

Respiratory: upper respiratory tract infection, bronchitis

Skin: acne, increased pigmentation, urticaria, pruritus, erythema nodosum, hemorrhagic eruption, alopecia, hirsutism

Other: increased appetite, weight changes, edema, flulike symptoms, **hypersensitivity reactions**

Interactions

Drug-drug. *Corticosteroids:* enhanced corticosteroid effects

CYP450 inducers (such as barbiturates, rifampin): decreased estrogen efficacy

Hypoglycemics, warfarin: altered requirement for these drugs

Phenytoin: loss of seizure control

Tamoxifen: interference with tamoxifen efficacy

Tricyclic antidepressants: reduced antidepressant effect

Drug-diagnostic tests. *Antithrombin III, folate, low-density lipoproteins, pyridoxine, total cholesterol, urine pregnanediol:* decreased values

Cortisol; factors VII, VIII, IX, and X; glucose; high-density lipoproteins; phospholipids; prolactin; prothrombin; sodium; triglycerides: increased values

Metyrapone test: false decrease

Thyroid function tests: false interpretation

Drug-food. *Caffeine:* increased caffeine levels

Drug-herb. *Black cohosh:* increased risk of adverse reactions

---

Red clover: interference with estrogen therapy

Saw palmetto: antiestrogenic effects

St. John's wort: decreased drug blood level and effects

Drug-behaviors. *Smoking:* increased risk of adverse cardiovascular reactions

Precautions

Use cautiously in:
- cardiovascular disease, severe hepatic or renal disease, asthma, bone disease, migraines, seizures, breast nodules, fibrocystic breasts, abnormal mammograms
- family history of breast or genital tract cancer
- breastfeeding.

Patient monitoring

- Monitor fluid intake and output; weigh patient daily.
- Evaluate patient for breast tenderness and swelling; as needed, administer analgesics and apply cool compresses.
- ◀ Know that drug increases risk of thromboembolism, CVA, and MI.
- Monitor liver function test results and assess abdomen for liver enlargement.
- Check serum phosphatase levels in patients with prostate cancer.
- Monitor calcium and glucose levels.

Patient teaching

- Instruct patient to recognize and immediately report signs and symptoms of thrombophlebitis and thromboembolism.
- Teach patient how to perform breast self-examination; emphasize importance of monthly checks.
- Tell patient to report breakthrough vaginal bleeding.
- Mention that drug may cause contact lens intolerance; advise patient to report vision changes.
- Inform men that drug may cause gynecomastia.
- As appropriate, review all other significant and life-threatening adverse reactions and interactions, especially those related to the drugs, tests, foods, herbs, and behaviors mentioned above.

etanercept
Enbrel

Pharmacologic class: Immunomodulator

Therapeutic class: Antiarthritic

Pregnancy risk category B

Action

Reacts with and deactivates free-floating tumor necrosis factor responsible for inflammation

Availability

Powder for injection: 25 mg

Indications and dosages

➤ To reduce signs and symptoms of moderately to severely active rheumatoid arthritis; to delay structural damage related to rheumatoid arthritis; to treat polyarticular-course juvenile rheumatoid arthritis; to reduce signs and symptoms of psoriatic arthritis or psoriasis

Adults: 25 mg S.C. twice weekly 72 to 96 hours apart

Children ages 4 to 17: 0.4 mg/kg S.C. twice weekly 72 to 96 hours apart, to a maximum of 25 mg/dose

Contraindications

- Hypersensitivity to drug
- Sepsis or risk of sepsis

Administration

- Inject S.C. into thigh, abdomen, or upper arm.
- Rotate injection sites.

Route	Onset	Peak	Duration
S.C.	Slow	72 hr	Unknown

♣ Canada   ◀ Clinical alert   Reactions in **bold** are life-threatening

Adverse reactions
CNS: demyelinating disorders (such as multiple sclerosis and myelitis), asthenia, headache, depression, dizziness, paresthesias, fatigue, **cerebral hemorrhage, seizures, cerebrovascular accident (CVA)**

CV: thrombophlebitis, myocardial ischemia, hypotension, hypertension, chest pain, deep vein thrombosis, **myocardial infarction (MI), heart failure**

EENT: ocular inflammation, pharyngitis, rhinitis, cough, bronchitis, sinusitis

GI: nausea, vomiting, abdominal pain, diarrhea, abdominal abscess, dyspepsia, altered taste, anorexia, cholecystitis, **GI hemorrhage, intestinal perforation, pancreatitis**

GU: pyelonephritis, membranous glomerulonephropathy

Hematologic: anemia, **aplastic anemia, leukopenia, pancytopenia, thrombocytopenia**

Metabolic: hypomagnesemia

Musculoskeletal: bursitis, polymyositis, joint pain

Respiratory: congestion, pneumonia, dyspnea, **pulmonary embolism, interstitial lung disease**

Skin: flushing, cellulitis, pruritus, rash, cutaneous vasculitis, urticaria, alopecia, angioedema

Other: adenopathy, weight gain, fever, irritation at injection site, peripheral edema, flulike symptoms

Interactions
None significant

Precautions
Use cautiously in:
• preexisting or recent onset of demyelinating disorders, including multiple sclerosis and myelitis.

Patient monitoring
• Watch for signs and symptoms of pancytopenia and infection.

• Monitor patient for signs and symptoms of GI bleeding; stop therapy immediately if these occur.

• Monitor complete blood count and coagulation studies.

• Check for signs and symptoms of cardiac compromise.

• Monitor pulmonary function test results periodically to assess lung status.

• Assess patient's ability to self-administer drug.

• Check for irritation at injection site; apply cool compresses as needed.

• Monitor patient for conjunctival dryness; apply artificial tears as needed.

Patient teaching
• Tell patient to withhold dose and notify prescriber if he develops an infection or is exposed to persons with chickenpox.

• Teach patient to expect redness, swelling, and pain at injection site; assure him that these problems will diminish over time.

• As appropriate, review all other significant and life-threatening adverse reactions mentioned above.

ethambutol hydrochloride
Etibi ♣, Myambutol

Pharmacologic class: Synthetic antitubercular

Therapeutic class: Antituberculotic, antileprotic

Pregnancy risk category B

Action
Unknown; thought to interfere with RNA synthesis of metabolites of bacteria, decreasing replication

Availability
Tablets: 100 mg, 400 mg

Indications and dosages

➤ Adjunct in tuberculosis and atypical mycobacterial infection caused by *Mycobacterium tuberculosis*

Adults and adolescents: 15 mg/kg P.O. daily in patients who haven't received previous antitubercular therapy; 25 mg/kg P.O daily, decreased to 15 mg/kg daily after 60 days, in patients who have received previous antitubercular therapy

Contraindications
• Hypersensitivity to drug
• Children younger than age 13

Administration
• Obtain specimen for culture and sensitivity testing as necessary before starting therapy.
• Give with food.

Route	Onset	Peak	Duration
P.O.	Rapid	2-4 hr	24 hr

Adverse reactions
CNS: confusion, disorientation, dizziness, hallucinations, headache, peripheral neuritis, malaise
EENT: optic neuritis, blurred vision, decreased visual acuity, eye pain, red-green color blindness
GI: nausea, vomiting, abdominal pain, GI upset, anorexia
Hematologic: eosinophilia, **thrombocytopenia**
Hepatic: transient hepatic impairment; elevated aspartate aminotransferase (AST), alanine aminotransferase (ALT), and bilirubin levels
Metabolic: hyperuricemia, hypoglycemia
Musculoskeletal: joint pain, gouty arthritis
Respiratory: bloody sputum, **pulmonary infiltrates**
Skin: rash, pruritus, toxic epidermal necrolysis
Other: fever, **anaphylactoid reactions**

Interactions
Drug-drug. *Aluminum salts:* delayed and reduced ethambutol absorption
Other neurotoxic drugs: increased risk of neurotoxicity
Drug-diagnostic tests. *AST, ALT, bilirubin, uric acid:* increased levels
Glucose: decreased level

Precautions
Use cautiously in:
• impaired renal and hepatic function, cataracts, recurrent eye inflammation, gout, diabetic retinopathy.

Patient monitoring
• Monitor liver function test results, complete blood count, and blood urea nitrogen, creatinine glucose, and serum uric acid levels.
• Give analgesics for drug-induced pain, as prescribed.
• Monitor blood cultures and sensitivity test results periodically throughout therapy.
• Observe for signs and symptoms of gout.

Patient teaching
• Instruct patient to take drug with 8 oz of water; if stomach upset occurs, advise him to take it with food.
• If patient must take antacids, advise him to take only aluminum-free antacids.
• Advise patient to report vision changes and to have annual eye examinations. Reassure him that visual disturbances will subside within several weeks to months after drug is discontinued.
• As appropriate, review all other significant and life-threatening adverse reactions and interactions, especially those related to the drugs and tests mentioned above.

e

etidronate disodium
Didronel, Didronel IV

Pharmacologic class: Bisphosphonate
Therapeutic class: Bone resorption inhibitor, hypocalcemic agent
Pregnancy risk category B (oral use), *C* (I.V. use)

Action
Blocks calcium absorption, slowing bone metabolism, thereby decreasing bone resorption and new bone formation

Availability
Injection: 300 mg/ampule in 6-ml ampules
Tablets: 200 mg, 400 mg

Indications and dosages
➤ Paget's disease
Adults: 5 to 10 mg/kg P.O. daily as a single dose for up to 6 months, or 11 to 20 mg/kg P.O. daily for no more than 3 months
➤ Heterotopic ossification after hip replacement
Adults: 20 mg/kg P.O. daily for 1 month before surgery and 3 months afterward
➤ Heterotopic ossification in spinal cord injury
Adults: Initially, 20 mg/kg P.O. daily for 2 weeks, decreased to 10 mg/kg P.O. daily for 10 weeks
➤ Hypercalcemia related to cancer
Adults: 7.5 mg/kg/day I.V. infused over at least 2 hours for 3 consecutive days; may continue infusion for up to 7 days if necessary. May start P.O. dosing after last infusion.

Contraindications
• Hypersensitivity to drug
• Severe renal impairment

Administration
• For I.V. use, dilute with 250 ml of normal saline solution; infuse slowly over at least 2 hours.
• Give oral dose with water or juice 2 hours before meals.
• Don't allow patient to eat for 2 hours after dose.

Route	Onset	Peak	Duration
P.O. (Paget's)	1 mo	Unknown	1 yr
P.O. (ossif.)	Unknown	Unknown	Several mo
I.V. (hypercalc.)	24 hr	3 days	11 days

Adverse reactions
All reactions occur only with I.V. use unless otherwise noted.
CNS: seizures
GI: nausea, constipation, stomatitis, loss of taste, metallic taste
Hematologic: anemia
Hepatic: elevated liver function test results
Metabolic: hypomagnesemia, hypophosphatemia
Musculoskeletal: bone pain and tenderness, fractures (all with oral use)
Respiratory: dyspnea
Skin: rash (with oral use)
Other: fever, fluid overload

Interactions
Drug-drug. *Antacids; buffers containing aluminum, calcium, iron, or magnesium; mineral supplements:* decreased etidronate absorption
Calcitonin: additive hypocalcemic effect
Warfarin: increased prothrombin time
Drug-diagnostic tests. *Blood urea nitrogen (BUN), creatinine:* increased levels
Calcium, magnesium: decreased levels
Liver function tests: abnormal results
Drug-food. *Foods high in aluminum, calcium, iron, or magnesium:* decreased etidronate absorption

---

Precautions

Use cautiously in:
• moderate renal impairment, long bone fractures, heart failure, hypocalcemia, hypovitaminosis D
• pregnant or breastfeeding patients
• children (safety not established).

Patient monitoring

• Monitor fluid intake and output.
◀≋ Watch for seizures.
• Monitor patient for GI discomfort; divide dose as needed to alleviate symptoms.
• Assess bowel pattern; increase fluids and administer stool softeners, as prescribed, to ease constipation.
• Monitor calcium, phosphorus, magnesium, creatinine, and BUN levels; liver function test results; and bone scans.

Patient teaching

• Instruct patient not to take drug with food because of decreased drug absorption.
• Teach patient not to consume high-calcium products, such as milk products or antacids, within 2 hours of taking dose.
• Stress importance of eating diet high in vitamin D and calcium.
• Teach patient to report bone pain or decreased range of motion.
• As appropriate, review all other significant and life-threatening adverse reactions and interactions, especially those related to the drugs, tests, and foods mentioned above.

etodolac
Apo-Etodolac✚, Lodine, Lodine XL, Ultradol✚

Pharmacologic class: Pyranocarboxylic acid, nonsteroidal anti-inflammatory drug (NSAID)

Therapeutic class: Nonopioid analgesic

Pregnancy risk category C (third trimester: *D*)

Action

Blocks activity of cyclooxygenase (needed for prostaglandin synthesis), thereby easing pain and reducing inflammation

Availability

Capsules: 200 mg, 300 mg
Tablets: 400 mg, 500 mg
Tablets (extended-release): 400 mg, 500 mg, 600 mg

Indications and dosages

➤ Osteoarthritis, rheumatoid arthritis
Adults: 300 mg P.O. two or three times daily, or 400 P.O. mg b.i.d., or 500 mg P.O. b.i.d, or 400 to 1,200 mg P.O. (extended-release tablets) once daily
➤ Mild to moderate pain
Adults: 200 to 400 mg P.O. q 6 to 8 hours, not to exceed 1,200 mg/day

Contraindications

• Hypersensitivity to drug
• Concurrent use of other NSAIDs
• Active GI bleeding or ulcer disease

Administration

• Give with food or antacids to reduce GI upset.
• Ensure patient swallows extended-release tablets whole without crushing or chewing.

• Withhold drug several days before invasive surgery, as ordered.

Route	Onset	Peak	Duration
P.O.	30 min	1-2 hr	4-12 hr
P.O. (extended)	Unknown	3-12 hr	6-12 hr

Adverse reactions

CNS: dizziness, malaise, weakness, depression, nervousness
CV: hypertension, fluid retention
EENT: blurred vision, tinnitus
GI: nausea, vomiting, constipation, diarrhea, flatulence, peptic ulcer, duodenitis, intestinal ulceration, dyspepsia, gastritis, melena
GU: dysuria, urinary frequency, polyuria, **renal failure**
Hematologic: thrombocytopenia
Hepatic: cholestatic jaundice, **cholestatic hepatitis, liver necrosis**
Skin: rash, cutaneous vasculitis with purpura, hyperpigmentation, skin peeling
Other: chills, fever, allergic reaction

Interactions

Drug-drug. *Aminoglycosides:* elevated aminoglycoside blood level in premature infants
Anticoagulants: prolonged prothrombin time
Beta blockers: reduced antihypertensive effect
Bisphosphonates: increased risk of gastric ulcers
Cholestyramine: decreased etodolac absorption
Cyclosporine: increased risk of nephrotoxicity
Diuretics: decreased diuretic effect
Lithium: increased lithium blood level, greater risk of toxicity
Methotrexate: increased risk of methotrexate toxicity
Phenylbutazone: increased etodolac effects
Phenytoin: increased phenytoin blood level

Salicylates: decreased etodolac blood level
Drug-diagnostic tests. *Bleeding time:* prolonged
Blood urea nitrogen (BUN), creatinine, hepatic enzymes: increased levels
Urine bilirubin, urine ketones: false-positive results
Drug-herb. *Arnica, chamomile, clove, dong quai, feverfew, garlic, ginkgo, ginseng:* increased risk of bleeding
White willow: increased etodolac effects
Drug-behaviors. *Alcohol use:* increased risk of adverse effects
Sun exposure: phototoxicity

Precautions

Use cautiously in:
• severe cardiovascular, renal, or hepatic disease
• elderly patients
• breastfeeding patients
• children (safety not established).

Patient monitoring

• Assess for GI bleeding and gastric upset; administer antacids as needed and prescribed.
• Know that drug may cause false-positive results in urine bilirubin and urine ketone tests.
◀ Monitor patient for signs and symptoms of thrombocytopenia and increased bleeding time.
• Assess for fluid retention and weigh patient daily.
• Watch for decreased blood pressure control in hypertensive patients.
• Monitor complete blood count, liver function test results, BUN and creatinine levels, and coagulation studies.

Patient teaching

• Instruct patient to take drug with meals if possible.
• Instruct patient to immediately report unusual bleeding or bruising.
• Tell patient to avoid activities that can cause injury.

• As appropriate, review all other significant and life-threatening adverse reactions and interactions, especially those related to the drugs, tests, herbs, and behaviors mentioned above.

etonogestrel and ethinyl estradiol vaginal ring
NuvaRing

Pharmacologic class: Sex hormone
Therapeutic class: Contraceptive
Pregnancy risk category X

Action
Inhibits ovulation by altering cervical mucosa and endometrium of uterus, which reduces likelihood of sperm entering uterus and becoming implanted

Availability
Vaginal ring: delivers 0.12 mg etonogestrel and 0.015 mg ethinyl estradiol per day over 3 weeks

Indications and dosages
➤ Prevention of pregnancy
Adults: Place one ring into vagina and leave in place for 3 weeks, then remove for 1 week. Insert next ring on same day of week as in previous cycle.

Contraindications
• Hypersensitivity to drug or its components
• Breast and uterine cancers or other known or suspected estrogen-dependent neoplasms
• Thromboembolic disease (current or previous)
• Diabetes with vascular involvement
• Headache with focal neurologic symptoms
• Hepatic tumors or active hepatic disease, cholestatic jaundice

• Major surgery with prolonged immobilization
• Severe hypertension
• Undiagnosed vaginal bleeding
• Valvular heart disease with complications
• Patients older than age 35 who smoke more than 15 cigarettes daily
• Pregnancy or breastfeeding

Administration
• Be aware that best way to insert ring is with patient lying down, squatting, or standing with one leg raised.

Route	Onset	Peak	Duration
Vaginal	Rapid	Unknown	Unknown

Adverse reactions
CNS: headache, dizziness, lethargy, depression, **increased risk of cerebrovascular accident, seizures**
CV: hypertension, **myocardial infarction, thromboembolism**
EENT: contact lens intolerance, worsening of myopia or astigmatism
GI: nausea, vomiting, abdominal cramps, bloating, anorexia, gallbladder disease, **pancreatitis**
GU: amenorrhea, dysmenorrhea, cervical erosion, loss of libido, vaginal candidiasis, impotence, testicular atrophy, breast tenderness, breast enlargement or secretion, **increased risk of endometrial and breast cancer**
Hepatic: cholestatic jaundice, **hepatic adenoma**
Metabolic: hyperglycemia, hypercalcemia, sodium and water retention
Musculoskeletal: leg cramps
Respiratory: pulmonary embolism
Skin: acne, oily skin, increased pigmentation, urticaria
Other: edema, increased appetite, weight changes

Interactions
Drug-drug. *Acetaminophen:* decreased acetaminophen blood level

Anti-infectives, barbiturates, carbamazepine, fosphenytoin, rifampin: decreased contraceptive efficacy
Corticosteroids: increased corticosteroid effects
Cyclosporine: increased risk of cyclosporine toxicity
CYP3A4 inhibitors (such as itraconazole, ketoconazole): increased hormone levels
Dantrolene, other hepatotoxic drugs: increased risk of hepatotoxicity
Hypoglycemics, warfarin: altered requirements for these drugs
Miconazole (vaginal capsules): increased hormone blood levels
Phenytoin: loss of seizure control
Protease inhibitors: increased contraceptive metabolism
Tamoxifen: interference with tamoxifen efficacy
Tricyclic antidepressants: reduced antidepressant effects
Drug-diagnostic tests. *Antithrombin III, folate, low-density lipoproteins, pyridoxine, total cholesterol:* decreased levels
Cortisol; factors VII, VIII, IX, and X; glucose; high-density lipoproteins; phospholipids; prolactin; prothrombin; sodium; triglycerides: increased levels
Drug-food. *Caffeine:* increased caffeine blood level
Drug-herb. *Black cohosh:* increased risk of adverse reactions
Red clover: interference with contraceptive action
Saw palmetto: antiestrogenic effects
St. John's wort: decreased contraceptive blood level and effects
Drug-behaviors. *Smoking:* increased risk of adverse cardiovascular reactions

Precautions
Use cautiously in:
• underlying cardiovascular disease, severe hepatic or renal disease, asthma, bone disease, migraines, breast disease, seizures, sexually transmitted disease
• family history of breast or genital tract cancers.

Patient monitoring
◀£ Monitor CNS status; report adverse CNS reactions immediately.
• Assess blood pressure frequently.
• Monitor patient for depression.
• Assess for yellowing of skin or eyes.
• Evaluate for liver engorgement.
• Check for dry eyes; administer artificial tears as needed.
• Monitor glucose, calcium, and electrolyte levels and lipid profile.

Patient teaching
• Teach patient to insert and remove ring on same day of week and at same time of day.
• Inform patient that smoking during therapy may increase risk of blood clots, phlebitis, and stroke.
• Explain that for continued contraception, new implant must be inserted exactly 1 week after old one is removed, even if patient is menstruating.
• Tell patient that if ring slips out, pregnancy protection remains adequate provided ring is replaced within 3 hours.
• Tell patient to report signs and symptoms of depression.
• Teach patient how to perform breast self-examinations; emphasize importance of monthly checks.
• As appropriate, review all other significant and life-threatening adverse reactions and interactions, especially those related to the drugs, tests, foods, herbs, and behaviors mentioned above.

etoposide (VP-16-213)
Etopophos, Toposar, VePesid, VP-16

Pharmacologic class: Podophyllotoxin derivative
Therapeutic class: Antineoplastic
Pregnancy risk category D

Action
Damages DNA before mitosis by inhibiting topoisomerase II enzyme; this action impairs ability to repair DNA, thus inhibiting selected cancer cell growth. Cell-cycle-phase specific.

Availability
Capsules: 50 mg
Injection: 20 mg/ml
Powder for injection: 100 mg in single-dose vials

Indications and dosages
➣ Testicular cancer
Adults: 50 to 100 mg/m² I.V. daily for 5 days. Or 100 mg/m² I.V. on days 1, 3, and 5, with course of treatment repeated q 3 to 4 weeks.
➣ Small-cell carcinoma of lung
Adults: 70 mg/m² P.O. (rounded up or down to nearest 50 mg) daily for 4 days, then give maximum of 100 mg/m² P.O. (rounded up or down to nearest 50 mg) daily for 5 days every 3 to 4 weeks; alternatively 35 mg/m² I.V. daily for 4 days, then a maximum of 50 mg/m² I.V. daily for 5 days q 3 to 4 weeks
Dosage adjustment
• Renal impairment

Off-label uses
• AIDS-related Kaposi's sarcoma
• Wilms' tumor
• Neuroblastoma
• Malignant lymphomas
• Hodgkin's disease
• Ovarian neoplasms

Contraindications
• Hypersensitivity to drug
• Pregnancy or breastfeeding

Administration
• For I.V. concentrations above 0.4 mg/ml, mix each 100 mg with 250 to 500 ml of dextrose 5% in water or normal saline solution to help prevent crystallization.

• Give I.V. infusion over 30 to 60 minutes. Don't use in-line filter.
◀€ Avoid rapid infusion, which may cause severe hypotension and bronchospasm.
• Administer with antiemetics, as prescribed.
• Wear disposable gloves when handling. If drug comes into contact with skin, wash thoroughly with soap and water.

Route	Onset	Peak	Duration
P.O., I.V.	7-14 days	9-16 days	20 days

Adverse reactions
CNS: drowsiness, fatigue, headache, vertigo, peripheral neuropathy
CV: hypotension (with I.V. use), **heart failure, myocardial infarction**
GI: nausea, vomiting, stomatitis
GU: sterility
Hematologic: anemia, **leukopenia, thrombocytopenia, bone marrow depression**
Hepatic: hepatotoxicity
Metabolic: hyperuricemia
Musculoskeletal: muscle cramps
Respiratory: pulmonary edema, bronchospasm
Other: alopecia, fever, phlebitis at I.V. site, allergic reactions including **anaphylaxis**

Interactions
Drug-drug. *Antineoplastics:* additive bone marrow depression
Live-virus vaccines: increased risk of adverse reactions
Drug-diagnostic tests. *Hemoglobin, neutrophils, platelets, red blood cells, while blood cells:* decreased values
Uric acid: increased level

Precautions
Use cautiously in:
• active infections, decreased bone marrow reserve, renal or hepatic impairment
• patients with childbearing potential.

Patient monitoring

• Monitor blood pressure during and after infusion; stop infusion if severe hypotension occurs.
• With I.V. use, monitor infusion rate closely to prevent infusion reactions.
• Throughout infusion, check I.V. site for extravasation, which may cause thrombophlebitis.
• Keep diphenhydramine, hydrocortisone, epinephrine, and artificial airway at hand in case anaphylaxis occurs.
• Assess for CNS adverse effects; assist patient during ambulation as needed.
• Monitor for signs and symptoms of bone marrow depression.
• Monitor complete blood count, liver function test results, and blood urea nitrogen and creatinine levels. Report platelet count below 50,000/mm³ or neutrophil count below 500/mm³.

Patient teaching

• Teach patient to inspect mouth daily for ulcers and bleeding gums.
• Instruct patient to move slowly when rising to avoid light-headedness or dizziness from sudden blood pressure decrease.
• Tell patient that drug may cause hair loss.
• As appropriate, review all other significant and life-threatening adverse reactions and interactions, especially those related to the drugs and tests mentioned above.

---

exemestane
Aromasin

Pharmacologic class: Aromatase inhibitor

Therapeutic class: Hormonal antineoplastic

Pregnancy risk category D

Action

Lowers estrogen concentration, thereby limiting breast cancer cell growth due to estrogen-dependent tumors

Availability

Tablets: 25 mg

Indications and dosages

➤ Advanced breast cancer in postmenopausal women after tamoxifen therapy
Adults: 25 mg P.O. once daily after a meal

Contraindications

• Hypersensitivity to drug

Administration

• Administer after meals with a full glass of water.
• Know that drug shouldn't be taken by premenopausal women or patients taking other drugs that contain estrogen.

Route	Onset	Peak	Duration
P.O.	Unknown	1-2 hr	24 hr

Adverse reactions

CNS: confusion, asthenia, generalized weakness, hypoesthesia, paresthesia, headache, dizziness, pain, fatigue, anxiety, insomnia, depression
CV: hypertension, chest pain
EENT: sinusitis
GI: nausea, vomiting, diarrhea, constipation, abdominal pain, dyspepsia, anorexia
GU: urinary tract infection
Musculoskeletal: pathologic fractures, arthritis, back pain, skeletal pain
Respiratory: dyspnea, bronchitis, cough, upper respiratory tract infection
Skin: rash, itching, alopecia, diaphoresis
Other: increased appetite, fever, hot flashes, edema, infection, flulike symptoms, lymphedema

---

Interactions
Drug-drug. *CYP3A4 inducers:* decreased exemestane blood level

Precautions
None

Patient monitoring
• Monitor vital signs, especially blood pressure.
• Check for adverse GI effects; give antiemetics, as prescribed, for nausea and vomiting.
• Assess bowel elimination pattern; increase fluids and administer stool softeners, as needed, to ease constipation.
• Monitor pain level; administer analgesics as prescribed to relieve pain.
• Monitor liver function test results, complete cell blood count, and blood urea nitrogen, creatinine, and electrolyte levels.

Patient teaching
• Teach patient to report depression, insomnia, or excessive anxiety.
• Advise patient to take drug with full glass of water after breakfast, lunch, or dinner.
• Instruct patient to wear cotton clothing to let skin breathe if drug causes increased sweating or hot flashes.
• As appropriate, review all other significant adverse reactions and interactions, especially those related to the drugs mentioned above.

ezetimibe
Zetia

Pharmacologic class: Cholesterol absorption inhibitor
Therapeutic class: Antihyperlipidemic
Pregnancy risk category C

Action
Inhibits the absorption of cholesterol in the intestine, resulting in decreased intestinal delivery to the liver and increased systemic clearance. Net effect is decreased serum cholesterol level.

Availability
Tablets: 10 mg

💊 Indications and dosages
➤ Adjunct to diet and exercise to lower cholesterol, low-density lipoprotein, and apolipoprotein B levels in patients with primary hypercholesterolemia; adjunct to other lipid-lowering drugs to treat homozygous familial hypercholesterolemia; adjunct to diet for treatment of homozygous sitosterolemia
Adults: 10 mg/day P.O.

Contraindications
• Hypersensitivity to drug
• Active hepatic disease
• Pregnancy or breastfeeding

Administration
• Be aware that drug may be given concurrently with HMG-CoA reductase inhibitor, atorvastatin, or simvastatin.
• When giving with bile acid sequestrant, administer ezetimibe at least 2 hours before or 4 hours after that drug.
• Give with or without food.

Route	Onset	Peak	Duration
P.O.	Moderate	4-12 hr	Unknown

Adverse reactions
CNS: headache, dizziness, fatigue
GI: nausea, vomiting, diarrhea, abdominal pain, flatulence, dyspepsia, dry mouth, anorexia
Hepatic: abnormal liver function test results

Musculoskeletal: back pain, myalgia, joint pain
Respiratory: pneumonia, pharyngitis, sinusitis, upper respiratory tract infection
Other: viral infection

Interactions
Drug-drug. *Cholestyramine:* decreased ezetimibe blood level
Cyclosporine, fenofibrate, gemfibrozil: increased ezetimibe blood level
Fibrates: increased risk of cholesterol excretion into gallbladder
Immunosuppressants: increased immunosuppression and bone marrow depression
Drug-diagnostic tests. *Liver function tests:* increased values

Precautions
Use cautiously in:
• renal or hepatic impairment
• elderly patients.

Patient monitoring
• Monitor hepatic and lipid profiles.
• Give at least 2 hours before or 4 hours after bile acid sequestrant (if prescribed).
• Assess for unexplained muscle pain; report this finding to prescriber.

Patient teaching
• Teach patient about appropriate cholesterol-lowering diet as well as role of exercise and weight loss.
• Instruct patient to report GI upset.
• Caution women not to become pregnant during therapy.
• Advise patient to relieve dry mouth with hard candy or gum.
• As appropriate, review all other significant adverse reactions and interactions, especially those related to the drugs and tests mentioned above.

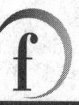

factor IX (human)
AlphaNine SD, Mononine

factor IX (recombinant)
BeneFix

factor IX complex
Bebulin VH, Profilnine SD, Proplex T (heat-treated)

Pharmacologic class: Blood modifier
Therapeutic class: Antihemophilic
Pregnancy risk category C

Action
Converts fibrinogen to fibrin, increasing clotting factors

Availability
Powder for injection: Various strengths; units specified on label

Indications and dosages
➤ Factor IX deficiency (hemophilia B or Christmas disease); anticoagulant overdose
Adults and children: Dosage individualized. Use following equations to calculate approximate units of factor IX needed:
Human product—1 unit/kg times body weight (in kg) times desired increase in factor IX level expressed as percentage of normal
Recombinant product—1.2 units/kg times body weight (in kg) times desired increase in factor IX level expressed as percentage of normal
Proplex T—0.5 unit/kg times body weight (in kg) times desired increase in factor IX level expressed as percentage of normal

---

Off-label uses
- Hepatic dysfunction
- Esophagitis
- Unspecified GI hemorrhage (with human product)

Contraindications
- Hypersensitivity to mouse or hamster protein (with BeneFix)
- Fibrinolysis

Administration
◀╲ Administer by slow I.V. infusion.
- If prescribed, administer hepatitis B vaccine before giving factor IX.
- Know that dosage is highly individualized according to degree of factor IX deficiency, patient's weight, and bleeding severity.
- Warm drug to room temperature before reconstitution; use within 3 hours of reconstitution.
- Don't use glass syringes. Don't shake reconstituted solution or mix with other I.V. solutions.

Route	Onset	Peak	Duration
I.V.	Immediate	10-30 min	Unknown

Adverse reactions
CNS: light-headedness, paresthesia, headache
CV: blood pressure changes, **thromboembolic reactions, myocardial infarction**
EENT: allergic rhinitis
GI: nausea, vomiting, altered taste
Hematologic: disseminated intravascular coagulation
Respiratory: pulmonary embolism
Skin: rash, flushing, diaphoresis, pruritus, urticaria
Other: fever, chills, burning sensation in jaw and skull, pain at I.V. injection site

Interactions
Drug-drug. *Aminocaproic acid:* increased risk of thrombosis

Precautions
Use cautiously in:
- recent surgery
- neonates and infants (safety and efficacy not established).

Patient monitoring
- Be aware that factor IX complex may transmit hepatitis.
- Closely monitor vital signs during infusion.
◀╲ Observe for hemolytic reaction; if it occurs, stop infusion, flush line with saline solution, and notify prescriber immediately.
- Monitor I.V. injection site closely.
- Monitor coagulation studies.

Patient teaching
- Inform patient that drug is capable of transmitting diseases.
- Teach patient to report unusual bleeding or bruising.
- Caution patient to avoid activities that can cause injury.
- Teach patient to wear medical identification specifying that he has a blood-clotting disorder.
- Instruct patient to notify surgeon or dentist of his blood-clotting disorder before surgery or invasive dental procedures.
- As appropriate, review all other significant and life-threatening adverse reactions and interactions, especially those related to the drugs mentioned above.

famciclovir
Famvir

Pharmacologic class: Synthetic nucleoside
Therapeutic class: Antiviral
Pregnancy risk category B

Action
After conversion to penciclovir, famciclovir selectively inhibits DNA polymerase and viral DNA synthesis.

Availability
Tablets: 125 mg, 250 mg, 500 mg

⚠ Indications and dosages
➤ Acute herpes zoster infection (shingles)
Adults: 500 mg P.O. q 8 hours for 7 days
➤ Recurrent genital herpes
Adults: 125 mg P.O. b.i.d. for 5 days; start therapy as soon as symptoms appear
➤ Suppression of recurrent genital herpes
Adults: 250 mg P.O. b.i.d. up to 1 year
➤ Recurrent herpes simplex infection in patients with human immunodeficiency virus (HIV)
Adults: 500 mg P.O. b.i.d. for 7 days
Dosage adjustment
• Renal impairment

Contraindications
• Hypersensitivity to drug

Administration
• Know that for best response, therapy should begin within 6 hours after onset of genital herpes symptoms or lesions.
• Give drug with or without food.

Route	Onset	Peak	Duration
P.O.	Unknown	1 hr	Unknown

Adverse reactions
CNS: headache, fatigue, dizziness, drowsiness, paresthesia, insomnia
EENT: pharyngitis, sinusitis
GI: diarrhea, nausea, vomiting, constipation, abdominal pain, anorexia
Musculoskeletal: back pain, joint pain
Skin: pruritus
Other: fever

Interactions
Drug-drug. *Digoxin:* increased digoxin blood level, increased risk of toxicity
Probenecid: increased blood level of penciclovir (active antiviral compound of famciclovir)

Precautions
Use cautiously in:
• renal or hepatic impairment
• elderly patients
• pregnant or breastfeeding patients
• children younger than age 18.

Patient monitoring
• When giving digoxin concurrently, monitor digoxin blood level and evaluate for digoxin toxicity.
• Monitor complete blood count and electrolyte, blood urea nitrogen, and creatinine levels.
• Be aware that drug may take several weeks to reach therapeutic level.
• Know that renal failure may raise drug blood level, increasing risk of adverse reactions.
• Avoid direct contact with infected areas; wash hands frequently and wear gloves.

Patient teaching
• Instruct patient to take with food or milk to avoid upset stomach.
• Inform patient that drug doesn't cure herpes; it only decreases pain and itching by allowing sores to heal and preventing new ones from forming.
• Advise patient to wear loose-fitting clothing to avoid irritating lesions.
• Tell patient to report rash or itching.
• As appropriate, review all other significant adverse reactions and interactions, especially those related to the drugs mentioned above.

famotidine

Apo-Famotidine✲, Gen-Famotidine✲, Mylanta AR, Novo-Famotidine✲, Nu-Famotidine✲, Pepcid, Pepcid AC, Pepcid AC Acid Controller, Pepcid RPD, Rhoxal-Famotidine✲

Pharmacologic class: Histamine$_2$-receptor antagonist
Therapeutic class: Antiulcer drug
Pregnancy risk category B

Action

Blocks action of histamine at histamine$_2$-receptor sites located in gastric parietal cells, inhibiting gastric acid secretion and stabilizing pepsin

Availability

Gelcaps: 10 mg
Oral suspension (cherry-banana-mint flavor): 40 mg/5 ml
Solution for injection: 10 mg/ml, 20 mg/ 50 ml of normal saline solution
Tablets: 10 mg, 20 mg, 40 mg
Tablets (chewable, mint flavor with aspartame): 10 mg
Tablets (orally disintegrating, mint flavor): 20 mg, 40 mg

🖊 Indications and dosages

➢ Short-term treatment of active duodenal ulcers and benign gastric ulcers
Adults: 40 mg P.O. once daily at bedtime, or 20 mg P.O. b.i.d. for up to 8 weeks
➢ Prophylaxis of duodenal ulcers
Adults: 20 mg P.O. once daily at bedtime
➢ Gastroesophageal reflux disease
Adults: 20 mg P.O. b.i.d. for up to 6 weeks; maximum dosage of 40 mg b.i.d. for up to 12 weeks

Children ages 1 to 16: 1 mg/kg P.O. daily in two divided doses up to a maximum of 40 mg twice daily
➢ Gastric hypersecretory conditions (such as Zollinger-Ellison syndrome)
Adults: Initially, 20 mg P.O. q 6 hours, increased as needed to 160 mg q 6 hours
➢ Hospitalized patients with pathologic hypersecretory conditions or ulcers; patients who can't take oral drugs
Adults: 20 mg I.V. q 12 hours
➢ Prevention or treatment of heartburn, acid indigestion, and sour stomach (Pepcid AC only)
Adults: For prevention, 10 mg P.O. 60 minutes before eating, or 10-mg chewable tablet 15 minutes before eating, to a maximum of 20 mg/24 hours for up to 2 weeks. For symptomatic treatment, 10 mg P.O. once or twice daily.
Dosage adjustment
• Renal impairment

Contraindications

• Hypersensitivity to drug or other histamine$_2$-receptor antagonists
• Alcohol intolerance (some oral liquid products)

Administration

• Be aware that drug usually is given in one daily dose to patients with renal insufficiency.
• Give P.O. with food or liquids unless otherwise recommended.
• Dilute I.V. form with 10 ml dextrose 5% in water or normal saline solution (100 ml) for I.V. piggyback administration.
• Administer by I.V. push over 2 minutes or I.V. piggyback over 30 minutes.
• Know that drug may cause transient irritation at I.V. site.

Route	Onset	Peak	Duration
P.O.	Within 60 min	1-4 hr	6-12 hr
I.V.	Rapid	0.5-3 hr	8-15 hr

Adverse reactions
CNS: dizziness, headache, paresthesia, asthenia
CV: palpitations
GI: nausea, diarrhea, constipation, altered taste, dry mouth, anorexia
EENT: orbital edema, conjunctival redness, tinnitus
Musculoskeletal: musculoskeletal pain
Skin: flushing, acne, dry skin
Other: fever, pain at injection site, **hypersensitivity reactions**

Interactions
Drug-food. *Caffeine-containing foods:* increased gastric irritation
Drug-herb. *Yerba maté:* decreased famotidine clearance
Drug-behaviors. *Alcohol use, smoking:* increased gastric irritation

Precautions
Use cautiously in:
• renal impairment
• elderly patients
• pregnant or breastfeeding patients.

Patient monitoring
• Assess patient for GI signs and symptoms.
• Monitor blood urea nitrogen and creatinine levels in patients with renal impairment.

Patient teaching
• Teach patient that drug is most effective when taken at bedtime.
• Inform patient that pain relief may not begin for several days after therapy starts.
• Caution patient to avoid alcohol, caffeine, and smoking because they may increase gastric irritation.
• As appropriate, review all other significant adverse reactions and interactions, especially those related to the foods, herbs, and behaviors mentioned above.

fat emulsions (I.V.)
Intralipid 10%, Intralipid 20%, Liposyn II 10%, Liposyn II 20%, Liposyn III 10%, Liposyn III 20%

Pharmacologic class: Lipid
Therapeutic class: Nutritional caloric agent and fatty acid
Pregnancy risk category C

Action
Raise plasma triglyceride levels and convert triglycerides to free fatty acids, resulting in increases in oxygen, calories, and heat production

Availability
Injection: 50 ml (10%, 20%), 100 ml (10%, 20%), 200 ml (10%, 20%), 250 ml (10%, 20%), 500 ml (10%, 20%)

Indications and dosages
➢ To prevent fatty acid deficiency
Adults: 500 ml (10% of total caloric intake) I.V. twice weekly, infused initially at 1 ml/minute for 30 minutes, not to exceed 500 ml over 4 to 6 hours
➢ Treatment of fatty acid deficiency
Adults and children: 8% to 10% of total caloric intake I.V.
➢ Adjunct to total parenteral nutrition (TPN)
Adults: 1 ml/minute I.V. for 15 to 30 minutes (10% emulsion), or 0.5 ml/minute I.V. for 15 to 30 minutes (20% emulsion). If no adverse effects, increase rate to 500 ml over 4 to 8 hours, not to exceed 2.5 g/kg/day.
Children: 0.1 ml/minute I.V. for 10 to 15 minutes (10% emulsion), or 0.05 ml/minute I.V. for 10 to 15 minutes (20% emulsion). If no adverse effects, increase rate to 1 g/kg over 4 hours, not to exceed 3 g/kg/day. Fat emulsion provides up to 60% of daily caloric intake;

protein-carbohydrate TPN should supply remaining 40%.

Contraindications

- Hypersensitivity to drug
- Allergy to eggs
- Acute pancreatitis

Administration

◀€ Ask patient if he's allergic to eggs before starting therapy.

- Infuse over 24 hours using administration pump. Don't use in-line filter; drug particles are bigger than filter.
- Drug may be piggybacked into TPN proximal to infusion site but past hyperalimentation filter. Hang drug higher than TPN bag to prevent backup into bag.
- Change I.V. tubing with each new bottle to prevent bacterial growth.
- Be aware that moisture causes drug to break down.

Route	Onset	Peak	Duration
I.V.	Rapid	Immediate	Unknown

Adverse reactions

GI: splenomegaly (with prolonged use)
Hematologic: leukocytosis, **thrombocytopenia, leukopenia** (with prolonged use)
Hepatic: abnormal liver function test results, jaundice, **hepatomegaly** (with prolonged use)
Metabolic: metabolic acidosis
Respiratory: impaired pulmonary diffusion capacity, **pulmonary edema**
Other: "fat overload" with too-rapid infusion (causing dilution of electrolyte concentration, irritation at injection site), overloading syndrome with prolonged use (causing **focal seizures, fever, leukocytosis, splenomegaly, shock**), **sepsis, hypersensitivity reaction**

Interactions

Drug-diagnostic tests. *Bilirubin, lipids, hepatic enzymes:* increased levels
Platelets, white blood cells: decreased counts

Precautions

Use cautiously in:
- renal impairment, severe hepatic impairment, pulmonary disease, anemia
- pregnant patients
- premature infants.

Patient monitoring

- Observe closely for adverse reactions during first few hours of transfusion.
- Monitor I.V. site closely; change site as needed.
- Assess for hepatomegaly and splenomegaly; report positive findings.
- Monitor lipid and hepatic profile, electrolyte and glucose levels, complete blood count, and coagulation studies.
- Monitor fluid intake and output; assess for fluid overload (caused by osmotic pull of fat emulsion).

Patient teaching

- Teach patient to report shortness of breath, persistent nausea, or headache.
- As appropriate, review all other significant and life-threatening adverse reactions and interactions, especially those related to the tests mentioned above.

felodipine
Plendil, Renedil✢

Pharmacologic class: Calcium channel blocker
Therapeutic class: Antihypertensive, antianginal
Pregnancy risk category C

Action
Impedes extracellular calcium ion movement across membranes of myocardial muscle cells, which depresses myocardial contractility and impulse formation in pacemaker cells; slows impulse conduction velocity; and dilates coronary arteries and peripheral arterioles. Net effect is reduced cardiac workload and decreased blood pressure.

Availability
Tablets (extended-release): 2.5 mg, 5 mg, 10 mg

⚠ Indications and dosages
➤ Hypertension
Adults: Initially, 5 mg P.O. daily; depending on response, may decrease to 2.5 mg or increase to a maximum of 10 mg P.O. daily at 2-week intervals
Dosage adjustment
• Hepatic impairment
• Elderly patients

Off-label uses
• Heart failure
• Angina pectoris or vasospastic (Prinzmetal's) angina

Contraindications
• Hypersensitivity to drug

Administration
• Make sure patient swallows tablets whole without crushing or chewing.
• Give without regard to meals.

Route	Onset	Peak	Duration
P.O.	1 hr	2-4 hr	Up to 24 hr

Adverse reactions
CNS: headache, syncope, dizziness, nervousness, psychiatric disturbances, paresthesia, drowsiness, insomnia, asthenia, anxiety, confusion, irritability
CV: chest pain, peripheral edema, hypotension, palpitations, tachycardia, angina, **arrhythmias, myocardial infarction, atrioventricular (AV) block**
EENT: pharyngitis, rhinorrhea
GI: nausea, vomiting, diarrhea, constipation, abdominal discomfort, dyspepsia, cramps, flatulence, dry mouth, dysgeusia
Hematologic: anemia
Musculoskeletal: back pain
Respiratory: bronchitis, sneezing
Skin: dermatitis, rash, pruritus, urticaria, erythema
Other: facial edema, thirst, warm sensation

Interactions
Drug-drug. *Antifungals, cimetidine, erythromycin, propranolol, ranitidine:* increased felodipine blood level, increased risk of toxicity
Barbiturates, hydantoins: decreased felodipine blood level
Beta blockers, digoxin, disopyramide, phenytoin: bradycardia, conduction defects, heart failure
Fentanyl, nitrates, other antihypertensives, quinidine: additive hypotension
Nonsteroidal anti-inflammatory drugs: decreased antihypertensive effects
Drug-food. *Grapefruit juice:* increased felodipine blood level and effects
Drug-behaviors. *Acute alcohol ingestion:* additive hypotension

Precautions
Use cautiously in:
• cardiac disease, arrhythmias, severe hepatic or renal impairment
• elderly patients
• pregnant or breastfeeding patients
• children (safety not established).

Patient monitoring
◄€ Don't give to patient with heart block unless he has a pacemaker.
◄€ Use extreme caution when administering to patients with pulmonary hypertension, renal insufficiency, heart failure, or compromised ventricular

function (especially those receiving beta blockers concurrently).
• Monitor fluid intake and output; obtain daily weight.
• Monitor ECG and vital signs; assess for signs and symptoms of heart block.
• Assess for reflex tachycardia, angina, and sustained hypotension.
• Check hepatic profile and alkaline phosphatase level in patients with hepatic impairment.

Patient teaching
• Inform patient that drug controls high blood pressure but doesn't cure it, so he should continue to take drug even if he feels well.
• Instruct patient to move slowly when rising to avoid light-headedness or dizziness from sudden blood pressure decrease.
• Explain that exercise and hot weather may increase drug's hypotensive effects.
• Tell patient to report peripheral edema, persistent headache, or flushing.
• Recommend that patient use hard candy or gum if dry mouth or thirst occurs.
• As appropriate, review all other significant and life-threatening adverse reactions and interactions, especially those related to the drugs, foods, and behaviors mentioned above.

fenofibrate
Apo-Fenofibrate✦, Lofibra, Nu-Fenofibrate✦, Tricor

Pharmacologic class: Fibric acid derivative
Therapeutic class: Antihyperlipidemic
Pregnancy risk category C

Action
Inhibits triglyceride synthesis in liver, reducing number of low- and very-low-density lipoproteins. Also increases uric acid secretion.

Availability
Capsules (micronized): 67 mg, 134 mg, 200 mg
Tablets: 54 mg, 160 mg

Indications and dosages
➤ Adjunct to dietary therapy to decrease low-density lipoprotein, total cholesterol, triglyceride, and apolipoprotein B levels
Adults: 200-mg capsule or 160-mg tablet P.O. daily
➤ Hypertriglyceridemia
Adults: Initially, 67 to 200 mg/day P.O. (capsules) or 54 to 160 mg/day (tablets); may be increased as needed q 4 to 8 weeks up to 200 mg/day (capsules) or 160 mg/day (tablets)
Dosage adjustment
• Renal impairment
• Elderly patients

Off-label uses
• Hyperlipoproteinemia types III, IIa, and IIb (adjunct to diet)
• Polymetabolic syndrome X

Contraindications
• Hypersensitivity to drug
• Hepatic and severe renal impairment
• Gallbladder disease
• Breastfeeding

Administration
◀€ Before giving drug, be aware of potentially serious interactions, such as with nephrotoxic drugs.
• Administer with meals for best response.
• Give bile acid sequestrants (resins) at least 1 hour before or 4 to 6 hours after fenofibrate.

Route	Onset	Peak	Duration
P.O.	Variable	6-8 hr	Unknown

Adverse reactions

CNS: fatigue, headache, migraine, drowsiness, dizziness, insomnia, depression, vertigo, anxiety, paresthesia, hypotonia, nervousness, neuralgia

CV: ventricular extrasystole, tachycardia, varicose veins, phlebitis, angina, hypertension, hypotension, peripheral vascular disease, vasodilation, abnormal ECG, coronary artery disease, **arrhythmias, myocardial infarction, atrial fibrillation**

EENT: conjunctivitis, abnormal vision, cataracts, refraction disorder, otitis media, pharyngitis, laryngitis, sinusitis

GI: nausea, vomiting, diarrhea, constipation, abdominal pain, flatulence, dyspepsia, gastritis, gastroenteritis, esophagitis, duodenal or peptic ulcer, colitis, rectal disorder, rectal hemorrhage, cholelithiasis, cholecystitis

GU: urinary frequency, dysuria, prostatic disorder, abnormal renal function, urolithiasis, gynecomastia, vaginal candidiasis, cystitis, decreased libido

Hematologic: eosinophilia, anemia, lymphadenopathy, **thrombocytopenia, leukopenia**

Hepatic: abnormal liver function test results, fatty liver deposits

Metabolic: increased creatinine level, hypoglycemia, hyperuricemia, gout

Musculoskeletal: back, muscle, or joint pain; myositis; arthritis; tenosynovitis; arthrosis; bursitis

Respiratory: respiratory disorders, rhinitis, bronchitis, increased cough, dyspnea, asthma, pneumonia

Skin: rash, pruritus, urticaria, bruising, acne, eczema, diaphoresis, dermatitis, herpes simplex, herpes zoster, alopecia, nail disorder

Other: weight loss or gain, edema, fever, flulike symptoms, hypersensitivity reactions

Interactions

Drug-drug. *Bile acid sequestrants (resin):* decreased absorption and efficacy of fenofibrate
Immunosuppressants, other nephrotoxic drugs: increased risk of renal toxicity
Oral anticoagulants: increased risk of bleeding
Statins: rhabdomyolysis, acute renal failure

Drug-diagnostic tests. *Alanine aminotransferase, alkaline phosphatase, aspartate aminotransferase, blood urea nitrogen, creatinine, gamma-glutamyltransferase, uric acid:* increased levels
Granulocytes, hemoglobin, neutrophils, platelets, white blood cells (WBCs): decreased values

Drug-food. *Any food:* increased drug absorption

Drug-behaviors. *Alcohol use:* elevated triglyceride levels

Precautions

Use cautiously in:
• pancreatitis, cholelithiasis
• patients receiving warfarin concurrently
• pregnant patients
• children.

Patient monitoring

• Assess creatine kinase and lipid levels and hepatic function test results.
• Monitor complete blood count and WBC count; expect decreases at start of therapy, then stabilization.

Patient teaching

• Instruct patient to take drug with meals for best effect.
• Remind patient that he still needs to follow a triglyceride-lowering diet.
• Teach patient to report unexplained muscle pain, tenderness, or weakness, particularly if associated with malaise or fever.
• Advise patient to avoid driving and other hazardous activities until he

knows how drug affects concentration and alertness.

• Teach patient to minimize GI upset by eating frequent, small servings of healthy food and drinking plenty of fluids.

• Tell patient that drug may take up to 2 months to alter lipid values.

• Inform breastfeeding patient that she must choose between taking fenofibrate and breastfeeding.

• Inform patient that he'll undergo regular blood testing.

• As appropriate, review all other significant and life-threatening adverse reactions and interactions, especially those related to the drugs, tests, foods, and behaviors mentioned above.

fenoldopam mesylate
Corlopam

Pharmacologic class: Dopamine receptor agonist (vasodilator)
Therapeutic class: Emergency antihypertensive
Pregnancy risk category B

Action

Stimulates dopamine$_1$ postsynaptic receptors, thereby decreasing blood pressure and total peripheral resistance and increasing renal blood flow

Availability

Ampules: 10 mg/ml in single-dose, 5-ml ampules

⚠ Indications and dosages

➤ Severe or malignant hypertension when rapid blood pressure reduction is indicated
Hospitalized adults: Initially, give 0.025 to 0.3 mcg/ kg/minute I.V.; titrate upward or downward no more often than q 15 minutes to achieve desired blood pressure, at recommended increments of 0.05 to 0.1 mcg/kg/ minute.

Contraindications

• Hypersensitivity to drug or sulfites

Administration

◀ἔ Don't give as I.V. bolus. Give only by continuous I.V. infusion, using infusion pump, at a concentration of 40 mcg/ml or less.

• Begin infusion at a rate no faster than 0.1 mcg/kg/minute, to avoid tachycardia.

Route	Onset	Peak	Duration
I.V.	15 min	20 min	Unknown

Adverse reactions

CNS: anxiety, dizziness, headache, light-headedness, insomnia, nervousness

CV: angina pectoris, nonspecific chest pain, hypotension, flushing, palpitations, ST-wave and T-wave changes, tachycardia, bradycardia, **heart failure, ischemic heart disease, myocardial infarction**

EENT: increased intraocular pressure, nasal congestion

GI: nausea, vomiting, diarrhea, constipation, abdominal pain and fullness

GU: oliguria, urinary tract infection

Hematologic: leukocytosis, bleeding

Metabolic: hypokalemia; increased blood urea nitrogen (BUN), glucose, aminotransferase, lactate dehydrogenase (LD), and creatinine levels

Musculoskeletal: leg cramps, back pain

Respiratory: dyspnea, upper respiratory tract infection

Skin: diaphoresis

Other: injection site pain, fever, hypersensitivity reactions including **anaphylaxis**

Interactions

Drug-drug. *Beta blockers:* increased hypotension

Dopamine antagonists, metoclopramide: decreased fenoldopam effects
Drug-diagnostic tests. *Aminotransferase, BUN, creatinine, glucose, LD, potassium:* decreased levels

Precautions

Use cautiously in:
- glaucoma, intraocular hypertension, tachycardia, hypotension, hypokalemia, liver disease
- patients receiving concurrent beta blockers.

Patient monitoring

- Watch closely for signs and symptoms of anaphylaxis or severe asthma.
◀€ Monitor blood pressure carefully at least every 15 minutes to detect hypotension, especially in patients with acute cerebral infarction or hemorrhage.
- When desired blood pressure decrease occurs, discontinue therapy or taper dosage as ordered.
- Know that patients with asthma are at higher risk for sulfite sensitivity.
- Assess respiratory and cardiac status regularly.
- Assess potassium levels closely.
- Evaluate fluid intake and urinary output.

Patient teaching

◀€ Tell patient to immediately report signs or symptoms of anaphylaxis or breathing problems.
- Refer patient to dietitian if adverse GI effects significantly limit food intake.
- Teach patient that drug may cause rapid heart rate and lower blood pressure, possibly resulting in dizziness.

fentanyl citrate
Sublimaze

fentanyl transdermal system
Duragesic, Duragesic 25, Duragesic 50, Duragesic 75, Duragesic 100

fentanyl transmucosal
Actiq, Fentanyl Oralet

Pharmacologic class: Opioid agonist
Therapeutic class: Opioid analgesic, anesthesia adjunct
Controlled substance schedule II
Pregnancy risk category C

Action

Binds to specific opioid receptors in CNS, producing analgesia

Availability

Injection: 0.05 mg/ml
Transmucosal lozenges: 200 mcg, 400 mcg, 600 mcg, 800 mcg, 1,200 mcg, 1,600 mcg
Transdermal system: 25 mcg/hour, 50 mcg/hour, 75 mcg/hour, 100 mcg/hour

⊘ Indications and dosages

➤ Breakthrough pain in opioid-tolerant cancer patients
Adults: One 200-mcg lozenge dissolved in mouth over 15 minutes; additional unit may be given 15 minutes later. If patient requires more than 1 unit per episode (as evaluated over several episodes), dosage may be increased; for optimal use or titration, don't exceed 4 units/day.
➤ Management of chronic pain in patients requiring opioid analgesics
Adults: Initially, 25 mcg/hour transdermal system; no more than 25 mcg/hour in patients who haven't been re-

ceiving opioids. To calculate dosage for patients already receiving opioids, assess 24-hour requirement for current opioid. Using recommended equianalgesic table, convert to an equivalent amount of morphine/24 hours. Then use recommended fentanyl conversion table to convert to fentanyl transdermal. During dosage titration, keep additional short-acting opioids at hand to treat breakthrough pain; morphine 10 mg I.M. or 60 mg P.O. q 4 hours (60 mg/24 hours I.M. or 360 mg/24 hours P.O.) is roughly equivalent to transdermal fentanyl 100 mcg/hour. Transdermal patch lasts 72 hours in most patients, but some patients require new patch q 48 hours. Titrate up by 25 mcg/hour q 72 hours.

➤ Short-term analgesia during anesthesia and immediate preoperative and postoperative periods

Adults: 0.05 to 0.1 mg I.M. 30 to 60 minutes before surgery and as adjunct to general anesthesia; total dosage is 0.002 mg/kg. Maintenance dosage during surgery is 0.025 to 0.1 mg I.V. or I.M. Postoperatively, 0.05 to 0.1 mg I.M. to control pain, tachypnea, or emergence delirium; repeat in 1 to 2 hours if needed.

Children ages 2 to 12: 2 to 3 mcg/kg I.V., depending on vital signs; or 5 to 15 mcg/kg transmucosally

➤ General anesthesia (with oxygen only)

Adults: 0.05 to 0.1 mg/kg I.V. for high-dose therapy; up to 0.12 mg/kg may be necessary.

➤ Adjunct to regional anesthesia

Adults: 0.05 to 0.1 mg I.M. or slow I.V. over 1 to 2 minutes

Dosage adjustment
• Elderly patients

Contraindications
• Hypersensitivity to drug or transdermal adhesive
• Alcohol intolerance
• Acute bronchial asthma

• Pregnancy (transdermal system)
• Breastfeeding
• Children under age 12; children under age 18 weighing less than 50 kg (110 lb)

Administration
• Before applying transdermal patch, clip hair at site; don't use razor. Wash area with clean water only; dry well.
• Apply transdermal patch to nonirritated, nonirradiated flat surface; press firmly in place for 30 seconds.
• In elderly patients, don't initiate fentanyl patch at dosages above 25 mcg/hour unless patient is already receiving more than 135 mg/day of oral morphine or equivalent.
• Know that patients receiving lozenge form may get second dose 30 minutes after first lozenge is placed in mouth.
• Inject I.V. dose slowly over 1 to 2 minutes.
• Have narcotic antagonist (naloxone) and emergency equipment available when giving drug I.V.
• Drug isn't recommended for control of mild or intermittent pain.

Route	Onset	Peak	Duration
I.V.	1-2 min	3-5 min	0.5-1 hr
I.M.	7-8 min	20-30 min	1-2 hr
Transdermal	6 hr	12-24 hr	72 hr
Transmucosal	Rapid	15-30 min	Several hr

Adverse reactions
CNS: sedation, headache, vertigo, floating feeling, dizziness, lethargy, confusion, light-headedness, nervousness, hallucinations, delirium, insomnia, anxiety, fear, coma, mood changes, tremor, **seizures**
CV: palpitations, hypotension, hypertension, tachycardia, bradycardia, **arrhythmias, circulatory depression, cardiac arrest, shock**
EENT: blurred vision, diplopia, **laryngospasm**

GI: nausea, vomiting, constipation, dry mouth, biliary tract spasm, anorexia
GU: ureteral or vesical sphincter spasm, urinary retention or hesitancy, oliguria, decreased libido or potency
Hematologic: decreased hemoglobin value; decreased granulocyte, platelet, neutrophil, and white blood cell counts
Hepatic: increased lipase and amylase levels
Musculoskeletal: skeletal and thoracic muscle rigidity
Respiratory: slow and shallow respirations, suppression of cough reflex, **apnea, bronchospasm**
Skin: local skin irritation (transdermal system), rash, urticaria, pruritus, diaphoresis, flushing, erythema, cold sensitivity
Other: physical or psychological drug dependence, drug tolerance, pain or phlebitis at injection site

Interactions
Drug-drug. *Barbiturate anesthetics:* decreased effects of both drugs
Buprenorphine, dezocine, nalbuphine: decreased analgesic effect
CNS depressants (including antidepressants, other opioid analgesics, sedating antihistamines, sedative-hypnotics, skeletal muscle relaxants): profound sedation, hypoventilation, and hypotension
Erythromycin, ketoconazole, some protease inhibitor antiretrovirals: decreased metabolism and increased effects of fentanyl, possibly leading to profound sedation, hypoventilation, and hypotension
Monoamine oxidase inhibitors: severe, unpredictable reactions
Partial-antagonist opioid analgesics, opioid antagonists: withdrawal in physically dependent patients
Drug-diagnostic tests. *Amylase, lipase:* increased levels
Drug-food. *Grapefruit juice:* decreased drug metabolism, increased risk of toxicity

Drug-herb. *Chamomile, hops, kava, skullcap, valerian:* increased CNS depression
Drug-behaviors. *Alcohol use:* profound sedation, hypoventilation, and hypotension

Precautions
Use cautiously in:
• diabetes mellitus, severe or chronic pulmonary or hepatic disease, cardiovascular disease, CNS tumors, adrenal insufficiency, hypothyroidism, renal impairment
• alcoholism or drug abuse
• elderly patients
• pregnant patients
• children younger than age 2 (safety not established).

Patient monitoring
• Assess for muscle rigidity in patients receiving high doses, and discuss need for neuromuscular blockers with prescriber. Patient will need ventilator if blocker is given.
• Monitor respiratory and cardiovascular function and urinary output.
• In patients using transdermal system, monitor pain level often to determine whether patch is effective for 72 hours or needs to be replaced after 48 hours. Know that drug level rises gradually for first 24 hours after patch is applied; supplemental analgesics may be needed during this period.
• If patient develops fever, assess for signs and symptoms of opioid toxicity because more drug is absorbed at higher body temperatures.
• If patient has adverse reactions to transdermal system, monitor him for at least 12 hours after patch removal.
• Carefully monitor hematologic studies and hepatic enzyme levels.

Patient teaching
◀€ Caution patient to keep transmucosal (lozenge) form out of reach of children even though it's supplied in

individually sealed, child-resistant pouches. One lozenge can be fatal to a child.

• Instruct patient to place lozenge between cheek and gum and suck on it over 15 minutes without chewing or swallowing.

• Teach patient proper technique for applying and disposing of transdermal patch.

• Tell patient that transdermal form is absorbed more rapidly if skin becomes warm by fever or hot environment. Instruct him to avoid electric blankets, heating pads, heat lamps, hot tubs, and heated water beds and to promptly report fever or a move to a hot climate.

• Instruct patient to avoid driving and other hazardous activities until he knows how drug affects concentration and alertness.

• As appropriate, review all significant and life-threatening adverse reactions and interactions, especially those related to the drugs, tests, foods, herbs, and behaviors mentioned above.

fexofenadine hydrochloride
Allegra

Pharmacologic class: Peripherally selective piperidine, selective histamine$_1$-receptor antagonist
Therapeutic class: Antihistamine (nonsedating type), second-generation
Pregnancy risk category C

Action
Blocks effects of histamine at peripheral histamine$_1$-receptor sites, decreasing allergic effects

Availability
Capsules: 60 mg
Tablets: 30 mg, 60 mg, 180 mg

⚕ Indications and dosages
➤ Seasonal allergic rhinitis, management of chronic idiopathic urticaria
Adults and children older than age 12: 60 mg P.O. b.i.d or 180 mg once daily
Children ages 6 to 11: 30 mg P.O. b.i.d.
Dosage adjustment
• Renal impairment

Contraindications
• Hypersensitivity to fexofenadine, terfenadine, or their components

Administration
• Don't give with apple, orange, or grapefruit juice.
• Don't give antacids within 2 hours of fexofenadine.

Route	Onset	Peak	Duration
P.O.	Within 1 hr	2-3 hr	12-24 hr

Adverse reactions
CNS: drowsiness, fatigue, headache
EENT: otitis media
GI: nausea, dyspepsia
Metabolic: dysmenorrhea
Respiratory: upper respiratory tract infection
Other: viral infection

Interactions
Drug-drug. *Antacids containing aluminum and magnesium:* decreased absorption and efficacy of fexofenadine
Drug-diagnostic tests. *Skin allergy tests:* false-negative results
Drug-food. *Apple, orange, and grapefruit juice:* decreased absorption and efficacy of fexofenadine

Precautions
Use cautiously in:
• renal impairment
• concurrent ketoconazole or erythromycin therapy
• elderly patients

• pregnant or breastfeeding patients
• children younger than age 12 (safety not established).

Patient monitoring
• Monitor renal function.
• Watch for signs and symptoms of viral infection.

Patient teaching
• Teach patient to stop drug 4 days before diagnostic skin tests to avoid interference with test results.
• Advise patient to report signs or symptoms of viral infection, especially upper respiratory tract infection.
• Instruct patient to avoid driving and other hazardous activities until he knows how drug affects concentration and alertness.
• As appropriate, review all other significant adverse reactions and interactions, especially those related to the drugs, tests, and foods mentioned above.

filgrastim
Neupogen

Pharmacologic class: Granulocyte colony–stimulating factor
Therapeutic class: Hematopoietic stimulator, antineutropenic
Pregnancy risk category C

Action
Induces formation of neutrophil progenitor cells by binding directly to receptor on surface granulocyte; also potentiates effects of mature neutrophils and reduces fever and risk of infection associated with severe neutropenia

Availability
Singleject prefilled syringes: 300 mcg, 480 mcg

Vial for injection: 300 mcg/ml, 480 mcg/1.6 ml

Indications and dosages
➤ To prevent infection after myelosuppressive chemotherapy
Adults: 5 mcg/kg/day S.C. injection or I.V. infusion over 15 to 30 minutes or continuous S.C. or I.V. infusion, increased by 5 mcg/kg with each chemotherapy cycle if needed
➤ To reduce duration of neutropenia after bone marrow transplantation
Adults: 10 mcg/kg/day I.V. over 4 or 24 hours or as a continuous S.C. infusion over 24 hours
➤ To enhance peripheral blood progenitor cell collection in autologous hematopoietic stem cell transplantation
Adults: 10 mcg/kg S.C. injection or as continuous S.C. infusion daily, beginning 4 days before first leukapheresis and continuing until last day of leukapheresis
➤ To reduce occurrence and duration of neutropenia in congenital neutropenia
Adults: 6 mcg/kg S.C. b.i.d.
➤ To reduce occurrence and duration of neutropenia in idiopathic or cyclic neutropenia
Adults: 5 mcg/kg S.C. daily

Off-label uses
• AIDS
• Aplastic anemia
• Hairy cell leukemia
• Myelodysplasia

Contraindications
• Hypersensitivity to drug, its components, or *Escherichia coli*–derived proteins

Administration
◀ Give I.V. injection directly without diluting.

• Know that drug may be injected into venous return line of dialysis tubing after dialysis is completed.

◀€ If drug must be diluted, use dextrose 5% in water; never use saline solution, which may cause drug to precipitate.

• Don't mix filgrastim with other drugs, and don't shake.

• Don't give within 24 hours of chemotherapy, bone marrow transplantation, or radiation therapy.

Route	Onset	Peak	Duration
I.V.	5-60 min	24 hr	1-7 days
S.C.	5-60 min	2-8 hr	1-7 days

Adverse reactions

CNS: headache, fever, weakness
CV: chest pain, hypotension, transient supraventricular tachycardia, **myocardial infarction, arrhythmias**
EENT: sore throat, stomatitis
GI: nausea, vomiting, diarrhea, constipation, abdominal pain, splenomegaly
GU: bleeding
Hematologic: leukocytosis, sickle cell crisis, **thrombocytopenia, splenic rupture**
Metabolic: hyperuricemia, elevated lactate dehydrogenase (LD) and alkaline phosphatase levels
Musculoskeletal: bone, joint, muscle, arm, and leg pain
Respiratory: dyspnea, cough
Skin: pruritus, rash, alopecia, cutaneous necrotic vasculitis, erythema
Other: fever, mucositis, pain at injection site, edema, hypersensitivity reactions

Interactions

Drug-drug. *Lithium:* increased neutrophil production
Topotecan: prolonged neutropenia duration
Vincristine: increased risk of severe atypical peripheral neuropathy

Drug-diagnostic tests. *Alkaline phosphatase, creatinine, LD, uric acid:* increased levels
Platelets: decreased count

Precautions

Use cautiously in:
• patients taking lithium or other drugs that may potentiate neutrophil release
• breastfeeding patients.

Patient monitoring

• Obtain complete blood count and platelet count before initiating therapy, and monitor these counts often thereafter.
• Monitor cardiovascular status carefully.
• Assess for signs and symptoms of sickle cell crisis or splenic rupture.

Patient teaching

• Teach patient to recognize and promptly report signs and symptoms of allergic response.
• Instruct patient to avoid driving and other hazardous activities until he knows how drug affects concentration and alertness.
• Advise patient to discuss with prescriber need for iron supplements, vitamin B_{12}, and folic acid.
• Teach patient how to monitor blood pressure at home.
• Tell patient to minimize GI upset by eating small, frequent servings of healthy foods and drinking adequate fluids.
• Inform patient that he'll undergo regular blood testing during therapy.
• As appropriate, review all other significant and life-threatening adverse reactions and interactions, especially those related to the drugs and tests mentioned above.

finasteride
Propecia, Proscar

Pharmacologic class: Androgen inhibitor

Therapeutic class: Sex hormone, hair regrowth stimulant

Pregnancy risk category X

Action
Inhibits enzyme 5-alpha reductase, which converts testosterone to metabolite 5-alpha dihydrotestosterone in prostate, liver, and skin

Availability
Tablets: 1 mg (Propecia), 5 mg (Proscar)

Indications and dosages
➤ Symptomatic benign prostatic hypertrophy (BPH)
Adults: 5 mg P.O. daily
➤ Male pattern baldness
Adults: 1 mg P.O. daily

Off-label uses
• Acne in women
• Hirsutism

Contraindications
• Hypersensitivity to drug
• Females
• Children

Administration
• Give with or without food.
• Know that female patients who are or may be pregnant shouldn't handle crushed or broken tablets. (Tablets are coated, so normal handling doesn't pose a problem).

Route	Onset	Peak	Duration
P.O. (BPH)	Unknown	8 hr	24 hr
P.O. (baldness)	3 mo	Unknown	Unknown

Adverse reactions
CNS: dizziness, headache, asthenia
EENT: lip swelling
GU: impotence, decreased ejaculate volume, decreased libido, testicular pain, gynecomastia
Musculoskeletal: back pain
Skin: rash

Interactions
Drug-drug. *Theophylline:* increased theophylline clearance
Drug-diagnostic tests. *Prostate-specific antigen (PSA):* 50% decrease

Precautions
Use cautiously in:
• hepatic impairment, obstructive uropathy.

Patient monitoring
• Carefully evaluate sustained increases in PSA level during therapy.
• Monitor fluid intake and output carefully.

Patient teaching
• Tell patient that drug may be taken with or without food.
• Teach patient to avoid driving and other hazardous activities until he knows how drug affects concentration and alertness.
• Inform patient that he may experience impotence and decreased ejaculate; advise him to discuss these issues with prescriber.
• Advise female caregivers who are or may be pregnant not to handle crushed or broken tablets.
• Tell patient that he may need at least 6 months of therapy for BPH treatment and at least 3 months to see improvement in male pattern baldness.
• Teach patient taking drug for BPH that he'll undergo periodic digital rectal exams.
• Instruct patient not to donate blood for at least 1 month after last dose.

• As appropriate, review all other significant adverse reactions and interactions, especially those related to the drugs and tests mentioned above.

flecainide acetate
Tambocor

Pharmacologic class: Cardiac benzamide local anesthetic

Therapeutic class: Antiarrhythmic (class IC)

Pregnancy risk category C

Action
Inhibits fast sodium channels of myocardial cell membrane, depressing action potential. Also slows conduction, shortens action potential, inhibits extracellular calcium influx, stops paroxysmal reentrant supraventricular tachycardia, and decreases conduction in accessory pathways in Wolff-Parkinson-White syndrome.

Availability
Tablets: 50 mg, 100 mg, 150 mg

🕖 Indications and dosages
➤ Supraventricular tachyarrhythmias (including paroxysmal supraventricular tachycardia and paroxysmal atrial fibrillation or flutter)

Adults: Initially, 50 mg P.O. q 12 hours, increased by 50 mg b.i.d. q 4 days until desired response occurs or maximum daily dosage of 300 mg is reached; some patients require dosing q 8 hours.

➤ Sustained, life-threatening ventricular tachycardia

Adults: Initially, 100 mg P.O. q 12 hours, increased by 50 mg b.i.d. q 4 days until desired response occurs or maximum daily dosage of 400 mg is reached; some patients may require dosing q 8 hours.

Dosage adjustment
• Heart failure
• Renal impairment

Off-label uses
• Ventricular arrhythmias
• Wolff-Parkinson-White syndrome

Contraindications
• Hypersensitivity to drug
• Preexisting atrioventricular block or right bundle-branch block
• Recent myocardial infarction

Administration
• Initiate therapy only in a hospital setting with trained personnel and continuous ECG monitoring.
• Before giving, correct hypokalemia or hyperkalemia.
• Once arrhythmias have been adequately controlled, dosage may be reduced.

Route	Onset	Peak	Duration
P.O.	Unknown	2-3 hr	12 hr

Adverse reactions
CNS: dizziness, anxiety, fatigue, headache, depression, malaise, tremor, weakness, hypoesthesia, paresthesia
CV: chest pain, palpitations, second- or third-degree heart block, **heart failure, new or worsening arrhythmias**
EENT: blurred vision, visual disturbances, corneal deposits
GI: nausea, vomiting, constipation, abdominal pain, dyspepsia, anorexia
Hepatic: drug-induced hepatitis
Respiratory: dyspnea
Skin: rash, diaphoresis
Other: edema, fever

Interactions
Drug-drug. *Acidifying drugs:* increased renal elimination, decreased efficacy of flecainide (with urine pH below 5)
Alkalinizing drugs: increased flecainide blood level, possible toxicity

Amiodarone: doubling of flecainide blood level

Beta blockers: increased blood levels of both drugs

Beta blockers, disopyramide, verapamil: additive myocardial depressant effects

Digoxin: 15% to 25% increase in digoxin blood level

Other antiarrhythmics (including calcium channel blockers): increased risk of arrhythmias

Drug-diagnostic tests. *Alkaline phosphatase:* increased levels (with prolonged therapy)

Drug-food. *Foods that increase urine pH above 7 (as in strict vegetarian diets):* increased drug blood level

Foods that decrease urine pH below 5 (such as acidic juices): increased renal elimination and possibly decreased efficacy of drug

Drug-behaviors. *Smoking:* increased plasma clearance and decreased efficacy of drug

Precautions

Use cautiously in:
- heart failure, renal impairment
- patients taking concurrent disopyramide, beta blockers, verapamil, or amiodarone
- pregnant or breastfeeding patients
- children (safety not established).

Patient monitoring

◀€ Monitor ECG for worsening arrhythmias.
- Measure pacing threshold 1 week before and after starting drug.
- Monitor potassium and flecainide levels.
- Assess respiratory status regularly.

Patient teaching

- Instruct patient to immediately report cardiac or respiratory symptoms.
- Instruct patient to avoid driving and other hazardous activities until he knows how drug affects concentration, alertness, and vision.

- Teach patient that drug may cause numbness; advise him to avoid injuries to areas of sensory impairment.
- Teach patient to minimize GI upset by eating small, frequent servings of healthy food and drinking adequate fluids.
- Inform patient that he'll undergo regular blood testing during therapy.
- As appropriate, review all other significant and life-threatening adverse reactions and interactions, especially those related to the drugs, tests, foods, and behaviors mentioned above.

fluconazole
Diflucan

Pharmacologic class: Synthetic azole
Therapeutic class: Systemic antifungal
Pregnancy risk category C

Action

Alters cellular membrane, increasing permeability and leakage of essential elements needed for fungal growth; at higher levels, may be fungicidal

Availability

Injection: 2 mg/ml in 100- or 200-ml bottles or containers
Powder for oral suspension: 50 mg/5 ml in 35-ml bottle, 200 mg/5 ml in 35-ml bottle
Tablets: 50 mg, 100 mg, 150 mg, 200 mg

🕖 Indications and dosages

➤ Oropharyngeal candidiasis
Adults: 200 mg P.O. or I.V. on first day, followed by 100 mg daily for at least 2 weeks
Children: 6 mg/kg P.O. or I.V. on first day, followed by 3 mg/kg/day for at least 2 weeks
➤ Esophageal candidiasis
Adults: 200 mg P.O. or I.V. on first day,

followed by 100 mg/day for 3 weeks and then for 2 weeks after symptom resolution. Up to 400 mg/ day may be used in severe cases.

Children: 6 mg/kg P.O. or I.V. on first day, followed by 3 mg/kg/day for 3 weeks and for at least 2 weeks after symptom resolution

➤ Systemic candidiasis

Adults: 400 mg P.O. or I.V. on first day, followed by 200 mg/day for 4 weeks and at least 2 weeks after resolution

Children: 6 to 12 mg/kg/day P.O. or I.V. daily

➤ Vaginal candidiasis

Adults: 150 mg P.O. as a single dose

➤ Cryptococcal meningitis

Adults: 400 mg P.O. or I.V. on first day, followed by 200 or 400 mg/day for 10 to 12 weeks after cerebrospinal fluid (CSF) is negative

Children: 12 mg/kg P.O. or I.V. on first day, followed by 6 mg/kg/day for 10 to 12 weeks after CSF is negative

➤ Suppression of cryptococcal meningitis in patients with AIDS

Adults: 200 mg daily P.O. or I.V.

➤ To prevent candidiasis after bone marrow transplantation

Adults: 400 mg P.O. or I.V. daily for several days before and 7 days after neutrophil count rises above 1,000 cells/mm³

Dosage adjustment
• Renal impairment
• Elderly patients

Contraindications
• Hypersensitivity to drug

Administration
◄€ Limit I.V. infusion to 200 mg/hour or less, using an infusion pump.
• Don't piggyback with other I.V. infusions.
• Keep overwrap on I.V. bag until just before use.
• Know that plastic container may be opaque (from moisture absorbed dur-

ing sterilization); this doesn't affect drug and will decrease over time.

Route	Onset	Peak	Duration
P.O.	Slow	1-2 hr	2-4 days
I.V.	Rapid	1 hr	2-4 days

Adverse reactions
CNS: headache, dizziness
GI: nausea, vomiting, diarrhea, dyspepsia, abdominal discomfort, altered taste
Hematologic: leukopenia, thrombocytopenia
Hepatic: increased hepatic enzyme levels, **hepatotoxicity**
Skin: rash, pruritus, exfoliative skin disorders (including **Stevens-Johnson syndrome**)
Other: anaphylaxis

Interactions
Drug-drug. *Alfentanil, cyclosporine, phenytoin, rifabutin, tacrolimus, theophylline, zidovudine:* increased blood levels of these drugs, greater risk of toxicity

Benzodiazepines, buspirone, losartan, nisoldipine, tricyclic antidepressants, zolpidem: increased blood levels and effects of these drugs

CYP3A4 inducers: inhibition of CYP3A4 enzyme system and alteration in actions of drugs metabolized by this system (with fluconazole dosage above 200 mg/day)

Glipizide, glyburide, tolbutamide: increased hypoglycemic effects of these drugs

Rifampin: increased rifampin blood level, decreased fluconazole blood level

Thiazide diuretics: increased fluconazole blood level

Warfarin: increased warfarin activity

Drug-diagnostic tests. *Alanine aminotransferase, alkaline phosphatase, bilirubin, gamma-glutamyltransferase:* increased levels

Platelets, white blood cells: decreased counts

Precautions
Use cautiously in:
- hypersensitivity to other azole antifungals
- renal impairment or hepatic disease
- pregnant or breastfeeding patients
- children (safety not established below age 6 months).

Patient monitoring
◀≶ Stay alert for signs and symptoms of anaphylaxis and stop drug immediately if these occur.
- Monitor liver function test results and hematologic studies.
◀≶ Assess for rash; monitor patient if lesions develop. Stop drug and notify prescriber if lesions progress (may signal Stevens-Johnson syndrome).
- Be aware that patients with human immunodeficiency virus have greater risk of adverse reactions.

Patient teaching
- Teach patient to recognize and immediately report signs and symptoms of allergic response.
- Emphasize importance of contacting prescriber if rash occurs to determine whether patient is developing Stevens-Johnson syndrome.
- Instruct patient to avoid driving and other hazardous activities until he knows how drug affects concentration and alertness.
- Teach patient to minimize GI upset by eating frequent, small servings of healthy food and drinking adequate fluids.
- As appropriate, review all other significant and life-threatening adverse reactions and interactions, especially those related to the drugs and tests mentioned above.

flucytosine
Ancobon

Pharmacologic class: Fluorinated pyrimidine analog
Therapeutic class: Antifungal
Pregnancy risk category C

Action
Unclear; thought to act by converting to fluorouracil in cells of susceptible fungi and interfering with protein synthesis

Availability
Capsules: 250 mg, 500 mg

🕖 Indications and dosages
➢ Severe fungal infections caused by susceptible strains of *Candida* species (including septicemia, endocarditis, urinary tract infections [UTIs]), and pulmonary infections) and *Cryptococcus* species (including meningitis, pulmonary infections, and UTIs)
Adults: 50 to 150 mg/kg P.O. daily in four equally divided doses q 6 hours
Dosage adjustment
- Renal impairment (glomerular filtration rate below 50 ml/minute)

Off-label uses
- Chromomycosis

Contraindications
- Hypersensitivity to flucytosine or other antifungals

Administration
- Give capsules a few at a time over 15 minutes to minimize nausea and vomiting.
- Be aware that flucytosine is rarely used alone. Expect to give another antifungal or amphotericin B concurrently.

Route	Onset	Peak	Duration
P.O.	Variable	2 hr	10-12 hr

Adverse reactions

CNS: headache, dizziness, confusion, hallucinations, vertigo, psychosis, ataxia, paresthesia, parkinsonism, peripheral neuropathy

CV: chest pain, **cardiac arrest**

EENT: hearing loss

GI: nausea, vomiting, diarrhea, dyspepsia, ulcerative colitis, abdominal discomfort, anorexia, duodenal ulcer, **hemorrhage**

GU: azotemia, crystalluria, **renal failure**

Hematologic: eosinophilia, anemia, leukopenia, **aplastic anemia, thrombocytopenia, bone marrow depression, agranulocytosis**

Hepatic: jaundice, increased hepatic enzyme levels

Metabolic: hypoglycemia, hypokalemia

Respiratory: dyspnea, **respiratory arrest**

Skin: rash, pruritus, urticaria, photosensitivity

Interactions

Drug-drug. *Amphotericin B:* synergistic effects, increased risk of toxicity

Drug-diagnostic tests. *Alanine aminotransferase, alkaline phosphatase, aspartate aminotransferase, bilirubin, gamma-glutamyltransferase:* increased levels

Glucose, granulocytes, hemoglobin, platelets, potassium, white blood cells: decreased values

Precautions

Use cautiously in:
• renal impairment, underlying hepatic disease, bone marrow depression
• pregnant or breastfeeding patients
• children (safety not established).

Patient monitoring

• Monitor renal and liver function test results.
• Carefully monitor blood glucose level and hematologic test results.
◀€ Assess for serious cardiovascular, renal, respiratory, and hematologic adverse reactions.
• Evaluate serum electrolyte levels, particularly potassium.
• Assess for signs and symptoms of bleeding.

Patient teaching

• Teach patient to take capsules over 15-minute period to reduce GI upset.
• Instruct patient to immediately report unusual bleeding or bruising.
• Tell patient to avoid driving and other hazardous activities until he knows how drug affects concentration and alertness.
• Instruct patient to minimize GI upset by eating frequent, small servings of healthy food and drinking adequate fluids.
• Inform patient that he'll undergo regular blood testing during therapy.
• As appropriate, review all other significant and life-threatening adverse reactions and interactions, especially those related to the drugs and tests mentioned above.

fludrocortisone acetate
Florinef Acetate

Pharmacologic class: Adrenocortical steroid

Therapeutic class: Synthetic mineralocorticoid and glucocorticoid

Pregnancy risk category C

Action
Acts on distal renal tubule, increasing sodium reabsorption and potassium excretion

Availability
Tablets: 0.1 mg

🚺 Indications and dosages
➤ Addison's disease (adrenocortical insufficiency)
Adults: 0.1 mg P.O. daily; typical dosage range is 0.1 mg three times weekly to 0.2 mg daily.
➤ Salt-losing adrenogenital syndrome
Adults: 0.1 to 0.2 mg P.O. daily

Off-label uses
• Hyponatremia
• Severe orthostatic hypotension

Contraindications
• Hypersensitivity to drug, tartrazine (some products), or sulfites (some products)
• Systemic fungal infection

Administration
• Give single daily doses in morning; spread multiple doses evenly throughout day.
• Administer with food to reduce GI upset.
• Avoid abrupt discontinuation; taper dosage when withdrawing.
• Reduce dosage, as ordered, if transient hypertension develops.

Route	Onset	Peak	Duration
P.O.	Variable	2 hr	1-2 days

Adverse reactions
CNS: headache, vertigo, **seizures**
CV: hypertension, cardiac hypertrophy, increased blood volume, **heart failure**
GU: glycosuria
Metabolic: hypernatremia, hypokalemia, hyperglycemia, decreased thyroid hormone levels, increased serum cholesterol level

Musculoskeletal: joint pain, tendon contractures, arm and leg weakness
Skin: urticaria, allergic rash, bruising, diaphoresis
Other: edema, infection, impaired wound healing, **anaphylaxis**

Interactions
Drug-drug. *Amphotericin B, potassium-depleting diuretics:* enhanced hypokalemia
Anabolic steroids: increased risk of edema
Aspirin: increased ulcerogenic effect; decreased pharmacologic effect of aspirin; rarely, salicylate toxicity (in patients who discontinue steroids after concurrent high-dose aspirin therapy)
Barbiturates, phenytoin, rifampin: decreased effect of fludrocortisone
Cardiac glycosides: increased risk of arrhythmias or digitalis toxicity associated with hypokalemia
Estrogen: increased risk of toxicity
Insulin, oral hypoglycemics: decreased hypoglycemic effect
Oral anticoagulants: decreased prothrombin time
Vaccines: neurologic complications and lack of antibody response to vaccine
Drug-diagnostic tests. *Cholesterol, urine glucose:* increased levels
Nitroblue-tetrazolium test (for bacterial infection): false-negative result
Potassium, thyroxine, triiodothyronine: decreased levels
Drug-food. *Sodium-containing foods:* increased blood pressure
Drug-herb. *Echinacea:* antagonism of fludrocortisone's immunosuppressive effect

Precautions
Use cautiously in:
• cardiovascular disease, cirrhosis, diverticulitis, ulcerative colitis, peptic ulcer, renal insufficiency, hypertension, myasthenia gravis, adrenal insufficiency
• pregnant or breastfeeding patients.

Patient monitoring

• Monitor blood pressure; report hypertension immediately.

• Assess for serious adverse reactions, particularly hypersensitivity and cardiovascular effects.

• Monitor sodium, potassium, and glucose levels carefully.

• Assess for signs and symptoms of infection.

• Weigh patient daily; report sudden weight gain.

Patient teaching

• Tell patient to take drug with meals or snack to minimize GI upset.

• Instruct patient on long-term therapy not to stop drug therapy abruptly.

• Advise patient on long-term therapy to wear or carry identification stating that he is receiving this drug.

◄ Teach patient to recognize and report signs and symptoms of adrenal insufficiency: fatigue, appetite loss, nausea, vomiting, diarrhea, weight loss, weakness, dizziness, and low blood glucose level.

• Advise patient to consume a diet low in sodium and high in potassium and protein.

• As appropriate, review all other significant and life-threatening adverse reactions and interactions, especially those related to the drugs, tests, foods, and herbs mentioned above.

flumazenil
Anexate✚, Romazicon

Pharmacologic class: Benzodiazepine receptor antagonist
Therapeutic class: Antidote
Pregnancy risk category C

Action

Antagonizes the CNS-depressant effects of benzodiazepines and inhibits activity at gamma-aminobutyric acid–benzodiazepine receptor sites

Availability

Injection: 0.1 mg/ml in 5- and 10-ml vials

ⓕ Indications and dosages

➤ Reversal of conscious sedation or general anesthesia

Adults: 0.2 mg I.V. given over 15 seconds. Additional doses may be given at 1-minute intervals until desired results occur, up to a total dosage of 1 mg. If resedation occurs, regimen may be repeated at 20-minute intervals, not to exceed 3 mg/hour.

Children: 0.01 mg/kg I.V. (up to 0.2 mg) given over 15 seconds; if desired results don't occur after 45 seconds, further injections of 0.01 mg/kg (up to 0.2 mg) may be given at 1-minute intervals (up to four additional doses) to a maximum total dosage of 0.05 mg/kg or 1 mg, whichever is lower.

➤ Suspected benzodiazepine overdose

Adults: 0.2 mg I.V. given over 30 seconds. If desired results don't occur after 30 seconds, 0.3 mg may be given over 30 seconds. Further doses of 0.5 mg may be given at 1-minute intervals, if necessary, to a total dosage of 3 mg; usual required dosage is 1 to 3 mg. If resedation occurs, additional doses of 0.5 mg/minute over 2 minutes may be given at 20-minute intervals (no more than 1 mg at a time or 3 mg/hour).

Children: 10 mcg/kg (0.01 mg/kg) I.V., up to a maximum of 0.2 mg (200 mcg)

Contraindications

• Hypersensitivity to drug or benzodiazepines

Administration

• Confirm airway is stable before giving drug.
• Dilute with dextrose 5% in water, lactated Ringer's solution, or normal saline solution.
• Inject into large vein through free-flowing I.V. solution over 15 to 30 seconds.
• Store in vial until ready for use. Drug remains stable in syringe for 24 hours.

Route	Onset	Peak	Duration
I.V.	1-2 min	6-10 min	1-2 hr

Adverse reactions

CNS: dizziness, vertigo, ataxia, agitation, confusion, drowsiness, fatigue, headache, sleep disorders, paresthesia, rigors, **seizures**
CV: chest pain, hypertension, palpitations, **arrhythmias**
EENT: blurred or abnormal vision, abnormal hearing
GI: nausea, vomiting
Respiratory: hyperventilation
Skin: flushing, sweating
Other: shivering, pain at injection site

Interactions

Drug-drug. *Tricyclic antidepressants:* reversal of benzodiazepine effect, leading to arrhythmias or seizures (when given for mixed overdose)

Precautions

Use cautiously in:
• head injury
• history of seizures
• pregnant or breastfeeding patients
• children younger than age 2 (safety not established).

Patient monitoring

• Be aware that drug has short duration of action; monitor patient for sedation and give additional doses as needed.
• Assess neurologic status frequently; watch for seizures.

• Monitor cardiovascular status, watching closely for arrhythmias.
• Watch for extravasation into surrounding tissue.

Patient teaching

• Before giving drug and on discharge, inform patient that although he may feel alert, resedation may recur.
• Inform patient that drug may impair memory and judgment.
• Instruct patient not to drive or engage in other hazardous activities requiring complete alertness for at least 24 hours after discharge.
• Tell patient to avoid alcohol and over-the-counter drugs for at least 24 hours after receiving drug.

fluorouracil
(5-fluorouracil, 5-FU)
Adrucil, Efudex, Fluoroplex

Pharmacologic class: Antimetabolite
Therapeutic class: Antineoplastic
Pregnancy risk category D

Action

Inhibits DNA and RNA synthesis and prevents thymidine production, leading to death of neoplastic cells; cell-cycle S-phase specific

Availability

Cream: 1%, 5%
Injection: 50 mg/ml in 10-ml ampules and 10-, 20-, and 100-ml vials
Solution: 1%, 2%, 5%

⏺ Indications and dosages

➢ Advanced colorectal cancer
Adults: 370 mg/m² I.V. for 5 days, preceded by leucovorin 200 mg/m² daily for 5 days; may be repeated q 4 to 5 weeks

➢ Other cancers
Adults: Initially, 12 mg/kg/day I.V. for 4 days, then 1 day of rest, then 6 mg/kg I.V. every other day for four to five doses. Or 7 to 12 mg/kg/day I.V. for 4 days, followed by 3-day rest, then 7 to 10 mg/kg I.V. q 3 to 4 days for three doses. As maintenance dose, 7 to 12 mg/kg I.V. q 7 to 10 days, or 300 to 500 mg/m²/day I.V. for 4 to 5 days, repeated monthly (no single daily dose should exceed 800 mg).
Poor-risk patients: 3 to 6 mg/kg/day I.V. for 3 days, then 3 mg/kg/day I.V. on days 5, 7, and 9 (not to exceed 400 mg/dose)
➢ Actinic (solar) keratoses
Adults: 1% solution or cream applied once or twice daily to lesions on head, neck, or chest; 2% to 5% solution or cream may be needed for other areas.
➢ Superficial basal cell carcinoma
Adults: 5% solution or cream applied b.i.d. for 3 to 6 weeks (up to 12 weeks)

Contraindications
• Hypersensitivity to drug
• Bone marrow depression
• Pregnancy or breastfeeding

Administration
◄€ Consult facility's cancer protocols to ensure that drug is being given appropriately. Protocols vary in dosage, administration technique, and cycle length.
• Follow facility policy for handling and preparing carcinogenic, mutagenic, and teratogenic drugs.
• Give antiemetic before fluorouracil to reduce GI upset.
• Know that drug may be given by direct I.V. injection without dilution.
• For I.V. infusion, dilute with dextrose 5% in water, sterile water, or normal saline solution in plastic bags (not glass bottles).
◄€ Be aware of importance of leucovorin rescue if prescribed with fluorouracil therapy.

• Check infusion site frequently to detect extravasation.
• Use nonmetal applicator or appropriate gloves to apply topical forms.
• Avoid applying topical product to mucous membranes or irritated skin.
• Don't use occlusive dressings over topical forms.
• Know that pyridoxine may be given with fluorouracil to reduce risk of palmar-plantar erythrodysesthesia (hand-foot syndrome).

Route	Onset	Peak	Duration
I.V.	1-9 days	9-21 days	30 days
Topical	Unknown	Unknown	Unknown

Adverse reactions
CNS: acute cerebellar syndrome or dysfunction, confusion, disorientation, euphoria, ataxia, headache, weakness, malaise
CV: angina, myocardial ischemia, **thrombophlebitis**
EENT: visual changes, photophobia, lacrimation, lacrimal duct stenosis, nystagmus, epistaxis
GI: nausea, vomiting, diarrhea, stomatitis, anorexia, GI ulcer or bleeding
Hematologic: anemia, **leukopenia, thrombocytopenia**
Hepatic: elevated hepatic enzyme levels
Metabolic: decreased plasma albumin level
Skin: alopecia, maculopapular rash, melanosis of nails, nail loss, palmar-plantar erythrodysesthesia, photosensitivity, local inflammation reaction (with cream), dermatitis
Other: fever, **anaphylaxis**

Interactions
Drug-drug. *Bone marrow depressants (including other antineoplastics):* additive bone marrow depression
Irinotecan: dehydration, neutropenia, sepsis

Leucovorin calcium: increased risk of fluorouracil toxicity

Live-virus vaccines: decreased antibody response to vaccine, increased risk of adverse reactions

Drug-diagnostic tests. *Alanine aminotransferase, alkaline phosphatase, aspartate aminotransferase, bilirubin, lactate dehydrogenase, urinary 5-hydroxyindoleacetic acid:* increased levels

Albumin, granulocytes, platelets, red blood cells, white blood cells (WBCs): decreased levels

Drug-behaviors. *Sun exposure:* increased risk of phototoxicity

Precautions

Use cautiously in:
• renal and hepatic impairment, infections, edema, ascites
• obese patients.

Patient monitoring

◀€ Watch for signs and symptoms of toxicity, especially stomatitis and diarrhea; stop drug and notify prescriber if these occur. Note that toxicity may take 1 to 3 weeks to develop.
• Monitor complete blood count, WBC and platelet counts, and kidney and liver function test results.
• Assess fluid intake and output.
• With long-term use, watch for serious rash on hands and feet; notify prescriber and discuss need for pyridoxine.
• Assess for bleeding tendencies.
• Monitor blood glucose level in patients at risk for hyperglycemia.

Patient teaching

◀€ Teach patient importance of taking leucovorin as prescribed with high-dose therapy.

◀€ Instruct patient to report signs and symptoms of toxicity, particularly stomatitis and diarrhea; inform him that these may not occur for 1 to 3 weeks.

• Advise patient to avoid driving and other hazardous activities until he knows how drug affects concentration and alertness.
• Teach patient to avoid activities that can cause injury. Tell him to use soft toothbrush and electric razor to avoid gum and skin injury.
• Advise patient to minimize GI upset by eating frequent, small servings of healthy food and drinking adequate fluids.
• Tell patient that drug may cause reversible hair loss.
• Inform patient that he'll undergo regular blood testing during therapy.
• As appropriate, review all other significant and life-threatening adverse reactions and interactions, especially those related to the drugs, tests, and behaviors mentioned above.

fluoxetine hydrochloride
Prozac, Prozac Weekly, Sarafem

Pharmacologic class: Selective serotonin reuptake inhibitor (SSRI)
Therapeutic class: Antidepressant
Pregnancy risk category B

Action

Selectively inhibits serotonin reuptake in CNS neurons; has a weak effect on norepinephrine and dopamine uptake

Availability

Capsules: 10 mg, 20 mg, 40 mg
Capsules (delayed-release): 90 mg
Oral solution: 20 mg/5 ml
Tablets: 10 mg

🖊 Indications and dosages

➤ Depression, obsessive-compulsive disorder
Adults: 20 mg/day P.O. in morning. After several weeks, may increase by 20 mg/day at weekly intervals. Give

dosages above 20 mg/day in two divided doses (morning and noon); don't exceed 80 mg/day. In depression, patients stabilized on 20 mg/day may be switched to 90-mg/week delayed-release capsules (Prozac Weekly) 7 days after last 20-mg dose.

➤ Bulimia nervosa

Adults: 60 mg/day P.O.; may be titrated upward over several days

➤ Premenstrual dysphoric disorder

Adults: 20 mg/day P.O., not to exceed 80 mg/day

Dosage adjustment

• Hepatic impairment
• Elderly patients

Off-label uses

• Alcoholism
• Bipolar II disorder
• Borderline personality disorder
• Diabetic peripheral neuropathy
• Narcolepsy
• Posttraumatic stress disorder
• Schizophrenia
• Social phobia

Contraindications

• Hypersensitivity to drug
• Monoamine oxidase (MAO) inhibitor use within past 14 days

Administration

◀◊ Be aware that drug should be discontinued 5 weeks before MAO inhibitor therapy begins.
• Give drug before 2 P.M. to prevent nighttime insomnia.

Route	Onset	Peak	Duration
P.O.	Unknown	6-8 hr	Unknown

Adverse reactions

CNS: anxiety, drowsiness, headache, insomnia, nervousness, abnormal dreams, dizziness, fatigue, hypomania, mania, weakness, tremor, **seizures**
CV: chest pain, palpitations, prolonged QTc interval

EENT: visual disturbances, stuffy nose, sinusitis, pharyngitis
GI: nausea, vomiting, diarrhea, constipation, abdominal pain, dyspepsia, abnormal taste, dry mouth, anorexia
GU: sexual dysfunction, dysmenorrhea, urinary frequency, increased blood urea nitrogen (BUN)
Hepatic: elevated alanine aminotransferase and creatine kinase levels
Metabolic: hypouricemia, hypocalcemia, hypoglycemia, hyperglycemia, hyponatremia
Musculoskeletal: joint, back, or muscle pain
Respiratory: cough, upper respiratory tract infection, dyspnea, respiratory distress
Skin: diaphoresis, pruritus, erythema nodosum, flushing, rash
Other: allergic reactions, weight loss, fever, flulike symptoms, hot flashes, hypersensitivity reactions

Interactions

Drug-drug. *Adrenergics:* increased sensitivity to adrenergics, increased risk of serotonin syndrome
Alprazolam: decreased metabolism and increased effects of alprazolam
Antidepressants, phenothiazines, risperidone, tryptophan: increased risk of adverse reactions
Antihistamines, opioids, other antidepressants, sedative-hypnotics: additive CNS depression
Buspirone: potentiation of fluoxetine effects, increased risk of seizures
Carbamazepine, clozapine, digoxin, haloperidol, lithium, phenytoin, warfarin: increased levels of these drugs, increased risk of adverse reactions
Cyproheptadine: decrease in or reversal of fluoxetine effects
Digoxin, warfarin, other highly protein-bound drugs: increased risk of adverse reactions to either drug
Drugs that induce CYP450-2D6: increased effects of these drugs

Efavirenz, ritonavir, saquinavir, other CYP450 inhibitors: increased risk of serotonin syndrome
MAO inhibitors: confusion, agitation, seizures, hypertension, and hyperpyrexia (serotonin syndrome)
Ritonavir: increased ritonavir blood level

Drug-diagnostic tests. *Alanine aminotransferase, alkaline phosphatase, BUN, creatine kinase, electrolytes, glucose:* increased levels

Drug-herb. *S-adenosimethionine (SAM-e), St. John's wort:* increased risk of serotonin syndrome

Drug-behaviors. *Alcohol use:* additive CNS depression

Precautions

Use cautiously in:
• hepatic or renal impairment, diabetes mellitus, cardiovascular disease
• history of seizures
• pregnant or breastfeeding patients.

Patient monitoring

◀€ Monitor patient for signs and symptoms of depression; assess for suicidal ideation.
• Evaluate neurologic status, watching especially for seizures.
• Monitor cardiovascular status, particularly for prolonged QTc interval.
• Assess weight regularly; watch for signs of eating disorders.

Patient teaching

• Teach patient to establish effective bedtime routine to minimize sleep disorders.
• Tell patient that drug may take 4 weeks or longer to be fully effective.
• Instruct patient to contact prescriber if he develops worsening depression or has suicidal thoughts.
• Tell patient to avoid driving and other hazardous activities until he knows how drug affects concentration and alertness.

• Instruct patient to minimize adverse GI effects by eating frequent, small servings of healthy food and drinking adequate fluids.
• Advise patient to discuss anti-itching medicines with prescriber if rash develops.
• As appropriate, review all other significant and life-threatening adverse reactions and interactions, especially those related to the drugs, tests, herbs, and behaviors mentioned above.

fluoxymesterone
Halotestin

Pharmacologic class: Androgen, anabolic steroid
Therapeutic class: Sex hormone
Controlled substance schedule III
Pregnancy risk category X

Action

Hormone responsible for normal growth and development of male sex organs; accelerates growth rate in children. Also has antiestrogen effect, which may be helpful in treating estrogen-dependent tumors.

Availability

Tablets: 2 mg, 5 mg, 10 mg

🖉 Indications and dosages

➤ Hypogonadism caused by testicular deficiency
Adults: 5 to 20 mg P.O. daily
➤ Delayed puberty in boys
Adolescents: 2.5 to 10 mg P.O. daily in divided doses for 4 to 6 months; individualize dosages and reduce to minimum when desired effects occur.
➤ Inoperable metastatic breast carcinoma
Adults: 10 to 40 mg/day P.O. in divided doses

Contraindications

• Hypersensitivity to drug, its components, or tartrazine
• Prostate cancer or breast cancer (other than inoperable breast cancer in women)
• Cardiac, renal, or hepatic disease
• Pregnancy or breastfeeding

Administration

• Give drug with food if it causes GI upset.
• Drug may contain tartrazine; check for allergies.

Route	Onset	Peak	Duration
P.O.	Unknown	2 hr	9 hr

Adverse reactions

CNS: headache, anxiety, depression, paresthesia
GI: nausea
GU: fluid retention, decreased urinary output, increased libido, menstrual irregularities, gynecomastia
Hematologic: polycythemia, **leukopenia**
Hepatic: hepatic dysfunction, **peliosis hepatitis, hepatocellular carcinoma**
Metabolic: androgenic effects, hypoestrogenic effects, hypercalcemia, altered serum cholesterol level, sodium and chloride retention
Skin: acne, hirsutism, male pattern baldness, seborrhea
Other: hypersensitivity reactions, chills, premature epiphyseal closure, edema, virilization (females)

Interactions

Drug-drug. *Cyclosporine:* increased cyclosporine blood level
Hepatotoxic drugs: increased risk of hepatotoxicity
Insulin, oral antidiabetics: decreased blood glucose level
Oral anticoagulants: increased sensitivity to coagulants

Drug-diagnostic tests. *Calcium, creatinine, creatinine clearance, lipids, hepatic enzymes, red blood cells:* increased values
Drug-herb. *Chaparral, comfrey, eucalyptus, germander, pennyroyal, skullcap, valerian:* increased risk of hepatotoxicity

Precautions

Use cautiously in:
• benign prostatic hypertrophy
• prepubertal boys.

Patient monitoring

• Watch for jaundice and monitor liver function tests.
• Monitor hemoglobin, hematocrit, and serum cholesterol level.
• Evaluate for weight gain and edema.
• Monitor skeletal maturation by X-ray in prepubertal males.
• Assess prepubertal males for excess hormonal effects (acne, priapism, increased body and facial hair, and phallic enlargement).
• Monitor postpubertal males for excess hormonal effects (testicular atrophy, erectile dysfunction, enlarged breasts, and epididymitis).
• Monitor serum calcium level; watch for signs and symptoms of hypercalcemia.

Patient teaching

• Advise patient to take drug with food to minimize GI upset.
• Advise patient to consume high-calorie, high-protein diet and eat frequent, small meals.
• Instruct patient to weigh himself regularly and report sudden increases.
• Tell women to stop drug and contact prescriber if menstrual irregularities develop.
• Instruct women to avoid pregnancy during therapy by using nonhormonal contraceptives.

• As appropriate, review all other significant and life-threatening adverse reactions and interactions, especially those related to the drugs, tests, and herbs mentioned above.

fluphenazine decanoate
Modecate, Modecate Concentrate, Prolixin Decanoate, Rho-Fluphenazine Decanoate✦

fluphenazine hydrochloride
Anatensol✦, Apo-Fluphenazine✦, Moditen HCl✦, Permitil✦, Permitil Concentrate, PMS-Fluphenazine✦, Prolixin, Prolixin Concentrate

Pharmacologic class: Phenothiazine, dopaminergic blocker
Therapeutic class: Anxiolytic, antipsychotic
Pregnancy risk category C

Action
Unclear; thought to alter postsynaptic dopamine receptors in brain, thereby preventing psychotic symptoms

Availability
fluphenazine decanoate
Depot injection: 25 mg/ml
fluphenazine hydrochloride
Elixir: 2.5 mg/5ml
Injection: 2.5 mg/ml
Oral concentrate: 5 mg/ml
Tablets: 1 mg, 2.5 mg, 5 mg, 10 mg

🚺 Indications and dosages
➢ Psychotic disorders
Adults: 2.5 to 10 mg/day (hydrochloride) P.O. in divided doses q 6 to 8 hours; typical daily dosage is 1 to 5 mg; give oral doses above 20 mg/day with caution. Or initially, 1.25 mg I.M., di-

vided and given q 6 to 8 hours. Parenteral (hydrochloride) dosage is one-third to one-half of oral dosage. Or 12.5 to 25 mg I.M. or S.C. (decanoate); base subsequent dosage and dosing intervals on patient response, not to exceed 100 mg.
Dosage adjustment
• Elderly patients

Contraindications
• Hypersensitivity to drug, sulfites (with injectable form), or benzyl alcohol
• Narrow-angle glaucoma
• Bone marrow depression
• Severe hepatic or cardiovascular disease

Administration
• Don't give parenteral form to comatose or severely depressed patient.
• Use gloves when handling; keep drug away from clothing or skin to prevent contact dermatitis.
• Dilute concentrated forms in juice, milk, or semisolid food just before giving to patient.
• Give long-acting, oil-based preparations with dry needle of at least 21G.
• Be aware that antacids and adsorbent antidiarrheals may decrease adsorption of fluphenazine; give 1 hour before or 2 hours after fluphenazine.

Route	Onset	Peak	Duration
P.O.	<1 hr	0.5 hr	6-8 hr
I.M. (HCl)	1 hr	1-5-2hr	6-8 hr
I.M.	24-72 hr	Unknown	1-6 wk
S.C.	Unknown	Unknown	Unknown

Adverse reactions
CNS: sedation, extrapyramidal reactions, tardive dyskinesia, drowsiness, pseudoparkinsonism, **neuroleptic malignant syndrome, seizures**

CV: hypotension, tachycardia
EENT: blurred vision, dry eyes, lens opacities, nasal congestion
GI: constipation, dry mouth, anorexia, **paralytic ileus**
GU: urinary retention, menstrual irregularities, inhibited ejaculation, priapism, gynecomastia, lactation
Hematologic: hemolytic anemia, eosinophilia, **aplastic anemia, agranulocytosis, leukopenia, thrombocytopenia**
Hepatic: jaundice, elevated hepatic enzyme levels, **hepatitis**
Metabolic: galactorrhea, hyperthermia
Skin: photosensitivity, rash
Other: allergic reactions, pain at injection site, sterile abscess

Interactions
Drug-drug. *Activated charcoal, adsorbent antidiarrheals, antacids:* decreased fluphenazine adsorption
Anticholinergics: decreased fluphenazine effects
Antidepressants, antihistamines, general anesthetics, monoamine oxidase inhibitors, opioid analgesics, sedative-hypnotics: additive CNS depression
Antihistamines, disopyramide, quinidine, tricyclic antidepressants (TCAs): increased risk of anticholinergic effects
Antihypertensives: additive hypotension
Barbiturates: increased fluphenazine metabolism, decreased efficacy
Bromocriptine: decreased bromocriptine efficacy
Guanethidine: inhibition of antihypertensive effects
Lithium: disorientation, unconsciousness, extrapyramidal symptoms
Meperidine: excessive sedation and hypotension
Ofloxacin: increased QTc interval
Phenytoin: increased or decreased phenytoin blood level
Pimozide: increased risk of potentially serious cardiovascular reactions
Propranolol: increased blood levels of both drugs

TCAs: increased blood levels and effects of TCAs
Drug-diagnostic tests. *Alanine aminotransferase, alkaline phosphatase, aspartate aminotransferase, bilirubin:* increased levels
Granulocytes, hematocrit, hemoglobin, leukocytes, platelets: decreased values
Pregnancy tests: false-positive or false-negative results
Urine bilirubin: false-positive results
Drug-herb. *Angel's trumpet, jimsonweed, scopolia:* increased anticholinergic effects
Chamomile, hops, kava, skullcap: increased CNS depression
St. John's wort: photosensitivity
Yohimbe: fluphenazine toxicity
Drug-behaviors. *Alcohol use:* increased CNS depression
Sun exposure: increased risk of photosensitivity

Precautions
Use cautiously in:
• diabetes, respiratory disease, prostatic hypertrophy, CNS tumors
• elderly patients
• pregnant or breastfeeding patients (safety not established)
• children with acute illnesses, infections, gastroenteritis, or dehydration.

Patient monitoring
◀ℰ Monitor patient for signs and symptoms of neuroleptic malignant syndrome (extrapyramidal symptoms, hyperthermia, autonomic symptoms).
◀ℰ Stop drug and notify prescriber immediately if patient shows signs or symptoms of blood dyscrasias (fever, infection, sore throat, cellulitis, or weakness).
• Observe for tardive dyskinesia.
• Watch for bleeding tendencies.
• Monitor bilirubin level, complete blood count, and liver function test results.

• Assess renal function and ophthalmic test results in patients on long-term therapy.

Patient teaching

• Caution patient that stopping drug suddenly may cause serious adverse effects.

• Instruct patient to avoid driving and other hazardous activities until he knows how drug affects concentration, alertness, and vision.

• Teach patient to report urinary retention or constipation.

• Instruct patient to report unusual bleeding or bruising.

• Teach patient to avoid activities that can cause injury. Tell him to use soft toothbrush and electric razor to avoid gum and skin injury.

• Inform patient that he'll undergo regular blood testing during therapy.

• As appropriate, review all other significant and life-threatening adverse reactions and interactions, especially those related to the drugs, tests, herbs, and behaviors mentioned above.

flurazepam hydrochloride
Apo-Flurazepam✦, Dalmane, Novo-Flupam✦, Somnol✦

Pharmacologic class: Benzodiazepine
Therapeutic class: Sedative-hypnotic
Controlled substance schedule IV
Pregnancy risk category X

Action

Depresses CNS at the limbic, thalamic, and hypothalamic levels, probably by potentiating gamma-aminobutyric acid (GABA), an inhibitory neurotransmitter

Availability

Capsules: 15 mg, 30 mg

Indications and dosages

➤ Short-term management of insomnia (less than 4 weeks)
Adults: 15 to 30 mg P.O. at bedtime
Dosage adjustment
• Elderly or debilitated patients

Contraindications

• Hypersensitivity to drug or other benzodiazepines
• Preexisting CNS depression
• Narrow-angle glaucoma
• Pregnancy or breastfeeding

Administration

• Evaluate patient's mental status and check kidney and liver function test results and complete blood count (CBC) before starting drug.

Route	Onset	Peak	Duration
P.O.	15-45 min	0.5-1 hr	7-8 hr

Adverse reactions

CNS: confusion, poor concentration, dizziness, daytime drowsiness, headache, lethargy, depression, paradoxical excitation, ataxia
EENT: blurred vision, abnormal taste
GI: nausea, vomiting, diarrhea, constipation, dyspepsia, abdominal pain
Hepatic: increased hepatic enzyme levels, hyperbilirubinemia
Respiratory: sleep apnea
Skin: rash
Other: physical or psychological drug dependence, drug tolerance, hangover

Interactions

Drug-drug. *Antidepressants, antihistamines, opioids:* additive CNS depression
Barbiturates, rifampin: increased flurazepam metabolism, decreased efficacy
Cimetidine, disulfiram, fluoxetine, hormonal contraceptives, isoniazid, ketoconazole, metoprolol, propoxyphene, propranolol, valproic acid: decreased

flurazepam metabolism, enhanced efficacy
Levodopa: decreased levodopa efficacy
Theophylline: decreased sedative effects of flurazepam
Drug-diagnostic tests. *Alanine aminotransferase, alkaline phosphatase, aspartate aminotransferase, total and direct bilirubin:* increased levels
Drug-herb. *Chamomile, hops, kava, skullcap, valerian:* additive CNS depression
Drug-behaviors. *Alcohol use:* additive CNS depression
Smoking: increased drug metabolism and clearance

Precautions

Use cautiously in:
• hepatic dysfunction
• history of suicide attempt or drug dependence
• elderly patients
• children younger than age 15 (safety not established).

Patient monitoring

• With long-term use, watch for signs and symptoms of physical or psychological dependence.
• Monitor patient's mental status, especially for depression and suicidal ideation.
• Watch for signs of drug hoarding or overuse.
• Monitor CBC and liver and kidney function test results.

Patient teaching

• Tell patient that drug is more effective over several days because it builds up in body.
• Teach patient (and significant others as appropriate) to report signs of depression or suicidal thoughts or actions.
• Inform patient that drug may cause physical or psychological dependence; instruct him to take only prescribed amount of drug.

• Teach patient to minimize GI upset by eating frequent, small servings of healthy food and drinking adequate fluids.
• As appropriate, review all other significant adverse reactions and interactions, especially those related to the drugs, tests, herbs, and behaviors mentioned above.

flutamide
Euflex✤, Eulexin, Novo-Flutamide✤

Pharmacologic class: Antiandrogen
Therapeutic class: Antineoplastic
Pregnancy risk category D

Action
Exerts potent antiandrogenic activity at the cellular level by inhibiting androgen uptake or nuclear binding of androgen

Availability
Capsules: 125 mg

Indications and dosages
➤ Metastatic prostatic cancer
Adults: 250 mg P.O. t.i.d. q 8 hours, given with luteinizing hormone-releasing hormone (LHRH) analog; total daily dosage is 750 mg.

Off-label uses
• Benign prostatic hypertrophy

Contraindications
• Hypersensitivity to drug
• Severe hepatic impairment
• Women

Administration
• Be aware that leuprolide acetate is the most common LHRH analog given with flutamide.

Route	Onset	Peak	Duration
P.O.	Variable	2 hr	72 hr

Adverse reactions

CNS: drowsiness, confusion, depression, anxiety, nervousness, paresthesia

CV: peripheral edema, hypertension

GI: nausea, vomiting, diarrhea, constipation, abdominal pain, dyspepsia, anorexia, dry mouth

GU: impotence, loss of libido, gynecomastia, hot flashes

Hematologic: anemia, **leukopenia, thrombocytopenia**

Hepatic: elevated alanine aminotransferase (ALT) and aspartate aminotransferase levels, **hepatitis**

Skin: rash, photosensitivity

Interactions

Drug-drug. *Warfarin:* increased prothrombin time

Drug-diagnostic tests. *Alkaline phosphatase, ALT, blood urea nitrogen, creatine kinase:* increased levels

Hemoglobin, platelets, white blood cells: decreased counts

Drug-herb. *Chaparral, comfrey, eucalyptus, germander, pennyroyal, skullcap, valerian:* increased risk of hepatotoxicity

Drug-behaviors. *Sun exposure:* increased risk of photosensitivity

Precautions

None

Patient monitoring

• Monitor complete blood count and liver function test results.

• Watch for bleeding tendencies and signs of liver damage (jaundice, vomiting, or dark yellow or brown urine).

• Monitor blood pressure.

Patient teaching

• Instruct patient to report unusual bleeding or bruising.

• Advise patient to avoid activities that can cause injury. Tell him to use soft toothbrush and electric razor to avoid gum and skin injury.

• Instruct patient to avoid driving and other hazardous activities until he knows how drug affects concentration and alertness.

• Instruct patient to minimize GI upset by eating frequent, small servings of healthy food.

• Inform patient that he'll undergo regular blood testing during therapy.

• As appropriate, review all other significant and life-threatening adverse reactions and interactions, especially those related to the drugs, tests, herbs, and behaviors mentioned above.

fluvastatin sodium
Lescol, Lescol XL

Pharmacologic class: HMG-CoA reductase inhibitor

Therapeutic class: Antihyperlipidemic

Pregnancy risk category X

Action

Competitively inhibits HMG-CoA reductase, an enzyme needed to synthesize cholesterol; inhibition of cholesterol synthesis reduces cholesterol concentration in hepatic cells, in turn increasing synthesis of low-density lipoprotein (LDL) receptors and increasing LDL uptake. Net effect is reduction in plasma cholesterol concentration.

Availability

Capsules: 20 mg, 40 mg

Tablets (extended-release): 80 mg

Indications and dosages

➤ Adjunctive therapy to control low-density lipoprotein, total cholesterol, apolipoprotein B, and triglyceride levels

Adults: 20 mg once daily at bedtime; may increase to 40 mg once daily, 20 mg b.i.d., or 80 mg extended-release at bedtime. Maximum dosage is 80 mg/day.

Contraindications
- Hypersensitivity to drug
- Active hepatic disease
- Pregnancy or breastfeeding

Administration
- Give with or without food.
- Know that drug works better when taken in evening.
- If patient's also receiving bile-acid resin, give fluvastatin at bedtime, at least 4 hours after resin.

Route	Onset	Peak	Duration
P.O.	1-2 wk	4-6 wk	Unknown
P.O. (extended)	2 wk	4 wk	Unknown

Adverse reactions
CNS: amnesia, emotional lability, facial paralysis, syncope, headache, hyperkinesia, poor coordination, malaise, paresthesia, peripheral neuropathy, drowsiness, weakness
CV: orthostatic hypotension, palpitations, phlebitis, **arrhythmias**
EENT: amblyopia, altered refraction, dry eyes, eye hemorrhage, glaucoma, hearing loss, tinnitus, epistaxis, gingival hemorrhage, sinusitis, pharyngitis
GI: nausea, vomiting, diarrhea, constipation, dyspepsia, flatulence, abdominal pain or cramps, stomatitis, colitis, stomach ulcers, dysphagia, esophagitis, gastroenteritis, melena, tenesmus, **rectal hemorrhage, pancreatitis**
GU: urinary frequency, urinary retention, cystitis, decreased libido, dysuria, epididymitis, hematuria, impotence, nephritis, nocturia, renal calculi

Hematologic: anemia, **thrombocytopenia**
Hepatic: jaundice, elevated hepatic enzyme levels, **hepatitis**
Metabolic: hyperglycemia, hypoglycemia, increased creatine kinase level
Musculoskeletal: joint pain, back pain, leg cramps, gout, bursitis, myasthenia gravis, myositis, torticollis
Respiratory: dyspnea, pneumonia, bronchitis
Skin: acne, alopecia, contact dermatitis, eczema, diaphoresis, rash, urticaria, skin ulcers, seborrhea, photosensitivity
Other: appetite changes, weight gain, allergic reaction, fever, facial or generalized edema, flulike symptoms, infection

Interactions
Drug-drug. *Antacids, cholestyramine, colestipol:* decreased fluvastatin blood level
Antifungals, cyclosporine, erythromycin, niacin, other HMG-CoA inhibitors: increased risk of myopathy
Cimetidine, omeprazole, ranitidine: increased fluvastatin blood level
Digoxin: increased digoxin blood level
Phenytoin: increased blood levels of both drugs
Rifampin: increased fluvastatin metabolism, decreased blood level
Drug-diagnostic tests. *Alanine aminotransferase, aspartate aminotransferase:* increased levels
Drug-herb. *Comfrey, germander, jin bu huan, pennyroyal, skullcap, valerian:* increased risk of hepatotoxicity
Red yeast rice: increased risk of adverse reactions
Drug-behaviors. *Alcohol use:* increased risk of hepatotoxicity

Precautions
Use cautiously in:
- alcoholism, hypotension, renal impairment, visual disturbances, severe metabolic disorders

- patients receiving concurrent azole antifungals
- women of childbearing age
- children younger than age 18 (safety not established).

Patient monitoring
- Watch for allergic response to drug.
- Assess for myositis and monitor creatine kinase level if patient has muscle pain.
- Monitor liver function test results and lipid levels.
- Watch for bleeding tendencies.
- Monitor patients receiving phenytoin when fluvastatin therapy is initiated or when fluvastatin dosage is changed.

Patient teaching
- Teach patient to recognize and report signs and symptoms of allergic response.
- Instruct patient to avoid driving and other hazardous activities until he knows how drug affects concentration, alertness, and vision.
- Advise patient to minimize GI upset by eating frequent, small servings of healthy food and drinking adequate fluids.
- Inform male patient drug may cause erectile dysfunction (impotence) and abnormal ejaculation.
- Tell patient that full effect of drug may take up to 4 weeks.
- Teach patient to report unusual bleeding or bruising.
- Instruct patient to move slowly when rising to avoid light-headedness or dizziness from sudden blood pressure decrease.
- Tell patient that he'll undergo regular blood testing during therapy.
- As appropriate, review all other significant and life-threatening adverse reactions and interactions, especially those related to the drugs, tests, herbs, and behaviors mentioned above.

fluvoxamine maleate
Apo-Fluvoxamine ❖, Luvox

Pharmacologic class: Selective serotonin reuptake inhibitor (SSRI)

Therapeutic class: Antidepressant, antiobsessive

Pregnancy risk category C

Action
Selectively inhibits serotonin reuptake in CNS, which relieves depression and reduces behaviors related to obsessive-compulsive disorder

Availability
Tablets: 25 mg, 50 mg, 100 mg

🖊 Indications and dosages
➣ Obsessive-compulsive disorder, depression

Adults: Initially, 50 mg daily at bedtime; may increase by 50 mg q 4 to 7 days until desired effect occurs (not to exceed 300 mg/day). If daily dosage exceeds 100 mg, give in two equally divided doses; if doses aren't equal, give larger dose at bedtime. Periodic adjustments to dosage are made to maintain lowest dosage that controls symptoms.

Children ages 8 to 17: Initially, 25 mg at bedtime; may increase by 25 mg/day q 4 to 7 days until desired effect occurs (up to 200 mg/day). If daily dosage exceeds 50 mg, give in divided doses, with larger dose at bedtime.

Dosage adjustment
- Hepatic impairment
- Elderly patients

Off-label uses
- Autism
- Anxiety disorders

Contraindications

• Hypersensitivity to drug or other SSRIs
• Monoamine oxidase (MAO) inhibitor use within past 14 days

Administration

• Be aware that fluvoxamine should be discontinued 5 weeks before MAO therapy begins.
• Give with or without food.

Route	Onset	Peak	Duration
P.O.	Rapid	2-8 hr	Unknown

Adverse reactions

CNS: dizziness, drowsiness, headache, insomnia, nervousness, anxiety, apathy, manic reactions, depression, psychotic reactions, hypokinesia or hyperkinesia, tremor
CV: hypertension, palpitations, orthostatic hypotension, tachycardia
EENT: sinusitis, abnormal taste, tooth disorder, dental caries
GI: nausea, vomiting, diarrhea, constipation, dyspepsia, flatulence, dry mouth, dysphagia, anorexia
GU: decreased libido, sexual dysfunction, anorgasmia
Hepatic: elevated hepatic enzyme levels
Musculoskeletal: hypertonia, myoclonus, twitching
Respiratory: cough, dyspnea
Skin: diaphoresis
Other: edema, weight gain or loss, chills, fever, flulike symptoms, yawning, hot flashes, allergic reactions, hypersensitivity reaction

Interactions

Drug-drug. *Beta blockers (such as propranolol), carbamazepine, lithium, L-tryptophan, methadone, some benzodiazepines, theophylline, tolbutamide, warfarin:* decreased fluvoxamine metabolism, increased effects
Clozapine: increased clozapine blood level and risk of toxicity

MAO inhibitors: serotonin syndrome
Tricyclic antidepressants: increased fluvoxamine blood level
Drug-behaviors. *Smoking:* decreased fluvoxamine efficacy

Precautions

Use cautiously in:
• cardiovascular disease, hepatic or renal impairment, mania, seizures, suicidal tendency
• labor and delivery
• elderly patients
• pregnant or breastfeeding patients.

Patient monitoring

◄╡ Watch for depression and suicidal ideation.
• Assess patient's appetite; report weight gain or loss.
• Monitor liver function test results.
• Monitor cardiovascular status, particularly blood pressure.

Patient teaching

◄╡ Instruct patient to contact prescriber if his depression worsens or he believes he may harm himself.
• Advise patient to avoid driving and other hazardous activities until he knows how drug affects concentration and alertness.
• Tell patient to minimize GI upset by eating frequent, small servings of healthy food and drinking adequate fluids.
• Teach patient to establish effective bedtime routine to minimize sleep disorders.
• Instruct female patient to notify prescriber immediately if she thinks she may be pregnant.
• Inform patient that drug may take several weeks to be fully effective.
• As appropriate, review all other significant adverse reactions and interactions, especially those related to the drugs and behaviors mentioned above.

fondaparinux sodium
Arixtra

Pharmacologic class: Selective factor Xa inhibitor

Therapeutic class: Anticoagulant, antithrombotic

Pregnancy risk category B

Action
Selectively inhibits factor Xa, which disrupts blood coagulation and inhibits thrombin formation and thrombus development

Availability
Injection: 2.5 mg/0.5 ml in single-dose syringe

🕖 Indications and dosages
➤ To prevent deep vein thrombosis and pulmonary emboli after hip or knee surgery

Adults: 2.5 mg S.C. 6 to 8 hours after surgery and hemostasis has been established; then, once daily for 5 to 7 days

Dosage adjustment
• Renal impairment

Contraindications
• Hypersensitivity to drug
• Bacterial endocarditis
• Hemophilia
• Bleeding disorders
• Severe renal disease

Administration
◀€ Don't give until 6 to 8 hours after surgery, to minimize risk of major bleeding.

◀€ Give by S.C. injection only—don't give I.M.

• Rotate injection sites among fatty tissue areas on left and right anterolateral and posterolateral abdominal wall.

• Don't expel air bubble from syringe; doing so may reduce amount of drug delivered.

• Listen for slight click when plunger is fully released. After drug has been injected, needle retracts and white safety indicator is visible.

• Don't mix with other injections or infusions.

Route	Onset	Peak	Duration
S.C.	Rapid	3 hr	72 hr

Adverse reactions
CNS: depression, dizziness, asthenia, headache, abnormal thinking, neuropathy, confusion, insomnia

CV: hypotension

GI: nausea, vomiting, diarrhea, constipation, abdominal pain, dyspepsia, dry mouth, anorexia

GU: urinary tract infection, urinary retention

Hematologic: anemia, minor bleeding, hematoma, purpura, **thrombocytopenia, major bleeding, retroperitoneal hemorrhage, postoperative hemorrhage**

Metabolic: hypokalemia

Other: increased wound drainage, injection site bleeding, bullous eruption, pain, edema, fever

Interactions
Drug-drug. *Anticoagulants:* increased risk of bleeding

Drug-herb. *Anise, astragalus, bilberry, black currant, bladder wrack, bogbean, boldo, borage, buchu, capsaicin, cat's claw, celery, chaparral, cinchona, clove oil, dandelion, dong quai, fenugreek, feverfew, garlic, ginger, ginkgo, papaya, red clover, rhubarb, safflower oil, skullcap, tan-shen:* additive anticoagulant effect

St. John's wort: reduced anticoagulant effect

Precautions
Use cautiously in:
• diabetic retinopathy, hepatic disease, blood dyscrasias, heparin-induced thrombocytopenia, severe hypertension, alcoholism
• patients older than age 75.

Patient monitoring
• Monitor complete blood count, platelet count, creatinine level, and renal function; assess stools for occult blood.
• Watch for bleeding tendencies, especially postoperative hemorrhage.
• Check for increased wound drainage after surgery.
• Monitor vital signs, temperature, and fluid intake and output.
• In patients undergoing concomitant neuraxial anesthesia or spinal puncture, watch for neurologic impairment (indicating possible spinal or epidural hematoma).

Patient teaching
• Instruct patient to avoid hazardous activities until he knows how drug affects concentration and alertness.
• Teach patient to minimize GI upset by eating frequent, small servings of healthy food and drinking adequate fluids.
• Caution patient to avoid activities that can cause injury. Tell him to use soft toothbrush and electric razor to avoid gum and skin injury.
• Tell patient that he'll undergo regular blood testing during therapy.
• As appropriate, review all other significant and life-threatening adverse reactions and interactions, especially those related to the drugs and herbs mentioned above.

foscarnet sodium
Foscavir

Pharmacologic class: Organic analog of inorganic pyrophosphate
Therapeutic class: Antiviral
Pregnancy risk category C

f

Action
Inhibits replication of pyrophosphate binding sites on virus-specific DNA polymerases and reverse transcriptases

Availability
Injection: 24 mg/ml in 250-ml and 500-ml bottles

Indications and dosages
➤ Acyclovir-resistant herpes simplex virus infection
Adults: 40 mg/kg I.V. over 1 hour q 8 to 12 hours for 2 to 3 weeks
➤ Cytomegalovirus retinitis in patients with AIDS
Adults: 90 mg/kg I.V. given over 1 to 2 hours q 12 hours for 2 to 3 weeks, depending on clinical response; follow with maintenance infusion of 90 to 120 mg/kg daily over 2 hours.
Dosage adjustment
• Renal impairment

Contraindications
• Hypersensitivity to drug

Administration
• Don't give by rapid I.V. infusion or bolus injection.
• Administer by controlled I.V. infusion through central or peripheral line with good blood flow.
• For peripheral administration, dilute with dextrose 5% in water or normal saline solution to a concentration of 12 mg/ml.

• Know that induction treatments are given over at least 1 hour and maintenance infusions, over 2 hours.

Route	Onset	Peak	Duration
I.V.	Unknown	Unknown	Unknown

Adverse reactions
CNS: vertigo, abnormal gait, hypertonia, hemiparesis, hyperreflexia, speech disorders, headache, fatigue, tremor, ataxia, dementia, EEG abnormalities, hyporeflexia, neuralgia, neuritis, paresthesia, depression, confusion, anxiety, insomnia, amnesia, hallucinations, agitation, **coma, seizures, paralysis, tetany, cerebral edema**
CV: hypertension, hypotension, palpitations, ECG abnormalities, nonspecific ST-T segment changes
EENT: visual field defects, eye pain, conjunctivitis, tinnitus, otitis, sinusitis, pharyngitis, vocal cord paralysis
GI: nausea, vomiting, diarrhea, constipation, duodenal ulcer, dyspepsia, dysphagia, flatulence, esophageal ulceration, ulcerative stomatitis, glossitis, melena, enterocolitis, proctitis, gastroenteritis, cholecystitis, tenesmus, **rectal hemorrhage, pseudomembranous colitis, paralytic ileus, ulcerative colitis, pancreatitis**
GU: decreased creatinine clearance, dysuria, polyuria, glomerulonephritis, toxic nephropathy, nephrosis, renal tubular disorders, pyelonephritis, uremia, hematuria, albuminuria, **acute renal failure**
Hepatic: jaundice, hepatomegaly, **hepatitis**
Metabolic: hypokalemia, hypocalcemia, hypomagnesemia, acidosis, hypophosphatemia, hyperphosphatemia, dehydration, glycosuria, hypervolemia, hyponatremia, hypochloremia, hypercalcemia
Musculoskeletal: joint, back, or muscle pain
Respiratory: hemoptysis, cough, dyspnea, pneumonia, bronchitis, pneumothorax, **respiratory depression, pleural effusion, pulmonary hemorrhage, bronchospasm, pulmonary infiltration**
Skin: rash, diaphoresis, pruritus, skin ulceration, seborrhea, skin discoloration, alopecia, acne, dermatitis, facial edema, dry skin, urticaria
Other: fever, infection, ascites, pain and inflammation at injection site

Interactions
Drug-drug. *Aminoglycosides, amphotericin, other nephrotoxic drugs:* increased risk of nephrotoxicity
Pentamidine: severe hypocalcemia
Zidovudine: increased risk of severe anemia
Drug-diagnostic tests. *Alkaline phosphatase, ALT, amylase, AST, bilirubin, creatinine, platelets:* increased levels
Calcium, granulocytes, hemoglobin, magnesium, phosphate, potassium, red blood cells, sodium, white blood cells: decreased values

Precautions
Use cautiously in:
• hepatic or renal impairment, severe anemia
• history of seizures
• elderly patients
• breastfeeding or pregnant patients
• children.

Patient monitoring
• Monitor fluid intake and output and renal function test results (especially 24-hour creatinine clearance) carefully.
• Assess hematocrit, hemoglobin, and electrolyte levels.
• Monitor cardiovascular and respiratory status regularly.
• Evaluate neurologic status closely.
• Assess frequently for signs and symptoms of infection, including sepsis.

Patient teaching
• Teach patient to report signs or symptoms of infection, numbness and

---

tingling, especially around mouth or in arms or legs.

• Instruct patient to report unusual pain, redness, swelling, or other changes at infusion site.

• Inform patient that he'll undergo regular blood testing during therapy.

• As appropriate, review all other significant and life-threatening adverse reactions and interactions, especially those related to the drugs and tests mentioned above.

fosfomycin tromethamine
Monurol Sachet

Pharmacologic class: Phosphoric acid derivative

Therapeutic class: Antibacterial, urinary tract anti-infective

Pregnancy risk category B

Action
Interferes with bacterial cell wall synthesis, blocking binding of bacteria to cells in urinary epithelium, thereby preventing and curing infections

Availability
Granule packet: 3 g

✒ Indications and dosages
➣ Uncomplicated urinary tract infections (UTIs) in women
Women over age 18: One packet dissolved in water P.O. as a single dose

Contraindications
• Hypersensitivity to drug

Administration
• Obtain specimens for urine culture and sensitivity testing, as prescribed, before giving.

• Give with or without food.

• Mix with 90 to 120 ml of cool water and stir to dissolve; administer immediately after dissolving.

• Don't give more than one dose per episode of UTI.

Route	Onset	Peak	Duration
P.O.	Rapid	2-4 hr	Unknown

Adverse reactions
CNS: dizziness, headache, paresthesia, weakness
EENT: rhinitis, pharyngitis
GI: nausea, vomiting, diarrhea, constipation, abdominal pain, dysphagia, dyspepsia, anorexia
GU: vaginitis, dysmenorrhea
Musculoskeletal: back pain
Skin: rash
Other: fever

Interactions
Drug-drug. *Metoclopramide, other drugs that increase GI motility:* decreased fosfomycin blood level and urinary excretion, increased GI motility

Precautions
Use cautiously in:
• acute cystitis
• pregnant or breastfeeding patients
• children (safety and efficacy not established).

Patient monitoring
• Monitor patient for resolution of UTI symptoms within 2 to 3 days.

Patient teaching
• Teach patient proper technique for dissolving and taking drug.

• Instruct patient to take only one dose per UTI episode.

• Advise patient to contact prescriber if symptoms don't resolve in 2 to 3 days.

• Instruct patient to avoid driving and other hazardous activities until she knows how drug affects concentration and alertness.

• Teach patient to minimize GI upset by eating frequent, small servings of healthy food and drinking adequate fluids.

• As appropriate, review all other significant adverse reactions and interactions, especially those related to the drugs mentioned above.

fosinopril sodium
Monopril

Pharmacologic class: Angiotensin-converting enzyme (ACE) inhibitor

Therapeutic class: Antihypertensive

Pregnancy risk category C (first trimester), *D* (second and third trimesters)

Action
Prevents conversion of angiotensin I to the vasoconstrictor angiotensin II, reduces sodium and water retention, and enhances blood flow in circulatory system

Availability
Tablets: 10 mg, 20 mg

Indications and dosages
➤ Hypertension
Adults: 10 mg P.O. once daily; may be increased as required up to 80 mg/day. (Typical range is 20 to 40 mg P.O. once daily.)
➤ Heart failure
Adults: 10 mg P.O. once daily (5 mg in patients who've had vigorous diuresis); may be increased over several weeks up to 40 mg/day. (Typical range is 20 to 40 mg/day.)
Dosage adjustment
• Renal impairment

Off-label uses
• Adjunct in myocardial infarction
• Nephropathy

Contraindications
• Hypersensitivity to drug or other ACE inhibitors
• Angioedema (hereditary or idiopathic)
• Pregnancy

Administration
• Don't give within 2 hours of antacid use.
• Give with or without food, but avoid giving with high-potassium foods or potassium supplements.

Route	Onset	Peak	Duration
P.O.	Within 1 hr	2-6 hr	24 hr

Adverse reactions
CNS: dizziness, fatigue, headache, insomnia, weakness, drowsiness, vertigo
CV: hypotension, angina pectoris, tachycardia
EENT: sinusitis
GI: nausea, vomiting, diarrhea, altered taste, anorexia
GU: proteinuria, impotence, decreased libido, **renal failure**
Hematologic: agranulocytosis, bone marrow depression
Metabolic: hyperkalemia
Respiratory: cough, eosinophilic pneumonitis, asthma, bronchitis, dyspnea
Skin: angioedema, rash
Other: fever

Interactions
Drug-drug. *Allopurinol:* increased risk of hypersensitivity reactions
Antacids: decreased fosinopril absorption
Antihypertensives, diuretics, general anesthetics, nitrates, phenothiazines: additive hypotension
Cyclosporine, indomethacin, potassium-sparing diuretics, potassium supplements: hyperkalemia
Digoxin, lithium: increased blood levels of these drugs, greater risk of toxicity

---

Indomethacin: decreased hypotensive effects

Drug-diagnostic tests. *Alanine aminotransferase, alkaline phosphatase, aspartate aminotransferase, bilirubin, blood urea nitrogen, creatinine, potassium:* increased levels

Antinuclear antibody titer: false-positive results

Sodium: decreased level

Drug-food. *Salt substitutes containing potassium:* hyperkalemia

Drug-herb. *Capsaicin:* increased incidence of cough

Drug-behaviors. *Acute alcohol ingestion:* additive hypotension

Precautions

Use cautiously in:
• aortic stenosis, cardiomyopathy, cerebrovascular or cardiac insufficiency, renal or hepatic impairment, hyponatremia, hypovolemia
• blacks with hypertension
• patients receiving diuretics concurrently
• elderly patients
• breastfeeding patients (safety not established)
• children (safety not established).

Patient monitoring

• Monitor complete blood count and liver and kidney function test results.
• Measure blood pressure to assess drug's efficacy and detect hypotension.
• Assess patient's potassium intake; monitor potassium level.
• Monitor cardiovascular, respiratory, and neurologic status.

Patient teaching

• Instruct patient to avoid driving and other hazardous activities until he knows how drug affects concentration and alertness.
• Encourage patient to drink enough fluids to remain well hydrated.

• Tell patient to report dizziness, fainting, bleeding tendencies, swelling, or persistent cough.
• Teach patient to minimize GI upset by eating frequent, small servings of healthy food and drinking adequate fluids.
• Instruct female patient to notify prescriber if she thinks she may be pregnant.
• Tell patient that he'll undergo regular blood testing during therapy.
• As appropriate, review all other significant and life-threatening adverse reactions and interactions, especially those related to the drugs, tests, foods, herbs, and behaviors mentioned above.

fosphenytoin sodium
Cerebyx

Pharmacologic class: Hydantoin
Therapeutic class: Anticonvulsant
Pregnancy risk category D

Action

Regulates neuronal membrane and prevents hyperexcitability caused by excessive stimulation; limits spread of seizure activity from active focus. Exerts antiseizure activity without causing general CNS depression.

Availability

Injection: 150 mg in 2-ml vials (100 mg phenytoin sodium), 750 mg in 10-ml vials (500 mg phenytoin sodium)

⚕ Indications and dosages

➢ Status epilepticus
Adults: 15 to 20 mg phenytoin sodium equivalent (PE)/kg I.V. at 100 to 150 mg PE/minute as a loading dose, then 4 to 6 mg (PE)/kg I.V. daily as a maintenance dose
➢ To prevent seizures during neurosurgery

Adults: 10 to 20 mg PE/kg I.M. or I.V. as a loading dose. Maintenance dosage is 4 to 6 mg PE/kg/day I.M. or I.V.
Dosage adjustment
- Hepatic disease
- Renal impairment
- Elderly patients

Contraindications
- Hypersensitivity to drug
- Alcohol intolerance
- Adams-Stokes syndrome
- Arrhythmias

Administration
- Know that drug is a phenytoin pro-drug and is given in phenytoin sodium equivalent (PE) units to avoid the need to perform molecular weight-based adjustments when converting between fosphenytoin and phenytoin sodium doses.
- For I.V. use, dilute in dextrose 5% in water or normal saline solution.
- Don't give faster than 150 mg PE/minute.
- When giving I.M., rotate injection sites.

Route	Onset	Peak	Duration
I.V.	Rapid	Unknown	Up to 24 hr
I.M.	Unknown	30 min	Up to 24 hr

Adverse reactions
CNS: ataxia, agitation, dizziness, drowsiness, dysarthria, dyskinesia, extrapyramidal syndrome, headache, nervousness, weakness, confusion, hyperesthesia, paresthesia, speech disorder, **cerebral edema, coma, intracranial hypertension**
CV: hypotension, tachycardia
EENT: diplopia, nystagmus, tinnitus, gingival hyperplasia
GI: nausea, vomiting, constipation, altered taste, dry mouth, anorexia
GU: pink, red, or reddish brown urine
Hematologic: lymphadenopathy, **aplastic anemia, agranulocytosis,** leukopenia, megaloblastic anemia, thrombocytopenia
Hepatic: increased hepatic enzyme levels, **drug-induced hepatitis**
Metabolic: hypocalcemia, hypokalemia, decreased thyroid function test results, hyperglycemia, increased glucose tolerance
Musculoskeletal: back or pelvic pain, osteomalacia
Skin: hypertrichosis, rash, pruritus, exfoliative dermatitis
Other: fever, facial edema, weight loss, injection site pain, allergic reactions including **Stevens-Johnson syndrome**

Interactions
Drug-drug. *Amiodarone, benzodiazepines, chloramphenicol, cimetidine, disulfiram, estrogens, felbamate, fluconazole, fluoxetine, halothane, influenza vaccine, isoniazid, itraconazole, ketoconazole, methylphenidate, miconazole, omeprazole, phenothiazines, phenylbutazone, salicylates, sulfonamides, tolbutamide, trazodone:* increased fosphenytoin blood level
Antidepressants, antihistamines, opioids, sedative-hypnotics: additive CNS depression
Barbiturates, carbamazepine, reserpine: decreased fosphenytoin blood level
Corticosteroids, cyclosporine, doxycycline, estrogens, felbamate, methadone, quinidine, rifampin: altered effects of these drugs
Dopamine: additive hypotension
Lidocaine, propranolol: additive cardiac depression
Streptozocin, theophylline: decreased efficacy of these drugs
Warfarin: initially, increased warfarin effects in patients stabilized on warfarin therapy, followed by decreased response to warfarin
Drug-diagnostic tests. *Alkaline phosphatase, glucose, glucose tolerance:* increased
Dexamethasone, metyrapone: test interference

Potassium, thyroxine: decreased levels
Drug-behaviors. *Acute alcohol ingestion:* increased drug blood level, additive CNS depression
Chronic alcohol ingestion: decreased drug blood level

Precautions
Use cautiously in:
• hepatic or renal impairment, severe cardiac or respiratory disease
• elderly patients
• pregnant or breastfeeding patients (safety not established).

Patient monitoring
◀€ Monitor electrocardiogram, vital signs, and overall patient status continuously during infusion and for 10 to 20 minutes afterward.
• Be prepared to slow administration or stop therapy if significant cardiovascular reactions occur.
• Monitor neurologic status carefully, especially for signs of increasing intracranial pressure.
◀€ Assess for rash; stop drug and notify prescriber if it occurs.
• Monitor phenytoin blood level after drug has metabolized to phenytoin (about 2 hours after I.V. dose or 4 hours after I.M. dose).
• Monitor electrolyte levels.
• Evaluate blood glucose level; watch for hyperglycemia in patients with diabetes.

Patient teaching
• Inform patient that he may experience sensory disturbances during I.V. administration.
• Teach patient to immediately report adverse effects, particularly rash.
• Tell patient that drug may turn his urine pink, red, or reddish brown.
• As appropriate, review all other significant and life-threatening adverse reactions and interactions, especially those related to the drugs, tests, and behaviors mentioned above.

frovatriptan succinate
Frova

Pharmacologic class: Serotonin 5-hydroxytryptamine $(5\text{-}HT)_1$-receptor agonist
Therapeutic class: Antimigraine agent
Pregnancy risk category C

Action
Binds to selective serotonin receptors on cranial arteries, causing vasoconstriction and decreased blood flow, which relieves migraine in selected patients

Availability
Tablets: 2.5 mg

⚕ Indications and dosages
➤ Acute migraine headache
Adults: 2.5 mg P.O. as a single dose at first sign of migraine; if headache returns, may be repeated after 2 hours. Maximum dosage is three doses in 24 hours.

Contraindications
• Ischemic heart disease
• Uncontrolled hypertension
• Peripheral vascular disease
• Cerebrovascular disorders

Administration
• Give one tablet with plenty of fluids at first sign of migraine.
• If headache returns, administer another tablet after 2 hours.
• Don't exceed three tablets in 24-hour period.
• Give first dose under close supervision if patient has coronary artery disease or other risk factors.

Route	Onset	Peak	Duration
P.O.	Variable	2-4 hr	Unknown

Adverse reactions

CNS: dizziness, headache, anxiety, malaise, fatigue, weakness, drowsiness, paresthesia, sensation loss

CV: palpitations, tightness in chest, **myocardial infarction (MI)**

EENT: abnormal vision, tinnitus, rhinitis

GI: nausea, diarrhea, dyspepsia, abdominal pain, altered taste

Musculoskeletal: skeletal or muscle pain

Skin: flushing, diaphoresis, photosensitivity

Other: hot or cold sensations

Interactions

Drug-drug. *Ergot alkaloids, other serotonin 5-HT$_1$-receptor agonists:* prolonged vasoactive reactions

Hormonal contraceptives, propranolol: increased frovatriptan bioavailability

Selective serotonin reuptake inhibitors: weakness, hyperreflexia, incoordination

Drug-behaviors. *Sun exposure:* increased risk of photosensitivity

Precautions

Use cautiously in:

• patients taking monoamine therapy or selective serotonin reuptake inhibitors.

Patient monitoring

• Assess for cardiovascular reactions, especially signs or symptoms of MI.

• Monitor neurologic status, particularly for indications of stroke.

• Check for rash and itching.

Patient teaching

• Instruct patient to take one tablet with plenty of fluids at first sign of migraine.

• Tell patient he may take second tablet 2 hours after first dose if headache returns.

• Instruct patient to avoid driving and other hazardous activities until he knows how drug affects concentration and alertness.

• Teach patient to minimize GI upset by eating frequent, small servings of healthy food and drinking adequate fluids.

• As appropriate, review all other significant and life-threatening adverse reactions and interactions, especially those related to the drugs and behaviors mentioned above.

fulvestrant
Faslodex

Pharmacologic class: Estrogen receptor antagonist

Therapeutic class: Antineoplastic

Pregnancy risk category D

Action

Inhibits cell division by binding with and downgrading estrogen receptor protein in breast cancer cells

Availability

Prefilled syringes: 125 mg/2.5 ml, 250 mg/5 ml

Indications and dosages

➤ Hormone receptor–positive advanced metastatic breast cancer after antiestrogen therapy

Adults: 250 mg I.M. q month as a single 5-ml injection, or two concomitant 2.5-ml injections

Contraindications

• Hypersensitivity to drug

• Pregnancy

Administration

• Expel air bubble from syringe before giving injection.

• Administer I.M. injection slowly.

• Know that drug may be given as one 5-ml injection or as two concomitant 2.5-ml injections.

Route	Onset	Peak	Duration
I.M.	Slow	2-3 days	Unknown

Adverse reactions

CNS: depression, light-headedness, dizziness, headache, hallucinations, vertigo, insomnia, paresthesia, anxiety, weakness
CV: chest pain, vasodilation, peripheral edema
EENT: pharyngitis
GI: nausea, vomiting, diarrhea, constipation, abdominal pain, food distaste, anorexia
GU: urinary tract infection, pelvic pain
Hematologic: anemia
Musculoskeletal: back pain, bone pain, arthritis
Respiratory: dyspnea, increased cough
Skin: flushing, rash, diaphoresis
Other: fever, hot flashes, injection site reactions, pain, flulike symptoms

Interactions

Drug-drug. *Anticoagulants:* increased bleeding risk

Precautions

Use cautiously in:
• bleeding disorders, hepatic dysfunction, thrombocytopenia
• breastfeeding patients.

Patient monitoring

• Monitor complete blood count.
• Assess liver function test results.

Patient teaching

• Advise patient to report signs and symptoms of infection, especially urinary tract infection.
• Instruct patient to avoid driving and other hazardous activities until she knows how drug affects concentration and alertness.

• Tell patient to notify prescriber immediately if she thinks she may be pregnant.
• Teach patient comfort measures to minimize hot flashes and rash.
• Instruct patient to minimize GI upset and sore throat by eating frequent, small servings of healthy food and drinking adequate fluids.
• Tell patient that drug may cause headache, muscle aches, or bone pain. Encourage her to discuss activity recommendations and pain management with prescriber.
• Advise patient to establish effective bedtime routine to minimize sleep disorders.
• As appropriate, review all other significant adverse reactions and interactions, especially those related to the drugs mentioned above.

furosemide
Apo-Furosemide✤, Furoside✤, Lasix, Lasix Special✤, Novosemide✤

Pharmacologic class: Sulfonamide loop diuretic
Therapeutic class: Diuretic, antihypertensive
Pregnancy risk category C

Action

Inhibits sodium and chloride reabsorption from ascending loop of Henle and distal renal tubules; increases plasma volume, promoting renal excretion of water, sodium, chloride, magnesium, hydrogen, and calcium

Availability

Injection: 10 mg/ml
Oral solution: 10 mg/ml
Tablets: 20 mg, 40 mg, 80 mg, 500 mg

⏺ Indications and dosages

➤ Acute pulmonary edema

Adults: 40 mg I.V. given over 1 to 2 minutes; if adequate response doesn't occur within 1 hour, give 80 mg. I.V. over 1 to 2 minutes.

➤ Edema secondary to heart failure, hepatic or renal disease, or hypertension

Adults: Initially, 20 to 80 mg/day P.O. as a single dose; may be increased by 20 to 40 mg P.O. q 6 to 8 hours (up to 600 mg/day has been used in heart failure and renal failure). When maintenance dosage is determined, may give every other day or two to three times weekly. Or 20 to 40 mg. I.M. or I.V. q 2 hours until desired response occurs.

Children: 2 mg/kg P.O. as a single dose; may be increased by 1 to 2 mg/kg q 6 to 8 hours, up to 5 to 6 mg/kg/day

Neonates: (Longer dosage intervals recommended.) 1 mg/kg I.V. or I.M.; may increase by 1 mg/kg q 2 hours (not to exceed 6 mg/kg)

➤ Hypertension

Adults: 40 mg P.O. b.i.d. (up to 200 mg P.O. if accompanied by pulmonary edema or acute renal failure)

Off-label uses

- Bronchopulmonary dysplasia
- Hypercalcemia associated with cancer

Contraindications

- Hypersensitivity to drug, thiazides, or sulfonamides

Administration

- Know that I.V. dose may be given by direct injection over 1 to 2 minutes.
- For I.V. infusion, dilute in dextrose 5% in water, normal saline solution, or lactated Ringer's solution.

◀◉ Don't infuse more than 4 mg/minute.

- Give oral doses in morning with food. If second dose is prescribed, give it in afternoon.

Route	Onset	Peak	Duration
P.O.	30-60 min	1-2 hr	6-8 hr
I.V.	5 min	30 min	2 hr
I.M.	10-30 min	Unknown	4-8 hr

Adverse reactions

CNS: dizziness, encephalopathy, headache, insomnia, nervousness, vertigo, weakness, asterixis, paresthesia, confusion, fatigue, nystagmus, drowsiness

CV: ECG changes, chest pain, hypotension, volume depletion, thrombophlebitis, **arrhythmias**

EENT: blurred vision, hearing loss, tinnitus

GI: nausea, vomiting, diarrhea, constipation, dyspepsia, gastric irritation, anorexia, dry mouth, **acute pancreatitis**

GU: excessive urination, nocturia, glycosuria, oliguria, nipple tenderness, premature ejaculation, difficulty maintaining erection, **renal failure**

Hematologic: purpura, **blood dyscrasias, leukopenia**

Hepatic: jaundice

Metabolic: hyperglycemia, hyperuricemia, dehydration, hypokalemia, hypochloremic alkalosis, hypomagnesemia

Musculoskeletal: joint pain, myalgia, muscle cramps or tenderness

Skin: photosensitivity, rash, diaphoresis, urticaria, pruritus

Other: pain, weight gain

Interactions

Drug-drug. *Activated charcoal:* decreased furosemide absorption

Aminoglycosides, cisplatin, ethacrynic acid: increased risk of ototoxicity

Amphotericin B, cisplatin, corticosteroids, diuretics, mezlocillin, piperacillin, stimulant laxatives: additive hypokalemia

Anticoagulants: increased anticoagulant effect

Antihypertensives, nitrates: additive hypotension

Cardiac glycosides: arrhythmias

Chloral hydrate: transient diaphoresis, hot flashes, hypertension, tachycardia, weakness, and nausea

Clofibrate: exaggerated diuretic response, muscle pain and stiffness

Hydantoins, nonsteroidal anti-inflammatory drugs, probenecid: diuresis inhibition

Lithium: decreased lithium excretion, possible toxicity

Neuromuscular blockers: prolonged neuromuscular blockade

Propranolol: increased propranolol blood level

Salicylic acid: salicylate toxicity (at lower dosages), decreased furosemide efficacy

Sucralfate: decreased naturietic and antihypertensive effects of furosemide

Sulfonylureas: decreased glucose tolerance, resulting in hyperglycemia

Theophyllines: altered, enhanced, or inhibited theophylline effect

Drug-diagnostic tests. *Calcium, magnesium, platelets, potassium, sodium:* decreased values

Cholesterol, creatinine, glucose, nitrogenous compounds: increased levels

Drug-herb. *Dandelion:* interference with drug's diuretic effect

Ephedra (ma huang), ginseng: decreased furosemide efficacy

Licorice: rapid potassium loss

Drug-behaviors. *Acute alcohol ingestion:* additive hypotension

Sun exposure: increased risk of photosensitivity

Precautions

Use cautiously in:
• diabetes mellitus, severe hepatic disease
• elderly patients
• pregnant or breastfeeding patients
• neonates.

Patient monitoring

• Watch for signs and symptoms of ototoxicity.

• Assess for other indications of drug toxicity (abdominal pain, sore throat, fever).

• Monitor complete blood count, blood urea nitrogen, and electrolyte, uric acid, and CO_2 levels.

• Monitor blood pressure, pulse, fluid intake and output, and weight.

• Assess blood glucose levels in patients with diabetes mellitus.

• Monitor dietary potassium intake; watch for signs and symptoms of hypokalemia.

Patient teaching

• Instruct patient to take drug in morning with food (and second dose, if prescribed, in afternoon) to prevent nocturia.

• Teach patient that drug may cause serious interactions with many common drugs; instruct him to tell all prescribers he's taking furosemide.

• Instruct patient to report signs and symptoms of ototoxicity (hearing loss, ringing in ears, vertigo) and other drug toxicities.

• Advise patient to avoid driving and other hazardous activities until he knows how drug affects concentration and alertness.

• Instruct patient to move slowly when rising to avoid light-headedness or dizziness from sudden blood pressure decrease.

• Tell patient to discuss need for potassium and magnesium supplements with prescriber.

• Advise patient to minimize GI upset by eating frequent, small servings of healthy food and drinking plenty of fluids.

• Inform patient that he'll under regular blood testing during therapy.

• As appropriate, review all other significant and life-threatening adverse reactions and interactions, especially those related to the drugs, tests, herbs, and behaviors mentioned above.

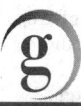

gabapentin
Neurontin

Pharmacologic class: 1-amino-methyl cyclohexoneacetic acid
Therapeutic class: Anticonvulsant
Pregnancy risk category C

Action
Unknown; studies show that drug has similar properties to those of other anticonvulsants.

Availability
Capsules: 100 mg, 300 mg, 400 mg
Oral solution: 250 mg/5 ml
Tablets: 600 mg, 800 mg

Indications and dosages
➤ Adjunctive treatment of partial seizures
Adults and children older than age 12: Initially, give 300 mg P.O. t.i.d. Usual range is 900 to 1,800 mg/day in three divided doses. (Some patients have tolerated dosages up to 2,400 to 3,600 mg/day.)
Children ages 5 to 12: Initially, give 10 to 15 mg/kg/day P.O. in three divided doses, titrated upward over 3 days to 25 to 35 mg/kg/day in three divided doses. (Some patients have tolerated dosages up to 50 mg/kg/day.)
Children ages 3 to 4: Initially, give 10 to 15 mg/kg/day P.O. in three divided doses, titrated upward over 3 days to 40 mg/kg/day in three divided doses. (Some patients have tolerated dosages up to 50 mg/kg/day.)
Dosage adjustment
• Renal impairment

Off-label uses
• Bipolar disorder
• Migraine prophylaxis
• Tremor associated with multiple sclerosis

Contraindications
• Hypersensitivity to drug

Administration
• Give with or without food.
• Administer first dose at bedtime to reduce adverse effects.
• Don't give within 2 hours of antacids.
• Schedule daily doses no more than 12 hours apart.

Route	Onset	Peak	Duration
P.O.	Rapid	2-4 hr	8 hr

Adverse reactions
CNS: drowsiness, anxiety, dizziness, hostility, malaise, vertigo, weakness, ataxia, altered reflexes, hyperkinesia, paresthesia, tremor, amnesia, abnormal thinking, difficulty concentrating, emotional lability
CV: hypertension, peripheral edema
EENT: abnormal vision, nystagmus, diplopia, amblyopia rhinitis, pharyngitis, dry throat, dental abnormalities
GI: nausea, vomiting, constipation, flatulence, dyspepsia, anorexia, increased appetite, dry mouth, gingivitis
GU: impotence
Hematologic: leukopenia
Musculoskeletal: joint, back, or muscle pain; fractures
Respiratory: cough
Skin: pruritus, abrasion
Other: facial edema, weight gain

Interactions
Drug-drug. *Antacids:* decreased gabapentin absorption
Antihistamines, CNS depressants, sedative-hypnotics: increased risk of CNS depression

---

✚ Canada   ◀€ Clinical alert   Reactions in **bold** are life-threatening

Drug-diagnostic tests. *Urinary protein dipstick test:* false-positive result (use sulfosalicylic acid precipitation procedure)

White blood cells: decreased count

Drug-herb. *Chamomile, hops, kava, skullcap, valerian:* increased risk of CNS depression

Drug-behaviors. *Alcohol use:* increased risk of CNS depression

Precautions

Use cautiously in:
- renal insufficiency
- elderly patients
- pregnant or breastfeeding patients
- children younger than age 3 (safety not established).

Patient monitoring

- Evaluate neurologic status and motor function.
- Assess white blood cell count.
- Monitor blood pressure.

Patient teaching

- ◀╎ Instruct patient not to stop taking drug suddenly; it must be tapered to minimize seizure risk.
- Teach patient to take first dose at bedtime to reduce adverse effects.
- Tell patient he may take drug with or without food.
- Instruct patient to avoid driving and other hazardous activities until he knows how drug affects concentration, alertness, motor function, and vision.
- Teach patient to minimize GI upset by eating frequent, small servings of healthy food and drinking adequate fluids.
- Tell patient that drug may cause joint pain, muscle aches, or bone pain. Encourage him to discuss activity recommendations and pain management with prescriber.
- Advise parents that drug may cause emotional lability and concentration problems in children; tell them to notify prescriber if these occur.

- Instruct female patients to report possible pregnancy to prescriber.
- As appropriate, review all other significant and life-threatening adverse reactions and interactions, especially those related to the drugs, tests, herbs, and behaviors mentioned above.

galantamine hydrobromide
Reminyl

g

Pharmacologic class: Cholinesterase inhibitor

Therapeutic class: Anti-Alzheimer's agent

Pregnancy risk category B

Action

Unclear; may reversibly inhibit acetylcholinesterase, which increases concentration of acetylcholine (necessary for nerve impulse transmission) in synapses of the brain

Availability

Oral solution: 4 mg/ml
Tablets: 4 mg, 8 mg, 12 mg

⚠ Indications and dosages

➤ Mild to moderate dementia of Alzheimer's disease

Adults: Initially, 4 mg P.O. b.i.d. If patient tolerates dosage well after at least 4 weeks of therapy, increase to 8 mg P.O. b.i.d. May increase to 12 mg P.O. b.i.d. after at least 4 weeks at previous dosage. Range of recommended dosage is 16 to 24 mg daily in two divided doses.

Dosage adjustment
- Moderate hepatic or renal impairment

Off-label uses

- Vascular dementia

Contraindications

- Hypersensitivity to drug
- Severe hepatic or renal impairment
- Pregnancy or breastfeeding
- Children

Administration

- Give with morning and evening meals.
- Before giving, make sure patient is well hydrated to minimize GI upset.
- Give with antiemetics as needed.
- Use pipette to add oral solution to beverage, and have patient drink it right away.

Route	Onset	Peak	Duration
P.O.	Unknown	1 hr	Unknown

Adverse reactions

CNS: depression, dizziness, headache, tremor, insomnia, drowsiness, fatigue, syncope
CV: bradycardia
EENT: rhinitis
GI: nausea, vomiting, diarrhea, abdominal pain, dyspepsia, anorexia
GU: urinary tract infection, hematuria
Hematologic: anemia
Other: weight loss

Interactions

Drug-drug *Anticholinergics:* antagonism of anticholinergic activity
Cholinergics: synergistic effects
Cimetidine, erythromycin, ketoconazole, paroxetine: increased galantamine bioavailability

Precautions

Use cautiously in:
- asthma, chronic obstructive pulmonary disease, GI bleeding, moderate renal or hepatic impairment, Parkinson's disease, seizures.

Patient monitoring

- Assess fluid intake and output to ensure adequate hydration, which helps reduce GI upset.
- Monitor cognitive status.
- Evaluate patient for cardiac conduction abnormalities; assess pulse regularly for bradycardia.
- Observe for bleeding tendencies.
- Assess for depression and suicidal ideation.

Patient teaching

- Instruct caregiver in proper technique for using oral pipette.
- Teach caregiver how to measure pulse rate; advise him to report slow pulse right away.
- Tell caregiver to prevent patient from performing hazardous activities until adverse reactions are known.
- Recommend frequent, small servings of healthy food and adequate fluids to minimize GI upset.
- Tell caregiver to watch for and report signs of depression.
- Teach patient and caregiver to establish an effective bedtime routine.
- As appropriate, review all other significant adverse reactions and interactions, especially those related to the drugs mentioned above.

---

ganciclovir (DHPG)
Cytovene, Vitrasert

Pharmacologic class: Acyclic purine nucleoside analog of 2'-deoxyguanosine
Therapeutic class: Antiviral
Pregnancy risk category C

Action

Inhibits binding of deoxyguanosine triphosphate to DNA polymerase by terminating DNA synthesis, thereby inhibiting viral replication

Availability

Capsules: 250 mg, 500 mg
Injection: 500 mg/vial

🖊 Indications and dosages

➤ Prevention of cytomegalovirus (CMV) in patients with advanced human immunodeficiency virus (HIV) infection

Adults: 1,000 mg P.O. t.i.d.

➤ Prevention of CMV disease in transplant recipients

Adults: 5 mg/kg I.V. q 12 hours for 7 to 14 days; then 5 mg/kg daily or 6 mg/kg daily five times weekly

➤ CMV retinitis in immunocompromised patients

Adults and children older than age 3 months: Initially, 5 mg/kg I.V. q 12 hours for 14 to 21 days, followed by a maintenance dosage of 5 mg/kg/day or 6 mg/kg five times weekly. For oral maintenance therapy, give 1,000 mg P.O. t.i.d. or 500 mg P.O. q 3 hours while patient is awake.

Dosage adjustment
• Renal impairment
• Elderly patients

Off-label uses
• CMV gastroenteritis and CMV pneumonia

Contraindications
• Hypersensitivity to drug or acyclovir
• Neutropenia or thrombocytopenia
• Breastfeeding

Administration
• Reconstitute 500 mg with 10 ml of sterile water. Shake vial to dissolve drug. Dilute drug again in 50 to 250 ml of I.V. solution.
• If patient is on fluid restriction, dilute to a concentration of 10 mg/ml or less.
◀❚ Administer I.V. infusion slowly over at least 60 minutes using infusion pump.
◀❚ Don't give by I.V. bolus or by I.M. or S.C. route.

• Give I.V. solution within 24 hours of dilution to reduce risk of bacterial contamination.
• Administer oral dose with food.

Route	Onset	Peak	Duration
P.O.	Slow	2-4 hr	Unknown
I.V.	Unknown	Unknown	Unknown

Adverse reactions

CNS: ataxia, coma, confusion, dizziness, headache, drowsiness, tremor, abnormal thinking, agitation, amnesia, neuropathy, paresthesia, **seizures**

CV: hypertension, hypotension, phlebitis, **arrhythmias**

GI: nausea, vomiting, diarrhea, abdominal pain, dyspepsia, flatulence, anorexia, dry mouth

Hematologic: anemia, **agranulocytosis, thrombocytopenia, leukopenia**

Hepatic: abnormal liver function test results

Respiratory: pneumonia

Skin: rash, diaphoresis, pruritus

Other: fever; infection; chills; inflammation, pain, phlebitis at injection site; **sepsis**

Interactions

Drug-drug. *Amphotericin B, cyclosporine, other nephrotoxic drugs:* increased risk of renal impairment and ganciclovir toxicity

Cilastatin, imipenem: heightened seizure activity

Cytotoxic drugs: increased toxic effects

Immunosuppressants: increased immunologic and bone marrow depression

Probenecid: increased ganciclovir blood level

Zidovudine: increased risk of agranulocytosis

Drug-diagnostic tests. *Alanine aminotransferase, alkaline phosphatase, aspartate aminotransferase, creatinine, gamma-glutamyltransferase:* increased levels

g

Granulocytes, hemoglobin, neutrophils, platelets, white blood cells: decreased values

Precautions

Use cautiously in:
• renal impairment
• history of cytopenic reactions.

Patient monitoring

• Monitor kidney function test results.
• Monitor neutrophil and platelet counts.
• Assess fluid intake and output to ensure adequate hydration.
• Monitor neurologic status closely, watching for seizures or coma.
• Check for signs and symptoms of infection, particularly sepsis.

Patient teaching

• Teach patient to report signs and symptoms of infection, including those at infusion site.
• Instruct patient to avoid driving and other hazardous activities until he knows how drug affects concentration and alertness.
• Inform patient that drug may cause birth defects. Tell female patients to use effective birth control during therapy; advise male patients to use barrier contraception during and for 90 days after therapy.
• Instruct patient to minimize GI upset by eating frequent, small servings of healthy food.
• Tell patient that he'll undergo regular blood testing during therapy.
• As appropriate, review all other significant and life-threatening adverse reactions and interactions, especially those related to the drugs and tests mentioned above.

gatifloxacin
Tequin

Pharmacologic class: Fluoroquinolone
Therapeutic class: Anti-infective
Pregnancy risk category C

Action

Inhibits bacterial DNA gyrase, an enzyme involved in replication, transcription, and repair of bacterial DNA, in susceptible gram-negative and gram-positive aerobic and anaerobic bacteria

Availability

Injection: 200 mg/20-ml vial, 400 mg/20-ml vial
Tablets: 200 mg, 400 mg

🖊 Indications and dosages

➤ Acute chronic bronchitis, urinary tract infections (UTIs), or acute pyelonephritis; complicated UTIs; uncomplicated skin and skin-structure infections
Adults: 400 mg P.O. or I.V. q 24 hours for 7 to 10 days
➤ Acute sinusitis
Adults: 400 mg P.O. or I.V. q 24 hours for 10 days
➤ Community-acquired pneumonia
Adults: 400 mg P.O. or I.V. q 24 hours for 7 to 14 days
➤ Uncomplicated UTIs, cystitis
Adults: 400 mg P.O. or I.V. as a single dose, or 200 mg P.O. or I.V. q 24 hours for 3 days
➤ Uncomplicated urethral gonorrhea (in men), endocervical or rectal gonorrhea (in women)
Adults: 400 mg P.O. or I.V. as a single dose
Dosage adjustment
• Renal impairment

Off-label uses
- Chronic prostatitis
- Atypical pneumonia

Contraindications
- Hypersensitivity to drug
- Prolonged QTc interval
- Concurrent disopyramide or amiodarone therapy
- Pregnancy
- Children younger than age 18 (except in postexposure inhalation or cutaneous anthrax)

Administration
◄€ Administer I.V. over 60 minutes; avoid rapid or bolus I.V. infusion.
- Don't dilute with sterile water for injection. Dilute with compatible solution, such as dextrose 5% in water, normal saline solution, or dextrose 5% and 0.9% sodium chloride injection.
- Be aware that parenteral solution is for I.V. use only.
- Give oral doses at least 4 hours before ferrous sulfate, aluminum- or magnesium-containing antacids, or buffered tablets or solutions.

Route	Onset	Peak	Duration
P.O.	Rapid	1-2 hr	24 hr
I.V.	Rapid	End of infusion	24 hr

Adverse reactions
CNS: dizziness, headache
EENT: pharyngitis
GI: diarrhea, abdominal pain or discomfort, abdominal cramps, abnormal taste
GU: vaginitis
Hematologic: increased platelet count
Hepatic: elevated hepatic enzyme levels, hyperbilirubinemia
Metabolic: hyperglycemia, hypoglycemia
Respiratory: dyspnea
Skin: photosensitivity, rash
Other: pain or phlebitis at injection site, hypersensitivity reactions

Interactions
Drug-drug. *Amiodarone, bepridil, disopyramide, erythromycin, pentamidine, phenothiazines, pimozide, procainamide, quinidine, sotalol, tricyclic antidepressants:* increased risk of serious cardiovascular reactions
Antacids, bismuth subsalicylate, iron salts, sucralfate, zinc salts: decreased gatifloxacin absorption
Antineoplastics: decreased gatifloxacin blood level
Corticosteroids: increased risk of tendon rupture
Drug-diagnostic tests. *Alanine aminotransferase, alkaline phosphatase, aspartate aminotransferase, bilirubin, lactate dehydrogenase, platelets:* increased levels
Hematocrit, hemoglobin: decreased values
Drug-food. *Milk, yogurt:* impaired drug absorption (but drug doesn't interact with other dietary calcium sources)
Tube feedings: impaired drug absorption
Drug-herb. *Dong quai, St. John's wort:* phototoxicity
Fennel: decreased drug absorption
Drug-behaviors. *Sun exposure:* phototoxicity

Precautions
Use cautiously in:
- acute myocardial ischemia, arrhythmias, cirrhosis, renal impairment, CNS disease
- elderly patients
- breastfeeding patients.

Patient monitoring
◄€ Stop drug and immediately report signs or symptoms of hypersensitivity reaction, including fever, rash, fatigue, nausea, vomiting, diarrhea, or abdominal pain.
- Monitor renal function test results in patients with renal insufficiency.

• Assess blood glucose levels in patients with diabetes mellitus.

Patient teaching
• Advise patient to take drug at least 4 hours before ferrous sulfate, antacids containing aluminum or magnesium, or buffered tablets and solutions.
◀◣ Instruct patient to stop taking drug and contact prescriber immediately if he experiences fever, rash, nausea, vomiting, diarrhea, or abdominal pain.
• Instruct patient to avoid driving and other hazardous activities until he knows how drug affects concentration and alertness.
• As appropriate, review all other significant adverse reactions and interactions, especially those related to the drugs, tests, foods, herbs, and behaviors mentioned above.

gemcitabine hydrochloride
Gemzar

Pharmacologic class: Antimetabolite (pyrimidine analog)
Therapeutic class: Antineoplastic
Pregnancy risk category D

Action
Kills malignant cells undergoing DNA synthesis; arrests progression of cells at the G1/S border

Availability
Powder for injection: 200 mg in 10-ml vial, 1 g in 50-ml vial

🕒 Indications and dosages
➤ Pancreatic cancer
Adults: 1,000 mg/m^2 I.V. q week for 7 weeks, followed by 1 week of rest. May continue with cycles of once-weekly administration for 3 weeks, followed by 1 week of rest.

➤ Non-small-cell lung cancer (given with cisplatin)
Adults: 1,000 mg/m^2 I.V. on days 1, 8, and 15 of each 28-day cycle (cisplatin also given on day 1); or 1,250 mg/m^2 on days 1 and 8 of each 21-day cycle (cisplatin also given on day 1)

Off-label uses
• Breast and bladder cancer

Contraindications
• Hypersensitivity to drug

Administration
• Follow facility policy for preparing, handling, and administering carcinogenic, mutagenic, and teratogenic drugs.
• Add 5 ml of preservative-free normal saline solution to 200-mg vial, or add 25 ml of solution to 1-g vial. Shake vial to dissolve drug.
• Reconstitute drug to 40 mg/ml. If necessary, dilute it further to 1 mg/ml.
◀◣ Infuse over 30 minutes; infusions longer than 60 minutes and more frequently than weekly increase risk of toxicity.

Route	Onset	Peak	Duration
I.V.	Unknown	Unknown	Unknown

Adverse reactions
CNS: paresthesia
GI: nausea, vomiting, diarrhea, stomatitis
GU: hematuria, proteinuria, **hemolytic uremic syndrome, renal failure**
Hematologic: anemia, **leukopenia, thrombocytopenia**
Hepatic: transient elevation of transaminase and bilirubin levels
Respiratory: dyspnea, **bronchospasm**
Skin: alopecia, rash, cellulitis
Other: flulike symptoms, fever, edema, injection site reactions, **anaphylactoid reactions**

Interactions

Drug-drug. *Live-virus vaccines:* decreased antibody response to vaccine, increased risk of adverse reactions
Other antineoplastics: additive bone marrow depression

Drug-diagnostic tests. *Alanine aminotransferase, alkaline phosphatase, aspartate aminotransferase, bilirubin:* transient increase
Blood urea nitrogen, serum creatinine: increased levels

Precautions

Use cautiously in:
• hepatic or renal impairment
• women of childbearing age
• pregnant or breastfeeding patients.

Patient monitoring

◀€ Stop infusion and notify prescriber immediately if patient has signs or symptoms of allergic reaction.
• Monitor liver and kidney function test results.
• Monitor complete blood count and white cell differential, particularly neutrophil and platelet counts.
• Assess degree of bone marrow depression; expect dosage changes based on blood counts.
• Watch for signs and symptoms of infection and bleeding tendencies, even after drug therapy ends.
• Evaluate respiratory status regularly.
• Monitor temperature, especially during first 12 hours of therapy.

Patient teaching

◀€ Instruct patient to stop taking drug and immediately report signs or symptoms of allergic reaction.
◀€ Advise patient to watch for and immediately report signs or symptoms of infection (especially flulike symptoms).
• Instruct patient to report unusual bleeding or bruising.
• Teach patient to avoid driving and other hazardous activities until he

knows how drug affects concentration and alertness.
• Advise patient to avoid activities that can cause injury. Tell him to use soft toothbrush and electric razor to avoid gum and skin injury.
• Teach patient to minimize GI upset by eating frequent, small servings of healthy food.
• Inform patient that he'll undergo blood testing periodically throughout therapy.
• As appropriate, review all other significant and life-threatening adverse reactions and interactions, especially those related to the drugs and tests mentioned above.

g

gemfibrozil
Apo-Gemfibrozil✤, Gen-Fibro✤, Lopid, Novo-Gemfibrozil✤, Nu-Gemfibrozil✤

Pharmacologic class: Fibric acid derivative
Therapeutic class: Antihyperlipidemic
Pregnancy risk category C

Action

Inhibits peripheral lipolysis, resulting in decreased triglyceride levels; also inhibits synthesis and increases clearance of very-low-density lipoproteins (LDLs)

Availability

Capsules: 300 mg
Tablets: 600 mg

⌀ Indications and dosages

➢ Type IIb hyperlipidemia in patients without coronary artery disease who are unresponsive to other treatment measures; adjunctive therapy for types IV and V hyperlipidemia

Adults: 1,200 mg P.O. daily in divided doses

Contraindications
- Hypersensitivity to drug
- Gallbladder disease
- Severe renal dysfunction
- Hepatic dysfunction

Administration
- Before starting drug and throughout therapy, patient should use dietary measures and exercise to control hyperlipidemia.
- Give 30 minutes before meal.

Route	Onset	Peak	Duration
P.O.	2-5 days	4 wk	Unknown

Adverse reactions
CNS: fatigue, hypoesthesia, paresthesia, drowsiness, syncope, vertigo, dizziness, headache, **seizures**
CV: vasculitis
EENT: cataracts, blurred vision, retinal edema, abnormal taste, hoarseness
GI: nausea, vomiting, diarrhea, abdominal or epigastric pain, heartburn, flatulence, gallstones, dry mouth
GU: decreased male fertility, dysuria, impotence
Hematologic: eosinophilia, anemia, bone marrow hypoplasia, **leukopenia, thrombocytopenia**
Hepatic: increased alanine aminotransferase (ALT), alkaline phosphatase (ALP), aspartate aminotransferase (AST), bilirubin, and lactate dehydrogenase (LD) levels; **hepatotoxicity**
Metabolic: hypoglycemia
Musculoskeletal: joint, back, or muscle pain; myasthenia; myopathy; synovitis; myositis; **rhabdomyolysis**
Respiratory: cough
Skin: alopecia, rash, urticaria, eczema, pruritus, angioedema
Other: chills, weight loss, increased risk of bacterial and viral infection, lupus-like syndrome, **anaphylaxis**

Interactions
Drug-drug. *Chenodiol, ursodiol:* decreased gemfibrozil efficacy
Cyclosporine: decreased cyclosporine effects
HMG-CoA reductase inhibitors: increased risk of rhabdomyolysis
Sulfonylureas: increased hypoglycemic effects
Warfarin: increased bleeding risk
Drug-diagnostic tests. *ALP, ALT, AST, bilirubin, creatine kinase (CK), glucose, LD:* increased levels
Hematocrit, hemoglobin, leukocytes, potassium: slightly decreased values

Precautions
Use cautiously in:
- renal impairment, cholelithiasis, diabetes, hypothyroidism
- pregnant or breastfeeding patients
- children (safety not established).

Patient monitoring
- Monitor kidney and liver function test results and serum lipid levels.
- ◄€ Watch for signs and symptoms of adverse reactions, especially bleeding tendency.
- Take periodic blood counts during first year of therapy.
- Check CK level if myopathy occurs.

Patient teaching
- Tell patient to take drug 30 minutes before breakfast and dinner.
- ◄€ Advise patient to immediately report signs or symptoms of anaphylaxis or other allergic reactions.
- Instruct patient to report unusual bleeding or bruising.
- Tell patient to avoid driving and other hazardous activities until he knows how the drug affects concentration and alertness.
- Stress importance of diet and exercise in lowering lipid levels.
- Advise patient to minimize GI upset by eating frequent, small servings of healthy food.

• Inform patient that he'll undergo regular blood testing during therapy.
• As appropriate, review all other significant and life-threatening adverse reactions and interactions, especially those related to the drugs and tests mentioned above.

gemifloxacin mesylate
Factive

Pharmacologic class: Quinolone antibiotic
Therapeutic class: Broad-spectrum anti-infective
Pregnancy risk category C

Action
Inhibits DNA synthesis by inhibiting DNA gyrase and topoisomerase IV (enzymes needed for bacterial growth)

Availability
Tablets: 320 mg

Indications and dosages
➤ Acute exacerbation of chronic bronchitis caused by *Streptococcus pneumoniae, Haemophilus influenzae, H. parainfluenzae,* or *Moraxella catarrhalis*
Adults: 320 mg P.O. daily for 5 days
➤ Mild to moderate community-acquired pneumonia caused by *S. pneumoniae, H. influenzae, M. catarrhalis, Mycoplasma pneumoniae, Chlamydia pneumoniae,* or *Klebsiella pneumoniae*
Adults: 320 mg P.O. daily for 7 days
Dosage adjustment
• Renal impairment

Contraindications
• Hypersensitivity to drug
• History of prolonged Qtc interval

Administration
• Advise patient to swallow tablet whole without chewing.
• Give at same time every day with plenty of fluids, with or without food.
• Don't give iron, multivitamins, didanosine, sucralfate, or antacids containing magnesium or aluminum within 3 hours of drug.

Route	Onset	Peak	Duration
P.O.	Unknown	0.5-2 hr	Unknown

Adverse reactions
CNS: fatigue, headache, insomnia, drowsiness, nervousness, dizziness, tremor, vertigo, **seizures, loss of consciousness**
CV: hypotension, prolonged QTc interval, **cardiovascular collapse, shock**
EENT: vision abnormality, pharyngitis
GI: nausea, vomiting, diarrhea, constipation, abdominal pain, dyspepsia, gastritis, gastroenteritis, flatulence, anorexia, altered taste, dry mouth, **pseudomembranous colitis**
GU: genital candidiasis, vaginitis, **acute renal insufficiency or failure, interstitial nephritis**
Hematologic: eosinophilia, anemia, **leukopenia, granulocytopenia, thrombocytopenia**
Hepatic: jaundice, bilirubinemia, **hepatitis, acute hepatic necrosis, hepatic failure**
Metabolic: hyperglycemia
Musculoskeletal: joint, back, or muscle pain; leg cramps; tendinitis; rupture of shoulder, hand, or Achilles tendon
Respiratory: dyspnea, pneumonia
Skin: rash, urticaria, photosensitivity, pruritus, eczema, flushing, angioedema
Other: hot flashes, fungal infection, hypersensitivity reactions

Interactions
Drug-drug. *Antacids containing aluminum or magnesium, didanosine, iron, multivitamins, sucralfate:* reduced gemifloxacin absorption

Antiarrhythmics (class IA, such as quinidine and procainamide, and class III, such as amiodarone and sotalol), antipsychotics, erythromycin, tricyclic antidepressants: increased risk of prolonged QTc interval

Sucralfate: decreased gemifloxacin bioavailability

Drug-diagnostic tests. *Alanine aminotransferase, aspartate aminotransferase:* increased levels

Sun exposure: increased risk of photosensitivity

Precautions

Use cautiously in:
• epilepsy or history of seizures
• pregnant or breastfeeding patients
• children younger than age 18 (safety not established).

Patient monitoring

• Stay alert for signs and symptoms of hypersensitivity reaction.
• Monitor ECG in patients at risk for prolonged QTc interval.
• Watch for signs and symptoms of tendon rupture.

Patient teaching

• Instruct patient to take drug at same time each day, with or without food.
• Teach patient to recognize and report signs and symptoms of allergic response.
• Advise patient to take iron, vitamins, antacids, didanosine, or sucralfate 3 hours before or 2 hours after drug.
• Instruct patient to stop taking drug and contact prescriber immediately if signs or symptoms of hypersensitivity reaction occur.
• Tell patient that drug may cause tendon rupture; encourage him to immediately report sudden severe pain in shoulder, hand, or Achilles tendon.
• Advise patient to avoid driving and other hazardous activities until he knows how drug affects concentration and alertness.

• Teach patient to minimize GI upset by eating frequent, small servings of healthy food and drinking adequate fluids.
• As appropriate, review all other significant and life-threatening adverse reactions and interactions, especially those related to the drugs and tests mentioned above.

gemtuzumab ozogamicin
Mylotarg

Pharmacologic class: Monoclonal antibody
Therapeutic class: Antineoplastic
Pregnancy risk category D

Action

Binds to CD33 antigen on surface of leukemic blasts, leading to formation of complex that's internalized by cell. Derivative is released inside myeloid cell lysosomes and binds to DNA, causing DNA double-strand breakage and cell death.

Availability

Powder for injection: 5 mg

Indications and dosages

➤ CD33-positive acute myeloid leukemia (confirmed by bone marrow aspirate); patients who are in first relapse and don't qualify for other cytotoxic chemotherapy

Adults ages 60 and older: 9 mg/m^2 I.V. infusion over 2 hours q 14 days for up to two doses. Give with diphenhydramine and acetaminophen 1 hour before infusion, as prescribed.

Contraindications

• Hypersensitivity to drug

Administration

◀𝄞 Premedicate as prescribed to prevent postinfusion symptom complex (fever, chills, and possibly hypotension and dyspnea), which may occur 24 hours after administration.

• Prepare drug under biological safety hood with fluorescent light off.

• Reconstitute with 5 ml of sterile water for injection. Gently swirl vial to mix.

• Withdraw prescribed dose and inject into 100-ml I.V. bag of normal saline solution. Place bag into ultraviolet protectant bag.

• Administer immediately through separate peripheral or central line over 2 hours, using 1.2-micron terminal filter in infusion line.

◀𝄞 Don't give by I.V. push or bolus.

• Monitor vital signs during infusion.

Route	Onset	Peak	Duration
I.V.	Unknown	Unknown	Unknown

Adverse reactions

CNS: depression, dizziness, headache, insomnia, pain, weakness

CV: hypertension, hypotension, tachycardia, peripheral edema

EENT: epistaxis, rhinitis, pharyngitis

GI: nausea, vomiting, diarrhea, constipation, dyspepsia, abdominal pain, enlarged abdomen, anorexia, stomatitis

GU: hematuria, **vaginal hemorrhage**

Hematologic: anemia, **hemorrhage,** leukopenia, **neutropenia, neutropenic fever, thrombocytopenia**

Hepatic: elevated hepatic enzyme and bilirubin levels, **hepatotoxicity**

Metabolic: hyperglycemia, hypokalemia, hypomagnesemia

Musculoskeletal: joint or back pain

Respiratory: cough, dyspnea, hypoxia, pneumonia

Skin: ecchymosis, petechiae, rash

Other: chills, fever, herpes simplex, injection site reaction, tumor lysis syndrome, **sepsis**

Interactions

Drug-diagnostic tests. *Alanine aminotransferase, aspartate aminotransferase, bilirubin, glucose:* increased levels
Hematocrit, hemoglobin, magnesium, platelets, potassium, white blood cells: decreased values

Precautions

Use cautiously in:

• renal or hepatic impairment, bone marrow depression

• patients receiving aspirin or anticoagulants concurrently

• pregnant or breastfeeding patients

• children (safety and efficacy not established).

Patient monitoring

• Monitor vital signs every 4 hours after infusion.

◀𝄞 Observe for postinfusion syndrome for up to 24 hours after drug is infused.

• Assess complete blood cell and platelet counts daily for 14 days or until neutrophil and platelets recover.

• Monitor electrolyte levels and liver function test results.

• Check for bleeding tendency.

Patient teaching

• Instruct patient to report unusual bleeding or bruising and signs and symptoms of infection.

• Teach patient to avoid driving and other hazardous activities until he knows how drug affects concentration and alertness.

• Advise patient to minimize GI upset by eating frequent, small servings of healthy food.

• Inform patient that he'll undergo regular blood testing during therapy.

• As appropriate, review all other significant and life-threatening adverse reactions and interactions, especially those related to the tests mentioned above.

gentamicin sulfate
Cidomycin✤, Garamycin, Genoptic, Gentacidin, Gentak, G-Mycin, Jenamicin

Pharmacologic class: Aminoglycoside
Therapeutic class: Anti-infective
Pregnancy risk category D (parenteral), *C* (topical)

Action
Destroys gram-negative bacteria by irreversibly binding to 30S subunit of bacterial ribosomes and blocking protein synthesis, resulting in misreading of genetic code that causes ribosomes to separate from messenger RNA

Availability
Cream: 0.1%
Injection: 40 mg/ml (adult), 10 mg/ml (pediatric)
I.V. infusion (premixed): 40 mg, 60 mg, 70 mg, 80 mg, 90 mg, 100 mg, 120 mg (in normal saline solution)
Ointment: 0.1%
Ointment (ophthalmic): 0.3% (base)
Solution (ophthalmic): 0.3% (base)

⁄ Indications and dosages
➤ Serious infection caused by *Pseudomonas aeruginosa*, *Escherichia coli*, and *Proteus, Klebsiella, Serratia, Enterobacter, Citrobacter,* and *Staphylococcus* species
Adults: 3 mg/kg daily in three divided doses I.M. or I.V. infusion q 8 hours. For serious infections, up to 5 mg/kg/day in three to four divided doses; reduce dosage to 3 mg/kg/day as indicated.
Children: 2 to 2.5 mg/kg q 8 hours I.M. or I.V. infusion
Infants older than age 1 week: 2.5 mg/kg q 8 hours I.M. or I.V. infusion

Neonates younger than 1 week, pre-term infants: 2.5 mg/kg q 12 hours I.M. or I.V. infusion
➤ Prevention of endocarditis before surgery
Adults: 1.5 mg/kg I.M. or I.V. 30 minutes before surgery, to a maximum dosage of 80 mg; given with ampicillin or vancomycin, as ordered
Children: 2 mg/kg I.M. or I.V. 30 minutes before surgery, to a maximum dosage of 80 mg
➤ External ocular infections caused by susceptible organisms, especially *P. aeruginosa, Proteus* species, *Klebsiella pneumoniae, E. coli,* and other gram-negative bacteria
Adults and children: One to two drops in eye q 4 hours. For serious infections, up to 2 drops q hour, or apply ophthalmic ointment to lower conjunctival sac b.i.d. or t.i.d.
➤ Treatment and prevention of superficial burns caused by susceptible bacteria
Adults and children older than age 1: Gently rub small amount of drug on affected area three or four times daily .
Dosage adjustment
• Renal impairment
• Cystic fibrosis

Off-label uses
• Pelvic inflammatory disease

Contraindications
• Hypersensitivity to drug or other aminoglycosides

Administration
• Before starting drug, obtain specimens as needed for culture and sensitivity testing.
• For I.V. infusion, dilute with 50 to 200 ml of dextrose 5% in water (D_5W) or normal saline solution, and give over 30 minutes to 2 hours.
• After infusion, flush line with normal saline solution or D_5W.

• For intrathecal use, use only preservative-free form of drug.
• Obtain peak blood drug level 30 minutes after 30-minute infusion; obtain trough level within 30 minutes of next scheduled dose.
• Give cephalosporins or parenteral penicillin 1 hour before or after gentamicin, as prescribed.
• For topical treatment of burns, gauze dressings may or may not be applied.

Route	Onset	Peak	Duration
I.V.	Immediate	30-90 min	Unknown
I.M.	Unknown	30-90 min	Unknown
Topical, ophthalmic	Unknown	Unknown	Unknown

Adverse reactions

CNS: dizziness, vertigo, muscle twitching, tremors, numbness, depression, confusion, lethargy, headache, paresthesia, **neuromuscular blockade, seizures, neurotoxicity**
CV: hypotension, hypertension, palpitations
EENT: visual disturbances, dry eyes, nystagmus, photophobia, ototoxicity, deafness, tinnitus
GI: nausea, vomiting, stomatitis, increased salivation, splenomegaly, anorexia
GU: azotemia, increased urinary casts, polyuria, dysuria, impotence, **nephrotoxicity**
Hematologic: eosinophilia, leukemoid reaction, increased or decreased reticulocyte count, hemolytic anemia, **aplastic anemia, neutropenia, agranulocytosis, leukopenia, thrombocytopenia, pancytopenia**
Hepatic: elevated alanine aminotransferase (ALT), aspartate aminotransferase (AST), and bilirubin levels; hepatomegaly; **hepatotoxicity; hepatic necrosis**
Musculoskeletal: joint pain
Respiratory: apnea

Skin: exfoliative dermatitis, rash, pruritus, urticaria, purpura, alopecia
Other: weight loss, superinfection, pain and irritation at I.M. site

Interactions

Drug-drug. *Acyclovir, amphotericin B, carboplatin, cephalosporins, cisplatin, loop diuretics, vancomycin, other ototoxic or nephrotoxic drugs:* increased risk of ototoxicity and nephrotoxicity
Dimenhydrinate, other antiemetics: masking of ototoxicity symptoms
General anesthetics, neuromuscular blockers: increased activity of these drugs
Indomethacin: increased gentamicin peak and trough levels
Penicillins (such as ampicillin, ticarcillin): synergistic effect
Tacrolimus: nephrotoxicity
Drug-diagnostic tests. *ALT, AST, bilirubin, blood urea nitrogen (BUN), creatinine, lactate dehydrogenase:* increased levels
Granulocytes, hemoglobin, platelets, white blood cells: decreased values

Precautions

Use cautiously in:
• renal impairment, neuromuscular diseases, hearing impairment
• sulfite sensitivity (with parenteral use)
• obese patients
• elderly patients
• pregnant or breastfeeding patients
• infants, neonates, premature infants.

Patient monitoring

• Watch for signs and symptoms of hypersensitivity reactions.
◀ᚖ Be aware that monitoring of drug blood level is especially important when therapy lasts more than 5 days, in acute or chronic renal impairment, in infants younger than 3 months, in concomitant use of nephrotoxic drugs, in patients requiring higher doses or interval adjustments (such as those with

cystic fibrosis, endocarditis, or critical illness), in those with signs of nephrotoxicity or ototoxicity, in obese patients, and in patients with extracellular fluid volume changes.
• Assess fluid intake and output, urine specific gravity, and urinalysis for signs of nephrotoxicity.
• Monitor complete blood count, BUN, creatinine level, and creatinine clearance.
• Weigh patient regularly.
• Assess for signs and symptoms of ototoxicity (hearing loss, tinnitus, ataxia, and vertigo).

Patient teaching
• Teach patient to recognize and immediately report signs and symptoms of hypersensitivity reactions.
• Advise patient to report signs and symptoms of ototoxicity (hearing loss, ringing in ears, vertigo).
• Instruct patient to drink plenty of fluids to ensure adequate urine output.
• Teach patient to monitor urine output and report significant changes.
• Instruct patient to avoid driving and other hazardous activities until he knows how drug affects concentration and alertness.
• As appropriate, review all other significant and life-threatening adverse reactions and interactions, especially those related to the drugs and tests mentioned above.

glatiramer acetate
Copaxone

Pharmacologic class: Immunomodulator

Therapeutic class: Multiple sclerosis agent

Pregnancy risk category B

Action
Unknown; thought to alter the immune processes responsible for pathogenesis of multiple sclerosis

Availability
Injection: 20 mg lyophilized glatiramer acetate and 40 mg mannitol in single-use 2-ml vial; 1-ml vial of sterile water for injection included for reconstitution

⃰ Indications and dosages
➤ To reduce frequency of relapse in patients with relapsing-remitting multiple sclerosis
Adults: 20 mg/day S.C.

Contraindications
• Hypersensitivity to drug

Administration
• Give only by S.C. injection into arms, abdomen, hips, or thighs.
• Use immediately after preparation; discard unused portion.

Route	Onset	Peak	Duration
S.C.	Slow	Unknown	Unknown

Adverse reactions
CNS: abnormal dreams, agitation, anxiety, confusion, emotional lability, migraine, nervousness, speech disorder, stupor, tremor, weakness, vertigo
CV: chest pain, hypertension, palpitations, tachycardia, peripheral edema
EENT: eye disorder, nystagmus, ear pain, rhinitis, dental caries
GI: nausea, vomiting, diarrhea, anorexia, gastroenteritis, GI disorder, oral candidiasis, salivary gland enlargement, ulcerative stomatitis
GU: amenorrhea, dysmenorrhea, hematuria, impotence, menorrhagia, abnormal Papanicolaou smear, urinary urgency, vaginal candidiasis, **vaginal hemorrhage**
Hematologic: ecchymosis, lymphadenopathy

♣ Canada ◀≣ Clinical alert Reactions in **bold** are life-threatening

Musculoskeletal: joint, back, or neck pain; foot drop; hypertonia
Respiratory: bronchitis, dyspnea, hyperventilation
Skin: eczema, facial edema, erythema, diaphoresis, pruritus, rash, skin atrophy, skin nodules, urticaria, warts
Other: weight gain, herpes simplex, herpes zoster, chills, cysts, flulike symptoms, pain at injection site

Interactions
None reported

Precautions
Use cautiously in:
• pregnant or breastfeeding patients
• children (safety and efficacy not established).

Patient monitoring
◀€ Assess for immediate postinjection reaction, including flushing, chest pain, anxiety, breathing problems, and hives.
• Monitor patient for transient chest pain, but be aware that this problem doesn't seem to be clinically significant.
• Check for vaginal bleeding.
• Watch for signs and symptoms of infection.

Patient teaching
• Teach patient how to prepare and self-administer drug; supervise him the first time he does so.
• Teach patient to recognize and immediately report signs and symptoms of postinjection reaction. Tell him this reaction may occur right away or several months after first dose.
• Instruct patient to avoid driving and other hazardous activities until he knows how drug affects concentration and alertness.
• Instruct patient to notify prescriber of signs or symptoms of infection.
• Provide dietary counseling; refer patient to dietitian if adverse GI effects significantly affect food intake.

• As appropriate, review all other significant and life-threatening adverse reactions.

glimepiride
Amaryl

Pharmacologic class: Sulfonylurea
Therapeutic class: Hypoglycemic
Pregnancy risk category C

Action
Lowers blood glucose level by stimulating insulin release from pancreas, increasing insulin sensitivity at receptor sites, and decreasing hepatic glucose production; also increases peripheral tissue sensitivity to insulin and causes mild diuresis

Availability
Tablets: 1 mg, 2 mg, 4 mg

🕖 Indications and dosages
➤ Adjunct to diet and exercise to lower blood glucose level in patients with type 2 diabetes mellitus when diet and exercise alone prove ineffective
Adults: Initially, 1 to 2 mg P.O. once daily given with first main meal; usual maintenance dosage is 1 to 4 mg P.O. once daily. When patient reaches 2 mg/day, raise dosage no more than 2 mg q 1 to 2 weeks, depending on glycemic control. Maximum dosage is 8 mg/day.
➤ Adjunct to insulin therapy in patients with type 2 diabetes mellitus when diet, exercise, or glimepiride alone prove ineffective
Adults: 8 mg P.O. once daily with low-dose insulin, given with first main meal. Based on glycemic control, raise insulin dosage weekly as indicated.
➤ Adjunct to metformin therapy in patients with type 2 diabetes mellitus when diet, exercise, and glimepiride or metformin alone prove ineffective

Adults: 1 to 4 mg/day P.O. given with first main meal, increased gradually to a maximum of 8 mg/day P.O.; give with metformin if patient's response to glimepiride monotherapy isn't adequate; adjust dosages based on glycemic response to determine minimum effective dosage.

Dosage adjustment
• Renal or hepatic impairment
• Adrenal or pituitary insufficiency

Contraindications
• Hypersensitivity to drug or sulfonamides
• Diabetic coma or ketoacidosis
• Severe renal, hepatic, or endocrine disease
• Pregnancy or breastfeeding

Administration
• Check baseline creatinine level for normal renal function before giving first dose.
• Give with first meal of day.

Route	Onset	Peak	Duration
P.O.	1 hr	2-3 hr	>24 hr

Adverse reactions
CNS: dizziness, drowsiness, headache, weakness
CV: increased CV mortality risk
EENT: blurred vision
GI: nausea, vomiting, diarrhea, constipation, cramps, heartburn, epigastric distress, anorexia, increased appetite
Hematologic: aplastic anemia, leukopenia, pancytopenia, thrombocytopenia, agranulocytosis
Hepatic: cholestatic jaundice, elevated liver function test results, **hepatitis**
Metabolic: hypoglycemia, hyponatremia, elevated cholesterol level
Skin: angioedema, photosensitivity, rash, erythema, urticaria, eczema, maculopapular eruptions

Interactions
Drug-drug. *Androgens (such as testosterone), chloramphenicol, clofibrate, guanethidine, monoamine oxidase inhibitors, nonsteroidal anti-inflammatory drugs (except diclofenac), salicylates, sulfonamides, tricyclic antidepressants:* increased risk of hypoglycemia
Beta blockers: altered response to glimepiride, necessitating dosage change; prolonged hypoglycemia (with nonselective agents)
Calcium channel blockers, corticosteroids, estrogens, hydantoins, hormonal contraceptives, isoniazid, nicotinic acid, phenothiazines, phenytoin, rifampin, sympathomimetics, thiazide diuretics, thyroid preparations: decreased hypoglycemic effect of glimepiride
Warfarin: initially increased, then decreased, effects of both drugs
Drug-diagnostic tests. *Alanine aminotransferase, alkaline phosphatase, aspartate aminotransferase, bilirubin, blood urea nitrogen, cholesterol:* increased levels
Glucose, granulocytes, hemoglobin, platelets, white blood cells: decreased levels
Drug-herb. *Agoral marshmallow, aloe (oral), bitter melon, burdock, chromium, coenzyme Q10, dandelion, eucalyptus, fenugreek:* additive hypoglycemic effects
Glucosamine: impaired glycemic control
Drug-behaviors. *Alcohol use:* disulfiram-like reaction
Sun exposure: increased risk of photosensitivity

Precautions
Use cautiously in:
• hepatic or renal disease; cardiovascular disease; impaired thyroid, pituitary, or adrenal function
• elderly patients.

Patient monitoring
- Monitor complete blood count with white cell differential, electrolyte levels, and blood chemistry results.
- Monitor blood glucose level regularly; assess HbA1c level every 3 to 6 months.
- Evaluate kidney and liver function test results frequently, especially in patients with impairments.
- Assess neurologic status; report cognitive or sensory impairment.

Patient teaching
- Instruct patient to self-monitor his blood glucose level as prescribed.
- Teach patient signs and symptoms of hypoglycemia and hyperglycemia.
- Stress importance of diet and exercise to help control diabetes.
- Instruct patient to wear or carry medical identification describing his condition.
- Advise patient to keep sugar source readily available at all times in case of hypoglycemia.
- Instruct patient to avoid driving and other hazardous activities until he knows how drug affects concentration and alertness.
- Tell patient that he'll undergo regular blood testing during therapy.
- As appropriate, review all other significant and life-threatening adverse reactions and interactions, especially those related to the drugs, tests, herbs, and behaviors mentioned above.

glipizide
Glucotrol, Glucotrol XL

Pharmacologic class: Sulfonylurea
Therapeutic class: Hypoglycemic
Pregnancy risk category C

Action
Lowers blood glucose level by stimulating insulin release from pancreas, increasing insulin sensitivity at receptor sites, and decreasing hepatic glucose production; also increases peripheral tissue sensitivity to insulin and causes mild diuresis

Availability
Tablets: 5 mg, 10 mg
Tablets (extended-release): 5 mg, 10 mg

🖊 Indications and dosages
➤ Control of blood glucose level in patients with type 2 diabetes mellitus who have some pancreatic function and don't respond to diet therapy
Adults: 5 mg/day P.O. initially, increased as needed after several days (range is 2.5 to 40 mg/day). Give extended-release tablet once daily; give daily dosages over 15 mg in two divided doses.
➤ Conversion from insulin therapy
Adults: With insulin dosages exceeding 20 units/day, start patient with usual glipizide dosage and reduce insulin dosage by 50%; with insulin dosages of 20 units/day or less, insulin may be discontinued when glipizide is started.
Dosage adjustment
- Hepatic or renal impairment
- Elderly patients

Contraindications
- Hypersensitivity to drug
- Severe renal, hepatic, thyroid, or other endocrine disease
- Uncontrolled infection, serious burns, or trauma
- Patients taking sulfonamides
- Pregnancy or breastfeeding

Administration
- Check baseline creatinine level for normal renal function before giving first dose.

g

- Give daily dose at breakfast (if patient takes two daily doses, give second dose at dinner).
- Give drug 30 minutes before a meal—preferably breakfast.

Route	Onset	Peak	Duration
P.O.	15-30 min	1-2 hr	Up to 24 hr

Adverse reactions

CNS: dizziness, drowsiness, headache, weakness
CV: increased CV mortality risk
EENT: blurred vision
GI: nausea, vomiting, diarrhea, constipation, cramps, heartburn, epigastric distress, anorexia, increased appetite
Hematologic: aplastic anemia, agranulocytosis, leukopenia, pancytopenia, thrombocytopenia
Hepatic: cholestatic jaundice, elevated liver function test results, **hepatitis**
Metabolic: hypoglycemia, hyponatremia, elevated cholesterol level
Skin: angioedema, photosensitivity, rash, pruritus, erythema, urticaria, eczema

Interactions

Drug-drug. *Androgens (such as testosterone), chloramphenicol, clofibrate, guanethidine, monoamine oxidase inhibitors, nonsteroidal anti-inflammatory drugs (except diclofenac), salicylates, sulfonamides, tricyclic antidepressants:* increased risk of hypoglycemia
Beta blockers: altered response to glipizide, requiring dosage change; prolonged hypoglycemia (with nonselective agents)
Calcium channel blockers, corticosteroids, estrogens, hydantoins, hormonal contraceptives, isoniazid, nicotinic acid, phenothiazines, phenytoin, rifampin, sympathomimetics, thiazide diuretics, thyroid preparations: decreased hypoglycemic effect
Warfarin: initially increased, then decreased, effects of both drugs

Drug-diagnostic tests. *Alanine aminotransferase, alkaline phosphatase, aspartate aminotransferase, bilirubin, blood urea nitrogen, cholesterol:* increased levels
Glucose, granulocytes, hemoglobin, platelets, white blood cells: decreased levels
Drug-herb. *Aloe (oral), bitter melon, burdock, chromium, coenzyme Q10, dandelion, eucalyptus, fenugreek:* additive hypoglycemic effects
Glucosamine: impaired glycemic control
Drug-behaviors. *Alcohol use:* disulfiram-like reaction

Precautions

Use cautiously in:
- hepatic, renal, or cardiovascular disease; impaired thyroid, pituitary, or adrenal function
- elderly patients.

Patient monitoring

- Monitor blood glucose level, especially during periods of increased stress.
- Evaluate complete blood count and renal function test results.
- Check for signs and symptoms of lactic acidosis (malaise, muscle pain, respiratory distress, drowsiness, and abdominal distress).
- If patient is ill or has abnormal laboratory values, monitor electrolyte, ketone, glucose, pH, lactate dehydrogenase, pyruvate, and metformin levels.
- Monitor cardiovascular status.

Patient teaching

- Advise patient to take daily dose with breakfast (and second dose, if prescribed, with dinner).
- Teach patient to immediately report signs and symptoms of lactic acidosis and to stop drug (unless prescriber directs otherwise).
- Advise patient to monitor blood glucose level as instructed by prescriber.

• Tell patient he may need supplemental insulin during times of stress or when he can't maintain adequate oral intake.

• Instruct patient to avoid driving and other hazardous activities until he knows how drug affects concentration and alertness.

• Teach patient to minimize GI upset by eating frequent, small servings of healthy food.

• Tell patient that he'll undergo regular blood testing during therapy.

• As appropriate, review all other significant and life-threatening adverse reactions and interactions, especially those related to the drugs, tests, herbs, and behaviors mentioned above.

glucagon
GlucaGen Diagnostic Kit

Pharmacologic class: Antihypoglycemic

Therapeutic class: Insulin antagonist
Pregnancy risk category B

Action
Increases blood glucose concentrations by converting glycogen in the liver to glucose; also relaxes GI smooth muscle

Availability
Powder for injection: 1-mg vial

Indications and dosages
➤ Hypoglycemia

Adults and children weighing more than 20 kg (44 lb): 1 mg S.C., I.M., or I.V. Give I.V. glucose if patient fails to respond.

Children weighing 20 kg (44 lb) or less: 20 to 30 mcg/kg or 0.5-mg dose S.C., I.M., or I.V. Give I.V. glucose if patient fails to respond.

➤ Diagnostic aid for radiologic examination

Adults: 0.25 to 2 mg I.V. or I.M. before radiologic procedure

Contraindications
• Hypersensitivity to drug
• Insulinoma
• Pheochromocytoma

Administration
◀ Use only in hypoglycemic emergencies for patients with diabetes mellitus.

◀ Patient should respond within 15 minutes. Because of potential serious adverse reactions associated with prolonged cerebral hypoglycemia, give I.V. glucose if patient fails to respond to glucagon.

• Mix drug in 1-unit vial with 1 ml of diluent supplied by manufacturer.
• Dilute doses over 2 mg with sterile water for injection.
• Use drug immediately; discard unused portion.
• Give patient carbohydrate-rich foods as soon as he's alert.

Route	Onset	Peak	Duration
I.V.	Immediate	30 min	60-90 min
I.M., S.C.	4-10 min	Unknown	12-32 min

Adverse reactions
CV: hypotension
GI: nausea, vomiting
Metabolic: hypokalemia (with overdose)
Respiratory: bronchospasm, respiratory distress
Skin: urticaria, rash

Interactions
Drug-drug. *Anticoagulants:* enhanced anticoagulant effects
Drug-diagnostic tests. *Potassium:* decreased levels

Precautions
Use cautiously in:
• cardiac disease, adrenal insufficiency, chronic hypoglycemia
• history suggesting insulinoma or pheochromocytoma
• elderly patients
• pregnant or breastfeeding patients.

Patient monitoring
• Monitor blood glucose level.
• Assess blood pressure, electrolyte levels, and respiratory status.

Patient teaching
• Teach patient and significant others the proper time and technique for using this emergency drug.
◀ Emphasize importance of contacting prescriber right away if hypoglycemic emergency occurs.
◀ Teach caregiver or significant other to arouse patient immediately and give additional carbohydrate by mouth as soon as patient can tolerate it.
• As appropriate, review all other significant and life-threatening adverse reactions and interactions, especially those related to the drugs and tests mentioned above.

glyburide
Albert Glyburide✤, Apo-Glyburide✤, DiaBeta, Euglucon✤, Gen-Glybe✤, Glynase PresTab, Micronase, Novo-Glyburide✤, Nu-Glyburide✤

Pharmacologic class: Sulfonylurea
Therapeutic class: Hypoglycemic
Pregnancy risk category B

Action
Increases insulin binding and sensitivity at receptor sites, stimulating its release from beta cells in the pancreas, and reducing blood glucose concentration levels; also decreases the production of basal glucose in the liver, enhances sensitivity and action of peripheral tissue to insulin, inhibits platelet aggregation, and causes mild diuresis

Availability
Tablets: 1.25 mg, 2.5 mg, 5 mg
Tablets (micronized): 1.5 mg, 3 mg, 6 mg

⊘ Indications and dosages
➤ Control of blood glucose level in patients with type 2 diabetes mellitus who have some pancreatic function and don't respond to diet therapy
Adults: Initially, 2.5 to 5 mg regular tablets P.O. once daily (range is 1.25 to 20 mg/day). Or initially, 1.5 to 3 mg micronized tablets P.O. once daily (range is 0.75 to 12 mg/day); divide daily dosages above 6 mg.
Dosage adjustment
• Elderly patients
➤ Conversion from insulin therapy
Adults: With insulin dosage below 20 units/day, give 2.5 to 5 mg glyburide daily; with insulin dosages of 20 to 40 units/day, give 5 mg glyburide; with insulin dosage above 40 units/day, give 5 mg glyburide daily or 3 mg (micronized formulation) P.O. once daily and reduce insulin dosage by 50%
Dosage adjustment
• Hepatic or renal failure

Contraindications
• Hypersensitivity to drug or sulfonamides
• Type 1 (insulin-dependent) diabetes
• Severe renal, hepatic, thyroid, or other endocrine disease
• Patients taking sulfonamides (including thiazide diuretics)
• Pregnancy or breastfeeding

Administration

🔈 Be aware that micronized glyburide is not bioequivalent to regular glyburide.

• Check baseline creatinine level for normal renal function before giving first dose.

• Give daily dose at breakfast (for patient receiving drug b.i.d., give second dose at dinner).

• Adjust dosage slowly if patient is using metformin.

Route	Onset	Peak	Duration
P.O.	45-60 min	1.5-3 hr	24 hr

Adverse reactions

CNS: dizziness, drowsiness, headache, weakness

CV: increased CV mortality risk

EENT: changes in visual accommodation, blurred vision

GI: nausea, vomiting, diarrhea, constipation, cramps, heartburn, epigastric distress, anorexia

Hematologic: aplastic anemia, leukopenia, thrombocytopenia, agranulocytosis, pancytopenia

Hepatic: cholestatic jaundice, elevated liver function test results, **hepatitis**

Metabolic: hyponatremia, **hypoglycemia**

Skin: photosensitivity, rash, pruritus, urticaria, angioedema, eczema, erythema

Other: increased appetite

Interactions

Drug-drug. *Androgens (such as testosterone), chloramphenicol, clofibrate, guanethidine, monoamine oxidase inhibitors, nonsteroidal anti-inflammatory drugs (except diclofenac), salicylates, sulfonamides, tricyclic antidepressants:* increased risk of hypoglycemia

Beta blockers: altered response to glyburide, requiring increased or decreased dosage; prolonged hypoglycemia (with nonselective agents)

Calcium channel blockers, corticosteroids, estrogens, hydantoins, hormonal contraceptives, isoniazid, nicotinic acid, phenothiazines, phenytoin, rifampin, sympathomimetics, thiazide diuretics, thyroid preparations: decreased hypoglycemic effect of glyburide

Warfarin: initially increased, then decreased, effects of both drugs

Drug-diagnostic tests. *Alanine aminotransferase, alkaline phosphatase, aspartate aminotransferase, bilirubin, blood urea nitrogen, cholesterol:* increased levels

Glucose, granulocytes, hemoglobin, platelets, white blood cells: decreased values

Drug-herb. *Agoral marshmallow, aloe (oral), bitter melon, burdock, chromium, coenzyme Q10, dandelion, eucalyptus, fenugreek:* increased hypoglycemic effects

Glucosamine: impaired glycemic control

Drug-behaviors. *Alcohol use:* disulfiram-like reaction

Precautions

Use cautiously in:

• hepatic, renal, or cardiovascular disease; impaired thyroid, pituitary, or adrenal function

• infection, stress, or changes in diet

• elderly patients.

Patient monitoring

• Monitor blood glucose level, especially during periods of increased stress.

• Monitor complete blood count and renal function test results.

• Assess for signs and symptoms of lactic acidosis (malaise, muscle pains, respiratory distress, drowsiness, abdominal distress).

• If patient is ill or has abnormal laboratory findings, monitor electrolyte, ketone, glucose, pH, lactate dehydrogenase, and pyruvate levels.

• Evaluate cardiovascular status.

Patient teaching
• Advise patient to take daily dose with breakfast (and second dose, if prescribed, with dinner).
• Instruct patient in glucose self-monitoring as prescribed; teach him to report significant changes in glucose level.
• Inform patient that he may need supplemental insulin during times of stress or when he can't maintain adequate oral intake.
• Teach patient signs and symptoms of hypoglycemia and hyperglycemia.
• Instruct patient to keep sugar source available at all times.
• Encourage patient to drink plenty of fluids daily.
• Stress importance of diet and exercise in helping to control diabetes.
• Advise patient to wear or carry medical identification about his condition.
• Instruct patient to avoid driving and other hazardous activities until he knows how drug affects concentration and alertness.
• Tell patient that he'll undergo regular blood testing during therapy.
• As appropriate, review all other significant and life-threatening adverse reactions and interactions, especially those related to the drugs, tests, herbs, and behaviors mentioned above.

glycopyrrolate
Robinul, Robinul Forte

Pharmacologic class: Anticholinergic
Therapeutic class: Antispasmodic, antimuscarinic, parasympatholytic
Pregnancy risk category B

Action
Inhibits action of acetylcholine on muscarinic receptors that mediate effects of parasympathetic postganglionic impulses. This actions causes relaxation of cardiac smooth muscle, inhibition of vagal reflexes, and a decrease in tracheal and bronchial secretions.

Availability
Injection: 0.2 mg/ml
Tablets: 1 mg, 2 mg

⚕ Indications and dosages
➤ Adjunct therapy in peptic ulcer disorders
Adults: 1 mg P.O. t.i.d. or 2 mg (Forte) two to three times daily to a maximum dosage of 8 mg/day P.O.; or 0.1 to 0.2 mg I.M. or I.V. three or four times daily
➤ To diminish secretions and block cardiac vagal reflexes before surgery
Adults and children ages 2 and older: 0.0044 mg/kg I.M. 30 to 60 minutes before surgery
Children ages 1 month to 2 years: 0.0088 mg/kg I.M. 30 to 60 minutes before surgery
➤ To diminish or block cholinergic effects caused by anticholinesterase
Adults and children: 0.2 mg I.V. for each 1 mg of neostigmine or 5 mg of pyridostigmine; may give I.V. undiluted or with dextrose injection by infusion
➤ Bradycardia
Adults: 0.1 mg I.V., repeated q 2 to 3 minutes p.r.n.

Off-label uses
• Sweating

Contraindications
• Hypersensitivity to drug
• Arrhythmias
• COPD
• GI disease, infection, atony or ileus
• Myasthenia gravis
• Glaucoma
• Obstructive uropathy
• Severe prostatic hypertrophy

Administration

- Give oral dose 30 to 60 minutes before meals.
- Have resuscitation equipment on hand to treat curare-like effects of overdose.

Route	Onset	Peak	Duration
P.O.	Unknown	Unknown	8-12 hr
I.V.	1 min	Unknown	3-7 hr
I.M., S.C.	15-30 min	30-45 min	3-7 hr

Adverse reactions

CNS: weakness, nervousness, insomnia, drowsiness, dizziness, headache, confusion, excitement
CV: palpitations, tachycardia
EENT: blurred vision, photophobia, mydriasis, increased intraocular pressure, cycloplegia
GI: nausea, vomiting, constipation, abdominal distention, epigastric distress, heartburn, gastroesophageal reflux, dry mouth, loss of taste, **paralytic ileus**
GU: urinary hesitancy or retention, lactation suppression, impotence
Skin: urticaria, decreased sweating or anhidrosis
Other: allergic reaction, fever, irritation at I.M. site, **anaphylaxis, malignant hyperthermia**

Interactions

Drug-drug. *Amantadine, antihistamines, antiparkinsonian drugs, disopyramide, glutethimide, meperidine, phenothiazines, procainamide, quinidine, tricyclic antidepressants:* additive anticholinergic effects

Precautions

Use cautiously in:
- cardiovascular disease, heart failure, hypertension, renal or hepatic disease, Down syndrome, hyperthyroidism, hiatal hernia, ulcerative colitis, prostatic hypertrophy, autonomic neuropathy, spasticity, suspected brain damage
- pregnant patients.

Patient monitoring

- Check for signs and symptoms of anaphylaxis and malignant hyperthermia.
- Monitor neurologic and cardiovascular status.
- Assess for curare-like effects (neuromuscular blockade leading to muscle weakness and possible paralysis) from overdose.
- Assess fluid intake and output.

Patient teaching

- Advise patient to take oral dose 30 to 60 minutes before meals.
- Teach patient to report signs and symptoms of adverse effects, especially anaphylaxis or muscle weakness.
- Instruct patient to avoid driving and other hazardous activities until he knows how drug affects concentration, vision, and alertness.
- Teach patient to minimize GI upset by eating frequent, small servings of healthy food and drinking adequate fluids.
- Tell patient to report urinary hesitancy or retention.
- As appropriate, review all other significant and life-threatening adverse reactions and interactions, especially those related to the drugs mentioned above.

goserelin acetate
Zoladex, Zoladex LA✦, Zoladex 3-Month

Pharmacologic class: Gonadotropin-releasing hormone analog
Therapeutic class: Antineoplastic, hormone
Pregnancy risk category D (breast cancer), *X* (endometriosis)

Action

Synthetic form of luteinizing hormone-releasing hormone (LHRH); inhibits gonadotropin production by acting directly on the pituitary gland. Increases the release of luteinizing hormone (LH), follicle-stimulating hormone (FSH), and testosterone, resulting in decreased testosterone and estradiol levels.

Availability

Implant: 3.6 mg, 10.8 mg (in preloaded syringes)

🖊 Indications and dosages

➤ Palliative treatment of prostate cancer in patients who can't tolerate orchiectomy or estrogen therapy; treatment of locally confined prostate cancer (given with flutamide and radiation therapy)
Adult males: 3.6 mg (implant) S.C. q 12 weeks into upper abdominal wall
➤ Palliative treatment of advanced breast cancer; management of endometriosis
Adults: 3.6 mg S.C. q 4 weeks; may increase dosage to 7.2 mg q 4 weeks (breast cancer). Or 3.6 mg S.C. q 4 weeks continued for 6 months (endometriosis).
➤ Endometrial thinning before endometrial ablation for dysfunctional uterine bleeding
Adults: One or two 3.6-mg implants given 4 weeks apart; if one implant is used, surgery is performed at 4 weeks; if two implants are used, surgery is performed 2 to 4 weeks after second implant.

Contraindications

• Hypersensitivity to drug or its components, other LHRHs, or other LHRH-agonist analogs
• Undiagnosed vaginal bleeding
• Pregnancy or breastfeeding

Administration

• Administer pretreatment pregnancy test to women of childbearing age.
• Administer S.C. into upper abdominal wall using aseptic technique.
• Give local anesthetic and stretch skin with one hand. Insert needle into S.C. fat, then change angle of needle until it parallels abdominal wall. Push needle in until hub touches patient's skin, and withdraw about 1 ml before depressing plunger all the way.
• Don't aspirate after inserting needle; blood will be visible in syringe if needle enters blood vessel.
🔊 Don't give by I.V. route.
• Be aware that if implant must be removed, it can be located by ultrasound.

Route	Onset	Peak	Duration
S.C.	Unknown	2-4 wk	End of therapy

Adverse reactions

CNS: headache, anxiety, depression, dizziness, fatigue, insomnia, lethargy, pain, emotional lability, weakness, **cerebrovascular accident**
CV: vasodilation, chest pain, hypertension, palpitations, peripheral edema, **myocardial infarction, arrhythmias**
EENT: blurred vision
GI: nausea, vomiting, diarrhea, constipation, ulcer, anorexia
GU: renal insufficiency, urinary obstruction, decreased libido, impotence, breast swelling or tenderness, infertility, sexual dysfunction, lower urinary tract symptoms, vaginitis, amenorrhea, decreased testicular size
Hematologic: anemia
Musculoskeletal: increased bone pain, joint pain, decreased bone density
Metabolic: gout, hyperglycemia, increased lipid levels, hypercalcemia
Respiratory: dyspnea, chronic obstructive pulmonary disease, upper respiratory tract infection

Skin: rash, acne, diaphoresis, seborrhea
Other: hirsutism, chills, fever, hot flashes, infection, weight gain

Interactions
Drug-diagnostic tests. *Calcium, glucose, high-density lipoproteins, low-density lipoproteins, triglycerides:* increased levels
FSH, LH: initially increased, then decreased, levels

Precautions
Use cautiously in:
• risk factors for osteoporosis
• chronic alcohol or tobacco use
• patients receiving drugs that affect bone density
• children younger than age 18 (safety not established).

Patient monitoring
• Assess menstrual symptoms and watch for breakthrough bleeding.
• Monitor neurologic status, checking especially for signs and symptoms of cerebrovascular accident.
• Monitor cardiovascular and respiratory status.

Patient teaching
• Advise female patients to avoid pregnancy and to use a nonhormonal contraception method.
• Instruct patient to call prescriber if menstrual bleeding persists or if she experiences breakthrough bleeding.
• Advise patient that menstruation may be delayed after therapy ends.
• As appropriate, review all other significant and life-threatening adverse reactions and interactions, especially those related to the tests mentioned above.

granisetron hydrochloride
Kytril

Pharmacologic class: 5-hydroxy-tryptamine$_3$ antagonist
Therapeutic class: Antiemetic
Pregnancy risk category B

Action
Binds to serotonin receptors in chemoreceptor trigger zone and in vagal nerve treminals, blocking serotonin release and controlling nausea and vomiting

Availability
Injection: 1 mg/ml
Oral solution: 2 mg/10 ml in 30-ml bottles
Tablets: 1 mg

Indications and dosages
➤ To prevent nausea and vomiting caused by emetogenic chemotherapy
Adults and children ages 2 to 16: For I.V. use, 10 mcg/kg I.V. within 30 minutes before chemotherapy. For P.O. use (adults only), 1 mg P.O. b.i.d., with first dose given at least 60 minutes before chemotherapy and second dose given 12 hours later on days when chemotherapy is administered; or 2 mg P.O. once daily at least 60 minutes before chemotherapy.
➤ To prevent nausea and vomiting associated with radiation therapy
Adults: 2 mg P.O. once daily within 1 hour of radiation therapy
➤ Acute nausea and vomiting after surgery
Adults: 1 mg I.V. undiluted and administered over 30 seconds

Contraindications
• Hypersensitivity to drug

Administration
• For I.V. infusion, dilute drug with normal saline solution or dextrose 5% in water.
• Infuse I.V. over 5 minutes, starting 30 minutes before chemotherapy.
• For direct I.V. injection, give undiluted over 30 seconds.
• Don't mix I.V. form with other drugs.
• For oral drug, give first dose 60 minutes before chemotherapy and second dose 12 hours after first.

Route	Onset	Peak	Duration
P.O.	Rapid	60 min	24 hr
I.V.	Rapid	30 min	Up to 24 hr

Adverse reactions
CNS: headache, anxiety, CNS stimulation, weakness, drowsiness, dizziness
CV: hypertension
GI: nausea, vomiting, diarrhea, constipation, abdominal pain, altered taste
Hematologic: anemia, **leukopenia, thrombocytopenia**
Hepatic: elevated hepatic enzyme levels
Skin: alopecia
Other: fever, chills, shivering, decreased appetite

Interactions
Drug-diagnostic tests. *Alanine aminotransferase, aspartate aminotransferase:* increased levels
Electrolytes: altered levels
Hemoglobin, platelets, white blood cells: decreased values
Drug-herb. *Horehound:* enhanced serotonergic effects

Precautions
Use cautiously in:
• pregnant or breastfeeding patients
• children younger than age 18 (safety of P.O. use not established)
• children younger than age 2 (safety of I.V. use not established).

Patient monitoring
• Monitor complete blood count with white cell differential, as well as hepatic enzymes.
• Monitor blood pressure and temperature.

Patient teaching
• Instruct patient to avoid driving and other hazardous activities until he knows how drug affects concentration and alertness.
• Teach patient to minimize GI upset by eating frequent, small servings of healthy food.
• Tell patient that he'll undergo regular blood testing during therapy.
• As appropriate, review all other significant and life-threatening adverse reactions and interactions, especially those related to the tests and herbs mentioned above.

guaifenesin (glyceryl guaiacolate)
Anti-Tuss, Benylin-E✦, Breonesin, Calmylin Expectorant✦, Diabetic Tussin EX, Duratuss G, Gee-Gee, Genatuss, GG-Cen, Glyate, Glycotuss, Glytuss, Guiatuss, Hytuss, Hytuss-2X, Monafed, Mucinex, Mytussin, Naldecon Senior EX, Organidin NR, Pneumomist, Resyl✦, Robitussin, Scot-tussin Expectorant, Siltussin SA, Tusibron, Uni-tussin

Pharmacologic class: Propanediol derivative
Therapeutic class: Expectorant
Pregnancy risk category C

Action
Exerts vasoconstrictive action, leading to decreased edema and congestion;

also increases respiratory secretions and reduces mucus viscosity

Availability

Capsules: 200 mg
Oral solution: 100 mg/5 ml, 200 mg/5 ml
Syrup: 100 mg/5 ml
Tablets: 100 mg, 200 mg, 1,200 mg
Tablets (extended-release): 600 mg

🖊 Indications and dosages

➤ Cough associated with upper respiratory tract infections
Adults: 200 to 400 mg P.O. q 4 hours, or 600 to 1,200 mg P.O. extended-release tablets q 12 hours (not to exceed 2,400 mg/day)
Children ages 6 to 12: 100 to 200 mg P.O. q 4 hours, or 600 mg P.O. extended-release tablets q 12 hours (not to exceed 1,200 mg/day)
Children ages 2 to 6: 50 to 100 mg P.O. q 4 hours (not to exceed 600 mg/day)

Contraindications

• Hypersensitivity to drug
• Alcohol intolerance (with some products)

Administration

• Give with a full glass of water.

Route	Onset	Peak	Duration
P.O.	30 min	Unknown	4-6 hr
P.O. (extended)	Unknown	Unknown	12 hr

Adverse reactions

CNS: headache, dizziness
GI: nausea, vomiting, diarrhea, stomach pain
Skin: rash, urticaria

Interactions

Drug-diagnostic tests. *Urinary 5-hydroxyindoleacetic acid, vanillylmandelic acid:* inaccurate results

Precautions

Use cautiously in:
• diabetes mellitus, cough lasting more than 1 week or accompanied by fever, rash, or headache
• patients receiving disulfiram concurrently
• pregnant patients.

Patient monitoring

• Assess cough quality and productivity. Reevaluate treatment if cough persists and is accompanied by fever or headache.
• Monitor patient for drug efficacy.

Patient teaching

• Advise patient to take the drug with 8 oz of water and to drink plenty of fluids.
• Instruct patient to contact prescriber if cough lasts more than 1 week.
• Tell patient to avoid driving and other hazardous activities until he knows how drug affects concentration and alertness.
• Teach patient to minimize GI upset by eating frequent, small servings of healthy food.
• As appropriate, review all other significant adverse reactions and interactions, especially those related to the tests mentioned above.

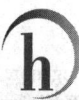

haloperidol
Apo-Haloperidol✦, Haldol, Novo-Peridol✦, Peridol✦, PMS Haloperidol✦

haloperidol decanoate
Haldol Decanoate 50, Haldol Decanoate 100, Haldol LA✦

haloperidol lactate
Haldol, Haldol Concentrate, Haloperidol Intensol

Pharmacologic class: Butyrophenone
Therapeutic class: Antipsychotic
Pregnancy risk category C

Action
Unknown; thought to block postsynaptic dopamine receptors in brain and increase dopamine turnover rate, inhibiting signs and symptoms of psychosis

Availability
Injection (decanoate): 50 mg/ml, 100 mg/ml
Injection (lactate): 5 mg/ml
Oral concentrate (lactate): 2 mg/ml
Tablets: 0.5 mg, 1 mg, 2 mg, 5 mg, 10 mg, 20 mg

⏃ Indications and dosages
➢ Acute or chronic psychosis, Tourette syndrome, severe behavioral problems in children
Adults: 0.5 to 5 mg P.O. two to three times daily, up to 100 mg/day for severe symptoms. Or 2 to 5 mg I.M. (lactate) q 1 to 8 hours, not to exceed 100 mg/day. For patients previously maintained on low oral dosages, initial dose of I.M. decanoate form is 10 to 15 times the previous daily oral haloperidol equivalent.
Children ages 3 to 12 or weighing 15 to 40 kg (33 to 88 lb): 50 mcg/kg/day P.O. in two to three divided doses; may increase by 500 mcg (0.5 mg)/day q 5 to 7 days as needed, up to 150 mcg/kg/day for psychosis or 75 mcg/kg/day for Tourette syndrome and nonpsychotic disorders
Dosage adjustment
• Elderly patients

Off-label uses
• Antiemetic
• Infantile autism
• Intractable hiccups

Contraindications
• Hypersensitivity to drug, tartrazine, sesame oil, or benzyl alcohol (with some products)
• Severe CNS depression

Administration
◀⏃ Don't give decanoate form I.V.
• Using 21G needle, administer decanoate by deep I.M. injection. Two injections may be necessary; maximum volume shouldn't exceed 3 ml.
• Be aware that recommended interval between I.M. injections of decanoate is 4 weeks.
• Dilute oral concentrate in water, soda, or juice (orange, apple, tomato) immediately before giving to patient.

Route	Onset	Peak	Duration
P.O.	Unknown	3-6 hr	Unknown
I.V. (lactate)	Unknown	Unknown	Unknown
I.M. (decanoate)	20-30 min	30-45 min	4-8 hr

Adverse reactions
CNS: confusion, drowsiness, restlessness, extrapyramidal reactions, tardive dyskinesia, sedation, lethargy, insom-

nia, vertigo, **seizures, neuroleptic malignant syndrome**

CV: hypotension, hypertension, tachycardia, ECG changes, **torsades de pointes** (with I.V. use)

EENT: blurred vision, dry eyes

GI: constipation, ileus, dry mouth, anorexia

GU: urinary retention, menstrual irregularities, gynecomastia, priapism

Hematologic: leukocytosis, anemia, **leukopenia**

Hepatic: jaundice, elevated hepatic enzyme levels, **drug-induced hepatitis**

Metabolic: elevated thyroid function test results, galactorrhea

Respiratory: dyspnea, respiratory depression, **bronchospasm, laryngospasm**

Skin: diaphoresis, photosensitivity, rash

Other: hyperpyrexia, hypersensitivity reactions

Interactions

Drug-drug. *Antidepressants, antihistamines, atropine, disopyramide, phenothiazines, quinidine, other anticholinergics:* additive anticholinergic effects

Antihypertensives, nitrates: additive hypotension

CNS depressants (including antihistamines, opioid analgesics, sedativehypnotics): additive CNS depression

Epinephrine: severe hypotension and tachycardia

Levodopa, pergolide: decreased therapeutic effects of haloperidol

Lithium: acute encephalopathic syndrome

Methyldopa: dementia

Drug-diagnostic tests. *Alanine aminotransferase, aspartate aminotransferase, thyroid function studies:* increased levels

Arterial blood gases, bicarbonate: altered levels

White blood cells: increased or decreased count

Drug-herb. *Angel's trumpet, jimsonweed, scopolia:* antagonism of cholinergic effects

Chamomile, hops, kava, skullcap, valerian: increased CNS depression

Nutmeg: reduced haloperidol efficacy

Drug-behaviors. *Acute alcohol ingestion:* additive hypotension

Precautions

Use cautiously in:

• hepatic disease, bone marrow depression, cardiac disease, respiratory insufficiency, CNS tumors, seizures, diabetes mellitus, narrow-angle glaucoma, prostatic hypertrophy

• elderly patients

• pregnant or breastfeeding patients.

Patient monitoring

• Monitor CNS status closely, especially for seizures and neuroleptic malignant syndrome (extrapyramidal symptoms, hyperthermia, autonomic disturbances).

◀≋ Monitor cardiovascular status, particularly for ECG changes, blood pressure changes, torsades de pointes, and atypical rapid ventricular tachycardia that may progress to ventricular fibrillation (with I.V. use).

• Assess respiratory status.

• Monitor complete blood count with white cell differential and liver function test results.

• With prolonged use, monitor patient for tardive dyskinesia (months or even years after starting drug).

Patient teaching

• Instruct patient to dilute oral concentrate with water, cola, or juice immediately before taking drug.

• Advise patient to minimize GI upset by eating frequent, small servings of healthy food and drinking adequate fluids.

• As appropriate, review all other significant and life-threatening adverse reactions and interactions, especially

h

---

those related to the drugs, tests, herbs, and behaviors mentioned above.

heparin sodium
Calcilean, Calciparine, Hepalean✦, Heparin Leo✦, Hep-Lock✦, Hep-Lock U/P, Hep-Pak, Uniparin

Pharmacologic class: Antithrombotic
Therapeutic class: Anticoagulant
Pregnancy risk category C

Action
Inhibits thrombus by blocking conversion of prothrombin to thrombin and fibrinogen to fibrin, preventing clots from forming

Availability
Solution for injection: 10 units/ml, 100 units/ml, 1,000 units/ml, 5,000 units/ml, 7,500 units/ml, 10,000 units/ml, 20,000 units/ml, 40,000 units/ml

⚕ Indications and dosages
➣ Therapeutic anticoagulation
Adults: 10,000 units I.V by intermittent bolus, followed by 5,000 to 10,000 units q 4 to 6 hours I.V. Or 5,000 units I.V. by continuous infusion, followed by 20,000 to 40,000 units I.V. over 24 hours (about 1,000 units/hour or 15 to 18 units/kg/hour). Or 5,000 units I.V., followed by initial S.C. dose of 10,000 to 20,000 units, then 8,000 to 10,000 units q 8 hours or 15,000 to 20,000 units q 12 hours.
Children: 50 units/kg I.V. by intermittent bolus, followed by 50 to 100 units/kg I.V. q 4 hours. Or 50 units/kg I.V. by continuous infusion, followed by 100 units/kg/4 hours or 20,000 units/m²/24 hours.
➣ To prevent thromboembolism
Adults: 5,000 units S.C. q 8 to 12 hours

(may be started 2 hours before surgery)
➣ To prevent blood clotting during cardiovascular surgery
Adults: At least 150 units/kg I.V. (300 units/kg if procedure is less than 60 minutes; 400 units/kg if more than 60 minutes)
➣ I.V. flush
Adults and children: 10 to 100 units/ml I.V. heparin sodium solution to fill heparin lock set

Off-label uses
• Prophylaxis of left ventricular thrombi
• Prophylaxis of cerebrovascular accident after myocardial infarction

Contraindications
• Hypersensitivity to drug
• Bleeding disorders
• Severe thrombocytopenia
• Patients who cannot have regular blood coagulation tests

Administration
• Draw baseline blood sample for clotting studies before starting drug.
◀≋ Be aware that USP units and IU are not equivalent for this drug.
◀≋ Use infusion pump to administer I.V. dose; check regularly to ensure that infusion rate is correct.
• Draw blood for partial thromboplastin time from opposite arm 4 hours after start of continuous I.V. infusion.
• Put note at patient's bedside to remind personnel to apply pressure dressings after taking blood.
• With intermittent I.V. drug infusion, draw blood 30 minutes before dose, using arm that doesn't have I.V. infusion.
• Don't mix heparin with other drugs or piggyback other drugs into heparin infusion line.
• For S.C. dose, inject slowly between iliac crests in lower abdomen, deep into S.C. fat layer. Leave needle in place for 10 seconds before withdrawing.

Don't massage area after injection. Alternate S.C. sites every 12 hours.
• Have protamine available as heparin agonist.

◀₹ Don't give heparin I.M.

◀₹ Be aware that heparin products containing benzyl alcohol shouldn't be used in premature infants.

Route	Onset	Peak	Duration
I.V.	Immediate	5-10 min	2-6 hr
S.C.	20-60 min	2-4 hr	8-12 hr

Adverse reactions

EENT: rhinitis
Hematologic: anemia, **bleeding, thrombocytopenia, severely prolonged clotting time**
Hepatic: elevated alanine aminotransferase (ALT) and aspartate aminotransferase (AST) levels, **hepatitis**
Metabolic: hyperkalemia
Musculoskeletal: osteoporosis (in long-term use)
Skin: irritation, rash, urticaria, hematoma, ulceration, cutaneous or subcutaneous necrosis, pruritus, alopecia (in long-term use)
Other: fever, pain at injection site, hypersensitivity reactions, **white clot syndrome, anaphylactoid reactions**

Interactions

Drug-drug. *Antihistamines, digoxin, nicotine, tetracyclines:* decreased anticoagulant effect of heparin
Cefamandole, cefmetazole, cefoperazone, cefotetan, plicamycin, quinidine, valproic acid, other drugs that cause hypoprothrombinemia: increased bleeding risk
Drugs that affect platelet function (including abciximab, aspirin, clopidogrel, dextran, dipyridamole, eptifibitide, nonsteroidal anti-inflammatory drugs, some penicillins, thrombolytics, ticlopidine, tirofiban): increased bleeding risk
Drug-diagnostic tests. *ALT, AST, free fatty acids, thyroxine, triiodothyronine resin:* increased levels

Cholesterol, triglycerides: decreased levels
125I fibrinogen uptake: false-negative results
Prothrombin time: prolonged
Drug-herb. *Anise, arnica, chamomile, clove, dong quai, feverfew, garlic, ginger, ginseng:* increased bleeding risk
Drug-behaviors. *Smoking:* increased bleeding risk

Precautions

Use cautiously in:
• severe hepatic or renal disease, bacterial endocarditis, hypertension, brain injury, retinopathy, ulcer disease
• recent CNS or ophthalmologic surgery
• immediate postpartum period
• women older than age 60
• pregnant patients.

Patient monitoring

• Monitor infusion rate closely, even when using infusion pump.
• Evaluate vital signs.

◀₹ Watch for signs and symptoms of anaphylactoid reaction.

◀₹ Assess for white clot syndrome (new thrombus formation in association with thrombocytopenia caused by irreversible platelet aggregation).

◀₹ Stay alert for signs and symptoms of bleeding tendency.

• Check partial thromboplastin time and platelet count frequently.
• Monitor liver function test results.
• In long-term therapy, periodically assess stool for occult blood.

Patient teaching

• If patient is self-administering drug, teach proper technique and emphasize need to rotate injection sites.

◀₹ Tell patient that nosebleeds, blood in urine, or black stools may be first signs of overdose and should be reported immediately.

• Instruct patient to report other unusual bleeding or bruising.

• Urge patient to avoid activities that can cause injury. Tell him to use soft toothbrush and electric razor to avoid gum and skin injury.

• Tell patient that he'll undergo regular blood testing during therapy.

• As appropriate, review all other significant and life-threatening adverse reactions and interactions, especially those related to the drugs, tests, herbs, and behaviors mentioned above.

hetastarch
Hespan

Pharmacologic class: Nonprotein colloid

Therapeutic class: Plasma volume expander

Pregnancy risk category C

Action
Expands plasma volume when given I.V. as a result of its osmotic effect. Increases erythrocyte sedimentation rate when added to whole blood.

Availability
Injection: 500 ml (6 g/100 ml in normal saline solution)

Indications and dosages
➤ Adjunctive therapy for plasma volume expansion in shock caused by hemorrhage, burns, surgery, sepsis, or other trauma
Adults: 500 to 1,000 ml I.V., depending on blood lost and hemoconcentration; total daily dosage shouldn't exceed 1,500 ml.
➤ Continuous flow centrifugation leukapheresis
Adults: 250 to 700 ml I.V. infused at a constant fixed ratio to venous whole blood (usually 1 to 8) up to twice weekly for a total of 7 to 10 treatments

Contraindications
• Hypersensitivity to drug
• Severe bleeding disorders
• Severe heart failure
• Renal failure

Administration
• Give by I.V. infusion only.
• Be aware that drug can be given at rates up to 20 ml/kg/hour for patients in acute hemorrhagic shock.

Route	Onset	Peak	Duration
I.V.	Immediate	Immediate	24-36 hr

Adverse reactions
CNS: headache
CV: peripheral edema of legs
EENT: periorbital edema
GI: nausea, vomiting, submaxillary and parotid glandular enlargement
Hematologic: prolonged prothrombin time (PT) and partial thromboplastin time (PTT), dilution of clotting factors, **increased bleeding and clotting times**
Musculoskeletal: muscle pain
Metabolic: fluid overload
Respiratory: wheezing
Skin: rash, urticaria
Other: chills, fever, flulike symptoms, hypersensitivity reaction

Interactions
None significant

Precautions
Use cautiously in:
• hepatic disorders
• pregnant patients.

Patient monitoring
• Stay alert for signs and symptoms of hypersensitivity reaction.
• Monitor vital signs and temperature.
• Assess for signs and symptoms of fluid overload, including peripheral edema of legs and periorbital edema.
• Check for adverse reactions, especially bleeding tendency.

• Monitor complete blood cell, leukocyte, and platelet counts as well as hemoglobin, hematocrit, PT, and PTT.

Patient teaching
• Teach patient to recognize and report signs and symptoms of allergic response and other adverse reactions.
• Advise patient to minimize GI upset by eating frequent, small servings of healthy food.
• Instruct patient to report unusual bleeding or bruising.
• Teach patient to avoid activities that can cause injury. Tell him to use soft toothbrush and electric razor to avoid gum and skin injury.
• Tell patient that he'll undergo regular blood testing during therapy.
• As appropriate, review all other significant and life-threatening adverse reactions.

histrelin acetate
Supprelin

Pharmacologic class: Hormone
Therapeutic class: Gonadotropin-releasing hormone (GnRH) agonist
Pregnancy risk category X

Action
Inhibits gonadotropin secretion; with daily therapy, desensitizes responsiveness of pituitary gonadotropin and decreases synthesis of ovarian and testicular hormones

Availability
Injection: 120 mcg/0.6 ml, 300 mcg/0.6 ml, 600 mcg/0.6 ml

Indications and dosages
➤ Centrally mediated (idiopathic or neurogenic) precocious puberty

Girls up to age 8, boys up to age 9½: 10 mcg/kg S.C. daily; if no response in 3 months, reevaluate therapy.

Off-label uses
• Endometriosis
• Uterine fibroids

Contraindications
• Hypersensitivity to drug
• Congenital adrenal hyperplasia
• Steroid-secreting tumors
• Pregnancy or breastfeeding

Administration
• Administer by S.C. route only.
• Know that each vial is for one-time use; discard any leftover drug.
• Rotate injection site daily.

Route	Onset	Peak	Duration
S.C.	Slow	3 mo	Unknown

Adverse reactions
CNS: malaise, nervousness, dizziness, depression, headache, insomnia, anxiety, paresthesia, mood changes, drowsiness, lethargy, fatigue, tremor, hyperkinesia, **seizures**
CV: vasodilation, hypertension, palpitations, tachycardia
EENT: vision disturbances, diplopia, photophobia, hearing loss, otalgia, ear congestion, nasal infections, epistaxis, sinusitis, rhinorrhea
GI: nausea, vomiting, diarrhea, constipation, abdominal pain, dyspepsia, altered taste, anorexia, dry mouth
GU: nocturia, dysuria, urinary incontinence, glycosuria, hematuria, menstrual changes, vaginal dryness, leukorrhea, hypermenorrhea, dysmenorrhea, vaginal bleeding, decreased breast size, nipple discharge
Hematologic: anemia, purpura
Metabolic: hyperlipidemia
Musculoskeletal: joint pain, back pain, myalgia, muscle cramps

h

Respiratory: cough, asthma, bronchitis, dyspnea, upper respiratory tract infection, hyperventilation

Skin: pallor, pruritus, erythema, urticaria, diaphoresis, rash, acne, swelling, alopecia, angioedema

Other: weight gain; hot flashes; chills; thirst; fever; **acute hypersensitivity reaction; anaphylaxis**

Interactions

Drug-diagnostic tests. *Hemoglobin:* decreased value
Lipids: increased levels

Precautions

None

Patient monitoring

• Monitor for acute hypersensitivity reaction.

• Evaluate patient's response to drug; if desired response doesn't occur within 3 months, prescriber should consider alternative therapy.

• Monitor GnRH level.

• Rotate injection sites; monitor sites for pain, inflammation, or infection. Apply heat or administer steroids, as needed and prescribed.

Patient teaching

• Teach patient or parents proper method of preparing and injecting drug.

• Instruct patient or parents to warm drug to room temperature before injecting.

• Teach patient or parents to rotate injection sites, keep track of sites on calendar, and assess sites closely for pain, swelling, redness, and infection.

• Advise parents that patient will need to undergo regular blood tests, X-rays, and monitoring of sexual development.

• Instruct parents to notify prescriber if patient experiences dyspnea or rapid heartbeat.

• As appropriate, review all other significant and life-threatening adverse reactions and interactions, especially those related to the tests mentioned above.

hydralazine hydrochloride
Apo-Hydralazine✣, Apresoline, Novo-Hylazin✣, Nu-Hydral✣

Pharmacologic class: Peripheral vasodilator

Therapeutic class: Antihypertensive

Pregnancy risk category C

Action

Relaxes vascular smooth muscle, thereby reducing blood pressure, decreasing peripheral vascular resistance, and increasing heart rate, stroke volume, and cardiac output

Availability

Injection: 20 mg/ml
Tablets: 10 mg, 25 mg, 50 mg, 100 mg

Indications and dosages

➤ Hypertension

Adults: Initially, 10 mg P.O. q.i.d. After 2 to 4 days, may increase to 25 mg P.O. q.i.d. for remainder of first week; then may increase further to 50 mg P.O q.i.d., up to 300 mg/day. Once maintenance dosage is established, drug may be given in two daily doses.

Children: Initially, 0.75 to 1 mg/kg/day P.O. in four divided doses; may increase gradually over 3 to 4 weeks to 7.5 mg/kg or 200 mg daily

Neonates: 0.5 mg/kg P.O., I.M., or I.V. q 4 to 6 hours

➤ Heart failure

Adults: Initially, 25 to 50 P.O. q.i.d.; may increase up to 300 mg/day given in three to four divided doses. Or 5 to 40 mg I.V. or I.M., repeated p.r.n.

➤ Eclampsia
Adults: 5 mg I.V., followed by another 5 mg I.V. q 15 to 20 minutes until blood pressure decreases adequately; if no response occurs after a total dose of 20 mg, prescriber may consider alternative drug.

Contraindications
• Hypersensitivity to drug or tartrazine

Administration
• Administer oral form with food.
• Inject I.V. form slowly over 1 minute; monitor blood pressure response continuously.
• Draw up and use parenteral drug immediately; solution changes color after coming in contact with metal needle.

Route	Onset	Peak	Duration
P.O.	45 min	2 hr	3-8 hr
I.V.	10-20 min	15-30 min	3-8 hr
I.M.	10-30 min	1 hr	3-8 hr

Adverse reactions
CNS: dizziness, drowsiness, headache, peripheral neuritis
CV: tachycardia, angina, orthostatic hypotension, **arrhythmias**
EENT: lacrimation, nasal congestion
GI: nausea, vomiting, diarrhea, constipation, anorexia
Metabolic: sodium retention
Musculoskeletal: joint pain, arthritis
Skin: rash, blisters, flushing, pruritus, urticaria
Other: chills, fever, lymphadenopathy, edema, lupuslike syndrome

Interactions
Drug-drug. *Antihypertensives, nitrates:* additive hypotension
Beta-adrenergic blockers: decreased risk of hydralazine-induced tachycardia
Epinephrine: reduced pressor response to epinephrine
Metoprolol, propranolol: increased blood levels of both drugs
Monoamine oxidase inhibitors: increased hypotension
Nonsteroidal anti-inflammatory drugs: decreased antihypertensive response
Drug-diagnostic tests. *Coombs' test:* positive results
Granulocytes, hemoglobin, neutrophils, platelets, red blood cells, white blood cells: decreased levels
Drug-behaviors. *Alcohol use:* additive hypotensive response

Precautions
Use cautiously in:
• cardiovascular or cerebrovascular disease, severe renal or hepatic disease
• pregnant or breastfeeding patients
• children.

Patient monitoring
• Monitor complete blood count, lupus erythematosus cell studies, and antinuclear antibody titers before therapy and periodically throughout.
• Monitor blood pressure, pulse rate and regularity, and daily weight.
• To avoid rapid blood pressure drop, withdraw drug gradually when discontinuing.
◀ Assess for lupuslike signs and symptoms, including joint pain, fever, myalgia, pharyngitis, and splenomegaly.
• Watch for peripheral neuritis; if it occurs, expect to give pyridoxine.

Patient teaching
• Tell patient to take tablets with food.
• Instruct patient to move slowly when sitting up or standing (especially in morning on awakening) to avoid dizziness or light-headedness from sudden blood pressure decrease.
◀ Instruct patient to contact prescriber immediately if fever, muscle and joint aches, or sore throat occurs.
• Teach patient to report chest pain or numbness or tingling of hands or feet.
• To minimize GI upset, advise patient to eat small, frequent meals.

• Instruct patient not to discontinue drug abruptly because severe hypertension may result.

• As appropriate, review other significant and life-threatening adverse reactions and interactions, especially those related to the drugs, tests, and behaviors mentioned above.

hydrochlorothiazide

Apo-Hydro✤, Dichlotride, Diuchlor H✤, Esidrix, Ezide, Hydrochlor, Hydro-D, HydroDIURIL, Hydro-Par, Microzide, Neo-Codema✤, Novo-Hydrazide✤, Oretic, Urozide✤

Pharmacologic class: Thiazide diuretic
Therapeutic class: Diuretic, antihypertensive
Pregnancy risk category B

Action

Increases sodium and water excretion by inhibiting sodium reabsorption in distal tubules; promotes excretion of chloride, potassium, magnesium, and bicarbonate. Also may produce arteriolar dilation, thereby reducing blood pressure.

Availability

Capsules: 12.5 mg
Oral solution: 10 mg/ml, 100 mg/ml
Tablets: 25 mg, 50 mg, 100 mg

🖊 Indications and dosages

➤ Edema associated with heart failure, renal dysfunction, cirrhosis, corticosteroid therapy, or estrogen therapy
Adults: 25 to 100 mg P.O. daily or intermittently, to a maximum dosage of 200 mg/day

➤ Mild to moderate hypertension
Adults: Initially, 12.5 mg daily P.O., then 12.5 to 50 mg/day P.O. Higher-than-recommended dosages may be given in refractory cases.
Children ages 6 months to 12 years: 60 mg/m^2 or 2.2 mg/kg P.O. daily in two divided doses
Children under age 6 months: Up to 3.3 mg/kg P.O. daily in two divided doses

Off-label uses

• Hypercalcemia
• Ménière's disease

Contraindications

• Hypersensitivity to drug, other thiazides, sulfonamides, or tartrazine

Administration

• Give with food or milk if GI upset occurs.
• Administer early in day so diuretic effect doesn't interfere with sleep.

Route	Onset	Peak	Duration
P.O.	2 hr	3-6 hr	6-12 hr

Adverse reactions

CNS: dizziness, drowsiness, lethargy, headache, insomnia, nervousness, vertigo, asthenia, asterixis, paresthesias, confusion, fatigue, encephalopathy
CV: chest pain, orthostatic hypotension, ECG changes, thrombophlebitis, **arrhythmias**
EENT: nystagmus
GI: nausea, vomiting, epigastric distress, anorexia, **pancreatitis**
GU: polyuria, nocturia, impotence, loss of libido, **renal failure**
Hematologic: anemia, hemolytic anemia, **agranulocytosis, leukopenia, thrombocytopenia**
Hepatic: jaundice, hepatitis
Metabolic: dehydration, gout, hyperglycemia, hypokalemia, hypocalcemia, hypochloremic alkalosis, hypomagnesemia, hyponatremia, hypophosphatemia, hypovolemia, hyperuricemia, hyperlipidemia

---

Musculoskeletal: muscle cramps
Skin: photosensitivity, urticaria, rash, dermatitis, purpura, alopecia, flushing
Other: fever, weight loss, **anaphylaxis**

Interactions

Drug-drug. *Allopurinol:* increased risk of hypersensitivity reaction
Amphotericin B, corticosteroids, digoxin, mezlocillin, piperacillin, ticarcillin: increased risk of hypokalemia
Antihypertensives, barbiturates, nitrates, opioids: increased hypotension
Cholestyramine, colestipol: decreased hydrochlorothiazide absorption
Digoxin: increased risk of hypokalemia
Lithium: decreased lithium excretion, increased blood level
Nonsteroidal anti-inflammatory drugs: decreased hydrochlorothiazide efficacy
Drug-diagnostic tests. *Bilirubin, blood and urine glucose (in diabetic patients), calcium, creatinine, uric acid:* increased levels
Cholesterol, low-density lipoproteins, magnesium, potassium, protein-bound iodine, sodium, triglycerides, urinary calcium: decreased levels
Drug-herb. *Dandelion:* interference with diuretic activity
Ginkgo: decreased antihypertensive effects
Licorice, stimulant laxative herbs (aloe, cascara sagrada, senna): increased risk of hypokalemia
Drug-behaviors. *Alcohol use:* increased hypotension
Sun exposure: increased risk of photosensitivity

Precautions

Use cautiously in:
• renal or severe hepatic impairment, fluid or electrolyte imbalances, gout, systemic lupus erythematosus, hyperparathyroidism, glucose tolerance abnormalities, bipolar disorder
• pregnant or breastfeeding patients.

Patient monitoring

• Monitor blood pressure, fluid intake and output, and daily weight.
• Assess electrolyte levels, especially potassium; monitor for signs and symptoms of hypokalemia.
• Monitor blood urea nitrogen and creatinine levels.
• Check blood glucose level in diabetic patients.
• Assess for signs and symptoms of gout attacks in patients with gouty arthritis.

Patient teaching

• Advise patient to take drug with food or milk if GI upset occurs.
• Instruct patient to take drug early in day to avoid nighttime urination.
• Teach patient to track intermittent doses on calendar.
• Tell patient to weigh himself daily, at same time on same scale and wearing same clothes.
• Instruct patient to report decreased urination, swelling, unusual bleeding or bruising, dizziness, numbness, muscle weakness or cramping, or fatigue.
• Instruct patient to move slowly when sitting up or standing to avoid dizziness or light-headedness from sudden blood pressure decrease.
• Tell patient to avoid driving and other hazardous activities until he knows how drug affects concentration and alertness.
• As appropriate, review all other significant and life-threatening adverse reactions and interactions, especially those related to the drugs, tests, herbs, and behaviors mentioned above.

h

hydrocodone bitartrate
Hycodan ✦, Robidone ✦, Tussinex

hydrocodone bitartrate and acetaminophen
Anexsia, Bancap-HC, Ceta-Plus, Co-Gesic, Dolacet, Duocet, Hydrocet, Hydrogesic, Hy-Phen, Lorcet-HD, Lortab, Margesic-H, Norco, Oncet, Panacet, Stagesic, T-Gesic, Vanacet, Vicodin, Zydone

hydrocodone bitartrate and aspirin
Alor, Azdone, Damason-P, Lortab ASA, Panasal

hydrocodone bitartrate and ibuprofen
Vicoprofen

Pharmacologic class: Opioid agonist/nonopioid analgesic combination

Therapeutic class: Opioid analgesic; allergy, cold, and cough remedy (antitussive)

Controlled substance schedule III

Pregnancy risk category C

Action
Blocks the release of inhibitory neurotransmitters, altering perception of and emotional response to pain. Hydrocodone combined with ibuprofen raises pain threshold at CNS level by nonselectively inhibiting cyclooxygenase; as a result, prostaglandin synthesis decreases and anti-inflammatory and analgesic effects occur.

Availability
hydrocodone bitartrate
Suspension: 5 mg/5 ml, 10 mg/5 ml
Syrup: 5 mg/ml

Tablets: 5 mg
hydrocodone and acetaminophen
Capsules: 5 mg hydrocodone/500 mg acetaminophen
Elixir/oral solution: 2.5 mg hydrocodone/167 mg acetaminophen/5 ml
Tablets: 2.5 mg hydrocodone/500 mg acetaminophen; 5 mg hydrocodone/400 mg acetaminophen; 5 mg hydrocodone/500 mg acetaminophen; 7.5 mg hydrocodone/400 mg acetaminophen; 7.5 mg hydrocodone/500 mg acetaminophen; 7.5 mg hydrocodone/650 mg acetaminophen; 7.5 mg hydrocodone/750 mg acetaminophen; 10 mg hydrocodone/325 mg acetaminophen; 10 mg hydrocodone/500 mg acetaminophen; 10 mg hydrocodone/650 mg acetaminophen; 10 mg hydrocodone/660 mg acetaminophen
hydrocodone and aspirin
Tablets: 5 mg hydrocodone/500 mg aspirin
hydrocodone and ibuprofen
Tablets: 7.5 mg hydrocodone/200 mg ibuprofen

💊 Indications and dosages
➤ Moderate to severe pain
Adults: 2.5 to 10 mg P.O. q 3 to 6 hours p.r.n.; with combination products, don't exceed 4 g/day
Children: 0.15 to 0.2 mg/kg P.O. q 3 to 6 hours
➤ Cough
Adults: 5 mg P.O. q 4 to 6 hours p.r.n. (usually given with decongestants)

Contraindications
• Hypersensitivity to hydrocodone, acetaminophen, aspirin, or ibuprofen (for corresponding combination products) or to alcohol, aspartame, saccharine, sugar, or tartrazine (with some products)

Administration
• In patients receiving concurrent monoamine oxidase (MAO) inhibitors, know that hydrocodone may pro-

duce severe, unpredictable reactions.
Initial dosage may need to be 25% lower than usual dosage.

Route	Onset	Peak	Duration
P.O.	10-30 min	30-60 min	4-6 hr

Adverse reactions
CNS: confusion, drowsiness, sedation, dysphoria, euphoria, floating feeling, hallucinations, headache, anxiety, depression, fatigue, insomnia, lethargy, nervousness, slurred speech, tremor, asthenia, unusual dreams
CV: orthostatic hypotension, bradycardia, peripheral edema, palpitations, **arrhythmias**
EENT: blurred vision, vision changes, diplopia, miosis, tinnitus, pharyngitis, rhinitis, sinusitis
GI: nausea, vomiting, constipation, dysphagia, esophagitis, dyspepsia, flatulence, gastritis, gastroenteritis, mouth ulcers, dry mouth, anorexia
GU: urinary retention or frequency, impotence
Respiratory: respiratory depression, bronchitis, dyspnea
Skin: pruritus, urticaria, diaphoresis, flushing
Other: physical or psychological drug dependence, drug tolerance

Interactions
Drug-drug. *Angiotensin-converting enzyme inhibitors:* decreased therapeutic effects of these drugs
Antihistamines, sedative-hypnotics: additive CNS depression
Buprenorphine, butorphanol, nalbuphine, pentazocine: precipitation of opioid withdrawal in physically dependent patients
Buprenorphine, pentazocine: decreased analgesia
Lithium: increased lithium blood level (with hydrocodone and ibuprofen only)
MAO inhibitors: severe, unpredictable reactions

Methotrexate: increased methotrexate blood level
Naloxone: withdrawal symptoms
Oral anticoagulants: increased risk of GI bleeding (with hydrocodone and ibuprofen only)
Drug-diagnostic tests. *Amylase, lipase:* increased levels
Drug-herb. *Chamomile, hops, kava, skullcaps, valerian:* increased CNS depression
Drug-behaviors. *Alcohol use:* increased CNS depression

Precautions
Use cautiously in:
• severe renal, hepatic, or pulmonary disease; increased intracranial pressure; hypothyroidism; adrenal insufficiency; prostatic hypertrophy; thrombocytopenia; alcoholism
• elderly patients
• pregnant or breastfeeding patients.

Patient monitoring
• In prolonged use, monitor for psychological and physical dependence.
• Watch closely for withdrawal symptoms when drug is discontinued.
• Assess carefully for adverse reactions in elderly patients.
◀ Monitor for signs and symptoms of drug overdose, including nausea, vomiting, blurred vision, cool and clammy skin, dizziness, confusion, dyspnea, respiratory depression, bradycardia, hearing loss, tinnitus, headache, and mood or behavior changes.

Patient teaching
• Inform patient that drug may cause drowsiness; advise him to avoid driving and other hazardous activities until CNS effects are known.
• Tell patient that prolonged use may lead to physical or psychological dependence.
• Caution patient to avoid alcohol during therapy.

• Instruct patient to move slowly when sitting up or standing to avoid dizziness or light-headedness from sudden blood pressure decrease.

• As appropriate, review all other significant and life-threatening adverse reactions and interactions, especially those related to the drugs, tests, herbs, and behaviors mentioned above.

hydrocortisone
Cortef, Cortenema, Hycort✦, Hydrocortone

hydrocortisone acetate
Cortifoam

hydrocortisone butyrate
Locoid

hydrocortisone cypionate
Aquacort✦, Cortate✦, Cortef, Texacort✦

hydrocortisone sodium phosphate
Hydrocortone Phosphate

hydrocortisone sodium succinate
A-hydroCort, Solu-Cortef

Pharmacologic class: Short-acting corticosteroid

Therapeutic class: Anti-inflammatory (steroidal)

Pregnancy risk category C

Action
Suppresses inflammatory and immune responses, mainly by inhibiting migration of leukocytes and phagocytes and by decreasing inflammatory mediators

Availability
Cream, gel, lotion, ointment, solution: various strengths
Injection: 50 mg/ml; 100 mg/vial, 250 mg/vial, 500 mg/vial, 1,000 mg/vial
Intrarectal aerosol foam: 90 mg
Oral suspension: 10 mg/5 ml
Retention enema: 100 mg/60 ml
Tablets: 5 mg, 10 mg, 20 mg

🖊 Indications and dosages
➤ Replacement therapy in adrenocortical insufficiency, hypercalcemia associated with cancer, rheumatoid arthritis, other types of arthritis, collagen diseases, dermatologic diseases, autoimmune disorders, hematologic disorders, trichinosis, ulcerative colitis, multiple sclerosis, proctitis, nephrotic syndrome, aspiration pneumonia
hydrocortisone, hydrocortisone cypionate—
Adults and children: 20 to 240 mg/day P.O.
hydrocortisone acetate (suspension)—
Adults and children: 5 to 75 mg by intra-articular injection (depending on joint size) q 2 to 3 weeks (with local anesthetic, if desired)
hydrocortisone acetate (intrarectal foam)—
Adults and children: One applicatorful of intrarectal foam daily or b.i.d. for 2 to 3 weeks; thereafter, one applicatorful every other day
hydrocortisone sodium phosphate—
Adults and children: 15 to 240 mg/day S.C., I.M., or I.V., with dosage adjusted according to response
hydrocortisone sodium succinate—
Adults and children: 100 to 500 mg I.M. or I.V.; may repeat at 2-, 4-, or 6-hour intervals, depending on patient response and clinical condition
hydrocortisone retention enema—
Adults and children: 100 mg P.R. at bedtime for 21 nights or until desired response occurs; patient should retain enema for at least 1 hour.

Off-label uses
- Bell's palsy
- Phlebitis
- Stomatitis

Contraindications
- Hypersensitivity to drug, alcohol, bisulfites, or tartrazine (with some products)
- Systemic fungal infections
- Concurrent use of immunosuppressive corticosteroids
- Concurrent administration of live-virus vaccines

Administration
- Give oral form with food or milk to avoid GI upset.
- Give I.V. hydrocortisone sodium succinate over 30 seconds to a few minutes; also may be given as intermittent infusion. For continuous infusion, dilute in normal saline solution, dextrose 5% in water, or dextrose 5% in normal saline solution.
- Inject I.M. dose deep into gluteal muscle; rotate injection sites to prevent muscle atrophy.
- Be aware that S.C. administration may cause muscle atrophy or sterile abscess.
- ◀€ Never abruptly discontinue high-dose or long-term systemic therapy.
- Know that systemic forms typically are used for adrenal replacement rather than inflammation because of their potent mineralocorticoid activity.

Route	Onset	Peak	Duration
P.O.	1-2 hr	1-2 hr	1-1.5 days
I.V.	Immediate	Unknown	1-1.5 days
I.M.	Rapid	4-8 hr	1-1.5 days
P.R.	Slow	3-5 days	4-6 days
S.C., topical	Unknown	Unknown	Unknown

Adverse reactions
CNS: meningitis, headache, nervousness, depression, euphoria, personality changes, psychoses, vertigo, paresthesia, insomnia, restlessness, conus medullaris syndrome, **increased intracranial pressure, seizures**
CV: hypotension, thrombophlebitis, hypertension, **heart failure, shock, fat embolism, thromboembolism, arrhythmias**
EENT: cataracts, glaucoma, increased intraocular pressure, epistaxis, nasal congestion, nasal septum perforation, anosmia, dysphonia, hoarseness, nasopharyngeal or oropharyngeal fungal infections
GI: nausea, vomiting, rectal bleeding, esophageal candidiasis or ulcer, abdominal distention, dry mouth, altered taste, **peptic ulceration, pancreatitis**
Hematologic: purpura
Metabolic: sodium and fluid retention, hypokalemia, hypocalcemia, hyperglycemia, hypercholesterolemia, decreased thyroxine level, immunosuppression, adrenal insufficiency, cushingoid appearance, amenorrhea, growth retardation, diabetes mellitus, **adrenal-pituitary suppression**
Musculoskeletal: osteoporosis, aseptic joint necrosis, muscle pain or weakness, steroid myopathy, loss of muscle mass, tendon rupture, spontaneous fractures
Respiratory: cough, wheezing, rebound congestion, **bronchospasm**
Skin: facial edema, rash, pruritus, urticaria, contact dermatitis, acne, bruising, hirsutism, petechiae, striae, acneiform lesions, skin fragility and thinness, angioedema
Other: appetite changes; weight gain; increased susceptibility to infection; masking or aggravation of infection; adhesive arachnoiditis; injection site pain, burning, or atrophy; hypersensitivity reactions including **anaphylaxis**

Interactions
Drug-drug. *Amphotericin B, loop and thiazide diuretics, mezlocillin, piperacillin, ticarcillin:* additive hypokalemia

Fluoroquinolones: increased risk of tendon rupture

Hormonal contraceptives: prolonged half-life and increased effects of hydrocortisone

Insulin, oral hypoglycemics: increased requirements for these drugs

Live-virus vaccines: decreased antibody response to vaccine, increased risk of adverse reactions

Nonsteroidal anti-inflammatory drugs: increased risk of adverse GI reactions

Phenobarbital, phenytoin, rifampin: decreased hydrocortisone efficacy

Somatrem: inhibition of growth-promoting effect

Drug-diagnostic tests. *Calcium, potassium, thyroxine, triiodothyronine:* decreased levels

Cholesterol, glucose: increased levels

Digoxin assays: false elevations (with some methods)

Nitroblue tetrazolium test: false-negative results

Drug-herb. *Echinacea:* increased immunostimulation

Ginseng: potentiation of immunomodulation

Drug-behaviors. *Alcohol use:* increased risk of gastric irritation and GI ulcers

Precautions

Use cautiously in:
• hypertension, osteoporosis, glaucoma, renal disease, hypothyroidism, cirrhosis, GI disease, thromboembolic disorders, myasthenia gravis, heart failure
• pregnant or breastfeeding patients
• children ages 6 and younger (safety not established).

Patient monitoring

• In high-dose therapy (which should not exceed 48 hours), watch closely for signs and symptoms of depression or psychotic episodes.
• Monitor blood pressure, weight, and electrolyte levels regularly.

• Assess blood glucose levels in diabetic patients; expect to increase insulin or oral hypoglycemic dosage.
• Monitor patient's response to weaning; watch for adrenal crisis, which may occur if drug is discontinued too quickly.

Patient teaching

• Instruct patient to take daily dose with food by 8 A.M.
◀🔊 Urge patient to immediately report unusual weight gain, face or leg swelling, epigastric burning, vomiting of blood, black tarry stools, irregular menstrual cycles, fever, prolonged sore throat, cold or other infection, or worsening of symptoms.
• Teach patient to eat small, frequent meals and to take antacids as needed to minimize GI upset.
• Advise patient that response to drug will be monitored regularly.
• In long-term use, instruct patient to have regular eye examinations.
• Instruct patient to wear medical identification stating that he's taking this drug.
• As appropriate, review all other significant and life-threatening adverse reactions and interactions, especially those related to the drugs, tests, herbs, and behaviors mentioned above.

hydromorphone hydrochloride
Dilaudid, Dilaudid-5, Dilaudid-HP, Hydrostat IR, PMS-Hydromorphone✤

Pharmacologic class: Opioid agonist

Therapeutic class: Opioid analgesic, antitussive

Controlled substance schedule II

Pregnancy risk category C (at term with high doses or long-term use: *D*)

Action
Binds to opiate receptors in the spinal cord and CNS, altering perception of and response to painful stimuli while producing generalized CNS depression. Also subdues cough reflex and decreases GI motility.

Availability
Injection: 1 mg/ml, 2 mg/ml, 3 mg/ml, 4 mg/ml, 10 mg/ml
Oral solution: 5 mg/5 ml
Rectal suppositories: 3 mg
Tablets: 1 mg, 2 mg, 3 mg, 4 mg, 8 mg

Indications and dosages
➤ Moderate to severe pain
Adults weighing more than 50 kg (110 lb): 2 to 10 mg P.O. (tablets) q 3 to 6 hours p.r.n. or 2.5 to 10 mg P.O. (oral solution) q 4 to 6 hours p.r.n.; or 1 to 2 mg S.C., I.M., or I.V. q 4 to 6 hours p.r.n. (with I.V. dose given over 2 to 3 minutes), increased to 3 to 4 mg q 4 to 6 hours p.r.n. for severe pain; or 3 mg P.R. q 6 to 8 hours p.r.n.

Contraindications
• Hypersensitivity to narcotics or bisulfites
• Acute or severe bronchial asthma or upper respiratory tract obstruction
• Premature neonates

Administration
• For maximal analgesic effect, give before pain becomes severe.
• For I.V. infusion, mix with dextrose 5% in water, normal saline solution, or lactated Ringer's solution.
• Administer I.V. form slowly, over at least 2 minutes.
• Rotate I.M. and S.C. sites to prevent muscle atrophy.
• Give oral form with food to avoid GI upset.

Route	Onset	Peak	Duration
P.O.	30 min	90-120 min	4 hr
I.V.	10-15 min	15-30 min	2-3 hr
I.M., S.C.	15 min	30-60 min	4-5 hr
P.R.	15-30 min	30-90 min	4-5 hr

Adverse reactions
CNS: confusion, sedation, dysphoria, euphoria, floating feeling, hallucinations, headache, unusual dreams, anxiety, dizziness, drowsiness
CV: hypotension, hypertension, palpitations, bradycardia, tachycardia
EENT: blurred vision, diplopia, miosis, nystagmus, tinnitus, laryngeal edema, **laryngospasm**
GI: nausea, vomiting, constipation, abdominal cramps, biliary tract spasm, anorexia
GU: urinary retention, dysuria
Hepatic: hepatotoxicity
Respiratory: dyspnea, wheezing, **bronchospasm, respiratory depression**
Skin: flushing, diaphoresis
Other: physical or psychological drug dependence; drug tolerance; injection site pain, redness, or swelling

Interactions
Drug-drug. *Antidepressants, antihistamines, monoamine oxidase (MAO) inhibitors, sedative-hypnotics:* additive CNS depression
Antihypertensives, diuretics, guanadrel, guanethidine, mecamylamine: increased risk of hypotension
Atropine, belladonna alkaloids, difenoxin, diphenoxylate, kaolin and pectin, loperamide, paregoric: increased risk of CNS depression, severe constipation
Barbiturates: increased sedation
Buprenorphine, butorphanol, nalbuphine, pentazocine: precipitation of opioid withdrawal in physically dependent patients
Nalbuphine, pentazocine: decreased analgesia

Drug-diagnostic tests. *Amylase, lipase:* increased levels

Drug-herb. *Chamomile, hops, kava, skullcap, valerian:* increased CNS depression

Drug-behaviors. *Alcohol use:* increased CNS depression

Precautions

Use cautiously in:
• increased intracranial pressure; severe renal, hepatic, or pulmonary disease; hypothyroidism; adrenal insufficiency; prostatic hypertrophy; alcoholism
• concurrent use of MAO inhibitors
• elderly patients
• pregnant or breastfeeding patients.

Patient monitoring

◀ᚷ With I.V. use, monitor for respiratory depression; keep resuscitation equipment and naloxone available.
• Assess for signs and symptoms of physical or psychological drug dependence.
• Monitor for constipation.

Patient teaching

• Instruct patient to take drug as prescribed before pain becomes severe.
• Teach patient to take oral form with food to avoid GI upset.
• Advise patient to report difficulty breathing, nausea, vomiting, or dizziness.
• Instruct patient to avoid driving and other hazardous activities until he knows how drug affects concentration and alertness.
• As appropriate, review all other significant and life-threatening adverse reactions and interactions, especially those related to the drugs, tests, herbs, and behaviors mentioned above.

hydroxychloroquine sulfate
Plaquenil

Pharmacologic class: 4-amino-quinolone

Therapeutic class: Antimalarial, antirheumatic, anti-inflammatory (disease-modifying)

Pregnancy risk category C

Action

Unknown; thought to interfere with inhibition of protein synthesis and DNA replication, leading to parasitic death

Availability

Tablets: 200 mg (155 mg base); 200 mg hydroxychloroquine sulfate is equivalent to 155 mg of hydroxychloroquine base

🕖 Indications and dosages

➤ Prophylaxis of malaria (dosages expressed as mg of base)
Adults: 310 mg P.O. q week, starting 1 to 2 weeks before entering endemic area and continuing for 4 weeks after leaving area
Children: 5 mg/kg P.O. q week, starting 1 to 2 weeks before entering endemic area and continuing for 4 weeks after leaving area
➤ Malaria (dosages expressed as mg of base)
Adults: Initially, 620 mg P.O., then 310 mg 6 hours, 24 hours, and 48 hours later
Children: Initially, 10 mg/kg P.O., then 5 mg/kg 6 hours, 24 hours, and 48 hours later
➤ Rheumatoid arthritis
Adults: 400 to 600 mg/day P.O. for 4 to 12 weeks, then reduced by 50%
➤ Systemic lupus erythematosus
Adults: 400 mg P.O. once or twice daily

for several months, then reduced to 200 to 400 mg daily, depending on response

Contraindications
• Hypersensitivity to drug or chloroquine
• Retinal or visual field changes
• Long-term therapy in children

Administration
• Give with food or milk.
• For patients receiving doses to prevent malaria, schedule doses on same day of week.

Route	Onset	Peak	Duration
P.O.	Unknown	2-4.5 hr	Unknown

Adverse reactions
CNS: anxiety, apathy, confusion, fatigue, headache, psychoses, mood swings, irritability, neuromyopathy, peripheral neuritis, **seizures**
CV: ECG changes, hypotension
EENT: visual disturbances, retinopathy, keratopathy, ototoxicity, tinnitus
GI: nausea, vomiting, diarrhea, abdominal cramps, anorexia
Hematologic: leukopenia, agranulocytosis, aplastic anemia, thrombocytopenia
Hepatic: jaundice, hepatotoxicity
Musculoskeletal: muscle weakness
Skin: dermatoses, rash, pruritus, pigmentation changes, pleomorphic skin eruption, worsened psoriasis, alopecia, bleaching of hair
Other: weight loss

Interactions
Drug-drug. *Aluminum salts, kaolin, magnesium salts:* decreased hydroxychloroquinine absorption
Cimetidine: decreased hepatic metabolism of hydroxychloroquinine
Hepatotoxic drugs: increased risk of hepatotoxicity
Drug-diagnostic tests. *Granulocytes, hemoglobin, platelets:* decreased values

Drug-behaviors. *Sun exposure:* exacerbation of drug-induced dermatoses

Precautions
Use cautiously in:
• hepatic or renal impairment, glucose-6-phosphate dehydrogenase (G6PD) deficiency, psoriasis, bone marrow depression, alcoholism
• obese patients
• pregnant or breastfeeding patients
• children.

Patient monitoring
◀️ Monitor for signs and symptoms of overdose, such as nausea, vomiting, drowsiness, visual disturbances, cardiovascular collapse, and seizures.
• Watch for adverse reactions.

Patient teaching
• Advise patient to take drug with food or milk.
◀️ Instruct patient to immediately report vision changes, nausea, vomiting, drowsiness, or headache.
• Tell patient to report such adverse reactions as hearing loss, ringing in ears, muscle weakness, rash, bleeding, bruising, yellowing of skin and sclera, mental changes, and mood swings.
• In long-term therapy, advise patient to have regular eye exams.
• As appropriate, review all other significant and life-threatening adverse reactions and interactions, especially those related to the drugs, tests, and behaviors mentioned above.

hydroxyurea
Droxia, Hydrea, Mylocel

Pharmacologic class: Antimetabolite
Therapeutic class: Antineoplastic
Pregnancy risk category D

Action
Unknown; may inhibit enzyme necessary for DNA synthesis and RNA or protein synthesis

Availability
Capsules: 200 mg, 250 mg, 300 mg, 400 mg, 500 mg
Tablets: 100 mg, 1,000 mg

💊 Indications and dosages
➤ Head and neck cancer, ovarian cancer, malignant melanoma
Adults: 60 to 80 mg/kg (2 to 3 g/m²) P.O. as a single daily dose q 3 days, or 20 to 30 mg/kg/day P.O. as a single dose. Therapy should begin 7 days before radiation.
➤ Resistant chronic myelogenous leukemia
Adults: 20 to 30 mg/kg/day P.O. in one or two divided doses
➤ Sickle cell anemia
Adults and children: 15 mg/kg/day P.O. as a single dose; may increase by 5 mg/kg/day P.O. q 12 weeks, up to 35 mg/kg/day

Off-label uses
• Thrombocythemia
• Human immunodeficiency virus

Contraindications
• Hypersensitivity to drug or tartrazine
• Bone marrow depression
• Severe anemia or thrombocytopenia

Administration
• Provide frequent mouth care.

Route	Onset	Peak	Duration
P.O.	Unknown	2 hr	24 hr

Adverse reactions
CNS: drowsiness, malaise, confusion, dizziness, headache
GI: nausea, vomiting, diarrhea, constipation, stomatitis, anorexia
GU: dysuria, renal tubular dysfunction, hyperuricemia, elevated blood urea nitrogen (BUN) and creatinine levels, infertility
Hematologic: megaloblastosis, anemia, **leukopenia, thrombocytopenia, bone marrow depression**
Hepatic: hepatitis
Metabolic: hyperuricemia
Skin: alopecia, erythema, exacerbation of post-radiation erythema, pruritus, rash, urticaria
Other: chills, fever

Interactions
Drug-drug. *Myelosuppressants:* additive bone marrow depression
Live-virus vaccines: decreased antibody response to vaccine, increased risk of adverse reactions
Drug-diagnostic tests. *Mean corpuscular volume (MCV):* transient increase
BUN, creatinine, uric acid: increased levels
Hemoglobin, platelets, red blood cells, white blood cells: decreased values

Precautions
Use cautiously in:
• renal or hepatic impairment
• obese patients
• females of childbearing age
• elderly patients.

Patient monitoring
• Assess complete blood count weekly.
• Closely monitor patients with renal or hepatic impairment; check kidney or liver function test results frequently.
• Assess fluid status; make sure patient drinks 10 to 12 glasses of water daily.

Patient teaching
• Teach patient to mark dates for drug doses, diagnostic tests, and treatments on calendar.
• Instruct patent to report such adverse effects as appetite loss, nausea, vomiting, oral lesions, constipation, diarrhea, confusion, dizziness, headache, and rash.

• Instruct female patients to use barrier method of birth control.

• Tell patient he'll need to undergo regular blood tests to monitor drug effects.

• As appropriate, review all other significant and life-threatening adverse reactions and interactions, especially those related to the drugs and tests mentioned above.

hydroxyzine hydrochloride
Apo-Hydroxyzine✦, Atarax, Novo-Hydroxyzin✦, Vistaril

hydroxyzine pamoate
Vistaril

Pharmacologic class: Piperazine derivative

Therapeutic class: Anxiolytic, antihistamine, sedative-hypnotic

Pregnancy risk category NR

Action
Unknown; anxiolytic and sedative effects may be due to suppression of activity in the subcortical levels of the CNS. Antihistamine effects may result from suppression of histamine at cellular receptor sites.

Availability
Capsules: 25 mg, 50 mg, 100 mg (pamoate)
Injection: 25 mg/ml, 50 mg/ml
Oral suspension: 25 mg/5 ml (pamoate)
Syrup: 10 mg/5 ml
Tablets: 10 mg, 25 mg, 50 mg, 100 mg

ⓘ Indications and dosages
➤ Psychiatric emergencies; acute and chronic alcoholism
Adults: 50 to 100 mg I.M. immediately, then q 4 to 6 hours p.r.n.

➤ Nausea and vomiting; adjunct in preoperative and postoperative sedation
Adults: 25 to 100 mg I.M. q 4 to 6 hours
Children: 1.1 mg/kg I.M. q 4 to 6 hours
➤ Anxiety
Adults and children ages 6 and older: 50 to 100 mg P.O. q.i.d.
Children younger than age 6: 50 mg P.O. daily in divided doses
➤ Pruritus
Adults: 25 mg P.O. three or four times daily
Children ages 6 and older: 50 to 100 mg P.O. daily in divided doses
Children younger than age 6: 50 mg P.O. daily in divided doses

Off-label uses
• Seasonal allergic rhinitis

Contraindications
• Hypersensitivity to drug or cetirizine

Administration
◀€ Don't administer I.V. or S.C. because tissue necrosis may occur.
• Use Z-track method for I.M. injection; inject deep into large muscle (preferably, upper outer quadrant of buttock).

Route	Onset	Peak	Duration
P.O., I.M.	15-30 min	2-4 hr	4-6 hr

Adverse reactions
CNS: drowsiness, agitation, dizziness, headache, asthenia, ataxia
GI: nausea, constipation, dry mouth, bitter taste
GU: urinary retention
Respiratory: wheezing
Skin: flushing
Other: hypersensitivity reaction, pain or abscess at I.M. injection site

h

Interactions
Drug-drug. *Anticholinergics, antidepressants, antihistamines, phenothiazines, quinidine:* additive effects of these drugs

Antidepressants, antihistamines, opioids, other CNS depressants, sedative-hypnotics: additive CNS depression

Drug-diagnostic tests. *Skin tests using allergen extracts:* false-negative results

Drug-herb. *Angel's trumpet, jimsonweed, scopolia:* increased anticholinergic effects

Chamomile, hops, kava, skullcap, valerian: increased CNS depression

Drug-behaviors. *Alcohol use:* increased CNS depression

Precautions
Use cautiously in:
• severe hepatic dysfunction
• elderly patients.

Patient monitoring
• Monitor closely for CNS depression and oversedation, especially if patient is receiving other CNS depressants.
• Assess for drug effects, especially in elderly patients.
• Monitor liver function test results in patients with hepatic impairment.

Patient teaching
• Instruct patient to avoid driving and other hazardous activities until he knows how drug affects his concentration and alertness.
• Advise patient to contact prescriber if he experiences difficulty breathing, muscle spasms, or incoordination.
• As appropriate, review all other significant adverse reactions and interactions, especially those related to the drugs, tests, herbs, and behaviors mentioned above.

hyoscyamine
Cystospaz

hyoscyamine sulfate
Anaspaz, A-Spas S/L, Cystospaz-M, Donnamar, ED-SPAZ, Gastrosed, Levbid, Levsin, Levsin Drops, Levsinex, Levsinex Timecaps, Levsin/SL, Neoquess, NuLev

Pharmacologic class: Anticholinergic
Therapeutic class: Antispasmodic
Pregnancy risk category C

Action
Competitively inhibits the action of acetylcholine at autonomic nerve sites, relaxing smooth muscle and decreasing gland secretions

Availability
Capsules (timed-release): 0.375 mg
Elixir: 0.125 mg/5 ml
Injection: 0.5 mg/ml
Oral solution: 0.125 mg/ml
Tablets: 0.125 mg, 0.15 mg
Tablets (extended-release): 0.375 mg
Tablets (orally disintegrating): 0.125 mg
Tablets (sublingual): 0.125 mg

⏀ Indications and dosages
➢ Adjunct in GI tract disorders; pain and hypersecretion in pancreatitis; cystitis; renal colic; infant colic; acute rhinitis; anticholinesterase poisoning; rigidity, tremors, and hyperhidrosis in Parkinson's disease; partial heart block associated with vagal activity
Adults: 0.125 to 0.25 mg P.O. or S.L. three to four times daily, or 0.375 to 0.75 mg P.O. (extended-release) q 12 hours, or 0.25 to 0.5 mg S.C., I.M., or I.V. three to four times daily p.r.n.
Children ages 2 to 12: 0.0625 to 0.125 mg (one-half to one whole NuLev

tablet) P.O. q 4 hours p.r.n., not to exceed six tablets in 24 hours

Contraindications

• Hypersensitivity to anticholinergics, alcohol, sulfites, or tartrazine
• Narrow-angle glaucoma, synechia
• GI obstructive disease, severe ulcerative colitis
• Renal or hepatic disease
• Neonates or premature infants

Administration

• Administer 30 to 60 minutes before meals and at bedtime.
• Give bedtime dose at least 2 hours after last evening meal or snack.

Route	Onset	Peak	Duration
P.O.	20-30 min	0.5-1 hr	4-12 hr
P.O. (extended)	20-30 min	40-90 min	12 hr
I.V.	2 min	15-30 min	4 hr
I.M., S.C.	Unknown	15-30 min	4-12 hr
S.L.	5-20 min	0.5-1 hr	4 hr

Adverse reactions

CNS: confusion, excitement, nervousness, dizziness, light-headedness, headache, insomnia,
CV: palpitations, tachycardia
EENT: blurred vision, cycloplegia, increased intraocular pressure, mydriasis, photophobia
GI: nausea, vomiting, constipation, bloating, dry mouth, altered taste, **paralytic ileus**
GU: urinary hesitancy or retention, impotence, lactation suppression
Skin: flushing, decreased sweating, urticaria, local irritation (with I.M., I.V., or S.C. use)
Other: allergic reactions, including fever; heat intolerance; **anaphylaxis**

Interactions

Drug-drug. *Amantadine, antihistamines, antiparkinsonian agents, disopyramide, glutethimide, meperidine, procainamide, quinidine, tricyclic antidepressants:* increased anticholinergic effects
Antacids: decreased hyoscyamine absorption
Atenolol: increased atenolol effects
Ketoconazole: interference with absorption of both drugs
Methotrimeprazine: increased risk of extrapyramidal effects
Phenothiazines: decreased phenothiazine effects, increased anticholinergic effects
Drug-herb. *Jimsonweed:* adverse cardiovascular effects

Precautions

Use cautiously in:
• cardiovascular disease, prostatic hypertrophy, reflux esophagitis, brain damage, autonomic neuropathy, hyperthyroidism, glaucoma, Down syndrome, spastic paralysis
• elderly patients
• pregnant patients (safety not established) or breastfeeding patients
• infants and small children.

Patient monitoring

• Monitor for adverse reactions.
• Assess for mental status changes, such as confusion.
• Evaluate fluid intake and output.
• Assess patient's response to temperature changes (especially hot weather); drug raises risk of heat intolerance, predisposing patient to heat stroke.

Patient teaching

• Teach patient to take drug on empty stomach 30 to 60 minutes before meals and at least 2 hours after last evening meal or snack.
• Instruct patient with urinary hesitancy to empty bladder before taking drug.
• Advise patient to avoid driving and other hazardous activities until he knows how drug affects concentration and alertness.

• As appropriate, review all other significant and life-threatening adverse reactions and interactions, especially those related to the drugs and herbs mentioned above.

ibritumomab tiuxetan
Zevalin

Pharmacologic class: Monoclonal antibody
Therapeutic class: Antineoplastic
Pregnancy risk category D

Action
Binds indium-111 (In-111) or yttrium-90 (Y-90) with free amino groups of lysines and arginines within antibody; binds specifically to CD20 antigen, found on surface of normal and malignant B lymphocytes. Radioactive component of Y-90 causes cellular damage due to free radicals in target cells.

Availability
Injection: 3.2 mg/2 ml (two Zevalin kits containing four vials each)

Indications and dosages
➤ Non-Hodgkin's lymphoma
Adults: Given in two-step regimen that includes pre-dose of rituximab
Step 1: Single I.V. infusion of 250 mg/m² rituximab (not included in Zevalin kit) at 50 mg/hour; increase rate by 50 mg/hour q 30 minutes, up to a maximum of 400 mg/hour. If hypersensitivity or infusion-related reaction occurs, temporarily slow or interrupt infusion; if symptoms improve, may continue infusion at 50% of previous rate. Within 4 hours of rituximab dose,

5 mCi of In-111 Zevalin I.V. should be given over 10 minutes.
Step 2: 7 to 9 days after step 1, I.V. infusion of 250 mg/m² rituximab (not included in Zevalin kit) at 100 mg/hour (50 mg/hour if infusion-related reaction occurred during first rituximab dose); increase by 100 mg/hour q 30 minutes, to a maximum of 400 mg/hour, as tolerated. Within 4 hours of rituximab dose, 0.3 to 0.4 mCi/kg (depending on platelet count) of Y-90 Zevalin given I.V. over 10 minutes, not to exceed absolute maximum allowable dose of 32 mCi, regardless of patient's weight.

Contraindications
• Hypersensitivity to any drugs in therapeutic regimen, components of these drugs, or murine products
• Pregnancy or breastfeeding

Administration
◀♪ Assess for human antimurine antibody before treatment. If positive, patient may have hypersensitivity reaction.
• Premedicate patient with acetaminophen and diphenhydramine before each rituximab infusion, as prescribed.
• Be aware that ibritumomab should be used only as part of a regimen that consists of a combination of ibritumomab and rituximab.
◀♪ Administer ibritumomab by slow I.V. infusion over 10 minutes; monitor closely.
◀♪ Don't give by I.V. push.
◀♪ Take steps to prevent extravasation of Y-90 Zevalin. If extravasation occurs, immediately stop infusion and restart in another vein.
• Don't give Y-90 Zevalin if patient's platelet count is below 100,000/mm³.
• Follow facility policy on radiation precautions to protect patients, visitors, and medical personnel from radiation exposure.

Route	Onset	Peak	Duration
I.V.	Unknown	Unknown	Unknown

Adverse reactions
CNS: dizziness, anxiety, headache, insomnia, asthenia
CV: hypotension, peripheral edema
EENT: rhinitis, epistaxis, throat irritation
GI: nausea, vomiting, diarrhea, constipation, anorexia, dyspepsia, abdominal pain or enlargement, melena
Hematologic: anemia, **thrombocytopenia, neutropenia, pancytopenia, hemorrhage**
Musculoskeletal: joint pain, myalgia, back pain
Respiratory: increased cough, dyspnea, **apnea, bronchospasm**
Skin: flushing, bruising, diaphoresis, petechiae, pruritus, rash, urticaria, angioedema
Other: bacterial infection, I.V. site irritation, fever, chills, generalized pain, tumor pain, hypersensitivity reactions including **anaphylaxis, myeloid malignancies, dysplasias**

Interactions
None significant

Precautions
Use cautiously in:
• cardiac conditions
• elderly patients.

Patient monitoring
◀€ Institute infection control protocols; protect patient from potential sources of infection.
◀€ Assess complete blood count and platelet count before starting therapy; monitor both counts regularly during and after therapy.
◀€ Monitor for hypersensitivity reactions, which can be fatal; know that these usually occur within 30 minutes to 2 hours of administration.

• Watch for unusual bleeding or bruising.

Patient teaching
◀€ Instruct patient to promptly report difficulty breathing, rash, fever, chills, severe GI distress, black tarry stools, illness or injury, or unusual bleeding or bruising.
• Inform patient that drug increases his risk of infection; instruct him to avoid crowds and potential or known sources of infection.
• Instruct patient to eat small, frequent meals and take antiemetic drugs for nausea and vomiting, as needed and prescribed.
• Advise patient that he'll undergo blood testing during therapy to monitor drug effects.
• As appropriate, review all other significant and life-threatening adverse reactions mentioned above.

ibuprofen
Actiprofen Caplets♣, Advil, Advil Migraine, Apo-Ibuprofen♣, Children's Advil, Children's Motrin, Excedrin IB, Genpril, Haltran, Junior Strength Advil, Junior Strength Motrin, Medipren, Menadol, Midol IB, Motrin IB, Novo-Profen♣, Nu-Ibuprofen♣, Nuprin

Pharmacologic class: Nonsteroidal anti-inflammatory drug (NSAID)
Therapeutic class: Analgesic, antipyretic, anti-inflammatory
Pregnancy risk category B (third trimester: *D*)

Action
Unknown; thought to inhibit cyclooxygenase, an enzyme needed for prostaglandin synthesis

Availability
Capsules (liquigels): 200 mg
Oral suspension: 100 mg/2.5 ml,
100 mg/5 ml
Pediatric drops: 50 mg/1.25 ml
Tablets: 100 mg, 200 mg, 300 mg,
400 mg, 600 mg, 800 mg
Tablets (chewable): 50 mg, 100 mg

⚕ Indications and dosages
➣ Rheumatoid arthritis, osteoarthritis
Adults: 1.2 to 3.2 g/day P.O. in two to
four divided doses
➣ Mild to moderate pain
Adults: 400 mg P.O. q 4 to 6 hours
p.r.n.
➣ Primary dysmenorrhea
Adults: 400 mg P.O. q 4 hours p.r.n.
➣ Juvenile arthritis
Children: 30 to 40 mg/kg/day P.O. in
three or four divided doses; daily
dosages above 50 mg aren't recom-
mended.
➣ Fever reduction, pain relief
Children ages 6 to 12: 5 mg/kg P.O. if
temperature is below 102.5° F (39.2° C)
or 10 mg/kg if temperature is above
102.5° F; maximum daily dosage is
40 mg/kg.

Off-label uses
• Migraine and tension headaches

Contraindications
• Hypersensitivity to drug or other
NSAIDs
• Pregnancy

Administration
• Ideally, give drug 1 hour before or 2
hours after meal. If GI upset occurs,
give with meals.

Route	Onset	Peak	Duration
P.O. (analgesic)	30 min	1-2 hr	4-6 hr
P.O. (anti-inflam.)	7 days	1-2 wk	Unknown

Adverse reactions
CNS: headache, dizziness, drowsiness,
nervousness, **aseptic meningitis**
CV: arrhythmias
EENT: amblyopia, blurred vision, tin-
nitus
GI: nausea, vomiting, constipation,
dyspepsia, abdominal discomfort, **GI
bleeding**
GU: cystitis, hematuria, azotemia,
renal failure
Hematologic: anemia, prolonged
bleeding time, **aplastic anemia, neutropenia, pancytopenia, thrombocytopenia, leukopenia, agranulocytosis**
Hepatic: hepatitis
Metabolic: hypoglycemia, hyperglycemia
Respiratory: bronchospasm
Skin: rash, pruritus, urticaria
Other: edema, allergic reactions including **anaphylaxis, Stevens-Johnson
syndrome**

Interactions
Drug-drug. *Acetaminophen:* increased
risk of adverse renal reactions
Antihypertensives, diuretics: decreased
efficacy of these drugs
Antineoplastics: increased risk of adverse hematologic reactions
*Aspirin and other NSAIDs, corticoste-
roids:* additive adverse GI effects
*Cefamandole, cefoperazone, cefotetan,
drugs affecting platelet function (including abciximab, clopidogrel, eptifibatide,
ticlopidine, tirofiban), plicamycin,
thrombolytics, valproic acid, warfarin:*
increased risk of bleeding
Cyclosporine: increased risk of nephrotoxicity
Digoxin: slightly increased digoxin
blood level
Lithium: increased lithium blood level,
greater risk of lithium toxicity
Methotrexate: increased risk of methotrexate toxicity
Probenecid: increased risk of ibuprofen
toxicity

Drug-diagnostic tests. *Alanine aminotransferase, alkaline phosphatase, aspartate aminotransferase, blood urea nitrogen, creatinine, lactate dehydrogenase, potassium:* increased levels
Bleeding time: prolonged
Creatinine clearance: decreased
Glucose, hematocrit, hemoglobin: decreased levels
Platelets, white blood cells: decreased counts
Drug-herb. *Anise, arnica, chamomile, clove, dong quai, fenugreek, feverfew, garlic, ginger, ginkgo, ginseng, licorice:* increased risk of bleeding
White willow: additive adverse GI effects
Drug-behaviors. *Alcohol use:* additive adverse GI effects
Sun exposure: phototoxicity

Precautions

Use cautiously in:
• severe cardiovascular, renal, or hepatic disease; GI disease; asthma; chronic alcohol use
• elderly patients
• breastfeeding patients.

Patient monitoring

• Monitor for desired effect (analgesic, anti-inflammatory, or antipyretic).
• Watch for GI upset and adverse CNS effects, such as headache and drowsiness.
• Closely monitor for GI bleeding and ulcer development, especially in long-term therapy.
• In long-term therapy, assess renal and hepatic function regularly.

Patient teaching

• Teach patient to take drug with full glass of water, with food, or after meals to minimize GI upset.
• To help prevent esophageal irritation, instruct patient to avoid lying down for 30 to 60 minutes after taking dose.
• Teach patient to report black tarry stools, vision changes, finger or ankle swelling, weight gain, itching, rash, fever, or sore throat.
• Instruct patient to avoid driving and other hazardous activities until he knows how drug affects concentration, alertness, and balance.
• As appropriate, review all other significant and life-threatening adverse reactions and interactions, especially those related to the drugs, tests, herbs, and behaviors mentioned above.

ibutilide fumarate
Corvert

Pharmacologic class: Ibutilide derivative

Therapeutic class: Antiarrhythmic (class III)

Pregnancy risk category C

Action

Prolongs myocardial action potential by slowing repolarization and atrioventricular (AV) conduction

Availability

Solution: 0.1 mg/ml in 10-ml vials

Indications and dosages

➤ To convert atrial fibrillation or flutter to sinus rhythm
Adults weighing more than 60 kg (132 lb): 1 vial (1 mg) by I.V. infusion over 10 minutes; may repeat after 10 minutes if arrhythmia persists
Adults weighing less than 60 kg (132 lb): 0.1 ml/kg (0.01 mg/kg) by I.V. infusion over 10 minutes; may repeat after 10 minutes if arrhythmia persists

Contraindications

• Hypersensitivity to drug or its components

Administration

◀€ Stop infusion immediately if patient develops sustained or nonsustained ventricular tachycardia.

• As appropriate, administer diluted or undiluted. To dilute, add 10-ml vial to 50 ml of normal saline solution or dextrose 5% in water to yield a concentration of 0.017 mg/ml.

• Infuse drug over 10 minutes.

• Don't give with amiodarone, disopyramide, quinidine, procainamide, or sotalol because of increased risk of dangerous arrhythmias.

Route	Onset	Peak	Duration
I.V.	Immediate	10 min	Unknown

Adverse reactions

CNS: headache, light-headedness, dizziness, numbness or tingling in arms
CV: hypotension, hypertension, ventricular extrasystoles, nonsustained ventricular tachycardia, bundle-branch block, bradycardia, **ventricular arrhythmias, ventricular tachycardia, AV heart block, heart failure**
GI: nausea
GU: renal failure

Interactions

Drug-drug. *Amiodarone, disopyramide, quinidine, procainamide, sotalol:* increased risk of dangerous arrhythmias
Antihistamines, phenothiazines, tricyclic antidepressants: increased proarrhythmic effect (prolonged QT interval)

Precautions

Use cautiously in:
• ventricular and atrioventricular arrhythmias
• pregnant or breastfeeding patients.

Patient monitoring

• Assess electrolyte levels before giving drug. Expect to correct electrolyte abnormalities (especially involving potassium and magnesium) because hypo-

kalemia and hypomagnesemia can lead to arrhythmias.

• Monitor the patient for premature ventricular contractions, sinus tachycardia, sinus bradycardia, and heart block.

• Monitor ECG during infusion and for at least 4 hours afterward.

• Keep emergency equipment (defibrillator, emergency cart and drug box, oxygen, suction, and intubation equipment) at hand during administration and for at least 4 hours afterward.

• Monitor prothrombin time, International Normalized Ratio, and activated partial thromboplastin time if anticoagulant therapy is concurrent.

Patient teaching

• Tell patient he'll be monitored closely for at least 4 hours after drug administration.

• Instruct patient to immediately report chest pain, dizziness, numbness, palpitations, headache, or difficulty breathing.

• As appropriate, review all other significant and life-threatening adverse reactions and interactions, especially those related to the drugs mentioned above.

idarubicin hydrochloride
Idamycin, Idamycin PFS

Pharmacologic class: Anthracycline antibiotic
Therapeutic class: Antineoplastic
Pregnancy risk category D

Action

Unknown; may inhibit nucleic acid synthesis

Availability

Injection: 1 mg/ml

Powder for injection: 5 mg, 10 mg, 20 mg

Route	Onset	Peak	Duration
I.V.	Immediate	Several min	Unknown

⚕ Indications and dosages
➢ Acute myeloid leukemia given with other antileukemic drugs
Adults: 12 mg/m^2/day by slow I.V. injection over 10 to 15 minutes for 3 days. As prescribed, give with cytarabine by continuous I.V. infusion for 7 days, or give cytarabine as I.V. bolus followed by 5 days of cytarabine by continuous I.V. infusion. Second course may be ordered, depending on response.
Dosage adjustment
• Renal or hepatic impairment
• Severe mucositis

Off-label uses
• Acute nonlymphocytic and chronic myelogenous leukemias
• Non-Hodgkin's lymphoma
• Breast cancer

Contraindications
• Hypersensitivity to drug
• Cardiac disease
• Pregnancy or breastfeeding

Administration
• When preparing drug, wear goggles and gloves because exposure may cause severe skin reaction. If exposure occurs, wash affected area immediately with soap and water. If drug contacts eyes, follow standard eye irrigation procedure.
• Reconstitute 5-, 10-, or 20-mg vial with 5, 10, or 20 ml of normal saline solution, respectively, to yield concentration of 1 mg/ml.
• Administer slowly over 10 to 15 minutes into I.V. tubing that's infusing normal saline solution or dextrose 5% in water.
• Don't administer drug S.C. or I.M. because this may cause tissue necrosis.

Adverse reactions
CNS: headache, mental status changes, peripheral neuropathy, **seizures**
CV: chest pain, **heart failure, atrial fibrillation, myocardial infarction, arrhythmias**
GI: nausea, vomiting, diarrhea, cramps, mucositis, **GI hemorrhage**
GU: red urine, **renal failure**
Hematologic: bone marrow depression
Hepatic: hepatic function changes
Metabolic: hyperuricemia
Skin: alopecia, urticaria, bullous erythematous rash on palms and soles, erythema at previously irradiated sites, tissue necrosis or urticaria at injection site
Other: fever, infection, hypersensitivity reaction

Interactions
Drug-drug. *Alkaline solutions, heparin:* incompatibility

Precautions
Use cautiously in:
• renal or hepatic impairment
• bone marrow depression
• previous treatment with anthracyclines or cardiotoxic drugs.

Patient monitoring
• Evaluate injection site for burning, stinging, and extravasation. If extravasation occurs, stop infusion and restart in another vein; rinse area with normal saline solution and apply cold compresses. (Local infiltration with corticosteroids may be indicated.)
• Monitor patient's response to therapy regularly.
• Assess serum uric acid level and complete blood count.

• Monitor hemodynamic status and cardiac output; assess for S_3 heart sound (which signals heart failure).
• Assess fluid intake and output; make sure patient is adequately hydrated to prevent hyperuricemia.

Patient teaching

• Instruct patient to report unusual bleeding or bruising, difficulty breathing, or sudden weight gain.
• Teach patient to eat small, frequent meals.
• Advise patient to keep follow-up appointments for assessment, regular blood testing, and monitoring of drug effects.
• As appropriate, review all other significant and life-threatening adverse reactions and interactions.

ifosfamide
Iflex

Pharmacologic class: Alkylating agent, nitrogen mustard
Therapeutic class: Antineoplastic
Pregnancy risk category D

Action
Alkylates DNA, interfering with replication and synthesis of susceptible cells, which results in cell death

Availability
Injection: 1 g, 3 g in single-dose vials

🕖 Indications and dosages
➢ Germ-cell testicular cancer (given with other antineoplastics and an agent for hemorrhagic cystitis)
Adults: 1.2 g/m²/day by I.V. infusion over 30 minutes for 5 days; therapy may be repeated q 3 weeks or following recovery from hematologic toxicity.

Off-label uses
• Acute leukemia
• Breast, lung, ovarian, and pancreatic cancer
• Malignant lymphomas
• Sarcomas

Contraindications
• Hypersensitivity to drug
• Severe bone marrow depression
• Pregnancy or breastfeeding

Administration
• To reconstitute, add sterile water or bacteriostatic water to vial and shake gently.
• Mix 20 ml of diluent with 1-g vial or 60 ml of diluent with 3-g vial to a concentration of 50 mg/ml. For smaller concentrations, dilute solution further with normal saline solution, dextrose 5% in water, lactated Ringer's solution, or sterile water.
• Administer I.V. slowly over at least 30 minutes.

Route	Onset	Peak	Duration
I.V.	Immediate	Unknown	Unknown

Adverse reactions
CNS: drowsiness, confusion, ataxia, hallucinations, depressive psychosis, dizziness, disorientation, cranial nerve dysfunction, **coma, seizures**
CV: phlebitis
GI: nausea, vomiting, diarrhea, anorexia, stomatitis
GU: hematuria, bladder fibrosis, gonadal suppression, **nephrotoxicity, hemorrhagic cystitis**
Hematologic: anemia, **leukopenia, thrombocytopenia, bone marrow depression**
Hepatic: elevated hepatic enzyme levels
Metabolic: metabolic acidosis, increased uric acid level
Skin: alopecia
Other: infection, **secondary neoplasms**

Interactions
Drug-drug. *Anticoagulants, aspirin, nonsteroidal anti-inflammatory drugs:* increased risk of bleeding
Barbiturates, chloral hydrate, fosphenytoin, phenytoin: increased toxicity
Corticosteroids: decreased ifosfamide effects
Cyclophosphamide: increased risk of cardiac tamponade
Myelosuppressants: increased hematologic toxicity
Drug-diagnostic tests. *Hepatic enzymes:* increased levels
Platelets, white blood cells: decreased counts

Precautions
Use cautiously in:
• impaired renal and hepatic function, bone marrow depression.

Patient monitoring
• Monitor hematopoietic function test results (such as complete blood count with white cell differential) before therapy and weekly during therapy.
• Assess fluid intake and output; ensure intake of at least 2 L of fluids daily to prevent bladder toxicity.
◀ Monitor urine output for hematuria and hemorrhagic cystitis; administer mesna (protective drug), as indicated and prescribed.

Patient teaching
• Teach patient to report jaundice, unusual bleeding or bruising, blood in urine, pain on urination, fever, chills, sore throat, cough, difficulty breathing, unusual lumps or masses, mouth sores, or pain in flank, stomach, or joints.
• Instruct patient to maintain adequate hydration and nutrition; advise him to drink 10 to 12 glasses of fluid daily.
• Inform patient that drug may cause hair loss.
• Advise both male and female patients to use reliable birth control during and

immediately after therapy because drug may cause severe birth defects.
• Urge patient to keep regular follow-up appointments for blood testing and monitoring of drug effects.
• As appropriate, review other significant and life-threatening adverse reactions and interactions, especially those related to the drugs and tests mentioned above.

imatinib mesylate
Gleevec

Pharmacologic class: Protein-tyrosine kinase inhibitor
Therapeutic class: Antineoplastic
Pregnancy risk category D

Action
Inhibits proliferation of Bcr-Abl tyrosine kinase, an abnormal chromosome protein found in most patients with chronic myeloid leukemia (CML). As a result, tumor growth in CML patients is suppressed.

Availability
Capsules: 100 mg

Indications and dosages
➣ CML in chronic phase, accelerated phase, or blast crisis phase (after failure of interferon alpha therapy)
Adults: During chronic phase, 400 mg P.O. daily as a single dose; during accelerated phase or blast crisis, 600 mg P.O. daily as a single dose. Daily dosage may be increased to 600 mg P.O. in chronic phase or to 800 mg P.O. (400 mg b.i.d.) in accelerated phase or blast crisis.
➣ Kit (CD117)-positive unresectable or metastatic malignant GI stromal tumors
Adults: 400 to 600 mg P.O. daily

Dosage adjustment
• Renal, hepatic, or hematologic impairment

Contraindications
• Hypersensitivity to drug or its components

Administration
• Give with a meal and large glass of water.

Route	Onset	Peak	Duration
P.O.	Unknown	2-4 hr	Unknown

Adverse reactions
CNS: headache, fatigue, asthenia, malaise, insomnia, headache, **cerebral hemorrhage**
GI: nausea, vomiting, diarrhea, constipation, anorexia, abdominal pain or cramps, dyspepsia, **GI hemorrhage**
GU: elevated creatinine level
Hematologic: anemia, **hemorrhage, neutropenia, thrombocytopenia**
Hepatic: elevated hepatic enzyme levels, hyperbilirubinemia
Metabolic: hypokalemia
Musculoskeletal: myalgia, muscle cramps, musculoskeletal or joint pain
Respiratory: cough, dyspnea, pneumonia
Skin: rash, pruritus, night sweats, petechiae
Other: weight gain, fluid retention, edema, fever

Interactions
Drug-drug. *Cyclosporine, dihydropyridine calcium channel blockers, pimozide, some HMG-CoA reductase inhibitors, triazolobenzodiazepines:* increased blood levels of these drugs
CYP450-3A4 inducers (such as carbamazepine, dexamethasone, phenobarbital, phenytoin, rifampin): increased metabolism and decreased blood level of imatinib
CYP450-3A4 inhibitors (such as clarithromycin, erythromycin, itraconazole, ketoconazole): decreased metabolism and increased blood level of imatinib
Warfarin: altered warfarin metabolism
Drug-diagnostic tests. *Alanine aminotransferase, alkaline phosphatase, aspartate aminotransferase, bilirubin, creatinine:* increased levels
Hemoglobin, neutrophils, platelets, potassium: decreased values
Drug-herb. *St. John's wort:* decreased imatinib effects

Precautions
Use cautiously in:
• renal or hepatic impairment
• pregnant or breastfeeding patients.

Patient monitoring
• Assess for GI distress. Provide small, frequent meals; consult dietitian if nausea and vomiting persist.
◀❦ Monitor complete blood count before therapy and regularly during therapy; expect to adjust dosage if bone marrow depression occurs.
• Evaluate for edema and fluid retention.
• Measure daily weight and fluid intake and output.

Patient teaching
• Instruct patient to avoid potential sources of infection, such as crowds and people with known infections.
• Tell patient that drug may cause sudden weight gain and fluid retention; teach him to weigh himself daily.
• Instruct patient to contact prescriber if he develops sudden weight gain, swelling, difficulty breathing, signs or symptoms of infection, unusual bleeding or bruising, or jaundice.
• Tell patient that he'll need to undergo frequent blood testing to monitor drug effects.
• As appropriate, review all other significant and life-threatening adverse reactions and interactions, especially those related to the drugs, tests, and herbs mentioned above.

---

imipenem and cilastatin sodium

Primaxin

Pharmacologic class: Carbapenem
Therapeutic class: Anti-infective
Pregnancy risk category C

Action

Imipenem acts against a variety of gram-positive and gram-negative organisms by binding to bacterial cell wall, resulting in cell death. Addition of cilastatin prevents renal inactivation of imipenem, resulting in increased urinary concentration. Imipenem resists actions of many enzymes that degrade most other penicillins and penicillin-like agents.

Availability

Powder for I.M. injection: 500 mg imipenem/500 mg cilastatin, 750 mg imipenem/750 mg cilastatin
Powder for I.V. injection: 250 mg imipenem/250 mg cilastatin, 500 mg imipenem/500 mg cilastatin

Indications and dosages

➤ Lower respiratory tract infections, urinary tract infections, abdominal infections, gynecologic infections, skin infections, bone and joint infections, endocarditis, and polymicrobial infections
Adults: For mild infections, 250 to 500 mg I.V. q 6 hours; for moderate infections, 500 mg I.V. q 6 to 8 hours or 1 g I.V. q 8 hours; for serious infections, 500 mg I.V. q 6 hours to 1 g q 6 to 8 hours or 500 to 750 mg I.M. q 12 hours
Children: 15 to 25 mg/kg I.V. q 6 hours or 10 to 15 mg/kg I.M. q 6 hours
Infants ages 4 weeks to 3 months: 25 mg/kg I.V. q 6 hours

Infants ages 1 to 4 weeks: 25 mg/kg I.V. q 8 hours
Infants age 1 week and younger: 25 mg/kg I.V. q 12 hours
Dosage adjustment
• Renal impairment

Contraindications

• Hypersensitivity to drug, penicillins, or cephalosporins

Administration

• For I.V. use, reconstitute each 250- or 500-mg vial with 10 ml of diluent; shake well.
• For piggyback infusion, add 250- or 500-mg I.V. dose to 100 ml of diluent; shake solution until clear and drug is completely dissolved.
• Infuse doses of 500 mg or less over 20 to 30 minutes; infuse doses of 750 to 1,000 mg over 40 to 60 minutes.
• For I.M. use, inject into large muscle.

Route	Onset	Peak	Duration
I.V.	Rapid	End of infusion	6-8 hr
I.M.	Rapid	1-2 hr	12 hr

Adverse reactions

CNS: dizziness, drowsiness, **seizures**
CV: hypotension
GI: nausea, vomiting, diarrhea, **pseudomembranous colitis**
GU: elevated blood urea nitrogen and creatinine levels
Hematologic: eosinophilia
Hepatic: elevated hepatic enzyme levels, hyperbilirubinemia
Skin: rash, pruritus, diaphoresis, urticaria
Other: phlebitis at I.V. site, fever, superinfection, allergic reactions including **anaphylaxis**

Interactions

Drug-drug. *Aminoglycosides:* interference with imipenem effects
Cyclosporine, ganciclovir: increased risk of seizures

Probenecid: decreased renal excretion of imipenem

Drug-diagnostic tests. *Alanine aminotransferase, alkaline phosphatase, aspartate aminotransferase, bilirubin, blood urea nitrogen, creatinine, lactate dehydrogenase:* increased levels

Direct Coombs' test: positive results

Hematocrit, hemoglobin: decreased levels

Precautions

Use cautiously in:
- seizure disorders, renal impairment
- history of multiple hypersensitivity reactions
- elderly patients
- pregnant or breastfeeding patients
- children (safety not established).

Patient monitoring

◀€ Stay alert for seizures in patients with brain lesions, head trauma, or other CNS disorders and in those receiving more than 2 g daily.
- Assess tissue or fluid culture results obtained before and during therapy.
- Monitor for signs and symptoms of infection, such as fever and elevated white blood cell count. Also evaluate for bacterial and fungal superinfection.

Patient teaching

- Caution patient to report discomfort at I.V. site.
- Instruct patient to report rash, hives, or difficulty breathing, as well as signs or symptoms of superinfection (such as diarrhea, mouth sores, and vaginal itching or discharge).
- As appropriate, review all other significant and life-threatening adverse reactions and interactions, especially those related to the drugs and tests mentioned above.

imipramine hydrochloride
Apo-Imipramine♣, Impril♣, Norfranil, Novopramine♣, Tipramine, Tofranil

imipramine pamoate
Tofranil-PM

Pharmacologic class: Dibenzazepine derivative

Therapeutic class: Tricyclic antidepressant

Pregnancy risk category C

Action

Unknown; may block reuptake of norepinephrine and serotonin at neuronal membrane, potentiating their effects

Availability

Capsules: 75 mg, 100 mg, 125 mg, 150 mg (pamoate)
Tablets: 10 mg, 25 mg, 50 mg, 75 mg (hydrochloride)

🕖 Indications and dosages

➤ Endogenous depression

Adults: 75 to 100 mg P.O. daily in divided doses (not to exceed 200 mg/day for outpatients or 300 mg/day for inpatients)

Elderly patients, adolescents: 30 to 40 mg P.O. daily in divided doses, up to 100 mg/day

➤ Functional enuresis

Children: 25 mg P.O. once daily 1 hour before bedtime. If necessary, increase by 25 mg/day at weekly intervals, up to 75 mg P.O. once daily in children ages 12 and older or up to 50 mg P.O. once daily in children under age 12.

➤ Attention-deficit/hyperactivity disorder

Children ages 6 and older: 2 to 5 mg/ kg P.O. daily in two or three divided doses

---

Off-label uses

• Diabetic neuropathy

Contraindications

• Hypersensitivity to drug or bisulfites
• Untreated narrow-angle glaucoma
• Monoamine oxidase (MAO) inhibitor use within past 14 days

Administration

◀€ Don't give concurrently with MAO inhibitors; interaction may lead to hypotension, tachycardia, and potentially fatal reactions.
• Give with food or milk if GI upset occurs.

Route	Onset	Peak	Duration
P.O.	Unknown	30 min-2 hr	2-6 wk

Adverse reactions

CNS: fatigue, sedation, agitation, confusion, hallucinations, drowsiness, dizziness, extrapyramidal effects, syncope, poor concentration, **cerebrovascular accident, seizures**
CV: hypotension, ECG changes, hypertension, palpitations, tachycardia, **arrhythmias, myocardial infarction, heart block**
EENT: blurred vision, increased intraocular pressure, lacrimation, tinnitus, nasal congestion
GI: nausea, constipation, dry mouth, **paralytic ileus**
GU: urinary retention, urinary tract dilation, gynecomastia, menstrual irregularities, galactorrhea, testicular swelling, libido changes, impotence
Hematologic: eosinophilia, purpura, **bone marrow suppression, agranulocytosis, thrombocytopenia, leukopenia**
Hepatic: elevated alkaline phosphatase (ALP) level, hyperbilirubinemia, **hepatitis**
Metabolic: hyperthermia, hypoglycemia, hyperglycemia

Skin: flushing, diaphoresis, photosensitivity, rash, urticaria, pruritus, vasculitis, petechiae, alopecia
Other: increased appetite, edema, weight gain or loss, drug fever, chills, hypersensitivity reactions

Interactions

Drug-drug. *Adrenergics:* increased hypertensive effect
Carbamazepine, class IC antiarrhythmics, other antidepressants, phenothiazines: additive effects of imipramine
CNS depressants: additive CNS depression
Clonidine: decreased clonidine effects
CYP450-2D6 inhibitors (such as amiodarone, cimetidine, quinidine, ritonavir): increased imipramine effects
Guanethidine: prevention of therapeutic response to imipramine
Levodopa: delayed or decreased levodopa absorption, hypertension
MAO inhibitors: hypotension, tachycardia, potentially fatal reactions
Selective serotonin reuptake inhibitors: increased imipramine blood level
Sparfloxacin: increased risk of cardiovascular reactions
Drug-diagnostic tests. *ALP, bilirubin:* elevated levels
Glucose: increased or decreased levels
Liver function tests: changes in values
Drug-herb. *Angel's trumpet, jimsonweed, scopolia:* increased anticholinergic effects
Chamomile, hops, kava, skullcap, valerian: increased CNS depression
Evening primrose oil: additive or synergistic effects
S-adenosylmethionine (SAM-e), St. John's wort: serotonin syndrome
Drug-behaviors. *Alcohol use:* increased CNS depression
Smoking: increased metabolism and altered effects of imipramine
Sun exposure: increased risk of photosensitivity reaction

Precautions
Use cautiously in:
• cardiovascular disease, prostatic enlargement, seizures, urinary retention
• elderly patients
• pregnant or breastfeeding patients.

Patient monitoring
◀﹦ Closely monitor patient's mood and risk of harming himself; limit drug access if patient may be suicidal.
• Assess for urinary retention and increased intraocular pressure in patients with history of urinary retention or narrow-angle glaucoma.
◀﹦ Monitor blood pressure before and during therapy and before dosage increases.
• Watch for arrhythmias in patients with a history of cardiac disease.
• During withdrawal, monitor for adverse effects, such as headache, malaise, nausea, vomiting, and sleep disturbances (may occur with abrupt withdrawal).
• Assess for signs and symptoms of infection; obtain complete blood count with white cell differential.

Patient teaching
• Instruct patient to eat small, frequent meals to minimize GI upset.
• Inform patient that he may experience changes in sexual function, such as impotence and decreased libido.
• Advise patient to report fever, chills, sore throat, dry mouth, excessive sedation, difficulty urinating, or palpitations.
• Teach patient to avoid driving and other hazardous activities until he knows how drug affects concentration and alertness.
• As appropriate, review all other significant and life-threatening adverse reactions and interactions, especially those related to the drugs, tests, herbs, and behaviors mentioned above.

immune globulin for I.M. use (IGIM)
BayGam

immune globulin for I.V. use, human (IGIV)
Carimune, Gamimune N 5% S/D, Gamimune N 10% S/D, Gammagard S/D, Gammagard S/D 0.5 g, Gammar-P IV, Iveegam EN, Panglobulin, Polygam S/D, Sandoglobulin, Venoglobulin-I, Venoglobulin-S

Pharmacologic class: Immune serum
Therapeutic class: Antibody production stimulator
Pregnancy risk category C

Action
Improves immunity by increasing antibodies against bacterial, viral, parasitic, and mycoplasmic antigens; acts through antimicrobial and antitoxin neutralization

Availability
Injection: 2- and 10-ml vials (IGIM)
Solution (5%): 10-, 50-, 100-, 200-, and 250-ml vials (IGIV)
Solution (10%): 10-, 50-, 100-, and 200-ml vials (IGIV)

⑪ Indications and dosages
➤ To prevent hepatitis A
Adults traveling to areas where hepatitis A is common: 0.02 ml/kg I.M. if staying less than 3 months; 0.06 ml/kg repeated q 4 to 6 months if staying 3 months or longer
Adults with household or institutional contacts: 0.02 ml/kg I.M.
➤ To prevent or reduce severity of measles in susceptible persons
Adults and children: 0.2 ml/kg to

0.25 ml/kg I.M. within 6 days of exposure to measles

➤ Exposure to measles in immunocompromised children

Children: 0.5 ml/kg I.M. as soon as possible after exposure

➤ Varicella in immunocompromised patients

Adults: 0.6 to 1.2 ml/kg I.M. as soon as possible if varicella-zoster immune globulin is unavailable

➤ To reduce risk of infection and fetal damage in women exposed to rubella during early pregnancy

Adults: 0.55 ml/kg I.M.

➤ Immunoglobulin deficiency

Adults: Initially, 1.3 ml/kg I.M., followed in 3 to 4 weeks by 0.66 ml/kg, up to 100 mg/kg q 3 to 4 weeks

➤ Immunodeficiency

Gamimune N—

Adults and children: 100 to 200 mg/kg I.V. or 2 to 4 ml/kg (10%) I.V. monthly

Gammagard S/D—

Adults and children: 200 to 400 mg/kg I.V., then in monthly doses based on clinical response

Gammar-P IV—

Adults: 200 to 400 mg/kg I.V. q 3 to 4 weeks

Children and adolescents: 200 mg/kg I.V. q 3 to 4 weeks

Iveegam EN—

Adults and children: 200 mg/kg I.V. monthly; may be increased up to 800 mg/kg/month based on clinical response

Panglobulin—

Adults and children: 200 mg/kg I.V. monthly, increased to 300 mg/kg/month (or infusion may be repeated more frequently than monthly)

Polygam S/D—

Adults and children: 100 to 400 mg/kg I.V. monthly

Sandoglobulin—

Adults and children: 100 to 400 mg/kg I.V. monthly. In patients with previously untreated agammaglobulinemia or hypogammaglobulinemia, first infu-

sion may be increased to 300 mg/kg or infusion frequency may be increased.

Venoglobulin—

Adults and children: 200 mg/kg I.V. monthly, increased up to 400 mg/kg/month (or infusion may be repeated more frequently than monthly)

➤ Idiopathic thrombocytopenic purpura

Gamimune N—

Adults and children: 400 mg/kg I.V. for 5 consecutive days, or 1,000 mg/kg/day for 1 day or for 2 consecutive days

Gammagard S/D—

Adults and children: 1,000 mg/kg I.V.; up to three doses may be given on alternating days, dependent on platelet count

Polygam S/D—

Adults and children: 1 g/kg I.V. (additional doses may be given, depending on clinical response); or 2,000 mg/kg I.V. over approximately 5 days for induction, with maintenance dosage of 1,000 mg/kg as needed to maintain platelet count of 30,000/mm^3 in children and 20,000/mm^3 in adults or to prevent bleeding between infusions

➤ Kawasaki disease

Gammagard S/D—

Adults and adolescents: 1 g/kg I.V. as a single dose; alternatively, 400 mg/kg/day for 4 consecutive days with aspirin

Iveegam EN—

Adults and children: 400 mg/kg/day I.V. with aspirin

Sandoglobulin—

Adults and children: 400 mg/kg I.V. for 2 to 5 consecutive days; if platelet count falls below 30,000/mm^3 or patient has significant bleeding, 0.4 g/kg may be given as a single infusion, increased up to 0.8 or 1g/kg as a single infusion, depending on clinical response

Venoglobulin S—

Adults and children: 2 g/kg I.V. infused over 10 to 12 hours with aspirin

➤ To prevent bacterial infection in patients with hypogammaglobulinemia or recurrent bacterial infection associated with B-cell chronic lymphocytic leukemia

Adults and adolescents: 400 mg/kg I.V. (Gammagard S/D or Polygam S/D) q 3 to 4 weeks

➤ To reduce the risk of graft-versus-host disease, interstitial pneumonia, septicemia, and other infections during first 100 days after bone marrow transplantation

Adults ages 20 and older: 500 mg/kg I.V. (Gamimune N) 7 days before and 2 days before transplantation and weekly through 90th day after transplantation

➤ To prevent bacterial infection in children with human immunodeficiency virus

Children: 400 mg/kg I.V. (Gamimune N) q 28 days

Off-label uses
• Chronic inflammatory demyelinating polyneuropathy
• Guillain-Barré syndrome

Contraindications
• Hypersensitivity to drug or its components
• Selective immunoglobulin A (IgA) deficiency

Administration
• Before initiating therapy, determine if patient has risk factors for acute renal failure (such as history of diabetes mellitus, renal insufficiency, sepsis, volume depletion, or paraproteinemia; use of nephrotoxic drugs; or age 65 or older).
• Give IGIM by I.M. route only; give IGIV by I.V. route only.
• If sterile laminar airflow conditions aren't available for drug reconstitution, administer immediately; discard unused portion.
• Don't shake vigorously because foaming may occur. Know that cold drug or diluent may take up to 20 minutes to dissolve.

Route	Onset	Peak	Duration
I.V.	Unknown	Unknown	21-28 days
I.M.	Unknown	2 days	Unknown

Adverse reactions
CNS: headache, malaise
CV: chest pain, tachycardia, **thromboembolism**
GI: nausea, vomiting, abdominal pain
Musculoskeletal: joint pain, back pain, myalgia
Respiratory: dyspnea
Skin: pruritus
Other: chills, lymphadenopathy, pain at injection site, **anaphylaxis**

Interactions
Drug-drug. *Live-virus vaccines:* decreased antibody response to vaccine

Precautions
Use cautiously in:
• bleeding disorders, renal impairment
• pregnant patients.

Patient monitoring
◀€ Monitor for acute inflammatory reaction in patients receiving drug for first time (usually appears within 30 to 60 minutes after infusion begins), in those whose last treatment was more than 8 weeks earlier, and when the initial infusion rate exceeds 1 ml/minute.
• Assess fluid volume status and blood urea nitrogen and creatinine levels.
• After infusion is completed, monitor patient closely for nausea, vomiting, drowsiness, and severe headache.

Patient teaching
• Instruct patient to report symptoms that occur during or after drug therapy.
• Advise patient to avoid live-virus vaccines for 3 months after therapy; drug may delay or inhibit body's response to vaccine.
• As appropriate, review all significant and life-threatening adverse reactions

and interactions, especially those related to the drugs mentioned above.

inamrinone lactate
Inocor

Pharmacologic class: Bipyridine derivative

Therapeutic class: Inotropic, vasodilator

Pregnancy risk category C

Action
Inhibits phosphodiestrase enzyme that causes degradation of cyclic adenosine monophosphate (cAMP), thus increasing concentrations of cAMP, which regulates intracellular and extracellular calcium levels; this results in increased myocardial contraction force. Also relaxes and dilates vascular smooth muscle, decreasing preload and afterload.

Availability
Injection: 5 mg/ml in 20-ml ampules

Indications and dosages
➤ Short-term management of heart failure

Adults: Initially, 0.75 mg/kg I.V. bolus over 2 to 3 minutes; may give additional bolus of 0.75 mg/kg over 30 minutes. Then begin maintenance infusion of 5 to 10 mcg/kg/minute. Maximum daily dosage is 10 mg/kg.

Off-label uses
• Open-heart surgery

Contraindications
• Hypersensitivity to drug or bisulfites

Administration
• Administer either undiluted or diluted in normal or half-normal saline solution to yield a concentration of 1 to 3 mg/ml, as prescribed. Don't mix with solutions containing dextrose.
• Give I.V. bolus over 2 to 3 minutes, followed by maintenance infusion.
• Protect drug from exposure to light.

Route	Onset	Peak	Duration
I.V.	2-5 min	10 min	30-120 min

Adverse reactions
CV: hypotension, **arrhythmias**
GI: nausea, vomiting
Hematologic: thrombocytopenia
Hepatic: hepatotoxicity
Other: hypersensitivity reaction

Interactions
Drug-drug. *Cardiac glycosides:* increased inotropic effects
Disopyramide: excessive hypotension
Drug-herb. *Aloe, buckthorn bark, cascara sagrada, ephedra, senna leaf:* increased drug action

Precautions
Use cautiously in:
• renal or hepatic disease, atrial fibrillation or flutter, severe aortic or pulmonic valvular disease, acute phase of myocardial infarction
• elderly patients
• pregnant or breastfeeding patients
• children.

Patient monitoring
◀€ Monitor vital signs frequently; expect to slow or stop infusion if significant hypotension occurs.
• Monitor hemodynamic indicators (including cardiac output, cardiac index, central venous pressure, and pulmonary artery wedge pressure) to assess drug efficacy.
• Assess daily weight and fluid intake and output.
◀€ Watch closely for ventricular arrhythmias, especially if patient has atrial flutter or atrial fibrillation.

• Assess for signs and symptoms of thrombocytopenia, such as bleeding or bruising.
• Monitor platelet count and electrolyte levels.

Patient teaching
• Instruct patient to report dizziness or light-headedness.
• As appropriate, review all other significant and life-threatening adverse reactions and interactions, especially those related to the drugs and herbs mentioned above.

indapamide
Lozide✤, Lozol

Pharmacologic class: Thiazide-like diuretic

Therapeutic class: Diuretic, antihypertensive

Pregnancy risk category B

Action
Increases sodium and water excretion by inhibiting sodium reabsorption in distal tubule; enhances excretion of sodium, chloride, potassium, and water. Also may cause arteriolar vasodilation.

Availability
Tablets: 1.25 mg, 2.5 mg

Indications and dosages
➤ Edema associated with heart failure
Adults: 2.5 mg P.O. daily in morning; after 1 week, may increase to 5 mg/day
➤ Mild to moderate hypertension
Adults: 1.25 mg P.O. daily in morning; may increase q 4 weeks, up to 5 mg/day

Contraindications
• Hypersensitivity to drug, other thiazide-like drugs, or tartrazine
• Anuria

Administration
• Administer with food or milk to reduce GI upset.
• Give early in day to avoid nocturia.

Route	Onset	Peak	Duration
P.O. (single dose)	1-2 hr	2 hr	36 hr

Adverse reactions
CNS: dizziness, light-headedness, headache, restlessness, insomnia, lethargy, fatigue, drowsiness, asthenia, depression, anxiety, nervousness, paresthesia, irritability, agitation
CV: orthostatic hypotension, palpitations, premature ventricular contractions, **arrhythmias**
EENT: blurred vision, rhinorrhea
GI: nausea, vomiting, diarrhea, constipation, bloating, epigastric distress, gastric irritation, abdominal pain or cramps, anorexia, dry mouth
GU: nocturia, polyuria, elevated blood urea nitrogen (BUN) and creatinine levels, glycosuria, impotence
Metabolic: dehydration, gout, hyperglycemia, hypokalemia, hypocalcemia, hypochloremic alkalosis, hypomagnesemia, hyponatremia, hypovolemia, hypophosphatemia, hyperuricemia, hyperlipidemia, decreased protein-bound iodine levels
Musculoskeletal: muscle cramps and spasms
Skin: flushing, rash, urticaria, pruritus, photosensitivity, necrotizing or cutaneous vasculitis
Other: weight loss

Interactions
Drug-drug. *Amphotericin B, corticosteroids:* additive hypokalemia
Antihypertensives, nitrates: additive hypotension
Cholestyramine, colestipol: decreased indapamide absorption
Lithium: decreased lithium excretion, increased risk of lithium toxicity

Sulfonylureas: decreased hypoglycemic efficacy

Drug-diagnostic tests. *Cholesterol, low-density lipoproteins, magnesium, potassium, protein-bound iodine, sodium, triglycerides, urinary calcium:* decreased levels

Bilirubin, blood and urine glucose (in diabetic patients), BUN, calcium, creatinine, uric acid: increased levels

Drug-herb. *Ginkgo:* decreased antihypertensive effects

Licorice, stimulant laxative herbs (aloe, cascara sagrada, senna): increased risk of hypokalemia

Drug-behaviors. *Acute alcohol ingestion:* additive hypotension

Sun exposure: increased risk of photosensitivity

Precautions

Use cautiously in:
• renal or severe hepatic impairment, ascites, fluid or electrolyte imbalances, gout, systemic lupus erythematosus, impaired glucose tolerance, hyperparathyroidism, bipolar disorder
• pregnant or breastfeeding patients.

Patient monitoring

◀≋ Assess for signs and symptoms of hypokalemia, including ventricular arrhythmias, muscle weakness, and cramping.
• Monitor BUN, creatinine, and electrolyte levels.
• Assess daily weight and fluid intake and output.
• Monitor blood pressure response to drug.
• Watch for signs and symptoms of orthostatic hypotension.

Patient teaching

• Advise patient to consume potassium-rich foods, such as oranges, bananas, potatoes, and spinach.
• Instruct patient to move slowly when sitting up or standing to avoid dizziness or light-headedness from sudden blood pressure decrease.
• Teach patient to weigh himself daily on the same scale at the same time of day and wearing similar clothing. Instruct him to report a gain of more than 2 lb (0.9 kg) in 1 day or 5 lb (2.2 kg) in 1 week.
• Instruct patient to avoid driving and other hazardous activities until he knows how drug affects concentration and alertness.
• As appropriate, review all other significant and life-threatening adverse reactions and interactions, especially those related to the drugs, tests, herbs, and behaviors mentioned above.

i

indinavir sulfate
Crixivan

Pharmacologic class: Protease inhibitor

Therapeutic class: Antiretroviral

Pregnancy risk category C

Action

Inhibits replication, function, and maturation of human immunodeficiency virus (HIV) protease, an essential enzyme needed in formation of infectious virus. As a result, further spread of virus is limited.

Availability

Capsules: 100 mg, 200 mg, 333 mg, 400 mg

🕖 Indications and dosages

➤ HIV infection (usually given with other antiretrovirals)

Adults: 800 mg P.O. q 8 hours

Dosage adjustment
• Mild to moderate hepatic insufficiency secondary to cirrhosis

Contraindications

- Hypersensitivity to drug or its components
- Concurrent use of cisapride, triazolam, midazolam, pimozide, or ergot derivatives

Administration

- Give with full glass of water on empty stomach 1 hour before or 2 hours after meals.
- If GI upset occurs, give with a light meal

Route	Onset	Peak	Duration
P.O.	Rapid	0.8 hr	8 hr

Adverse reactions

CNS: depression, dizziness, headache, drowsiness, malaise, asthenia
CV: angina, **myocardial infarction**
EENT: oral paresthesia, abnormal taste
GI: nausea, vomiting, diarrhea, abdominal pain or distention, dyspepsia, acid regurgitation, **pancreatitis**
GU: dysuria, crystalluria, nephrolithiasis or urolithiasis leading to **renal insufficiency or failure, interstitial nephritis**
Hematologic: anemia, acute hemolytic anemia, **increased spontaneous bleeding** (in hemophiliacs)
Hepatic: hepatic dysfunction, jaundice, **hepatic failure**
Metabolic: elevated triglyceride and cholesterol levels, new onset or exacerbation of diabetes mellitus, hyperglycemia
Musculoskeletal: joint or back pain
Respiratory: cough, dyspnea
Skin: urticaria, rash, pruritus
Other: increased or decreased appetite, body fat redistribution or accumulation, fever, **anaphylactoid reactions**

Interactions

Drug-drug. *Azole antifungals, delavirdine, interleukins:* elevated indinavir blood level, greater risk of toxicity

Cisapride, ergot derivatives, midazolam, pimozide, triazolam: CYP-3A4 inhibition by indinavir, leading to increased blood levels of these drugs and dangerous reactions
Didanosine, efavirenz, rifamycins: decreased indinavir effects
Drug-diagnostic tests. *Alanine aminotransferase, amylase, aspartate aminotransferase, bilirubin, glucose:* increased levels
Hemoglobin, neutrophils, platelets: decreased values
Drug-food. *Any food:* decreased indinavir absorption
Drug-herb. *St. John's wort:* decreased indinavir blood level

Precautions

Use cautiously in:

- renal or severe hepatic impairment, history of renal calculi
- pregnant or breastfeeding patients
- children.

Patient monitoring

- Assess fluid intake and output to ensure adequate hydration and prevent nephrolithiasis or urolithiasis.
- Monitor for adverse GI and CNS effects.
- Evaluate liver function test results; assess for hyperbilirubinemia.
- Monitor complete blood count with white cell differential; also assess cholesterol and glucose levels.

Patient teaching

- Teach patient to take drug 1 hour before or 2 hours after meals with a full glass of water.
- If GI upset occurs, advise patient to take drug with a light meal
◀╠ Instruct patient to report severe nausea or diarrhea, fever, chills, flank pain, urine or stool color changes, yellowing of skin or eyes, or personality changes.

• Tell patient that drug doesn't cure HIV infection and that its long-term effects are largely unknown.

• As appropriate, review all other significant and life-threatening adverse reactions and interactions, especially those related to the drugs, tests, foods, and herbs mentioned above.

indomethacin
Apo-Indomethacin✦, Indameth✦, Indochron ER, Indocid✦, Indocin, Indocin SR, Indotec✦, Novo-Methacin✦, Nu-Indo✦, Rhodacine✦

indomethacin sodium trihydrate
Indocin I.V.

Pharmacologic class: Nonsteroidal anti-inflammatory drug (NSAID)

Therapeutic class: Anti-inflammatory, analgesic, antipyretic

Pregnancy risk category B (third trimester: *D*)

Action
Unknown; thought to inhibit cyclooxygenase, an enzyme needed for prostaglandin synthesis

Availability
Capsules: 25 mg, 50 mg
Capsules (sustained-release): 75 mg
Oral suspension: 25 mg/5 ml
Powder for injection: 1-mg vials (sodium trihydrate)
Suppositories: 50 mg, 100 mg

⚠ Indications and dosages
➤ Rheumatoid arthritis; ankylosing spondylitis
Adults: 25 to 50 mg P.O. two or three times daily, not to exceed 200 mg daily; or one 75-mg sustained-release capsule P.O. once or twice daily

➤ Acute gouty arthritis
Adults: 50 mg P.O. t.i.d. until pain is tolerable; then reduce dosage rapidly and, finally, discontinue drug. Don't give sustained-release form.
➤ Acute bursitis or tendinitis of shoulder
Adults: 75 to 150 mg P.O. daily in three or four divided doses; discontinue once inflammation is controlled.
➤ Patent ductus arteriosus (PDA) in premature neonates weighing 500 to 1,750 g (when usual medical management is ineffective after 48 hours)
Neonates: In neonates less than 48 hours old, initially 0.2 mg/kg I.V.; then two subsequent doses of 0.1 mg/kg I.V. at 12- to 24-hour intervals. In neonates 2 to 7 days old, initially 0.2 mg/kg I.V., followed by two subsequent doses of 0.2 mg/kg I.V. at 12- to 24-hour intervals.

Off-label uses
• Bartter's syndrome
• Pericarditis

Contraindications
• Hypersensitivity to drug, its components, or other NSAIDs
• Active GI bleeding
• Concurrent diflunisal use
• Neonates with bleeding, coagulation defects, congenital heart disease, necrotizing enterocolitis, significant renal impairment, thrombocytopenia, or untreated infections

Administration
• Give oral form with food, a full glass of water, or antacids to reduce GI upset.
• Don't open or crush capsules.
• For arthritis, give up to 100 mg of daily dose at bedtime as needed to reduce nighttime pain and morning stiffness.
• Don't administer sustained-release form to patients with gouty arthritis.

✦ Canada   ◀€ Clinical alert   Reactions in **bold** are life-threatening

• Reconstitute I.V. form with 1 or 2 ml of preservative-free normal saline solution or preservative-free sterile water. Solution made with 1 ml of diluent yields a concentration of 100 mcg (0.1 mg) of indomethacin/0.1 ml; solution made with 2 ml of diluent yields a concentration of 50 mcg (0.05 mg) of indomethacin/0.1 ml.

• Give reconstituted solution I.V. over 5 to 10 seconds.

Route	Onset	Peak	Duration
P.O. (analgesic)	30 min	0.5-2 hr	4-6 hr
P.O. (sustained, analgesic)	30 min	Unknown	4-6 hr
P.O. (regular or sustained, anti-inflam.)	Up to 7 days	1-2 wk	Unknown
I.V. (PDA closure)	Up to 48 hr	Unknown	Unknown

Adverse reactions

CNS: headache, dizziness, drowsiness, fatigue, vertigo, depression, epilepsy, Parkinson's disease
EENT: tinnitus
GI: nausea, vomiting, diarrhea, constipation, abdominal pain or cramps, dyspepsia, ulcers, **GI bleeding**
Other: edema, phlebitis at I.V. site, allergic reactions including **anaphylaxis**

Interactions

Drug-drug. *Aminoglycosides, cardiac glycosides:* increased blood levels of these drugs (in infants)
Antihypertensives, diuretics: decreased efficacy of these drugs
Corticosteroids, other NSAIDs: additive adverse GI reactions
Cyclosporine: increased risk of nephrotoxicity
Diflunisal: potentially fatal GI hemorrhage
Lithium, zidovudine: increased risk of toxicity from these drugs

Methotrexate: increased risk of methotrexate toxicity
Probenecid: increased risk of indomethacin toxicity
Drug-diagnostic tests. *Dexamethasone suppression test:* false-negative result
Drug-herb. *Anise, arnica, chamomile, clove, dong quai, feverfew, garlic, ginger, ginkgo, ginseng:* increased risk of bleeding

Precautions

Use cautiously in:
• severe cardiovascular, renal, or hepatic disease
• history of ulcer disease
• elderly patients
• pregnant or breastfeeding patients.

Patient monitoring

• Assess for dizziness, drowsiness, headache, fatigue, and exacerbation of depression, epilepsy, or Parkinson's disease.
• Monitor for drug efficacy, indicated by improved joint mobility, pain relief, and decreased inflammation.
• Watch for signs and symptoms of GI bleeding and ulceration.
• With I.V. use, assess I.V. site for extravasation.

Patient teaching

• Teach patient to take drug with food, full glass of water, or an antacid to reduce GI upset.
• Advise patient not to open or crush capsules.
• Inform breastfeeding patient that indomethacin enters breast milk and may cause seizures in infant. Advise her to use a different infant feeding method during therapy.
• Instruct patient to avoid driving and other hazardous activities until he knows how drug affects concentration, balance, and alertness.
• As appropriate, review all other significant and life-threatening adverse

reactions and interactions, especially those related to the drugs, tests, and herbs mentioned above.

infliximab
Remicade

Pharmacologic class: Monoclonal antibody

Therapeutic class: Antirheumatic, GI anti-inflammatory

Pregnancy risk category C

Action
Neutralizes and prevents activity of tumor necrosis factor-alpha (TNF-alpha), resulting in anti-inflammatory and antiproliferative activity. Also decreases pain and swelling, reduces rate of joint destruction in rheumatoid arthritis, and eases symptoms of Crohn's disease.

Availability
Powder for injection: 100 mg/vial

Indications and dosages
➤ Rheumatoid arthritis (given with methotrexate)
Adults: Initially, 3 mg/kg I.V., followed by 3 mg/kg 2 and 6 weeks after initial dose, then q 8 weeks; in partial responders, dosage may be adjusted up to 10 mg/kg or treatment may be repeated as often as every 4 weeks.
➤ Moderate to severe active Crohn's disease
Adults: 5 mg/kg I.V. as a single infusion over at least 2 hours
➤ To reduce the number of draining enterocutaneous fistulas in patients with fistulizing Crohn's disease
Adults: 5 mg/kg by I.V. infusion, repeated 2 and 6 weeks after initial infusion

Off-label uses
• Complicated ankylosing spondylitis
• Sarcoidosis

Contraindications
• Hypersensitivity to drug, murine proteins, or other drug components
• Heart failure (NYHA class III or IV)

Administration
• Know that latent tuberculosis (TB) should be treated before infliximab therapy begins.
• To reconstitute, use 21G or smaller needle to add 10 ml of sterile water to each vial. To mix, swirl (don't shake); solution may foam and appear clear or light yellow.
• Withdraw volume equal to amount of reconstituted drug from 250-ml polypropylene or polyolefin infusion bag or glass bottle. Add reconstituted drug to infusion bag or bottle; use within 3 hours.
• Administer I.V. infusion over at least 2 hours. Use polyethylene-lined infusion set equipped with in-line, filter with pore size of 1.2 microns or less.

Route	Onset	Peak	Duration
I.V.	1-2 wk	Unknown	12-48 wk

Adverse reactions
CNS: fatigue, headache, anxiety, depression, dizziness, insomnia
CV: chest pain, hypertension, hypotension, tachycardia, peripheral edema, **worsening of heart failure**
EENT: conjunctivitis, rhinitis, sinusitis, laryngitis, pharyngitis, oral pain, tooth pain, moniliasis
GI: nausea, vomiting, diarrhea, constipation, abdominal pain, dyspepsia, flatulence, ulcerative stomatitis, **intestinal obstruction**
GU: dysuria, urinary frequency, urinary tract infection
Hematologic: hematoma, **pancytopenia**

Hepatic: increased hepatic enzyme levels

Musculoskeletal: arthritis, joint pain, back pain, involuntary muscle contractions, myalgia

Respiratory: upper respiratory tract infection, bronchitis, cough, dyspnea

Skin: acne, diaphoresis, dry skin, bruising, eczema, erythema, flushing, pruritus, urticaria, rash, alopecia

Other: chills, hot flashes, flulike symptoms, herpes simplex, herpes zoster, lupuslike syndrome, infections, hypersensitivity reactions, **anaphylaxis**

Interactions

Drug-drug. *Vaccines:* decreased antibody response to vaccine

Drug-diagnostic tests. *Antinuclear antibodies:* positive titers

Hemoglobin: decreased value

Precautions

Use cautiously in:
• history of TB or exposure to TB
• elderly patients
• pregnant or breastfeeding patients
• children (safety not established).

Patient monitoring

• Monitor for signs and symptoms of hypersensitivity reaction, including fever, chills, itching, rash, chest pain, dyspnea, facial flushing, and headache.

• Watch for evidence of infection, especially in patients who are receiving immunosuppressant therapy or have chronic infections. Drug increases risk of life-threatening opportunistic infections (histoplasmosis, listeriosis, pneumocystosis) and TB.

• Assess for heart failure in patients with history of cardiac disease.

• Monitor complete blood count with white cell differential and platelets.

Patient teaching

• Instruct patient to report signs or symptoms of infusion reaction, such as fever, chills, itching, rash, chest pain, dyspnea, facial flushing, and headache; these may occur up to 12 days after therapy.

• Teach patient to report infection symptoms, such as fever, burning on urination, cough, or sore throat.

• Advise patient to avoid potential infection sources, such as crowds and people with known illness or infection.

• As appropriate, review all other significant and life-threatening adverse reactions and interactions, especially those related to the drugs and tests mentioned above.

insulin, regular (insulin injection)

Humulin R, Humulin-R Regular U-500 (concentrate), Iletin II Regular, Insulin-Toronto✚, Novolin ge Toronto✚, Novolin R, Novolin R PenFill, Velosulin BR

insulin (lispro)

Humalog Mix, Humalog Pen

insulin lispro protamine, human

Humalog Mix 50/50, Humalog Mix 75/25 Z

insulin zinc suspension (lente insulin)

Humulin L, Lente Iletin II, Novolin ge Lente✚, Novolin L

insulin zinc suspension, extended (ultralente insulin)

Humulin U, Novolin ge Ultralente, Novolin U, Ultralente U

isophane insulin suspension (NPH insulin)
Humulin N, Novolin N, NPH-N, NPH Iletin II

isophane insulin suspension (NPH) and insulin injection (regular)
Humulin 50/50 (50% isophane insulin and 50% insulin injection), Humulin 70/30 (70% isophane insulin and 30% insulin injection), Humulin 70/30 PenFill, Novolin 70/30, Novolin 70/30 PenFill

Pharmacologic class: Pancreatic hormone
Therapeutic class: Hypoglycemic
Pregnancy risk category B

Action
Promotes glucose transport, which causes stimulation of carbohydrate metabolism in skeletal and cardiac muscle and adipose tissue. Also facilitates phosphorylation of glucose in the liver, where it's converted to glycogen. Directly affects fat and protein metabolism, stimulates protein synthesis, inhibits release of free fatty acids, and indirectly decreases phosphate and potassium.

Availability
Isophane suspension, injection (regular): 70 units NPH and 30 units regular insulin/ml (100 units/ml total), 50 units NPH and 50 units regular insulin/ml (100 units/ml total)
Isophane suspension (NPH insulin): 100 units/ml
Lispro: 100 units/ml in 10-ml vials and 1.5-ml cartridges
Lispro 75/25: insulin lispro/protamine insulin lispro mixture
Regular insulin injection: 100 units/ml
Regular U-500 (concentrated), insulin human injection: 500 units/ml
Zinc suspension, extended (ultralente): 100 units/ml
Zinc suspension (lente insulin): 100 units/ml

Indications and dosages
➤ Type 1 (insulin-dependent) diabetes mellitus, type 2 (non-insulin-dependent) diabetes mellitus unresponsive to dietary modifications and oral hypoglycemics
Adults and children: Individualized dosage given S.C. based on patient's glucose level, adjusted to premeal and bedtime glucose levels. Reserve concentrated insulin (500 units/ml) for patients requiring more than 200 units/day.
➤ Diabetic ketoacidosis (regular insulin)
Adults and children: Loading dose of 0.15 units/kg I.V. bolus, followed by continuous infusion of 0.1 unit/kg/hour until glucose level drops; then S.C. insulin with dosage adjustments according to glucose level

Contraindications
• Hypersensitivity to drug or its components
• Hypoglycemia

Administration
◀ Don't give insulin I.V. (except for nonconcentrated regular insulin) because anaphylactic reactions may occur.
• When mixing two types of insulin, draw up regular insulin into syringe first.
• For I.V. infusion, mix regular insulin only with normal or half-normal saline solution, as prescribed, for a concentration of 1 unit/ml.
• Rotate S.C. injection sites to prevent lipodystrophy.

• Use mixtures of regular and NPH or regular and lente insulins within 5 to 15 minutes of mixing.

Route	Onset	Peak	Duration
I.V. (regular)	10-30 min	15-30 min	Unknown
S.C. (lente)	1-2.5 hr	7-15 hr	24 hr
S.C. (lispro)	15 min	30-90 min	6-8 hr
S.C. (lispro/ protamine mix; regular U-500 conc.)	Unknown	Unknown	Unknown
S.C. (NPH)	1-1.5 hr	4-12 hr	24 hr
S.C. (regular)	30-60 min	2-4 hr	Unknown
S.C. (ultralente)	8 hr	10-30 hr	>36 hr

Adverse reactions

Metabolic: hypokalemia, sodium retention, **hypoglycemia, rebound hyperglycemia (Somogyi effect)**
Skin: urticaria, rash, pruritus
Other: edema; lipodystrophy; lipohypertrophy; erythema, stinging, or warmth at injection site; allergic reactions including **anaphylaxis** (with S.C. injection)

Interactions

Drug-drug. *Acetazolamide, albuterol, antiretrovirals, asparaginase, calcitonin, corticosteroids, cyclophosphamide, danazol, dextrothyroxine, diazoxide, diltiazem, diuretics, dobutamine, epinephrine, estrogens, hormonal contraceptives, isoniazid, morphine, niacin, phenothiazines, phenytoin, somatropin, terbutaline, thyroid hormones:* decreased hypoglycemic effect
Anabolic steroids, angiotensin-converting enzyme inhibitors, calcium, chloroquine, clofibrate, clonidine, disopyramide, fluoxetine, guanethidine, mebendazole, monoamine oxidase inhibitors, *octreotide, oral hypoglycemics, phenylbutazone, propoxyphene, pyridoxine, salicylates, sulfinpyrazone, sulfonamides, tetracyclines:* increased hypoglycemic effect
Beta-adrenergic blockers (nonselective): masking of some hypoglycemia symptoms, delayed recovery from hypoglycemia
Lithium carbonate: decreased or increased hypoglycemic effect
Pentamidine: increased hypoglycemic effect, possibly followed by hyperglycemia
Drug-diagnostic tests. *Glucose, inorganic phosphate, magnesium, potassium:* decreased levels
Liver and thyroid function tests: interference with test results
Urine vanillylmandelic acid: increased level
Drug-herb. *Basil, burdock, glucosamine, sage:* altered glycemic control
Chromium, coenzyme Q10, dandelion, eucalyptus, fenugreek, marshmallow: increased hypoglycemic effect
Garlic, ginseng: decreased blood glucose level
Drug-behaviors. *Alcohol use:* increased hypoglycemic effect
Marijuana use: increased blood glucose level
Smoking: increased blood glucose level, decreased response to insulin

Precautions

Use cautiously in:
• hepatic or renal impairment, hypothyroidism, hyperthyroidism
• elderly patients
• pregnant or breastfeeding patients
• children.

Patient monitoring

• Monitor glucose level frequently to assess drug efficacy and appropriateness of dosage.
• Watch blood glucose level closely in patients converting from one insulin type to another and in patients under

unusual stress, as from surgery or trauma.

• Monitor for signs and symptoms of hypoglycemia (such as CNS changes); keep glucose source at hand in case hypoglycemia occurs.

• Assess for signs and symptoms of hyperglycemia, such as polydipsia, polyphagia, polyuria, and diabetic ketoacidosis (including blood and urinary ketones, metabolic acidosis, extremely elevated blood glucose level, and hypovolemia).

• Monitor for glycosuria.

• Closely evaluate kidney and liver function test results in patients with renal or hepatic impairment.

Patient teaching

• Teach patient how to administer insulin S.C. as appropriate.

• Advise patient to draw up regular insulin into syringe first when mixing two types of insulin. Caution him not to change order of mixing insulins.

• Advise patient to rotate S.C. injection sites and keep a record of sites used, to prevent fatty tissue breakdown.

• Teach patient to recognize and report signs and symptoms of hypoglycemia and hyperglycemia; advise him to carry a glucose source at all times.

• Explain to patient how to monitor and record blood glucose level and, if indicated, urine glucose and ketone levels.

• Instruct patient to store insulin in refrigerator (not freezer) away from direct sunlight.

• Teach patient that dietary changes, activity, and stress can alter blood glucose level and insulin requirement.

• Instruct patient to wear medical identification stating that he is diabetic and takes insulin.

• Advise patient to have regular medical examinations, including eye and dental checkups.

• As appropriate, review all other significant and life-threatening adverse reactions and interactions, especially those related to the drugs, tests, herbs, and behaviors mentioned above.

insulin aspart (rDNA origin)
NovoLog

Pharmacologic class: Pancreatic hormone
Therapeutic class: Hypoglycemic
Pregnancy risk category B

Action
Short-acting insulin form; promotes glucose transport, which causes stimulation of carbohydrate metabolism in skeletal and cardiac muscle and adipose tissue. Also facilitates phosphorylation of glucose in the liver, where it's converted to glycogen. Directly affects fat and protein metabolism, stimulates protein synthesis, inhibits release of free fatty acids, and indirectly decreases phosphate and potassium.

Availability
Injection: 100 units/ml in 10-ml vials and 3-ml PenFill cartridges

Indications and dosages
➣ Type 1 (insulin-dependent) diabetes mellitus, type 2 (non-insulin-dependent) diabetes mellitus
Adults and children ages 6 and older:
Dosage tailored to patient's needs and given in divided doses related to meals; insulin asparte provides 50% to 70% of dose and intermediate or long-acting insulin provides remainder. Dosage range is 0.5 to 1 unit/kg daily in divided doses based on meals.

Contraindications

• Hypersensitivity to drug or its components
• Hypoglycemia

Administration

• Be aware that drug is bioavailable as regular human insulin but has a faster onset and shorter duration.
• Give S.C only, 5 to 10 minutes before a meal.
• When mixing with intermediate or long-acting insulin, draw up insulin aspart into syringe first.
• When giving by pump, don't mix with other insulins.
• Rotate injection sites to prevent lipodystrophy.

Route	Onset	Peak	Duration
S.C.	15 min	1-3 hr	3-5 hr

Adverse reactions

Metabolic: hypokalemia, sodium retention, **hypoglycemia, rebound hyperglycemia (Somogyi effect)**
Musculoskeletal: myalgia
Skin: urticaria, rash, pruritus
Other: edema; lipodystrophy; lipohypertrophy; redness, warmth, or stinging at injection site; allergic reactions including **anaphylaxis**

Interactions

Drug-drug. *Acetazolamide, albuterol, antiretrovirals, asparaginase, calcitonin, corticosteroids, cyclophosphamide, danazol, dextrothyroxine, diazoxide, diltiazem, diuretics, dobutamine, epinephrine, estrogens, hormonal contraceptives, isoniazid, morphine, niacin, phenothiazines, phenytoin, somatropin, terbutaline, thyroid hormones:* decreased hypoglycemic effect
Anabolic steroids, angiotensin-converting enzyme inhibitors, calcium, chloroquine, clofibrate, clonidine, disopyramide, fluoxetine, guanethidine, mebendazole, monoamine oxidase inhibitors, octreotide, oral hypoglycemics, phenyl-

butazone, propoxyphene, pyridoxine, salicylates, sulfinpyrazone, sulfonamides, tetracyclines: increased hypoglycemic effect
Beta-adrenergic blockers (nonselective): masking of some hypoglycemia signs and symptoms, delayed recovery from hypoglycemia
Lithium carbonate: decreased or increased hypoglycemic effect
Pentamidine: increased hypoglycemic effect, possibly followed by hyperglycemia
Drug-diagnostic tests. *Glucose, inorganic phosphate, magnesium, potassium:* decreased levels
Liver and thyroid function studies: test interference
Urine vanillylmandelic acid: increased level
Drug-herb. *Basil, bee pollen, burdock, glucosamine, sage:* altered glycemic control
Chromium, coenzyme Q10, dandelion, eucalyptus, fenugreek, marshmallow: increased hypoglycemic effect
Garlic, ginseng: decreased blood glucose level
Drug-behaviors. *Alcohol use:* increased hypoglycemic effect
Marijuana use: increased blood glucose level
Smoking: increased blood glucose level, decreased response to insulin

Precautions

Use cautiously in:
• hepatic or renal impairment, hypothyroidism, hyperthyroidism
• elderly patients
• pregnant or breastfeeding patients
• children.

Patient monitoring

• Monitor blood glucose level frequently to gauge drug efficacy and appropriateness of dosage.
• Watch blood glucose level closely in patients converting from one insulin type to another and in patients under

unusual stress, as from surgery or trauma.
• Be alert for signs and symptoms of hypoglycemia (such as CNS changes); keep glucose source at hand.
• Assess for evidence of hyperglycemia, such as polydipsia, polyphagia, polyuria, and diabetic ketoacidosis (including urine and blood ketones, metabolic acidosis, extremely elevated blood glucose level, and hypovolemia).
• Monitor for glycosuria.
• Closely monitor kidney and liver function test results in patients with renal or hepatic impairment.

Patient teaching
• Teach patient how to administer insulin S.C. or by injection pen.
• If patient must mix insulin aspart with intermediate or long-acting insulin, instruct him to draw up insulin aspart into syringe first.
• Advise patient to rotate S.C. injection sites and keep a record of sites used, to prevent fatty tissue breakdown.
• Teach patient to recognize and report signs and symptoms of hypoglycemia and hyperglycemia. Advise him to always carry a glucose source.
• Explain to patient how to monitor and record blood glucose level and, if indicated, urine glucose and ketone levels.
• Inform patient that changes in diet, activity, and stress level affect blood glucose levels and insulin requirements.
• Teach patient to wear medical identification stating that he is diabetic and takes insulin.
• Instruct patient to have regular medical, vision, and dental examinations.
• Advise patient to store insulin in refrigerator; tell him not to freeze it.
• As appropriate, review all other significant and life-threatening adverse reactions and interactions, especially those related to the drugs, tests, herbs, and behaviors mentioned above.

insulin glargine (rDNA origin)
Lantus

Pharmacologic class: Pancreatic hormone
Therapeutic class: Hypoglycemic
Pregnancy risk category C

Action
Long-acting insulin form; promotes glucose transport, which causes stimulation of carbohydrate metabolism in skeletal and cardiac muscle and adipose tissue. Also facilitates phosphorylation of glucose in the liver, where it's converted to glycogen. Directly affects fat and protein metabolism, stimulates protein synthesis, inhibits release of free fatty acids, and indirectly decreases phosphate and potassium.

Availability
Injection: 100 units/ml in 10-ml vials and 3-ml cartridges

⚠ Indications and dosages
➤ Type 1 insulin-dependent diabetes mellitus in patients needing long-acting insulin
Adults and children ages 6 and older: For patients taking once-daily NPH or ultralente human insulin, start at same dosage as current insulin dosage. For patients taking twice-daily NPH or ultralente human insulin, the initial dose of glargine should be reduced by approximately 20% of the current insulin dosage for the first week; then adjust based on blood glucose levels.
➤ Type 2 non-insulin-dependent diabetes mellitus in patients treated with oral antidiabetics
Adults: Highly individualized dosage based on glucose levels and response to therapy

---

Contraindications

- Hypersensitivity to drug or its components
- Hypoglycemia

Administration

- Give by S.C. route only, 30 to 60 minutes before a meal or evening snack.
- Don't mix in solution with other drugs, including other insulins.
- Before drawing up insulin into syringe, roll vial between hands to ensure uniform dispersion; don't shake.
- Rotate injection sites to prevent lipodystrophy.

Route	Onset	Peak	Duration
S.C.	1.1 hr	5 hr	24 hr

Adverse reactions

Metabolic: rebound hyperglycemia **(Somogyi effect), hypoglycemia**
Skin: urticaria, rash, pruritus, redness, stinging, or warmth at injection site
Other: edema, lipodystrophy, lipohypertrophy, allergic reactions including **anaphylaxis**

Interactions

Drug-drug. *Acetazolamide, albuterol, antiretrovirals, asparaginase, calcitonin, corticosteroids, cyclophosphamide, danazol, dextrothyroxine, diazoxide, diltiazem, diuretics, dobutamine, epinephrine, estrogens, hormonal contraceptives, isoniazid, morphine, niacin, phenothiazines, phenytoin, somatropin, terbutaline, thyroid hormones:* decreased hypoglycemic effect
Anabolic steroids, angiotensin-converting enzyme inhibitors, calcium, chloroquine, clofibrate, clonidine, disopyramide, fluoxetine, guanethidine, mebendazole, monoamine oxidase inhibitors, octreotide, oral hypoglycemics, phenylbutazone, propoxyphene, pyridoxine, salicylates, sulfinpyrazone, sulfonamides, tetracyclines: increased hypoglycemic effect

Beta-adrenergic blockers (nonselective): masking of some hypoglycemia signs and symptoms, delayed recovery from hypoglycemia
Lithium carbonate: altered hypoglycemic effect
Pentamidine: increased hypoglycemic effect, possibly followed by hyperglycemia
Drug-diagnostic tests. *Glucose, inorganic phosphate, magnesium, potassium:* decreased levels
Liver and thyroid function studies: test interference
Urine vanillylmandelic acid: increased level
Drug-herb. *Basil, bee pollen, burdock, glucosamine, sage:* altered glycemic control
Chromium, coenzyme Q10, dandelion, eucalyptus, fenugreek, marshmallow: increased hypoglycemic effect
Garlic, ginseng: decreased blood glucose level
Drug-behaviors. *Alcohol use:* increased hypoglycemic effect
Marijuana use: increased blood glucose level
Smoking: increased blood glucose level, decreased response to insulin

Precautions

Use cautiously in:
- pregnant or breastfeeding patients
- children.

Patient monitoring

- Monitor blood glucose level frequently to assess drug efficacy and appropriateness of dosage.
- Watch blood glucose level closely in patients converting from one insulin type to another and in patients under unusual stress, as from surgery or trauma.
- Check for signs and symptoms of hypoglycemia (such as CNS changes); keep glucose source at hand.
- Monitor for signs and symptoms of hyperglycemia, such as polydipsia,

polyphagia, polyuria, and diabetic ketoacidosis (including blood and urine ketones, metabolic acidosis, extremely elevated blood glucose level, and hypovolemia).

• Monitor for glycosuria.

• Closely monitor kidney and liver function test results in patients with renal or hepatic impairment.

Patient teaching

• Instruct patient how to administer insulin S.C.

• Teach patient to recognize and report signs and symptoms of hypoglycemia and hyperglycemia. Advise him to always carry glucose source.

• Explain to patient how to monitor and record blood glucose level and, if indicated, urine glucose and ketone levels.

• Advise patient to rotate S.C. injection sites and keep a record of sites used.

• Inform patient that changes in diet, activity, and stress level can affect blood glucose level and insulin requirements.

• Teach patient to wear medical identification stating that he is diabetic and takes insulin.

• As appropriate, review all other significant and life-threatening adverse reactions and interactions, especially those related to the drugs, tests, herbs, and behaviors mentioned above.

interferon alfa-2a, recombinant
Roferon-A

interferon alfa-2b, recombinant
Intron A

Pharmacologic class: Biological response modifier

Therapeutic class: Antineoplastic, antiviral

Pregnancy risk category C

Action

Unknown; antitumor and antiviral activity may be related to drug's direct antiproliferative action against tumor or viral cells, inhibition of viral replication, and modulation of host immune response.

Availability
alfa-2a

Injection (single-use vials): 3 million IU, 9 million IU, 36 million IU

Injection (multidose vials): 9 million IU, 18 million IU

Sterile powder for injection: 18 million IU with diluent

alfa-2b

Injection: 3 million IU/0.5-ml vial, 5 million IU/0.5-ml vial, 1 million IU/ 1-ml vial, 10 million IU/1-ml vial; 18 million IU/3.2-ml vial, 25 million IU/ 3.2 ml vial

Powder for injection (vial with diluent): 3 million IU, 5 million IU, 10 million IU, 18 million IU, 25 million IU, 50 million IU

⚕ Indications and dosages
➢ Chronic hepatitis C

alfa-2a—

Adults: 3 million IU S.C. or I.M. three times weekly for 48 to 52 weeks. As alternative regimen, give induction dose of 6 million IU S.C. or I.M. three times weekly for first 12 weeks; then give 3 million IU three times weekly for 36 weeks. Lack of response after 3 months warrants drug withdrawal; prescriber may order 6 to 12 months of retreatment with either 3 or 6 million IU three times weekly.

alfa-2b—

Adults: 3 million IU I.M. or S.C. three times weekly. If patient tolerates therapy and alanine aminotransferase (ALT) level is normal after 16 weeks, continue for 18 to 24 weeks. If ALT doesn't normalize, drug may be withdrawn.

➤ Chronic hepatitis B

alfa-2b—

Adults: 30 to 35 million IU S.C. or I.M. weekly for 16 weeks, given as 5 million IU daily or 10 million IU three times weekly

➤ Hairy cell leukemia

alfa-2a—

Adults: 3 million IU S.C. or I.M. daily for 16 to 24 weeks; maintenance dosage is 3 million IU S.C. or I.M. three times weekly.

alfa-2b—

Adults: 2 million IU/m² I.M. or S.C. three times weekly for 6 months or longer

➤ AIDS-related Kaposi's sarcoma

alfa-2a—

Adults: 36 million IU S.C. or I.M. daily for 10 to 12 weeks; maintenance dosage is 36 million IU S.C. or I.M. three times weekly. Dosage may start at 3 million IU and increase q 3 days until reaching daily dosage of 36 million IU.

alfa-2b—

Adults: 30 million IU/m² S.C. or I.M. three times weekly; continue dosage unless patient becomes intolerant or disease advances rapidly.

➤ Chronic myelogenous leukemia (Philadelphia chromosome–positive)

alfa-2a—

Adults: Initially, 3 million IU S.C. or I.M. daily for 3 days, then 6 million IU for 3 days, then 9 million IU daily for duration of treatment

➤ Malignant melanoma (as adjunct to surgery in patients at high risk for systemic recurrence for up to 8 weeks after surgery)

alfa-2b—

Adults: 20 million IU/m² I.V. for 5 consecutive days per week for 4 weeks; then a maintenance dosage of 10 million IU/m² S.C. three times weekly for 48 weeks. Stop drug if patient has adverse reactions. When reactions ease, resume therapy at half of previous dosage. Withdraw drug if reactions persist.

➤ Condyloma acuminatum (genital or venereal warts)

alfa-2b—

Adults: 1 million IU/lesion intralesionally three times weekly for 3 weeks

➤ Initial treatment of clinically aggressive follicular non-Hodgkin's lymphoma

alfa-2b—

Adults: 5 million IU S.C. three times weekly for up to 18 months (given with chemotherapy regimen containing anthracycline)

Off-label uses
• Adjuvant treatment of malignant melanoma
• Hepatitis D

Contraindications
• Hypersensitivity to drug or its components
• Autoimmune disorders
• Pregnant women or female partners of males receiving drug

Administration
• Administer alfa-2a by S.C or I.M. route. Reconstitute with 3 ml of dilu-

ent provided by manufacturer; swirl gently to dissolve.

• Administer alfa-2b by S.C., I.M., or I.V. route. For I.V. use, reconstitute with diluent provided by manufacturer (bacteriostatic water for injection), according to chart provided. Mix gently, draw drug up into sterile syringe, and inject into 100 ml of normal saline solution. Infuse dose slowly over 20 minutes.

• Give antiemetics, as needed and prescribed, for nausea and vomiting.

Route	Onset	Peak	Duration
I.V. (alfa-2b)	Unknown	15-60 min	4 hr
I.M.	Unknown	2-12 hr	Unknown
S.C.	Unknown	3-12 hr	Unknown

Adverse reactions

CNS: dizziness, confusion, paresthesia, rigors, lethargy, depression, difficulty thinking or concentrating, insomnia, anxiety, fatigue, asthenia, amnesia, malaise, nervousness, drowsiness, **suicidal ideation**

CV: chest pain, hypertension, palpitations, **arrhythmias**

EENT: visual disturbances, stye, hearing disorders, nasal congestion, sinusitis, rhinitis, pharyngitis

GI: nausea, vomiting, diarrhea, constipation, abdominal pain, dyspepsia, flatulence, intestinal obstruction, eructation, stomatitis, gingivitis, dry mouth

GU: elevated blood urea nitrogen and creatinine levels, gynecomastia, impaired fertility in women, transient impotence

Hematologic: anemia, decreased hemoglobin, **leukopenia, thrombocytopenia, neutropenia**

Hepatic: elevated ALT, alkaline phosphatase (ALP), and aspartate aminotransferase (AST) levels; hyperbilirubinemia

Metabolic: hyperglycemia; hypocalcemia; elevated lactate dehydrogenase (LD), phosphorus, neutralizing antibodies, and uric acid levels

Musculoskeletal: joint pain, back pain, myalgia

Respiratory: cough, dyspnea

Skin: flushing, rash, dry skin, pruritus, alopecia, candidiasis, dermatitis, diaphoresis

Other: flulike symptoms, edema, weight loss

Interactions

Drug-drug. *Aminophylline, theophylline:* reduced clearance of these drugs
CNS depressants: additive CNS effects
Live-virus vaccines: decreased antibody response to vaccine, increased risk of adverse reactions
Zidovudine: synergistic effects

Drug-diagnostic tests. *ALP, ALT, AST, calcium, fasting glucose, LD, phosphate:* increased levels
Hemoglobin, platelets, white blood cells: decreased values
International Normalized Ratio, partial thromboplastin time, prothrombin time: increased values

Precautions

Use cautiously in:
• cardiac or pulmonary disease; bone marrow, autoimmune, seizure, or psychiatric disorders
• diabetic patients prone to ketoacidosis
• pregnant or breastfeeding patients
• children.

Patient monitoring

◀€ Before therapy and monthly during therapy, assess complete blood count with white cell differential, granulocyte count, bone marrow hairy cells, glucose and electrolyte levels, and liver and kidney function test results.
• Monitor fluid intake and output; keep patient well hydrated.
• Assess for GI upset; provide small, frequent meals, and give antiemetics to ease severe nausea and vomiting.

◀€ Monitor for mental status changes, depression, and suicidal ideation.

• Assess for bleeding and bruising.
• Institute infection-control measures; monitor for signs and symptoms of infection.

Patient teaching

• Teach patient or caregiver how to prepare and administer drug S.C. or I.M., rotate injection sites, and track dosing schedule and injection sites on calendar.
• Instruct patient to avoid driving and other hazardous activities until he knows how drug affects concentration, alertness, and vision.
• Inform female patients that drug has been linked to fetal abnormalities. Caution them not to get pregnant during therapy; advise them to use barrier birth-control method.
• Advise patient to avoid potential infection sources, such as crowds and people with known infections.
• Teach patient to eat small, frequent meals to combat nausea, vomiting, and loss of appetite.
• Advise male patients that drug may cause transient impotence.
• Teach patient to immediately report depression, suicidal thoughts, mental status changes, signs or symptoms of infection (such as fever, chills, sore throat), unusual bleeding or bruising, dizziness, palpitations, or chest pain.
• Tell patient he'll need regular follow-up examinations and blood tests to gauge drug effects.
• As appropriate, review all other significant and life-threatening adverse reactions and interactions, especially those related to the drugs and tests mentioned above.

interferon alfacon-1
Infergen

Pharmacologic class: Biological response modifier
Therapeutic class: Antiviral
Pregnancy risk category C

Action
Blocks viral replication and stimulates host immunomodulatory activity

Availability
Injection: 9-mcg/0.3-ml vials, 15-mcg/0.5-ml vials

🖊 Indications and dosages
➤ Chronic hepatitis C
Adults: 9 mcg S.C. as a single injection three times weekly for 24 weeks; wait at least 48 hours between doses.

Off-label uses
• Hairy cell leukemia

Contraindications
• Hypersensitivity to drug or *Escherichia coli*–derived products

Administration
• Administer by S.C. route.
• Give antiemetics for nausea and vomiting, as needed and prescribed.

Route	Onset	Peak	Duration
S.C.	Unknown	24-36 hr	Unknown

Adverse reactions
CNS: dizziness, confusion, rigors, paresthesia, lethargy, depression, difficulty thinking or concentrating, insomnia, anxiety, fatigue, amnesia, nervousness, drowsiness, asthenia, malaise, **suicidal ideation**
CV: chest pain, hypertension, palpitations, **arrhythmias**

EENT: visual disturbances, stye, hearing disorders, nasal congestion, rhinitis, sinusitis, pharyngitis

GI: nausea, vomiting, diarrhea, constipation, abdominal pain, dyspepsia, flatulence, eructation, anorexia, intestinal obstruction, stomatitis, gingivitis, dry mouth

GU: elevated blood urea nitrogen and creatinine levels, impaired fertility in women, gynecomastia, transient impotence

Hematologic: anemia, decreased hemoglobin, **leukopenia, thrombocytopenia, neutropenia**

Hepatic: increased alkaline phosphatase (ALP), aspartate aminotransferase (AST), and bilirubin levels

Metabolic: hyperglycemia; hypocalcemia; increased lactate dehydrogenase, phosphorus, neutralizing antibodies, and uric acid levels

Musculoskeletal: joint pain, back pain, myalgia

Respiratory: cough, dyspnea

Skin: rash, dryness, pruritus, flushing, alopecia, candidiasis, dermatitis, diaphoresis

Other: flulike symptoms, edema, weight loss

Interactions

Drug-drug. *Drugs metabolized by CYP450:* altered blood levels of both drugs

Drug-diagnostic tests. *Granulocytes, hemoglobin, platelets, white blood cells:* decreased values

ALP, AST, International Normalized Ratio, prothrombin time, triglycerides: increased values

Precautions

Use cautiously in:
• thyroid disorders, bone marrow depression, hepatic or cardiac disease, seizure disorders, compromised CNS function, severe psychiatric disorders
• pregnant or breastfeeding patients
• children age 18 and younger.

Patient monitoring

◀€ Before and regularly during therapy, assess complete blood count with white cell differential and hepatitis C virus antibody levels.

• Assess fluid intake and output; keep patient well hydrated.

• Monitor for GI upset; provide small, frequent meals and give antiemetics, as prescribed, to ease severe nausea and vomiting.

◀€ Stay alert for depression, mental status changes, psychosis, and suicidal ideation (especially in patients with history of mental illness).

• Assess for bleeding and bruising.

• Institute infection-control measures; monitor for signs and symptoms of infection.

• Monitor for flulike symptoms.

Patient teaching

• Teach patient or caregiver how to administer drug S.C., rotate injections sites, and track dosing schedule and injection sites on calendar.

• Advise patient to avoid sources of potential infection, such as crowds and people with known infections.

• Teach patient to eat small, frequent meals to combat nausea, vomiting, and appetite loss.

• Instruct patient to avoid driving and other hazardous activities until he knows how drug affects concentration, alertness, and vision.

• Inform female patients that drug has been linked to fetal abnormalities. Caution them not to get pregnant during therapy. Advise them to use barrier birth-control method.

• Instruct patient to report signs of symptoms of infection (such as fever, chills, sore throat), unusual bleeding or bruising, mental status changes, dizziness, palpitations, or chest pain.

• Tell patient he'll need regular follow-up examinations and blood tests to gauge drug effects.

• As appropriate, review all other significant and life-threatening adverse reactions and interactions, especially those related to the drugs and tests mentioned above.

interferon beta-1a
Avonex, Rebif

interferon beta-1b
Betaseron

Pharmacologic class: Biological response modifier

Therapeutic class: Antiviral, immunoregulator

Pregnancy risk category C

Action
Binds and competes with specific receptors on cell surface, inducing various interferon-induced gene products; also inhibits proliferation of T cells

Availability
Lyophilized powder for injection (beta-1a): 22 mcg (6 million IU; Rebif), 33 mcg (6.6 million IU; Avonex), 44 mcg (12 million IU; Rebif)
Powder for injection (beta-1b): 0.3 mg (9.6 million IU)
Prefilled syringes (beta-1a): 30 mcg/0.5 ml (Avonex)

⚕ Indications and dosages
➤ To reduce frequency of exacerbations in relapsing-remitting multiple sclerosis
Adults ages 18 and older: 8.8 mcg (Rebif) S.C. three times weekly, increased over 4-week period to 44 mcg S.C. three times weekly. Or 30 mcg (Avonex) I.M. once a week. Or 8 million IU (0.25 mg) S.C. (Betaseron) every other day.

Contraindications
• Hypersensitivity to drug, its components, or albumin

Administration
• Reconstitute Avonex (I.M. injection) and Rebif (S.C. injection) using diluent provided by manufacturer, according to instructions provided.
• Reconstitute Betaseron (S.C. injection) using 1.2 ml of diluent supplied by manufacturer, to yield a concentration of 0.25 mg/ml. Swirl gently to mix; don't shake. Use reconstituted drug within 3 hours; discard unused portion.

Route	Onset	Peak	Duration
I.M.	Unknown	Unknown	Unknown
S.C.	Unknown	1-8 hr	Unknown

Adverse reactions
CNS: dizziness, confusion, rigors, paresthesia, lethargy, depression, difficulty thinking or concentrating, insomnia, anxiety, fatigue, amnesia, nervousness, drowsiness, asthenia, malaise, **suicidal ideation**
CV: chest pain, hypertension, palpitations, **arrhythmias**
EENT: visual disturbances, stye, hearing disorders, nasal congestion, sinusitis, rhinitis, pharyngitis
GI: nausea, vomiting, diarrhea, constipation, abdominal pain, dyspepsia, flatulence, intestinal obstruction, eructation, stomatitis, gingivitis, dry mouth
GU: elevated blood urea nitrogen and creatinine levels, gynecomastia, breast pain, early or delayed menses, menstrual bleeding or spotting, shortened duration of menstrual flow, menorrhagia
Hematologic: decreased hemoglobin, anemia, **neutropenia, leukopenia, thrombocytopenia**
Hepatic: increased alanine aminotransferase (ALT), alkaline phosphatase (ALP), aspartate aminotransferase (AST), and bilirubin levels

Metabolic: increased glucose, lactate dehydrogenase, neutralizing antibodies, phosphorus, and uric acid levels; hypocalcemia

Musculoskeletal: joint pain, back pain, myalgia, myasthenia

Respiratory: cough, dyspnea

Skin: rash, dry skin, pruritus, flushing, alopecia, candidiasis, dermatitis, diaphoresis

Other: flulike symptoms, weight loss, edema, lymphadenopathy, inflammation, pain

Interactions

Drug-diagnostic tests. *ALP, ALT, AST, bilirubin:* increased levels
Neutrophils, white blood cells: decreased counts

Precautions

Use cautiously in:
• cardiac disease, seizure disorders, mental disorders, depression, suicidal tendencies
• women of childbearing age
• pregnant or breastfeeding patients
• children ages 18 and younger.

Patient monitoring

◀⁞ Before therapy and monthly during therapy, assess complete blood count with white cell differential, granulocyte count, bone marrow hairy cells, glucose and electrolyte levels, and liver and kidney function test results.
• Assess fluid intake and output; keep patient well hydrated.
• Watch for GI upset; provide small, frequent meals to minimize nausea and vomiting.
◀⁞ Monitor patient for mental status changes, depression, and suicidal ideation.
• Evaluate for bleeding and bruising.
• Institute infection-control measures; monitor for signs and symptoms of infection.

Patient teaching

• Teach patient or caregiver how to administer drug S.C. or I.M., rotate injection sites, and track dosing schedule and injection sites on calendar.
• Advise patient to avoid sources of potential infection, such as crowds and people with known infections.
• Teach patient to eat small, frequent meals to combat nausea, vomiting, and appetite loss.
• Instruct patient to avoid driving and other hazardous activities until he knows how drug affects concentration, alertness, and vision.
• Tell patient to contact prescriber immediately if depression and suicidal ideation occur.
• Inform female patients that drug has been linked to fetal abnormalities. Caution them not to get pregnant during therapy; advise them to use barrier birth-control method.
• Instruct patient to report signs of symptoms of infection (such as fever, chills, sore throat, achiness), unusual bleeding or bruising, mental status changes, dizziness, palpitations, or chest pain.
• Tell patient he'll need regular follow-up examinations and blood tests to monitor drug effects.
• As appropriate, review significant and life-threatening adverse reactions and interactions, especially those related to the tests mentioned above.

interferon gamma-1b
Actimmune

Pharmacologic class: Biological response modifier
Therapeutic class: Antineoplastic
Pregnancy risk category C

Action
Produced by human leukocytes in response to infectious stimuli. Enhances cellular toxicity and killer cell activity and promotes generation of oxygen metabolites in phagocytes, resulting in destruction of microorganisms.

Availability
Injection: 100 mcg (2 million IU)/0.5-ml vial

Indications and dosages
➤ Chronic granulomatous disease, severe malignant osteopetrosis
Adults with body surface area (BSA) greater than 0.5 m²: 50 mcg/m² (1 million IU/m²) S.C. three times weekly at bedtime
Adults with BSA of 0.5 m² or less: 1.5 mcg/kg S.C. three times weekly in deltoid or anterior thigh

Contraindications
• Hypersensitivity to drug, its components, or *Escherichia coli*–derived products

Administration
• Administer by S.C. route only and into the deltoid muscle.
• Give at bedtime if flulike symptoms occur.
• Provide antiemetics to ease nausea and vomiting, as prescribed.

Route	Onset	Peak	Duration
S.C.	Unknown	7 hr	Unknown

Adverse reactions
CNS: dizziness, confusion, paresthesia, lethargy, depression, difficulty thinking or concentrating, insomnia, anxiety, fatigue, amnesia, nervousness, drowsiness, asthenia, malaise
CV: chest pain, hypertension, palpitations, **arrhythmias**
GI: nausea, vomiting, diarrhea, constipation, abdominal pain, **pancreatitis**
GU: proteinuria

Hematologic: anemia, **leukopenia, thrombocytopenia, neutropenia**
Musculoskeletal: joint pain, back pain, myalgia
Skin: flushing, rash, dry skin, erythema
Other: flulike symptoms, weight loss, edema

Interactions
Drug-drug. *Bone marrow depressants:* increased bone marrow depression
Zidovudine: increased zidovudine blood level
Drug-diagnostic tests. *Hepatic enzymes:* increased levels
Neutrophils, platelets: decreased counts

Precautions
Use cautiously in:
• thyroid disorders, bone marrow depression, hepatic or cardiac disease, seizure disorders, compromised CNS function
• children ages 18 and younger.

Patient monitoring
◀€ Before therapy begins and monthly during therapy, assess complete blood count with white cell differential, granulocyte count, bone marrow hairy cells, glucose and electrolyte levels, and liver and kidney function tests results.
• Assess fluid intake and output; keep patient well hydrated to reduce risk of hypotension.
• Monitor for GI upset; provide small, frequent meals or antiemetics to ease severe nausea and vomiting.
◀€ Monitor patient for mental status changes and depression.
• Assess for flulike symptoms; if present, give drug at bedtime and provide supportive care, such as rest and acetaminophen for headache and fever.

Patient teaching
• Teach patient or caregiver how to give drug S.C., rotate injection sites,

and track dosing schedule and injection sites on calendar.

• Tell patient to contact prescriber immediately if depression occurs.

• Teach patient to eat small, frequent meals to combat nausea, vomiting, and appetite loss.

• Instruct patient to avoid driving and other hazardous activities until he knows how drug affects concentration and alertness.

• Inform female patients that drug has been linked to fetal abnormalities. Caution them not to get pregnant during therapy; advise them to use barrier birth-control method.

• Tell patient he'll need regular follow-up examinations and blood tests to monitor drug effects.

• As appropriate, review all other significant and life-threatening adverse reactions and interactions, especially those related to the drugs and tests mentioned above.

ipecac syrup
PMS-Ipecac✣

Pharmacologic class: Antidote
Therapeutic class: Emetic
Pregnancy risk category C

Action
Stimulates chemoreceptor trigger zone in CNS to induce vomiting; acts by irritating gastric mucosa

Availability
Syrup: 1.5% to 2% alcohol in 15-ml and 30-ml solution

⚕ Indications and dosages
➤ To induce vomiting in overdose or poisoning

Adults and children ages 12 and older: 15 to 30 ml P.O., followed by three to four 8-oz glasses of water; repeat 15-ml dose if patient doesn't vomit within 20 minutes. If patient doesn't vomit within 45 minutes after second dose, gastric lavage smay be ordered.

Children ages 1 to 12: 15 ml P.O., followed by one to two 4- to 8-oz glasses of water; repeat dose if patient doesn't vomit within 20 minutes. If patient doesn't vomit within 45 minutes after second dose, gastric lavage or activated charcoal may be ordered.

Infants ages 6 months to 1 year: 5 to 10 ml P.O., followed by one-half to one full glass of water

Contraindications
• Severe inebriation
• Anaphylaxis
• Seizures
• Shock
• Severe hypotension
• Poisoning with petroleum distillates, alkalis, strong acids, or strychnine

Administration
• Give orally to conscious patient as soon as possible after poisoning or overdose.

• Administer with adequate amounts of water.

• If vomiting doesn't occur within 20 minutes, repeat dose. If vomiting doesn't occur within 45 minutes after second dose, gastric lavage or activated charcoal is indicated. (If poisoning occurs in settings outside medical facilities, consult poison control center if patient doesn't vomit within 45 minutes after second dose.)

Route	Onset	Peak	Duration
P.O.	20 min	Unknown	20-25 min

Adverse reactions
Note: Most adverse reactions result from significant absorption and occur only if patient does not vomit.
CNS: nervousness, headache, fatigue, insomnia, depression, **seizures, coma**

CV: hypotension, bradycardia, palpitations, **arrhythmias, myocarditis**
EENT: blurred vision
GI: nausea, diarrhea, bloody diarrhea

Interactions
Drug-drug. *Activated charcoal:* neutralization of emetic effects

Precautions
Use cautiously in:
• pregnant or breastfeeding patients.

Patient monitoring
• Monitor vital signs and neurologic, respiratory, and cardiac status.
• Keep emergency equipment at hand in case of respiratory or cardiac arrest.
• Monitor parameters as applicable to specific toxic agent or drug ingested.

Patient teaching
• Instruct adults to drink at least 8 oz of water after taking ipecac and children to drink at least 4 to 8 oz of water after taking ipecac.
◀ Caution patient or parents not to confuse ipecac syrup with ipecac fluid extract, which is much stronger and potentially fatal.
• As appropriate, review all significant and life-threatening adverse reactions and interactions, especially those related to the drugs mentioned above.

ipratropium bromide
Alti-Ipratropium✢, Apo-Ipravent✢, Atrovent, Novo-Ipramide✢

Pharmacologic class: Anticholinergic
Therapeutic class: Allergy, cold, and cough remedy; bronchodilator
Pregnancy risk category B

Action
Inhibits cholinergic receptors in bronchial smooth muscle, decreasing level of cyclic guanosine monophosphate (cGMP), decreasing level of cGMP and causing bronchioles to dilate. Also inhibits secretions from glands lining the nasal mucosa when used locally.

Availability
Aerosol inhaler: 18 mcg/spray in 14-g canister (200 inhalations)
Nasal spray: 0.03% solution (21 mcg/spray in 30-ml bottle, 345 sprays/bottle); 0.06% solution (42 mcg/spray in 15-ml bottle, 165 sprays/bottle)
Solution for inhalation: 0.0125%, 0.02% in single-dose vials

ⓘ Indications and dosages
➤ Chronic obstructive pulmonary disease; bronchospasm, asthma, and allergic and nonallergic perennial rhinitis or common cold
aerosol—
Adults: Two inhalations (36 mcg) q.i.d.; not to exceed 12 inhalations in 24 hours
inhalation solution—
Adults: 500 mcg three to four times daily by oral nebulizer; space doses 6 to 8 hours apart as needed.
nasal spray (0.03% solution)—
Adults and children ages 6 and older: Two sprays (42 mcg) per nostril two to three times daily (total daily dosage of 168 to 252 mcg)
nasal spray (0.06% solution)—
Adults and children ages 12 and older: Two sprays (84 mcg) per nostril three to four times daily (total daily dosage of 504 to 672 mcg)

Contraindications
• Hypersensitivity to drug, its components, atropine, belladonna alkaloids, bromide, or fluorocarbons

---

✢ Canada　　　◀ Clinical alert　　　Reactions in **bold** are life-threatening

Administration

• Give by inhalation or intranasal route as directed.
• When using nasal spray, prime with seven actuations to initiate pump; give two actuations if spray hasn't been used for 24 hours.
• With aerosol inhaler, prime new inhaler with three sprays; also prime with three sprays if inhaler hasn't been used within past 24 hours.

Route	Onset	Peak	Duration
Inhalation	5-15 min	1-2 hr	3-4 hr (up to 8 hr)
Intranasal	15 min	Unknown	6-12 hr

Adverse reactions

CNS: dizziness, headache, nervousness
CV: hypotension, palpitations, chest pain
EENT: blurred vision, epistaxis, nasal dryness and irritation (with nasal spray), sore throat
GI: nausea, vomiting, GI irritation
Musculoskeletal: back pain
Respiratory: cough, upper respiratory tract infection, bronchitis, increased sputum, oropharyngeal edema, **bronchospasm**
Skin: rash
Other: flulike symptoms, hypersensitivity reactions including **anaphylaxis**

Interactions

Drug-drug. *Antihistamines, disopyramide, phenothiazines:* additive anticholinergic effects
Drug-herb. *Jaborandi, pill-bearing spurge:* decreased drug effects

Precautions

Use cautiously in:
• acute bronchospasm, bladder neck obstruction, prostatic hypertrophy, glaucoma, urinary retention, undiagnosed abdominal pain
• elderly patients
• pregnant or breastfeeding patients
• children ages 5 and younger (safety not established).

Patient monitoring

• Evaluate for urinary retention; have patient void before giving drug.
• Ensure proper fit of mouthpiece or face mask.
• Monitor patient's response to therapy, vital signs, and neurologic, cardiovascular, and respiratory status.
• Monitor fluid intake and output; keep patient well hydrated.
• Closely monitor for hypersensitivity reaction.

Patient teaching

• Teach patient how to use nasal spray or inhaler.
• Advise patient to rinse mouth after each dose to minimize throat irritation and dryness.
• Caution patient to keep drug out of eyes; if contact does occur, instruct him to rinse eyes with cool water and call prescriber.
• Instruct patient to avoid driving and other dangerous activities if drug causes dizziness or blurred vision.
• Tell patient drug may cause GI upset, nausea, vomiting, or cough.
• Instruct patient to report rash, palpitations, or vision changes.
• As appropriate, review all other significant and life-threatening adverse reactions and interactions, especially those related to the drugs and herbs mentioned above.

irbesartan
Avapro

Pharmacologic class: Angiotensin II receptor antagonist
Therapeutic class: Antihypertensive
Pregnancy risk category C (second and third trimesters: ***D***)

Action
Blocks aldosterone-secreting and potent vasoconstricting effects of angiotensin II at tissue receptor sites, which reduces vasoconstriction and lowers blood pressure

Availability
Tablets: 75 mg, 150 mg, 300 mg

Indications and dosages
➤ Hypertension
Adults: 150 mg P.O. once daily; may be increased to 300 mg P.O. once daily
Children ages 13 to 16: 150 mg/day P.O.; may be increased to 300 mg/day
Children ages 6 to 12: 75 mg/day P.O.; may be increased to 150 mg/day
➤ Hypertension in volume-depleted or hemodialysis patients who are receiving diuretics
Adults: Initially, 75 mg/day P.O.

Off-label uses
• Nephropathy in patients with type 2 diabetes and hypertension

Contraindications
• Hypersensitivity to drug
• Bilateral renal artery stenosis
• Pregnancy (second and third trimesters)

Administration
• Administer with or without food.
• Know that drug may be given with other antihypertensive drugs.

Route	Onset	Peak	Duration
P.O.	Unknown	Within 2 hr	24 hr

Adverse reactions
CNS: dizziness, fatigue, headache, syncope
CV: orthostatic hypotension, chest pain, peripheral edema
EENT: sinus disorders, dental pain
GI: nausea, diarrhea, constipation, abdominal pain, dry mouth

GU: albuminuria, **renal failure**
Metabolic: hyperkalemia, gout
Musculoskeletal: joint pain, back pain, muscle weakness
Respiratory: upper respiratory tract infection, cough, bronchitis

Interactions
Drug-drug. *Diuretics, other antihypertensives:* increased risk of hypotension
Lithium: increased lithium blood level
Nonsteroidal anti-inflammatory drugs: decreased antihypertensive effects
Potassium-sparing diuretics, potassium supplements: increased risk of hyperkalemia
Drug-diagnostic tests. *Albumin:* increased level
Drug-food. *Salt substitutes containing potassium:* increased risk of hyperkalemia

Precautions
Use cautiously in:
• heart failure, volume or sodium depletion, renal disease, hepatic impairment
• blacks
• women of childbearing age
• breastfeeding patients
• children ages 18 and younger (safety not established).

Patient monitoring
• Monitor vital signs, especially blood pressure.
• Watch blood pressure closely in situations where volume depletion may cause hypotension (such as diaphoresis, nausea, vomiting, diarrhea, and postoperative period).
• Assess fluid intake and output; keep patient well hydrated, especially if he's receiving diuretics concurrently.
• Watch for signs and symptoms of orthostatic hypotension.
• Monitor blood urea nitrogen and creatinine levels.

Patient teaching

• Tell patient he may take drug with or without food.

• Instruct patient to change positions slowly when sitting or standing and to stay well hydrated to minimize orthostatic hypotension.

• Advise patient to avoid driving and other hazardous activities until he knows how drug affects concentration and alertness.

• Tell female patient that drug has been linked to fetal injury and deaths. Caution her not to get pregnant during therapy; recommend barrier birth-control method.

• Instruct patient to report fever, chills, dizziness, or pregnancy.

• Tell patient to report severe vomiting or diarrhea or dehydration.

• As appropriate, review all other significant and life-threatening adverse reactions and interactions, especially those related to the drugs, tests, and foods mentioned above.

irinotecan hydrochloride
Camptosar

Pharmacologic class: Topoisomerase inhibitor

Therapeutic class: Hormonal antineoplastic

Pregnancy risk category D

Action

Inhibits topoisomerase 1, an enzyme that allows DNA replication by inducing reversible single-strand breaks that relieve torsional strain. By binding to topoisomerase 1, drug prevents religation of DNA strand, resulting in breakage of double-stranded DNA and cell death.

Availability

Injection: 20 mg/ml in 2-ml and 5-ml vials

Indications and dosages

➤ Recurrence or progression of metastatic colorectal carcinoma after fluorouracil (5-FU) therapy

Adults: 125 mg/m^2 I.V. infusion over 90 minutes on days 1, 8, 15, and 22 followed by a 2-week rest. Adjust dosage in increments based on patient tolerance. Use lower dosages when giving drug in combination with both leucovorin and 5-FU.

Off-label uses

• Most cancers

Contraindications

• Hypersensitivity to drug
• Concurrent atazanavir use
• Pregnancy or breastfeeding

Administration

• Dilute in dextrose 5% in water or normal saline solution to a concentration of 0.12 to 1.1 mg/ml.

• Infuse within 6 hours if stored at room temperature or within 24 hours if refrigerated.

• Give I.V. infusion over 90 minutes.

• Administer antiemetics to ease nausea and vomiting, as needed and prescribed.

Route	Onset	Peak	Duration
I.V.	Immediate	1-2 hr	Unknown

Adverse reactions

CNS: insomnia, dizziness, asthenia, headache, akathisia

CV: vasodilation, orthostatic hypotension

EENT: rhinitis

GI: nausea, vomiting, constipation, diarrhea, anorexia, stomatitis, flatulence, dyspepsia, abdominal pain or enlargement

Hematologic: anemia, **neutropenia, leukopenia, thrombocytopenia**
Hepatic: hepatotoxicity
Metabolic: dehydration
Musculoskeletal: back pain
Respiratory: dyspnea, increased cough
Skin: alopecia, diaphoresis, rash
Other: weight loss, edema, fever, pain, chills, minor infections

Interactions
Drug-drug. *Dexamethasone:* increased risk of lymphocytopenia
Diuretics: increased risk of dehydration
Laxatives: increased risk of diarrhea
Other antineoplastics: additive adverse effects
Drug-diagnostic tests. *Alkaline phosphatase:* increased level
Hemoglobin, neutrophils, white blood cells: decreased values

Precautions
Use cautiously in:
• bone marrow depression, severe diarrhea
• patients undergoing radiation therapy
• elderly patients
• children.

Patient monitoring
• Assess complete blood count before each infusion; don't give drug if neutrophil count is below 1,500 cells/mm².
• Monitor infusion site for extravasation; if it occurs, flush with sterile water and apply ice.
• Assess fluid intake and output; keep patient well hydrated.
• Monitor oral intake; evaluate for nausea and vomiting.
• Assess for diarrhea; expect to decrease dosage or withhold dose in severe diarrhea.
• Institute infection-control protocols to help protect patient from infection sources.
• Monitor liver function test results.

Patient teaching
• Inform patient that blood tests will be done before each dose.
• Teach patient that drug increases his risk of infection; advise him to avoid crowds and other potential infection sources.
• Caution female patient not to become pregnant during therapy; recommend barrier birth-control method.
• Instruct patient to report pain at infusion site; severe nausea or vomiting; severe, increased, or bloody diarrhea; infection; injury; or fatigue.
• As appropriate, review all other significant and life-threatening adverse reactions and interactions, especially those related to the drugs and tests mentioned above.

iron dextran
DexFerrum, InFeD

Pharmacologic class: Trace element
Therapeutic class: Iron supplement
Pregnancy risk category C

Action
Replenishes depleted stores of iron (a component of hemoglobin) in bone marrow

Availability
Injection: 50 mg/ml

Indications and dosages
➤ Iron deficiency anemia in patients who can't tolerate oral iron
Adults and children weighing more than 15 kg (33 lb): Dosage individualized based on patient's weight and hemoglobin (Hgb) value, using the following formula: Dosage (ml) = 0.0442 (desired Hgb minus patient's Hgb) times lean body weight (LBW) plus the product of 0.26 times LBW

Give test dose before initiating either I.V. or I.M. therapy: For I.V. use, administer test dose of 0.5 ml (25 mg) I.V. over 30 seconds to 5 minutes; if no reactions occur within 1 hour, give remainder of therapeutic dose I.V.; repeat this dose daily. For I.M. use, give 0.5-ml test dose by Z-track method; if no reactions occur, give daily doses not exceeding 100 mg I.M. in adults, 50 mg I.M. in children weighing more than 10 kg (22 lb), or 25 mg in infants weighing less than 5 kg (11 lb).

➤ Iron replacement for blood loss
Adults: Dosage individualized based on the following formula: Replacement iron (in mg) = blood loss (in ml) times hematocrit

Contraindications
• Hypersensitivity to drug, alcohol, tartrazine, or sulfites
• Acute phase of infectious kidney disease and hemolytic anemias

Administration
• For I.M. administration, inject by Z-track method into upper outer quadrant of gluteal muscle. Give test dose of 0.5 ml before starting therapy.
• For intermittent I.V. infusion, give test dose of 0.5 ml before starting therapy. Administer undiluted at a slow rate (no faster than 1 ml/minute).
• Don't give with oral iron preparations.

Route	Onset	Peak	Duration
I.V., I.M.	4 days	1-2 wk	Wks-mos

Adverse reactions
CNS: dizziness, headache, syncope, **seizures**
CV: chest pain, tachycardia, hypotension
EENT: metallic taste, tooth discoloration
GI: nausea, vomiting, abnormal taste
Hematologic: hemochromatosis, hemolysis, hemosiderosis

Musculoskeletal: joint pain, myalgia
Respiratory: dyspnea
Other: fever, lymphadenopathy, hypersensitivity reactions including **anaphylaxis**

Interactions
None significant

Precautions
Use cautiously in:
• autoimmune disorders, arthritis, severe hepatic impairment
• elderly patients
• breastfeeding patients
• children.

Patient monitoring
◀≶ Monitor for hypersensitivity reaction. Keep epinephrine and other emergency supplies on hand in case this reaction occurs.
• Assess serum ferritin levels regularly because these levels correlate with iron stores.
• In patients with rheumatoid arthritis, monitor for acute exacerbation of joint pain and swelling; provide appropriate comfort measures.
• Watch for signs and symptoms of iron overload, including decreased activity, sedation, and GI or respiratory tract bleeding.

Patient teaching
• Caution patient not to take oral iron preparations or vitamins containing iron during I.V. iron therapy.
• Instruct patient to report difficulty breathing, itching, or rash.
• Tell patient that he'll undergo periodic blood testing to monitor his response to therapy.
• As appropriate, review all other significant and life-threatening adverse reactions mentioned above.

iron sucrose
Venofer

Pharmacologic class: Trace element
Therapeutic class: Iron supplement
Pregnancy risk category B

Action
Replenishes depleted iron stores in bone marrow when iron is incorporated into hemoglobin

Availability
Aqueous complex for injection: 20 mg elemental iron/ml in 5-ml single-use vials (100 mg)

💊 Indications and dosages
➣ Iron deficiency anemia in patients undergoing chronic hemodialysis who are concurrently receiving erythropoietin
Adults: 100 mg (5 ml) I.V. directly into dialysis line or by slow injection or infusion during dialysis session (up to three times weekly) for 10 doses (total of 1,000 mg); no test dose needed

Off-label uses
• Autologous blood donation
• Bloodless surgery

Contraindications
• Hypersensitivity to drug, alcohol, tartrazine, or sulfites
• Primary hemochromatosis
• Hemolytic anemias, other anemias not caused by iron deficiency

Administration
• Dilute 100 mg of elemental iron in a maximum of 100 ml of normal saline solution; infuse slowly I.V. over at least 15 minutes.

• Administer I.V. directly into dialysis line or by infusion of 20 mg/minute, not to exceed 100 mg/injection.
• Don't give with oral iron preparations.

Route	Onset	Peak	Duration
I.V.	4 days	1-2 wk	Wks-mos

Adverse reactions
CNS: dizziness, headache, syncope, **seizures**
CV: chest pain, tachycardia, hypotension
EENT: metallic taste, tooth discoloration
GI: nausea, vomiting, abnormal taste
Hematologic: hemochromatosis, hemolysis, hemosiderosis
Musculoskeletal: muscle cramps, aches, or weakness; joint pain
Respiratory: dyspnea
Other: fever, lymphadenopathy, allergic reactions including **anaphylaxis**

Interactions
None significant

Precautions
Use cautiously in:
• autoimmune disorders, arthritis, severe hepatic impairment
• elderly patients
• breastfeeding patients
• children.

Patient monitoring
◀≷ Monitor for hypersensitivity reaction. Keep epinephrine and other emergency supplies available in case this reaction occurs.
• Assess hemoglobin, hematocrit, serum ferritin, and transferrin saturation levels before, during, and after therapy.
◀≷ Monitor blood pressure; stay alert for hypotension.
• Watch for signs and symptoms of iron overload, such as decreased activi-

ty, sedation, and bleeding in GI or respiratory tract.

Patient teaching

• Caution patient not to take oral iron preparations or vitamin supplements containing iron during I.V. iron therapy.

• Instruct patient to report dyspnea, itching, or rash.

• Advise patient that he'll undergo periodic blood testing to monitor his response to therapy.

• As appropriate, review all other significant and life-threatening adverse reactions mentioned above.

isoniazid (INH)

Isotamine♣, Laniazid, Nydrazid, PMS Isoniazid♣

Pharmacologic class: Isonicotinic acid hydrazide
Therapeutic class: Antitubercular
Pregnancy risk category C

Action

Inhibits cell wall biosynthesis by interfering with lipid and nucleic acid DNA synthesis in tubercle bacilli cells; bacteriostatic action is dependant on location

Availability

Injection: 100 mg/ml
Syrup: 50 mg/5 ml
Tablets: 100 mg, 300 mg

🖋 Indications and dosages

➤ First-line therapy for active tuberculosis (given with other agents)
Adults: 5 mg/kg P.O. or I.M. (maximum of 300 mg/day) once daily as a single dose, or 15 mg/kg (maximum of 900 mg/day) two to three times weekly

Children: 10 to 15 mg/kg P.O. or I.M. (maximum of 300 mg/day) once daily as a single dose, or 20 to 40 mg/kg (maximum of 900 mg/day) two to three times weekly

➤ To prevent tuberculosis in patients exposed to active disease (monotherapy)
Adults: 300 mg P.O. daily as a single dose for 6 to 12 months
Children and infants: 10 mg/kg P.O. daily as a single dose for up to 12 months

Off-label uses

• *Mycobacterium kansasii* infection

Contraindications

• Hypersensitivity to drug
• Acute hepatic disease or previous hepatitis caused by isoniazid therapy

Administration

• Give on empty stomach, either 1 hour before or 2 hours after meals. If GI upset occurs, administer with food.

• Administer parenterally only if patient can't take oral form.

• Use cautiously in diabetic or alcoholic patients and those at risk for neuropathy.

Route	Onset	Peak	Duration
P.O., I.M.	Rapid	1-2 hr	Up to 24 hr

Adverse reactions

CNS: peripheral neuropathy, dizziness, memory impairment, slurred speech, psychosis, **toxic encephalopathy, seizures**
EENT: visual disturbances
GI: nausea, vomiting
GU: gynecomastia
Hematologic: hemolytic anemia, eosinophilia, methemoglobinemia, **aplastic anemia, agranulocytosis, thrombocytopenia**
Hepatic: hepatitis
Metabolic: pyridoxine deficiency, hyperglycemia, metabolic acidosis

Respiratory: dyspnea
Other: fever, pellagra, lupuslike syndrome, injection site irritation, hypersensitivity reaction

Interactions

Drug-drug. *Aluminum-containing antacids:* decreased isoniazid absorption

Bacille Calmette-Guérin vaccine: ineffective vaccination

Carbamazepine: increased carbamazepine blood level

Disulfiram: psychotic reactions, incoordination

Hepatotoxic drugs: increased risk of hepatotoxicity

Ketoconazole: decreased ketoconazole blood level and efficacy

Other antituberculars: additive CNS toxicity

Phenytoin: inhibition of phenytoin metabolism

Drug-diagnostic tests. *Albumin:* increased level

Drug-food. *Foods containing tyramine:* hypertensive crisis, other severe reactions

Drug-behaviors. *Alcohol use:* increased risk of hepatitis

Precautions

Use cautiously in:
• severe renal impairment, diabetic retinopathy, ocular defects, diabetes, chronic alcoholism, hepatic damage
• Black and Hispanic women
• pregnant or breastfeeding patients
• children ages 13 and younger.

Patient monitoring

• Assess hepatic enzyme levels.
• Watch for adverse reactions, such as peripheral neuropathy.

Patient teaching

• Advise patient to take drug once daily on an empty stomach, 1 hour before or 2 hours after meals. If GI upset oc-

curs, tell him to take drug with small amount of food.
• Caution patient to avoid cheese, fish, salami, red wine, and yeast extracts because chills, diaphoresis, and palpitations may occur.
• Teach patient with peripheral neuropathy to take care to prevent burns and other injuries.
• Instruct patient to report anorexia, nausea, vomiting, jaundice, dark urine, and numbness or tingling of hands or feet.
• Tell patient he'll need periodic medical and eye examinations and blood tests to gauge drug effects.
• As appropriate, review all other significant and life-threatening adverse reactions and interactions, especially those related to the drugs, tests, foods, and behaviors mentioned above.

isoproterenol
Isuprel

isoproterenol hydrochloride
Isuprel, Isuprel Mistometer

isoproterenol sulfate
Medihaler-Iso

Pharmacologic class: Sympathomimetic, beta$_1$-adrenergic and beta$_2$-adrenergic agonist

Therapeutic class: Vasopressor, bronchodilator, antiasthmatic

Pregnancy risk category C

Action

Relaxes bronchial smooth muscle by acting on beta$_2$-adrenergic receptors; acts on beta$_1$-adrenergic receptors in heart, causing positive inotropic and chronotropic effects and increasing cardiac output. Also lowers peripheral vascular resistance in skeletal muscle and inhibits antigen-induced histamine release.

Availability
isoproterenol
Nebulizer inhaler: 0.25%, 0.5%, 1%
Solution for inhalation: 0.125%, 0.5%, 1%
isoproterenol hydrochloride
Aerosol inhaler: 131 mcg/metered spray
Injection: 20 mcg/ml, 200 mcg/ml
isoproterenol sulfate
Aerosol inhaler: 80 mcg/metered spray

🔷 Indications and dosages
➤ Bronchospasm

Adults and children: Three to six inhalations of aerosol inhaler daily. Or three to seven deep inhalations of isoproterenol 1% solution by nebulizer inhaler; may repeat in 5 to 10 minutes up to five times daily
➤ Acute dyspneic episodes

Adults and children: Initially, one inhalation of isoproterenol sulfate; may repeat after 2 to 5 minutes if needed. Maintenance dosage is one to two inhalations four to six times daily, to a maximum of six inhalations in 24 hours.
➤ Bronchospasm in chronic obstructive pulmonary disease (COPD)

Adults: 2 ml of 0.125% or 2.5 ml of 1% isoproterenol solution given by intermittent positive-pressure breathing (IPPB) device or nebulizer inhaler up to five times daily
➤ Asthma

Adults and children: One or two inhalations of isoproterenol hydrochloride or Medihaler-Iso; wait 1 to 5 minutes between inhalations. May repeat up to six times daily.
➤ Shock

Adults and children: 0.5 to 5 mcg/minute of isoproterenol hydrochloride by continuous I.V. infusion.
➤ Heart block, ventricular arrhythmias

Adults: Initially, 0.02 to 0.06 mg of isoproterenol hydrochloride I.V., with subsequent doses of 0.01 to 0.2 mg I.V. or 5 mcg/minute I.V. Or initially, 0.2 mg I.M, then 0.02 to 1 mg I.M., depending on clinical response. Or initially, 0.2 mg S.C., then 0.15 to 0.2 mg S.C., depending on clinical response.
Children: 2.5 mcg/minute or 0.1 mcg/kg/minute of isoproterenol hydrochloride I.V.; dosage adjusted based on clinical response.

Contraindications
• Angina pectoris
• Narrow-angle glaucoma
• Labor and delivery, breastfeeding

Administration
• Give I.V. form by direct injection or I.V. infusion. Always use continuous infusion pump to deliver infusion.

Route	Onset	Peak	Duration
Inhalation	2-5 min	Unknown	0.5-2 hr
I.V.	Immediate	Unknown	<1 hr

Adverse reactions
CNS: tremors, anxiety, insomnia, headache, dizziness, asthenia
CV: palpitations, tachycardia, angina, rapid blood pressure changes, **arrhythmias, cardiac arrest, Stokes-Adams attacks**
EENT: pharyngitis
GI: nausea, vomiting, heartburn
Metabolic: hyperglycemia
Respiratory: bronchitis, increased sputum, **pulmonary edema, bronchospasm**
Skin: diaphoresis
Other: parotid gland swelling (with prolonged use)

Interactions
Drug-drug. *Cyclopropane, epinephrine, halogenated general anesthetics:* increased risk of arrhythmias

Propranolol, other beta-adrenergic blockers: antagonism of bronchodilating effects

Drug-diagnostic tests. *Glucose:* increased level

Precautions

Use cautiously in:
• renal impairment, unstable vasomotor disorders, hypertension, coronary insufficiency, COPD, diabetes mellitus, hyperthyroidism
• history of cerebrovascular accident or seizures
• elderly patients.

Patient monitoring

• During I.V. administration, monitor ECG and vital signs carefully.
• Assess patient's response to drug and adjust I.V. infusion rate accordingly.
• Closely monitor arterial blood gas values, urine output, and central venous pressure.
• Be alert for rebound bronchospasm.

Patient teaching

• Teach patient using inhaler to exhale first, place mouthpiece well into mouth, and inhale deeply while releasing dose from inhaler. Instruct him to hold his breath for several seconds before slowly exhaling. Caution him to wait 2 minutes between inhalations.
• If patient also uses steroid inhaler, instruct him to use isoproterenol first, then wait 5 minutes before using steroid inhaler.
• Teach patient to clean inhaler by washing in soapy water weekly.
• Inform patient that drug may disturb sleep pattern. Discourage use before bedtime.
• As appropriate, review all other significant and life-threatening adverse reactions and interactions, especially those related to the drugs and tests mentioned above.

isosorbide dinitrate
Apo-ISDN✤, Cedocard-SR✤, Dilatrate-SR, Isordil, Isordil Tembids, Isordil Titradose, Isotrate, Sorbitrate

isosorbide mononitrate
Imdur, ISMO, Isotrate ER, Monoket

Pharmacologic class: Nitrate
Therapeutic class: Antianginal
Pregnancy risk category C

Action

Causes peripheral vasodilation, which leads to reduced preload and afterload and a subsequent decrease in myocardial oxygen consumption and increase in cardiac output. Also dilates the coronary arteries, thereby increasing blood flow and improving collateral circulation.

Availability
isosorbide dinitrate
Capsules: 40 mg
Capsules (extended-release): 40 mg
Tablets: 2.5 mg, 5 mg, 10 mg, 20 mg, 30 mg, 40 mg
Tablets (chewable): 5 mg, 10 mg
Tablets (extended-release): 20 mg, 40 mg
Tablets (sublingual): 2.5 mg, 5 mg, 10 mg
isosorbide mononitrate
Tablets: 10 mg, 20 mg
Tablets (extended-release): 30 mg, 60 mg, 120 mg

🖊 Indications and dosages
➢ Acute angina pectoris
Adults: 2.5 to 5 mg S.L.; may repeat dose q 5 to 10 minutes for a total of three doses in 15 to 30 minutes. Or 5-mg chewable tablet q 2 to 3 hours p.r.n.

> To prevent angina pectoris

Adults: 2.5 to 5 mg S.L.; may repeat dose q 2 to 3 hours or 15 minutes before activity that provokes angina. Or initially, 5 to 20 mg P.O.; usual maintenance dosage is 10 to 40 mg P.O. (regular-release) q 6 hours or 40 to 80 mg P.O. (extended-release) q 8 to 12 hours. Or 5- to 10-mg chewable tablet q 2 to 3 hours p.r.n.

> Chronic heart failure

Adults: 20 mg P.O. (ISMO, Monoket regular-release tablets) b.i.d. 7 hours apart; or 30 to 60 mg P.O. (Imdur sustained-release) once daily; may increase to 120 mg P.O. once daily (up to 240 mg/day)

Contraindications

- Hypersensitivity to drug
- Severe anemia
- Acute myocardial infarction
- Narrow-angle glaucoma
- Concurrent sildenafil therapy

Administration

- Give oral form 30 minutes before or 1 to 2 hours after a meal. Make sure patient swallows tablets or capsules whole.
- Have patient wet S.L. tablet with saliva before placing it under tongue. To avoid tingling sensation, advise him to place tablet in buccal pouch.

Route	Onset	Peak	Duration
P.O. (dinitrate)	15-40 min	Unknown	4 hr
P.O. (dinitrate, extended)	30 min	Unknown	≤12 hr
P.O. (mono-nitrate)	30-60 min	Unknown	7 hr
P.O. (mono-nitrate, extended)	Unknown	Unknown	12 hr
S.L. (dinitrate)	2-5 min	Unknown	1-2 hr

Adverse reactions

CNS: dizziness, headache, apprehension, asthenia, syncope
CV: orthostatic hypotension, tachycardia, paradoxical bradycardia
EENT: sublingual burning
GI: nausea, vomiting, abdominal pain
Skin: flushing

Interactions

Drug-drug. *Aspirin:* increased isosorbide blood level and effects
Beta-adrenergic blockers, calcium channel blockers, phenothiazines: additive hypotension
Dihydroergotamine: antagonism of dihydroergotamine effects
Sildenafil: potentially fatal hypotension
Drug-diagnostic tests. *Cholesterol:* decreased level
Methemoglobin, urine vanillylmandelic acid: increased levels

Precautions

Use cautiously in:
- head trauma, volume depletion
- elderly patients
- pregnant or breastfeeding patients
- children.

Patient monitoring

- Monitor ECG and vital signs closely (especially blood pressure).
- In suspected overdose, assess for signs and symptoms of increased intracranial pressure.
- Check arterial blood gas values and methemoglobin levels.

Patient teaching

- Teach patient to take oral drug 30 minutes before or 1 to 2 hours after a meal.
- Inform patient that drug may cause headache. Advise him to treat headache as usual and not to alter drug schedule; if headache persists, tell him to contact prescriber.
- Instruct patient to move slowly when sitting up or standing to avoid dizzi-

ness or light-headedness from sudden blood pressure decrease.

• As appropriate, review all other significant adverse reactions and interactions, especially those related to the drugs and tests mentioned above.

isradipine
DynaCirc, DynaCirc CR

Pharmacologic class: Calcium channel blocker
Therapeutic class: Antihypertensive
Pregnancy risk category C

Action
Inhibits calcium ion movement across cell membranes of cardiac and arterial muscles, causing relaxation of coronary and peripheral vascular smooth muscle. This action reduces diastolic blood pressure, enhances left ventricular function, and improves ejection rates; it also reduces mean vascular and systemic vascular resistance, increasing cardiac index and improving stroke volume.

Availability
Capsules: 2.5 mg, 5 mg
Tablets (controlled-release): 5 mg, 10 mg

⍟ Indications and dosages
➤ Hypertension
Adults: Initially, 2.5 mg P.O. b.i.d. (regular-release capsules); may increase in increments of 5 mg/day at 2- to 4-week intervals, to a maximum dosage of 20 mg/day. Or, 5 to 10 mg P.O. (controlled-release) daily as monotherapy or in combination with thiazide diuretic.

Contraindications
• Hypersensitivity to drug or other calcium channel blockers

Administration
• Give with or without food.
• Don't give with grapefruit juice.
• Don't crush or break controlled-release tablets; make sure patient swallows them whole.

Route	Onset	Peak	Duration
P.O.	2 hr	Unknown	Unknown
P.O. (controlled)	Unknown	Unknown	Unknown

Adverse reactions
CNS: dizziness, headache, fatigue, syncope, sleep disturbances
CV: peripheral edema, tachycardia, hypotension, chest pain, **arrhythmias**
GI: nausea, vomiting, constipation, abdominal pain or distention, dry mouth
GU: nocturia, urinary frequency
Hematologic: leukopenia
Hepatic: hepatitis
Skin: rash, pruritus, urticaria
Other: flushing

Interactions
Drug-drug. *Atracurium, gallamine, pancuronium, tubocurarine, vecuronium:* increased respiratory depression
Beta-adrenergic blockers: increased cardiac depression
Carbamazepine, digoxin, prazosin, quinidine: increased blood levels of these drugs
Drug-food. *Grapefruit juice:* increased drug absorption

Precautions
Use cautiously in:
• heart disease, hypotension, hepatic or renal disease, GI hypermotility or obstruction (controlled-release form)
• concurrent use of beta-adrenergic blockers
• elderly patients
• pregnant or breastfeeding patients
• children.

Patient monitoring

• Monitor vital signs closely, especially blood pressure.

• Assess liver function test results.

• Monitor for signs and symptoms of heart failure, such as dyspnea and peripheral edema.

Patient teaching

• Tell patient he may take drug with or without food, but not with grapefruit juice.

• Instruct patient to avoid driving and other hazardous activities until he knows how drug affects concentration and alertness.

• Caution patient to move slowly when sitting up or standing to avoid dizziness or light-headedness from sudden blood pressure decrease.

• Teach patients with heart failure to watch for and promptly report adverse reactions.

• As appropriate, review all other significant and life-threatening adverse reactions and interactions, especially those related to the drugs and foods mentioned above.

itraconazole
Sporanox

Pharmacologic class: Synthetic triazole
Therapeutic class: Antifungal
Pregnancy risk category C

Action
Prevents ergosterol synthesis in fungal cell membranes, altering membrane permeability

Availability
Capsules: 100 mg
Injection: 10 mg/ml
Oral solution: 10 mg/ml

Indications and dosages

➤ Aspergillosis, blastomycosis, histoplasmosis

Adults: 200 to 400 mg P.O. daily for at least 3 months until clinically cured. In life-threatening infections, give loading dose of 200 mg P.O. t.i.d. for 3 days, followed by 200 to 400 mg P.O. daily until clinically cured. Or 200 mg I.V. b.i.d. for four doses, followed by 200 mg P.O. daily; continue combination of I.V. and P.O. regimen for at least 3 months until clinically cured.

➤ Esophageal candidiasis

Adults: 100 to 200 mg of oral solution daily, swished in mouth for several seconds and swallowed, for at least 3 weeks; continue for 2 weeks after symptoms resolve.

➤ Oropharyngeal candidiasis

Adults: 200 mg of oral solution daily, swished in mouth for several seconds and swallowed, for 1 to 2 weeks

➤ Empiric therapy in febrile, neutropenic patients with suspected fungal infections

Adults: 200 mg I.V. b.i.d. for four doses, followed by 200 mg daily for up to 14 days. Continue 200 mg of oral solution b.i.d. until neutropenia resolves.

➤ Onychomycosis, tinea unguium

Adults: For toenails, 200 mg P.O. daily for 12 weeks. For fingernails, 200 mg b.i.d. for 1 week; wait 3 weeks, then repeat dosage for 1 week.

Contraindications

• Hypersensitivity to drug or its components

• Fungal meningitis

• Ventricular dysfunction, heart failure

• Concomitant use of astemizole, cisapride, dofetilide, midazolam, pimozide, quinidine, lovastatin, simvastatin, or triazolam

• Pregnancy or breastfeeding

Administration

• Obtain specimens for fungal cultures, as needed, before starting therapy.
• Administer oral solution without food when possible.
• For I.V. use, dilute contents of 250-mg ampule in 50-ml bag of normal saline solution to yield a final concentration of 75 ml of 3.33 mg/ml. Infuse over 1 hour. Don't mix with other drugs or give in same I.V. line with other drugs. After infusion, flush through two-way stopcock with 15 to 20 ml of normal saline solution for 30 seconds to 15 minutes.

Route	Onset	Peak	Duration
P.O.	Slow	4-6 hr	4-6 days
I.V.	Rapid	Unknown	End of infusion

Adverse reactions

CNS: dizziness, headache, fatigue, malaise
CV: peripheral edema, hypertension, **heart failure**
EENT: tinnitus
GI: nausea, vomiting, constipation, abdominal pain, flatulence, anorexia, **GI bleeding**
GU: albuminuria, impotence, gynecomastia, decreased libido
Hepatic: hepatic impairment
Metabolic: hypokalemia
Musculoskeletal: myalgia, bursitis, rhabdomyolysis
Respiratory: pulmonary edema
Skin: flushing, rash, pruritus, urticaria, herpes zoster infection
Other: fever

Interactions

Drug-drug. *Antacids, histamine$_2$-receptor blockers, isoniazid, phenytoin, rifampin:* decreased itraconazole blood level
Cyclosporine, digoxin, tacrolimus: increased blood levels of these drugs
HMG-CoA reductase inhibitors (such as astemizole, cisapride, dofetilide, midazo-lam, pimozide, quinidine, lovastatin, simvastatin): increased blood levels of these drugs, possibly causing serious cardiovascular reactions
Oral anticoagulants: enhanced anticoagulant effects
Oral hypoglycemics: additive hypoglycemia

Drug-diagnostic tests. *Alanine aminotransferase, alkaline phosphatase, aspartate aminotransferase, gamma-glutamyltransferase, potassium:* increased levels

Drug-food. *Any food, cola:* increased itraconazole blood level
Grapefruit juice: decreased blood level and reduced therapeutic effects of itraconazole

Precautions

Use cautiously in:
• hypersensitivity to drug or other azole derivatives
• renal impairment (with I.V. use), hepatic disorders, achlorhydria, hypochlorhydria
• children.

Patient monitoring

• In patients with hepatic dysfunction, monitor hepatic enzyme levels.
• Monitor for signs and symptoms of hepatic dysfunction (jaundice, fatigue, nausea, vomiting, dark urine, pale stools), heart failure, and pulmonary or peripheral edema.

Patient teaching

• Tell patient he may take drug with or without food but should avoid grapefruit juice and colas during therapy.
• Inform patient that drug interacts with many other drugs; advise him to tell all prescribers that he's taking it.
◀€ Teach patient to recognize and immediately report signs and symptoms of liver dysfunction and heart failure.
• Teach patient to avoid driving and other hazardous activities until he knows how drug affects concentration and alertness.

• As appropriate, review all other significant and life-threatening adverse reactions and interactions, especially those related to the drugs, tests, and foods mentioned above.

kanamycin sulfate
Kantrex

Pharmacologic class: Aminoglycoside
Therapeutic class: Anti-infective
Pregnancy risk category D

Action
Interferes with protein synthesis in bacterial cells by binding to 30S ribosomal subunit, causing misreading of genetic code; formation of inaccurate peptide sequence in protein chain leads to bacterial death

Availability
Capsules: 500 mg
Injection: 75 mg/2 ml, 500 mg/2 ml, 1,000 mg/3 ml

Indications and dosages
➤ Serious infections caused by susceptible strains of *Pseudomonas aeruginosa, Escherichia coli, Proteus, Klebsiella, Serratia, Enterobacter, Citrobacter,* and *Staphylococcus*
Adults and children: 5 mg/kg I.V. or I.M. q 8 hours, or 7.5 mg/kg I.V. or I.M. q 12 hours, or 15 mg/kg I.V. or I.M. once daily for 7 to 10 days, to a maximum dosage of 1.5 g/day
➤ Hepatic coma
Adults: 8 to 12 g/day P.O. in divided doses

➤ Bowel sterilization
Adults: 1 g P.O. q hour for 4 hours, then 1 g q 6 hours for 36 to 72 hours
Dosage adjustment
• Renal impairment
• Elderly patients

Contraindications
• Hypersensitivity to drug, other aminoglycosides, or bisulfites
• Intestinal obstruction

Administration
• Collect specimens for culture and sensitivity testing before therapy starts.
• Keep patient well hydrated; drug may cause nephrotoxicity.
• Administer I.M. injection deep into a large muscle.
• Reconstitute I.V. dose by mixing 500 mg in 100 to 200 ml of normal saline solution or dextrose 5% in water or by adding 1 g to 200 to 400 ml of either solution.
• Infuse I.V. solution over 30 to 60 minutes.

Route	Onset	Peak	Duration
P.O.	Slow	Unknown	Unknown
I.V.	Immediate	15-30 min	Unknown
I.M.	Rapid	30-90 min	Unknown

Adverse reactions
CNS: dizziness, vertigo, tremors, numbness, depression, confusion, lethargy, headache, paresthesia, **neuromuscular blockade, seizures, neurotoxicity**
CV: hypotension, hypertension, palpitations
EENT: visual disturbances, dry eyes, nystagmus, photophobia, hearing loss, tinnitus, ototoxicity
GI: nausea, vomiting, anorexia, splenomegaly, stomatitis, increased salivation
GU: polyuria, dysuria, azotemia, increased urinary excretion of casts, elevated blood urea nitrogen (BUN) and

creatinine levels, impotence, **nephro-toxicity**

Hematologic: purpura, increased or decreased reticulocyte count, eosino-philia, leukemoid reaction, hemolytic anemia, **aplastic anemia, neutropenia, agranulocytosis, leukopenia, thrombocytopenia, pancytopenia**

Hepatic: hepatomegaly, elevated alanine aminotransferase (ALT) and aspartate aminotransferase (AST) levels, hyperbilirubinemia, **hepatic necrosis, hepatotoxicity**

Musculoskeletal: joint pain, muscle twitching

Respiratory: apnea

Skin: rash, urticaria, pruritus, exfoliative dermatitis, alopecia

Other: weight loss, superinfection, pain and irritation at I.M. site

Interactions

Drug-drug. *Acyclovir, amphotericin B, cisplatin, potent diuretics, vancomycin:* increased risk of ototoxicity and nephrotoxicity

Dimenhydrinate: masking of ototoxicity symptoms

General anesthetics, neuromuscular junction blockers: increased neuromuscular blockade

Indomethacin: increased kanamycin peak and trough levels

Parenteral penicillins (such as ampicillin, ticarcillin), cephalosporins: kanamycin inactivation

Drug-diagnostic tests. *ALT, AST, bilirubin, BUN, creatinine, low-density lipoproteins, nonprotein nitrogen:* increased levels

Granulocytes, hemoglobin, platelets, white blood cells: decreased values

Precautions

Use cautiously in:
• renal impairment, neuromuscular diseases (such as myasthenia gravis), hearing impairment, obesity
• elderly patients

• pregnant or breastfeeding patients
• infants and neonates (safety not established).

Patient monitoring

• Monitor urine output, BUN and creatinine levels, and urinalysis.
• Evaluate cardiovascular status carefully.
• Assess neurologic status; institute safety measures as needed to prevent injury.
• Monitor peak and trough drug levels.
• Check for hearing loss based on baseline audiogram recorded before first dose.
• Assess for bleeding tendency.

Patient teaching

• Advise patient to minimize GI upset by eating small, frequent servings of healthy food.
◀◊ Instruct patient to report unusual bleeding or bruising immediately.
• Teach patient to promptly report tinnitus or difficulty hearing.
• Advise patient to maintain adequate hydration.
• Tell patient to avoid activities that can cause injury. Advise him to use soft-bristled toothbrush and electric razor to avoid gum and skin injury.
• Instruct patient to avoid driving and other hazardous activities until he knows how drug affects concentration and alertness.
• Tell patient he'll undergo regular blood testing during therapy.
• As appropriate, review all other significant and life-threatening adverse reactions and interactions, especially those related to the drugs and tests mentioned above.

ketoconazole
Nizoral

Pharmacologic class: Imidazole
Therapeutic class: Antifungal
Pregnancy risk category C

Action
Alters cell membranes, resulting in increased permeability and growth inhibition; also impedes ergosterol synthesis

Availability
Cream: 2%
Oral suspension: 100 mg/5 ml
Shampoo: 2%
Tablets: 200 mg

Indications and dosages
➤ Blastomycosis
Adults: 200 to 400 mg P.O. daily
Children ages 2 and older: 3.3 to 6.6 mg/kg P.O. as a single daily dose
➤ Mucocutaneous or vaginal candidiasis
Adults: 200 to 400 mg P.O. daily for 1 to 2 weeks
Children ages 2 and older: 3.3 to 6.6 mg/kg P.O. as a single daily dose
➤ Scaling secondary to dandruff or seborrheic dermatitis
Adults: 2% shampoo applied topically twice weekly for 4 weeks, then as needed to control symptoms
➤ Tinea corporis, tinea cruris, tinea versicolor
Adults: 2% cream applied topically to affected areas once daily for 2 weeks

Contraindications
• Hypersensitivity to drug or its components
• Fungal meningitis
• Concurrent oral triazolam therapy

Administration
• Apply cream to damp skin of affected area and a wide surrounding area.
• To use shampoo, wet hair, then apply shampoo and massage into scalp for 1 minute. Leave on hair for 5 minutes before rinsing. Rinse and repeat, leaving shampoo on scalp for 3 minutes this time before rinsing.
• Don't apply shampoo to broken or inflamed skin.
• For patients with achlorhydria, dissolve 200-mg tablet in 4 ml of 0.2N hydrochloric acid solution.
• Withhold antacids for at least 2 hours after giving oral ketoconazole.

Route	Onset	Peak	Duration
P.O.	Unknown	1-2 hr	Unknown
Topical	Unknown	Unknown	Unknown

Adverse reactions
CNS: headache, nervousness, dizziness, drowsiness, severe depression, **suicidal ideation**
EENT: photophobia
GI: nausea, vomiting, diarrhea, abdominal pain, anorexia
GU: impotence, gynecomastia
Hematologic: purpura, hemolytic anemia, **thrombocytopenia, leukopenia**
Hepatic: elevated alanine aminotransferase (ALT), alkaline phosphatase (ALP), and aspartate aminotransferase (AST) levels; **hepatotoxicity**
Metabolic: hyperlipidemia
Skin: pruritus, rash, dermatitis, urticaria, severe irritation, stinging (with cream), alopecia, abnormal hair texture, scalp pustules, oily skin, dry hair and scalp
Other: fever, chills, allergic reaction

Interactions
Drug-drug. *Antacids, anticholinergics, histamine₂-receptor antagonists:* decreased ketoconazole absorption
Cyclosporine: increased cyclosporine blood level

k

Isoniazid, rifampin: increased keto-conazole metabolism

Theophylline: decreased theophylline blood level

Topical corticosteroids: increased corticosteroid absorption

Triazolam (oral): increased triazolam effects

Drug-diagnostic tests. *ALP, ALT, AST:* increased levels

Hemoglobin, platelets, white blood cells: decreased values

Drug-herb. *Yew:* inhibited ketoconazole metabolism

Precautions

Use cautiously in:
- renal or hepatic disease, achlorhydria
- pregnant or breastfeeding patients
- children younger than age 2.

Patient monitoring

◀≶ Assess for suicidal ideation and signs and symptoms of depression.

◀≶ Monitor for signs and symptoms of hepatotoxicity, including nausea, fatigue, jaundice, dark urine, and pale stools.

- With long-term therapy, monitor patient for adrenal crisis

Patient teaching

◀≶ Advise patient to watch for signs and symptoms of depression and to immediately report suicidal thoughts.

◀≶ Teach patient to recognize and immediately report signs and symptoms of hepatotoxicity.

- Advise patient not to take antacids for at least 2 hours after oral ketoconazole.

- Instruct patient to apply cream to damp skin of affected area and a wide surrounding area.

- Tell patient to wet hair before applying shampoo and to massage into scalp for 1 minute; then leave shampoo on hair for 5 minutes before rinsing off. Teach him to shampoo again, leaving

shampoo on scalp for 3 minutes this time before rinsing.

- Caution patient not to apply shampoo to broken or inflamed skin.

- As appropriate, review all other significant and life-threatening adverse reactions and interactions, especially those related to the drugs, tests, and herbs mentioned above.

ketoprofen

Actron, Apo-Keto✤, Apo-Keto-E✤, Orudis, Orudis-E, Orudis KT, Orudis-SR✤, Oruvail, Rhodis✤

Pharmacologic class: Nonsteroidal anti-inflammatory drug (NSAID)

Therapeutic class: Analgesic, antipyretic, anti-inflammatory

Pregnancy risk category B (third trimester: *D*)

Action

Unknown; thought to inhibit prostaglandin and leukotriene synthesis and possibly, exert lysosomal membrane-stabilizing activity; also inhibits platelet aggregation and platelet thromboxane synthesis

Availability

Capsules: 25 mg, 50 mg, 75 mg
Capsules (extended-release): 100 mg, 150 mg, 200 mg
Tablets: 12.5 mg

ⓛ Indications and dosages

➤ Rheumatoid arthritis

Adults: 75 mg P.O. t.i.d. or 50 mg q.i.d; maximum dosage is 200 mg/day (Oruvail) or 300 mg/day (Orudis).

➤ Dysmenorrhea

Adults: 25 to 50 mg P.O. q 6 to 8 hours p.r.n.; if optimal response doesn't occur, may give up to 75 mg as a single

---

dose. Maximum dosage is 300 mg/day
P.O.

➢ Fever

Adults: One 12.5-mg tablet P.O. q 4 to
6 hours; give second dose if fever persists after 1 hour. Or initially, two 12.5-mg tablets P.O. Maximum dosage is
two 12.5-mg tablets in 4 hours or six
12.5-mg tablets in 24 hours, continued
for no more than 3 days.

➢ Pain

Adults: 25 to 50 mg P.O. q 6 to 8 hours
p.r.n.

Dosage adjustment
• Renal impairment, cirrhosis
• Elderly patients

Contraindications
• Hypersensitivity to drug, its components, or other NSAIDs
• Severe renal or hepatic disease
• Bleeding disorders

Administration
• Give tablets either 30 minutes before
or 2 hours after meals.
• Administer capsules with food, milk,
or antacids to minimize GI upset.

Route	Onset	Peak	Duration
P.O.	Within 1 hr	1-2 hr	4-6 hr
P.O. (extended)	Unknown	6-7 hr	≤24 hr

Adverse reactions
CNS: headache, dizziness, irritability
EENT: visual disturbances, tinnitus
GI: nausea, vomiting, diarrhea, constipation, abdominal pain or cramps,
dyspepsia, flatulence, stomatitis,
anorexia, **GI bleeding**
GU: urinary tract infection, renal impairment, elevated blood urea nitrogen, **nephrotoxicity**
Hematologic: prolonged bleeding
time, **agranulocytosis**
Skin: rash
Other: edema

Interactions
Drug-drug. *Angiotensin-converting enzyme inhibitors, beta-adrenergic blockers:* decreased antihypertensive effect
Anticoagulants: prolonged prothrombin time
Aspirin: altered ketoprofen distribution, metabolism, and excretion; increased risk of serious adverse reactions
Cholestyramine: decreased ketoprofen
absorption
Corticosteroids, other NSAIDs: additive
adverse GI reactions
Diuretics: decreased diuretic effect
Hydantoins, lithium: increased blood
levels of these drugs and greater risk of
toxicity
Methotrexate: increased risk of methotrexate toxicity
Probenecid: increased risk of ketoprofen toxicity
Drug-diagnostic tests. *Bleeding time:*
prolonged
Drug-herb. *Anise, arnica, chamomile,
clove, dong quai, feverfew, garlic, ginger,
ginkgo, ginseng:* increased risk of bleeding

Precautions
Use cautiously in:
• tartrazine intolerance
• hepatic or renal disease (extended-release form), ulcer disease, GI bleeding or perforation, chronic alcohol use
or abuse, asthma, rhinitis, urticaria
• elderly patients (extended-release
form)
• pregnant patients in second or third
trimester, breastfeeding patients
• children.

Patient monitoring
• Monitor closely for fluid retention in
elderly patients and those with heart
failure.
• Watch for adverse renal effects.

Patient teaching
• Teach patient to consult prescriber
before taking over-the-counter prepa-

rations (especially aspirin-containing products) or herbs.

• Caution patient to avoid driving and other hazardous activities until he knows how drug affects concentration and alertness.

• As appropriate, review all significant and life-threatening adverse reactions and interactions, especially those related to the drugs, tests, and herbs mentioned above.

ketorolac tromethamine
Acular, Toradol

Pharmacologic class: Nonsteroidal anti-inflammatory drug (NSAID)
Therapeutic class: Analgesic, antipyretic, anti-inflammatory
Pregnancy risk category C (third trimester: *D*)

Action
Interferes with prostaglandin biosynthesis by inhibiting cyclooxygenase pathway of arachidonic acid metabolism; also acts as potent inhibitor of platelet aggregation

Availability
Injection: 15 mg/ml in 1-ml preloaded syringes, 30 mg/ml in 1- and 2-ml preloaded syringes
Ophthalmic solution: 0.5%
Tablets: 10 mg

✔ Indications and dosages
➢ Short-term management of moderately severe pain
Adults younger than age 65: Initially, 30 mg I.V. or 60 mg I.M. as a single dose, or 30 mg I.M. or I.V. q 6 hours, not to exceed 120 mg/day. To switch to P.O. dosing, give 20 mg P.O. initially to patients who received single 30-mg I.V. or 60-mg I.M. dose, followed by 10 mg

P.O. q 4 to 6 hours as needed (not to exceed 40 mg/day).
➢ Ocular itching caused by allergic conjunctivitis
Adults and children ages 3 and older: One drop of 0.5% ophthalmic solution instilled in affected eye q.i.d.
➢ Postoperative ocular inflammation related to cataract extraction
Adults and children ages 3 and older: One drop of 0.5% ophthalmic solution instilled in operative eye q.i.d., starting 24 hours after surgery and continuing for up to 3 days afterward
Dosage adjustment
• Mild to moderate renal impairment
• Elderly patients
• Patients weighing less than 50 kg (110 lb)

Contraindications
• Hypersensitivity to drug, its components, or other NSAIDs
• Concurrent use of aspirin, other NSAIDs, or probenecid
• Peptic ulcer disease
• GI bleeding or perforation (current or previous)
• Severe renal impairment or risk of renal failure
• Increased risk of bleeding
• Labor and delivery
• Breastfeeding

Administration
• Be aware that oral therapy is indicated only as a continuation of parenteral therapy.
◀€ Know that parenteral therapy shouldn't exceed 20 doses over 5 days.
• Dilute with normal saline solution, dextrose 5% in water, dextrose 5% and normal saline solution, Ringer's solution, or lactated Ringer's solution.
• Administer I.V. bolus over 15 seconds or longer.
• Inject I.M. dose slowly and deeply into muscle.

• Don't give by epidural or intrathecal injection; don't use as prophylactic analgesic before major surgery.

Route	Onset	Peak	Duration
P.O.	Unknown	2-3 hr	≥4-6 hr
I.V., I.M.	10 min	1-2 hr	≥6 hr
Ophthalmic	Unknown	Unknown	Unknown

Adverse reactions

CNS: drowsiness, headache, dizziness
CV: hypertension
EENT: tinnitus
GI: nausea, vomiting, diarrhea, constipation, flatulence, dyspepsia, epigastric pain, stomatitis
Hematologic: prolonged bleeding time, **thrombocytopenia**
Skin: rash, pruritus, diaphoresis
Other: excessive thirst, edema, injection site pain

Interactions

Drug-drug. *Angiotensin-converting enzyme inhibitors, beta-adrenergic blockers:* decreased antihypertensive effect
Anticoagulants: prolonged prothrombin time
Aspirin: altered ketorolac distribution, metabolism, and excretion; increased risk of serious adverse reactions
Cholestyramine: decreased ketorolac absorption
Corticosteroids, other NSAIDs: additive adverse GI effects
Diuretics: decreased diuretic effect
Hydantoins, lithium: increased blood levels and greater risk of toxicity of these drugs
Methotrexate: increased risk of methotrexate toxicity
Probenecid: increased risk of ketorolac toxicity
Drug-diagnostic tests. *Bleeding time:* prolonged for 24 to 48 hours after therapy ends
Drug-herb. *Anise, arnica, chamomile, clove, dong quai, feverfew, garlic, ginger,* *ginkgo, ginseng:* increased risk of bleeding

Precautions

Use cautiously in:
• mild to moderate renal impairment, cardiovascular disease
• elderly patients
• pregnant patients
• children.

Patient monitoring

• Monitor for adverse reactions, especially prolonged bleeding time and CNS reactions.
• Check I.M. injection site for hematoma or bleeding.
• Monitor fluid intake and output.

Patient teaching

• Inform patient that drug is meant only for short-term pain management.
◀͡€ Instruct patient to immediately report bleeding and adverse CNS reactions.
• Advise patient to minimize GI upset by eating small, frequent servings of healthy foods.
• Instruct patient to avoid aspirin products and herbs during therapy.
• Teach patient to avoid driving and other hazardous activities until he knows how drug affects concentration and alertness.
• As appropriate, review all other significant and life-threatening adverse reactions and interactions, especially those related to the drugs, tests, and herbs mentioned above.

k

labetalol hydrochloride
Normodyne, Trandate

Pharmacologic class: Beta-adrenergic blocker (nonselective), alpha-adrenergic blocker (selective)
Therapeutic class: Antihypertensive
Pregnancy risk category C

Action
Blocks stimulation of beta$_1$- and beta$_2$-adrenergic receptor sites and alpha$_1$-adrenergic receptors, thereby decreasing myocardial contractile force and enhancing coronary artery blood flow and myocardial perfusion. Net effect is decreased heart rate and blood pressure.

Availability
Injection: 5 mg/ml
Tablets: 100 mg, 200 mg, 300 mg

⊘ Indications and dosages
➤ Hypertension
Adults: Initially, 100 mg P.O. b.i.d., alone or combined with a diuretic; may be increased by 100 mg b.i.d. q 2 to 3 days as needed. Usual range is 400 to 800 mg/day in two to three divided doses; dosages up to 2.4 g/day have been used.
➤ Hypertensive crisis
Adults: Initially, 20 mg by I.V. bolus, followed by injections of 40 to 80 mg q 10 minutes until blood pressure decreases to desired level; maximum dosage is 300 mg. Alternatively, 50 to 200 mg by continuous I.V. infusion at 2 mg/minute (some patients may require total dosage of 300 mg); continue infusion until desired blood pressure is

reached. Follow I.V. administration with P.O. dosing.
➤ Conversion from I.V. to oral dosing
Hospitalized adults: Discontinue I.V. therapy when desired blood pressure is controlled; start P.O. dosing when supine diastolic blood pressure begins to rise. Initially, 200 mg P.O., followed 6 to 12 hours later with an additional dose of 200 to 400 mg P.O., depending on blood pressure response. Then titrate at 1-day intervals to dosages ranging from 400 to 2,400 mg/day P.O. in two or three divided doses.
Dosage adjustment
• Chronic hepatic disease
• Elderly patients

Off-label uses
• Hypertension secondary to pheochromocytoma or clonidine withdrawal

Contraindications
• Hypersensitivity to drug
• Bronchospastic disease
• Cardiac failure, cardiogenic shock
• Second- or third-degree atrioventricular block
• Severe bradycardia

Administration
• Know that drug may be given as I.V. bolus or continuous infusion.
• Give direct I.V. injection over 2 minutes at 10-minute intervals.
• Dilute in dextrose 5% in water or normal saline solution; use infusion control pump for continuous infusion.
• Don't mix with 5% sodium bicarbonate injection.

Route	Onset	Peak	Duration
P.O.	20 min-2 hr	1-4 hr	8-12 hr
I.V.	2-5 min	5 min	16-18 hr

Adverse reactions
CNS: fatigue, asthenia, anxiety, depression, dizziness, paresthesia, drowsiness,

insomnia, memory loss, nightmares, mental status changes

CV: orthostatic hypotension, peripheral vasoconstriction, bradycardia, **arrhythmias, heart failure**

EENT: blurred vision, dry eyes, nasal congestion

GI: nausea, diarrhea, constipation

GU: increased blood urea nitrogen (BUN), impotence, decreased libido

Hematologic: purpura, **agranulocytosis, thrombocytopenia**

Hepatic: elevated liver function test results

Metabolic: hyperglycemia, hypoglycemia, increased low-density lipoprotein (LDL) level

Musculoskeletal: joint pain, back pain, muscle cramps

Respiratory: wheezing, **bronchospasm, pulmonary edema**

Skin: rash, pruritus

Interactions

Drug-drug. *Adrenergic bronchodilators, theophylline:* decreased efficacy of these drugs

Antihypertensives, nitrates: additive hypotension

Cimetidine, propranolol: increased labetalol effects

Digoxin: additive bradycardia

Dobutamine, dopamine: decreased beneficial cardiovascular effects of these drugs

General anesthetics, verapamil: additive myocardial depression

Insulin, oral hypoglycemics: altered hypoglycemic efficacy

Monoamine oxidase inhibitors: hypertension

Nonsteroidal anti-inflammatory drugs: decreased antihypertensive action

Drug-diagnostic tests. *Alanine aminotransferase, alkaline phosphatase, antinuclear antibodies, aspartate aminotransferase, BUN, glucose, LDLs, potassium, triglycerides, uric acid:* increased levels

Precautions

Use cautiously in:
- hepatic impairment, pulmonary disease, diabetes mellitus, hyperthyroidism, thyrotoxicosis
- elderly patients
- pregnant or breastfeeding patients
- children.

Patient monitoring

- Monitor ECG and vital signs, especially blood pressure.
- Assess cardiovascular and neurologic status closely to detect adverse reactions.
- Monitor complete blood count, blood glucose level, and liver function test results.

Patient teaching

- Inform patient that he may experience dizziness when starting therapy, especially if he's also taking a diuretic.
- Advise patient to move slowly when sitting up or standing to avoid dizziness or light-headedness from sudden blood pressure decrease.
- Instruct patient to avoid driving and other hazardous activities until he knows how drug affects concentration, vision, and alertness.
- Emphasize need for follow-up care and regular blood pressure monitoring.
◀︎ Caution patient not to stop taking drug abruptly because this may cause myocardial infarction or worsen angina.
- As appropriate, review all other significant and life-threatening adverse reactions and interactions, especially those related to the drugs and tests mentioned above.

lactulose
Cephulac, Cholac, Chronulac,
Constilac, Constulose, Duphalac,
Enulose, Evalose, Heptalac,
Lactulax✢, PMS-Lactulose, Portalac

Pharmacologic class: Osmotic
Therapeutic class: Laxative
Pregnancy risk category B

Action
Produces osmotic effect, causing increased water content in the colon and increased peristalsis. Breakdown products in colon lead to acidification of colonic contents and softening of feces, and prevent absorption of ammonia. Ammonium ions are poorly absorbed from colon to circulation, leading to reduced blood ammonia level in portal-system encephalopathy.

Availability
Powder (single-use packets): 10 g, 20 g
Syrup (cola flavor): 10 g /15 ml

💋 Indications and dosages
➤ Constipation
Adults: 10 to 20 g (15 to 30 ml) P.O. daily, increased to 60 ml daily p.r.n.
➤ Portal-system encephalopathy
Adults: 20 to 30 g (30 to 45 ml) P.O. three or four times daily until two or three soft stools are produced daily. Therapy may continue on long-term basis.

Contraindications
• Hypersensitivity to drug
• Galactosemia
• Low-galactose diet

Administration
• Don't administer concurrently with other laxatives.

• Dissolve contents of single-use packet in 4 oz of water or juice.
• Dilute syrup with water or fruit juice to mask taste.

Route	Onset	Peak	Duration
P.O.	24-48 hr	Unknown	Unknown

Adverse reactions
GI: diarrhea, intestinal cramps, abdominal distention, flatulence
Metabolic: hyperglycemia (in diabetic patients)

Interactions
Drug-drug. *Anti-infectives:* decreased lactulose efficacy
Other laxatives: interference with response to lactulose (in patients with hepatic encephalopathy)
Drug-diagnostic tests. *Blood ammonia:* 25% to 50% decrease in level
Glucose: increased level (in diabetic patients)

Precautions
Use cautiously in:
• diabetes mellitus
• elderly patients
• pregnant or breastfeeding patients
• children.

Patient monitoring
• Monitor for adverse GI reactions.
• Check stool consistency and frequency.
• Monitor electrolyte levels, especially in elderly patients.
• Check blood glucose level in diabetic patients.

Patient teaching
• Instruct patient to dissolve contents of single-use packet in 4 oz of water or juice.
• Suggest that patient dilute syrup with water or juice to mask taste.
• Tell patient that drug initially may cause flatulence and intestinal cramps

---

but that these symptoms usually subside.

• Inform patient that excessive use of drug may cause diarrhea, which may induce excessive fluid loss.

• Encourage patient to drink adequate fluids and to report signs and symptoms of dehydration.

• As appropriate, review all other significant adverse reactions and interactions, especially those related to the drugs and tests mentioned above.

lamivudine
Epivir, Epivir-HBV, 3TC✤

Pharmacologic class: Nucleoside reverse transcriptase inhibitor
Therapeutic class: Antiretroviral
Pregnancy risk category C

Action
Inhibits human immunodeficiency virus (HIV) reverse transcription by viral DNA chain termination; impedes RNA-and DNA-dependent DNA polymerase activities of reverse transcriptase

Availability
Oral solution: 5 mg/ml and 10 mg/ml in 240-ml bottles
Tablets: 100 mg, 150 mg

💋 Indications and dosages
➢ HIV infection (given with other antiretrovirals)
Adults and children older than age 16: 150 mg P.O. b.i.d. or 300 mg P.O. daily
Children ages 3 months to 16 years: 4 mg/kg P.O. b.i.d. to a maximum of 150 mg P.O. b.i.d.
➢ Chronic hepatitis B virus (HBV)
Adults: 100 mg Epivir-HBV P.O. once daily

Children ages 2 to 17: 3 mg/kg Epivir-HBV P.O. once daily, to a maximum of 100 mg P.O. daily
Dosage adjustment
• Renal impairment

Contraindications
• Hypersensitivity to drug or its components
• Breastfeeding

Administration
• Give with or without food.
◀℥ Be aware that Epivir contains 150 mg lamivudine, whereas Epivir-HBV contains 100 mg lamivudine; strengths aren't interchangeable. When given to patients with unrecognized or untreated HIV, Epivir-HBV is likely to cause rapid emergence of HIV resistance.

Route	Onset	Peak	Duration
P.O.	Unknown	0.9 hr	12 hr

Adverse reactions
CNS: fatigue, headache, insomnia, malaise, asthenia, depression, dizziness, paresthesia, peripheral neuropathy, **seizures**
GI: nausea, vomiting, diarrhea, anorexia, abdominal discomfort, dyspepsia, splenomegaly, **pancreatitis**
Hematologic: anemia, **neutropenia**
Hepatic: increased liver function test results, hepatomegaly with steatosis
Metabolic: hyperglycemia, lactic acidosis
Musculoskeletal: muscle, joint, or bone pain; muscle weakness; myalgia; rhabdomyolysis
Respiratory: cough, abnormal breath sounds, wheezing
Skin: alopecia, rash, urticaria, erythema multiforme
Other: lymphadenopathy, body fat redistribution, hypersensitivity reactions including **Stevens-Johnson syndrome, anaphylaxis**

Interactions

Drug-drug. *Co-trimoxazole:* increased lamivudine blood level
Zalcitabine: interference with effects of both drugs
Drug-diagnostic tests. *Alanine aminotransferase, alkaline phosphatase, aspartate aminotransferase, bilirubin, creatine kinase:* increased levels
Hemoglobin, hematocrit, neutrophils: decreased levels

Precautions

Use cautiously in:
• impaired renal function, history of hepatic disease, obesity
• granulocyte count below 1,000/mm³
• long-term therapy
• elderly patients
• women (especially if pregnant)
• children.

Patient monitoring

• Check vital signs regularly.
• Monitor complete blood count and platelet count frequently; watch for signs and symptoms of bone marrow toxicity.
• Monitor blood glucose level and kidney and liver function test results.
• Assess neurologic and mental status; report signs or symptoms of depression.
• Monitor women, obese patients, and those with a history of hepatic disease closely; they're at increased risk for lactic acidosis and severe hepatomegaly with steatosis.
• Monitor patients with HIV for coinfection with HBV (which may recur after drug is discontinued).

Patient teaching

• Tell patient he may take drug with or without food.
• Advise patient to minimize GI upset by eating small, frequent servings of healthy food and drinking plenty of fluids.

• Instruct patient to avoid driving and other hazardous activities until he knows how drug affects concentration and alertness.
• Inform patients with HIV that drug doesn't cure virus or prevent its transmission and that opportunistic infections may occur. Advise them to take appropriate precautions during sex.
• As appropriate, review all other significant and life-threatening adverse reactions and interactions, especially those related to the drugs and tests mentioned above.

lamotrigine
Lamictal, Lamictal Chewable Dispersible

Pharmacologic class: Phenyltriazine
Therapeutic class: Anticonvulsant
Pregnancy risk category C

Action

Unknown; blocks sodium channel membranes, which in turn inhibits release of the neurotransmitters glutamate and aspartate in the brain

Availability

Tablets: 25 mg, 100 mg, 150 mg, 200 mg
Tablets (chewable): 2 mg, 5 mg, 25 mg

⟋ Indications and dosages

➤ Adjunctive treatment of partial seizures
Adults and children ages 16 and older: In patients receiving valproic acid, usual dosage is 100 to 200 mg P.O. daily. (However, combination regimen increases risk of Stevens-Johnson syndrome and other life-threatening dermatologic reactions.) In patients receiving enzyme-inducing anticonvulsants other than valproic acid, 50

mg P.O. daily for 2 weeks, then 100 mg P.O. daily in two divided doses for 2 weeks; increase by 100 mg/day q 1 to 2 weeks, as needed. Maintenance dosage is 300 to 500 mg P.O. daily in two divided doses.

For conversion to monotherapy in patients also receiving one enzyme-inducing anticonvulsant, 500 mg P.O. daily in two divided doses while maintaining current dosage of enzyme-inducing anticonvulsant. Withdraw first drug over 4 weeks.

➤ Adjunctive treatment of Lennox-Gastaut syndrome

Adults and children ages 12 and older: In patients receiving valproic acid, 25 mg P.O. every other day for 2 weeks, then 25 mg P.O. daily for 2 weeks. Maintenance dosage is 100 to 400 mg P.O. daily in one or two divided doses.

In patients receiving enzyme-inducing anticonvulsants other than valproic acid, 50 mg P.O. daily in two divided doses for 2 weeks, then 100 mg P.O. daily in two divided doses for 2 weeks. Maintenance dosage is 300 to 500 mg P.O. daily in two divided doses.

Children ages 2 to 12 who weigh 17 kg (37 lb) or more: In patients receiving valproic acid, 0.15 mg/kg P.O. daily as a single dose or in two divided doses for 2 weeks. Maintenance dosage is 1 to 5 mg/kg daily.

In patients receiving enzyme-inducing anticonvulsants other than valproic acid, 0.6 mg/kg P.O. daily in two divided doses for 2 weeks; then 1.2 mg/kg P.O. daily in two divided doses for 2 weeks. Maintenance dosage is 5 to 15 mg/kg daily.

Dosage adjustment
• Moderate or severe hepatic dysfunction
• Renal impairment
• Cardiac disease

Off-label uses
• Absence, generalized tonic-clonic, and myoclonic seizures
• Drug-resistant seizures
• Acute management of depression in bipolar I disorder
• Mood stabilization in rapid-cycling bipolar II disorder

Contraindications
• Hypersensitivity to drug or its components

Administration
• Give with or without food.
• Don't crush or break regular tablets; make sure patient swallows them whole.
• Crush chewable tablets or mix in diluted fruit juice if patient can't chew them.

◀◣ Be aware that abrupt drug withdrawal may induce seizures. If drug must be discontinued, decrease dosage by 50% per week over at least 2 weeks (unless patient safety warrants more rapid withdrawal).

Route	Onset	Peak	Duration
P.O.	Unknown	1.4-4.8 hr	Unknown

Adverse reactions
CNS: dizziness, headache, drowsiness, ataxia incoordination, insomnia, tremor, depression, anxiety, irritability, impaired memory, poor concentration, emotional lability, vertigo, racing thoughts, dysarthria, sleep disorders, malaise, **seizures**
CV: palpitations
GI: nausea, vomiting, diarrhea, constipation, abdominal pain, dyspepsia, dry mouth, anorexia
GU: dysmenorrhea, amenorrhea, vaginitis
Hepatic: hepatotoxicity
Musculoskeletal: muscle spasm, neck pain
Respiratory: cough, dyspnea

Skin: alopecia, rash, urticaria, erythema multiforme
Other: hypersensitivity reactions including **anaphylaxis, Stevens-Johnson syndrome**

Interactions
Drug-drug. *Carbamazepine, phenobarbital, phenytoin, primidone:* decreased lamotrigine steady-state level
Folate inhibitors (such as methotrexate, co-trimoxazole): additive effects of lamotrigine
Valproic acid: decreased lamotrigine clearance, increased steady-state level
Drug-behaviors. *Sun exposure:* photosensitivity

Precautions
Use cautiously in:
• renal or hepatic impairment
• concurrent use of other anticonvulsants
• pregnant or breastfeeding patients
• children.

Patient monitoring
• Monitor vital signs regularly.
• Monitor CNS status carefully, noting adverse reactions and changes in seizure pattern.
• Check liver function test results frequently; watch for signs and symptoms of hepatotoxicity.

Patient teaching
• Tell patient he may take drug with or without food.
• Teach patient taking regular tablets to swallow them whole without crushing or breaking.
• Advise patient taking chewable tablets to crush them or mix them in diluted fruit juice if he can't chew them.
• Inform patient that dosage is adjusted slowly, as indicated.
• Instruct patient to avoid driving and other hazardous activities until he knows how drug affects concentration and alertness.
• Teach patient to minimize GI upset by eating small, frequent servings of healthy food and drinking plenty of fluids.
• As appropriate, review all other significant and life-threatening adverse reactions and interactions, especially those related to the drugs and behaviors mentioned above.

lansoprazole
Prevacid, Prevpac

Pharmacologic class: Gastric acid pump inhibitor
Therapeutic class: Antiulcer drug
Pregnancy risk category B

Action
Inhibits activity of proton pump in gastric parietal cells, resulting in decreased gastric acid production

Availability
Capsules (delayed-release): 15 mg, 30 mg
Granules for oral suspension (delayed-release, enteric-coated): 15 mg, 30 mg
Prevpac (combination product for Helicobacter pylori *infection):* daily pack containing two 30-mg lansoprazole, four 500-mg amoxicillin, and two 500-mg clarithromycin tablets

Indications and dosages
➤ Short-term treatment of duodenal ulcer
Adults: 15 mg P.O. daily for 4 weeks
➤ *H. pylori* eradication to reduce risk of duodenal ulcer recurrence
Adults: As triple therapy, 30 mg lansoprazole P.O., 1 g amoxicillin P.O., and 500 mg clarithromycin P.O. q 12 hours for 10 or 14 days. As dual therapy, 30

mg lansoprazole P.O. and 1 g amoxicillin P.O. q 8 hours for 14 days.

➤ Short-term treatment of benign gastric ulcer

Adults: 30 mg P.O. once daily for up to 8 weeks

➤ Gastric ulcer associated with nonsteroidal anti-inflammatory drugs (NSAIDs)

Adults: For healing, 30 mg P.O. once daily for up to 8 weeks; for prevention, 15 mg P.O. once daily for up to 12 weeks

➤ Short-term treatment of symptomatic gastroesophageal reflux disease (GERD)

Adults: 15 mg P.O. once daily for up to 8 weeks

➤ Short-term treatment of erosive esophagitis

Adults: 30 mg P.O. once daily for up to 8 weeks; some patients require 8 additional weeks. Maintenance dosage is 15 mg P.O. once daily.

➤ Pathologic hypersecretory conditions (including Zollinger-Ellison syndrome)

Adults: Initially, 60 mg P.O. once daily, up to a maximum of 90 mg P.O. b.i.d. Divide daily dosages over 120 mg.

Dosage adjustment
• Significant hepatic insufficiency

Contraindications
• Hypersensitivity to drug or its components
• Creatinine clearance below 30 ml/minute

Administration
• Give before meals.
• If patient has difficulty swallowing delayed-release capsule, open it and sprinkle contents into small amount of soft food, such as applesauce or pudding, or give with a small amount of orange or tomato juice.
• When injecting through nasogastric (NG) tube, open delayed-release capsule and mix granules with 40 ml of apple juice. Then rinse tube with additional apple juice to clear.

Route	Onset	Peak	Duration
P.O.	Rapid	Unknown	>24 hr

Adverse reactions
CNS: headache, confusion, anxiety, malaise, paresthesia, abnormal thinking, depression, dizziness, syncope, **cerebrovascular accident**
CV: chest pain, hypertension, hypotension, **myocardial infarction, shock**
EENT: visual field deficits, otitis media, tinnitus, epistaxis
GI: nausea, diarrhea, abdominal pain, cholelithiasis, dysphagia, ulcerative colitis, esophageal ulcer, hematemesis, stomatitis, **GI hemorrhage**
GU: renal calculi, impotence, abnormal menses, breast tenderness, gynecomastia
Hematologic: anemia
Respiratory: cough, asthma, bronchitis
Skin: urticaria, alopecia, acne, pruritus, photosensitivity

Interactions
Drug-drug. *Drugs requiring acidic pH (including ampicillin esters, digoxin, iron salts, itraconazole, ketoconazole):* decreased absorption of these drugs
Sucralfate: decreased lansoprazole absorption
Theophylline: increased theophylline clearance
Drug-food. *Any food:* decreased rate and extent of GI drug absorption
Drug-herb. *Male fern:* inactivation of herb
St. John's wort: increased risk of photosensitivity

Precautions
Use cautiously in:
• severe hepatic impairment
• elderly patients
• pregnant or breastfeeding patients
• children younger than age 18.

Patient monitoring
• Monitor for adverse GI reactions.
• Assess nutritional status and fluid balance to identify significant problems.

Patient teaching
• Tell patient to take drug before meals.
• If patient has difficulty swallowing, advise him to open delayed-release capsule and sprinkle contents into small amount of soft food, such as applesauce or pudding, or to take drug with small amount of orange or tomato juice.
• Teach patient to minimize GI upset by eating small, frequent servings of healthy food and drinking plenty of fluids.
• As appropriate, review all other significant and life-threatening adverse reactions and interactions, especially those related to the drugs, foods, and herbs mentioned above.

leflunomide
Arava

Pharmacologic class: Immune modulator

Therapeutic class: Antirheumatic (disease-modifying)

Pregnancy risk category X

Action
Inhibits T-cell pyrimidine biosynthesis, tyrosine kinases, and dihydroorotate dehydrogenase (DHODH). DHODH blockage relieves inflammation and blocks structural damage caused by inflammatory response to autoimmune process. Also shows analgesic, antipyretic, anti-inflammatory, and histamine-blocking activity.

Availability
Tablets: 10 mg, 20 mg, 100 mg

ⓘ Indications and dosages
➤ Active rheumatoid arthritis
Adults: 100 mg P.O. daily for 3 days, followed by a maintenance dosage of 20 mg daily. If intolerance occurs, decrease to 10 mg daily.
Dosage adjustment
• Elevated hepatic enzyme levels

Contraindications
• Hypersensitivity to drug or its components
• Immunocompromised state, including bone marrow dysplasia and severe uncontrolled infection
• Hepatic impairment or evidence of hepatitis B or C
• Live-virus vaccination
• Pregnancy or breastfeeding
• Children younger than age 18

Administration
• Give with or without food.
• Be aware that drug has a long half-life. To eliminate drug from bloodstream, give 8 g cholestyramine P.O. t.i.d. for 11 days to clear primary metabolite from plasma.

Route	Onset	Peak	Duration
P.O.	1 mo	3-6 mo	Unknown

Adverse reactions
CNS: headache, dizziness, asthenia
CV: chest pain, hypertension
EENT: rhinitis, sinusitis, pharyngitis
GI: nausea, vomiting, diarrhea, abdominal pain, dyspepsia, gastroenteritis, mouth ulcers, anorexia
GU: urinary tract infection
Hepatic: elevated hepatic enzyme levels, **hepatotoxicity**
Metabolic: hypokalemia
Musculoskeletal: joint pain or disorders, back pain, leg cramps, synovitis, tenosynovitis

---

Respiratory: bronchitis, increased cough, pneumonia, respiratory infection

Skin: alopecia, rash, dry skin, eczema, pruritus

Other: weight loss, pain, infection, allergic reactions, flulike symptoms

Interactions

Drug-drug. *Activated charcoal, cholestyramine:* rapid, steep drop in blood level of active leflunomide metabolite

Methotrexate, other hepatotoxic drugs: increased risk of hepatotoxicity

Rifampin: increased blood level of active leflunomide metabolite

Drug-diagnostic tests. *Alanine aminotransferase, aspartate aminotransferase:* increased levels

Precautions

Use cautiously in:
• renal insufficiency
• men attempting to father a child.

Patient monitoring

• Check vital signs closely.
◀︎€ Watch for signs and symptoms of hepatotoxicity.
• Assess cardiovascular and respiratory status carefully to detect adverse reactions.
• Monitor liver function test results and electrolyte levels.
• Stay alert for signs and symptoms of urinary tract infection.
• Observe patient closely after dosage reduction; metabolite levels may take several weeks to decrease.

Patient teaching

• Tell patient he may take drug with or without food.
• Instruct patient to avoid driving and other hazardous activities until he knows how drug affects concentration and alertness.
• Teach patient to minimize GI upset by eating small, frequent servings of healthy food and drinking plenty of fluids.
• Inform women of childbearing age that drug may harm fetus; tell her to contact prescriber immediately if she suspects pregnancy.
• Advise men planning to father a child to consult prescriber because of drug's harmful effects on fetus.
• Inform patient that he'll undergo regular blood testing to check hepatic function.
• As appropriate, review all other significant and life-threatening adverse reactions and interactions, especially those related to the drugs and tests mentioned above.

lepirudin
Refludan

Pharmacologic class: Thrombin inhibitor
Therapeutic class: Anticoagulant
Pregnancy risk category B

Action
Binds with thrombin, blocking its thrombogenic activity

Availability
Powder for injection: 50 mg

Indications and dosages
➢ Heparin-induced thrombocytopenia and associated thromboembolic disease
Adults: Initially, 0.4 mg/kg by I.V. bolus over 15 to 20 seconds (to a maximum of 44 mg), followed by 0.15 mg/kg by continuous I.V. infusion for 2 to 10 days or longer if needed

Dosage adjustment
• Renal impairment
• Elderly patients

Contraindications

• Hypersensitivity to drug, its components, or hirudin

Administration

• Check activated partial thromboplastin time (APTT) before initiating therapy.

◀€ Administer I.V. bolus slowly over at least 15 to 20 seconds.

• Follow bolus with continuous I.V. infusion lasting 2 to 10 days.

◀€ Be aware that dosage adjustments are based on APTT measured 4 hours after drug initiation and then at least once daily.

• To reconstitute, mix with sterile water for injection or 0.9% sodium chloride injection.

• For further dilution, use 0.9% sodium chloride injection or 5% dextrose injection.

Route	Onset	Peak	Duration
I.V.	Immediate	Unknown	Unknown

Adverse reactions

CNS: chills, fever
CV: heart failure, pericardial effusion, ventricular fibrillation
GI: GI bleeding
GU: hematuria, abnormal renal function
Hematologic: hemorrhage, thrombocytopenia
Hepatic: increased liver function test results
Respiratory: pneumonia, hemoptysis
Skin: rash, pruritus, urticaria
Other: bleeding at injection site, excessive bleeding from wounds, **multisystem failure, sepsis, anaphylaxis**

Interactions

Drug-drug. *Cefamandole, cefoperazone, cefotetan, clopidogrel, eptifibatide, nonsteroidal anti-inflammatory drugs, oral anticoagulants, platelet aggregation inhibitors, plicamycin, thrombolytics,* *ticlopidine, tirofiban, valproic acid:* increased risk of bleeding

Precautions

Use cautiously in:
• renal or hepatic disease, bleeding, bacterial endocarditis
• recent cerebrovascular accident or neurosurgery
• pregnant or breastfeeding patients
• children.

Patient monitoring

• Check vital signs frequently.

◀€ Monitor APTT at least daily; target range is 1.5 to 2.5.

• Assess fluid intake and output.

◀€ Watch closely for signs and symptoms of bleeding.

• Monitor complete blood count with white cell differential; assess liver function test results.

◀€ Monitor for adverse effects, particularly signs and symptoms of infection, multisystem failure, and cardiorespiratory problems.

Patient teaching

• Explain bleeding precautions that patient should take during therapy.

◀€ Teach patient to recognize and immediately report signs and symptoms of bleeding.

• Inform patient that he'll undergo frequent blood testing during therapy.

• As appropriate, review all significant and life-threatening adverse reactions and interactions, especially those related to the drugs mentioned above.

letrozole
Femara

Pharmacologic class: Aromatase inhibitor

Therapeutic class: Antineoplastic
Pregnancy risk category D

Action
Inhibits aromatase, an enzyme that promotes conversion of estrogen precursors to estrogen; this causes reduction of circulating estrogen levels, stopping progression of estrogen-sensitive breast cancer

Availability
Tablets: 2.5 mg

🕭 Indications and dosages
➤ Hormone-receptor–positive or hormone-receptor–unknown metastatic or advanced breast cancer in postmenopausal women; advanced breast cancer in postmenopausal women with disease progression despite antiestrogen therapy
Adults: 2.5 mg P.O. daily

Contraindications
• Hypersensitivity to drug or its components
• Pregnancy

Administration
• Give without regard to meals.

Route	Onset	Peak	Duration
P.O.	Unknown	2-3 days	Unknown

Adverse reactions
CNS: anxiety, depression, dizziness, drowsiness, fatigue, headache, vertigo, asthenia
CV: chest pain, hypertension
GI: nausea, vomiting, diarrhea, constipation, abdominal pain, dyspepsia, anorexia
Metabolic: hypercholesterolemia, hypercalcemia
Musculoskeletal: musculoskeletal or joint pain, fractures
Respiratory: cough, dyspnea, pleural effusion
Skin: alopecia, pruritus, rash, diaphoresis
Other: hot flashes, edema, weight gain

Interactions
Drug-diagnostic tests. *Cholesterol, gamma-glutamyltransferase:* increased levels

Precautions
Use cautiously in:
• severe hepatic impairment
• breastfeeding patients
• children (safety not established).

Patient monitoring
• Check vital signs; assess cardiovascular and respiratory status.
• Monitor renal and hepatic function, electrolyte levels, and lipid panels.
• Assess for adverse CNS effects, including depression; institute safety measures as needed to prevent injury.

Patient teaching
• Tell patient she can take drug with or without food.
• Instruct patient to weigh herself regularly and report significant changes.
• Advise patient and family to watch for signs and symptoms of depression.
• Teach patient to minimize GI upset by eating small, frequent servings of healthy food and drinking plenty of fluids.
• Instruct patient to avoid driving and other hazardous activities until she knows how drug affects concentration and alertness.
• Inform patient that treatment is long term and she'll require follow-up appointments with prescriber.
• As appropriate, review all other significant adverse reactions and interactions, especially those related to the tests mentioned above.

leuprolide acetate

Eligard, Lupron, Lupron Depot,
Lupron Depot-Ped, Lupron Depot-3
Month, Lupron Depot-4 Month,
Lupron-3 Month SR Depot, Viadur

Pharmacologic class: Gonadotropin-
releasing hormone (GnRH) analog
Therapeutic class: Antineoplastic
Pregnancy risk category X

Action

Inhibits and desensitizes GnRH receptors, thereby inhibiting gonadotropin
secretion when given continuously.
This action results in an initial increase, then a profound decrease, in
luteinizing hormone (LH) and follicle-
stimulating hormone levels and a reduction in sex hormones released in
response to LH stimulation.

Availability

Implant (12-month): 72 mg
Injection: 5 mg/ml
Lupron Depot injection: 3.75 mg/ml,
7.5 mg/ml
Lupron Depot-3 month injection: 11.25
mg, 22.5 mg
Lupron Depot-4 month injection: 30 mg
Lupron Depot-Ped injection: 7.5 mg,
11.25 mg, 15 mg

⚕ Indications and dosages

➤ Advanced prostate cancer
Adults: 1 mg S.C. daily or 7.5 mg I.M.
monthly (depot injection). Or 22.5 mg
I.M. q 3 months, 30 mg I.M. q 4
months, or one 72-mg implant q 12
months.
➤ Endometriosis
Adults: 3.75 mg I.M. (depot injection)
as a single injection once monthly, or
11.25 mg I.M. q 3 months for up to 6
months

➤ Adjunct to iron therapy in anemia
secondary to uterine leiomyomas
Adults: 3.75 mg I.M. monthly or 11.25
mg I.M. q 3 months as a single dose,
given with iron therapy. Recommended duration of therapy is 6 months or
less.
➤ Central precocious puberty
Children: 50 mcg/kg S.C. daily as a
single injection, increased in increments of 10 mcg/kg daily as needed
**Children weighing more than 37.5 kg
(82.5 lb):** Initially, 15 mg of Depot-Ped
I.M. q 4 weeks, increased in increments
of 3.75 mg q 4 weeks as needed
**Children weighing 25 to 37.5 kg (55 to
82.5 lb):** Initially, 11.25 mg of Depot-
Ped I.M. q 4 weeks, increased in increments of 3.75 mg q 4 weeks as needed
**Children weighing less than 25 kg
(55 lb):** Initially, 7.5 mg of Depot-Ped
I.M. q 4 weeks, increased in increments
of 3.75 mg q 4 weeks as needed

Contraindications

• Hypersensitivity to drug, its components, GnRH, or other GnRH analogs
• Undiagnosed abnormal vaginal
bleeding
• Women (4-month, 30-mg depot
form not recommended)
• Women and children (implant not
recommended)
• Pregnancy or breastfeeding

Administration

• Administer Eligard within 30 minutes of mixing; otherwise, discard
drug.
• Once Lupron injection is mixed, administer immediately; otherwise, discard.
• Administer Lupron Depot-Ped only
under prescriber's supervision.

Route	Onset	Peak	Duration
I.M. depot	4 hr	Variable	1, 3, 4 mo
Implant	Unknown	Unknown	1 yr
S.C. (prec. puberty)	1 wk	Unknown	4-12 wk after therapy
S.C. (endo-metriosis, cancer)	2-4 wk	After 1-2 mo	2-3 mo after therapy

Adverse reactions

CNS: anxiety, depression, dizziness, drowsiness, asthenia, fatigue, headache, vertigo, syncope, mood changes
CV: palpitations, angina, **arrhythmias, myocardial infarction**
EENT: blurred vision
GI: nausea, vomiting, diarrhea, constipation, abdominal pain, dyspepsia, sour taste, anorexia
GU: urinary frequency, hematuria, increased blood urea nitrogen and creatinine levels, decreased testes size, impotence, decreased libido, gynecomastia
Hematologic: anemia, **thrombocytopenia**
Respiratory: dyspnea, pleural rub, **worsening of pulmonary fibrosis, pulmonary embolism**
Skin: alopecia, pruritus, rash, diaphoresis
Other: edema, hot flashes, **anaphylaxis**

Interactions

Drug-diagnostic tests. *Pituitary-gonadal system tests:* misleading results during therapy and for up to 3 months afterward

Precautions

Use cautiously in:
• renal, hepatic, or cardiac impairment.

Patient monitoring

• Observe injection site for local reactions.

• Monitor cardiovascular and respiratory status carefully to detect serious adverse reactions.
• Evaluate neurologic status; institute safety measures as needed to prevent injury.
• Monitor serum testosterone and prostate-specific antigen levels periodically.

Patient teaching

• Inform patient that localized reaction may occur at injection site; tell him to contact prescriber if symptoms don't resolve.
• Advise patient and family to watch for and report signs or symptoms of depression.
• Tell patient that drug may cause libido changes or erectile dysfunction; encourage him to discuss these problems with prescriber.
• Instruct patient to avoid driving and other hazardous activities until he knows how drug affects concentration and alertness.
• Teach patient to minimize GI upset by eating small, frequent servings of healthy food and drinking plenty of fluids.
• Instruct women of childbearing age to use reliable contraception during therapy and to inform prescriber if they suspect pregnancy.
• Inform patients with prostate cancer that treatment may temporarily aggravate symptoms.
• As appropriate, review all other significant and life-threatening adverse reactions and interactions, especially those related to the tests mentioned above.

Route	Onset	Peak	Duration
Inhalation	10-17 min	1.5 hr	5-6 hr

levalbuterol hydrochloride
Xopenex

Pharmacologic class: Adrenergic beta$_2$ agonist

Therapeutic class: Bronchodilator

Pregnancy risk category C

Action
Binds to beta$_2$ receptors on bronchial cell membrane, stimulating intracellular enzyme adenylate cyclase to convert adenosine triphosphate to cyclic-3',5'-adenosine monophosphate; net effect is relaxation of smooth muscles, dilation of bronchioles, and increased diuresis.

Availability
Solution for inhalation: 0.31 mg/3 ml, 0.63 mg/3 ml, 1.25 mg/3 ml

Indications and dosages
➤ Prevention and treatment of bronchospasm in reversible obstructive airway disease

Adults and children ages 12 and older: 0.63 to 1.25 mg by oral inhalation via nebulizer q 6 to 8 hours

Children ages 6 to 11: 0.31 to 0.63 mg by oral inhalation via nebulizer t.i.d.

Contraindications
• Hypersensitivity to drug or its components
• Severe cardiac disease

Administration
• Use only with nebulizer system designed for this drug.
• Keep unopened vials in foil pouch; once pouch is opened, use within 2 weeks.
• If vial is removed from pouch, protect from light and use within 1 week.

Adverse reactions
CNS: anxiety, dizziness, hypertonia, insomnia, migraine, headache, nervousness, paresthesia, syncope, tremor

CV: chest pain, hypertension, hypotension, tachycardia

EENT: rhinitis, sinusitis, dry throat

GI: nausea, vomiting, diarrhea, constipation, abdominal pain, dyspepsia, sour taste, anorexia, dry mouth

Metabolic: hypokalemia

Musculoskeletal: muscle cramps, myalgia

Respiratory: asthma exacerbation, cough, dyspnea, **paradoxical bronchospasm**

Other: flulike symptoms, lymphadenopathy, chills

Interactions
Drug-drug. *Aerosol bronchodilators:* increased action of both drugs

Antidepressants: increased risk of adverse cardiovascular effects

Beta-adrenergic blockers: inhibition of levalbuterol effect

Digoxin: decreased digoxin blood level

Loop and thiazide diuretics: increased risk of hypokalemia

Drug-food. *Caffeine-containing foods and beverages:* increased stimulation

Drug-herb. *Cola nut, ephedra, guarana, yerba maté:* increased stimulation

Precautions
Use cautiously in:
• renal, hepatic, or cardiac impairment; hyperthyroidism; diabetes mellitus; hypertension; prostatic hypertrophy; narrow-angle glaucoma; seizures
• pregnant patients.

Patient monitoring
• Monitor vital signs and ECG closely.
• Assess cardiovascular and neurologic

---

status; institute safety measures as needed to prevent injury.

🔊 Monitor for paradoxical broncho-spasm; if this occurs, stop drug therapy and notify prescriber immediately.

• Check electrolyte levels for hypo-kalemia.

• Assess patient's response to drug; contact prescriber if patient needs more frequent doses for same effect.

Patient teaching

• Teach patient how to prepare drug, administer it with nebulizer, and maintain and clean nebulizer.

• Advise patient to continue treatment for about 5 to 15 minutes or until mist no longer forms in nebulizer reservoir.

• Caution patient to avoid driving and other hazardous activities until he knows how drug affects concentration and alertness.

• Advise patient to minimize GI upset by eating small, frequent servings of healthy food and drinking plenty of fluids.

• As appropriate, review all other significant and life-threatening adverse reactions and interactions, especially those related to the drugs, foods, and herbs mentioned above.

levetiracetam
Keppra

Pharmacologic class: Pyrrolidine derivative

Therapeutic class: Anticonvulsant

Pregnancy risk category C

Action

Unknown; thought to prevent seizures by inhibiting nerve impulses in hip-pocampus of the brain. Chemically un-related to other anticonvulsants.

Availability

Tablets: 250 mg, 500 mg, 750 mg

💊 Indications and dosages

➤ Adjunctive treatment for partial seizures

Adults and children ages 16 and older: 500 mg P.O. b.i.d., increased by 1,000 mg/day q 2 weeks to a maximum daily dosage of 3,000 mg

Dosage adjustment

• Renal impairment (especially in dialysis patients)

Contraindications

• Hypersensitivity to drug or its components

Administration

• Give with or without food.

• Don't discontinue drug suddenly; taper dosage gradually.

Route	Onset	Peak	Duration
P.O.	Rapid	1 hr	Unknown

Adverse reactions

CNS: anger, asthenia, aggression, ataxia, dizziness, headache, irritability, mental or mood changes, paresthesia, drowsiness, vertigo

EENT: diplopia, pharyngitis, rhinitis, sinusitis

GI: anorexia, nausea, vomiting

Hematologic: neutropenia, leukopenia

Respiratory: cough, sinusitis

Other: infection

Interactions

Drug-drug. *Phenytoin:* increased phenytoin blood level

Drug-herb. *Evening primrose oil:* lowered seizure threshold

Precautions

Use cautiously in:

• renal, hepatic, or cardiac impairment

• psychosis

- pregnant or breastfeeding patients
- children.

Patient monitoring

- Measure temperature; watch for signs and symptoms of infection.
- ◀≶ Monitor neurologic status; report signs or symptoms that patient is dangerous to himself or others.
- Evaluate nutritional status; report signs of anorexia.

Patient teaching

- Tell patient he may take drug with or without food.
- ◀≶ Advise family to contact prescriber if patient poses a danger to himself or others.
- ◀≶ Caution patient not to stop taking drug abruptly because doing so may increase seizure activity.
- Teach patient and family about adverse CNS reactions. Tell them to report these promptly and institute safety measures to prevent injury.
- Instruct patient to avoid activities that require mental alertness until CNS reactions are known.
- Teach patient to minimize GI upset by eating small, frequent servings of healthy food and drinking plenty of fluids.
- Inform patient that he'll undergo periodic blood testing during therapy.
- As appropriate, review all other significant and life-threatening adverse reactions and interactions, especially those related to the drugs and herbs mentioned above.

levodopa
Dopar, Larodopa, L-dopa

Pharmacologic class: Dopamine precursor
Therapeutic class: Antidyskinetic
Pregnancy risk category NR

Action

Levodopa is converted to dopamine in CNS, serving as a neurotransmitter that crosses blood-brain barrier. Improves balance between cholinergic and dopaminergic activity, aiding control of voluntary muscle movements related to Parkinson's disease (such as tremors and rigidity).

Availability

Capsules, tablets: 100 mg, 250 mg, 500 mg

⚕ Indications and dosages

➤ Idiopathic Parkinson's disease, postencephalitic parkinsonism, or manganese intoxication
Adults: 250 mg P.O. two to four times daily; may increase in increments no greater than 750 mg/day q 3 to 7 days. Maximum recommended dosage is 8 g/day.

Dosage adjustment
- Elderly patients

Off-label uses

- Herpes zoster
- Restless leg syndrome

Contraindications

- Hypersensitivity to drug or tartrazine
- Narrow-angle glaucoma
- Current or previous malignant melanoma
- Undiagnosed skin lesions
- Monoamine oxidase inhibitor (MAO) use within past 14 days
- Breastfeeding

Administration

- Give 1 hour before or 2 hours after meals.
- If patient has difficulty swallowing tablets or capsules, sprinkle contents on applesauce.
- Know that unless contraindicated, drug should be used concomitantly with peripheral decarboxylase inhibitor, such as carbidopa, to enhance

efficacy, reduce dosage requirement, and minimize adverse effects.

◀ Be aware that dosage must be tapered gradually; with abrupt withdrawal, a condition resembling neuroleptic malignant syndrome may occur.

• Stop MAO inhibitor therapy at least 2 weeks before starting levodopa (except type B MAO inhibitors, such as selegiline).

Route	Onset	Peak	Duration
P.O.	Unknown	1-3 hr	5 hr

Adverse reactions

CNS: involuntary movements, anxiety, dizziness, hallucinations, memory loss, ataxia, increased hand tremor, bradykinesia, headache, numbness, asthenia, syncope, confusion, insomnia, nightmares, delusions, malaise, fatigue, euphoria, psychiatric problems, psychotic changes, depression, dementia, **suicidal ideation**
CV: cardiac irregularities, palpitations, orthostatic hypotension
EENT: blurred vision, diplopia, blepharospasm, mydriasis, trismus, bruxism
GI: nausea, vomiting, diarrhea, constipation, abdominal pain and distress, dysphagia, burning sensation, flatulence, bitter or abnormal taste, dry mouth, anorexia, **upper GI hemorrhage**
GU: urinary retention or incontinence, dark urine, elevated blood urea nitrogen
Hematologic: hemolytic anemia, **leukopenia**
Hepatic: elevated alanine aminotransferase (ALT), alkaline phosphatase (ALP), aspartate aminotransferase (AST), bilirubin, lactate dehydrogenase, and protein-bound iodine levels; **hepatotoxicity**
Metabolic: hyperuricemia
Musculoskeletal: muscle twitching
Respiratory: hiccups, hyperventilation

Skin: flushing, rash, dark sweat, **melanoma**
Other: hot flashes, weight changes

Interactions

Drug-drug. *Anticholinergics:* decreased levodopa absorption
Antihypertensives: additive hypotension
Haloperidol, papaverine, phenothiazines, phenytoin, pyridoxine, reserpine: reversal of levodopa's effects
Inhalation hydrocarbon anesthetics: increased risk of arrhythmias
MAO inhibitors (except type B): severe hypertensive reactions
Methyldopa: altered levodopa efficacy, increased risk of adverse CNS effects
Drug-diagnostic tests. *ALP, ALT, AST, bilirubin, low-density lipoproteins, uric acid:* increased levels
Coombs' test: false-positive results
Granulocytes, hemoglobin, platelets, white blood cells: decreased values
Urine glucose, urine ketones: interference with test results
Drug-food. *Pyridoxine-rich foods:* reversal of levodopa's effects
Drug-herb. *5-hydroxytryptophan (5-HTP):* harmful skin changes
Kava: decreased levodopa efficacy
Octacosanol: worsening dyskinesias

Precautions

Use cautiously in:
• cerebrovascular, renal, hepatic, or endocrine disease
• history of cardiac, ulcer, or psychiatric disease
• pregnant patients
• children younger than age 18 (safety not established).

Patient monitoring

• Check vital signs carefully; watch for orthostatic hypotension.
• Monitor fluid intake and output; report urinary retention or incontinence.
• Evaluate complete blood count periodically.

• In long-term therapy, monitor hepatic and renal function and watch for signs and symptoms of hepatotoxicty.

• Monitor for adverse CNS reactions; institute safety measures as needed to prevent injury.

• Assess for signs and symptoms of drug overdose (such as arrhythmias and muscle and eyelid twitching).

• Monitor nutritional status; report significant problems.

Patient teaching

• Teach patient that high-protein foods may impair drug absorption.

• Instruct patient or family to contact prescriber if parkinsonian symptoms worsen.

• Inform patient and family of possible adverse CNS reactions.

• Caution patient to avoid sudden position changes, driving, and other hazardous activities until he knows how drug affects concentration and alertness.

• Teach patient to minimize GI upset by eating small, frequent servings of healthy food and drinking plenty of fluids.

• As appropriate, review all other significant and life-threatening adverse reactions and interactions, especially those related to the drugs, tests, foods, and herbs mentioned above.

levofloxacin
Levaquin, Quixin

Pharmacologic class: Fluoroquinolone
Therapeutic class: Anti-infective
Pregnancy risk category C

Action

Inhibits the enzyme DNA gyrase in susceptible gram-negative and gram-positive aerobic and anaerobic bacteria, thereby interfering with bacterial DNA synthesis

Availability

Ophthalmic solution: 0.5% (5 mg/ml)
Premixed solution for injection: 250 mg/ 50 ml, 500 mg/100 ml, 750 mg/150 ml
Solution for injection (concentrated): 500 mg/20 ml
Tablets: 250 mg, 500 mg, 750 mg

🕭 Indications and dosages

➤ Bronchitis caused by *Staphylococcus aureus, Streptococcus pneumoniae, Haemophilus influenzae, H. parainfluenzae,* or *Moraxella catarrhalis*
Adults: 500 mg I.V. or P.O. q 24 hours for 7 days

➤ Community-acquired pneumonia caused by *S. aureus, S. pneumoniae* (including penicillin-resistant strains), *H. influenzae, H. parainfluenzae, Klebsiella pneumoniae, M. catarrhalis, Chlamydia pneumoniae, Legionella pneumophila,* or *Mycoplasma pneumoniae*
Adults: 500 mg I.V. or P.O. q 24 hours for 7 to 14 days

➤ Nosocomial pneumonia caused by methicillin-susceptible strains of *S. aureus, Pseudomonas aeruginosa, Serratia marcescens, Escherichia coli, K. pneumoniae, H. influenzae,* and *S. pneumoniae;* complicated skin and skin-structure infections caused by *S. aureus, Enterococcus faecalis, Streptococcus pyogenes,* or *Proteus mirabilis*
Adults: 750 mg I.V. or P.O. q 24 hours for 7 to 14 days

➤ Acute maxillary sinusitis
Adults: 500 mg I.V. or P.O. q 24 hours for 10 to 14 days

➤ Uncomplicated skin and skin-structure infections caused by *S. aureus* or *S. pyogenes*
Adults: 500 mg I.V. or P.O. q 24 hours for 7 to 10 days

➤ Complicated urinary tract infections caused by *E. coli, Enterobacter cloacae, E. faecalis, K. pneumoniae,*

P. mirabilis, or *P. aeruginosa;* pyelonephritis caused by *E. coli*

Adults: 250 mg I.V. or P.O. q 24 hours for 10 days

➤ Uncomplicated urinary tract infections caused by *E. coli, K. pneumoniae,* or *Staphylococcus saprophyticus*

Adults: 250 mg I.V. or P.O. q 24 hours for 3 days

➤ Severe infectious diarrhea, diarrhea with fever or bloody stools

Adults: 500 mg P.O. q 24 hours for a maximum of 3 days

➤ Prophylaxis of traveler's diarrhea

Adults: 500 mg P.O. daily during risk period for a maximum of 3 weeks

➤ Gonorrhea

Adults and adolescents: For uncomplicated gonorrhea, 250 mg P.O. as a single dose. For disseminated gonococcal infection, 250 mg/day I.V. for 24 to 48 hours, followed by 500 mg/day P.O. to complete 1 week of therapy. If chlamydia is suspected along with either gonorrhea form, also give doxycycline for 7 days or oral azithromycin as a single dose, as prescribed.

➤ Pelvic inflammatory disease

Adults and adolescents: 500 mg I.V. or P.O. q 24 hours with or without metronidazole, followed by oral doxycycline to complete 14 days of therapy; or 500 mg P.O. daily for 14 days with or without metronidazole

➤ Chlamydia

Adults: 500 mg P.O. once daily for 7 days

➤ Conjunctivitis caused by *S. aureus, Corynebacterium* species, methicillin-susceptible strains of *Staphylococcus epidermidis, S. pneumoniae,* viridans-group streptococci, *Acinetobacter lwoffi, H. influenzae,* and *S. marcescens*

Adults and children ages 1 and older: One or two drops of 0.5% solution into affected eye q 2 hours while awake on days 1 and 2 (up to eight times daily); then one or two drops q 4 hours while awake on days 3 through 7 (up to four times daily)

Dosage adjustment
• Renal impairment

Contraindications
• Hypersensitivity to drug or other fluoroquinolones

Administration
• Be aware that oral and I.V. dosages are identical.
• Give parenteral form by I.V. route only; drug isn't for I.M., S.C., intrathecal, or intraperitoneal use.
• To prepare I.V. infusion, use compatible solution, such as 0.9% sodium chloride injection, dextrose 5% and 0.9% sodium chloride injection, dextrose 5% in water, or dextrose 5% in lactated Ringer's solution.
• Infuse over 60 to 90 minutes, depending on dosage. Don't infuse with other drugs
• Flush I.V. line before and after infusing drug.
◀€ Avoid rapid or bolus I.V. administration.
• Give oral doses 2 hours before or after sucralfate, iron, antacids containing magnesium or aluminum, or multivitamins with zinc.
• Give oral drug without regard to food, but don't give it with milk or yogurt alone.

Route	Onset	Peak	Duration
P.O.	Rapid	1–2 hr	24 hr
I.V.	Rapid	End of infusion	24 hr

Adverse reactions
CNS: dizziness, headache, insomnia, **seizures**
CV: chest pain, palpitations, hypotension
EENT: sinusitis, photophobia, pharyngitis
GI: nausea, vomiting, diarrhea, constipation, abdominal pain, dyspepsia, flatulence, altered taste, **pseudomembranous colitis**

GU: vaginitis
Hematologic: lymphocytopenia
Metabolic: hyperglycemia, hypoglycemia
Musculoskeletal: back pain, tendon rupture, tendinitis
Skin: photosensitivity
Other: reaction and pain at I.V. site, hypersensitivity reactions including **Stevens-Johnson syndrome**

Interactions

Drug-drug. *Antacids containing aluminum or magnesium, didanosine (tablets), iron salts, sucralfate, zinc salts:* decreased levofloxacin absorption
Cimetidine: interference with levofloxacin elimination
Nonsteroidal anti-inflammatory drugs: increased risk of CNS stimulation and seizures
Drug-diagnostic tests. *Glucose:* increased or decreased level
Lymphocytes: decreased count
EEG: abnormal findings
Drug-food. *Concurrent tube feedings, milk, yogurt:* impaired levofloxacin absorption
Drug-herb. *Dong quai, St. John's wort:* phototoxicity
Fennel: decreased levofloxacin absorption
Drug-behaviors. *Sun exposure:* phototoxicity

Precautions

Use cautiously in:
• bradycardia, acute myocardial ischemia, prolonged QTc interval, cirrhosis, renal impairment, underlying CNS disease, uncorrected hypocalcemia
• elderly patients
• pregnant or breastfeeding patients
• children younger than age 18.

Patient monitoring

• Check vital signs, especially blood pressure; too-rapid infusion can cause hypotension.

• Closely monitor patients with renal insufficiency
• Monitor blood glucose level closely in diabetic patients.
◀ Assess for hypersensitivity reaction; discontinue drug immediately if rash or other signs or symptoms occur.

Patient teaching

◀ Instruct patient to stop taking drug and contact prescriber if he experiences signs or symptoms of hypersensitivity reaction (rash, hives, or other skin reactions).
• Caution patient to avoid driving and other activities that require mental alertness until CNS effects of drug are known.
• Instruct patient not to take drug with milk, yogurt, multivitamins containing zinc or iron, or antacids containing aluminum or magnesium.
• As appropriate, review all other significant and life-threatening adverse reactions and interactions, especially those related to the drugs, tests, foods, herbs, and behaviors mentioned above.

levorphanol tartrate
Levo-Dromoran

Pharmacologic class: Synthetic opioid agonist
Therapeutic class: Opioid analgesic
Controlled substance schedule II
Pregnancy risk category C

Action

Inhibits adenylate cyclase, which regulates release of pain neurotransmitters (such as acetylcholine, dopamine, substance P, and gamma-aminobutyric acid). Also stimulates mu and kappa opioid receptors, altering the perception of and emotional response to pain.

Availability
Injection: 2 mg/ml
Tablets: 2 mg

⚕ Indications and dosages
➢ Moderate to severe pain
Adults: 2 mg P. O. q 6 to 8 hours; may
increase to 3 mg P.O. q 6 to 8 hours as
necessary, not to exceed 12 mg in 24
hours. Or 1 to 2 mg I.M. or S.C. q 6 to
8 hours, not to exceed 8 mg in 24
hours. Or 1 mg I.V. by slow injection;
may repeat in 3 hours, but don't exceed
8 mg in 24 hours.
Dosage adjustment
• Hepatic or renal insufficiency
• Elderly patients

Off-label uses
• Preoperative sedation

Contraindications
• Hypersensitivity to drug, other opi-
oid agonists, or sulfites
• Bronchial asthma
• Head injury, increased intracranial
pressure
• Respiratory depression
• Acute alcoholism
• Pregnancy or breastfeeding

Administration
• Make sure resuscitation equipment is
available before starting therapy.
• Give I.V. injection slowly; monitor
patient response.
• Know that I.V. route is preferred in
emergencies only.
• After parenteral administration,
place patient in supine position with
legs elevated to minimize adverse reactions.
• Be aware that 2 mg of levorphanol
tartrate is analgesically equivalent to 10
to 15 mg of morphine and 100 mg of
meperidine.

Route	Onset	Peak	Duration
P.O.	10-60 min	90-120 min	4-5 hr
I.V.	Unknown	20 min	4-5 hr
I.M.	Unknown	60 min	4-5 hr
S.C.	Unknown	60-90 min	4-5 hr

Adverse reactions
CNS: personality disorders, nervousness, insomnia, hypokinesia, dyskinesia, drowsiness, light-headedness, dizziness, depression, delusions, confusion,
amnesia, sedation, euphoria, delirium,
mood changes, **coma, seizures**
CV: tachycardia, palpitations, hypotension, bradycardia, facial flushing,
**shock, peripheral circulatory collapse,
cardiac arrest**
EENT: diplopia, abnormal vision
GI: nausea, vomiting, constipation,
abdominal pain, dyspepsia, increased
colonic motility (in patients with
chronic ulcerative colitis), dry mouth
GU: dysuria, urinary retention or hesitancy, ureteral or vesicle sphincter
spasms, oliguria, decreased libido
Hepatic: biliary tract spasms, elevated
amylase and lipase levels, **hepatic failure**
Respiratory: suppressed cough reflex,
hyperventilation, periods of apnea
Skin: urticaria, rash, pruritus, cyanosis
Other: injection site pain, redness, or
swelling; physical or psychological
drug dependence

Interactions
Drug-drug. *Alfentanil, fentanyl, sufentanil, other CNS depressants:* increased
CNS and respiratory depression, increased risk of hypotension
Anticholinergics: increased risk of severe constipation
*Antidiarrheals (such as atropine, difen-
oxin, kaolin, loperamide), antihypertensives:* increased risk of hypotension
Buprenorphine, naloxone, naltrexone:
decreased levorphanol efficacy

Metoclopramide: antagonism of metoclopramide effects

Neuromuscular blockers: increased risk
of prolonged CNS and respiratory depression

Drug-diagnostic tests. *Amylase, lipase:*
increased levels

Drug-behaviors. *Alcohol use:* increased
CNS depression

Precautions

Use cautiously in:

• renal or hepatic dysfunction, chronic
obstructive pulmonary disease, acute
abdominal conditions, cardiovascular
disease, seizure disorders, cerebral arteriosclerosis, Addison's disease, prostatic
hypertrophy, toxic psychosis

• children.

Patient monitoring

• Check vital signs and respiratory
status, and monitor ECG carefully.

• Evaluate fluid intake and output.

• Assess neurologic status; institute
safety precautions as needed to prevent
injury.

• Watch for signs and symptoms of
depression.

• Monitor liver and kidney function
test results.

Patient teaching

• With parenteral administration, explain need for continuous vital sign
and ECG monitoring.

• To minimize adverse effects, instruct
patient to lie supine after parenteral
administration, if possible.

◀€ Instruct patient or caregiver to report adverse reactions immediately.

• Teach caregiver to institute safety
measures as needed to prevent injury,
and to report significant problems.

• Instruct patient to minimize GI upset
by eating small, frequent servings of
healthy food and drinking plenty of
fluids.

• Caution patient to avoid driving and
other hazardous activities until he

knows how drug affects concentration
and alertness.

• As appropriate, review all other significant and life-threatening adverse
reactions and interactions, especially
those related to the drugs, tests, and
behaviors mentioned above.

levothyroxine sodium (L-thyroxine, T$_4$)

Eltroxin✦, Levo-T, Levothroid,
Levoxyl, PMS-Levothyroxine
Sodium✦, Synthroid, Thyro-Tabs,
Unithroid

Pharmacologic class: Synthetic thyroxine hormone

Therapeutic class: Thyroid hormone
replacement

Pregnancy risk category A

Action

Synthetic form of thyroxine that replaces endogenous thyroxine and increases thyroid hormone levels in body.
Thyroid hormones help regulate cell
growth and differentiation and increase metabolism of lipids, protein,
and carbohydrates.

Availability

Powder for injection: 200 mcg/vial in 6-
and 10-ml vials, 500 mcg/vial in 6- and
10-ml vials

Tablets: 25 mcg, 50 mcg, 75 mcg,
88 mcg, 100 mcg, 112 mcg, 125 mcg,
137 mcg, 150 mcg, 175 mcg, 200 mcg,
300 mcg

🕖 Indications and dosages

➤ Hypothyroidism; some types of
thyroid cancer

Adults: All dosages are highly individualized. Initially, 0.05 mg PO, increased
in increments of 0.025 mg q 2 to 3
weeks depending on cardiovascular

status. Maintenance dosage is 0.2 mg daily, adjusted within first 4 weeks of therapy. For patients who can't tolerate oral doses, adjust I.M. or I.V. dose to about one-half of oral dosage.

➤ Congenital hypothyroidism

Children over age 12: Up to 150 mcg or 2 to 3 mcg/kg P.O. daily

Children ages 6 to 12: 100 to 150 mcg P.O. daily

Children ages 1 to 6: 75 to 100 mcg P.O. daily

Infants ages 6 to 12 months: 50 to 75 mcg P.O. daily

Infants ages 3 to 6 months: 25 to 50 mcg P.O. daily

Infants up to 3 months: 10 to 15 mcg/kg P.O. daily

➤ Myxedema coma or stupor

Adults: Initially, 0.4 mg rapid I.V., followed by 0.1 to 0.2 mg I.V. daily; maintenance dosage is 0.05 to 0.1 mg I.V., adjusted based on T_4 level. Once patient is clinically stable, convert to P.O. therapy.

➤ Thyroid-stimulating hormone suppression

Adults: 2.6 mcg/kg P.O. daily for 7 to 10 days

Dosage adjustment

• Cardiovascular disease

• Psychosis or agitation

• Elderly patients

Contraindications

• Hypersensitivity to drug, its components, or tartrazine

• Acute myocardial infarction

• Thyrotoxicosis

• Adrenal insufficiency

Administration

• Be aware that all dosages are highly individualized.

• Give tablets on an empty stomach 30 minutes to 1 hour before first meal of day.

• If patient can't swallow tablets, crush them and sprinkle into a small amount of food, such as applesauce. For infants

and children, dissolve tablets in a small amount of water, non-soybean formula, or breast milk and administer immediately.

• Don't give oral form within 4 hours of bile acid sequestrants or antacids (which interfere with levothyroxine absorption).

• Reconstitute Synthroid powder for injection with 5 ml of 0.9% sodium chloride injection; shake until clear and use immediately.

• Be aware that levothyroxine sodium preparations aren't bioequivalent. Patient should consistently use same brand or generic product, with dosing based on weight, age, general physical condition, and duration of symptoms.

• Know that when drug is used for thyroid-stimulating hormone suppression test, radioactive iodine (^{131}I) is given before and after 7- to 10-day course.

Route	Onset	Peak	Duration
P.O.	Unknown	Unknown	Unknown
I.V.	6-8 hr	24 hr	Unknown
I.M.	Unknown	Unknown	Unknown

Adverse reactions

CNS: insomnia, irritability, nervousness, headache

CV: tachycardia, angina pectoris, hypotension, hypertension, increased cardiac output, **arrhythmias, cardiovascular collapse**

GI: vomiting, diarrhea, abdominal cramps

GU: menstrual irregularities

Metabolic: hyperthyroidism

Musculoskeletal: accelerated bone maturation (in children), decreased bone density (in women on long-term therapy)

Skin: alopecia (in children), diaphoresis

Other: heat intolerance, weight loss

Interactions

Drug-drug. *Aminoglutethimide, amiodarone, anabolic steroids, antithyroid drugs, asparaginase, barbiturates, carbamazepine, chloral hydrate, cholestyramine, clofibrate, colestipol, corticosteroids, danazol, diazepam, estrogens, ethionamide, fluorouracil, heparin (with I.V. use), insulin, lithium, methadone, mitotane, nitroprusside, oxyphenbutazone, perphenazine, phenylbutazone, phenytoin, propranolol, salicylates (large doses), sulfonylureas, thiazides:* altered thyroid function test results

Antacids, bile acid sequestrants: interference with levothyroxine absorption

Anticoagulants: increased anticoagulant action

Beta-adrenergic blockers (selected): decreased beta blocker action

Cardiac glycosides: decreased cardiac glycoside blood levels

Cholestyramine, colestipol: levothyroxine inefficacy

Theophyllines: decreased theophylline clearance

Drug-diagnostic tests. *Thyroid function tests:* decreased values

Drug-food. *Foods high in iron or fiber, soybeans:* decreased drug absorption

Precautions

Use cautiously in:
• cardiovascular disease, severe renal insufficiency, diabetes mellitus
• elderly patients
• pregnant or breastfeeding patients.

Patient monitoring

• Check vital signs and ECG routinely.
• Monitor thyroid and liver function test results.
• Evaluate for signs and symptoms of overdose, including those of hyperthyroidism (weight loss, cardiac symptoms, abdominal cramps).
• Monitor closely for drug efficacy.
• Monitor patients with Addison's disease or diabetes mellitus for worsening of these conditions.

• Watch for signs and symptoms of bleeding tendency, especially in patients receiving anticoagulants concurrently.

Patient teaching

• Caution patient or parent to avoid getting overheated, as in hot environment or during vigorous exercise.
• Tell patient or parent to report adverse effects, including signs or symptoms of hyperthyroidism or hypothyroidism.
• Instruct patient to minimize GI upset by eating small, frequent servings of healthy food.
• Instruct patient to avoid driving and other hazardous activities until he knows how drug affects concentration and alertness.
• Inform parents that child may lose hair during first few months of therapy; reassure them that this effect is usually transient.
• Tell patient he may require lifelong therapy and will undergo regular blood testing.
• As appropriate, review all other significant and life-threatening adverse reactions and interactions, especially those related to the drugs, tests, and foods mentioned above.

lidocaine hydrochloride

Anestacon, Dentipatch, DermaFlex, Lidoderm, LidoPen Auto-Injector, Xylocaine, Xylocaine-MPF, Xylocaine Viscous, Xylocard✤

Pharmacologic class: Amide
Therapeutic class: Antiarrhythmic (class IB), local anesthetic
Pregnancy risk category B

Action

Exerts antiarrhythmic action by suppressing automaticity of ventricular cells, decreasing diastolic depolarization, and increasing ventricular fibrillation threshold. Produces local anesthesia by reducing sodium permeability of sensory nerves, thereby blocking generation and conduction of impulses.

Availability

Injection for I.M. use: 300 mg/3 ml automatic injection device
Injection for direct I.V. use: 1% and 2% in syringes and vials
Injection for I.V. infusion: 2 mg/ml, 4 mg/ml, 8 mg/ml
Injection for I.V injection admixtures: 40 mg/ml, 100 mg/ml, 200 mg/ml
Patch: 5%
Topical cream: 0.5%, 4%
Topical gel: 0.5%, 2.5%
Topical jelly: 2%
Topical liquid, ointment: 2.5%, 5%
Topical solution: 2%, 4%
Topical spray: 0.5%, 10%

✒ Indications and dosages

➤ Ventricular tachycardia or ventricular fibrillation
Adults: Initially, 50 to 100 mg I.V. bolus given at 25 to 50 mg/minute. If desired response doesn't occur after 5 minutes, give second dose at 25 to 50 mg/minute; continue to give a repeat dose q 5 minutes until desired response occurs; maximum dosage is 300 mg given over 1 hour. Maintenance dosage is 20 to 50 mcg/kg/minute by continuous I.V. infusion, usually for no more than 24 hours.
Children: Initially, 0.5 to 1 mg/kg I.V. bolus, repeated based on patient response, not to exceed 5 mg/kg. Maintenance dosage is 10 to 50 mcg/kg/minute by continuous I.V. infusion.
➤ Caudal anesthesia (without epinephrine)
Adults: For obstetric analgesia, 200 to 300 mg administered caudally as 1%

solution; for surgical anesthesia, 225 to 300 mg as 1.5% solution. For continuous caudal anesthesia, don't repeat maximum dosage at intervals of less than 90 minutes.
➤ Epidural anesthesia (without epinephrine)
Adults: For lumbar analgesia, 250 to 300 mg administered epidurally as 1% solution, 225 to 300 mg as 1.5% solution, or 200 to 300 mg as 2% solution; for thoracic anesthesia, 200 to 300 mg as 1% solution. For continuous epidural anesthesia, don't repeat maximum dosage at intervals of less than 90 minutes.
➤ I.V. regional infiltration (without epinephrine)
Adults: 50 to 300 mg I.V. as 0.5% solution. For I.V. regional anesthesia, maximum dosage is 4 mg/kg.
➤ I.V. local infiltration (without epinephrine)
Children: Up to 5 mg/kg I.V. as a 0.25% to 1% solution
➤ Spinal anesthesia (without epinephrine)
Adults: For obstetric low-spinal or saddle-block anesthesia (normal vaginal delivery), 50 mg of 5% Xylocaine-MPF with glucose 7.5%, or 9 to 15 mg of 1.5% Xylocaine-MPF with dextrose 7.5%; for cesarean section, 75 mg of 5% Xylocaine-MPF with glucose 7.5%; for surgical anesthesia, 75 to 100 mg of 5% Xylocaine-MPF with glucose 7.5%.
➤ Paracervical anesthesia (without epinephrine)
Adults: For obstetric analgesia, 100 mg administered paracervically as 1% solution (each side); for paracervical block, maximum dosage of 200 mg over each 90-minute period (half administered on each side)
➤ Peripheral nerve block
Adults: For brachial nerve block, 225 to 300 mg as 1.5% solution; for dental nerve block, 20 to 100 mg as 2% solution with epinephrine 1:100,000 or 1:50,000; for intercostal nerve block, 30

mg as 1% solution; for pudendal nerve block, 100 mg as 1% solution; for paravertebral nerve block, 30 mg to 50 mg as 1% solution

➣ Sympathetic nerve block (without epinephrine)

Adults: For cervical nerve block, 50 mg as 1% solution; for lumbar nerve block, 50 to 100 mg as 1% solution

➣ Dental anesthesia

Adults: 1 to 5 ml of lidocaine 2% with epinephrine 1:50,000 or 1:100,000; maximum dosage is less than 500 mg (7 mg/kg).

Children: 20 to 30 mg as 2% solution with epinephrine 1:100,000

➣ Topical anesthesia for skin or mucous membranes

Adults: Apply a thin layer of gel, jelly, or ointment to skin or mucous membranes as needed before procedure; or apply lidocaine 5% patch to most painful areas and to intact skin (up to three patches at a time for up to 12 hours within a 24-hour period).

Off-label uses

• Pediatric patients with cardiac arrest who develop frequent premature ventricular contractions
• Status epilepticus

Contraindications

• Hypersensitivity to drug or other amide local anesthetics
• Heart failure, cardiogenic shock, second- or third-degree heart block
• Wolff-Parkinson-White or Adams-Stokes syndrome

Administration

• Make sure resuscitation equipment and oxygen are available before giving drug.
• Dilute injection in additive syringe and single-use vial according to manufacturer's instructions before administering as I.V. infusion.

• Add 1 g of lidocaine to 1 L of dextrose 5% in water to make a solution of 1 mg/ml.
• Deliver infusion by infusion pump no faster than 4 mg/minute.
• Be aware that drug can be given I.M. using 10% parenteral solution only.

Route	Onset	Peak	Duration
I.V.	45-90 sec	Immediate	10-20 min
I.M.	5-15 min	Unknown	60-90 min
Topical	2-5 min	Unknown	30-60 min

Adverse reactions

CNS: anxiety; confusion; difficulty speaking; dizziness; hallucinations; lethargy; paresthesia; light-headedness; fatigue; drowsiness; headache; persistent sensory, motor, or **autonomic deficit of lower spinal segment; septic meningitis; seizures**

CV: bradycardia, hypotension, new or worsening **arrhythmias, cardiac arrest**

EENT: diplopia, abnormal vision

GI: nausea, vomiting, dry mouth

GU: urinary retention

Metabolic: methemoglobinemia

Respiratory: suppressed cough reflex, respiratory depression, **respiratory arrest**

Skin: rash; urticaria; pruritus; erythema; contact dermatitis; cutaneous lesions; tissue irritation, sloughing, and necrosis

Other: fever; edema; infection, burning, stinging, tenderness, and swelling at injection site; **anaphylaxis**

Interactions

Drug-drug. *Beta-adrenergic blockers, cimetidine:* increased lidocaine blood level

Mexiletine, tocainide: additive cardiac effects

Monoamine oxidase inhibitors, tricyclic antidepressants: prolonged hypertension

---

Phenytoin, procainamide: increased cardiac depression
Drug-diagnostic tests. *Creatine kinase:* increased level (with I.M. use)

Precautions

Use cautiously in:
• renal or hepatic disorders, inflammation or sepsis in injection area
• labor or delivery
• breastfeeding patients.

Patient monitoring

◀€ Monitor vital signs and ECG continuously; watch for cardiac depression.
◀€ Evaluate level of consciousness closely.
◀€ Watch for localized and systemic adverse reactions, particularly anaphylaxis.
◀€ Stay alert for seizures.
◀€ Monitor neurologic status for deficits of lower spinal segment.
• Give supportive oxygen therapy, as indicated and prescribed.
• Monitor electrolyte, blood urea nitrogen, and creatinine levels.
• Assess topical site for adverse reactions.

Patient teaching

• Discuss reason for drug therapy with patient and family when appropriate.
• Explain that patient will be monitored continuously during therapy.
• Instruct patient to promptly report discomfort at I.V. site as well as adverse effects.
• As appropriate, review all other significant and life-threatening adverse reactions and interactions, especially those related to the drugs and tests mentioned above.

linezolid
Zyvox

Pharmacologic class: Oxazolidinone
Therapeutic class: Anti-infective
Pregnancy risk category C

Action

Selectively binds to bacterial 23S ribosomal RNA of 50S subunit, preventing formation of an essential component of bacterial translation process. Bacteriostatic or bactericidal against gram-positive and certain gram-negative bacteria.

Availability

Injection: 2 mg/ml
Powder for oral suspension: 100 mg/5 ml
Tablets: 400 mg, 600 mg

💊 Indications and dosages

➤ Vancomycin-resistant *Enterococcus faecium* infections
Adults and children ages 12 and older: 600 mg P.O. or I.V. infusion q 12 hours for 14 to 28 days
➤ Nosocomial pneumonia caused by *Staphylococcus aureus* (methicillin-susceptible and resistant strains) or *Streptococcus pneumoniae* (penicillin-susceptible strains only); community-acquired pneumonia; complicated skin and skin-structure infections
Adults and children ages 12 and older: 600 mg P.O. or I.V. infusion q 12 hours for 10 to 14 days
➤ Uncomplicated skin and soft-tissue infections caused by *S. aureus* (methicillin-susceptible strains only) or *Streptococcus pyogenes*
Adults and children ages 12 and older: 400 mg P.O. q 12 hours for 10 to 14 days

Contraindications
- Hypersensitivity to drug or its components
- Phenylketonuria (oral suspension only)
- Bone marrow depression
- Pseudomembranous colitis

Administration
- For I.V. injection, use single-use, ready-to-use infusion bag; check for particulate matter before giving. Infuse over 30 to 120 minutes.
- For I.V. infusion, mix with dextrose 5% in water, normal saline solution, or lactated Ringer's injection.
- Flush I.V. line before and after administering drug to avoid incompatibilities.
- Know that oral drug may be given with or without food.

Route	Onset	Peak	Duration
P.O.	Rapid	1-2 hr	Unknown
I.V.	Unknown	Unknown	Unknown

Adverse reactions
CNS: anxiety, confusion, difficulty speaking, dizziness, hallucinations, lethargy, paresthesia, light-headedness, fatigue, drowsiness, headache, **seizures**
GI: nausea, vomiting, diarrhea, gastritis, anorexia, dry mouth, **pseudomembranous colitis**
Hematologic: altered prothrombin time, **thrombocytopenia**
Skin: rash, photosensitivity, diaphoresis
Other: fever, fungal infections

Interactions
Drug-drug. *Antiplatelet drugs (such as aspirin, dipyridamole, nonsteroidal anti-inflammatory drugs):* increased risk of bleeding
Monoamine oxidase inhibitors, pseudoephedrine: increased risk of hypertension and associated adverse effects
Serotonergics: serotonin syndrome

Drug-food. *Tyramine-containing foods and beverages (such as beer; Chianti and certain other red wines; aged cheese; bananas; aged, cured, or spoiled meats; salted herring and other dried fish; avocado; bananas; bean curd; red plums; soy sauce; spinach; tofu, tomatoes; and yeast):* hypertension

Precautions
Use cautiously in:
- hepatic dysfunction, hypertension, hyperthyroidism, pheochromocytoma
- pregnant or breastfeeding patients.

Patient monitoring
- Monitor neurologic status; institute safety measures as needed to prevent injury.
- Check I.V. site for infiltration.
- Watch for adverse reactions.
- Monitor complete blood count, coagulation studies, and culture and sensitivity tests.

Patient teaching
- Tell patient he may take drug with or without food but should avoid foods containing tyramine.
- Instruct patient to minimize adverse GI effects by eating small, frequent servings of healthy foods.
- Caution patient to avoid driving and other hazardous activities until he knows how drug affects concentration and alertness.
- As appropriate, review all significant and life-threatening adverse reactions and interactions, especially those related to the drugs and foods mentioned above.

liothyronine sodium (T₃)

Cytomel, Tertroxin, Triostat

Pharmacologic class: Synthetic thyroxine hormone

Therapeutic class: Thyroid hormone replacement

Pregnancy risk category A

Action

Synthetic form of triiodothyronine (T_3); helps regulate cell growth and differentiation and increases metabolism of lipids, proteins, and carbohydrates. Also enhances aerobic mitochondrial function, thus stimulating myosin ATPase and reducing tissue lactic acidosis.

Availability

Injection: 10 mcg/ml in 1-ml vials
Tablets: 5 mcg, 25 mcg, 50 mcg

Indications and dosages

➢ Thyroid hormone replacement in mild hypothyroidism
Adults: All dosages are individualized. Initially, 25 mcg P.O. once daily; may increase in increments of 12.5 to 25 mcg/day q 1 to 2 weeks; usual maintenance dosage is 25 to 75 mcg P.O. daily.
➢ Myxedema
Adults: All dosages are individualized. Initially, 2.5 to 5 mcg P.O. once daily; increase in increments of 5 to 10 mcg/day q 1 to 2 weeks, up to 25 mcg/day. If response still not adequate, increase by 12.5 to 25 mcg P.O. daily q 1 to 2 weeks until desired response occurs. Usual maintenance dosage is 50 to 100 mcg/day P.O.
➢ Myxedema coma
Adults: Initially, 25 to 50 mcg I.V.; after 4 hours, reassess patient's need for subsequent doses (up to 65 mcg in 24 hours). In cardiovascular disease, initial dosage is 10 to 20 mcg I.V. Separate doses by at least 4 hours but no more than 12 hours.
➢ Simple goiter
Adults: All dosages are individualized. Initially, 5 mcg P.O. once daily; increase by 5 to 10 mcg/day q 1 to 2 weeks, up to 25 mcg/day, then increase by 12.5 to 25 mcg P.O. daily q week until desired effect occurs. Usual maintenance dosage is 50 to 100 mcg P.O. daily.
Children: Initially, 5 mcg P.O once daily; increase by 5 mcg weekly until desired effect occurs.
➢ T_3 suppression test to distinguish hyperthyroidism from euthyroidism
Adults: 75 to 100 mcg P.O. daily for 7 days
Dosage adjustment
• Severe, long-standing hypothyroidism
• Cardiovascular disease
• Psychosis or agitation
• Elderly patients

Contraindications

• Hypersensitivity to drug, its components, or tartrazine
• Acute myocardial infarction
• Thyrotoxicosis
• Adrenal insufficiency and coexisting hypothyroidism
• Uncontrolled hypertension

Administration

• Know that all dosages are highly individualized.
• Administer single oral dose in morning with or without food.
• Injectable drug is for I.V. use only; don't give I.M.
• Give repeat I.V. doses more than 4 hours but less than 12 hours apart.
• Be aware that in T_3 suppression test, radioactive iodine (^{131}I) is given before and after 7-day liothyronine course.

Route	Onset	Peak	Duration
P.O.	Unknown	24-72 hr	72 hr
I.V.	Unknown	Unknown	Unknown

Adverse reactions

CNS: insomnia, irritability, nervousness, headache

CV: tachycardia, angina pectoris, hypotension, hypertension, increased cardiac output, **arrhythmias, cardiovascular collapse**

GI: vomiting, diarrhea, cramps

GU: menstrual irregularities

Metabolic: hyperthyroidism, hyperglycemia

Musculoskeletal: accelerated bone maturation (in children), decreased bone density (in women with long-term use)

Skin: alopecia (in children), diaphoresis

Other: weight loss, heat intolerance

Interactions

Drug-drug. *Anabolic steroids, antithyroid drugs, asparaginase, barbiturates, carbamazepine, chloral hydrate, clofibrate, corticosteroids, danazol, estrogens, fluorouracil, heparin (with I.V. use), lithium, methadone, mitotane, oxyphenbutazone, perphenazine, phenylbutazone, phenytoin, propranolol, salicylates (large doses), sulfonylureas:* altered thyroid function test results

Anticoagulants: increased anticoagulant action

Beta-adrenergic blockers (selected): impaired beta blocker action

Cardiac glycosides: decreased cardiac glycoside blood level

Cholestyramine, colestipol: liothyronine inefficacy

Theophyllines: decreased theophylline clearance

Drug-diagnostic tests. *Thyroid function tests:* altered values

Drug-food. *Foods high in iron or fiber, soybeans:* decreased drug absorption

Precautions

Use cautiously in:
• cardiovascular disease, severe renal insufficiency, uncorrected adrenocortical disorders, diabetes mellitus
• elderly patients
• pregnant or breastfeeding patients.

Patient monitoring

• Monitor for evidence of overdose, including signs and symptoms of hyperthyroidism (weight loss, cardiac symptoms, abdominal cramps).

• In patients with Addison's disease or diabetes mellitus, assess for evidence that these conditions are worsening. In diabetic patients, monitor blood glucose level.

• Monitor vital signs and ECG routinely.

• Check thyroid and liver function test results.

• Monitor for signs and symptoms of bleeding tendency, especially if patient is taking anticoagulants.

Patient teaching

• Teach patient to take drug in morning with or without food.

• Instruct patient to minimize adverse GI effects by eating small, frequent servings of healthy food.

• Instruct patient to avoid driving and other hazardous activities until he knows how drug affects concentration and alertness.

• Teach parents that hair loss may occur in children during first few months but that this effect is usually transient.

• Tell patient that he may require lifelong therapy and will need to undergo regular blood testing.

• As appropriate, review all other significant and life-threatening adverse reactions and interactions, especially those related to the drugs, tests, and foods mentioned above.

liotrix
Thyrolar

Pharmacologic class: Synthetic thyroid hormone
Therapeutic class: Thyroid hormone replacement
Pregnancy risk category A

Action
Raises basal metabolic rate, helps regulate cell growth and differentiation, and increases metabolism of lipids, proteins, and carbohydrates

Availability
Tablets: 12.5 mcg levothyroxine sodium and 3.1 mcg liothyronine sodium (Thyrolar-¼); 25 mcg levothyroxine sodium and 6.25 mcg liothyronine sodium (Thyrolar-½); 50 mcg levothyroxine sodium and 12.5 mcg liothyronine sodium (Thyrolar-1); 100 mcg levothyroxine sodium and 25 mcg liothyronine sodium (Thyrolar-2); 150 mcg levothyroxine sodium and 37.5 mcg liothyronine sodium (Thyrolar-3)

Indications and dosages
➤ Hypothyroidism
Adults: All dosages are individualized. Initially, one tablet Thyrolar-½ P.O., increased by one tablet Thyrolar-¼ P.O. daily until desired effect occurs. Usual maintenance dosage is one tablet Thyrolar-1 or Thyrolar-2 P.O. daily, adjusted within first 4 weeks of therapy based on laboratory results.
➤ Congenital hypothyroidism
Children over age 12: 18.75/75 mcg P.O. daily
Children ages 6 to 11: 12.5/50 to 18.75/75 mcg P.O. daily
Children ages 1 to 5: 9.35/37.5 to 12.5/50 mcg P.O. daily
Children ages 6 to 12 months: 6.25/25 to 9.35/37.5 mcg P.O. daily
Children up to 6 months: 3.1/12.5 to 6.25/25 mcg (Thyrolar-¼) P.O. daily
Dosage adjustment
• Severe, long-standing hypothyroidism
• Cardiovascular disease
• Psychosis or agitation
• Elderly patients

Contraindications
• Hypersensitivity to drug, its components, or tartrazine
• Acute myocardial infarction
• Thyrotoxicosis
• Adrenal insufficiency and coexisting hypothyroidism

Administration
• Know that all dosages are highly individualized.
• Administer single daily oral dose in morning with or without food.

Route	Onset	Peak	Duration
P.O. (levothyroxine)	Unknown	Unknown	Unknown
P.O. (liothyronine)	Unknown	24-72 hr	72 hr

Adverse reactions
CNS: insomnia, irritability, nervousness, headache
CV: tachycardia, angina pectoris, hypotension, hypertension, increased cardiac output, **arrhythmias, cardiovascular collapse**
GI: vomiting, diarrhea, cramps
GU: menstrual irregularities
Metabolic: hyperthyroidism
Musculoskeletal: accelerated bone maturation (in children), decreased bone density (in women on long-term therapy)
Skin: alopecia (in children), diaphoresis
Other: weight loss, heat intolerance

Interactions

Drug-drug. *Aminoglutethimide, amiodarone, anabolic steroids, antithyroid drugs, asparaginase, barbiturates, carbamazepine, chloral hydrate, cholestyramine, clofibrate, colestipol, corticosteroids, danazol, diazepam, estrogens, ethionamide, fluorouracil, heparin (with I.V. use), insulin, lithium, methadone, mitotane, nitroprusside, oxyphenbutazone, P-aminosalicyclic acid, perphenazine, phenylbutazone, phenytoin, propranolol, salicylates (large doses), sulfonylureas, thiazides:* altered thyroid function test values

Anticoagulants: increased anticoagulant action

Beta-adrenergic blockers (selected): decreased beta blocker action

Cardiac glycosides: decreased cardiac glycoside blood level

Cholestyramine, colestipol: liotrix inefficacy

Theophyllines: decreased theophylline clearance

Drug-diagnostic tests. *Thyroid function tests:* decreased values

Drug-food. *Foods high in iron or fiber, soybeans:* decreased drug absorption

Precautions

Use cautiously in:
• cardiovascular disease, severe renal insufficiency, diabetes mellitus, uncorrected adrenocortical disorders
• elderly patients
• pregnant or breastfeeding patients.

Patient monitoring

• Monitor for evidence of overdose, such as signs and symptoms of hyperthyroidism (weight loss, cardiac symptoms, abdominal cramps).
• Watch closely for signs and symptoms of undertreatment.
• In patients with Addison's disease or diabetes mellitus, assess for signs that these conditions are worsening. In diabetic patients, monitor blood glucose level.

• Check vital signs and ECG routinely.
• Monitor thyroid and liver function test results.
• Assess for signs and symptoms of bleeding tendency, especially if patient is taking anticoagulants.

Patient teaching

• Tell patient or parents that drug should be taken in morning, with or without food.
• Advise diabetic patient or his parent to monitor blood glucose level closely.
• Teach patient to minimize GI upset by eating small, frequent servings of healthy food and drinking plenty of fluids.
• Caution patient to avoid driving and other hazardous activities until he knows how drug affects concentration and alertness.
• Inform parents that hair loss may occur in children during first few months of therapy but that this effect is usually transient.
• Explain that patient may require lifelong therapy and will need to undergo regular blood testing.
• As appropriate, review all other significant and life-threatening adverse reactions and interactions, especially those related to the drugs, tests, and foods mentioned above.

lisinopril
Prinivil, Zestril

Pharmacologic class: Angiotensin-converting enzyme (ACE) inhibitor

Therapeutic class: Antihypertensive

Pregnancy risk category C (second and third trimesters: *D*)

Action

Inhibits conversion of angiotensin I to angiotensin II (a potent vasoconstrictor), thereby decreasing systemic vascular resistance and reducing blood pressure, preload, and afterload. Also inactivates bradykinin (a vasodilator) and other vasodilatory prostaglandins, increases plasma renin levels, and reduces aldosterone levels, resulting in systemic vasodilation.

Availability
Tablets: 2.5 mg, 5 mg, 10 mg, 20 mg, 30 mg, 40 mg

Indications and dosages
➤ Hypertension
Adults: Initially, 10 mg P.O. daily, increased up to a maintenance dosage of 20 to 40 mg/day; maximum daily dosage is 80 mg. In patients taking diuretics, 5 mg/day P.O.
➤ Heart failure
Adults: 5 mg/day P.O. (Prinivil), increased in increments as ordered to a maximum of 20 mg/day as a single dose. Or 5 to 40 mg P.O. (Zestril) as a single daily dose given with digitalis and diuretics, increased in increments of no more than 10 mg at intervals of at least 2 weeks, to highest dosage tolerated; maximum dosage is 40 mg/day P.O.
➤ Adjunctive therapy after acute myocardial infarction
Adults: Initially, 5 mg P.O., followed by 5 mg after 24 hours, 10 mg after 48 hours, and then 10 mg daily for 6 weeks (given with standard thrombolytic, aspirin, or beta-adrenergic blocker therapy). If systolic pressure is 120 mm Hg or lower, initial dosage is 2.5 mg for 2 days, followed by 2.5 to 5 mg/day.
Dosage adjustment
• Impaired renal function
• Heart failure with hyponatremia

Contraindications
• Hypersensitivity to drug or other ACE inhibitors
• Angioedema (hereditary, idiopathic, or ACE-inhibitor induced)

• Pregnancy (second and third trimesters)

Administration
• Give once a day in morning, with or without food.
◀᷂ Measure blood pressure before administering; withhold drug if appropriate according to prescriber's blood pressure parameters. Adjust dosage according to blood pressure response.
• Expect prescriber to add low-dose diuretic if lisinopril alone doesn't control blood pressure.

Route	Onset	Peak	Duration
P.O.	1 hr	6 hr	24 hr

Adverse reactions
CNS: dizziness, fatigue, headache, asthenia
CV: hypotension, orthostatic hypotension, syncope, chest pain, angina pectoris
GI: nausea, diarrhea, abdominal pain, altered taste, anorexia
GU: increased blood urea nitrogen (BUN) and creatinine levels, impotence, decreased libido
Hematologic: increased hemoglobin and hematocrit
Hepatic: elevated liver function test results
Metabolic: hyperkalemia, hyponatremia
Musculoskeletal: myalgia
Respiratory: cough, upper respiratory tract infection, asthma, bronchitis, dyspnea
Skin: rash, pruritus, angioedema
Other: fever, **anaphylaxis**

Interactions
Drug-drug. *Cyclosporine, potassium-sparing diuretics, potassium supplements:* hyperkalemia
Diuretics, other antihypertensives: excessive hypotension
Indomethacin: reduced antihypertensive effect

Lithium: increased lithium blood level, greater risk of lithium toxicity
Nonsteroidal anti-inflammatory drugs: further renal deterioration in patients with renal compromise, decreased antihypertensive effects
Thiazides: hypokalemia
Drug-diagnostic tests. *BUN, creatinine, hematocrit, hemoglobin:* slightly increased levels
Liver function tests, potassium: increased values
Sodium: decreased level
Drug-food. *Salt substitutes containing potassium:* hyperkalemia
Drug-herb. *Capsaicin:* cough
Drug-behaviors. *Acute alcohol ingestion:* excessive hypotension

Precautions
Use cautiously in:
• renal impairment, hypertension, cerebrovascular or cardiac insufficiency
• family history of angioedema
• concurrent diuretic therapy
• elderly patients
• pregnant patients in first trimester
• breastfeeding patients
• children (safety not established).

Patient monitoring
• Before and periodically during therapy, monitor complete blood count with white cell differential, as well as kidney and liver function test results.
◀€ Monitor for signs and symptoms of angioedema or anaphylaxis. If these occur, discontinue drug and contact prescriber immediately.
• Check blood pressure frequently to assess drug efficacy. Monitor closely for hypotension, especially in patients also taking diuretics.
• Check vital signs and ECG regularly; assess cardiovascular status carefully.
• Monitor respiratory and neurologic status.
• Assess potassium intake and potassium level.

Patient teaching
• Teach patient to take drug once a day in morning, with or without food.
• Inform patient that drug may cause temporary blood pressure decrease if he stands up suddenly; advise him to rise slowly and carefully.
• Explain that drug may cause muscle aches or headache; encourage patient to discuss activity recommendations and pain relief with prescriber.
• Caution patient to avoid driving and other hazardous activities until he knows how drug affects concentration and alertness.
• Teach patient to minimize GI upset by eating small, frequent servings of healthy food.
• Tell patient that he'll undergo regular blood testing during therapy.
• As appropriate, review all other significant and life-threatening adverse reactions and interactions, especially those related to the drugs, tests, foods, herbs, and behaviors mentioned above.

lithium carbonate
Eskalith, Eskalith CR, Lithizine✿, Lithobid, Lithonate, Lithotabs

lithium citrate
Cibalith-S

Pharmacologic class: Miscellaneous CNS drug
Therapeutic class: Antimanic drug
Pregnancy risk category D

Action
Unknown; transforms sodium exchange and transport in nerves and muscles and controls reuptake of neurotransmitters, thereby influencing emotional responses

Availability
Capsules: 150 mg, 300 mg, 600 mg
Capsules (slow-release): 150 mg, 300 mg
Syrup (citrate): 300 mg (8 mEq lithium)/5 ml
Tablets: 300 mg
Tablets (controlled-release): 450 mg
Tablets (slow-release): 300 mg

🕖 Indications and dosages
➤ Acute mania
Adults and children ages 12 and older: 900 to 1,800 mg P.O. daily in divided doses (for example, 300 to 600 mg t.i.d. or 450 to 900 mg b.i.d. of controlled- or slow-release forms) to achieve blood level of 1 to 1.5 mEq/L; blood level measured b.i.d. until patient is stabilized. Maintenance dosage is 900 to 1,200 mg/day in divided doses (for example, 300 to 400 mg t.i.d. or 450 to 600 mg b.i.d. of controlled- or slow-release form) to maintain blood level of 0.6 to 1.2 mEq/L. Monitor blood level at least q 2 months.
Dosage adjustment
• Impaired renal function
• Elderly patients

Off-label uses
• Acute manic episodes in children
• Corticosteroid-induced psychosis
• Neutropenia secondary to antineoplastic therapy
• Tardive dyskinesia
• Alcoholism
• Bulimia

Contraindications
• Hypersensitivity to or intolerance of alcohol or tartrazine (with some products)
• Severe cardiovascular or renal disease
• Severe sodium depletion
• Pregnancy or breastfeeding
• When drug's therapeutic effects and blood level can't be monitored closely

Administration
◀🔊 Be aware that dosages are individualized according to lithium blood level and clinical response.
• Give with food or milk to minimize GI upset.
• Make sure patient swallows slow-release tablets whole without chewing or crushing them.
• When switching patient from the immediate-release to the controlled- or slow-release form, administer same total daily dosage.
• Know that immediate-release tablets typically are given three or four times daily, whereas controlled-release forms usually are given twice daily, roughly 12 hours apart.

Route	Onset	Peak	Duration
P.O.	Unknown	0.5-3 hr	Unknown
P.O. (controlled, slow-release)	Unknown	3-12 hr	Unknown

Adverse reactions
CNS: headache, tremor, tics, EEG changes, ataxia, choreoathetotic movements, tongue movements, extrapyramidal reactions, cogwheel rigidity, blackout spells, dizziness, drowsiness, psychomotor retardation, slow mental functioning, slurred speech, startled response, restlessness, agitation, confusion, stupor, hallucinations, poor memory, worsening of organic brain syndrome, **coma, epileptiform seizures**
CV: bradycardia, ECG changes, hypotension, sinus node dysfunction with severe bradycardia and syncope, **arrhythmias, peripheral circulatory collapse**
EENT: blurred vision, nystagmus, tinnitus
GI: nausea, vomiting, diarrhea, abdominal pain, fecal incontinence, gastritis, flatulence, dyspepsia, anorexia, metallic or salty taste, increased saliva-

tion, salivary gland swelling, altered taste, dry mouth

GU: urinary incontinence, glycosuria, decreased creatinine clearance, albuminuria, oliguria, polyuria or other signs of nephrogenic diabetes insipidus, impotence, sexual dysfunction

Hematologic: leukocytosis

Metabolic: hypothyroidism with decreased thyroxine (T_4) and triiodothyronine (T_3) levels, hyperthyroidism, goiter, hyperglycemia, hypercalcemia, hyponatremia, hyperparathyroidism

Musculoskeletal: muscle fasciculations and twitching, clonic arm or leg movements, hypertonicity, hyperactive deep tendon reflexes, swollen or painful joints, muscle weakness, polyarthralgia

Skin: dry thin hair, alopecia, diminished or absent skin sensation, chronic folliculitis, eczema with dry skin, new onset or exacerbation of psoriasis, pruritus with or without rash, cutaneous ulcers, angioedema

Other: weight gain; excessive thirst; polydipsia; fever; dental caries; edema of lips, ankles, and wrists

Interactions

Drug-drug. *Acetazolamide, alkalinizing agents (such as sodium bicarbonate), urea, verapamil, xanthines:* decreased lithium blood level

Calcium channel blockers, carbamazepine, haloperidol, methyldopa: increased risk of neurotoxicity

Diuretics: increased sodium loss, increased risk of lithium toxicity

Fluoxetine, loop diuretics, metronidazole, nonsteroidal anti-inflammatory drugs: increased risk of lithium toxicity

Iodide salts: synergistic effects, increased risk of hypothyroidism

Neuromuscular blockers: prolonged neuromuscular blockade, severe respiratory depression

Phenothiazines: decreased phenothiazine blood level or increased lithium level, greater risk of neurotoxicity

Selective serotonin reuptake inhibitors: increased risk of tremor, confusion, dizziness, agitation, and diarrhea

Sympathomimetics: decreased pressor sensitivity

Tricyclic antidepressants: increased antidepressant effects

Drug-diagnostic tests. *Albumin, creatinine, sodium, T_3, T_4:* decreased levels

Calcium, glucose, ^{131}I uptake, white blood cells (WBCs): increased levels

Drug-food. *Caffeine-containing foods and beverages:* decreased lithium blood level and efficacy

Drug-herb. *Caffeine-containing herbs (cola nut, guarana, yerba maté):* decreased lithium blood level and efficacy

Precautions

Use cautiously in:

• hepatic, cardiac, renal, or thyroid disease; diabetes mellitus; seizure disorders; systemic infections; urinary retention; brain trauma; organic brain syndrome

• elderly patients

• children (safety not established).

Patient monitoring

• Obtain baseline ECG and electrolyte levels before therapy and periodically during therapy.

• Assess neurologic and psychiatric status; institute safety measures as needed to prevent injury.

• Monitor lithium blood level, WBC count, and thyroid and kidney function test results.

• Assess cardiovascular status regularly.

• Monitor fluid intake and output; watch for edema and weight gain.

Patient teaching

• Encourage patient to take drug with food or milk to minimize GI upset.

• Instruct patient to swallow slow-release tablets whole without chewing or crushing them.

• Tell patient that beneficial effects may not occur for 1 to 3 weeks.

• Advise patient to limit foods and beverages containing caffeine because they may interfere with drug action.

• Teach patient to maintain adequate fluid intake.

• Explain that drug may cause adverse CNS effects; advise patient to avoid activities requiring mental alertness until effects are known.

◀⋐ Emphasize importance of having regular blood tests to help detect and prevent serious adverse reactions.

• Instruct patient to carry medical identification at all times.

• As appropriate, review all significant and life-threatening adverse reactions and interactions, especially those related to the drugs, tests, foods, and herbs mentioned above.

lomefloxacin hydrochloride
Maxaquin

Pharmacologic class: Fluoroquinolone
Therapeutic class: Anti-infective
Pregnancy risk category C

Action
Inhibits the enzyme DNA gyrase in susceptible gram-negative and gram-positive aerobic and anaerobic bacteria, thereby interfering with bacterial DNA synthesis

Availability
Tablets: 400 mg

❼ Indications and dosages
➤ Acute bacterial exacerbation of chronic bronchitis caused by *Haemophilus influenzae* or *Moraxella catarrhalis;* uncomplicated cystitis caused by *Klebsiella pneumoniae, Proteus mirabilis, Staphylococcus saprophyticus,* or *Escherichia coli*

Adults: 400 mg P.O. daily for 10 days
➤ Complicated urinary tract infections

Adults: 400 mg P.O. for 14 days
➤ Uncomplicated gonorrhea

Adults: 400 mg P.O. as a single dose
➤ Perioperative prophylaxis (transurethral surgery)

Adults: 400 mg P.O. 2 to 6 hours before surgery
➤ Perioperative prophylaxis (transrectal prostate biopsy)

Adults: 400 mg P.O. 1 to 6 hours before surgery

Dosage adjustment
• Renal impairment

Contraindications
• Hypersensitivity to drug or other fluoroquinolones

Administration
• Administer on empty stomach when possible.

• Know that drug shouldn't be used in *Streptococcus pneumoniae*–induced acute bacterial exacerbation of chronic bronchitis.

Route	Onset	Peak	Duration
P.O.	Rapid	Unknown	24 hr

Adverse reactions
CNS: dizziness, headache
CV: chest pain, **cardiopulmonary arrest, cerebral thrombosis**
Hematologic: agranulocytosis
Hepatic: hepatic disease
GI: nausea, diarrhea, constipation, abdominal pain, **pseudomembranous colitis**
Skin: photosensitivity
Other: hypersensitivity reactions including **anaphylaxis**

Interactions
Drug-drug. *Antacids, iron salts, sucralfate:* decreased lomefloxacin absorption

Nonsteroidal anti-inflammatory drugs: increased risk of CNS stimulation and seizures

Probenecid: decreased urinary excretion of lomefloxacin

Drug-food. *Any food:* delayed drug absorption

Drug-herb. *Dong quai, St. John's wort:* increased risk of photosensitivity

Fennel: decreased drug absorption

Precautions

Use cautiously in:
• bradycardia, acute myocardial ischemia, cirrhosis, renal impairment, underlying CNS disease
• elderly patients
• pregnant or breastfeeding patients
• children under age 18.

Patient monitoring

◀€ Watch for signs and symptoms of anaphylaxis.
• Assess for drug efficacy.
• Monitor vital signs and ECG; assess cardiovascular status carefully.
◀€ Monitor for signs and symptoms of serious reactions to quinolones (such as cardiopulmonary arrest, cerebral thrombosis, hepatic disease, agranulocytosis).
• Monitor liver and kidney function test results, complete blood count, blood glucose level, and urinalysis. Know that other quinolones have caused changes in hematologic, blood glucose, and kidney function test results.

Patient teaching

• Instruct patient to take drug on empty stomach, if possible.
◀€ Advise patient to report rash immediately so prescriber can determine if it reflects a hypersensitivity reaction.
◀€ Advise patient to report diarrhea, which may be first sign of pseudomembranous colitis.
• Teach patient to avoid driving and other hazardous activities until he

knows how drug affects concentration and alertness.
• Instruct patient to minimize GI upset by eating small, frequent servings of healthy food.
• Tell patient he'll need to undergo regular blood testing during therapy.
• As appropriate, review all other significant and life-threatening adverse reactions and interactions, especially those related to the drugs, foods, and herbs mentioned above.

lomustine
CeeNU

Pharmacologic class: Alkylating drug (nitrosourea)

Therapeutic class: Antineoplastic

Pregnancy risk category D

Action

Inactivates neoplastic cells by alkylating DNA, which causes DNA structural modification and fragmentation; thought to act in late G1 or early S phase of cell cycle

Availability

Capsules: 10 mg, 40 mg, 100 mg
Dose pack: two 100-mg capsules, two 40-mg capsules, and two 10-mg capsules

⊘ Indications and dosages

➤ Adjunctive therapy in primary and metastatic brain tumors and Hodgkin's disease

Adults and children: When used as monotherapy, 130 mg/m² P.O. as a single dose q 6 weeks in previously untreated patients. In bone marrow suppression, initial dosage is 100 mg/m² P.O. q 6 weeks; don't repeat dose until platelet count exceeds 100,000/mm³ and leukocyte count is higher than 4,000/mm³. When given with other cy-

totoxic drugs, dosage generally is reduced to 50% or 75% of monotherapy dosage.
Dosage adjustment
• Bone marrow depression (based on leukocyte and platelet counts)

Contraindications
• Hypersensitivity to drug

Administration
• Obtain complete blood count (CBC) with white cell differential before starting therapy.
• Give drug 2 to 4 hours after meals to enhance absorption.
• Administer antiemetic before giving drug, as prescribed, to minimize nausea.
• If vomiting occurs shortly after administration, notify prescriber.

Route	Onset	Peak	Duration
P.O.	10 min	3 hr	48 hr

Adverse reactions
CNS: anxiety, confusion, dizziness, hallucinations, lethargy, headache, paresthesia, light-headedness, drowsiness, fatigue, **seizures**
GI: nausea; vomiting; anorexia; sore mouth, lips, and throat; **GI bleeding**
GU: amenorrhea, azoospermia, progressive azotemia, **nephrotoxicity, renal failure**
Hematologic: anemia, **leukopenia, thrombocytopenia, bone marrow depression**
Hepatic: hepatotoxicity
Skin: alopecia
Other: secondary malignancies

Interactions
Drug-drug. *Anticoagulants, nonsteroidal anti-inflammatory drugs:* increased risk of bleeding
Myelosuppressants: increased bone marrow depression

Drug-diagnostic tests. *Hemoglobin, platelets, red blood cells, white blood cells:* decreased values
Liver function tests, nitrogenous compounds: increased values

Precautions
Use cautiously in:
• renal or hepatic dysfunction, bone marrow depression
• pregnant or breastfeeding patients.

Patient monitoring
• Watch for evidence of overdose, including bone marrow depression, nausea, and vomiting.
◀€ Monitor CBC and platelet counts closely; watch for signs of bleeding and bruising.
• Avoid I.M. injection if platelet count is below 100,000/mm³.
• Check kidney and liver function test results regularly.
• Assess neurologic status carefully; institute safety measures as needed to prevent injury.
• Watch for signs and symptoms of secondary malignancies.

Patient teaching
• Instruct patient to contact prescriber if he vomits shortly after taking drug.
◀€ Tell patient to immediately report easy bruising or bleeding, which may signal a low platelet count.
• Instruct patient to avoid exposure to people with infections because drug may increase susceptibility to infection.
◀€ Caution women of childbearing age to use reliable contraception and to immediately report suspected or confirmed pregnancy.
• Advise patient to avoid driving and other hazardous activities until he knows how drug affects concentration and alertness.
• Teach patient to minimize GI side effects by eating small, frequent servings of healthy food.

- Inform patient that drug may cause hair loss.
- Tell patient that he'll undergo frequent blood testing during therapy.
- As appropriate, review all other significant and life-threatening adverse reactions and interactions, especially those related to the drugs and tests mentioned above.

loperamide hydrochloride

Apo-Loperamide✤, Diarr-Eze✤, Imodium, Imodium A-D, Kaopectate II, Loperacap✤, Novo-Loperamide✤, Pepto Diarrhea Control, PMS-Loperamide✤, Rho-Loperamide✤, Riva-Loperamide✤

Pharmacologic class: Piperidine derivative
Therapeutic class: Antidiarrheal
Pregnancy risk category B

Action
Inhibits peristalsis of intestinal contents by direct effect on intestinal wall muscles; also reduces fecal volume, increases fecal bulk, and minimizes fluid and electrolyte loss

Availability
Capsules: 2 mg
Solution: 1 mg/5 ml
Tablets: 2 mg

🕖 Indications and dosages
➣ Acute diarrhea
Adults: Initially, 4 mg P.O., then 2 mg after each loose stool. Usual maintenance dosage is 4 to 8 mg P.O. daily in divided doses, not to exceed 16 mg daily.
Children ages 8 to 12 or weighing more than 30 kg (66 lb): Initially, 2 mg P.O. t.i.d., then 1 mg/kg after each loose stool, not to exceed 6 mg daily

Children ages 6 to 8 or weighing 20 to 30 kg (44 to 66 lb): Initially, 2 mg P.O. b.i.d., then 1 mg/kg after each loose stool, not to exceed 4 mg daily
Children ages 2 to 5 or weighing 13 to 20 kg (29 to 44 lb): Initially, 1 mg P.O. t.i.d., then 1 mg/kg after each loose stool, not to exceed 3 mg daily
➣ Chronic diarrhea
Adults: Initially, 4 mg P.O., then 2 mg after each loose stool; reduce dosage as tolerated. Don't exceed 16 mg daily for more than 10 days.

Contraindications
- Hypersensitivity to drug
- Abdominal pain of unknown cause (especially with fever)
- Acute diarrhea caused by enteroinvasive *Escherichia coli, Salmonella,* or *Shigella*
- Acute ulcerative colitis
- Bloody diarrhea with body temperature above 101º F (38.3º C) (with OTC products)
- Pseudomembranous colitis associated with broad-spectrum anti-infectives
- Children younger than age 6

Administration
- Use patient's weight to determine appropriate dosage (especially in children).

Route	Onset	Peak	Duration
P.O.	1 hr	2.5-5 hr	10 hr

Adverse reactions
CNS: drowsiness, dizziness
GI: nausea; vomiting; constipation; abdominal pain, distention, or discomfort; dry mouth; **toxic megacolon** (in patients with acute ulcerative colitis)
Other: allergic reactions

Interactions
Drug-drug. *Antidepressants, antihistamines, other anticholinergics:* additive anticholinergic effects

CNS depressants (including antihistamines, opioid analgesics, sedative-hypnotics): additive CNS depression
Drug-herb. *Chamomile, hops, kava, skullcap, valerian:* increased CNS depression
Drug-behaviors. *Alcohol use:* increased CNS depression

Precautions
Use cautiously in:
- hepatic disease
- elderly patients
- pregnant or breastfeeding patients
- children.

Patient monitoring
◀€ Watch for signs and symptoms of abdominal distention, which may signal toxic megacolon in patients with ulcerative colitis.
- Monitor bowel movements to evaluate drug efficacy and determine need for repeat doses.
- Monitor stool culture results as indicated.
- Check stool for occult blood as indicated.
- Evaluate fluid intake and output.
- Monitor patient (especially child) for CNS effects.

Patient teaching
- Teach patient or parent to maintain high fluid intake to prevent dehydration.
- Instruct patient or parents to report fever, mucus in stool, or history of hepatic disease before using drug.
- Caution patient or parents to discontinue drug if symptoms worsen or diarrhea lasts longer than 2 days.
- As appropriate, review all other significant and life-threatening adverse reactions and interactions, especially those related to the drugs, herbs, and behaviors mentioned above.

loracarbef
Lorabid

Pharmacologic class: Second-generation cephalosporin
Therapeutic class: Anti-infective
Pregnancy risk category B

Action
Binds to essential proteins of bacterial cell wall, interfering with cell-wall synthesis in susceptible strains of gram-positive and gram-negative bacteria; bactericidal

Availability
Capsules: 200 mg, 400 mg
Oral suspension: 100 mg/5 ml
Powder for oral solution: 100 mg/5 ml, 200 mg/5 ml

🖊 Indications and dosages
➤ Acute and secondary bacterial infections in acute and chronic bronchitis caused by *Streptococcus pneumoniae*
Adults and children ages 13 and older: 200 to 400 mg P.O. q 12 hours for 7 days
➤ Pneumonia, uncomplicated pyelonephritis caused by *Escherichia coli*
Adults and children ages 13 and older: 400 mg P.O. q 12 hours for 14 days
➤ Pharyngitis or tonsillitis caused by *Streptococcus pyogenes*
Adults and children ages 13 and older: 200 mg P.O. q 12 hours for 10 days
Infants and children ages 6 months to 12 years: 15 mg/kg/day P.O. (oral suspension) in divided doses q 12 hours for 10 days
➤ Sinusitis caused by *S. pneumoniae, Haemophilus influenzae,* or *Moxarella catarrhalis*
Adults and children ages 13 and older: 400 mg P.O. q 12 hours for 10 days

---

➤ Uncomplicated skin and skin-structure infections caused by *Staphylococcus aureus* or *S. pyogenes*

Adults and children ages 13 and older: 200 mg P.O. q 12 hours for 7 days

➤ Uncomplicated cystitis caused by *E. coli* or *Staphylococcus saprophyticus*

Adults and children ages 13 and older: 200 mg P.O. q 24 hours for 7 days

➤ Acute otitis media or acute maxillary sinusitis caused by *S. pneumoniae, H. influenzae, M. catarrhalis,* or *S. pyogenes*

Children ages 6 months to 12 years: 30 mg/kg/day P.O. (oral suspension) in divided doses q 12 hours for 10 days

➤ Impetigo caused by *S. aureus* or *S. pyogenes*

Children ages 6 months to 12 years: 15 mg/kg/day P.O. (oral suspension) in divided doses q 12 hours for 7 days

Dosage adjustment
• Renal impairment
• Elderly patients

Contraindications

• Hypersensitivity to drug or other cephalosporins

Administration

• Administer 1 hour before or 2 hours after a meal.

• Reconstitute oral suspension as follows: for 50-ml bottle, add 15 ml of water twice to dry mixture; shake well after each addition. For 100-ml bottle, add 30 ml of water twice; shake well after each addition.

• Use oral suspension for patients with otitis media because it's more rapidly absorbed than capsules.

Route	Onset	Peak	Duration
P.O.	Rapid	0.5-1.2 hr	12 hr

Adverse reactions

CNS: headache, nervousness, drowsiness, dizziness, insomnia
CV: vasodilation

GI: nausea, vomiting, diarrhea, epigastric distress, **pseudomembranous colitis**
GU: transient increases in blood urea nitrogen (BUN) and creatinine levels, vaginal candidiasis, vaginitis
Hematologic: eosinophilia, transient **thrombocytopenia, leukopenia**
Hepatic: transient increases in alanine aminotransferase (ALT), alkaline phosphatase (ALP), and aspartate aminotransferase (AST) levels
Skin: rash, urticaria, pruritus, erythema multiforme
Other: allergic reaction, superinfection, **anaphylaxis, Stevens-Johnson syndrome**

Interactions

Drug-drug. *Potent diuretics:* increased risk of renal dysfunction
Probenecid: increased loracarbef blood level

Drug-diagnostic tests. *ALP, ALT, AST, BUN, creatinine, eosinophils:* transient elevations
Coombs' test, urine glucose tests using Benedict's or Fehling's solution or Clinitest tablets: false-positive results
Platelets, white blood cells: transient decreases

Drug-food. *Moderate- or high-fat meal:* increased drug bioavailability
Drug herb. *Anise, arnica, asafetida, bogbean, boldo, celery, chamomile, clove, danshen, fenugreek, feverfew, garlic, ginger, ginkgo, ginseng, horse chestnut, horseradish, licorice, meadowsweet, onion, papain, passionflower, poplar, prickly ash, quassia, red clover, turmeric, wild carrot, wild lettuce, willow:* increased risk of bleeding

Precautions

Use cautiously in:
• renal impairment, phenylketonuria (with products containing aspartame)
• history of GI disease (especially colitis)

- elderly patients
- pregnant or breastfeeding patients.

Patient monitoring

◀€ Watch for signs and symptoms of anaphylaxis, Stevens-Johnson syndrome, and hepatic dysfunction; withhold drug and contact prescriber immediately if these occur.
- Monitor for signs and symptoms of toxicity, including rash, vomiting, diarrhea, and epigastric distress.
- Measure patient's temperature; watch for signs and symptoms of superinfection.
- Check bowel movements for early signs of pseudomembranous colitis.
- Monitor complete blood count with white cell differential as well as kidney function test results, as appropriate.
- Obtain and monitor cultures as indicated.

Patient teaching

- Teach patient or parents to monitor patient's bowel movements and report significant diarrhea.
- Instruct patient to increase fluid intake as tolerated.
◀€ Caution patient to stop taking drug and immediately report rash, yellowing of skin or eyes, or signs or symptoms of toxicity (such as vomiting, diarrhea, or epigastric distress).
- Advise patient to eat a low-fat diet because high-fat meals alter drug's action.
- Explain that many herbs may increase risk of bleeding from this drug; discourage their use.
- As appropriate, review all other significant and life-threatening adverse reactions and interactions, especially those related to the drugs, tests, foods, and herbs mentioned above.

loratadine
Alavert, Claritin, Claritin RediTabs

Pharmacologic class: Histamine$_1$-receptor antagonist (second-generation)
Therapeutic class: Antihistamine (nonsedating)
Pregnancy risk category B

Action
Selective histamine$_1$-receptor antagonist; blocks peripheral effects of histamine released during allergic reactions and decreases allergy symptoms

Availability
Syrup: 1 mg/ml
Tablets: 10 mg
Tablets (rapidly disintegrating): 10 mg

🖊 Indications and dosages
➤ Symptomatic treatment of seasonal allergies, chronic idiopathic urticaria
Adults and children ages 6 and older: 10 mg P.O. daily
Children ages 2 to 5: 5 mg P.O. daily
Dosage adjustment
- Renal or hepatic impairment

Contraindications
- Hypersensitivity to drug or sulfites

Administration
- To enhance drug absorption, give once a day on empty stomach when possible.
- Place rapidly disintegrating tablet on tongue; give with or without water.
- Use rapidly disintegrating tablets within 6 months of opening foil pouch and immediately after opening individual tablet blister.

Route	Onset	Peak	Duration
P.O.	1-3 hr	8-12 hr	>24 hr

Adverse reactions
CNS: headache, nervousness, insomnia
EENT: conjunctivitis, earache, epistaxis, pharyngitis
GI: abdominal pain, dry mouth; diarrhea, stomatitis, and tooth disorder in children
Skin: rash, photosensitivity, angioedema
Other: fever, flulike symptoms, viral infections

Interactions
Drug-food. *Any food:* increased drug absorption

Precautions
Use cautiously in:
- hepatic or renal impairment
- elderly patients
- pregnant patients
- children younger than age 2 (safety not established).

Patient monitoring
- Watch for adverse reactions, especially in children.
- Assess patient's response to drug.
- Watch for new symptoms or exacerbation of existing symptoms.

Patient teaching
- Advise patient to take drug exactly as prescribed, once a day on empty stomach.
- Teach patient to report persistent or worsening symptoms.
- Instruct patient to report adverse reactions, such as headache or nervousness.
- Caution patient to avoid driving and other hazardous activities until he knows how drug affects concentration and alertness.
- As appropriate, review all other significant adverse reactions and interactions, especially those related to the foods mentioned above.

lorazepam
Apo-Lorazepam✦, Ativan,
Novo-Lorazem✦, Nu-Loraz✦

Pharmacologic class: Benzodiazepine
Therapeutic class: Anxiolytic
Controlled substance schedule IV
Pregnancy risk category D

Action
Unknown; thought to depress CNS at limbic system and affect neurotransmission in reticular activating system

Availability
Injection: 2 mg/ml, 4 mg/ml
Solution (concentrated): 2 mg/ml
Tablets: 0.5 mg, 1 mg, 2 mg

🗲 Indications and dosages
➤ Anxiety
Adults: 2 to 3 mg P.O. daily in two or three divided doses, up to a maximum dosage of 10 mg daily
➤ Insomnia
Adults: 2 to 4 mg P.O. at bedtime
➤ Adjunctive treatment of delirium
Adults: 0.5 to 1 mg I.V. immediately after haloperidol I.V.; adjust dosage according to patient response
➤ Premedication before surgery
Adults: 0.05 mg/kg (not to exceed 4 mg) by deep I.M. injection at least 2 hours before surgery, or 0.044 mg/kg (not to exceed 2 mg) I.V. 15 to 20 minutes before surgery
➤ Nausea and vomiting secondary to cancer chemotherapy
Adults: 2.5 mg P.O. on evening before and just after initiation of chemotherapy, or 1.5 mg/m² I.V. over 5 minutes 45 minutes before chemotherapy begins, up to a maximum of 3 mg I.V.
Dosage adjustment
- Elderly or debilitated patients

Off-label uses
- Acute alcohol withdrawal syndrome
- Status epilepticus

Contraindications
- Hypersensitivity to drug, other benzodiazepines, polyethylene or propylene glycol, or benzyl alcohol
- Acute narrow-angle glaucoma
- Coma or CNS depression
- Hepatic or renal failure

Administration
- For I.V. use, dilute with equal volume of compatible diluent, such as normal saline solution or dextrose 5% in water. Keep resuscitation equipment and oxygen readily available.
- ◀ Give I.V. doses slowly over 5 minutes. Rate shouldn't exceed 2 mg/minute.
- Don't give parenteral form to children under age 18.

Route	Onset	Peak	Duration
P.O.	15-45 min	1-6 hr	Up to 48 hr
I.V.	Rapid	15-20 min	Up to 48 hr
I.M.	15-30 min	1-2 hr	Up to 48 hr

Adverse reactions
CNS: amnesia, agitation, ataxia, depression, disorientation, dizziness, drowsiness, headache, incoordination, asthenia
CV (with too rapid I.V. administration): bradycardia, hypotension, tachycardia, apnea, **cardiac arrest, cardiovascular collapse**
EENT: blurred vision, diplopia, nystagmus
GI: nausea, abdominal discomfort
Other: increased or decreased appetite

Interactions
Drug-drug. *CNS depressants (including antidepressants, antihistamines, benzodiazepines, sedative-hypnotics):* additive CNS depression

Hormonal contraceptives: increased lorazepam clearance
Drug-herb. *Chamomile, hops, kava, skullcap, valerian:* increased CNS depression
Drug-behaviors. *Alcohol use:* increased CNS depression
Smoking: increased metabolism and decreased efficacy of lorazepam

Precautions
Use cautiously in:
- hepatic or renal impairment
- history of suicide attempt, drug abuse, depressive disorder, or psychosis
- elderly patients
- pregnant or breastfeeding patients.

Patient monitoring
- During I.V. administration, monitor ECG and cardiovascular and respiratory status.
- Monitor vital signs closely.
- Evaluate for amnesia.
- Watch closely for CNS depression; institute safety precautions as needed to prevent injury.
- Monitor for signs and symptoms of overdose (such as confusion, hypotension, coma, and labored breathing).
- Assess liver function test results and complete blood count.

Patient teaching
- Teach patient and family about possible CNS effects of drug; recommend appropriate safety precautions.
- Explain that with long-term use, drug must be discontinued slowly (typically over 8 to 12 weeks).
- Instruct patient to avoid alcohol because it increases drowsiness and other CNS effects.
- Caution patient to avoid smoking because it speeds drug breakdown in body.
- As appropriate, review all significant and life-threatening adverse reactions and interactions, especially those relat-

ed to the drugs, herbs, and behaviors mentioned above.

losartan potassium
Cozaar

Pharmacologic class: Angiotensin II receptor antagonist
Therapeutic class: Antihypertensive
Pregnancy risk category C (first trimester), *D* (second and third trimesters)

Action
Blocks effects of angiotensin II at various receptor sites, including vascular smooth muscle and adrenal glands

Availability
Tablets: 25 mg, 50 mg, 100 mg

🧪 Indications and dosages
➤ Management of hypertension
Adults: Initially, 50 mg/day P.O.; range is 25 to 100 mg/day as a single dose or in two divided doses. May be used alone or with other drugs.
Dosage adjustment
• Hepatic impairment
• Concurrent diuretic therapy

Off-label uses
• Type 2 diabetes with nephropathy

Contraindications
• Hypersensitivity to drug or its components
• Pregnancy (second and third trimesters) or breastfeeding

Administration
• Administer with or without food.
• Know that if drug efficacy (measured at trough) is inadequate with once-daily dosing, prescriber may switch to twice-daily regimen using same or higher daily dosage.

• Be aware that drug may take 3 to 6 weeks to reach maximal efficacy.

Route	Onset	Peak	Duration
P.O.	Unknown	1 hr	Unknown

Adverse reactions
CNS: dizziness, insomnia, headache
EENT: sinus disorders
GI: nausea, vomiting, diarrhea, dyspepsia, abdominal pain
Metabolic: hyperkalemia
Musculoskeletal: joint pain, back pain, muscle cramps
Respiratory: symptoms of upper respiratory infection, cough
Other: hypersensitivity reactions

Interactions
Drug-drug. *Diuretics, other antihypertensives:* increased risk of hypotension
Fluconazole: inhibited losartan metabolism, increased antihypertensive effects
Potassium-sparing diuretics, potassium supplements: hyperkalemia
Phenobarbital, rifamycins: enhanced losartan metabolism, decreased antihypertensive effects
Drug-diagnostic tests. *Albumin:* increased level
Drug-food. *Salt substitutes containing potassium:* hyperkalemia

Precautions
Use cautiously in:
• heart failure, renal or hepatic impairment, obstructive biliary disorders
• high-dose diuretic therapy
• black patients
• pregnant patients
• children younger than age 18 (safety not established).

Patient monitoring
• Monitor blood pressure to evaluate drug efficacy.
• Assess liver and kidney function test results and electrolyte levels.

• Stay alert for oliguria, progressive azotemia, and renal failure in patients with severe heart failure and renal function that depends on renin-angiotensin-aldosterone system.

• Know that in black patients, losartan and other ACE inhibitors may be ineffective when used alone.

• Be aware that drug may cause fetal injury or death when used during second or third trimester of pregnancy.

Patient teaching

• Instruct patient to avoid potassium supplements or salt substitutes containing potassium, unless directed by physician.

• Caution female patients not to take drug during second or third trimesters of pregnancy. Advise them to contact prescriber immediately if they suspect pregnancy.

• As appropriate, review all other significant adverse reactions and interactions, especially those related to the drugs, tests, and foods mentioned above.

lovastatin

Altocor, Apo-Lovastatin✚,
Dom-Lovastatin✚, Gen-Lovastatin✚,
Mevacor, Novo-Lovastatin✚,
PMS-Lovastatin✚

Pharmacologic class: HMG-CoA reductase inhibitor
Therapeutic class: Antihyperlipidemic
Pregnancy risk category X

Action

Inhibits HMG-CoA reductase, an enzyme crucial to cholesterol synthesis pathway; decreases total cholesterol and low-density lipoprotein (LDL) level and increases high-density lipoprotein level

Availability

Tablets: 10 mg, 20 mg, 40 mg
Tablets (extended-release): 10 mg, 20 mg, 40 mg, 60 mg

Indications and dosages

➢ To reduce LDL, total cholesterol, apolipoprotein B, and triglyceride levels in patients with primary hypercholesterolemia (types IIa and IIb); to slow coronary artery disease progression
Adults: 20 mg P.O. daily, increased at 4-week intervals to a maximum of 80 mg/day as a single dose or in divided doses. Or, 20 mg P.O. (extended-release) daily, increased at 4-week intervals to a maximum daily dosage of 60 mg.
Dosage adjustment
• Severe renal insufficiency

Off-label uses

• High-risk patients with diabetic dyslipidemia, familial dysbetalipoproteinemia, familial combined hyperlipidemia, or nephrotic hyperlipidemia

Contraindications

• Hypersensitivity to drug, its components, or angiotensin-converting enzyme inhibitors
• Active hepatic disease or unexplained persistent hepatic enzyme elevation
• Concurrent gemfibrozil or azole antifungal therapy
• Females of childbearing age
• Pregnancy or breastfeeding

Administration

• Give daily dose with evening meal.
• Increase dosage at intervals of 4 weeks or longer, as ordered.
• Discontinue drug if alanine aminotransferase (ALT) or aspartate aminotransferase (AST) level remains more than three times the upper limit of normal.
• Be aware that drug may be used to treat heterozygous familial hypercholesterolemia in boys and postmenar-

chal girls ages 10 and older with high LDL and cholesterol levels (despite an adequate trial of diet therapy).

• Don't give with grapefruit juice; doing so may increase drug blood level.

Route	Onset	Peak	Duration
P.O.	Unknown	2 hr	Unknown
P.O. (extended)	Unknown	Unknown	Unknown

Adverse reactions

CNS: headache, dizziness, asthenia
EENT: blurred vision, eye irritation
GI: nausea, vomiting, constipation, diarrhea, abdominal pain or cramps, dyspepsia, flatulence
Musculoskeletal: myalgia, cramps, **rhabdomyolysis**
Skin: pruritus, rash
Other: hypersensitivity reaction

Interactions

Drug-drug. *Antifungals, cyclosporine, erythromycin, folic acid derivatives, gemfibrozil, niacin, other HMG-CoA inhibitors:* increased risk of myopathy and rhabdomyolysis
Bile acid sequestrants: decreased lovastatin blood level
Isradipine: increased lovastatin clearance
Warfarin: increased prothrombin time, bleeding
Drug-diagnostic tests. *ALT, AST:* increased levels
Drug-food. *Grapefruit juice:* increased lovastatin blood level
Drug-herb. *Red yeast rice:* increased risk of adverse reactions

Precautions

Use cautiously in:
• cerebral arteriosclerosis, heart disease, renal impairment, severe acute infection, severe hypotension or hypertension, uncontrolled seizures, myopathy, visual disturbances, major surgery, trauma, alcoholism

• severe metabolic, endocrine, or electrolyte problems
• children.

Patient monitoring

• Obtain liver function test results before starting therapy, 6 and 12 weeks after therapy begins or dosage is increased, and periodically thereafter.

Patient teaching

• Teach patient to take immediate-release tablets with evening meal or extended-release tablets at bedtime.
• Instruct patient not to break, crush, or chew extended-release tablets.
• Teach patient about importance of cholesterol-lowering diet and other therapies, such as exercise and weight control.
• Instruct patient to report unexplained muscle pain, tenderness, or weakness as well as signs or symptoms of hepatotoxicity (fever, malaise, abdominal pain, clay-colored stools, or tea-colored urine).
◀︎ Advise patient to contact prescriber immediately if she is breastfeeding or suspects pregnancy.
• As appropriate, review all other significant and life-threatening adverse reactions and interactions, especially those related to the drugs, tests, foods, and herbs mentioned above.

loxapine hydrochloride
Loxapac✿, Loxitane C, Loxitane IM

loxapine succinate
Apo-Loxapine✿, Loxapac✿, Loxitane, Nu-Loxapine✿

Pharmacologic class: Tricyclic dibenzoxazepine derivative
Therapeutic class: Antipsychotic
Pregnancy risk category C

Action
Unknown; thought to relieve psychotic symptoms by blocking neurotransmission of postsynaptic dopamine receptors in the brain

Availability
Capsules: 5 mg, 10 mg, 25 mg, 50 mg
Injection: 50 mg/ml
Oral concentrate: 25 mg/ml

🕖 Indications and dosages
➤ Psychotic disorders
Adults: 10 mg P.O. b.i.d.; increase over first 7 to 10 days, up to 100 mg/day P.O. in two to four divided doses. Or give 12.5 to 50 mg I.M. q 4 to 6 hours. Maximum dosage is 250 mg/day.
Dosage adjustment
• Elderly patients

Contraindications
• Hypersensitivity to drug or other dibenzoxazepines
• Coma or severe CNS depression
• Severe drug-induced depression

Administration
• Give loxapine hydrochloride orally or I.M. Don't administer I.V.
• Administer loxapine succinate by oral route only.
• Mix loxapine hydrochloride oral concentrate with grapefruit juice or orange juice just before administering.

Route	Onset	Peak	Duration
P.O.	30 min	1.5-3 hr	12 hr
I.M.	Rapid	Rapid	Unknown

Adverse reactions
CNS: drowsiness, insomnia, vertigo, headache, dizziness, weakness, akinesia, staggering or shuffling gait, slurred speech, agitation, extrapyramidal reactions, sedation, syncope, tardive dyskinesia, numbness, confusion, pseudoparkinsonism, EEG changes, **seizures, neuroleptic malignant syndrome**
CV: orthostatic hypotension, hypertension, ECG changes
EENT: blurred vision, ptosis, nasal congestion
GI: nausea, vomiting, constipation, dry mouth, **paralytic ileus**
GU: urinary retention
Hematologic: leukopenia, agranulocytosis, thrombocytopenia
Hepatic: hepatocellular injury with elevated hepatic enzyme levels
Metabolic: polydipsia
Musculoskeletal: muscle twitching
Skin: rash, pruritus, seborrhea, photosensitivity, alopecia
Other: weight gain or loss, hyperpyrexia, facial edema, hypersensitivity reactions

Interactions
Drug-drug. *Anticholinergics, CNS depressants:* additive effects
Epinephrine: severe hypotension, tachycardia, decreased epinephrine effects
Drug-diagnostic tests. *Liver function tests:* increased values
Granulocytes, platelets, white blood cells: decreased counts
Drug-behaviors. *Alcohol use:* increased CNS depression

Precautions
Use cautiously in:
• seizures, cardiovascular or respiratory disorders, circulatory collapse, cerebral arteriosclerosis, severe hypotension, hypertension, glaucoma, prostatic hypertrophy, breast cancer, thyrotoxicosis, peptic ulcer, impaired renal function, bone marrow depression, subcortical brain damage, Parkinson's disease, hepatic disease, blood dyscrasias
• pregnant or breastfeeding patients
• children younger than age 16.

Patient monitoring
• Measure blood pressure before drug therapy starts and periodically during therapy.

• Monitor hematologic studies and liver function tests.

◀€ Stay alert for evidence of neuroleptic malignant syndrome (extrapyramidal symptoms, hyperpyrexia, muscle rigidity, altered mental status, irregular pulse or blood pressure, tachycardia, arrhythmias, diaphoresis).

• Assess for tardive dyskinesia (involuntary jerky movements of the face, tongue, jaws, trunk, arms, and legs), especially in elderly women.

Patient teaching

• Inform patient that drug may cause tardive dyskinesia.

• Instruct patient to avoid activities requiring mental concentration until drug's effects are known.

◀€ Teach patient to immediately report sore throat, fever, rash, impaired vision, tremors, involuntary muscle twitching, muscle stiffness, or yellowing of eyes or skin.

• Instruct patient to move slowly when sitting up or standing to avoid dizziness or light-headedness from sudden blood pressure decrease.

• Caution patient to avoid alcohol use.

• As appropriate, review all other significant and life-threatening adverse reactions and interactions, especially those related to the drugs, tests, and behaviors mentioned above.

lymphocyte immune globulin (antithymocyte globulin equine, ATG, ATG equine, LIG)
Atgam

Pharmacologic class: Immunoglobulin

Therapeutic class: Immunosuppressant

Pregnancy risk category C

Action
Unknown; thought to inhibit cell-mediated immune response by altering the function of or eliminating T lymphocytes

Availability
Injection: 50 mg immunoglobulin G/ml in 5-ml ampules

🕖 Indications and dosages
➤ To prevent acute renal allograft rejection

Adults: 15 mg/kg/day I.V. for 14 days; then switch to alternate-day dosing for 14 days (for a total of 21 doses in 28 days). Give first dose within 24 hours of transplantation.

Children: 5 to 25 mg/kg/day I.V. for 14 days; then switch to alternate-day dosing for 14 days (for a total of 21 doses in 28 days). Give first dose within 24 hours of transplantation.

➤ Acute renal allograft rejection

Adults and children: 10 to 15 mg/kg/day I.V. for 14 days, then switch to alternate-day dosing for 14 days (for a total of 21 doses in 28 days). Start therapy at first sign of rejection.

➤ Aplastic anemia

Adults: 10 to 20 mg/kg/day I.V. for 8 to 14 days; then switch to alternate-day dosing. Total of 21 doses in 28 days can be given.

Off-label uses
• Bone marrow, liver, and heart transplantation
• Multiple sclerosis
• Myasthenia gravis
• Scleroderma

Contraindications
• Hypersensitivity to drug

Administration
◀€ Because of high risk of anaphylaxis, perform intradermal skin test before first dose. Inject 0.1-ml dose of 1:1,000 dilution of LIG intradermally; to aid

interpretation, a control test using 0.9% sodium chloride injection is injected contralaterally. Observe site every 15 to 20 minutes during first hour after injection, and monitor patient for systemic manifestations. Local reaction of 10 mm or greater with a wheal, erythema, or both, with or without pseudopod formation and itching or marked local swelling, indicates a positive test (which warrants consideration of alternate therapy). Systemic reaction (such as tachycardia, dyspnea, hypotension, or anaphylaxis) precludes drug therapy.

• Premedicate with an antipyretic, an antihistamine, or corticosteroids, as prescribed, to minimize febrile or other reactions.

• For I.V. infusion, dilute prescribed dose in 250 to 1,000 ml of 0.45% or 0.9% sodium chloride injection. (Don't dilute in dextrose solutions or highly acidic solutions.) Final concentration shouldn't exceed 4 mg/ml.

• When adding drug to infusion container, invert the container so that air doesn't enter it. Gently swirl or rotate container to mix solution.

• Using in-line filter with pore size of 0.2 to 1 micron, infuse into central vein, shunt, or arteriovenous fistula. Infuse over at least 4 hours.

Route	Onset	Peak	Duration
I.V.	Immediate	5 days	Unknown

Adverse reactions

CNS: malaise, agitation, headache, dizziness, weakness, syncope, **encephalitis, seizures**
CV: hypotension, hypertension, chest pain, phlebitis, thrombophlebitis, bradycardia, tachycardia, myocarditis, cardiac irregularities, **heart failure**
EENT: periorbital edema
GI: nausea, vomiting, diarrhea, stomatitis

GU: abnormal kidney function test results
Hematologic: leukopenia, agranulocytosis, thrombocytopenia, aplastic anemia
Hepatic: hepatosplenomegaly, abnormal liver function test results
Metabolic: hyperglycemia
Musculoskeletal: joint pain or stiffness, myalgia, back pain
Respiratory: dyspnea, pleural effusion
Skin: rash, pruritus, urticaria, diaphoresis, night sweats
Other: burning soles and palms, fever, chills, pain at infusion site, edema, lymphadenopathy, hypersensitivity reactions including serum sickness and **anaphylaxis**

Interactions

Drug-diagnostic tests. *Creatinine, glucose, hepatic enzymes:* increased values
Hemoglobin, platelets, white blood cells: decreased values

Precautions

Use cautiously in:
• severe renal or hepatic disease
• pregnant or breastfeeding patients
• children.

Patient monitoring

◀€ During infusion, watch for signs and symptoms of hypersensitivity reaction, such as rash, respiratory distress, or chest, flank, or back pain. Be aware that hypersensitivity reaction may occur even with a negative skin test.

• Monitor for signs and symptoms of infection, such as fever, malaise, and sore throat (caused by immunosuppression).

Patient teaching

• Teach patient to immediately report adverse reactions during infusion, such as pain at infusion site or systemic complaints.

• Instruct patient to avoid sources of infection, such as people with known infections. Instruct him to promptly report signs or symptoms of infection.
• Advise patient to immediately report evidence of serum sickness, including fever, malaise, joint pain, nausea, vomiting, lymphadenopathy, and rash.
• As appropriate, review all other significant and life-threatening adverse reactions and interactions, especially those related to the tests mentioned above.

magaldrate (aluminum magnesium hydroxide sulfate)
Lowsium, Lowsium Plus, Riopan, Riopan Plus, Riopan Plus Double Strength

Pharmacologic class: GI drug
Therapeutic class: Antacid
Pregnancy risk category NR

Action
Increases gastric pH and elasticity of esophageal sphincter, decreasing pepsin activity and acid production in the GI tract

Availability
Oral solution: 540 mg/5 ml, 1,080 mg/ 5 ml

Indications and dosages
➤ Antacid
Adults: 5 to 10 ml P.O.

Contraindications
• Hypersensitivity to drug or its components
• Severe renal disease

Administration
• Give drug between meals with water, or at bedtime.

Route	Onset	Peak	Duration
P.O.	20 min	Unknown	20-180 min

Adverse reactions
GI: mild constipation, diarrhea
GU: increased urine pH
Metabolic: hypermagnesemia, hypophosphatemia, hypokalemia

Interactions
Drug-drug. *Diazepam, digoxin, indomethacin, iron salts, isoniazid, pseudoephedrine, tetracycline:* decreased effects of these drugs
Enteric-coated drugs: premature gastric release of these drugs
Drug-diagnostic tests. *Gastrin:* increased level
Potassium: decreased level

Precautions
Use cautiously in:
• renal disease, fluid restriction, dehydration, decreased GI motility, GI obstruction
• sodium-restricted diet
• elderly patients
• pregnant patients.

Patient monitoring
◀𝄞 Stay alert for signs and symptoms of magnesium toxicity, including hypotension, nausea, vomiting, ECG changes, CNS or respiratory depression, and coma.
• With long-term or repeated use, assess potassium, phosphorus, and magnesium levels.

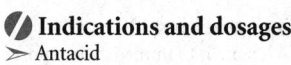

Patient teaching
- Teach patient to shake oral solution well before use and to drink water after taking dose.
- Instruct patient not to use drug for more than 2 weeks unless directed by prescriber.
- Advise patient to inform prescriber if he's taking other drugs; magaldrate may delay or enhance absorption of concurrently used drugs.
- Tell patient to report change in bowel habits.
- As appropriate, review all other significant adverse reactions and interactions, especially those related to the drugs and tests mentioned above.

magnesium citrate
Citro-Mag✦, Citroma, Evac-Q-Mag

magnesium hydroxide
Phillips Chewable, Phillips Milk of Magnesia, Phillips Milk of Magnesia Concentrate

magnesium sulfate
Epsom Salts

magnesium oxide
Mag-ox, Maox, Uro-Mag

Pharmacologic class: Mineral

Therapeutic class: Electrolyte replacement, laxative, antacid, anticonvulsant

Pregnancy risk category A (magnesium sulfate), *NR* (magnesium citrate, hydroxide, or oxide)

Action
Increases osmotic gradient in small intestine, which draws water into the intestines and causes distention; these effects stimulate peristalsis and bowel evacuation. Produces antacid action by reacting with hydrochloric acid in stomach to form water and increase gastric pH. Produces anticonvulsant action by depressing CNS and blocking transmission of peripheral neuromuscular impulses by decreasing amount of available acetylcholine.

Availability
magnesium citrate
Oral solution: 240-ml, 296-ml, and 300-ml bottles
magnesium hydroxide
Liquid: 400 mg/5 ml
Liquid concentrate: 800 mg/5 ml
Tablets (chewable): 300 mg, 600 mg
magnesium oxide
Capsules: 140 mg
Tablets: 400 mg, 420 mg, 500 mg
magnesium sulfate
Granules (for oral use): 120 g, 4 lb
Injection: 10%, 12.5%, 25%, 50%

Indications and dosages

➤ Mild magnesium deficiency
Adults: 1 g (2 ml of 50% sulfate solution) I.M. q 6 hours for four doses
➤ Severe hypomagnesemia
Adults: Up to 2 mEq/kg (0.5 ml/kg of 50% sulfate solution) I.M. over 4 hours, if necessary, or 5 g (approximately 40 mEq)/liter of 5% dextrose injection or sodium chloride solution by I.V. infusion over 3 hours
➤ To provide supplemental magnesium in total parenteral nutrition (TPN)
Adults: 8 to 24 mEq/day (sulfate) by I.V. infusion (added to TPN solution)
➤ Constipation; bowel evacuation
Adults and children ages 12 and older: Single dose of 5 to 10 ml P.O. (sulfate) in a half-glass of water; or 30 to 60 ml/day P.O. (hydroxide) given with water; or a single dose of 10 to 30 ml P.O. (hydroxide concentrate); or one-half to one whole bottle, as directed, of oral solution (citrate)

m

Children ages 6 to 12: Single dose of 2.5 to 5 ml P.O. (sulfate) in a half-glass of water; or 15 to 30 ml P.O. daily (hydroxide) given with water; or a single dose of 7.5 to 15 ml P.O. (hydroxide concentrate); or one-half to one whole bottle, as directed, of oral solution (citrate)

Children ages 2 to 5: Single dose of 5 to 15 ml P.O. (hydroxide); or 2.5 to 7.5 ml P.O. daily of Phillips' Milk of Magnesia (hydroxide concentrate)

➤ Indigestion associated with hyperacidity

Adults and children ages 12 and older: 5 to 15 ml P.O. (hydroxide liquid) up to q.i.d. with water; or 2.5 to 7.5 ml P.O. (hydroxide liquid concentrate) up to q.i.d. with water; or 622 mg to 1,244 mg P.O. (hydroxide tablets) up to q.i.d.; or 140 mg P.O. (oxide capsules) three or four times daily; or 400 to 800 mg P.O. (oxide tablets) daily

➤ To prevent and control seizures in preeclampsia or eclampsia

Adults: 4 to 5 g of 50% sulfate solution I.M. q 4 hours, as necessary; or 4 g of 10% to 20% sulfate solution I.V., not to exceed 1.5 ml/minute of 10% solution; or 4 to 5 g I.V. infusion in 250 ml of 5% dextrose or sodium chloride solution, not to exceed 3 ml /minute. (I.V. use is reserved for life-threatening seizures.)

➤ Acute nephritis to control hypertension, encephalopathy, and seizures in children

Children: 20 to 40 mg/kg I.M. of 20% solution, repeated as necessary

Off-label uses
• Bronchodilation in some asthmatic patients
• Post–myocardial infarction hypomagnesemia

Contraindications
• Hypermagnesemia
• Heart block
• Myocardial damage

• Active labor or within 2 hours of delivery

Administration
• When giving magnesium sulfate I.V., don't exceed a concentration of 20% or an infusion rate of 150 mg/minute except in seizures secondary to severe eclampsia.
• When giving magnesium sulfate I.M. to adults, use concentration of 25% to 50%; when giving to infants and children, don't exceed 20%.

Route	Onset	Peak	Duration
P.O.	3-6 hr	4 hr	Unknown
I.V.	Immediate	Unknown	30 min
I.M.	60 min	Unknown	3-4 hr

Adverse reactions
CNS (with I.V. use): confusion, decreased reflexes, dizziness, syncope, muscle weakness, sedation, hypothermia, flaccidity, **paralysis**
CV (with I.V. use): hypotension, **arrhythmias, circulatory collapse**
GI: nausea, vomiting, anorexia, cramps, flatulence
Metabolic: hypermagnesemia, hypocalcemia
Respiratory: respiratory paralysis
Skin: diaphoresis
Other: allergic reaction, injection site reaction, laxative dependence (with repeated or prolonged use)

Interactions
Drug-drug. *Aminoquinolones, nitrofurantoin, penicillamine, tetracyclines:* decreased absorption of these drugs (with oral magnesium)
CNS depressants: additive effects
Digoxin: heart block, conduction changes (with I.V. magnesium)
Enteric-coated drugs: faster dissolution of these drugs
Neuromuscular blockers: increased effects of these drugs (with I.V. use)

Drug-diagnostic tests. *Calcium, magnesium:* increased levels (with I.V. use)

Precautions

Use cautiously in:
• renal insufficiency, abdominal pain, nausea and vomiting, rectal bleeding, anuria, hypocalcemia
• pregnant patients.

Patient monitoring

◀≝ When giving prolonged or repeated I.V. infusions, assess patellar reflex and a respiratory rate of 16 breaths/minute or more.
• With I.V. use, monitor magnesium level (desired level is 3 to 6 mg/dl or 2.5 to 5 mEq/L). Check for indications of magnesium toxicity (hypotension, nausea, vomiting, ECG changes, muscle weakness, mental or respiratory depression, and coma). Have injectable calcium available to counteract magnesium toxicity.
• Monitor urine output, which should measure 100 ml or more every 4 hours.
• If I.V. magnesium was given before delivery, assess neonate for signs and symptoms of magnesium toxicity, such as neuromuscular or respiratory depression.
• Monitor electrolyte levels and liver function test results.

Patient teaching

• Teach patient about adverse reactions; instruct him to report symptoms that occur during I.V. administration.
• Advise patient to consult prescriber before using magnesium if he's taking other drugs; magnesium may delay or enhance drug absorption.
• Tell patient that repeated or prolonged use of magnesium citrate, hydroxide, or sulfate may cause laxative dependence. Inform him that a healthy diet and exercise will decrease need for laxatives.
• As appropriate, review all other significant and life-threatening adverse

reactions and interactions, especially those related to the drugs and tests mentioned above.

mannitol
Osmitrol, Resectisol

Pharmacologic class: Osmotic diuretic
Therapeutic class: Diuretic
Pregnancy risk category C, D (third trimester)

Action

Increases osmotic pressure of plasma in the glomerular filtrate of the kidney, inhibiting tubular reabsorption of water and electrolytes (including sodium and potassium), thereby enhancing water flow from tissues such as the brain and ultimately decreasing intracranial and intraocular pressures; serum sodium levels are increased, while potassium and blood urea levels are reduced. Also protects the kidneys by preventing toxins from forming and blocking the tubules.

m

Availability

Injection: 5%, 10%, 15%, 20%, 25%
Solution: 5 g/100 ml

Indications and dosages

➤ Test dose for marked oliguria or suspected inadequate renal function
Adults: 0.2 g/kg I.V. infusion (about 50 ml of 25% solution, 75 ml of 20% solution, or 100 ml of 15% solution) over 3 to 5 minutes. If urine flow doesn't increase, a second dose may be given; if response is inadequate after second dose, patient should be reevaluated.
➤ To prevent acute renal failure (oliguria) during cardiovascular and other surgeries
Adults: 50 to 100 g I.V. infusion as a 5% to 25% solution given over 90 minutes to several hours, up to 6 g/kg/day

➤ Acute renal failure (oliguria)
Adults: 50 to 100 g I.V. infusion as a 15% to 25% solution given over 90 minutes to several hours, up to 6 g/kg/day
➤ To reduce intracranial pressure and brain mass
Adults: 1.5 to 2 g/kg I.V. infusion as a 15% to 25% solution given over 30 to 60 minutes
➤ To reduce intraocular pressure
Adults: 1.5 to 2g/kg I.V. infusion as a 15% to 20% solution given over 30 minutes; for preoperative use, give 60 to 90 minutes before surgery.
➤ To promote diuresis in drug toxicity
Adults: 25 g I.V. infusion as a loading dose, followed by an infusion of 5% to 25% solution given continuously to maintain urine output of 100 to 500 ml/hour
➤ Irrigation during transurethral resection of prostate
Adults: 2.5% to 5% solution instilled into bladder by indwelling urethral catheter, as needed

Contraindications
• Hypersensitivity to drug
• Active intracranial bleeding
• Anuria secondary to severe renal disease
• Progressive heart failure, renal damage, or renal dysfunction
• Severe pulmonary congestion or pulmonary edema
• Severe dehydration

Administration
• Don't give drug until adequate renal function and urinary output have been established.
• Be aware that at low temperatures, mannitol solution may crystallize (especially concentrations above 15%).
• Don't give electrolyte-free mannitol solutions with blood; if blood is given

with mannitol, add 20 mEq or more of sodium chloride solution to each liter of mannitol solution to avoid pseudo-agglutination.
• Drug may be given as continuous or intermittent I.V. infusion; infuse at prescribed route using infusion device and in-line filter.
• Avoid extravasation; local edema and tissue necrosis may occur.

Route	Onset	Peak	Duration
I.V. (diuresis)	1-3 hr	Unknown	Up to 8 hr
I.V. (intraocular press.)	30-60 min	Unknown	4-8 hr
I.V. (intracranial press.)	15 min	Unknown	3-8 hr

Adverse reactions
CNS: dizziness, headache, **seizures**
CV: chest pain, hypotension, hypertension, tachycardia, thrombophlebitis, **heart failure, vascular overload**
EENT: blurred vision, rhinitis
GI: nausea, vomiting, diarrhea, dry mouth
GU: polyuria, urinary retention, osmotic nephrosis
Metabolic: dehydration, water intoxication, hypervolemia, hyperkalemia, hypernatremia, hypokalemia, hyponatremia, metabolic acidosis
Respiratory: pulmonary congestion
Skin: rash, urticaria, extravasation with edema and tissue necrosis
Other: chills, fever, thirst, edema

Interactions
Drug-drug. *Digoxin:* increased risk of digoxin toxicity
Diuretics: increased therapeutic effects of mannitol
Lithium: increased urinary excretion of lithium
Drug-diagnostic tests. *Electrolytes:* increased or decreased levels

Precautions

Use cautiously in:

- severe renal disease, heart failure, dehydration
- pregnant or breastfeeding patients.

Patient monitoring

- In comatose patient, insert indwelling urinary catheter as ordered to monitor urine output.
- Monitor renal function tests, urinary output, fluid balance, electrolyte levels (especially sodium and potassium), and central venous pressure.
- Watch for excessive fluid loss and signs and symptoms of hypovolemia and dehydration.
- Assess for evidence of circulatory overload, including pulmonary edema, water intoxication, and heart failure.
- Be aware that overhydration may be treated with diuretics or hemodialysis.

Patient teaching

- Teach patient about importance of monitoring exact urinary output.
- Advise patient to report pain at infusion site as well as adverse reactions, such as increased shortness of breath or pain in back, legs, or chest.
- Tell patient he may be thirsty or have a dry mouth; emphasize that fluid restrictions are necessary, but that frequent mouth care and comfort measures should help.
- As appropriate, review all other significant and life-threatening adverse reactions and interactions, especially those related to the drugs and tests mentioned above.

mebendazole
Vermox

Pharmacologic class: Benzimidazole
Therapeutic class: Antihelmintic
Pregnancy risk category C

Action

Blocks uptake of glucose and interferes with absorption of susceptible helminths

Availability

Tablets (chewable): 100 mg

Indications and dosages

➤ Pinworm (*Enterobius vermicularis*)
Adults and children over age 2: 100 mg P.O. as a single dose; repeat in 3 weeks, if necessary.
➤ Whipworm (*Trichuris trichiura*), roundworm (*Ascaris lumbricoides*), American hookworm (*Necator americanus*), common hookworm (*Ancylostoma duodenale*), and mixed infections
Adults and children over age 2: 100 mg P.O. in morning and evening for 3 days; repeat in 3 weeks, if necessary.

Contraindications

- Hypersensitivity to drug

Administration

- Know that tablets may be chewed, swallowed, or crushed and mixed with food.

Route	Onset	Peak	Duration
P.O.	Unknown	2-5 hr	Unknown

Adverse reactions

GI: abdominal pain, diarrhea
Other: fever

Interactions

Drug-drug. *Carbamazepine, phenytoin:* increased mebendazole metabolism and decreased efficacy (with high doses)
Cimetidine: inhibited mebendazole metabolism and increased blood level

Precautions

Use cautiously in:

- impaired hepatic function, Crohn's ileitis, ulcerative colitis

m

• pregnant patients (should be used in first trimester only if benefit justifies risk to fetus)
• breastfeeding patients
• children younger than age 2.

Patient monitoring
• With prolonged therapy, monitor hematologic and hepatic studies.
• Ask family members if they have signs or symptoms of pinworm; infection spreads easily.

Patient teaching
• Tell patient he may chew tablets, swallow them whole, or crush them and mix with food.
• Inform patient that parasite removal from GI tract may take up to 3 days after treatment. If he's not cured after 3 weeks, a second course may be necessary.
• Advise patient not to prepare food for others.
• Teach patient to maintain strict hygiene to prevent reinfection; instruct him to disinfect toilet facilities daily and to change and launder clothing, bed linens, and towels daily.
• Tell patient that dietary restrictions, fasting, and laxatives aren't necessary.
• As appropriate, review all other significant adverse reactions and interactions, especially those related to the drugs mentioned above.

mechlorethamine hydrochloride
(HN$_2$, mustine, nitrogen mustard)
Mustargen

Pharmacologic class: Alkylating agent, nitrogen mustard agent
Therapeutic class: Antineoplastic
Pregnancy risk category D

Action
Interferes with DNA and RNA synthesis by cross-linking strands of cellular DNA; cell-cycle-phase nonspecific

Availability
Powder for injection: 10 mg/vial

🖊 Indications and dosages
➤ Palliative combination therapy in chronic myelocytic or chronic lymphocytic leukemia, lymphosarcoma, polycythemia vera, mycosis fungoides, and bronchogenic carcinoma
Adults: 0.4 mg/kg I.V. given as a single dose or in divided doses of 0.1 to 0.2 mg/kg/day I.V., with subsequent doses given after hematologic recovery (usually 3 to 6 weeks)
➤ Palliative treatment in advanced Hodgkin's disease (stages III and IV)
Adults: 6 mg/m^2 I.V. on days 1 and 8 of 28-day cycle as part of MOPP regimen (mechlorethamine, vincristine, procarbazine, prednisone); in subsequent cycles, blood counts determine dosage.
➤ Palliative treatment of metastatic carcinoma with effusion
Adults: 0.4 mg/kg intrapleurally or intraperitoneally or 0.2 mg/kg intrapericardially

Off-label uses
• Cutaneous mycosis fungoides (topical solution)

Contraindications
• Hypersensitivity to drug
• Active infection

Administration
◀≣ Follow facility policy when handling and preparing; drug is carcinogenic, mutagenic, and teratogenic.
• Know that severe nausea and vomiting may occur 1 to 3 hours after administration; premedicate with antiemetics and sedatives, as prescribed.

◀€ Be aware that drug has a narrow margin of safety; use extreme caution with dosages.
• Reconstitute with 10 ml of sterile water or sodium chloride for injection, to yield a concentration of 1 mg/ml. Give immediately after reconstitution.
• Withdraw calculated dosage and inject either directly into a vein or into port of free-flowing I.V. line (preferred).
◀€ Monitor I.V. site for infiltration; drug is a potent vesicant.
• If extravasation occurs, infiltrate area with sterile isotonic sodium thiosulfate, apply ice compresses for 6 to 12 hours, and notify prescriber.
◀€ Neutralize equipment or unused solution in equal volumes of 5% sodium thiosulfate and 5% sodium bicarbonate; soak for 45 minutes, then discard unused solution according to facility policy.
• Consult current published protocols before intracavitary use.
• After intracavitary administration, change patient's position every 5 to 10 minutes to promote uniform drug distribution.

Route	Onset	Peak	Duration
I.V., intra-cavitary	Unknown	Unknown	Unknown

Adverse reactions
GI: nausea, vomiting, diarrhea
GU: infertility, delayed menses, oligomenorrhea, amenorrhea
Hematologic: anemia, **leukopenia, thrombocytopenia, lymphocytopenia, granulocytopenia, agranulocytosis, persistent pancytopenia**
Metabolic: hyperuricemia
Skin: rash, alopecia, erythema multiforme
Other: herpes zoster reactivation; chromosome abnormalities; tissue necrosis; phlebitis at I.V. site; hypersensitivity reactions, including **anaphylaxis; amyloidosis; secondary cancers**

Interactions
Drug-drug. *Other antineoplastics:* additive bone marrow depression
Live-virus vaccines: decreased antibody response to vaccine, increased risk of adverse reactions
Drug-diagnostic tests. *Granulocytes, lymphocytes, platelets, red blood cells:* decreased counts
Uric acid: increased level

Precautions
Use cautiously in:
• infections, chronic lymphocytic leukemia, decreased bone marrow reserve, hematopoietic depression, amyloidosis, severe edema, obesity
• previous radiation therapy or chemotherapy
• elderly or debilitated patients
• patients with childbearing potential
• pregnant or breastfeeding patients
• children (safety and efficacy not established).

Patient monitoring
• Monitor hematologic, kidney, and liver function studies.
• Watch for hyperuricemia; maintain adequate hydration to prevent elevated uric acid level.
• Monitor patient for infection. Lymphocytopenia occurs within 24 hours; significant granulocytopenia occurs in 6 to 8 days and lasts 10 to 21 days, with recovery within 2 weeks after nadir.

Patient teaching
• Teach patient to report pain or burning at injection site.
• Advise patient to immediately report signs or symptoms of infection, including fever, malaise, or sore throat.
• Instruct patient to avoid crowds and practice good handwashing.
◀€ Teach patient to report bleeding gums, dark stools, bruising, or bleeding.
• Tell patient to avoid pregnancy or breastfeeding.

• Inform patient that drug may cause sterility.

• As appropriate, review all other significant and life-threatening adverse reactions and interactions, especially those related to the drugs and tests mentioned above.

meclizine hydrochloride
Antivert, Bonamine♣, Bonine, Dramamine Less Drowsy Formula

Pharmacologic class: Anticholinergic
Therapeutic class: Antiemetic, antivertigo drug
Pregnancy risk category B

Action
Possesses anticholinergic, CNS depressant, and antihistaminic effects; decreases sensitivity of middle-ear labyrinth and depresses conduction in vestibular-cerebellar pathways

Availability
Capsules: 15 mg, 25 mg, 30 mg
Tablets: 12.5 mg, 25 mg, 50 mg
Tablets (chewable): 25 mg

💊 Indications and dosages
➢ Prevention and management of motion sickness
Adults: 25 to 50 mg P.O. 1 hour before travel; may repeat q 24 hours for duration of travel
➢ Prevention and management of vertigo
Adults: 25 to 100 mg P.O. daily in divided doses

Contraindications
• Hypersensitivity to drug
• Children younger than age 12

Administration
• Know that tablets may be chewed or swallowed whole.

Route	Onset	Peak	Duration
P.O.	1 hr	Unknown	8-24 hr

Adverse reactions
CNS: drowsiness, fatigue, confusion, euphoria, nervousness, restlessness, insomnia, excitement, vertigo, **seizures**
CV: hypotension, palpitations, tachycardia
EENT: blurred vision, diplopia, visual and auditory hallucinations, tinnitus, dry nose, dry throat
GI: nausea, vomiting, diarrhea, constipation, dry mouth, anorexia
GU: difficulty urinating, urinary retention, urinary frequency
Skin: rash, urticaria

Interactions
Drug-drug. *Anticholinergics (including some antihistamines, antidepressants, atropine, haloperidol, phenothiazines):* additive anticholinergic effects
Antihistamines, CNS depressants (such as opioids, sedative-hypnotics): additive CNS depression
Drug-diagnostic tests. *Skin tests using allergen extracts:* false-negative results
Drug-behaviors. *Alcohol use:* additive CNS depression

Precautions
Use cautiously in:
• prostatic hypertrophy, stenosing peptic ulcer, bladder neck obstruction, pyloroduodenal obstruction, arrhythmias, narrow-angle glaucoma, bronchial asthma
• pregnant or breastfeeding patients
• children.

Patient monitoring
• Discontinue drug, as ordered, at least 4 days before skin testing.
• Know that drug has anticholinergic effects.

Patient teaching

• Teach patient to take drug as prescribed to minimize adverse effects.

• Instruct patient to avoid driving and other hazardous activities until he knows how drug affects concentration and alertness.

• Teach patient to relieve dry mouth with hard candy or frequent sips of fluids.

• As appropriate, review all other significant and life-threatening adverse reactions and interactions, especially those related to the drugs, tests, and behaviors mentioned above.

medroxyprogesterone acetate
Alti-MPA♣, Amen, Curretab, Cycrin, Depo-Provera, Gen-Medroxy♣, Novo-Medrone♣, Provera

Pharmacologic class: Hormone
Therapeutic class: Progestin
Pregnancy risk category X

Action
Inhibits pituitary gonadotropin secretion, thus preventing follicular maturation, ovulation, and pregnancy

Availability
Suspension for depot injection: 50 mg/ml, 100 mg/ml, 150 mg/ml, 400 mg/ml
Tablets: 2.5 mg, 5 mg, 10 mg, 100 mg

💊 Indications and dosages
➢ Secondary amenorrhea
Adults: 5 to 10 mg/day P.O. for 5 to 10 days, starting at any time during menstrual cycle
➢ Dysfunctional uterine bleeding, menses induction
Adults: 5 to 10 mg/day P.O. for 5 to 10 days, starting on day 16 or 21 of menstrual cycle

➢ To prevent estrogen-related endometrial changes in postmenopausal women
Adults: 2.5 to 5 mg/day P.O. given with 0.625 mg conjugated estrogens P.O. (monophasic regimen); or 5 mg/day P.O. on days 15 to 28 of cycle, given with 0.625 mg conjugated estrogens P.O. daily throughout cycle (biphasic regimen)
➢ Renal or endometrial carcinoma
Adults: 400 to 1,000 mg I.M.; may repeat weekly. If improvement occurs, decrease dosage to 400 mg q month.

Off-label uses
• Advanced breast cancer
• Female contraception

Contraindications
• Hypersensitivity to drug or parabens (I.M. suspension)
• Cerebrovascular or thromboembolic disease
• Severe hepatic disease
• Breast or genital cancer
• Pregnancy (first 4 months)

Administration
• Before starting therapy, obtain thorough history and physical examination, with emphasis on breast and pelvic organs. Also obtain Pap smear, and repeat annually during therapy.
• With contraceptive use, rule out pregnancy before first dose and when more than 14 weeks have passed since previous dose.
• For I.M. injection, inject deep into gluteal, deltoid, or anterior thigh muscle; rotate injection sites.

Route	Onset	Peak	Duration
P.O.	Unknown	Unknown	Unknown
I.M.	Wks-1 mo	1 mo	Unknown

Adverse reactions
CNS: insomnia, migraine, nervousness, drowsiness, dizziness, fatigue, depression, mood changes

CV: thrombophlebitis, **thromboembolism**
EENT: diplopia, proptosis, papilledema, retinal vascular lesions
GI: abdominal pain, bloating
GU: amenorrhea, infertility, spotting, cervical secretions, galactorrhea, breast tenderness and secretion, cervical erosions, leukorrhea, pelvic pain
Hepatic: jaundice
Metabolic: fluid retention, hyperglycemia
Musculoskeletal: leg cramps, back pain
Respiratory: pulmonary embolism
Skin: pruritus, urticaria, rash, acne, alopecia, hirsutism, cholasma, melasma, sterile abscesses, induration at I.M. site
Other: weight and appetite changes, edema, angioneurotic edema, allergic reactions including **anaphylaxis**

Interactions

Drug-drug. *Bromocriptine:* decreased bromocriptine efficacy
Carbamazepine, phenobarbital, phenytoin, rifampin: decreased contraceptive efficacy
Drug-diagnostic tests. *Alkaline phosphatase, low-density lipoproteins:* increased levels
High-density lipoproteins, pregnanediol excretion: decreased levels
Thyroid hormone assays: altered results
Drug-behaviors. *Alcohol use:* additive CNS depression

Precautions

Use cautiously in:
• seizure disorder, renal or cardiovascular disease, asthma, diabetes mellitus, depression, migraine
• history of hepatic disease.

Patient monitoring

• Monitor patient for fluid retention and for signs and symptoms of thrombophlebitis, including pain, swelling, and redness of lower legs.

• Assess for visual disturbances and headache; if ocular examination shows papilledema or retinal vascular lesions, drug should be discontinued.
• Evaluate liver function test results.
• Watch for abdominal pain, fever, malaise, jaundice, darkened urine, and clay-colored stools.

Patient teaching

• Advise patient that drug may cause nausea, vomiting, headache, abdominal pain, painful breast swelling, and abnormal bleeding pattern. Instruct her to report these effects if they're pronounced.
• Teach patient to report bloating, swelling, appetite loss, rash, yellowed skin, mood changes or depression, nervousness, dizziness, chest pain, shortness of breath, visual disturbances, or severe headache.
• Teach patient how to perform breast self-examination.
• Tell patient she must undergo yearly physical examinations with Pap smear.
• As appropriate, review all other significant and life-threatening adverse reactions and interactions, especially those related to the drugs, tests, and behaviors mentioned above.

mefloquine hydrochloride
Lariam

Pharmacologic class: 4-quinolinemethanol derivative, quinine analog
Therapeutic class: Antimalarial
Pregnancy risk category C

Action

Unknown; thought to increase intravesicular pH in parasite acid vesicles and form complexes with hemin, inhibiting parasite development

Availability
Tablets: 250 mg

🕭 Indications and dosages
➤ Acute malarial infection caused by *Plasmodium falciparum* or *Plasmodium vivax*

Adults: 1,250 mg P.O. as a single dose, or 750 mg P.O. as a single dose followed by 500 mg P.O. 12 hours later
Children weighing more than 45 kg (99 lb): 20 to 25 mg/kg P.O. in two divided doses given 6 to 8 hours apart
Children weighing less than 45 kg (99 lb): Initially, 15 mg/kg P.O., followed by 10 mg/kg 8 to 12 hours later
➤ Malaria prophylaxis
Adults and children weighing more than 45 kg (99 lb): 250 mg P.O. once weekly on same day each week, starting 1 week before entering endemic area and continuing for 4 weeks after leaving area
Children weighing 31 to 45 kg (67 to 99 lb): 187.5 mg P.O. q week
Children weighing 20 to 30 kg (44 to 66 lb): 125 mg P.O. q week
Children weighing 15 to 19 kg (33 to 44 lb): 62.5 mg P.O. q week

Contraindications
• Hypersensitivity to drug or related agents

Administration
• After completing mefloquine therapy for acute malarial infection, patient should receive primaquine (or other 8-aminoquinolone) to prevent relapse.

Route	Onset	Peak	Duration
P.O.	Unknown	7-24 hr	Unknown

Adverse reactions
CNS: dizziness, syncope, headache, psychotic changes, depression, hallucinations, confusion, anxiety, fatigue, vertigo, **seizures**
EENT: blurred vision, tinnitus
GI: nausea, vomiting, diarrhea, loose stools, abdominal discomfort, anorexia
Hematologic: decreased hematocrit, **leukopenia, thrombocytopenia**
Hepatic: transaminase elevations
Musculoskeletal: myalgia
Skin: rash
Other: fever, chills

Interactions
Drug-drug. *Beta blockers, quinidine, quinine:* ECG abnormalities, cardiac arrest
Chloroquine, quinine: increased risk of seizures
Valproic acid: decreased valproic acid blood level, loss of seizure control
Drug-diagnostic tests. *Hematocrit, platelets, white blood cells:* decreased values
Transaminases: transient increases

Precautions
Use cautiously in:
• cardiac disorders and seizure disorders.

Patient monitoring
◀🕭 Monitor patients with acute *P. vivax* malaria who are at high risk for relapse. Because drug doesn't eliminate exoerythrocytic (hepatic-phase) parasites, patient should receive primaquine after mefloquine therapy.
• Watch for psychiatric symptoms, such as acute anxiety, depression, restlessness, or confusion; these may precede more serious psychiatric events.
• Evaluate hepatic function during prolonged prophylactic therapy.
• In patients receiving related drugs (such as quinine, quinidine, or chloroquine) concurrently, stay alert for increased risk of ECG abnormalities and seizures. Separate administration times by at least 12 hours.
• Closely monitor patients with serious or life-threatening *P. falciparum* infection; be aware that they should receive I.V. antimalarial drug and that meflo-

m

quine may be used to complete course
of therapy.

Patient teaching
• Teach patient to take drug with full
glass of water and not on empty stomach.
• In prophylactic use, teach patient to
take first dose 1 week before departure
and to continue therapy as prescribed
upon return; tell him to take drug on
same day each week.
• Advise patient to report fever after
returning from a malarious area.
• Inform patient that malaria prophylaxis also should include protective
clothing, insect repellent, and bed net-
ting.
◀﹦ Tell patient to immediately report
psychiatric symptoms (such as acute
anxiety, depression, restlessness, or
confusion) and to stop taking drug.
• Instruct patient to avoid driving and
other hazardous activities because drug
may cause dizziness.
• Instruct patient to have periodic
ophthalmic examinations because drug
may cause eye damage.
• As appropriate, review all other significant and life-threatening adverse
reactions and interactions, especially
those related to the drugs and tests
mentioned above.

megestrol acetate
Apo-Megestrol✽, Megace,
Megace-OS✽

Pharmacologic class: Hormone
Therapeutic class: Progestin, antineo-
plastic, appetite stimulant
Pregnancy risk category D (tablets),
X (suspension)

Action
Unknown; suppresses growth of pro-
gestin-sensitive breast and endometrial
tumors, possibly by inhibiting pituitary
and adrenal function

Availability
Oral suspension: 40 mg/ml
Tablets: 20 mg, 40 mg

⃠ Indications and dosages
➣ Breast carcinoma
Adults: 160 mg/day P.O. as a single
dose, or 40 mg P.O. q.i.d.
➣ Endometrial or ovarian carcinoma
Adults: 40 to 320 mg/day P.O. in divid-
ed doses
➣ AIDS wasting syndrome
Adults: 800 mg (suspension only) P.O.
daily; after 1 month, may decrease to
400 mg P.O. daily. Range is 400 to 800
mg P.O. daily.

Off-label uses
• Endometriosis, endometrial hyper-
plasia
• Prostatic hypertrophy
• Contraception

Contraindications
• Hypersensitivity to drug
• Alcohol intolerance (with suspen-
sion)
• Cancers other than breast and endo-
metrial
• Pregnancy (tablets in first 4 months;
suspension in all trimesters)
• Breastfeeding

Administration
• Give with meals if GI upset occurs.

Route	Onset	Peak	Duration
P.O.	Wks-1 mo	2 mo	Unknown

Adverse reactions
CNS: headache, insomnia, drowsiness,
asthenia, confusion, neuropathy, hyperesthesia, abnormal thinking, paresthesias, depression, **seizures**

CV: hypertension, thrombophlebitis, chest pain
EENT: amblyopia, retinal thrombosis, pharyngitis
GI: nausea, vomiting, flatulence, constipation, abdominal pain, dyspepsia, dry mouth, increased salivation, oral candidiasis
GU: breast tenderness, breakthrough bleeding, impotence, decreased libido
Hematologic: anemia, **leukopenia**
Hepatic: hepatomegaly
Metabolic: hyperglycemia, increased lactate dehydrogenase level
Musculoskeletal: carpal tunnel syndrome, back pain
Respiratory: dyspnea, cough, pneumonia, **pulmonary embolism**
Skin: alopecia, rash, pruritus, sweating
Other: edema, fever, weight gain, herpes infection

Interactions
None significant

Precautions
Use cautiously in:
• diabetes mellitus, severe hepatic disease, renal disease, cardiovascular disease, seizure disorders, migraine, asthma, cerebral hemorrhage, undiagnosed vaginal bleeding, depression
• history of thrombophlebitis.

Patient monitoring
• Monitor patient for signs and symptoms of thromboembolic disorders.
• Stay alert for visual disturbances, headache, abdominal pain, and indications of hepatomegaly.
• Monitor glucose level in diabetic patients.

Patient teaching
• Inform patient that drug may cause back or abdominal pain, headache, nausea, vomiting, or breast tenderness.
◀€ Instruct patient to immediately report pain, swelling, or redness of lower legs, chest or back pain, or shortness of breath.
• Advise patient to contact prescriber if adverse effects become pronounced or if other troublesome signs or symptoms occur.
• Teach patient to use reliable contraception.
◀€ Instruct patient to immediately report suspected pregnancy.
• Tell patient to avoid breastfeeding.
• Advise diabetic patients to monitor blood glucose level.
• As appropriate, review all other significant and life-threatening adverse reactions.

meloxicam
Mobic, Mobicox♣

Pharmacologic class: Nonopioid analgesic, nonsteroidal anti-inflammatory drug (NSAID)

Therapeutic class: Analgesic, anti-inflammatory drug

Pregnancy risk category C, D (third trimester)

Action
Unknown; thought to reduce inflammation and pain by inhibiting prostaglandin synthetase (cyclooxygenase)

Availability
Tablets: 7.5 mg

⍟ Indications and dosages
➤ Osteoarthritis
Adults: 7.5 mg P.O. once daily; may increase to 15 mg/day

Contraindications
• Hypersensitivity to drug, its components, or other NSAIDs
• Asthma
• Severe hepatic disease
• Severe renal impairment

- Peptic ulcer disease
- Concurrent aspirin use
- Pregnancy (third trimester), breast-feeding

Administration

- Before starting therapy, ask patient about aspirin sensitivity or allergies to other NSAIDs; if patient is dehydrated, provide adequate fluids.

Route	Onset	Peak	Duration
P.O.	Unknown	5-6 hr	24 hr

Adverse reactions

CNS: headache, dizziness, syncope, malaise, fatigue, asthenia, depression, confusion, nervousness, drowsiness, insomnia, vertigo, tremor, paresthesia, anxiety, **seizures**

CV: hypertension, hypotension, palpitations, angina, vasculitis, **heart failure, arrhythmias, myocardial infarction**

EENT: abnormal vision, conjunctivitis, hearing loss, tinnitus, pharyngitis

GI: nausea, vomiting, diarrhea, constipation, colitis, GI ulcers with perforation, abdominal pain, dyspepsia, gastroesophageal reflux, esophagitis, flatulence, altered taste, dry mouth, ulcerative stomatitis, **pancreatitis, GI hemorrhage**

GU: urinary frequency, urinary tract infection, increased blood urea nitrogen (BUN) and creatinine levels, albuminuria, hematuria, **renal failure**

Hematologic: anemia, purpura, **leukopenia, thrombocytopenia**

Hepatic: increased alanine aminotransferase (ALT), aspartate aminotransferase (AST), gamma-glutamyl transferase (GGT) and bilirubin levels; **hepatitis**

Musculoskeletal: joint pain, back pain

Metabolic: dehydration

Respiratory: upper respiratory infection, dyspnea, coughing, asthma, **bronchospasm**

Skin: rash, urticaria, pruritus, bullous eruption, sweating, alopecia, photosensitivity, angioedema

Other: hot flashes, increased appetite, weight gain or loss, fluid retention and edema, masking of infection symptoms, hypersensitivity reactions including **anaphylaxis**

Interactions

Drug-drug. *Angiotensin-converting enzyme inhibitors:* decreased antihypertensive effect

Anticoagulants: increased risk of bleeding

Aspirin: increased meloxicam blood level, increased risk of toxicity

Cholestyramine: decreased meloxicam blood level

Furosemide, thiazides: decreased diuretic effect

Lithium: increased lithium blood level

Drug-diagnostic tests. *ALT, AST, bilirubin, BUN, creatinine, GGT:* increased levels

Hemoglobin, platelets, white blood cells: decreased values

Drug-behaviors. *Alcohol use, smoking:* increased risk of GI irritation and bleeding

Precautions

Use cautiously in:
- bleeding disorders, GI or cardiac disorders, renal impairment
- concurrent oral anticoagulant or corticosteroid therapy
- elderly or debilitated patients
- patients in first or second trimester of pregnancy
- children younger than age 18 (safety and efficacy not established).

Patient monitoring

- Closely monitor patients with aspirin-sensitivity asthma because of risk of severe bronchospasm.
- In prolonged therapy, monitor complete blood count and kidney and liver function studies.

• Assess for cardiovascular disorders and hepatotoxicity.

• Monitor patient for fluid retention and weight gain.

Patient teaching

📢 Instruct patient to immediately report signs and symptoms of hepatotoxicity, including right upper quadrant pain, nausea, fatigue, lethargy, pruritus, and jaundice.

• Teach patient to report abdominal pain, blood in stool or emesis, or black tarry stools.

• Instruct patient to avoid alcohol and smoking.

• Advise pregnant patients to avoid drug, especially during third trimester.

• Teach patient to consult prescriber before taking over-the-counter preparations.

• As appropriate, review all other significant and life-threatening adverse reactions and interactions, especially those related to the drugs, tests, and behaviors mentioned above.

melphalan (L-PAM, L-phenylalanine mustard, L-sarcolysin)
Alkeran

melphalan hydrochloride
Alkeran

Pharmacologic class: Alkylator
Therapeutic class: Antineoplastic
Pregnancy risk category D

Action

Forms cross-links between strands of cellular DNA, causing disruption in DNA and RNA transcription, resulting in cell death

Availability

Powder for injection (melphalan hydrochloride): 50 mg
Tablets: 2 mg

🖊 Indications and dosages

➤ Multiple myeloma
Adults: Initially, 6 mg P.O. daily for 2 to 3 weeks, then discontinue drug for up to 4 weeks or until white blood cell (WBC) and platelet counts increase; then give maintenance dosage of 2 mg/day or 0.15 mg/kg/day P.O. for 7 days or 0.25 mg/kg for 4 days, repeated q 4 to 6 weeks. Or give 16 mg/m^2 by I.V. infusion over 15 to 20 minutes at 2-week intervals for four doses (usually with prednisone); I.V. dose can be repeated q 4 weeks after recovery from toxicity.

➤ Nonresectable advanced ovarian cancer
Adults: 0.2 mg/kg/day P.O. for 5 days q 4 to 5 weeks

Dosage adjustment
• Renal impairment

Contraindications

• Hypersensitivity to drug or chlorambucil

• Severe leukopenia, thrombocytopenia, or anemia

• Chronic lymphocytic leukemia

• Pregnancy or breastfeeding

Administration

• Before starting therapy, obtain complete blood count with white cell differential and platelet count; repeat periodically before each course.

• For I.V. use, reconstitute by rapidly injecting 10 ml of supplied diluent into vial with lyophilized powder; shake until solution is clear (yields a concentration of 5 mg/ml).

• Dilute desired dosage in 0.9% sodium chloride injection to a concentration no greater than 0.45 mg/ml. Administer over 15 minutes; be sure to

m

give entire dose within 60 minutes of reconstitution.

◄⧚ Minimize time between reconstitution, dilution, and administration because solution is unstable.

Route	Onset	Peak	Duration
P.O.	5 days	2-3 wk	5-6 wk
I.V.	Unknown	Unknown	Unknown

Adverse reactions

CV: hypotension, tachycardia, vasculitis

GI: nausea, vomiting, diarrhea, oral ulcers, stomatitis

GU: hyperuricemia, amenorrhea, gonadal suppression, infertility

Hematologic: anemia, purpura, **bone marrow depression, leukopenia, thrombocytopenia**

Hepatic: hepatotoxicity

Metabolic: hyperuricemia

Respiratory: dyspnea, **interstitial pneumonitis, bronchospasm, fibrosis**

Skin: rash, urticaria, pruritus, alopecia, sweating

Other: edema, extravasation at I.V. site, allergic reactions including **anaphylaxis**

Interactions

Drug-drug. *Carmustine:* increased pulmonary toxicity

Cimetidine: decreased GI absorption of melphalan

Cisplatin: increased risk of renal dysfunction, decreased melphalan clearance

Cyclosporine: increased risk of nephrotoxicity, severe renal failure

Interferon alfa: decreased melphalan blood level

Live-virus vaccines: decreased antibody response to vaccine

Myelosuppressants: additive toxicity

Nalidixic acid: increased risk of severe hemorrhagic necrotic enterocolitis (in children)

Drug-diagnostic tests. *Hemoglobin, platelets, red blood cells, white blood cells:* decreased values

Nitrogenous compounds: increased levels

Drug-food. *Any food:* decreased absorption of oral melphalan

Precautions

Use cautiously in:
• bone marrow depression, infection, renal disease
• previous radiation therapy
• patients with childbearing potential
• children (safety and efficacy not established).

Patient monitoring

• Check for thrombocytopenia and leukopenia; if platelet count exceeds 100,000/mm³ or WBC count drops below 3,000/mm³, discontinue drug until peripheral blood counts recover.

• Monitor patient closely for effects of bone marrow depression, including infections, anemia, and bleeding.

◄⧚ After multiple courses, watch for acute hypersensitivity reaction. If it occurs, discontinue drug and administer volume expanders, corticosteroids, or antihistamines, as prescribed.

• Watch for signs and symptoms of GI or pulmonary toxicity.

• Evaluate renal and hepatic function closely.

Patient teaching

• Teach patient to take oral tablets without food, because food may decrease drug absorption.

• Instruct patient to take entire daily oral dose at one time on empty stomach.

◄⧚ Teach patient to immediately report unusual bleeding or bruising, fever, chills, sore throat, shortness of breath, yellowing of skin or eyes, persistent cough, flank or stomach pain, joint pain, black tarry stools, rash, or unusual lumps or masses.

• Instruct patient to consult prescriber before using over-the-counter medications.

- Advise patient to use reliable contraception.
- Teach patient to avoid breastfeeding.
- As appropriate, review all other significant and life-threatening adverse reactions and interactions, especially those related to the drugs, tests, and foods mentioned above.

menotropins
Humegon, Pergonal, Repronex

Pharmacologic class: Hormone
Therapeutic class: Exogenous gonadotropin
Pregnancy risk category X

Action
Simulates action of follicle-stimulating hormone (FSH) by promoting follicular growth and maturation in females and by activating spermatogenesis in males

Availability
Injection: 75 IU luteinizing hormone (LH) and 75 IU FSH activity/ampule, 150 IU LH and 150 IU FSH activity/ampule

Indications and dosages
➤ To induce ovulation and pregnancy
Women: 75 IU each of FSH and LH I.M. daily for 9 to 12 days, then 10,000 units of human chorionic gonadotropin (hCG) I.M. 1 day after last menotropins dose. If ovulation doesn't occur, increase to 150 IU each of FSH and LH daily for 9 to 12 days, followed by 10,000 units of hCG I.M. 1 day after last menotropins dose. If ovulation does occur, repeat for two menstrual cycles.
➤ Infertility in men
Men: 5,000 units of hCG three times weekly for 4 to 6 months, then give 75 IU each of FSH and LH (Pergonal only) I.M. three times weekly with 2,000 USP units of hCG twice weekly for 4 months. If desired response isn't achieved, menotropins dosage only may be increased.

Contraindications
- Hypersensitivity to drug
- Abnormal uterine bleeding, uterine fibromas
- Thyroid or adrenal dysfunction
- Organic intracranial lesion
- Pituitary tumor
- Pregnancy

Administration
- Know that drug is given I.M. only, except Repronex, which may be prescribed for S.C. use.
- To reconstitute powder for injection, add 1 to 2 ml of 0.9% sodium chloride injection to ample.
- Inject immediately after reconstitution; discard unused drug portion.
- Rotate injection sites.
- Withhold hCG if serum estradiol level exceeds 2,000 pg/ml, or abdominal pain occurs.

Route	Onset	Peak	Duration
I.M.	9-12 days	Unknown	Unknown
S.C.	Unknown	Unknown	Unknown

Adverse reactions
CNS: headache, malaise, dizziness, **cerebrovascular accident**
CV: tachycardia, venous thrombophlebitis, **arterial occlusion, arterial thromboembolism**
GI: nausea, vomiting, diarrhea, abdominal cramps and distention, **hemoperitoneum**
GU: ovarian enlargement with pain, gynecomastia, multiple births, ovarian hyperstimulation syndrome (OHSS), ovarian cysts, hemoconcentration, **ectopic pregnancy**
Metabolic: electrolyte imbalance

m

♣ Canada   ◀€ Clinical alert   Reactions in **bold** are life-threatening

Musculoskeletal: muscle aches, joint pain
Respiratory: dyspnea, tachypnea, atelectasis, **adult respiratory distress syndrome, pulmonary embolism, pulmonary infarction**
Skin: rash
Other: fever, hypersensitivity reaction, **anaphylaxis**

Interactions
None significant

Patient monitoring
• Before starting menotropins/hCG therapy to induce ovulation and pregnancy, patient should undergo gynecologic and endocrine evaluation with hysterosalpingogram to rule out pregnancy and neoplastic lesions.
• Assess patient to confirm anovulation; obtain urinary gonadotropin levels as ordered to rule out primary ovarian failure. Male partner's fertility should be evaluated.
• In older females (who are at greater risk of anovulatory disorders and endometrial cancer), assess cervical dilation and curettage results.
• Evaluate patient for expected ovarian stimulation without hyperstimulation.
◀ Monitor for early indications of OHSS—severe pelvic pain, nausea, vomiting, and weight gain. OHSS usually occurs 2 weeks after treatment ends, peaks 7 to 10 days after ovulation, and resolves with menses onset.
• If OHSS occurs, drug is withdrawn and patient is hospitalized for bed rest, fluid and electrolyte management, and analgesics. Monitor daily fluid intake and output, weight, abdominal girth, hematocrit, serum and urinary electrolytes, urine specific gravity, blood urea nitrogen, and creatinine. Watch for hemoconcentration caused by fluid loss into peritoneal, pleural, and pericardial cavities.
• Stay alert for pulmonary and thromboembolic complications.

• Assess male patient for pituitary insufficiency as possible cause of infertility.

Patient teaching
• Before therapy, teach patient about duration of treatment and necessary monitoring.
• Inform patient about risk of multiple births with menotropins and hCG use.
• For infertile females, encourage daily intercourse starting on day before hCG administration.
• As appropriate, review all other significant and life-threatening adverse reactions.

meperidine hydrochloride (pethidine hydrochloride)
Demerol

Pharmacologic class: Opioid agonist
Therapeutic class: Analgesic, adjunct to anesthesia
Controlled substance schedule II
Pregnancy risk category C

Action
Binds to and depresses opiate receptors in spinal cord and CNS, altering perception of and response to pain

Availability
Injection: 10 mg/ml, 25 mg/ml, 50 mg/ml, 75 mg/ml, 100 mg/ml
Syrup: 50 mg/5 ml
Tablets: 50 mg, 100 mg

💊 Indications and dosages
➤ Moderate to severe pain
Adults: 50 to 150 mg P.O., I.M., or S.C. q 3 to 4 hours as needed
Children: 1 to 1.8 mg/kg P.O., I.M., or S.C. q 3 to 4 hours, not to exceed 100 mg/dose

➤ Preoperative sedation
Adults: 50 to 100 mg I.M. or S.C. 30 to 90 minutes before anesthesia, or 15 to 35 mg/hour I.V. as a continuous infusion

Children: 1 to 2.2 mg/kg P.O., I.M., or S.C. 30 to 90 minutes before anesthesia; don't exceed adult dosage.

➤ Analgesia during labor
Adults: 50 to 100 mg I.M. or S.C. when contractions are regular; may repeat q 1 to 3 hours

➤ Patient-controlled analgesia (PCA)
Adults: Initially, 10 mg I.V. With a range of 1 to 5 mg/incremental dose, recommended lockout interval is 6 to 10 minutes (minimum of 5 minutes).

Contraindications

• Hypersensitivity to drug or bisulfites (with some injectable products)
• Monoamine oxidase (MAO) inhibitor use within 14 days
• Pregnancy or breastfeeding (with long-term use)

Administration

• Give I.M. injection slowly into large muscle. Preferably, use diluted solution.
• Be aware that drug is compatible with 5% dextrose and lactated Ringer's solution; dextrose-saline solution combinations; and 2.5%, 5%, or 10% dextrose in water.
• Know that drug is incompatible with soluble barbiturates, aminophylline, heparin, morphine sulfate, methicillin, phenytoin, sodium bicarbonate, iodide, sulfadiazine, and sulfisoxazole.
• Don't give drug for chronic pain control because of potential toxicity and dependence.

Route	Onset	Peak	Duration
P.O.	15 min	60 min	2-4 hr
I.V.	Immediate	5-7 min	2-4 hr
I.M.	10-15 min	30-50 min	2-4 hr
S.C.	10-15 min	40-60 min	2-4 hr

Adverse reactions

CNS: confusion, sedation, dysphoria, euphoria, floating feeling, hallucinations, headache, unusual dreams, **seizures**
CV: hypotension, **bradycardia, cardiac arrest, shock**
EENT: blurred vision, diplopia, miosis
GI: nausea, vomiting, constipation, ileus, biliary tract spasms, increased amylase and lipase levels
GU: urinary retention
Respiratory: respiratory depression, respiratory arrest
Skin: flushing, sweating, induration
Other: pain at injection site, local irritation, physical or psychological drug dependence, drug tolerance

Interactions

Drug-drug. *Antihistamines, sedative-hypnotics:* additive CNS depression
Barbiturates, cimetidine, protease inhibitor antiretrovirals: increased respiratory and CNS depression
Chlorpromazine, thioridazine: increased risk of meperidine toxicity
MAO inhibitors, procarbazine: potentially fatal reaction
Opioid agonist-antagonists: precipitation of opioid withdrawal in physically dependent patients
Phenytoin: increased meperidine metabolism and decreased effects
Drug-diagnostic tests. *Amylase, lipase:* increased levels
Drug-herb. *Chamomile, hops, kava, skullcap, valerian:* increased CNS depression
Drug-behaviors. *Alcohol use:* increased CNS depression

Precautions

Use cautiously in:
• head trauma; increased intracranial pressure (ICP); severe renal, hepatic, or pulmonary disease; hypothyroidism; adrenal insufficiency; extensive burns; alcoholism

m

- undiagnosed abdominal pain or prostatic hyperplasia
- elderly or debilitated patients
- labor (drug may cause respiratory depression in neonates)
- children.

Patient monitoring
- Monitor vital signs and respiratory status; don't give drug if patient has significant respiratory or CNS depression.
- Reassess patient's pain level after administration.
- Watch for seizures, agitation, irritability, nervousness, tremors, twitches, and myoclonus in patients at risk for normeperidine accumulation (such as those with renal or hepatic impairment and patients with sickle-cell anemia, burns, or cancer who are receiving high doses).
- Use with extreme caution in patients with head injury; drug may increase ICP and cause adverse effects that obscure clinical course.
- Closely monitor patients with acute abdominal pain; drug may obscure diagnosis and clinical course.
- Evaluate bowel and bladder function.
- With long-term or repeated use, watch for psychological and physical drug dependence and tolerance.
- With pediatric patients, stay alert for increased risk of seizures.

Patient teaching
- Teach patient using oral syrup to take drug with a half-glass of water to minimize local anesthetic effect.
- Instruct patient to avoid driving and other hazardous activities because drug may cause dizziness or drowsiness.
- Advise patient to avoid alcohol.
- Teach ambulatory patient to change positions slowly to avoid orthostatic hypotension.
- Instruct patient to report adverse reactions promptly.

- As appropriate, review all other significant and life-threatening adverse reactions and interactions, especially those related to the drugs, tests, herbs, and behaviors mentioned above.

mercaptopurine
(6-mercaptopurine, 6-MP)
Purinethol

Pharmacologic class: Antimetabolite
Therapeutic class: Antineoplastic
Pregnancy risk category D

Action
Competes for an enzyme needed for purine synthesis; inhibits DNA and RNA synthesis and suppresses growth of certain cancer cells

Availability
Tablets: 50 mg

Indications and dosages
➣ Acute lymphatic (lymphocytic, lymphoblastic) leukemia, acute myelogenous and acute myelomonocytic leukemia
Adults and children: 2.5 mg/kg/day P.O. as a single dose, increased to 5 mg/kg/day after 4 weeks if toxicity or inadequate response occurs. When complete hematologic remission occurs, give a maintenance dosage of 1.5 to 2.5 mg/kg/day P.O. as a single dose (in combination with other agents as prescribed).

Contraindications
- Hypersensitivity to drug or thioguanine
- Breastfeeding

Administration
- Follow facility protocols regarding proper handling and disposal of drug.

• Be aware that total daily dosage is calculated to nearest multiple of 25 mg and given once daily.

◀℥ Withdraw drug immediately if leukocyte or platelet count falls rapidly or steeply.

Route	Onset	Peak	Duration
P.O.	Unknown	2 hr	Unknown

Adverse reactions

GI: nausea, vomiting, anorexia, diarrhea, GI ulcers, painful oral ulcers, **pancreatitis**

Hematologic: anemia, **leukopenia, thrombocytopenia**

Hepatic: jaundice, **hepatotoxicity**

Metabolic: hyperuricemia

Skin: rash, hyperpigmentation

Interactions

Drug-drug. *Allopurinol (dosages above 300 mg), aminosalicylate derivatives (mesalazine, olsalazine, sulfasalazine):* increased bone marrow depression

Coumadin: decreased anticoagulant effect

Drug-diagnostic tests. *Hemoglobin, platelets, red blood cells, uric acid, white blood cells:* increased values

Precautions

Use cautiously in:
• renal or hepatic impairment
• decreased platelet or neutrophil counts after chemotherapy or radiation
• pregnant patients.

Patient monitoring

◀℥ Watch for signs and symptoms of hepatotoxicity.

• Monitor weekly complete blood cell count with white cell differential and platelet count.

• Assess bone marrow aspiration and biopsy results, as necessary, to aid assessment of disease progression, resistance to therapy, and drug-induced marrow hypoplasia.

• Monitor serum uric acid level.

• Evaluate fluid intake and output.

• Monitor liver function test results and bilirubin level weekly at start of therapy, and then monthly.

Patient teaching

◀℥ Instruct patient to immediately report fever, sore throat, or increased bleeding or bruising as well as signs and symptoms of liver problems (right-sided abdominal pain, yellowing of skin or eyes, nausea, vomiting, flu-like symptoms, clay-colored stools, or dark urine).

• Advise both male and female patients to use reliable contraception.

• Encourage patient to maintain adequate fluid intake.

• As appropriate, review all other significant and life-threatening adverse reactions and interactions, especially those related to the drugs and tests mentioned above.

m

meropenem
Merrem I.V.

Pharmacologic class: Carbapenem
Therapeutic class: Anti-infective
Pregnancy risk category B

Action

Inhibits bacterial cell-wall synthesis and penetrates gram-negative and gram-positive bacteria

Availability

Powder for injection: 500-mg and 1-g vials

⏀ Indications and dosages

➤ Appendicitis and peritonitis caused by alpha-hemolytic streptococci, *Escherichia coli, Klebsiella pneumoniae, Pseudomonas aeruginosa, Bacteroides fragilis, Bacteroides thetaiotaomicron,* and *Peptostreptococcus* species

Adults: 1 g I.V. q 8 hours over 15 to 30 minutes by infusion or over 3 to 5 minutes as a bolus injection

Children weighing 50 kg (110 lb) or more: 1 g I.V. q 8 hours over 15 to 30 minutes by infusion or over 3 to 5 minutes as a bolus injection

Children ages 3 months and older weighing less than 50 kg (110 lb): 20 mg/kg q 8 hours over 15 to 30 minutes by infusion or over 3 to 5 minutes as a bolus injection

➤ Bacterial meningitis caused by *Streptococcus pneumoniae, Haemophilus influenzae,* or *Neisseria meningitides*

Children weighing 50 kg (110 lb) or more: 2 g I.V. q 8 hours over 15 to 30 minutes by infusion or over 3 to 5 minutes as a bolus injection

Children ages 3 month and older weighing less than 50 kg (110 lb): 40 mg/kg q 8 hours over 15 to 30 minutes by infusion or over 3 to 5 minutes as a bolus injection, up to a maximum of 2 g q 8 hours

Dosage adjustment
• Renal impairment

Off-label uses
• Acute pulmonary exacerbation caused by respiratory tract infection with susceptible organisms in cystic fibrosis patients

Contraindications
• Hypersensitivity to drug, its components, or other drugs in same class

Administration
• For I.V. bolus, add 10 or 20 ml to a 500-mg or 1-g vial, respectively, to yield a concentration of 50 mg/ml. Shake until clear. Administer over 3 to 5 minutes.
• For intermittent I.V. infusion, piggyback vials can be reconstituted with compatible I.V. solution (0.9% sodium chloride or 5% dextrose) to yield a concentration of 2.5 to 50 mg/ml. Or

vials can be reconstituted as for direct I.V. injection and added to compatible I.V. solution for further dilution. To reconstitute and administer ADD-Vantage systems, follow manufacturer's instructions. Infuse drug over 15 to 30 minutes.
• Use diluted solutions immediately if possible.

Route	Onset	Peak	Duration
I.V.	Unknown	1 hr	Unknown

Adverse reactions
CNS: headache, insomnia, dizziness, drowsiness, weakness, myoclonus, **seizures**
CV: hypotension, phlebitis, palpitations, **heart failure, cardiac arrest, myocardial infarction**
GI: nausea, vomiting, diarrhea, constipation, altered taste, tongue discoloration, oral candidiasis, glossitis, increased amylase and lipase levels, **pseudomembranous colitis**
GU: vaginal candidiasis
Hematologic: anemia, eosinophilia, decreased hemoglobin and hematocrit, **leukopenia, bone marrow depression, thrombocytopenia, neutropenia**
Respiratory: chest discomfort, dyspnea, hyperventilation
Skin: rash, urticaria, pruritus, erythema at injection site
Other: fever, pain, fungal infection, **anaphylaxis**

Interactions
Drug-drug. *Probenecid:* increased meropenem blood level
Drug-diagnostic tests. *Alanine aminotransferase, alkaline phosphatase, amylase, aspartate aminotransferase, bilirubin, blood urea nitrogen, eosinophils, gamma-glutamyl transpeptidase, lactate dehydrogenase, lipase:* increased values *Hematocrit, hemoglobin, platelets, neutrophils, white blood cells:* decreased values

International Normalized Ratio, partial thromboplastin time, prothrombin time: increased or decreased values

Precautions

Use cautiously in:

- sulfite sensitivity
- renal disease, seizure disorder
- pregnant or breastfeeding patients
- children.

Patient monitoring

- Collect specimens for culture and sensitivity testing as needed; however, drug therapy may begin pending results.

◀≋ Monitor patient for hypersensitivity reaction or anaphylaxis. If either occurs, stop infusion immediately and initiate emergency treatment.

- Monitor for CNS irritability and seizures.
- In prolonged therapy, evaluate hematopoietic, renal, and hepatic function and watch for overgrowth of nonsusceptible organisms.
- If diarrhea occurs, check for pseudomembranous colitis; obtain stool cultures.
- Obtain hearing tests in children being treated for bacterial meningitis.

Patient teaching

- Advise patient to report such adverse reactions as CNS irritability, diarrhea, rash, shortness of breath, or pain at infusion site.
- Instruct patient to contact prescriber if she's pregnant or breastfeeding; advise her to avoid breastfeeding.
- As appropriate, review all other significant and life-threatening adverse reactions and interactions, especially those related to the drugs and tests mentioned above.

mesalamine (5-aminosalicylic acid, 5-ASA, mesalazine)

Asacol, Canasa, Mesasal♣, Pentasa, Rowasa, Salofalk♣

Pharmacologic class: 5-amino-2-hydroxybenzoic acid

Therapeutic class: GI anti-inflammatory drug

Pregnancy risk category B

Action

Unknown; thought to act in colon, where it blocks cyclooxygenase and inhibits prostaglandin synthesis

Availability

Capsules (extended-release): 250 mg
Rectal suspension: 4 g/60 ml
Suppositories: 500 mg
Tablets (delayed-release): 250 mg, 400 mg, 500 mg
Tablets (extended-release): 250 mg, 500 mg

Indications and dosages

➢ Inflammatory bowel disease, including ulcerative colitis, proctitis, and proctosigmoiditis

Adults: 800 mg P.O. t.i.d. for 6 weeks (delayed-release tablets) or 1 g q.i.d. (extended-release capsules) for a total dosage of 4 g for up to 8 weeks; or 4-g enema (60 ml) P.R. at bedtime, retained for 8 hours, for 3 to 6 weeks; or 500 mg (suppository) P.R. b.i.d., increased to t.i.d. if inadequate response occurs after 2 weeks.

Contraindications

- Hypersensitivity to drug, its components (sulfite in rectal preparations), or salicylates

m

♣ Canada   ◀≋ Clinical alert   Reactions in **bold** are life-threatening

Administration

• Make sure patient swallows tablets whole without crushing or chewing.
• For best effect, have patient retain suppository for 1 to 3 hours.

Route	Onset	Peak	Duration
P.O.	Unknown	Unknown	6-8 hr
P.R.	Unknown	Unknown	24 hr

Adverse reactions

CNS: headache, dizziness, malaise, weakness
CV: chest pain
EENT: rhinitis, pharyngitis
GI: nausea, vomiting, diarrhea, eructation, flatulence, anal irritation (with rectal use), **pancreatitis**
GU: interstitial nephritis, **renal failure**
Musculoskeletal: back pain
Skin: alopecia, rash
Other: acute intolerance syndrome, fever, **anaphylaxis**

Interactions

None significant

Precautions

Use cautiously in:
• severe hepatic or renal impairment
• pregnant or breastfeeding patients.

Patient monitoring

◀€ Closely monitor patient with history of allergic reaction to sulfasalazine or sulfite sensitivity (if using enema).
• Assess renal and hepatic function before therapy starts and periodically during therapy.
• Monitor suppository efficacy, which should appear in 3 to 21 days; however, know that treatment usually continues for 3 to 6 weeks.
◀€ Watch for signs and symptoms of intolerance syndrome, such as cramping, acute abdominal pain, bloody diarrhea, fever, headache, and rash. If these occur, discontinue drug. Drug may be restarted later only if clearly

needed, under close medical supervision and at reduced dosage.

Patient teaching

• Instruct patient to swallow tablets or capsules whole.
• Tell patient to contact prescriber if partially intact tablets repeatedly appear in stools.
• Teach patient using suppository to avoid excessive handling and to retain suppository for 1 to 3 hours or longer for maximum benefit.
• Instruct patient on proper enema administration; tell him to stay in position for at least 30 minutes and, if possible, retain medication overnight.
◀€ Advise patient to promptly report cramping, acute abdominal pain, bloody diarrhea, fever, headache, or rash.
• As appropriate, review all other significant and life-threatening adverse reactions.

mesna
Mesnex, Uromitexan✤

Pharmacologic class: Detoxifying agent
Therapeutic class: Hemorrhagic cystitis inhibitor
Pregnancy risk category B

Action

Reacts in kidney with urotoxic ifosfamide metabolites (acrolein and 4-hydroxy-ifosfamide), resulting in their detoxification; also binds to double bonds of acrolein and to other urotoxic metabolites

Availability

Injection: 100 mg/ml in 2-ml and 10-ml vials
Tablets (coated): 400 mg

✒ Indications and dosages
➢ To prevent hemorrhagic cystitis in patients receiving ifosfamide
Adults: *Combination I.V. and P.O. regimen*—Single I.V. bolus dose of mesna at 20% of ifosfamide dosage, given at same time as ifosfamide, followed by two doses of mesna tablets P.O. at 40% of ifosfamide dosage given 2 and 6 hours after ifosfamide dose. *I.V. regimen*—I.V. bolus of mesna at 20% of ifosfamide dosage given at same time as ifosfamide, repeated 4 and 8 hours after each ifosfamide dose.
Dosage adjustment
• Children

Contraindications
• Hypersensitivity to drug or other thiol compounds

Administration
• Dilute ampules using dextrose 5% in water, dextrose 5% in normal saline solution, or lactated Ringer's solution for injection.
• Give I.V. bolus with ifosfamide dose and at prescribed intervals after ifosfamide doses.
◀€ Don't use multidose vial (contains benzyl alcohol) in neonates or infants; use in older children only with caution.
• If patient vomits within 2 hours of oral mesna dose, repeat oral dose or switch to I.V. route.

Route	Onset	Peak	Duration
P.O.	Unknown	4-8 hr	24 hr
I.V.	Unknown	1 hr	24 hr

Adverse reactions
CNS: fatigue, malaise, headache, dizziness, drowsiness, hyperesthesia, rigors, irritability
CV: hypertension, hypotension, ST-segment elevation, tachycardia
EENT: conjunctivitis, pharyngitis, rhinitis

GI: nausea, vomiting, diarrhea, constipation, anorexia, flatulence
Hematologic: hematuria
Hepatic: increased hepatic enzyme levels
Musculoskeletal: back pain, joint pain, myalgia
Respiratory: coughing, tachypnea, **bronchospasm**
Skin: flushing, rash
Other: arm or leg pain, injection site reactions, fever, flulike symptoms, allergic reactions

Interactions
Drug-diagnostic tests. *Urinary erythrocytes:* false-positive or false-negative results
Urine tests using Ames Multistix (during mesna/ifosfamide therapy): false-positive for ketonuria

Precautions
Use cautiously in:
• autoimmune disorders.

Patient monitoring
• Monitor nutritional and hydration status.
• Monitor vital signs and ECG; watch closely for blood pressure changes and tachycardia.
• Assess body temperature; stay alert for fever, flulike symptoms, and EENT infections.
• Monitor respiratory status carefully; especially for bronchospasm, cough, and tachypnea.

Patient teaching
• Inform patient that drug may cause significant adverse effects; reassure him that he'll be monitored closely.
• Encourage patient to request analgesics or other pain-relief measures for headache, back or joint pain, hyperesthesia, or muscle ache.
◀€ Advise patient to immediately report breathing difficulties and allergic symptoms.

m

• Inform patient about drug's adverse CNS effects; explain safety measures used to prevent injury.
• Teach patient to minimize GI upset by eating frequent, small servings of healthy food.
• As appropriate, review all other significant adverse reactions and interactions, especially those related to the tests mentioned above.

mesoridazine besylate
Serentil, Serentil Concentrate

Pharmacologic class: Phenothiazine, dopaminergic-blocking agent

Therapeutic class: Antipsychotic, anxiolytic

Pregnancy risk category C

Action
Unknown; thought to block postsynaptic dopamine receptors in brain, depressing the cerebral cortex, hypothalamus, and limbic system; also has anticholinergic and antihistaminic properties

Availability
Injection: 25 mg/ml
Oral concentrate: 25 mg/ml (0.6% alcohol)
Tablets: 10 mg, 25 mg, 50 mg, 100 mg

🕖 Indications and dosages
➤ Schizophrenia
Adults: Initially, 50 mg P.O. t.i.d. or 25 mg I.M.; repeat in 30 to 60 minutes as needed, to a maximum of 400 mg/day P.O. or 200 mg/day I.M.

Contraindications
• Hypersensitivity to drug or other phenothiazines
• Coma or severe CNS depression
• History of prolonged QTc interval

Administration
• Avoid skin contact with oral solution or injection; contact dermatitis may occur.
• Dilute oral concentrate in water, orange, or grape juice just before administering. Bulk dilutions are not recommended.
• Give I.M. injections deep into large muscle mass; massage to help prevent sterile abscess.
• Protect from light. Injection or concentrate may yellow slightly, but this doesn't affect potency. Don't use markedly discolored solution.

Route	Onset	Peak	Duration
P.O.	Variable	2-4 hr	4-6 hr
I.M.	Rapid	30 min	6-8 hr

Adverse reactions
CNS: drowsiness, insomnia, vertigo, headache, weakness, tremor, ataxia, slurred speech, exacerbation of psychotic symptoms, extrapyramidal syndrome, pseudoparkinsonism, dystonias, akathisia, tardive dyskinesia, **cerebral edema, seizures, neuroleptic malignant syndrome**
CV: hypotension, orthostatic hypotension, tachycardia, bradycardia, **cardiac arrest, heart failure, cardiomegaly, refractory arrhythmias, prolonged QTc interval, torsades de pointes**
GI: nausea, vomiting, constipation, dry mouth
GU: urinary retention, gynecomastia, breast engorgement (in breastfeeding patients), galactorrhea, menstrual irregularities, inhibited ovulation, libido changes, inhibited ejaculation
Hematologic: eosinophilia, leukocytosis, hemolytic anemia, **pancytopenia, leukopenia, agranulocytosis, aplastic anemia, thrombocytopenia**
Hepatic: jaundice
Metabolic: syndrome of inappropriate antidiuretic hormone secretion; hyperglycemia or hypoglycemia; glycosuria;

hyponatremia; pituitary tumor with hyperprolactinemia; decreased urinary levels of gonadotropins, estrogens, and progestins

Respiratory: dyspnea, cough reflex suppression with possible **aspiration, bronchospasm, laryngospasm, pulmonary edema**

Skin: rash, sterile abscess, mild photosensitivity reaction

Other: pain at I.M. injection site, allergic reaction

Interactions

Drug-drug. *Antacids:* inhibited mesoridazine absorption

Anticholinergic: increased anticholinergic effects

Antipsychotics, guanethidine: decreased antihypertensive effect

Barbiturates: decreased mesoridazine effects

CNS depressants: increased CNS depression

Disopyramide, fluoxetine, paroxetine, procainamide, quinidine: increased risk of serious or fatal arrhythmias

Lithium: increased CNS effects

Metrizamide: increased risk of seizures

Drug-diagnostic tests. *Blood glucose:* increased or decreased level

Eosinophils, liver function tests: increased values

Granulocytes, hemoglobin, platelets, sodium, white blood cells: decreased values

Drug-herb. *Kava:* increased risk of dystonic reactions

St. John's wort: increased risk of photosensitivity

Yohimbe: increased risk of toxicity

Drug-behaviors. *Alcohol use:* increased CNS depression

Sun exposure: increased risk of photosensitivity

Precautions

Use cautiously in:
• bone marrow depression, blood dyscrasias, circulatory collapse, subcortical brain damage, Parkinson's disease, hepatic damage, severe hypotension or hypertension
• history of seizure disorder
• pregnant or breastfeeding patients.

Patient monitoring

◖≋ Assess baseline ECG and potassium level before starting therapy. Correct potassium imbalance before giving first dose.
• Don't give to patients with QTc interval longer than 450 msec.
• Monitor ECG periodically, especially during dosage adjustment periods.
◖≋ Watch for dizziness, palpitations, and syncope; these symptoms warrant further cardiac evaluation (possibly with Holter monitoring).
• Monitor blood pressure before therapy starts and periodically during therapy.
• Monitor patients (especially elderly women) for signs of tardive dyskinesia.
• Evaluate hematologic studies and liver function tests.
◖≋ Monitor for neuroleptic malignant syndrome (extrapyramidal symptoms, hyperpyrexia, muscle rigidity, altered mental status, irregular pulse or blood pressure, tachycardia, diaphoresis, or arrhythmias).

Patient teaching

◖≋ Inform patient that drug may cause potentially fatal heart rhythm disturbances.
◖≋ Advise patient to promptly report such adverse reactions as fever, malaise, sore throat, jaundice, involuntary movements, dystonic reactions, dizziness, palpitations, or fainting.
• Tell patient that drug may cause tardive dyskinesia.
• Caution patient not to stop taking drug abruptly.
• Instruct patient to avoid driving and other hazardous activities until he knows how drug affects concentration and alertness.

• Instruct patient to move slowly when changing position, to avoid dizziness or light-headedness from sudden blood pressure decrease.

• As appropriate, review all other significant and life-threatening adverse reactions and interactions, especially those related to the drugs, tests, herbs, and behaviors mentioned above.

metaproterenol sulfate
Alupent, Arm-a-Med, Dey-Lute
Metaproterenol

Pharmacologic class: Sympathomimetic, selective beta$_2$-adrenergic agonist
Therapeutic class: Bronchodilator
Pregnancy risk category C

Action
Relaxes beta$_2$ receptors (pulmonary), causing bronchodilation and inhibiting histamine release; acts on beta$_1$ receptors (cardiac) with less effect

Availability
Aerosol solution for inhalation: 0.65 mg/metered spray
Nebulizer inhaler: 0.4%, 0.6%, or 5% solution
Syrup: 10 mg/5 ml
Tablets: 10 mg, 20 mg

🕖 Indications and dosages
➤ Bronchial asthma and reversible bronchospasm
Adults and children ages 9 and older or weighing more than 27 kg (59.5 lb): 20 mg P.O. three or four times daily
Children ages 6 to 9 or weighing less than 27 kg (59.5 lb): 10 mg P.O. three or four times daily
Aerosol solution for inhalation—
Adults and children ages 12 and older: Two or three inhalations by metered aerosol (1.3 or 1.9 mg) q 3 to 4 hours, to a maximum of 12 inhalations (7.8 mg) in 24 hours. Alternatively, 10 inhalations of undiluted 5% solution by hand-bulb nebulizer, or 0.3 ml of 5% solution diluted in 2.5 ml of 0.45% or 0.9% sodium chloride solution or 2.5 ml of commercial diluent 0.4% or 0.6% solution for nebulization given by intermittent positive-pressure breathing device.
Children ages 6 to 12: 0.1 ml of 5% solution diluted in 0.9% sodium chloride solution to a final volume of 3 ml, given by nebulizer three or four times daily as needed, but no more often than q 4 hours

Contraindications
• Hypersensitivity to drug
• Tachyarrhythmias
• Peripheral or mesenteric vascular thrombosis
• Profound hypoxia or hypercapnia
• General anesthesia

Administration
• If patient is using aerosol metered-dose inhaler, place mouthpiece well into his mouth and have him close lips tightly around it. Tell him to exhale completely through nose and then inhale slowly and deeply through mouth while activating inhaler. Have him hold his breath for a few seconds and then remove mouthpiece and exhale slowly. Wait roughly 2 minutes between inhalations. Rinse mouthpiece with water after use.
• Know that use of Aero-Chamber may aid proper drug delivery.

Route	Onset	Peak	Duration
P.O.	15 min	1 hr	4 hr or more
Inhalation (aerosol)	1 min	1 hr	4 hr or more
Inhalation (nebulizer)	5-30 min	Unknown	4 hr or more

Adverse reactions
CNS: nervousness, drowsiness, tremor, vertigo, headache, restlessness, apprehension, anxiety, fear, CNS stimulation, hyperkinesia, insomnia, irritability, weakness
CV: tachycardia, hypertension, palpitations, anginal pain, **cardiac arrest** (with excessive use)
GI: nausea, vomiting, diarrhea, heartburn, abnormal or bad taste, dry mouth
Respiratory: cough, respiratory difficulty, **bronchospasm, pulmonary edema, paradoxical bronchiolar constriction** (with excessive use)
Skin: rash, sweating, pallor, flushing
Other: hypersensitivity reaction

Interactions
Drug-drug. *Epinephrine, other sympathomimetics:* increased risk of arrhythmias
Monoamine oxidase inhibitors, tricyclic antidepressants: potentiation of metaproterenol effects
Propranolol and other beta blockers: inhibition of bronchodilating effect

Precautions
Use cautiously in:
• unstable vasomotor system disorders, hypertension, coronary artery disease, hyperthyroidism, chronic obstructive pulmonary disease complicated by degenerative heart disease
• history of cerebrovascular accident or seizure disorders
• labor and delivery
• pregnant or breastfeeding patients.

Patient monitoring
• If patient is using multiple drugs to control asthma, assess level of understanding regarding administration. Tell him to continue taking each drug as prescribed even if he feels better.
• Monitor patient for effective use of aerosol inhaler or hand-held nebulizer.

• Assess for drug efficacy; be aware that efficacy may decrease with prolonged use.
• Check for adverse effects.
◀❙ Monitor patient for hypersensitivity reaction or paradoxical bronchospasm. If either occurs, discontinue drug immediately, and implement alternative therapy and airway control measures.

Patient teaching
• Teach patient to take tablets with food if GI distress occurs.
• Instruct patient in proper use of metered-dose aerosol inhaler.
• Advise patient to remove canister and wash mouthpiece frequently.
◀❙ Caution patient not to increase number or frequency of inhalations without prescriber's consent; cardiac arrest may occur with excessive use.
• As appropriate, review all other significant and life-threatening adverse reactions and interactions, especially those related to the drugs mentioned above.

m

metformin hydrochloride
Apo-Metformin✦, Glucophage, Glucophage XR, Glycon✦, Novo-Metformin✦

Pharmacologic class: Biguanide
Therapeutic class: Hypoglycemic
Pregnancy risk category B

Action
Decreases production and absorption of glucose in the liver and intestines, increasing sensitivity to insulin

Availability
Tablets: 500 mg, 850 mg, 1,000 mg
Tablets (extended-release): 500 mg, 750 mg

✦ Canada   ◀❙ Clinical alert   Reactions in **bold** are life-threatening

⬛ Indications and dosages
➤ Adjunctive management of type 2 diabetes mellitus

Adults: Initially, 500 mg P.O. b.i.d.; may increase by 500 mg/week, up to 2,000 mg/day. If patient requires more than 2,000 mg/day, give in three divided doses (not to exceed 2,500 mg/day). Alternatively, 850 mg P.O. daily, increased by 850 mg q 2 weeks in divided doses, up to 2,550 mg/day in divided doses (850 mg t.i.d.). *Extended-release tablets*—500 mg/day P.O. with evening meal; may increase by 500 mg weekly, up to 2,000 mg/day. If 2,000 mg once daily is inadequate, 1,000 mg may be given b.i.d.

Dosage adjustment
• Elderly or debilitated patients

Contraindications
• Hypersensitivity to drug
• Metabolic acidosis
• Dehydration, sepsis, hypoxemia, impaired hepatic function, excessive alcohol use
• Underlying renal dysfunction
• Heart failure

Administration
• Know that drug is given in conjunction with diet therapy, sulfonylureas, or both.
• In patients on insulin, continue current insulin dosage and initiate metformin at 500 mg once daily (conventional or extended-release). Dosage may be raised 500 mg/week until glycemic control is adequate. Maximum dosage is 2,500 mg/day for conventional tablets and 2,000 mg/day for extended-release tablets. Reduce insulin dosage by 10% to 25% if fasting blood glucose is below 120 mg/dl.
• Administer with a meal.
• Make sure patient swallows extended-release tablets whole without crushing or chewing.

Route	Onset	Peak	Duration
P.O.	Unknown	2-4 hr	12 hr
P.O. (extended)	Unknown	4-8 hr	24 hr

Adverse reactions
GI: diarrhea, nausea, vomiting, abdominal bloating, unpleasant metallic taste
Metabolic: lactic acidosis
Other: decreased vitamin B_{12} level

Interactions
Drug-drug. *Amiloride, calcium channel blockers, digoxin, morphine, procainamide, quinidine, ranitidine, triamterene, trimethoprim, vancomycin:* altered response to metformin
Cimetidine, furosemide, nifedipine: increased metformin effects
Iodinated contrast media: increased risk of lactic acidosis
Drug-diagnostic tests. *Urine ketones:* false-positive results
Drug-herb. *Glucosamine:* decreased glycemic control
Chromium, coenzyme Q10, fenugreek: additive hypoglycemic effects
Drug-behaviors. *Alcohol use:* increased metformin effects

Precautions
Use cautiously in:
• renal impairment, myocardial infarction, cerebrovascular accident, hypoxia, pituitary deficiency or hyperthyroidism, chronic alcohol use
• elderly or debilitated patients
• pregnant or breastfeeding patients
• children (safety not established).

Patient monitoring
• When switching patient from chlorpropamide, stay alert for hypoglycemia during first 2 weeks of metformin therapy; chlorpropamide may stay in body for prolonged time. (Conversion from other standard oral hypoglycemics requires no transition period.)

• Monitor blood glucose level closely; if it isn't controlled after 4 weeks at maximum dosage, oral sulfonylurea may be added.

• Monitor kidney and liver function test results, particularly in elderly patients.

• Assess hematologic parameters and vitamin B_{12} levels at start of therapy and periodically throughout.

◀ Watch for signs and symptoms of lactic acidosis; stop drug if acidosis occurs. To aid differential diagnosis, check electrolyte, ketone, glucose, blood pH, lactate, and metformin levels.

• Periodically monitor glucose and glycosylated hemoglobin levels to evaluate drug efficacy.

Patient teaching

• Teach patient about diabetes and importance of proper diet, exercise, weight control, and blood glucose monitoring.

• Inform patient that drug may cause diarrhea, nausea, and upset stomach. Advise him to take it with meals to reduce these effects; inform him that adverse effects often subside over time.

◀ Teach patient to recognize and immediately report signs and symptoms of acidosis, such as weakness, fatigue, muscle pain, dyspnea, abdominal pain, dizziness, light-headedness, or slow or irregular heartbeat.

• Advise patient to report changes in health status (such as infection, persistent vomiting and diarrhea, or need for surgery); these may warrant dosage decrease or drug withdrawal.

• As appropriate, review all other significant and life-threatening adverse reactions and interactions, especially those related to the drugs, tests, herbs, and behaviors mentioned above.

methadone hydrochloride
Dolophine, Methadone HCl Diskets, Methadone HCl Intensol, Methadose

Pharmacologic class: Opioid agonist
Therapeutic class: Analgesic, opioid detoxification adjunct
Controlled substance schedule II
Pregnancy risk category C

Action
Binds to and depresses opiate receptors in spinal cord and CNS, altering perception of and response to pain

Availability
Injection: 10 mg/ml
Oral solution: 5 mg/5 ml, 10 mg/5 ml, 10 mg/ml (concentrate)
Tablets: 5 mg, 10 mg
Tablets (dispersible diskettes): 40 mg

m

⏀ Indications and dosages
➤ Opioid detoxification
Adults: Initially, 15 to 20 mg/day P.O. as needed, to a maximum of 120 mg/day. If patient can't tolerate oral doses, give I.M. or S.C. (usually at about 25% of total daily P.O. dosage) in two injections.
➤ To maintain opioid abstinence
Adults: Dosage highly individualized based on patient's weight, size, and response; maximum dosage is 120 mg/day.
➤ Chronic and severe pain
Adults: For chronic pain, 2.5 to 10 mg I.M. or S.C. q 3 to 4 hours as needed; adjust dosage and dosing interval as needed. For severe chronic pain (as in terminal illness), 5 to 20 mg P.O. q 6 to 8 hours; dosage may be increased or dosing interval may be shortened as needed, to a maximum dosage of 120 mg/day.

Children: Dosage individualized based on weight and size

Contraindications

• Hypersensitivity to drug or other opioid agonists
• Chronic obstructive pulmonary disease
• Cor pulmonale
• Increased intracranial pressure
• Severe inflammatory bowel disease
• Renal dysfunction
• Severe CNS depression
• Hypercapnia
• Seizures
• Acute alcoholism

Administration

• Mix dispersible tablets with 120 ml of water or orange juice, citrus Tang, or other acidic fruit beverages.
• Dilute 10 mg/ml of oral solution with water or other liquid to at least 30 ml. In detoxification and maintenance of opioid withdrawal, solution is usually diluted in at least 90 ml of fluid.
• When used parenterally, I.M. route is preferred. Rotate injection sites.
• For detoxification and maintenance, give oral liquid only to reduce potential for parenteral abuse, hoarding, and accidental ingestion.
• Patients who can't take oral drugs because of nausea or vomiting during detoxification or maintenance should be hospitalized and given methadone parenterally.

Route	Onset	Peak	Duration
P.O.	30-60 min	1.5-2 hr	4-6 hr
I.M., S.C.	10-20 min	1-2 hr	4-5 hr

Adverse reactions

CNS: amnesia, anxiety, coma, confusion, poor concentration, delirium, delusions, depression, dizziness, drowsiness, euphoria, fever, hallucinations, headache, insomnia, lethargy, light-headedness, malaise, psychosis, restlessness, sedation, clouded sensorium, syncope, tremor, **seizures**
CV: hypotension, palpitations, edema, bradycardia, **shock, cardiac arrest**
EENT: visual disturbances
GI: nausea, vomiting, constipation, ileus, biliary tract spasm, gastroesophageal reflux, indigestion, dysphagia, dry mouth, anorexia, increased amylase level
GU: urinary hesitancy, urinary retention, prolonged labor, difficult ejaculation, impotence
Hematologic: anemia, **leukopenia, thrombocytopenia**
Hepatic: elevated liver function test values
Musculoskeletal: joint pain
Respiratory: asthma exacerbation, atelectasis, depressed cough reflex, hypoventilation, wheezing, **pulmonary edema, bronchospasm, respiratory depression or arrest, apnea**
Skin: urticaria, pruritus, flushing, pallor, diaphoresis
Other: allergic reaction, hiccups, facial or injection site edema, pain, physical or psychological drug dependence, withdrawal symptoms

Interactions

Drug-drug. *Amitriptyline, antihistamines, chloral hydrate, clomipramine, glutethimide, methocarbamol, monoamine oxidase inhibitors, nortriptyline:* increased CNS and respiratory depression
Anticholinergics: increased risk of severe constipation leading to ileus
Antiemetics, general anesthetics, phenothiazines, sedative-hypnotics, tranquilizers: coma, hypotension, respiratory depression, severe sedation
Ascorbic acid, phenytoin, phosphate, potassium, rifampin: methadone precipitation
Cimetidine, fluvoxamine, protease inhibitors: increased analgesia, CNS and respiratory depression
Diuretics: increased diuresis

Hydroxyzine: increased analgesia, CNS depression, and hypotension
Paregoric, loperamide: increased CNS depression, severe constipation
Naloxone: antagonism of methadone's analgesic, CNS, and respiratory effects
Naltrexone: induction or worsening of withdrawal symptoms (when given within 7 days after methadone use)
Neuromuscular blockers: increased or prolonged respiratory depression
Drug-diagnostic tests. *Amylase:* increased level
Drug-behaviors. *Alcohol use:* increased CNS and respiratory depression

Precautions

Use cautiously in:
• head trauma; severe renal, hepatic, or pulmonary disease; hypothyroidism; adrenal insufficiency; undiagnosed abdominal pain; prostatic hypertrophy; urethral stricture; toxic psychosis; Addison's disease; fever; alcoholism
• recent renal or hepatic surgery
• elderly or debilitated patients
• pregnant patients, patients in labor, or breastfeeding patients.

Patient monitoring

• Assess patient for relief of severe chronic pain requiring around-the-clock dosing. Tailor dosage to patient's pain level and tolerance.
• Monitor CNS, respiratory, and cardiovascular status.
• Watch for deepening sedation, which may increase with successive doses.
• Evaluate bowel and bladder function. Give laxatives if appropriate.
• Monitor detoxification treatment closely. Short-term detoxification shouldn't exceed 30 days; long-term detoxification, 180 days.
• Assess patient on maintenance therapy for successful rehabilitation. Be aware that maintenance therapy should be part of a comprehensive treatment plan that encompasses medical, vocational rehabilitative, employ-

ment, educational, and counseling services.

Patient teaching

◀€ Instruct patient to promptly report severe adverse reactions.
• Tell patient he may take drug with food if GI upset occurs.
• Teach patient to avoid driving and other hazardous activities because drug may cause drowsiness and or dizziness.
• Teach ambulatory patient to change positions slowly to avoid orthostatic hypotension.
• Instruct patient not to discontinue drug abruptly.
• As appropriate, review all other significant and life-threatening adverse reactions and interactions, especially those related to the drugs, tests, and behaviors mentioned above.

methimazole

m

Tapazole

Pharmacologic class: Thiomidazole derivative
Therapeutic class: Antithyroid drug
Pregnancy risk category D

Action

Directly interferes with thyroid synthesis by preventing iodine from combining with thyroglobulin, leading to decreased thyroid hormone levels

Availability

Tablets: 5 mg, 10 mg

🕗 Indications and dosages

➤ Mild hyperthyroidism
Adults and adolescents: Initially, 15 mg P.O. daily as a single dose or in divided doses b.i.d. for 6 to 8 weeks or until response is adequate. Maintenance dosage is 5 to 30 mg/day as a single dose or in divided doses b.i.d.

Children: Initially, 0.4 mg/kg/day in three divided doses at 8-hour intervals. Maintenance dosage is 0.2 mg/kg/day in three divided doses at 8-hour intervals.

➤ Moderate hyperthyroidism

Adults and adolescents: Initially, 30 to 40 mg P.O. daily as a single dose or in divided doses for 6 to 8 weeks or until response is adequate. Maintenance dosage is 5 to 30 mg/day as a single dose or in divided doses.

Children: 0.4 mg/kg/day P.O. as a single dose or in divided doses at 8-hour intervals. Maintenance dosage is 0.2 mg/kg/day as a single dose or in three divided doses at 8-hour intervals.

➤ Severe hyperthyroidism

Adults and adolescents: Initially, 60 mg/day P.O. as a single dose or in divided doses for 6 to 8 weeks or until response is adequate. Maintenance dosage is 5 to 30 mg/day as a single dose or in divided doses.

Children: Initially, 0.4 mg/kg/day P.O. as a single dose or in three divided doses at 8-hour intervals. Maintenance dosage is 0.2 mg/kg/day as a single dose or in three divided doses at 8-hour intervals.

Contraindications

- Hypersensitivity to drug
- Breastfeeding

Administration

- Administer exactly as prescribed; total daily dosage usually is given in three equally divided doses at 8-hour intervals.
- Give with meals as needed to reduce GI upset.

Route	Onset	Peak	Duration
P.O.	30-40 min	60 min	2-4 hr

Adverse reactions

CNS: headache, vertigo, paresthesia, neuritis, depression, neuropathy, CNS stimulation

GI: nausea, vomiting, constipation, epigastric distress, ileus, salivary gland enlargement, dry mouth, anorexia

GU: nephritis

Hematologic: thrombocytopenia, agranulocytosis, leukopenia, aplastic anemia

Hepatic: jaundice, hepatic dysfunction, **hepatitis**

Metabolic: hypothyroidism

Musculoskeletal: joint pain, myalgia

Skin: rash, urticaria, skin discoloration, pruritus, erythema nodosum, exfoliative dermatitis, abnormal hair loss

Other: fever, lymphadenopathy, lupuslike syndrome

Interactions

Drug-drug. *Aminophylline, oxtriphylline, theophylline:* decreased clearance of both drugs

Amiodarone, iodine, potassium iodide: decreased response to methimazole

Anticoagulants: altered requirements of both drugs

Beta-adrenergic blockers: altered beta blocker clearance

Digoxin: increased digoxin blood level

Drug-diagnostic tests. *Granulocytes, hemoglobin, platelets, white blood cells:* decreased values

Precautions

Use cautiously in:
- bone marrow depression
- patients older than age 40
- pregnant patients.

Patient monitoring

- Check for agranulocytosis in patients older than age 40 and in those receiving more than 40 mg/day.
- Assess hematologic studies. Agranulocytosis usually occurs within first 2 months of therapy and is rare after 4 months.
- Monitor thyroid function tests periodically. After hyperthyroidism is controlled, elevated thyroid-stimulating

factor indicates need for dosage decrease.

• Assess liver function studies; check for signs and symptoms of hepatic dysfunction.

• Monitor patient for fever, sore throat, and other evidence of infection as well as for unusual bleeding or bruising.

• Assess patient for signs and symptoms of hypothyroidism, such as hard edema of subcutaneous tissue, drowsiness, slow mentation, dryness or loss of hair, decreased temperature, hoarseness, and muscle weakness.

Patient teaching

• Tell patient to take drug with meals if GI upset occurs.

• Advise patient to take drug exactly as prescribed to maintain constant blood level.

• Teach patient to report rash, fever, sore throat, unusual bleeding or bruising, headache, rash, yellowing of skin or eyes, abdominal pain, vomiting, or flulike symptoms.

• As appropriate, review all other significant and life-threatening adverse reactions and interactions, especially those related to the drugs and tests mentioned above.

methocarbamol

Carbacot, Methocarbamol♣,
Robaxin, Skelex

Pharmacologic class: Autonomic nervous system agent

Therapeutic class: Skeletal muscle relaxant (centrally acting)

Pregnancy risk category C

Action

Unknown; thought to depress central perception of pain without directly relaxing skeletal muscles or directly af-

fecting motor endplate or motor nerves

Availability

Injection: 100 mg/ml in 10-ml ampules, 100 mg/ml in 10-ml vials

Tablets: 500 mg, 750 mg

Indications and dosages

➤ Adjunct in muscle spasms associated with acute, painful musculoskeletal conditions

Adults: Initially, 1.5 g P.O. q.i.d. (up to 8 g/day) for 2 to 3 days, followed by 4 to 4.5 g/day P.O. in three to six divided doses; or 750 mg P.O. q 4 hours or 1 g P.O. q.i.d. or 1.5 g P.O. t.i.d. If oral dosing isn't feasible or if condition is severe, give 1 to 3 g/day I.M. or I.V. for a maximum of 3 days; course may be repeated after a 48-hour rest.

Off-label uses

• Tetanus

Contraindications

• Hypersensitivity to drug, its components, or polyethylene glycol (with parenteral form)

• Renal impairment (with parenteral form)

Administration

• Drug is usually given as part of regimen that includes rest and physical therapy.

• Don't give drug S.C.

• For direct I.V. injection, inject slowly; keep patient supine for 10 to 15 minutes afterward.

• For I.V. infusion, dilute 1 g with up to 250 ml of 5% dextrose or 0.9% sodium chloride injection.

• Avoid extravasation; drug is hypertonic.

• For I.M. use, inject no more than 500 mg (5 ml of 10% injection) into each gluteal area.

• Don't use parenteral form in patients with renal impairment; polyethylene

m

glycol vehicle may irritate kidneys.
• For tetanus management, crush and suspend tablets in water or saline solution, and give via nasogastric tube, if necessary.

Route	Onset	Peak	Duration
P.O.	30 min	2 hr	Unknown
I.V.	Immediate	End of infusion	Unknown
I.M.	Unknown	Unknown	Unknown

Adverse reactions

CNS: dizziness, light-headedness, drowsiness, syncope, **seizures** (with I.V. use)
CV: bradycardia or hypotension (with I.V. use)
EENT: blurred vision, conjunctivitis, nasal congestion
GI: nausea, GI upset, anorexia
GU: brown, black, or green urine
Musculoskeletal: mild muscle incoordination (with I.V. or I.M. use)
Skin: flushing (with I.V. use), pruritus, rash, urticaria
Other: fever, pain at I.M. injection site, phlebitis at I.V. site, allergic reactions including **anaphylaxis** (with I.M. or I.V. use)

Interactions

Drug-drug. *Antihistamines, CNS depressants (such as opioids, sedative-hypnotics):* additive CNS depression
Drug-diagnostic tests. *Urinary 5-hydroxyindoleacetic acid, urine vanillylmandelic acid:* false elevations
Drug-herb. *Chamomile, hops, kava, skullcap, valerian:* increased CNS depression
Drug-behaviors. *Alcohol use:* increased CNS depression

Precautions

Use cautiously in:
• seizure disorders (with parenteral use)
• pregnant or breastfeeding patients
• children (safety not established).

Patient monitoring

• Assess for orthostatic hypotension, especially with parenteral use. Keep patient supine for 10 to 15 minutes after I.V. administration.
• Watch for bradycardia and syncope after I.V. or I.M. administration. As needed and prescribed, give epinephrine, corticosteroids, or antihistamines to treat syncope.
• Monitor I.V. site for sloughing, pain, and thrombophlebitis.

Patient teaching

• Tell patient that drug may turn urine brown, black, or green.
• Advise patient to report adverse effects.
• Teach patient to avoid driving and other hazardous activities because drug may cause drowsiness or dizziness.
• Instruct patient to move slowly when changing position to avoid dizziness or light-headedness from sudden blood pressure decrease.
• As appropriate, review all other significant and life-threatening adverse reactions and interactions, especially those related to the drugs, tests, herbs, and behaviors mentioned above.

methotrexate
(amethopterin, MTX)

methotrexate sodium
Arbitrexate, Folex, Folex PFS, Mexate, Rheumatrex, Rheumatrex Dose Pack, Trexall

Pharmacologic class: Antimetabolite, folic acid antagonist
Therapeutic class: Antineoplastic
Pregnancy risk category X

Action

Reversibly binds to dihydrofolate reductase, interfering with folic acid metabolism and inhibiting DNA synthesis and cellular replication

Availability

Injection: 20-mg, 25-mg, 50-mg, 100-mg, 250-mg, and 1,000-mg vials *(lyophilized powder, preservative-free)*
Tablets: 2.5 mg, 5 mg, 7.5 mg, 10 mg, 15 mg

ⓘ Indications and dosages

➤ Acute lymphocytic leukemia
Adults and children: 3.3 mg/m^2 P.O. or I.M. for 4 to 6 weeks, then 20 to 30 mg/m^2 P.O. or I.M. weekly in two divided doses; given in combination with corticosteroid
➤ Meningeal leukemia
Adult and children: 12 mg/m^2 (maximum of 15 mg) intrathecally at intervals of 2 to 5 days, repeated until cerebrospinal fluid cell count is normal
➤ Burkitt's lymphoma
Adults: In stages I and II, 10 to 25 mg P.O. daily for 4 to 8 days; in stage III, combined with other neoplastic drugs. Patients in all stages usually require several courses of therapy, with 7- to 10-day rest periods between courses.
➤ Mycosis fungoides
Adults: 2.5 to 10 mg/day P.O., or 50 mg I.M. q week.
➤ Osteosarcoma
Adults: As part of adjunctive regimen with other antineoplastics, initially 12 g/m^2 I.V. as 4-hour infusion, then 12 to 15 g/m^2 I.V. as 4-hour infusion given at weeks 4, 5, 6, 7, 11, 12, 15, 16, 29, 30, 44, and 45 until peak blood level reaches 1,000 micromoles. Leucovorin rescue must start 24 hours after methotrexate infusion begins; if patient can't tolerate oral leucovorin, dose must be given I.M. or I.V. on same schedule.

➤ Trophoblastic tumors (choriocarcinoma, hydatidiform mole)
Adults: 15 to 30 mg P.O. or I.M. daily for 5 days. Repeat course three to five times as required, with rest periods of 1 week or more between courses, until toxic symptoms subside.
➤ Lymphosarcoma (stage III)
Adults: 0.625 to 2.5 mg/kg/day P.O., I.M., or I.V.
➤ Breast cancer
Adults: 40 mg/m^2 I.V. on days 1 and 8 of each treatment cycle, given with cyclophosphamide and fluorouracil; cycle is usually repeated monthly, with 2-week rest periods between cycles, for 6 to 12 months.
➤ Psoriasis
Adults: Give test dose of 5 to 10 mg P.O. 1 week before starting therapy to detect idiosyncratic reactions. Then give 2.5 to 5 mg P.O. at 12-hour intervals for three doses weekly or at 8-hour intervals for four doses weekly, to a maximum of 30 mg weekly. Alternatively, give 10 to 25 mg P.O., I.M., or I.V. as a single weekly dose, to a maximum dosage of 30 mg/week.
➤ Rheumatoid arthritis
Adults: 7.5 mg P.O. weekly as a single dose or divided as 2.5 mg q 12 hours for three doses. Gradually increase up to 20 mg/week; decrease dosage when adequate response occurs.
Dosage adjustment
• Renal or hepatic impairment
• Elderly patients

Off-label uses

• Relapsing-remitting multiple sclerosis
• Refractory Crohn's disease

Contraindications

• Hypersensitivity to drug
• Psoriasis or rheumatoid arthritis in pregnant patients
• Breastfeeding

m

Administration

◀€ Patient must be adequately hydrated before therapy, and urine must be alkalinized using sodium bicarbonate.

• Know that oral use is preferred. Give oral dose 1 hour before or 2 hours after meals; food decreases absorption of oral tablets and reduces peak blood level.

• Follow facility policy for handling, preparing, and administering carcinogenic, mutagenic, and teratogenic drugs.

• Reconstitute powder for injection with preservative-free solution, such as 5% dextrose solution or 0.9% sodium chloride injection. Reconstitute 20-mg and 50-mg vials to yield a concentration no greater than 25 mg/ml. Reconstitute 1-g vial with 19.4 ml to yield a concentration of 50 mg/ml.

• For high-dose I.V. infusion, dilute in 5% dextrose solution.

• For intrathecal use, reconstitute immediately before administration, using preservative-free solution (such as 0.9% sodium chloride for injection), to a concentration of 1 mg/ml.

◀€ For intrathecal or high-dose therapy, use preservative-free injection form.

• Avoid I.M. injections if platelet count is below 50,000/mm^3.

◀€ For osteosarcoma, ensure that leucovorin rescue is used appropriately in patients receiving high methotrexate doses, usually starting 24 hours after methotrexate infusion begins.

Route	Onset	Peak	Duration
P.O.	Unknown	1-2 hr	Unknown
I.V.	Immediate	Immediate	Unknown
I.M.	Unknown	0.5-1 hr	Unknown
Intrathecal	Unknown	Unknown	Unknown

Adverse reactions

CNS: demyelination, malaise, fatigue, dizziness, headache, aphasia, hemiparesis, drowsiness, **seizures, leukoencephalopathy, chemical arachnoiditis** (with intrathecal use)

EENT: blurred vision, pharyngitis

GI: nausea, vomiting, stomatitis, hematemesis, melena, GI ulcers, enteritis, gingivitis, pharyngitis, anorexia, **GI bleeding**

GU: hematuria, cystitis, infertility, menstrual dysfunction, defective spermatogenesis, abortion, **tubular necrosis, severe nephropathy, renal failure**

Hematologic: anemia, **leukopenia, thrombocytopenia, severe bone marrow depression**

Hepatic: elevated transaminase levels, **hepatotoxicity**

Metabolic: hyperuricemia, diabetes mellitus

Musculoskeletal: osteonecrosis, joint pain, myalgia, osteoporosis (with long-term use in children)

Respiratory: dry nonproductive cough, pneumonitis, **pulmonary fibrosis, pulmonary interstitial infiltrates**

Skin: pruritus, rash, urticaria, alopecia, painful plaque erosions, photosensitivity

Other: chills, fever, increased susceptibility to infection, **septicemia, anaphylaxis, sudden death**

Interactions

Drug-drug. *Activated charcoal:* decreased blood level of oral or I.V. methotrexate

Folic acid derivatives: antagonism of methotrexate effects

Fosphenytoin, phenytoin: decreased blood levels of these drugs

Hepatotoxic drugs: increased risk of hepatotoxicity

Nonsteroidal anti-inflammatory drugs, phenylbutazone, probenecid, salicylates, sulfonamides: increased methotrexate toxicity

Oral antibiotics: decreased methotrexate absorption

Penicillin, sulfonamide: increased methotrexate blood level
Procarbazine: increased nephrotoxicity
Theophylline: increased theophylline level
Vaccines: vaccine inefficacy
Drug-diagnostic tests. *Hemoglobin, platelets, red blood cells, white blood cells:* decreased values
Pregnancy tests: false-positive results
Protein-bound iodine, uric acid: increased levels
Drug-food. *Any food:* delayed methotrexate absorption and decreased peak blood level
Drug-herb. *Astragalus, echinacea, melatonin:* interference with methotrexate-induced immunosuppression
Drug-behaviors. *Alcohol use:* increased hepatotoxicity
Sun exposure: photosensitivity

Precautions

Use cautiously in:
• severe myocardial, hepatic, or renal disease; decreased bone marrow reserve; active infection; hypotension; coma
• elderly patients
• patients with childbearing potential
• young children.

Patient monitoring

• Watch for vomiting, diarrhea, or stomatitis, which may cause dehydration; discontinue therapy until these problems resolve.
◀≋ Know that high-dose therapy may cause nephrotoxicity. Monitor hydration status, urine alkalization (for pH above 6.5), methotrexate blood level, and renal function.
• Assess for fever, sore throat, bleeding, increased bruising, and other signs and symptoms of hematologic compromise or infection.
• With high-dose or intrathecal therapy, watch for CNS toxicity.
◀≋ Monitor creatinine and methotrexate blood levels 24 hours after ther-

apy starts and daily thereafter; adjust leucovorin dosage as prescribed.
• Check hematologic studies at least monthly; blood or platelet transfusions may be necessary.
• Monitor liver and kidney function studies every 1 to 3 months.
• Evaluate uric acid levels.
◀≋ Watch for signs and symptoms of pulmonary toxicity, such as fever, dry nonproductive cough, dyspnea, hypoxemia, and infiltrates on chest X-ray.
• Know that methotrexate exits slowly from third-space compartments (ascites, pleural effusions). Before therapy starts, fluid should be evacuated; during therapy, methotrexate blood level should be monitored.

Patient teaching

◀≋ Review dosing instructions carefully with patient to avoid toxicity. Tell patients with rheumatoid arthritis or psoriasis to take doses weekly.
• Teach patient to take oral doses 1 hour before or 2 hours after meals.
• Instruct patient to report diarrhea, abdominal pain, clay-colored or black tarry stools, fever, chills, sore throat, unusual bleeding or bruising, sores in or around mouth, cough or shortness of breath, yellowing of skin or eyes, dark or bloody urine, swelling of feet or legs, or joint pain.
• Teach patient to take temperature daily and to report fever or other signs or symptoms of infection.
• Instruct patient to drink 2 to 3 L of fluid each day.
• Advise male patients to use reliable contraception during therapy and for at least 3 months afterward; advise female patients to use reliable contraception during therapy and for one ovulatory cycle afterward.
• Teach patient not to take over-the-counter medications or herbal supplements without consulting prescriber.

m

• Advise patient to avoid sun exposure and to use sunscreen and protective clothing (especially if he has psoriasis).
• Instruct patient to avoid alcohol.
• Tell patient he'll need to undergo blood tests during therapy.
• As appropriate, review all other significant and life-threatening adverse reactions and interactions, especially those related to the drugs, tests, foods, herbs, and behaviors mentioned above.

methylcellulose
Citrucel, Entrocel✤, Prodiem✤

Pharmacologic class: Semisynthetic cellulose derivative
Therapeutic class: Bulk laxative
Pregnancy risk category NR

Action
Stimulates peristalsis by promoting water absorption into fecal matter and increasing bulk, resulting in bowel evacuation

Availability
Powder: 105 mg/g, 196 mg/g

🕖 Indications and dosages
➤ Chronic constipation
Adults and children older than age 12: Up to 6 g P.O. daily in divided doses of 0.45 g to 3 g
Children ages 6 to 12: Up to 3 g P.O. daily in divided doses of 0.45 g to 1.5 g

Contraindications
• Intestinal ulcers
• Hepatitis
• Signs or symptoms of appendicitis or acute surgical abdomen (such as abdominal pain, nausea, vomiting)

Administration
• Give with 8 oz of liquid.

• If patient is receiving maximum daily dosage, give in divided doses to reduce risk of esophageal obstruction.

Route	Onset	Peak	Duration
P.O.	12-24 hr	<3 days	Unknown

Adverse reactions
GI: nausea; vomiting; diarrhea; severe constipation; abdominal distention; cramps; esophageal, gastric, small intestinal, or colonic strictures (with dry form); **GI obstruction**
Other: laxative dependence (with long-term use)

Interactions
Drug-drug. *Antibiotics, digitalis, nitrofurantoin, oral anticoagulants, salicylates, tetracyclines:* decreased absorption and action of these drugs

Precautions
Use cautiously in:
• laxative-dependent patients.

Patient monitoring
• Assess patient's dietary habits; consider factors that promote constipation, such as certain diseases and medications.
• Monitor patient for signs and symptoms of esophageal obstruction.
• Evaluate fluid and electrolyte balance in patients using laxatives excessively.

Patient teaching
• Instruct patient to take drug with a full glass (8 oz) of water.
• Teach patient to prevent or minimize constipation through adequate fluid intake (four to six glasses of water daily), proper dietary habits, increased fiber intake, daily exercise, and responding promptly to urge to defecate.
◀€ Instruct patient to report chest pain or pressure, vomiting, and difficulty swallowing or breathing; these symptoms may indicate GI obstruction.

• Tell patient not to use drug for more than 1 week without prescriber's approval.

• Inform patient that chronic laxative use may lead to dependence.

• Teach patient to contact prescriber if constipation persists or if rectal bleeding or symptoms of electrolyte imbalance (muscle cramps, weakness, dizziness) occur.

• As appropriate, review all other significant and life-threatening adverse reactions and interactions, especially those related to the drugs mentioned above.

methyldopa
Aldomet, Apo-Methyldopa✤, Dopamet✤, Novomedopa✤, Nu-Medopa✤

methyldopate hydrochloride
Aldomet

Pharmacologic class: Centrally acting antiadrenergic
Therapeutic class: Antihypertensive
Pregnancy risk category B

Action
Stimulates CNS alpha-adrenergic receptors, decreasing sympathetic stimulation to the heart and blood vessels. Also reduces arterial pressure and plasma renin.

Availability
Injection: 50 mg/ml in 5- and 10-ml vials
Oral suspension (contains bisulfites): 250 mg/5 ml
Tablets: 125 mg, 250 mg, 500 mg

Indications and dosages
➤ Moderate to severe hypertension
Adults: 250 mg P.O. two to three times daily for 2 days (not to exceed 500 mg/day in divided doses if used with other agents); may be increased q 2 days as needed. Usual maintenance dosage is 500 mg to 2 g/day (not to exceed 3 g/day) P.O. in two to four divided doses or 250 to 500 mg I.V. q 6 hours (up to 1 g q 6 hours).
Children: 10 mg/kg/day (300 mg/m^2/day) P.O. in two to four divided doses; may be increased q 2 days up to 65 mg/kg/day (2 g/m^2/day), or 3 g/day in divided doses (whichever is lower) or 5 to 10 mg/kg I.V. q 6 hours; up to 65 mg/kg/day (2 g/m^2/day), or 3 g/day in divided doses (whichever is lower).

Contraindications
• Hypersensitivity to drug or its components
• Active hepatic disease or history of methyldopa-associated hepatic disorders
• Monoamine oxidase (MAO) inhibitor use within 14 days

Administration
• To prepare I.V. infusion, add required dosage to 100 ml of 5% dextrose injection. Or administer in 5% dextrose injection in a concentration of 100 mg/10 ml. Give over 30 to 60 minutes.
• Dilute and administer ADD-Vantage vials containing 50 mg/ml according to manufacturer's instructions.

Route	Onset	Peak	Duration
P.O.	Unknown	4-6 hr	24-48 hr
I.V.	Unknown	4-6 hr	10-16 hr

Adverse reactions
CNS: sedation, decreased mental acuity, depression, headache, asthenia, weakness, dizziness, paresthesia, parkinsonism, Bell's palsy, involuntary choreoathetotic movements

CV: bradycardia, edema, orthostatic hypotension, **myocarditis**
EENT: nasal congestion, sore black tongue
GI: nausea, vomiting, diarrhea, abdominal distention, colitis, dry mouth, sialadenitis, **pancreatitis**
GU: impotence, breast enlargement, gynecomastia, failure to ejaculate
Hematologic: eosinophilia, hemolytic anemia
Hepatic: abnormal liver function test results, **hepatitis**
Other: fever

Interactions
Drug-drug. *Adrenergics, MAO inhibitors:* excessive sympathetic stimulation
Amphetamines, barbiturates, nonsteroidal anti-inflammatory drugs, phenothiazines, tricyclic antidepressants: decreased antihypertensive effect
Anesthetics, antihypertensives, nitrates: additive hypotension
Ferrous gluconate, ferrous sulfate: decreased methyldopa blood level
Haloperidol: increased haloperidol effects, increased risk of psychoses
Levodopa: additive hypotension and CNS toxicity
Lithium: increased risk of lithium toxicity
Nonselective beta-adrenergic blockers: paradoxical hypertension
Tolbutamide: increased tolbutamide effects
Drug-diagnostic tests. *Alanine aminotransferase, alkaline phosphatase, aspartate aminotransferase, bilirubin, blood urea nitrogen, creatinine, potassium, prolactin, sodium, uric acid:* increased levels
Direct Coombs' test: positive results
Prothrombin time: prolonged
Drug-herb. *Capsicum:* reduced antihypertensive effects
Drug-behaviors. *Alcohol use:* increased hypotension

Precautions
Use cautiously in:
• elderly patients
• pregnant or breastfeeding patients.

Patient monitoring
• Monitor periodic blood counts to detect adverse hematologic reactions.
• Obtain direct Coombs' test before therapy starts and then 6 and 12 months later.
• Monitor hepatic function test results and check for signs and symptoms of hepatic dysfunction (particularly during first 6 to 12 weeks of therapy).
• Check for edema or weight gain. Diuretic may need to be added to regimen.
• Monitor blood pressure; drug tolerance may occur during second and third months of therapy.

Patient teaching
• Teach patient that sedation usually occurs when therapy starts and during dosage titration. To lessen this effect, advise him to initiate dosage titration in evening.
• Instruct patient to report fever, yellowing of skin or eyes, fatigue, abdominal pain, or flulike symptoms. Also tell him to report swelling or significant weight gain.
• Inform patient that urine may darken after exposure to air.
• Teach patient to move slowly when changing position to avoid dizziness or light-headedness from sudden blood pressure decrease.
• Advise patient to avoid driving and other hazardous activities until effects of drug are known or dosage titration is completed.
• As appropriate, review all other significant and life-threatening adverse reactions and interactions, especially those related to the drugs, tests, herbs, and behaviors mentioned above.

methylergonovine maleate
Methergine

Pharmacologic class: Ergot alkaloid
Therapeutic class: Oxytocic
Pregnancy risk category C

Action
Directly stimulates vascular smooth-muscle contractions in the uterus and cervix

Availability
Injection: 0.2 mg/ml
Tablets: 0.2 mg

💊 Indications and dosages
➤ Prevention and treatment of post-partum hemorrhage
Adults: 0.2 mg I.M.; repeat q 2 to 4 hours as needed to a total of five doses. Or, in emergencies, give 0.2 mg I.V. over 1 minute. After initial I.M. or I.V. dose, give 0.2 mg P.O. q 6 to 8 hours for 2 to 7 days; decrease dosage if cramping occurs.

Contraindications
• Hypersensitivity to drug
• Hypertension
• Toxemia
• Pregnancy (except in third stage of labor)

Administration
• Be aware that drug isn't routinely given I.V. because of risk of severe hypertension and cerebrovascular accident (CVA). Monitor blood pressure and uterine contractions during administration.
• If I.V. use is necessary, administer dose over 1 minute. Dose may be diluted in 5 ml of 0.9% sodium chloride injection.

• Know that reducing dosage may control severe uterine cramping.
• Be aware that prolonged therapy should be avoided because of risk of ergotism.

Route	Onset	Peak	Duration
P.O.	5-10 min	30 min	3 hr
I.V.	Immediate	Unknown	45 min
I.M.	2-5 min	Unknown	3 hr

Adverse reactions
CNS: dizziness, headache, hallucination, **seizures, CVA** (with I.V. use)
CV: hypertension, hypotension, transient chest pain, palpitations, thrombophlebitis
EENT: tinnitus, nasal congestion
GI: nausea, vomiting, diarrhea, foul taste
GU: hematuria
Musculoskeletal: leg cramps
Respiratory: dyspnea
Skin: diaphoresis, rash, allergic reactions

Interactions
Drug-drug. *Dopamine, ergot alkaloids, oxytocin, regional anesthetics, vasoconstrictors:* excessive vasoconstriction
Drug-diagnostic tests. *Prolactin:* increased level

Precautions
Use cautiously in:
• severe hepatic or renal disease, vascular disease, jaundice, sepsis
• patients in second stage of labor.

Patient monitoring
◀€ Know that if used during third stage of labor, drug increases risk for hemorrhage and infection.
• When giving drug I.V., closely monitor blood pressure and pulse, uterine contractions, and bleeding.
• Monitor patient for adverse effects.

Patient teaching
• Inform patient and family of reason for using drug; provide reassurance.
• Teach patient that drug may cause nausea, vomiting, dizziness, increased blood pressure, headache, ringing in ears, chest pain, or shortness of breath. Advise her to report severe or troublesome symptoms.
• As appropriate, review all other significant and life-threatening adverse reactions and interactions, especially those related to the drugs and tests mentioned above.

methylphenidate hydrochloride
Concerta, Focalin, Metadate CD, Metadate ER, Methylin, Methylin ER, PHL-Methylphenidate✦, PMS-Methylphenidate✦, Riphenidate✦, Ritalin, Ritalin LA, Ritalin-SR

Pharmacologic class: Piperidine derivative
Therapeutic class: CNS stimulant
Controlled substance schedule II
Pregnancy risk category C

Action
Increases release of norepinephrine, stimulating impulse transmission in the respiratory system and CNS and increasing mental alertness

Availability
Capsules (extended-release): 10 mg, 20 mg, 30 mg, 40 mg
Tablets (chewable): 2.5 mg, 5 mg, 10 mg
Tablets (extended-release): 10 mg, 18 mg, 20 mg, 27 mg, 36 mg, 54 mg
Tablets (prompt-release): 5 mg, 10 mg, 20 mg
Tablets (sustained-release): 20 mg

Indications and dosages
➤ Adjunctive treatment of attention deficit hyperactivity disorder (ADHD)
Adults: 5 to 20 mg P.O. (prompt-release tablets) two to three times daily; when maintenance dosage is determined, may switch to extended-release form.
Children older than age 6: Initially, 5 mg P.O. (prompt-release tablets) before breakfast and lunch; increase by 5 to 10 mg at weekly intervals, not to exceed 60 mg/day. When maintenance dosage is determined, may switch to extended-release form.

If previous methylphenidate dosage was 10 mg b.i.d. or 20 mg sustained-release, give Ritalin LA 20 mg P.O. once daily. If previous methylphenidate dosage was 15 mg b.i.d., give Ritalin LA 30 mg P.O. once daily. If previous methylphenidate dosage was 20 mg b.i.d. or 40 mg sustained-release, give Ritalin LA 40 mg P.O. once daily. If previous methylphenidate dosage was 30 mg b.i.d. or 60 mg sustained-release, give Ritalin LA 60 mg P.O. once daily.

In all patients, Ritalin-SR or Metadate ER may be used instead of prompt-release tablets when 8-hour dosage of those forms corresponds to titrated 8-hour dosage of prompt-release tablets.
Concerta—
Children ages 6 and older who haven't used methylphenidate previously: Initially, 18 mg P.O. once daily in morning; may be titrated weekly up to 54 mg/day
Children ages 6 and older using other methylphenidate forms: 18 mg P.O. once daily in morning if previous dosage was 5 mg two to three times daily, or 20 mg P.O. daily (sustained-release); 36 mg once daily in morning if previous dosage was 10 mg two to three times daily or 40 mg daily (sustained-release); or 54 mg once daily in

morning if previous dosage was 15 mg
two to three times daily or 60 mg once
daily (sustained-release)
Metadate CD—
Children ages 6 and older: Initially, 20
mg once daily; may be adjusted in
weekly 20-mg increments, to a maximum dosage of 60 mg/day taken once
daily in morning
➣ Narcolepsy
Adults: 10 mg P.O. (Ritalin, Ritalin SR,
or Metadate ER) two to three times
daily, 30 to 45 minutes before a meal.
Some patients may require up to 60 mg
daily.

Off-label uses
• Depression in ill, elderly patients
(such as those with cerebrovascular accident)
• To enhance analgesia and sedation in
patients receiving opioids

Contraindications
• Hypersensitivity to drug or its com-
ponents
• Glaucoma
• Motor tics, Tourette syndrome (or
family history of syndrome)
• Psychosis
• Suicidal or homicidal tendencies
• Monoamine oxidase (MAO) in-
hibitor use within 14 days

Administration
• Don't crush extended-release tablets
or extended-release trilayer core tablets
(Concerta).
• Have patient swallow extended-
release capsules (Metadate CD, Ritalin
LA) intact; or, if desired, sprinkle entire
contents onto small amount (1 tbsp)
of applesauce immediately before administration. (However, don't sprinkle
Ritalin LA onto warm applesauce because its release properties may be affected.) Give water after patient swallows dose.
• Don't give extended-release tablets to
initiate therapy or for daily use until

dosage has been titrated using conventional tablets.
• Give extended-release tablets at 8-
hour intervals if 8-hour dosage corresponds to titrated 8-hour dosage for
conventional tablets. Alternatively, extended-release capsules or extended-
release trilayer core tablets may be used
for initial dosing.
• To help prevent insomnia, give last
daily dose of conventional tablets several hours before bedtime.
• Discontinue drug periodically in
children who have responded to therapy, to assess patient's condition. After
withdrawal, improvement may be temporary or permanent.
• Be aware that therapy shouldn't continue indefinitely; it's usually discontinued by adolescence.

Route	Onset	Peak	Duration
P.O.	Unknown	1-3 hr	4-6 hr
P.O. (extended)	Unknown	Unknown	Up to 8 hr

Adverse reactions
CNS: hyperactivity, insomnia, restlessness, tremor, dizziness, headache, irritability, akathisia, dyskinesia, **toxic psychosis**
CV: hypertension, hypotension, palpitations, tachycardia
EENT: blurred vision
GI: nausea, vomiting, diarrhea, constipation, cramps, dry mouth, metallic
taste, anorexia
Skin: rash
Other: fever, suppression of weight
gain (in children), hypersensitivity reactions, physical or psychological drug
dependence, drug tolerance

Interactions
Drug-drug. *Anticonvulsants, selective
serotonin reuptake inhibitors, tricyclic
antidepressants, warfarin:* inhibited
metabolism and increased effects of
these drugs

Guanethidine: antagonism of hypotensive effect

MAO inhibitors, vasopressors: hypertensive crisis

Drug-food. *Caffeine-containing foods and beverages (coffee, cola, tea):* additive CNS stimulation

Drug-herb. *Ephedra, caffeine-containing herbs (cola nut, guarana, maté):* increased CNS stimulation

Drug-behaviors. *Alcohol use:* additive hypotension

Precautions

Use cautiously in:
• hypertension, cardiovascular disease, diabetes mellitus, seizure disorders
• elderly or debilitated patients
• pregnant or breastfeeding patients.

Patient monitoring

• Monitor patient periodically for drug tolerance and psychological dependence.
• Monitor patient for adverse effects; know that such effects usually can be controlled by adjusting schedule or dosage.
• Watch for tachycardia, abdominal pain, insomnia, anorexia, and weight loss (more common in children than adults).
• Consider periodic hematologic and hepatic studies, especially during prolonged therapy.
• Monitor blood pressure, especially in patients with history of hypertension.
• Evaluate child's weight and growth patterns.
• Assess child for tics, which may develop in 15% to 30% of children using drug.

Patient teaching

• Teach patient or parent that last daily dose should be taken several hours before bedtime to avoid insomnia.

• Make sure patient or parent understands how drug should be administered.
• Tell patients taking Concerta not to be concerned if tablet-like substance appears in stool.
• Teach patient or parent to report insomnia, palpitations, vomiting, fever, or rash.
• Caution patient or parent that continual use may lead to psychological or physical dependence.
• Instruct patient to avoid driving and other hazardous tasks until drug effects are known.
• As appropriate, review all other significant and life-threatening adverse reactions and interactions, especially those related to the drugs, foods, herbs, and behaviors mentioned above.

methylprednisolone
Medrol

methylprednisolone acetate
depMedalone, Depo-Medrol, Depoject, Depopred, Duralone, Medralone, M-Prednisol, M-Predrol, Medrol Dosepak, Meprolone Unipak, Methysone✚, Unimed✚

methylprednisolone sodium succinate
A-Methapred, Solu-Medrol

Pharmacologic class: Glucocorticoid

Therapeutic class: Antiasthmatic, antiinflammatory (steroidal), immunosuppressant

Pregnancy risk category C

Action

Unclear; reduces inflammation by stabilizing the membranes of leukocytic cells, reducing permeability and preventing edema; suppresses the immune system by reducing activity in the lymphatic system and interfering with antigen-antibody interactions of macrophages and T cells.

Availability
Enema: 40 mg
Solution for injection: 40 mg, 125 mg, 500 mg, 1 g, 2 g
Suspension for injection: 20 mg/ml, 40 mg/ml, 80 mg/ml
Tablets: 2 mg, 4 mg, 8 mg, 16 mg, 24 mg, 32 mg

⚕ Indications and dosages
➤ Diseases and disorders of the endocrine system, collagen, skin, eye, GI tract, and respiratory and hematologic systems; neoplastic diseases; allergies; edema; multiple sclerosis; tuberculous meningitis; trichinosis; rheumatic disorders; osteoarthritis; bursitis; localized inflammatory lesions
Adults: *Methylprednisolone*—2 to 60 mg P.O. daily in four divided doses, depending on disease or disorder.
Acetate—10 to 80 mg I.M., 4 to 80 mg by intra-articular or soft-tissue injection, or 20 to 60 mg intralesional injection (depending on type, size, and location of inflammation); may be repeated at 1 to 5 weeks.
Sodium succinate high-dose therapy—30 mg/kg I.V. given over at least 30 minutes; may be repeated q 4 to 6 hours. Doses may be administered by I.V. injection or infusion or by I.M. route.
➤ Life-threatening shock
Adults: Initially, 30 mg/kg (sodium succinate) I.V. given over 3 to 15 minutes, repeated q 4 to 6 hours as necessary; or 100 to 250 mg I.V. given over 3 to 15 minutes, repeated q 2 to 6 hours as necessary. High-dose therapy should end after 72 hours.

Off-label uses
• Lupus nephritis
• *Pneumocystis jiroveci* (formerly *Pneumocystis carinii*) pneumonia in AIDS patients

Contraindications
• Hypersensitivity to drug, its components, bisulfite, tartrazine
• Systemic fungal infections
• Idiopathic thrombocytopenic purpura

Administration
• As needed and prescribed, give prophylactic antacids to prevent peptic ulcers in patients receiving high doses.
• When methylprednisolone acetate is substituted for oral form, know that I.M. dosage should equal oral dosage and should be given once daily.
• Know that methylprednisolone acetate is not for I.V. use; it may be given I.M. or by intra-articular, intralesional, or soft-tissue injection.
• Be aware that methylprednisolone sodium succinate may be given I.M. or I.V. Reconstitute with bacteriostatic water for injection containing 0.9% benzyl alcohol, per manufacturer's instructions.
• When long-term methylprednisolone therapy is anticipated, alternate-day therapy should be considered.
• For direct I.V. injection, inject over at least 1 minute. For I.V. infusion, further dilute in compatible I.V. solution, such as 5% dextrose, 0.9% sodium chloride, or 5% dextrose in 0.9% sodium chloride injection. Use solution within 48 hours after mixing.

Route	Onset	Peak	Duration
P.O.	Rapid	2-3 hr	30-36 hr
I.M., I.V. (succinate)	Rapid	Unknown	Unknown
I.M. (acetate)	6-48 hr	4-8 days	1-4 wk

Adverse reactions

CNS: headache, restlessness, nervousness, depression, euphoria, personality changes, psychoses, vertigo, paresthesias, insomnia, meningitis, adhesive arachnoiditis, conus medullaris syndrome, **increased intracranial pressure, seizures**

CV: hypotension, thrombophlebitis, hypertension, **heart failure, arrhythmias, shock, fat embolism, thromboembolism**

EENT: cataracts, glaucoma, increased intraocular pressure, nasal irritation, nasal septum perforation, anosmia, sneezing, epistaxis, nasopharyngeal or oropharyngeal fungal infection, dysphonia, hoarseness, throat irritation

GI: nausea, vomiting, abdominal distention, rectal bleeding, bad taste, dry mouth, anorexia, esophageal ulcer or candidiasis, **peptic ulceration, pancreatitis**

GU: amenorrhea, irregular menses

Respiratory: cough, wheezing, **bronchospasm**

Metabolic: adrenal suppression (with long-term, high-dose use), decreased growth (in children), decreased carbohydrate tolerance, diabetes mellitus, hyperglycemia, sodium and fluid retention, hypokalemia, hypocalcemia, cushingoid state (with long-term use), hypothalamic-pituitary-adrenal suppression (with systemic use longer than 5 days), **acute adrenal insufficiency** (with abrupt withdrawal)

Musculoskeletal: muscle wasting, osteoporosis, osteonecrosis, tendon rupture, aseptic joint necrosis, muscle pain and weakness, steroid myopathy, spontaneous fractures (with long-term use)

Skin: facial edema, rash, pruritus, urticaria, contact dermatitis, acne, decreased wound healing, bruising, hirsutism, thin and fragile skin, petechiae, purpura, striae, subcutaneous fat atrophy, skin atrophy, acneiform lesions, angioedema

Other: increased appetite, weight gain (with long-term use), Churg-Strauss syndrome, increased susceptibility to infection, aggravation or masking of infections, impaired wound healing, atrophy at injection site, local pain and burning, irritation, hypersensitivity reaction

Interactions

Drug-drug. *Amphotericin B, mezlocillin, piperacillin, thiazide and loop diuretics, ticarcillin:* additive hypokalemia

Fluoroquinolones: increased risk of tendon rupture

Isoniazid, phenobarbital, phenytoin, rifampin: decreased methylprednisolone efficacy

Ketoconazole: decreased methylprednisolone clearance

Live-virus vaccines: decreased antibody response to vaccine, increased risk of adverse reactions

Nonsteroidal anti-inflammatory drugs: increased risk of adverse GI effects

Oral anticoagulants: altered anticoagulant requirements

Drug-diagnostic tests. *Calcium, potassium, thyroxine, triiodothyronine:* decreased levels

Cholesterol, glucose: increased levels

Nitroblue-tetrazolium test for bacterial infection: false-negative results

Drug-herb. *Echinacea:* increased immune stimulation

Ginseng: immunomodulation

Drug-behaviors. *Alcohol use:* increased risk of gastric irritation and ulcers

Precautions

Use cautiously in:
• cardiovascular, hepatic, renal, or GI disease; active untreated infections; thromboembolitic tendency; osteoporosis; myasthenia gravis; hypothyroidism; glaucoma; ocular herpes simplex; vaccinia or varicella; seizure disorders; metastatic carcinoma
• pregnant or breastfeeding patients
• children.

Patient monitoring
- Maintain patient on lowest effective dosage to minimize adverse effects.
- Monitor fluid and electrolyte balance, weight, and blood pressure.
- With long-term or high-dose use, assess patient for cushingoid effects, such as moon face, central obesity, acne, abdominal striae, hypertension, osteoporosis, myopathy, hyperglycemia, fluid and electrolyte imbalances, and increased susceptibility to infection.
- ◀€ Check for signs and symptoms of steroid-induced psychosis—delirium, euphoria, insomnia, mood swings, personality changes, and depression.
- Monitor growth and development in children on prolonged therapy.
- Know that long-term therapy (over 6 months) increases risk for osteoporosis. Obtain baseline bone density mass, and provide teaching about lifestyle factors (such as weight-bearing exercise, proper diet, moderation of alcohol intake, and smoking cessation) and possible need for calcium, vitamin D, or bisphosphonate therapy.
- With long-term use, withdraw drug gradually.
- ◀€ After dosage reduction or drug withdrawal, monitor patient for signs and symptoms of adrenal insufficiency.

Patient teaching
- Teach patient to take drug with food to minimize GI upset.
- Instruct patient on chronic therapy to have periodic eye examinations and to carry medical identification that states he's taking drug.
- Inform patient that drug increases risk for infection; advise him to avoid exposure to infections such as measles and chickenpox. Tell him to contact prescriber if exposure occurs.
- Teach patient to report unusual weight gain, leg or foot swelling, facial swelling, muscle weakness, black tarry stools, vomiting of blood, menstrual irregularities, sore throat, fever, or infection.
- ◀€ Tell patient to immediately report signs or symptoms of adrenal insufficiency (including fatigue, appetite loss, nausea, vomiting, diarrhea, weight loss, weakness, and dizziness) after dosage reduction or drug withdrawal.
- Advise diabetic patients to monitor blood glucose level carefully.
- As appropriate, review all other significant and life-threatening adverse reactions and interactions, especially those related to the drugs, tests, herbs, and behaviors mentioned above.

methysergide maleate
Sansert

Pharmacologic class: Ergot alkaloid
Therapeutic class: Serotonin antagonist, adrenergic blocker
Pregnancy risk category X

m

Action
Blocks the activity of serotonin, decreasing its vasoconstrictor effects in the brain

Availability
Tablets: 1 mg, 2 mg

Indications and dosages
➤ To prevent migraine or other vascular headaches
Adults: 4 to 8 mg P.O. daily in divided doses, with a 3- to 4-week rest period after each 6-month treatment

Contraindications
- Hypersensitivity to drug
- Coronary artery or valvular heart disease
- Hypertension
- Hepatic or renal disease

- Connective tissue disease
- Fibrotic pulmonary disease
- Phlebitis or cellulitis
- Pregnancy

Administration

- To minimize GI upset, give with food or milk, or initiate therapy gradually.
- Be aware that if drug is used for cluster headaches, it is usually given only during a cluster headache.
- After 6-month course, patient should discontinue therapy for 3 to 4 weeks. To avoid rebound headache, reduce dosage gradually over 2 to 3 weeks before withdrawal.

Route	Onset	Peak	Duration
P.O.	1-2 days	Unknown	1-2 days after last dose

Adverse reactions

CNS: rapid speech, hallucinations, euphoria, feelings of dissociation, weakness, hyperesthesia, light-headedness, ataxia, vertigo, drowsiness, insomnia
CV: vasoconstriction; chest pain; vascular insufficiency of legs; coldness, numbness, and pain in arms and legs; diminished or absent pulses; orthostatic hypotension; bruits; murmurs; peripheral edema; tachycardia; **fibrotic thickening of cardiac valves**
GI: nausea, vomiting, diarrhea, constipation, abdominal pain, heartburn, **retroperitoneal fibrosis**
Hematologic: eosinophilia, **neutropenia**
Musculoskeletal: joint pain, myalgia
Respiratory: pulmonary fibrosis
Skin: rash, flushing, alopecia
Other: weight gain

Interactions

Drug-drug. *Beta blockers:* increased peripheral ischemia, cold arms and legs
Drug-diagnostic tests. *Eosinophils:* increased count
Neutrophils: decreased count

Precautions

Use cautiously in:
- peptic ulcers
- breastfeeding
- children.

Patient monitoring

◀≋ Watch for fibrotic or vascular complications, including signs and symptoms of retroperitoneal fibrosis (malaise, fatigue, weight loss, backache, low-grade fever, urinary obstruction with flank pain, dysuria, polyuria, oliguria, elevated blood urea nitrogen, and vascular insufficiency of legs). I.V. pyelography is the most useful diagnostic test and should be repeated every 6 to 12 months during therapy.
◀≋ Monitor patient for signs and symptoms of pleuropulmonary fibrosis, including dyspnea, chest pain, pleural friction rub, and pleural effusion confirmed on chest X-ray.
◀≋ Check for signs and symptoms of cardiac fibrosis, including heart murmurs and dyspnea.

Patient teaching

- Tell patient to take oral doses with food or milk to minimize GI upset.
◀≋ Instruct patient to report signs or symptoms of impaired circulation (such as cold, numb, or painful hands and feet, leg cramps when walking, flank or chest pain, shortness of breath, or peripheral edema of ankle or hands).
- Teach patient that if his condition doesn't improve within 3 weeks, drug is unlikely to bring benefit.
- Advise patient to avoid driving and other activities that require mental alertness or coordination.
- As appropriate, review all other significant and life-threatening adverse reactions and interactions, especially those related to the drugs and tests mentioned above.

metoclopramide hydrochloride

Apo-Metoclop✦, Clopra, Emex, Maxeran✦, Maxolone, M-Predrol, Nu-Metoclopramide✦, Octamide, Octamide-PFS, Reglan

Pharmacologic class: Dopamine antagonist

Therapeutic class: Antiemetic, GI stimulant

Pregnancy risk category B

Action
Blocks dopamine receptors by disrupting the chemoreceptor trigger zone of the CNS, increasing peristalsis and promoting gastric emptying

Availability
Injection: 5 mg/ml
Solution (concentrated): 10 mg/ml
Syrup: 5 mg/5 ml
Tablets: 5 mg, 10 mg

Indications and dosages
➤ To prevent chemotherapy-induced vomiting
Adults: 1 to 2 mg/kg I.V. 30 minutes before chemotherapy. Two additional doses of 1 to 2 mg/kg may be given q 2 hours, then q 3 hours for three additional doses.
➤ To facilitate small-bowel intubation
Adults and children over age 14: 10 mg I.V.
Children ages 6 to 14: 2.5 to 5 mg I.V.
Children under age 6: 0.1 mg/kg I.V.
➤ Diabetic gastroparesis
Adults: 10 mg P.O. 30 minutes before meals and at bedtime for 2 to 8 weeks; if patient can't tolerate P.O. doses, give same dosage I.V. or I.M.
➤ Gastroesophageal reflux
Adults: 10 to 15 mg P.O. 30 minutes before meals and at bedtime (not to

exceed 0.5 mg/kg/day) for up to 12 weeks. For prevention, give a single dose of 20 mg (some patients may respond to doses as small as 5 mg).
➤ Postoperative nausea and vomiting
Adults: 10 to 20 mg I.M. near end of surgical procedure; repeat dose q 4 to 6 hours, as needed.
Dosage adjustment
• Renal impairment

Off-label uses
• Hiccups

Contraindications
• Hypersensitivity to drug
• Pheochromocytoma
• Parkinson's disease
• Suspected GI obstruction, perforation, or hemorrhage
• History of seizure disorders

Administration
• Mix oral solution with water, juice, carbonated beverages, or semisolid food (such as applesauce or pudding) just before administration.
• Give I.M. or direct I.V. without further dilution.
• Administer low doses (10 mg or less) by direct I.V. injection slowly over 1 to 2 minutes. (Rapid injection may cause intense anxiety and restlessness followed by drowsiness.)
• For I.V. infusion, dilute with 50 ml of 5% dextrose in 0.9% sodium chloride solution, 5% dextrose in 0.45% sodium chloride solution, or lactated Ringer's solution. Infuse over at least 15 minutes.

Route	Onset	Peak	Duration
P.O.	30-60 min	Unknown	1-2 hr
I.V.	1-3 min	Immediate	1-2 hr
I.M.	10-15 min	Unknown	1-2 hr

Adverse reactions
CNS: drowsiness, extrapyramidal reactions, restlessness, anxiety, depression,

m

irritability, tardive dyskinesia, fatigue, lassitude, insomnia, parkinsonian-like reactions, akathisia, dystonia

CV: hypertension, hypotension, **arrhythmias**

GI: nausea, constipation, diarrhea, dry mouth

GU: gynecomastia

Interactions

Drug-drug. *Anticholinergics, opioids:* antagonism of metoclopramide's effects on GI motility

Antidepressants, antihistamines, other CNS depressants (such as opioids, sedative-hypnotics): additive CNS depression

Cimetidine, digoxin: decreased blood levels of these drugs

General anesthestics: exaggerated hypotension

Haloperidol, phenothiazines: increased risk of extrapyramidal reactions

Levodopa: decreased metoclopramide efficacy

Monoamine oxidase inhibitors: increased catecholamine release

Drug-diagnostic tests. *Aldosterone, prolactin:* increased levels

Drug-behaviors. *Alcohol use:* increased blood alcohol level, increased CNS depression

Precautions

Use cautiously in:
• diabetes mellitus
• history of depression
• elderly patients
• pregnant or breastfeeding patients
• children.

Patient monitoring

• Monitor blood pressure during I.V. administration.

• Stay alert for depression and other adverse CNS effects.

◀€ Watch for extrapyramidal symptoms, which usually occur within first 24 to 48 hours of therapy. To reverse these symptoms, give diphenhydra-

mine 50 mg I.M. or benztropine 1 to 2 mg I.M., as prescribed.

• Check for development of parkinsonian-like symptoms, which may occur within first 6 months of therapy and usually subside within 2 to 3 months after withdrawal.

• With long-term use, assess patient for tardive dyskinesia.

• In diabetic patients, stay alert for gastric stasis; insulin dosage may need to be adjusted.

Patient teaching

• Teach patient to take drug 30 minutes before meals.

• Caution patient to avoid driving and other hazardous activities until drug's effects are known.

• Instruct patient to report involuntary movements of face, eyes, or limbs.

• As appropriate, review all other significant and life-threatening adverse reactions and interactions, especially those related to the drugs, tests, and behaviors mentioned above.

metolazone
Diulo, Mykrox, Zaroxolyn

Pharmacologic class: Thiazide-like diuretic

Therapeutic class: Diuretic, antihypertensive

Pregnancy risk category B

Action

Inhibits electrolyte reabsorption from ascending loop of Henle and decreases reabsorption of sodium and potassium in the distal renal tubules, increasing osmotic pressure in plasma and promoting diuresis

Availability

Tablets: 2.5 mg, 5 mg, 10 mg
Tablets (rapid-acting): 0.5 mg

⚕ Indications and dosages
➤ Hypertension
Adult: Initially, 0.5 mg (Mykrox) P.O., usually in morning, increased to 1 mg P.O. daily if necessary. Or 2.5 mg to 5 mg (Zaroxolyn) P.O. daily.
➤ Edema secondary to heart failure or renal disease
Adults: 5 to 20 mg (Zaroxolyn) P.O. daily

Contraindications
• Hypersensitivity to drug or other sulfonamide-derived drugs
• Anuria
• Hepatic coma

Administration
• Give drug in morning to avoid nighttime urination.
◀≣ Know that Mykrox and Zaroxoylin aren't equivalent and shouldn't be interchanged.
• Discontinue drug before parathyroid function tests are performed.
• Be aware that metolazone is the only thiazide-like diuretic that may produce diuresis in patients with glomerular filtration rates below 20 ml/minute.

Route	Onset	Peak	Duration
P.O.	1 hr	2 hr	12-24 hr

Adverse reactions
CNS: drowsiness, lethargy, vertigo, paresthesia, weakness, headache, fatigue
CV: chest pain, hypotension, palpitations, venous thrombosis, volume depletion, **arrhythmias**
GI: nausea, vomiting, bloating, cramping, anorexia, **pancreatitis**
GU: polyuria, nocturia, impotence, decreased libido
Hematologic: aplastic anemia, leukopenia, agranulocytosis
Hepatic: hepatitis
Metabolic: hypokalemia, dehydration, hypercalcemia, hypochloremic alkalosis, hypomagnesemia, hyponatremia, hypophosphatemia, hypovolemia, hyperglycemia, hyperuricemia
Musculoskeletal: muscle cramps
Skin: photosensitivity, rashes
Other: chills

Interactions
Drug-drug. *Amphotericin B, corticosteroids, mezlocillin, piperacillin, ticarcillin:* additive hypokalemia
Antigout drugs: increased uric acid level
Antihypertensives, nitrates: additive hypotension
Digoxin: increased risk of digoxin toxicity
Lithium: decreased lithium excretion, increased risk of lithium toxicity
Drug-diagnostic tests. *Bilirubin, calcium, cholesterol, creatinine, low-density lipoproteins, triglycerides, uric acid:* increased levels
Blood glucose, urine glucose: increased levels in diabetic patients
Magnesium, potassium, protein-bound iodine, sodium, urinary calcium: decreased levels
Drug-food. *Any food:* increased metolazone absorption
Drug-herb. *Aloe, cascara sagrada, senna:* increased risk of hypokalemia
Drug-behaviors. *Sun exposure:* increased risk of photosensitivity

Precautions
Use cautiously in:
• severe hepatic or renal impairment, gout, hyperparathyroidism, glucose tolerance abnormalities, fluid and electrolyte imbalances, bipolar disorders
• elderly patients
• pregnancy and breastfeeding
• children (safety not established).

Patient monitoring
• Monitor baseline and periodic electrolyte, blood urea nitrogen, glucose, and uric acid levels.
• Evaluate blood pressure regularly.
◀≣ Watch for signs and symptoms of hypokalemia, which may necessitate

m

---

potassium supplements, potassium-rich diet, or potassium-sparing diuretic. Hypokalemia is particularly dangerous to patients who are on digitalis or have had ventricular arrhythmias.

• Assess patient for fluid and electrolyte imbalances.

Patient teaching
• Advise patient to take drug in morning to avoid nighttime urination.
• Tell patient he may take drug with food or milk to prevent GI upset.
◀€ Instruct patient to report muscle pain, weakness, or cramps; nausea; vomiting; diarrhea; dizziness; restlessness; excessive thirst; fatigue; drowsiness; increased pulse; or irregular heart beats.
• Inform patient that drug may cause gout attacks. Advise him to report sudden joint pain.
• Teach patient to use sunscreen and protective clothing to avoid photosensitivity.
• As appropriate, review all other significant and life-threatening adverse reactions and interactions, especially those related to the drugs, tests, foods, herbs, and behaviors mentioned above.

metoprolol succinate
Toprol-XL

metoprolol tartrate
Apo-Metoprolol✤, Betaloc✤, Betaloc Durules✤, Lopresor, Lopresor SR✤, Lopressor, Novo-Metoprol✤, Nu-Metop✤, PMS-Metoprolol-L✤

Pharmacologic class: Beta-adrenergic blocker (selective)
Therapeutic class: Antihypertensive, antianginal
Pregnancy risk category C

Action
Blocks stimulation of beta$_1$ (myocardial)-adrenergic receptors, usually without affecting beta$_2$ (pulmonary, vascular, uterine)-adrenergic receptor sites

Availability
Injection (tartrate): 1 mg/ml
Tablets: 50 mg, 100 mg
Tablets (extended-release, succinate): 25 mg, 50 mg, 100 mg, 200 mg
Tablets (extended-release, tartrate): 100 mg

🕭 Indications and dosages
➢ Hypertension
Adults: 50 to 100 mg P.O. daily as a single dose or in two divided doses (conventional tablets) or once daily (extended-release tablets); may be increased q 7 days as needed, up to 450 mg/day (tartrate) or 400 mg (succinate extended-release)
➢ Angina pectoris
Adults: 100 mg P.O. daily as a single dose or in two divided doses (conventional tablets) or once daily (extended-release tablets); may be increased q 7 days as needed, up to 400 mg
➢ Acute myocardial infarction (MI)
Adults: As early treatment, 2.5 to 5 mg by rapid I.V. injection at approximately 2- to 5-minute intervals, to a total dosage of 15 mg over 10 to 15 minutes. If patient tolerates I.V. dose, give 50 mg P.O. 15 minutes after last I.V. dose, and continue P.O. doses q 6 hours for 48 hours. Maintenance dosage is 100 mg P.O. b.i.d. If patient doesn't tolerate I.V. dose, give 25 to 50 mg P.O. (depending on degree of intolerance), starting 15 minutes after last I.V. dose or when clinical condition allows; discontinue drug if patient shows severe intolerance. As late treatment, 100 mg P.O. b.i.d. when clinical condition allows, continued for at least 3 months.
➢ Symptomatic heart failure
Adults: 25 mg P.O. daily (extended-

release tablets) in patients with New York Heart Association Class II heart failure. Dosage may be doubled q 2 weeks, up to 200 mg/day or until highest tolerated dosage is reached. For patients with more severe heart failure, start with 12.5 mg P.O. daily.

Off-label uses
- Ventricular arrhythmias, tachycardia
- Tremors
- Anxiety

Contraindications
- Hypersensitivity to drug or other beta-adrenergic blockers
- Uncompensated heart failure (when used to treat hypertension or angina)
- Pulmonary edema or cardiogenic shock
- Bradycardia or heart block

Administration
- Be aware that food enhances metoprolol tartrate absorption; give drug with or immediately after meals.
- Know that succinate extended-release tablets are scored and can be divided; however, tablet or half-tablet should be swallowed whole and not crushed or chewed.
- For I.V. administration, give drug undiluted by direct injection.

Route	Onset	Peak	Duration
P.O.	15 min	1 hr	6-12 hr
P.O. (extended)	15 min	6-12 hr	24 hr
I.V.	Immediate	20 min	5-8 hr

Adverse reactions
CNS: fatigue, weakness, anxiety, depression, dizziness, drowsiness, insomnia, memory loss, mental status changes, nervousness, nightmares
CV: orthostatic hypotension, peripheral vasoconstriction, bradycardia, **heart failure, pulmonary edema**
EENT: blurred vision, stuffy nose

GI: nausea, vomiting, constipation, diarrhea, flatulence, gastric pain, heartburn, dry mouth
GU: urinary frequency, impotence, decreased libido
Hepatic: increased hepatic enzyme levels, **hepatitis**
Metabolic: hyperglycemia, hypoglycemia
Respiratory: wheezing, **bronchospasm**
Musculoskeletal: back pain, joint pain
Skin: rash
Other: drug-induced lupus syndrome

Interactions
Drug-drug. *Amphetamines, ephedrine, epinephrine, norepinephrine, phenylephrine, pseudoephedrine:* unopposed alpha-adrenergic stimulation (excessive hypertension, bradycardia)
Antihypertensives, nitrates: additive hypotension
Digoxin: additive bradycardia
Dobutamine, dopamine: reduced cardiovascular benefits from these drugs
General anesthetics, phenytoin (I.V.), verapamil: additive myocardial depression
Insulin, oral hypoglycemics: altered efficacy of these drugs
Monoamine oxidase (MAO) inhibitors: hypertension
Drug-diagnostic tests. *Blood urea nitrogen, lipoproteins, potassium, triglycerides, uric acid:* increased levels
Alanine aminotransferase, alkaline phosphatase, aspartate aminotransferase, glucose, lactate dehydrogenase: increased levels
Drug-food. *Any food:* enhanced drug absorption
Drug-behaviors. *Acute alcohol ingestion:* additive hypotension
Cocaine use: unopposed alpha-adrenergic stimulation (excessive hypertension, bradycardia)

Precautions
Use cautiously in:
- renal or hepatic impairment, pul-

m

monary disease, diabetes mellitus, thyrotoxicosis
- MAO inhibitor use within 14 days
- pregnant or breastfeeding patients
- children (safety not established).

Patient monitoring
- Measure blood pressure closely when starting therapy and titrating dosage. Once patient has stabilized, measure blood pressure every 3 to 6 months.
- Monitor blood pressure and pulse before I.V. administration; if patient is hypotensive or has bradycardia, notify prescriber before giving dose.
- Watch for orthostatic hypotension in at-risk patients, particularly elderly patients.
- Assess glucose levels in diabetic patients; be aware that drug may mask signs and symptoms of hypoglycemia.
- Monitor for signs and symptoms of hyperthyroidism; know that drug may mask these. Reduce dosage gradually in hyperthyroid patients.
- ◀℟ When discontinuing drug, reduce dosage gradually over 1 to 2 weeks.

Patient teaching
- Teach patient to take drug with or immediately after meals.
- Tell patient that extended-release tablets are scored and can be divided, but that he should swallow tablets or half-tablets whole and not crush or chew them.
- ◀℟ Advise patients with heart failure to report signs or symptoms of worsening condition, including weight gain and increasing shortness of breath.
- Advise patient to avoid driving and other hazardous activities until drug effects are known.
- Instruct patient to notify health care providers (including dentists) that he is taking drug before having surgery.
- As appropriate, review all other significant and life-threatening adverse reactions and interactions, especially those related to the drugs, tests, foods, and behaviors mentioned above.

metronidazole
Apo-Metronidazole✤, Flagyl, Flagyl ER, Flagyl IV RTU, Metric 21, Metro IV, MetroCream, MetroGel, MetroGel-Vaginal, MetroLotion, Metryl, Nidagel✤, PMS-Metronidazole✤, Protostat

metronidazole hydrochloride
Flagyl IV

Pharmacologic class: Nitroimidazole derivative
Therapeutic class: Anti-infective, antiprotozoal
Pregnancy risk category B

Action
Disturbs DNA synthesis in susceptible bacterial organisms

Availability
Capsules: 375 mg, 500 mg
Powder for injection: 5 mg/ml, 500-mg vials
Premixed injection: 500 mg/100 ml
Tablets: 250 mg, 500 mg
Tablets (extended-release): 750 mg
Topical cream, gel: 0.75% in 28.4-g tubes
Topical lotion: 0.75% in 59-ml bottle
Vaginal gel: 0.75% (37.5 mg/5-g applicator) in 70-g tubes

🖋 Indications and dosages
➤ Trichomoniasis
Adults: 2 g P.O. as a single dose or 500 mg P.O. b.i.d. for 7 days
➤ Bacterial infections caused by susceptible anaerobic organisms
Adults: Initially, 15 mg/kg I.V., fol-

lowed by 7.5 mg/kg I.V. q 6 to 8 hours or 500 mg I.V. q 6 hours or 7.5 mg/kg P.O. q 6 hours, not to exceed 4 g/day for 7 to 10 days.

➤ Amebiasis caused by *Entamoeba histolytica*

Adults: 750 mg P.O. q 8 hours for 5 to 10 days

➤ Amebic liver abscess

Adults: 500 to 700 mg P.O. t.i.d. for 5 to 10 days; if drug can't be given orally, administer 500 mg I.V. q 6 hours for 10 days.

Children: 35 to 50 mg/kg/day P.O. in three divided doses for 10 days, to a maximum of 750 mg/dose

➤ Bacterial vaginosis

Adults: In nonpregnant patients, 500 mg P.O. b.i.d. for 7 days or 750 mg/day P.O. (extended-release) for 7 days or 5 g of 0.75% vaginal gel b.i.d. for 5 days. In pregnant patients, 250 mg P.O. t.i.d. for 7 days.

➤ Pelvic inflammatory disease

Adults: 500 mg I.V. q 8 hours in conjunction with fluoroquinolone I.V., or 500 mg I.V. daily or 500 mg I.V. b.i.d. in conjunction with fluoroquinolone P.O., for 14 days

➤ Diarrhea and colitis associated with *Clostridium difficile*

Adults: 750 mg to 1 g/day P.O. in three or four divided doses for 7 to 14 days, or 250 mg P.O. q.i.d. or 500 mg P.O. t.i.d. for 10 days. If oral use isn't feasible, 500 to 750 mg I.V. q 6 to 8 hours.

➤ Giardiasis

Adults: 250 mg P.O. t.i.d. for 5 to 7 days

➤ Perioperative prophylaxis in colorectal surgery

Adults: Initially, 15 mg/kg I.V. infusion over 30 to 60 minutes 1 hour before surgery; if necessary, 7.5 mg/kg I.V. infusion over 30 to 60 minutes at 6 and 12 hours after initial dose

➤ Rosacea

Adults: Rub a thin layer of lotion, gel, or cream onto entire affected area

morning and evening; improvement should occur within 3 weeks.

Contraindications

• Hypersensitivity to drug, other nitroimidazole derivatives, or parabens (topical form only)

Administration

• Reconstitute powder for injection by adding 4.4 ml of sterile or bacteriostatic water for injection, 0.9% sodium chloride injection, or bacteriostatic sodium chloride injection to 500-mg vial. Further dilute resulting concentration (100 mg/ml) in 0.9% sodium chloride injection, 5% dextrose injection, or lactated Ringer's injection solution to a concentration of 8 mg/ml or less. Infuse I.V. over 1 hour.

• Be aware that when giving drug by I.V. injection, it need not be diluted or neutralized.

• Don't use equipment containing aluminum to reconstitute or transfer reconstituted solution to diluent; solution may turn reddish-brown.

• Don't interchange vaginal gel with topical gel, cream, or lotion.

m

Route	Onset	Peak	Duration
P.O.	Rapid	1-3 hr	8 hr
P.O. (extended)	Rapid	Unknown	Up to 24 hr
I.V.	Rapid	End of infusion	6-8 hr
Topical	Unknown	6-12 hr	Unknown
Vaginal	Unknown	6-12 hr	12 hr

Adverse reactions

CNS: dizziness, headache, ataxia, vertigo, incoordination, insomnia, fatigue
EENT: rhinitis, sinusitis, pharyngitis
GI: nausea, vomiting, diarrhea, abdominal pain, furry tongue, glossitis, unpleasant or metallic taste, dry mouth, anorexia
GU: dysuria, dark urine, incontinence
Hematologic: leukopenia

Skin: rash, urticaria, burning, mild skin dryness, skin irritation, transient redness (with topical forms)
Other: superinfection, phlebitis at I.V. site

Interactions
Drug-drug. *Azathioprine, fluorouracil:* increased risk of leukopenia
Cimetidine: decreased metronidazole metabolism, increased risk of toxicity
Disulfiram: acute psychosis and confusion
Lithium: increased lithium blood level
Phenobarbital: increased metronidazole metabolism, decreased efficacy
Warfarin: increased warfarin effects
Drug-diagnostic tests. *Alanine aminotransferase, aspartate aminotransferase, lactate dehydrogenase:* altered levels
Drug-behaviors. *Alcohol use:* disulfiram-like reaction

Precautions
Use cautiously in:
• severe hepatic impairment
• history of blood dyscrasias, seizures, or other neurologic problems
• breastfeeding patients
• children.

Patient monitoring
• Monitor I.V. site. Avoid prolonged use of indwelling catheter.
• Evaluate hematologic studies, especially in patients with history of blood dyscrasias.

Patient teaching
• Advise patient to take drug with food if it causes GI upset. However, instruct him to take extended-release tablets 1 hour before or 2 hours after meals.
• Teach patients with trichomoniasis to refrain from sexual intercourse or have male partner wear a condom to prevent reinfection. Explain that asymptomatic sex partners should be treated simultaneously.

• Advise patient to report fever, sore throat, bleeding, or bruising.
• Inform patient that drug may cause metallic taste and may discolor urine deep brownish-red.
• Tell patient using topical form to clean area thoroughly with mild cleanser before use and then wait 15 to 20 minutes before applying drug. Tell her she may apply cosmetics to skin after applying drug; with topical lotion, instruct her to let skin dry at least 5 minutes before applying cosmetics.
• As appropriate, review all other significant and life-threatening adverse reactions and interactions, especially those related to the drugs, tests, and behaviors mentioned above.

mexiletine hydrochloride
Mexitil, Novo-Mexiletine ✿

Pharmacologic class: Lidocaine-like agent
Therapeutic class: Antiarrhythmic (class IB)
Pregnancy risk category C

Action
Decreases duration of action potential and effective refractory period in cardiac conduction tissue by altering sodium transport across myocardial cell membranes

Availability
Capsules: 150 mg, 200 mg, 250 mg

⃠ Indications and dosages
➢ Serious ventricular arrhythmias, including ventricular tachycardia and premature ventricular contractions (PVCs)
Adults: Initially, 200 mg P.O. q 8 hours when rapid control isn't essential; may adjust dosage by 50 to 100 mg q 2 to 3 days. When rapid control is needed,

give initial loading dose of 400 mg P.O., followed by 200 mg in 8 hours.

Off-label uses
• Pain, dysesthesias, paresthesias associated with diabetes mellitus

Contraindications
• Hypersensitivity to drug
• Cardiogenic shock
• Second- or third-degree heart block (in patients without pacemakers)
• Breastfeeding

Administration
• Be aware that therapy should be initiated in hospital setting. Also, drug is reserved for life-threatening ventricular arrhythmias and shouldn't be used to treat asymptomatic PVCs.
• When switching patient to mexiletine from lidocaine, stop lidocaine infusion as soon as first oral mexiletine dose is given, but maintain I.V. line until heart rhythm is satisfactory.
• When switching patient to mexiletine from other class I oral antiarrhythmic agents, give mexiletine exactly as prescribed and titrate to patient's response.

Route	Onset	Peak	Duration
P.O.	30 min-2 hr	2-3 hr	8-12 hr

Adverse reactions
CNS: dizziness, nervousness, confusion, fatigue, headache, sleep disorder, tremor, poor coordination, paresthesia
CV: chest pain, edema, palpitations, **new or increased arrhythmias**
EENT: blurred vision, tinnitus
GI: nausea, vomiting, heartburn
Hematologic: leukopenia, neutropenia, agranulocytosis, thrombocytopenia
Hepatic: hepatic necrosis
Respiratory: dyspnea
Skin: rash

Interactions
Drug-drug. *Antacids, atropine, opioids:* slow mexiletine absorption
Cimetidine: increased or decreased mexiletine blood level
Metoclopramide: increased mexiletine absorption
Other antiarrhythmics: additive cardiac effects
Phenobarbital, phenytoin, rifampin: increased mexiletine metabolism, decreased efficacy
Theophylline: increased theophylline blood level, greater risk of toxicity
Urine acidifiers: increased mexiletine excretion, decreased blood level
Urine alkalinizers: decreased mexiletine excretion, increased blood level
Drug-diagnostic tests. *Antinuclear antibodies:* positive titers
Aspartate aminotransferase: transient increase
Platelets: decreased count (usually returns to normal within 1 month after drug withdrawal)
Drug-food. *Foods that drastically alter urine pH:* altered mexiletine blood level
Caffeine: 50% decrease in caffeine clearance
Drug-behaviors. *Cigarette smoking:* increased mexiletine metabolism, decreased efficacy

Precautions
Use cautiously in:
• sinus node or intraventricular conduction abnormalities, heart failure, hypotension, seizure disorder, severe hepatic impairment
• pregnant patients
• children (safety not established).

Patient monitoring
• Monitor vital signs and ECG frequently when initiating therapy.
• Evaluate liver function tests and hematologic studies.
• Watch for early evidence of toxicity (dizziness, tremor, poor coordination). With increasing toxicity, patient may

m

develop hypotension, sinus bradycardia, ventricular arrhythmias, and seizures. Therapeutic mexiletine blood level is 0.5 to 2 mcg/ml.

Patient teaching
• Tell patient to take drug with food or antacids if adverse GI reactions occur.
• Advise patient to avoid dietary changes that would markedly alter urine pH.
• Inform patient that drug may cause nausea, vomiting, diarrhea, constipation, heartburn, dizziness, tremor, nervousness, poor coordination, changes in sleep habits, headache, visual disturbances, tingling or numbness, ringing in ears, and palpitations or chest pain. Tell him to contact prescriber if these effects are bothersome or severe.
◀€ Tell patient to immediately report general tiredness, yellowing of skin or eyes, flulike symptoms, fever, or sore throat.
• As appropriate, review all other significant and life-threatening adverse reactions and interactions, especially those related to the drugs, tests, foods, and behaviors mentioned above.

midazolam hydrochloride
Apo-Midazolam✤, Versed, Versed Syrup

Pharmacologic class: Benzodiazepine
Therapeutic class: Anxiolytic, sedative-hypnotic, adjunct for general anesthesia induction
Controlled substance schedule IV
Pregnancy risk category D

Action
Unknown; thought to suppress CNS stimulation at the limbic and subcortical levels by potentiating the effects of gamma-aminobutyric acid, an inhibitory neurotransmitter

Availability
Injection: 1 mg/ml, 5 mg/ml
Syrup: 2 mg/ml

⚡ Indications and dosages
➤ To induce general anesthesia
Adults younger than age 55: 0.3 to 0.35 mg/kg I.V. over 20 to 30 seconds if patient hasn't received premedication, or 0.15 to 0.35 mg/kg (usual dosage of 0.25 mg/kg) I.V. over 20 to 30 seconds if patient has received premedication. Additional increments of 25% of initial dosage may be needed for induction completion.
➤ Sedation of intubated and mechanically ventilated patients
Adults: When rapid sedation is required, give loading dose of 0.01 to 0.05 mg/kg I.V. slowly; repeat dose q 10 to 15 minutes until adequate sedation occurs. To maintain sedation, infuse at initial rate of 0.02 to 0.10 mg/kg/hour (1 to 7 mg/hour). Adjust infusion rate as needed.
➤ Preoperative sedation
Adults: 0.07 to 0.08 mg/kg I.M. 30 minutes to 1 hour before surgery
➤ Sedation and amnesia before procedures or anesthesia induction
Children: 0.25 to 0.5 mg/kg P.O., up to 20 mg or 1 mg/kg
Dosage adjustment
• Elderly patients
• Children or neonates

Contraindications
• Hypersensitivity to drug or other benzodiazepines
• Shock or coma
• Uncontrolled severe pain
• Acute closed-angle glaucoma
• Pregnancy

Administration
◀€ Keep oxygen and resuscitation equipment at hand in case severe respi-

---

✤ Canada   ◀€ Clinical alert   Reactions in **bold** are life-threatening

ratory depression occurs.

• Inject I.M. dose deep into large muscle mass.

• Know that drug may be mixed in same syringe as meperidine, atropine, scopolamine, or morphine.

• Dilute concentrate for I.V. infusion to 0.5 mg/ml using dextrose 5% in water or normal saline solution. Infuse over at least 2 minutes; then wait at least 2 minutes before giving second dose. Be aware that excessive dosage or rapid I.V. delivery may cause severe respiratory depression.

• Give oral form with liquid, but never with grapefruit juice.

Route	Onset	Peak	Duration
P.O.	10-20 min	45-60 min	2-6 hr
I.V.	1.5-5 min	Rapid	2-6 hr
I.M.	15 min	15-60 min	2-6 hr

Adverse reactions

CNS: headache, oversedation, drowsiness, agitation and excitement (in children)

CV: hypotension, irregular pulse, bradycardia, **arrhythmias, cardiac arrest**

GI: nausea, vomiting

Respiratory: decreased respiratory rate, hiccups, **apnea, respiratory arrest**

Other: pain and tenderness at injection site

Interactions

Drug-drug. *CNS depressants (such as some antidepressants, antihistamines, barbiturates, opioids, tranquilizers) respiratory depressants:* potentiation of CNS effects of these drugs

Diltiazem, verapamil: increased midazolam blood level

Erythromycin: decreased midazolam clearance

Hormonal contraceptives: prolonged midazolam half-life

Rifampin: decreased midazolam blood level

Theophylline: increased sedative effect of midazolam

Drug-food. *Grapefruit juice:* increased bioavailability of oral midazolam

Drug-herb. *Chamomile, kava, skullcap, valerian:* increased CNS depression

Drug-behaviors. *Alcohol use:* potentiation of midazolam effects

Precautions

Use cautiously in:

• pulmonary disease, heart failure, renal impairment, severe hepatic impairment

• obese pediatric patients

• elderly or debilitated patients

• breastfeeding patients (safety not established)

• neonates.

Patient monitoring

• Monitor vital signs, ECG, respiratory status, and oxygen saturation.

• Assess neurologic status closely, especially in pediatric patients.

• Watch for nausea and vomiting.

Patient teaching

• Advise patient that drug causes perioperative amnesia.

• Instruct patient to avoid driving and other hazardous activities until he knows how drug affects concentration and alertness.

• If patient will take oral drug at home, instruct him to take it with liquid but never grapefruit juice.

midodrine hydrochloride
Amatine✚, ProAmatine

Pharmacologic class: Alpha$_1$-adrenergic agonist

Therapeutic class: Antihypotensive, vasopressor

Pregnancy risk category C

m

Action

Forms active metabolite, desglymidodrine, an alpha$_1$-adrenergic agonist that activates alpha-adrenergic receptors in arteriolar and venous vasculature. This activation increases blood pressure and vascular tone.

Availability

Tablets: 2.5 mg, 5 mg

⏐ Indications and dosages

➤ Symptomatic orthostatic hypotension

Adults: 10 mg P.O. t.i.d. during daytime hours with patient in an upright position. Give first dose when patient arises in the morning, second dose at midday, and third dose in late afternoon

Dosage adjustment
• Renal impairment

Contraindications

• Severe coronary artery disease or organic heart disease
• Acute renal disease
• Pheochromocytoma
• Hypertension

Administration

• Don't administer within 4 hours of bedtime.

Route	Onset	Peak	Duration
P.O.	Rapid	1-2 hr	Unknown

Adverse reactions

CNS: paresthesia
CV: vasodilation, bradycardia, **supine hypertension**
GI: abdominal pain, dry mouth
GU: urinary retention, frequency, or urgency
Skin: rash, pruritus, piloerection
Other: chills, increased pain

Interactions

Drug-drug. *Alpha- and beta-adrenergic blockers, cardiac glycosides, steroids:* increased risk of bradycardia, atrioventricular block
Alpha-adrenergic blockers, fludrocortisone: increased risk of supine hypertension

Precautions

Use cautiously in:
• renal or hepatic impairment, diabetes mellitus, vision problems
• pregnant or breastfeeding patients.

Patient monitoring

• Monitor supine and sitting blood pressure closely. Report marked rise in supine blood pressure.
• Stay alert for paresthesias.
• Monitor fluid intake and output; watch for urinary frequency, urgency, or retention.

Patient teaching

• Instruct patient to take drug while in upright position.
• Teach patient to take first dose as soon as he arises for the day, second dose at midday, and third dose in late afternoon (before 6 P.M.). Stress that doses must be taken at least 3 hours apart. Advise patient not to take drug after dinner or within 4 hours of bedtime.
◀ Instruct patient to promptly report symptoms of supine hypertension (pounding in ears, blurred vision, headache).
• Advise patient to avoid driving and other hazardous activities until he knows how drug affects concentration, vision, and alertness.
• As appropriate, review all other significant and life-threatening adverse reactions and interactions, especially those related to the drugs mentioned above.

---

mifepristone (RU-486)
Mifeprex

Pharmacologic class: Synthetic steroid
Therapeutic class: Antiprogestational agent, abortifacient
Pregnancy risk category NR

Action
Antagonizes progesterone receptor sites, inhibiting activity of endogenous and exogenous progesterone and stimulating uterine contractions, causing fetus to separate from placental wall

Availability
Tablets: 200 mg

🖊 Indications and dosages
➤ Termination of intrauterine pregnancy through day 49 of pregnancy
Adults: On day 1, mifepristone 600 mg P.O. as a single dose. On day 3, misoprostol 400 mcg P.O. (unless abortion has been confirmed).

Contraindications
• Hypersensitivity to drug
• Confirmed or suspected ectopic pregnancy
• Chronic adrenal failure
• Bleeding disorders or concurrent anticoagulant or corticosteroid therapy
• Presence of intrauterine device (IUD)

Administration
• Before giving dose, make sure patient doesn't have an IUD in place.
• Give only in a health care facility under supervision of health care provider qualified to assess pregnancy stage and rule out ectopic pregnancy.
• Administer with fluids, but not with grapefruit juice.

• Confirm termination of pregnancy 14 days after initial dose.

Route	Onset	Peak	Duration
P.O.	Rapid	90 min	11 days

Adverse reactions
CNS: dizziness, fainting, headache, weakness, fatigue, insomnia, asthenia, anxiety, syncope, rigors
EENT: sinusitis
GI: nausea, vomiting, diarrhea, abdominal cramping, dyspepsia
GU: vaginitis, leukorrhea, uterine cramping, pelvic pain, **uterine hemorrhage**
Hematologic: anemia, decreased hemoglobin
Musculoskeletal: leg pain, back pain
Skin: fever
Other: viral infections

Interactions
Drug-drug. *Carbamazepine, dexamethasone, phenobarbital, phenytoin, rifampin:* decreased mifepristone blood level and effects
Drugs metabolized by CYP450-3A4: decreased mifepristone metabolism and increased effects
Erythromycin, itraconazole, ketoconazole: inhibited mifepristone metabolism and increased blood level
Drug-diagnostic tests. *Hematocrit, hemoglobin:* decreased
Red blood cells: decreased count
Drug-food. *Grapefruit juice:* decreased mifepristone blood level and effects

Precautions
Use cautiously in:
• cardiovascular, respiratory, renal, or hepatic disorders; hypertension; type 1 diabetes mellitus; anemia; jaundice; seizure disorder; cervicitis; infected endocervical lesions, acute vaginitis; uterine scarring.

m

Patient monitoring
• Assess vital signs, breath sounds, and bowel sounds.
• Monitor uterine contractions and type and amount of vaginal bleeding.
• Evaluate complete blood count.

Patient teaching
• After administration, tell patient she'll need to return in 48 hours for a prostaglandin drug or to verify pregnancy termination.
• Tell patient she'll have contractions for 3 or more hours after receiving drug and that vaginal bleeding may last 9 to 16 days.
• Instruct patient to contact prescriber if she has persistent or extremely heavy vaginal bleeding, extreme fatigue, or orthostatic hypotension.
• Caution patient that vaginal bleeding does not prove that a complete abortion has occurred; tell her she'll need a follow-up appointment 2 weeks later to verify pregnancy termination.
• Teach patient that she's at risk for pregnancy right after abortion is complete; encourage appropriate contraceptive decisions.
• As appropriate, review all other significant and life-threatening adverse reactions and interactions, especially those related to the drugs, tests, and foods mentioned above.

miglitol
Glyset

Pharmacologic class: Alpha-glucosidase inhibitor
Therapeutic class: Hypoglycemic
Pregnancy risk category B

Action
Inhibits alpha-glucosidases, enzymes that convert oligosaccharides and di-saccharides to glucose; inhibition of these enzymes lowers blood glucose level, especially in postprandial hyper-glycemia

Availability
Tablets: 25 mg, 50 mg, 100 mg

Indications and dosages
➢ Adjunct to diet in management of non-insulin-dependent diabetes mellitus or in combination with a sulfonylurea when diet alone doesn't control hyperglycemia
Adults: 25 mg P.O. t.i.d. with first bite of each main meal; after 4 to 8 weeks, may increase to 50 mg P.O. t.i.d. After 3 months, adjust dosage further based on glycosylated hemoglobin (HbA1c) level, to a maximum of 100 mg P.O. t.i.d.

Contraindications
• Hypersensitivity to drug
• Type 1 diabetes mellitus, diabetic ketoacidosis
• Chronic intestinal disorder
• Cirrhosis
• Renal dysfunction
• Breastfeeding

Administration
• Give with first bite of three main meals.

Route	Onset	Peak	Duration
P.O.	Unknown	2-3 hr	Unknown

Adverse reactions
GI: abdominal pain, diarrhea, flatulence
Hematologic: below-normal serum iron level
Skin: rash

Interactions
Drug-drug. *Digestive enzyme preparations (such as amylase, pancreatin), intestinal absorbents (such as charcoal):* reduced miglitol efficacy

---

Digoxin, propranolol, ranitidine: decreased bioavailability of these drugs
Drug-food. *Carbohydrates:* increased diarrhea

Precautions
Use cautiously in:
- fever, infection, trauma, stress
- pregnant patients
- children (safety not established).

Patient monitoring
- Monitor blood glucose and HbA1c levels, complete blood count, and liver function test results.
- Watch for hyperglycemia or hypoglycemia, especially if patient also receives insulin or oral sulfonylureas.

Patient teaching
- Instruct patient to take drug three times daily with first bite of three main meals.
- Teach patient to take drug as prescribed; remind him that he may need insulin during periods of increased stress, infection, or surgery.
- Inform patient that sucrose (found in table sugar or cane sugar) and fruit juice are ineffective in treating hypoglycemia caused by miglitol. Advise him to use dextrose or glucagon instead if he must raise blood glucose level quickly.
- Reassure patient that GI effects usually subside after first few weeks.
- As appropriate, review all other significant adverse reactions and interactions, especially those related to the drugs and foods mentioned above.

milrinone lactate
Primacor

Pharmacologic class: Bipyridine phosphodiesterase inhibitor
Therapeutic class: Inotropic
Pregnancy risk category C

Action
Increases cellular levels of cyclic adenosine monophosphate, resulting in inotropic action; relaxes vascular smooth muscle and myocardial contractility

Availability
Injection: 1 mg/ml in 10-ml and 20-ml vials
Injection (premixed): 200 mcg/ml in dextrose 5% in water (D_5W)

Indications and dosages
➤ Heart failure
Adults: Initially, 50 mcg/kg I.V. bolus given slowly over 10 minutes, followed by a continuous I.V. infusion of 0.375 to 0.75 mcg/kg/minute. Don't exceed a total daily dosage of 1.13 mg/kg.
Dosage adjustment
- Renal impairment

Contraindications
- Hypersensitivity to drug
- Severe aortic or pulmonic valvular disease
- Acute phase of myocardial infarction

Administration
- Dilute 1 mg/ml solution with half-normal saline solution, normal saline solution, or D_5W, according to manufacturer's instructions.
- ◀ Don't administer in same I.V. line as furosemide or torsemide (precipitate will form).
- Expect to titrate infusion rate depending on patient's response.

m

Route	Onset	Peak	Duration
I.V.	5-15 min	1-2 hr	3-6 hr

Adverse reactions
CNS: headache
CV: hypotension, chest pain, angina, **ventricular or supraventricular arrhythmias, sustained ventricular tachycardia, ventricular fibrillation, death**

Interactions
Drug-drug. *Furosemide, torsemide:* precipitate formation when given in same I.V. line

Precautions
Use cautiously in:
• atrial flutter or fibrillation, renal impairment, electrolyte abnormalities, abnormal blood digoxin level
• elderly patients
• pregnant or breastfeeding patients
• children.

Patient monitoring
• Monitor vital signs and ECG; watch closely for evidence of ventricular arrhythmias, sustained tachycardia, or fibrillation.
• Assess cardiovascular status closely; stay alert for complaints of chest pain.
◀€ Stop drug and contact prescriber immediately if patient's systolic blood pressure drops 30 mm Hg or more.
• Assess patient for headache; provide analgesics as needed.

Patient teaching
• Instruct patient to change position slowly to avoid light-headedness or dizziness from hypotension.
• As appropriate, review all other significant and life-threatening adverse reactions and interactions, especially those related to the drugs mentioned above.

minocycline hydrochloride
Alti-Minocycline✤, Arestin, Dynacin, Gen-Minocycline✤, Minocin, Novo-Minocycline✤, Vectrin

Pharmacologic class: Tetracycline
Therapeutic class: Anti-infective
Pregnancy risk category D

Action
Binds reversibly to 30s ribosome, inhibiting bacterial protein synthesis

Availability
Capsules: 50 mg, 75 mg, 100 mg
Capsules (pellet-filled): 50 mg, 100 mg
Microspheres (sustained-release): 1 mg
Powder for injection: 100 mg/vial
Suspension: 50 mg/5 ml

⁄ Indications and dosages
➤ Infections caused by sensitive organisms, including *Mycoplasma, Chlamydia, rickettsiae,* and *Borrelia burgdorferi*
Adults: Initially, 200 mg P.O. or I.V., followed by 100 mg q 12 hours or 50 mg P.O. q 6 hours
➤ Gonorrhea
Adults: Initially, 200 mg P.O., followed by 100 mg q 12 hours for 4 days
➤ Syphilis
Adults: Initially, 200 mg P.O., followed by 100 mg q 12 hours for 10 to 15 days
➤ Acne
Adults: 50 mg P.O. one to three times daily
Dosage adjustment
• Children

Contraindications
• Hypersensitivity to drug, alcohol, or bisulfites
• Pregnancy or breastfeeding (except in treatment of anthrax infection)
• Children younger than age 8

Administration

• Used in patients allergic to penicillin.
• For I.V. use, add 5 ml of sterile water to 100 mg of powder for injection, then dilute further in 500 to 1,000 ml to a final concentration of 100 to 200 mcg/ml. Infuse over 6 hours.

Route	Onset	Peak	Duration
P.O.	Unknown	1-4 hr	Unknown
I.V.	Immediate	End of infusion	Unknown

Adverse reactions

CNS: headache
CV: pericarditis
EENT: pharyngitis; tooth disorder, pain, or discoloration; periodontitis; gingivitis; dental caries; dental infection
GI: nausea, vomiting, diarrhea, oral candidiasis, stomatitis, mouth ulcers
GU: bladder or vaginal yeast infections
Metabolic: eosinophilia, neutrophilia, hemolytic anemia, **thrombocytopenia**
Skin: photosensitivity, rash
Other: phlebitis at I.V. site, superinfection, hypersensitivity reactions including **anaphylaxis**

Interactions

Drug-drug. *Adsorbent antidiarrheals:* decreased minocycline absorption
Antacids containing aluminum, calcium, or magnesium; calcium, iron, and magnesium supplements; sodium bicarbonate: decreased minocycline absorption (with oral use)
Cholestyramine, colestipol: decreased oral absorption of minocycline
Hormonal contraceptives: decreased contraceptive efficacy
Methoxyflurane: nephrotoxicity
Penicillin: interference with bactericidal action of penicillin
Sucralfate: prevention of minocycline absorption
Warfarin: increased anticoagulant effect

Drug-diagnostic tests. *Alanine aminotransferase, alkaline phosphatase, amylase, aspartate aminotransferase, bilirubin, blood urea nitrogen:* increased levels
Hemoglobin, platelets, neutrophils, white blood cells: decreased counts
Urinary catecholamines: false elevation
Drug-food. *Dairy products:* decreased minocycline absorption
Drug-behaviors. *Alcohol use:* decreased antibiotic effect
Sun exposure: increased risk of photosensitivity reaction

Precautions

Use cautiously in:
• renal disease, hepatic impairment, nephrogenic diabetes insipidus
• cachectic or debilitated patients.

Patient monitoring

• Assess patient's oral health closely to identify dental problems.
• Monitor patient for superinfection, especially oral, bladder, and vaginal yeast infections.
• Evaluate complete blood count.

Patient teaching

• Tell patient he may take oral form with or without food, followed by a full glass of water. Instruct him to space doses evenly over 24 hours and to take one dose 1 hour before bedtime.
• Advise patient not to take oral form with iron, calcium, or magnesium products or with antacids.
• Inform female patients that drug may make hormonal contraceptives ineffective; recommend use of barrier birth control methods.
• Tell pregnant patients that drug may stain fetus' teeth if taken during last half of pregnancy.
• Emphasize importance of good oral hygiene to minimize adverse oral and dental effects.

m

• As appropriate, review all other significant and life-threatening adverse reactions and interactions, especially those related to the drugs, tests, foods, and behaviors mentioned above.

minoxidil
Apo-Gain✤, Gen-Minoxidil✤, Hairgro✤, Loniten, Minodyl, Minox✤, Minoxigaine✤, Rogaine, Rogaine Extra Strength

Pharmacologic class: Peripheral vaso-dilator (direct-acting)
Therapeutic class: Antihypertensive, hair growth stimulant
Pregnancy risk category C

Action
Reduces blood pressure by relaxing vascular smooth muscle, thus producing vasodilation. In hair growth stimulation, exact mechanism is unknown; may alter androgen metabolism in scalp or enhance microcirculation around hair follicles.

Availability
Tablets: 2.5 mg, 10 mg
Topical solution: 2%, 5%

🕖 Indications and dosages
➣ Severe symptomatic hypertension or hypertension associated with end-organ damage
Adults and children ages 12 and older: 2.5 to 5 mg/day as a single dose or in two divided doses; may double the dosage q 3 days. Usual range is 10 to 40 mg/day; for rapid blood pressure control with careful monitoring, dosage may be adjusted q 6 hr. Maximum dosage is 100 mg/day.
➣ Male pattern baldness, diffuse hair loss or thinning in women, adjunct to hair transplantation

Adults: Apply 1 ml of 2% or 5% topical solution to affected area b.i.d. for 4 months or longer.
➣ Alopecia areata
Adults: Apply 1 ml of 2% or 5% topical solution to scalp b.i.d.

Contraindications
• Hypersensitivity to drug
• Dissecting aortic aneurysm
• Concurrent guanethidine therapy
• Breastfeeding

Administration
• Give oral form with a beta-adrenergic blocker or diuretic, as prescribed, to control hypertension.
• Administer oral form with meals to decrease GI upset.
• If patient is receiving guanethidine, discontinue that drug 1 to 3 days before starting minoxidil to avoid severe orthostatic hypotension.

Route	Onset	Peak	Duration
P.O.	30 min	2-3 hr	2-5 days
Topical	Unknown	Unknown	Unknown

Adverse reactions
CV: ECG changes (such as T-wave changes), tachycardia, angina, **pericardial effusion, cardiac tamponade, heart failure**
GI: nausea, vomiting
Respiratory: pulmonary edema
Other: weight gain, edema

Interactions
Drug-drug. *Antihypertensives, nitrates:* additive hypotension
Guanethidine: severe orthostatic hypotension
Nonsteroidal anti-inflammatory drugs: decreased minoxidil efficacy
Drug-diagnostic tests. *Alkaline phosphatase, blood urea nitrogen, creatinine, plasma renin activity, sodium:* increased levels

---

Hematocrit, hemoglobin, red blood cells: decreased values

Precautions

Use cautiously in:
• recent MI, malignant hypertension, heart failure, angina pectoris, severe renal impairment
• pregnant patients.

Patient monitoring

• Monitor vital signs and ECG.
• Assess daily weight and fluid intake and output.
• Monitor cardiovascular status carefully; stay alert for signs and symptoms of heart failure.
• Evaluate patient for evidence of hypertrichosis.
• Be aware that hematologic and renal values usually return to pretreatment levels with continued therapy.

Patient teaching

• Instruct patient to take oral form with meals to decrease GI upset.
• Teach patient to weigh himself daily and report sudden weight gains.
• Tell patient taking oral form that drug may darken, lengthen, and thicken body hairs; tell him to shave or use depilatory to reduce unwanted hair growth. Reassure him that unwanted growth will disappear 1 to 6 months after he stops taking drug.
• Instruct patient not to use topical form on other body parts and not to let it contact mucous membranes.
• Teach patient using topical form that new scalp hair will be soft and barely visible. Caution him to use only 1 ml twice daily regardless of amount of balding. Remind him not to stop using drug suddenly; if he discontinues therapy, new hair growth will be lost.
• As appropriate, review all other significant and life-threatening adverse reactions and interactions, especially those related to the drugs and tests mentioned above.

mirtazapine
Remeron, Remeron RD✽, Remeron Soltab

Pharmacologic class: Piperazinoazepine

Therapeutic class: Tetracyclic antidepressant

Pregnancy risk category C

Action

Potentiates effects of norepinephrine and serotonin by blocking synapse reuptake in nerve cells. Also has anticholinergic action due to its disruption of muscarinic receptors.

Availability

Tablets: 15 mg, 30 mg
Tablets (orally disintegrating): 15 mg, 30 mg, 45 mg

Indications and dosages

➤ Depression (usually used in conjunction with psychotherapy)
Adults: Initially, 15 mg/day as a single dose at bedtime; may be increased q 1 to 2 weeks, up to 45 mg/day. Maintenance dosages range from 15 to 45 mg/day.

Dosage adjustment
• Renal or hepatic impairment

Contraindications

• Hypersensitivity to drug
• Monoamine oxidase (MAO) inhibitor use within 14 days

Administration

• Know that patient may take orally disintegrating tablet without water; have him place it on tongue until it melts. Make sure tablet isn't broken.

Route	Onset	Peak	Duration
P.O.	1-2 wk	≥6 wk	Unknown

Adverse reactions

CNS: drowsiness, dizziness, abnormal dreams, abnormal thinking, asthenia, tremor, confusion

CV: orthostatic hypotension, chest pain

EENT: sinusitis

GI: constipation, dry mouth

GU: urinary tract infection

Musculoskeletal: back pain, myalgia

Respiratory: increased cough, dyspnea

Other: flulike symptoms, increased appetite, weight gain, edema, increased thirst

Interactions

Drug-drug. *Benzodiazepines, other CNS depressants:* additive CNS depression

Drugs metabolized by CYP450 enzyme: altered metabolism of these drugs

MAO inhibitors: hypertension, seizures, death

Drug-herb. *Chamomile, hops, kava, skullcap, valerian:* increased CNS depression

S-adenosylmethionine (SAM-e), St. John's wort: increased risk of serotonergic adverse effects (including serotonin syndrome)

Drug-behaviors. *Alcohol use:* additive CNS effects

Precautions

Use cautiously in:

• hepatic or renal impairment; increased intraocular pressure

• history of seizures, psychiatric illnesses, cardiovascular or cerebrovascular disease

• elderly patients

• pregnant or breastfeeding patients

• children (safety not established).

Patient monitoring

• Monitor vital signs, especially for orthostatic hypotension.

• Assess neurologic status.

• Watch for weight gain caused by edema or increased appetite.

• Stay alert for urinary tract infection, sinusitis, and flulike symptoms.

Patient teaching

• Advise patient to take drug with food or milk to reduce GI upset.

• Tell patient he may crush conventional tablets if he can't swallow them whole.

• Inform patient that therapeutic effects may take 2 to 3 weeks

• Teach patient not to discontinue drug abruptly; dosage must be tapered.

• If drug causes oversedation, teach patient to consult prescriber about taking whole dose at bedtime.

• Instruct patient to avoid driving and other hazardous activities until he knows how drug affects concentration and alertness.

• As appropriate, review all other significant adverse reactions and interactions, especially those related to the drugs, herbs, and behaviors mentioned above.

misoprostol
Apo-Misoprostol✦, Cytotec

Pharmacologic class: Prostaglandin E$_1$ analog

Therapeutic class: Antiulcerative, cytoprotective agent

Pregnancy risk category X

Action

Reduces gastric acid secretion and increases gastric mucus and bicarbonate production, creating a protective coating on the gastric mucosa

Availability

Tablets: 100 mcg, 200 mcg

⃠ Indications and dosages

➤ To prevent gastric ulcers caused by nonsteroidal anti-inflammatory drugs

Adults: 200 mcg q.i.d. or 400 mcg b.i.d. with food; give last daily dose at bedtime. If intolerance occurs, decrease to 100 mcg q.i.d.

➤ Duodenal or gastric ulcer

Adults: 100 to 200 mcg P.O. q.i.d. with meals and at bedtime for 4 to 8 weeks

Off-label uses
• Pregnancy termination

Contraindications
• Hypersensitivity to prostaglandins
• Pregnancy or breastfeeding

Administration
◀€ Before starting therapy, make sure female patients are fully informed about dangers of taking drug when pregnant or breastfeeding.
• For antiulcerative use in female patients, start drug therapy on second or third day of normal menses.

Route	Onset	Peak	Duration
P.O.	Rapid	14-20 min	3-6 hr

Adverse reactions
CNS: headache
GI: nausea, vomiting, diarrhea, constipation, abdominal pain, dyspepsia, flatulence
GU: miscarriage, menstrual disorders, hypermenorrhea, dysmenorrhea, intermenstrual spotting, cramps, postmenopausal bleeding

Interactions
Drug-drug. *Magnesium-containing antacids:* increased risk of diarrhea

Precautions
Use cautiously in:
• women of childbearing age
• children younger than age 18 (safety not established).

Patient monitoring
• Assess GI status; report significant adverse effects.

• Monitor menstrual pattern or postmenopausal bleeding; report significant problems.

Patient teaching
• Instruct patient to take drug with food.
• Advise patient to report diarrhea, black tarry stools, cramping, abdominal pain, or menstrual irregularities.
• Inform patient that drug may cause spontaneous abortion; stress importance of using reliable contraception.
• Instruct female patients using drug for ulcer treatment to start therapy on second or third day of normal menses.
• Caution patient not to take antacids that contain magnesium; doing so worsens diarrhea.
• As appropriate, review all other significant adverse reactions and interactions, especially those related to the drugs mentioned above.

m

mitomycin
Mutamycin, Mytozytrex

Pharmacologic class: Antitumor antibiotic
Therapeutic class: Antineoplastic
Pregnancy risk category NR

Action
Selectively inhibits DNA synthesis by causing cross-linking of DNA strands and suppressing RNA and protein synthesis, resulting in cell death

Availability
Injection: 5-mg, 20-mg, and 40-mg vials

⦸ Indications and dosages
➤ Disseminated adenocarcinoma of stomach or pancreas; palliative treatment of colon and breast cancer, head,

and neck tumors, and advanced biliary, lung, and cervical squamous cell carcinomas

Adults: 20 mg/m² I.V. as a single dose; repeat cycle q 6 to 8 weeks, adjusting dosage if necessary.

➤ Bladder cancer

Adults: 20 to 60 mg intravesically q week for 8 weeks

Dosage adjustment

• Reduced white blood cell or platelet count

Contraindications

• Hypersensitivity to drug
• Thrombocytopenia, coagulation disorders, increased bleeding tendency
• Breastfeeding

Administration

◢℥ Follow facility policy for handling mutagenic, teratogenic, and carcinogenic drugs.

• Know that drug is usually administered with other agents.

• Reconstitute 5-mg vial with 10 ml of sterile water; shake, let mixture stand, and then administer by direct I.V. injection through Y-tube or three-way stopcock. Infuse over 5 to 10 minutes through I.V. line with running infusion of normal saline solution or dextrose 5% in water.

• Avoid extravasation and contact with skin, mucous membranes, and eyes.

Route	Onset	Peak	Duration
I.V.	Unknown	Unknown	Unknown

Adverse reactions

GI: nausea, vomiting, anorexia, mouth ulcers, stomatitis
GU: renal failure, **hemolytic uremic syndrome**
Hematologic: anemia, **leukopenia, thrombocytopenia**
Respiratory: pulmonary toxicity, interstitial pneumonitis

Skin: reversible alopecia; pruritus; desquamation; phlebitis, necrosis, and sloughing with extravasation at I.V. site
Other: fever

Interactions

Drug-drug. *Live-virus vaccines:* decreased antibody response to vaccine, increased risk of adverse reactions
Other antineoplastics: additive bone marrow depression
Vinca alkaloids: respiratory toxicity

Precautions

Use cautiously in:
• active infections, decreased bone marrow reserve, impaired hepatic function
• history of pulmonary disorders
• elderly patients
• pregnant patients.

Patient monitoring

• Monitor complete blood count with white cell differential and platelet count; watch for signs and symptoms of blood dyscrasias.

• Assess kidney function tests; measure fluid intake and output and evaluate fluid balance.

◢℥ Watch for signs and symptoms of hemolytic uremic syndrome (irritability, fatigue, pallor, and decreased urinary output).

• Monitor I.V. site, skin integrity, and oral health.

• Assess respiratory status carefully for severe pulmonary problems.

Patient teaching

• Teach patient to recognize and report signs and symptoms of hemolytic uremic syndrome, blood dyscrasias, and renal failure.

• Instruct patient to report cough or shortness of breath, even if it occurs several months after therapy ends.

• Teach patient to limit exposure to infections and avoid live vaccines.

• Tell patient that drug may cause hair loss; discuss options for dealing with this problem.

• As appropriate, review all other significant and life-threatening adverse reactions and interactions, especially those related to the drugs mentioned above.

mitoxantrone hydrochloride
Novantrone

Pharmacologic class: Antibiotic antineoplastic
Therapeutic class: Antineoplastic, immune modifier
Pregnancy risk category D

Action
Selectively inhibits DNA synthesis by causing cross-linking of DNA strands and suppressing RNA and protein synthesis, resulting in cell death

Availability
Injection: 2 mg/ml in 10-ml, 12.5-ml, and 15-ml vials

⚕ Indications and dosages
➤ Acute nonlymphocytic leukemia (given with other agents)
Adults: For induction, 12 mg/m²/day I.V. on days 1 to 3, with 100 mg/m² of cytosine arabinoside for 7 days as a continuous I.V. infusion (over 24 hours) on days 1 through 7. If remission doesn't occur, second induction course with mitoxantrone given for 2 days and cytosine arabinoside for 5 days at same daily dosages. For consolidation therapy, 12 mg/m²/day I.V. mitoxantrone on days 1 and 2 and 100 mg/m² I.V. cytosine arabinoside as a continuous infusion over 24 hours on

days 1 through 5, given 6 weeks following induction therapy.
➤ Bone pain in patients with advanced prostatic cancer
Adults: 12 to 14 mg/m² I.V. over 15 to 30 minutes q 21 days
➤ Multiple sclerosis
Adults: 12 mg/m² I.V. over 5 to 15 minutes q 3 months; maximum cumulative lifetime dosage is 140 mg/m².

Contraindications
• Hypersensitivity to drug
• Pregnancy

Administration
◀◎ Follow facility policy for handling mutagenic, teratogenic, and carcinogenic drugs.
• Dilute with 50 ml or more of normal saline solution or dextrose 5% in water (D₅W); infuse over 3 to 5 minutes into running I.V. line of normal saline solution or D₅W.
• Alternatively, dilute drug further in normal saline solution or D₅W and infuse intermittently over 15 to 30 minutes.
• If extravasation occurs, stop infusion immediately.
• Avoid contact with skin, mucous membranes, and eyes.
• Know that drug may be used to treat myelogenous, promyelocytic, monocytic, or erythroid acute leukemia.

Route	Onset	Peak	Duration
I.V.	Unknown	Unknown	Unknown

Adverse reactions
CNS: headache, **seizures**
CV: heart failure, arrhythmias, cardiotoxicity
EENT: conjunctivitis, stomatitis, mucositis
GI: nausea, vomiting, diarrhea, abdominal pain, **GI bleeding**
GU: urinary tract infection, **renal failure**

m

Hematologic: anemia, **bone marrow depression, leukopenia, thrombocytopenia**

Hepatic: jaundice, **hepatotoxicity**

Metabolic: hyperuricemia

Respiratory: cough, dyspnea

Skin: alopecia, petechiae, bruising, rashes

Other: fever, infection, hypersensitivity reaction

Interactions

Drug-drug. *Anthracycline antineoplastics (daunorubicin, doxorubicin, idarubicin):* increased risk of cardiomyopathy

Live-virus vaccines: decreased antibody response to vaccine

Other antineoplastics: additive bone marrow depression

Drug-diagnostic tests. *Alanine aminotransferase, aspartate aminotransferase, bilirubin, uric acid:* increased levels

Precautions

Use cautiously in:
• bone marrow depression, heart failure, chronic debilitating illness, hepatobiliary dysfunction
• elderly patients
• breastfeeding patients
• children.

Patient monitoring

• Monitor complete blood count with white cell differential; watch for signs and symptoms of blood dyscrasias.
• Assess vital signs, ECG, and respiratory and cardiovascular status.
• Monitor kidney and liver function tests; measure fluid intake and output and evaluate fluid balance.
• Measure temperature; stay alert for fever and signs and symptoms of urinary tract and other infections.

Patient teaching

• Advise patient to report chest pain, seizures, and trouble breathing.

• Instruct patient to limit exposure to infections and avoid live vaccines.
• Teach patient to minimize GI upset by eating small, frequent servings of healthy food and drinking plenty of fluids.
• As appropriate, review all other significant and life-threatening adverse reactions and interactions, especially those related to the drugs and tests mentioned above.

mivacurium chloride
Mivacron

Pharmacologic class: Nondepolarizing neuromuscular blocker

Therapeutic class: Skeletal muscle relaxant

Pregnancy risk category C

Action

Inhibits action of acetylcholine at motor endplate receptor sites, blocking neuromuscular transmission

Availability

Infusion: 0.5 mg/ml in 50 ml dextrose 5% in water (D_5W)
Injection: 2 mg/ml in 5 ml-vials, 2 mg/ml in 10-ml vials

Indications and dosages

➤ Adjunct to general anesthesia; to relax skeletal muscles to allow endotracheal intubation

Adults: 0.15 mg/kg I.V. bolus over 5 to 15 seconds. To maintain neuromuscular blockade after evidence of spontaneous recovery from initial dose, give 9 to 10 mcg/kg/ minute I.V. infusion.

Dosage adjustment
• End-stage renal or hepatic disease
• Asthma

- Obesity
- Children

Contraindications
- Hypersensitivity to drug, other benzylisoquinoliniums, or benzyl alcohol (multidose vials only)

Administration
- Before starting therapy, make sure emergency resuscitation equipment is available and patient is being monitored.
- Assess electrolyte levels; correct electrolyte imbalances before starting therapy.
- Keep in mind that when drug is used with isoflurane or enflurane, dosage is reduced 35% to 40%.
- Know that adequate muscle relaxation for endotracheal intubation usually occurs within 2 to 3 minutes of I.V. bolus and lasts 15 to 20 minutes.
- Expect to give a test dose.
- Dilute to 0.5 mg/ml using D_5W, normal saline solution, D_5W in normal saline solution, lactated Ringer's solution, or dextrose 5% in lactated Ringer's solution.
- Infuse at prescribed rate; if infusion begins with the initial dose of 0.15 mg/kg, use infusion rate of 4 mcg/kg/minute.
- Before giving premixed infusion, remove outer wrap and check contents for leaks by squeezing.
- Don't mix with other I.V. drugs
- Don't give I.M.

Route	Onset	Peak	Duration
I.V.	1-2 min	2-5 min	20-35 min

Adverse reactions
CNS: prolonged neuromuscular blockade, **paralysis**
CV: hypotension, tachycardia
Respiratory: apnea, **bronchospasm**
Skin: flushing

Interactions
Drug-drug. *Aminoglycosides (gentamicin, kanamycin, neomycin, streptomycin), bacitracin, colistimethate, colistin, lincomycin, magnesium salts, other nondepolarizing neuromuscular blockers, polymyxin B, tetracycline:* enhanced neuromuscular blockade, causing increased skeletal muscle relaxation and prolonged effects
Beta-adrenergic blockers, hormonal contraceptives, lithium, local anesthetics, procainamide, quinidine, quinine: enhanced neuromuscular blockade
Carbamazepine, phenytoin: delay of maximal blockade or shortened duration of action
Inhalation anesthetics: enhanced or prolonged mivacurium action

Precautions
Use cautiously in:
- renal, hepatic, neuromuscular, respiratory, or cardiovascular disease; fluid or electrolyte imbalances; metastatic cancer; obesity
- pregnant or breastfeeding patients
- elderly patients
- children younger than 3 months.

Patient monitoring
- During recovery and residual phase, watch for residual weakness, paralysis, and respiratory distress.
- Monitor recovery from neuromuscular blockade by checking patient's hand grip, head lift, and ability to cough voluntarily.

Patient teaching
- Explain all interventions to patient because he'll be conscious during procedure (unless anesthesia is given).
- Provide reassurance during recovery from neuromuscular blockade; tell patient that effects will wear off soon.

modafinil
Alertec✤, Provigil

Pharmacologic class: Nonamphetamine CNS stimulant
Therapeutic class: Analeptic
Controlled substance schedule IV
Pregnancy risk category C

Action
Unknown; stimulates CNS by decreasing release of gamma-aminobutyric acid, a CNS depressant, promoting wakefulness

Availability
Tablets: 100 mg, 200 mg

⬤ Indications and dosages
➤ Narcolepsy
Adults: 200 mg/day P.O. given as a single dose in the morning
Dosage adjustment
• Severe hepatic impairment

Contraindications
• Hypersensitivity to drug
• History of left ventricular hypertrophy, ischemic ECG changes, chest pain, arrhythmias, or mitral valve prolapse with previous CNS stimulant use

Administration
• Give without food (food delays drug absorption).

Route	Onset	Peak	Duration
P.O.	Unknown	2-4 hr	Unknown

Adverse reactions
CNS: headache, dizziness, nervousness, insomnia, depression, anxiety, amnesia, tremor, emotional lability
CV: hypertension, chest pain, vasodilation, hypotension, syncope, **arrhythmias**

EENT: abnormal vision, amblyopia, epistaxis, rhinitis, pharyngitis
GI: nausea, vomiting, diarrhea, dry mouth, anorexia
GU: abnormal urine, urinary retention, albuminuria, abnormal ejaculation
Hematologic: eosinophilia
Hepatic: abnormal hepatic enzyme levels
Metabolic: hyperglycemia
Musculoskeletal: joint disorders, neck pain and rigidity
Respiratory: lung disorder, dyspnea, asthma
Skin: dry skin
Other: fever, chills, herpes simplex infection

Interactions
Drug-drug. *Carbamazepine, phenobarbital, rifampin, other CYP3A4 inducers:* decreased modafinil blood level
Cyclosporine, theophylline: reduced blood levels of these drugs
Diazepam, phenytoin, propranolol, warfarin: increased blood levels of these drugs
Hormonal contraceptives: decreased contraceptive efficacy
Itraconazole, ketoconazole, other CYP3A4 inhibitors: increased modafinil blood level
Methylphenidate: delayed modafinil absorption
Tricyclic antidepressants (TCAs): increased TCA blood level
Drug-diagnostic tests. *Aspartate aminotransferase, eosinophils, gamma-glutamyl transferase, glucose:* increased values

Precautions
Use cautiously in:
• recent myocardial infarction, unstable angina, severe hepatic impairment, hyperthyroidism, hypertension, glaucoma, anxiety, drug abuse
• history of psychosis
• pregnant or breastfeeding patients.

✤ Canada   ◀€ Clinical alert   Reactions in **bold** are life-threatening

Patient monitoring
• Monitor cardiovascular status, including vital signs and ECG.
• Evaluate patient carefully to detect maximal improvement in wakefulness secondary to narcolepsy, compared to adverse CNS effects.
• Monitor neurologic status, including mood, motor function, cognition, and emotional lability.
• Assess blood glucose levels in diabetic patients.
• Evaluate respiratory status.
• Monitor patient carefully if he's receiving concurrent monoamine oxidase inhibitors.

Patient teaching
• Tell patient he may take drug with or without food, but that food may delay drug absorption up to 1 hour.
• Teach patient to immediately report chest pain or syncope.
• Instruct patient to avoid driving and other hazardous activities until he knows how drug affects concentration, vision, motor function, and alertness.
• Instruct female patients to use reliable nonhormonal birth-control method during therapy and for 1 month afterward.
• Advise diabetic patients to monitor blood glucose level closely and stay alert for hyperglycemia.
• As appropriate, review all other significant and life-threatening adverse reactions and interactions, especially those related to the drugs and tests mentioned above.

moexipril hydrochloride
Univasc

Pharmacologic class: Angiotensin-converting enzyme (ACE) inhibitor
Therapeutic class: Antihypertensive
Pregnancy risk category C, D (second and third trimesters)

Action
Inhibits conversion of angiotensin I to the vasoconstrictor angiotensin II; inactivates bradykinin and other vasodilatory prostaglandins. Increases plasma renin levels and reduces aldosterone levels, resulting in systemic vasodilation.

Availability
Tablets: 7.5 mg, 15 mg

Indications and dosages
➤ Hypertension
Adults: 7.5 mg P.O. daily 1 hour before a meal
Dosage adjustment
• Renal impairment
• Concurrent diuretic therapy

Contraindications
• Hypersensitivity to drug
• Angioedema secondary to ACE inhibitor use
• Pregnancy

Administration
• Know that dosage is adjusted according to blood pressure response.

Route	Onset	Peak	Duration
P.O.	30 min	6 hr	Up to 24 hr

Adverse reactions
CNS: dizziness, fatigue, headache
CV: hypotension, syncope
EENT: pharyngitis, sinusitis

GI: nausea, diarrhea, dyspepsia
GU: urinary frequency
Metabolic: hyperkalemia
Musculoskeletal: myalgia
Respiratory: upper respiratory infection, increased cough
Skin: rash, flushing, angioedema
Other: fever, flulike symptoms, hypersensitivity reactions including **anaphylaxis**

Interactions

Drug-drug. *Allopurinol:* increased risk of hypersensitivity reactions
Antacids: decreased moexipril absorption
Antihypertensives, general anesthetics, nitrates, phenothiazines: additive hypotension
Cyclosporine, indomethacin, potassium-sparing diuretics, potassium supplements, salt substitutes: hyperkalemia
Digoxin, lithium: increased blood levels of these drugs
Diuretics: excessive hypotension
Nonsteroidal anti-inflammatory drugs: blunted antihypertensive response
Drug-diagnostic tests. *Alanine aminotransferase, alkaline phosphatase, aspartate aminotransferase, bilirubin, blood urea nitrogen, creatinine, potassium:* increased levels
Antinuclear antibody: positive titer
Sodium: decreased level
Drug-food. *Salt substitutes containing potassium:* hyperkalemia
Drug-behaviors. *Acute alcohol ingestion:* additive hypotension

Precautions

Use cautiously in:
• renal or hepatic impairment, hypovolemia, hyponatremia, aortic stenosis or hypertrophic cardiomyopathy, cardiac or cerebrovascular insufficiency,
• family history of angioedema
• concurrent diuretic therapy
• black patients with hypertension
• elderly patients

• breastfeeding patients
• children (safety not established).

Patient monitoring

• Monitor vital signs, neurologic status, and cardiovascular status.
• Assess respiratory status; note whether patient has persistent dry cough.
• Evaluate for allergic reactions and angioedema.
• Be aware that moexipril monotherapy is less effective in black patients, who may need concurrent drugs.

Patient teaching

• Instruct patient to take drug 1 hour before a meal.
• Tell patient to report dry, persistent cough.
• Teach patient to change position slowly to minimize hypotension and syncope, especially during first few days of therapy.
• Advise patient to limit foods high in potassium and to avoid salt substitutes containing potassium.
• As appropriate, review all other significant and life-threatening adverse reactions and interactions, especially those related to the drugs, tests, foods, and behaviors mentioned above.

montelukast sodium
Singulair

Pharmacologic class: Leukotriene receptor antagonist
Therapeutic class: Antiasthmatic
Pregnancy risk category B

Action

Blocks the action of leukotrienes, decreasing smooth muscle contractions and edema in bronchial airways, pre-

venting inflammation and bronchospasm

Availability
Oral granules: 4-mg base/packet
Tablets: 10 mg
Tablets (chewable, cherry flavor): 4 mg,
5 mg

⚕ Indications and dosages
➤ Long-term management of asthma
Adults and children ages 15 and older:
10 mg/day P.O. in evening
Children ages 6 to 14: 5 mg/day P.O. in
evening
Children ages 2 to 5: 4 mg/day P.O. in
evening

Off-label use
• Chronic urticaria

Contraindications
• Hypersensitivity to drug or its components

Administration
• If desired, mix granules with applesauce or ice cream.

Route	Onset	Peak	Duration
P.O.	Unknown	3-4 hr	Unknown
P.O. (chewable)	Unknown	2-2.5 hr	Unknown
P.O. (granules)	Unknown	Unknown	Unknown

Adverse reactions
CNS: fatigue, headache, dizziness,
asthenia
EENT: nasal congestion, otitis and
sinusitis (in children)
GI: abdominal pain; nausea and diar-
rhea (in children); dyspepsia; infec-
tious gastroenteritis
Metabolic: eosinophilia
Respiratory: cough
Skin: rash
Other: influenza, fever, dental pain

Interactions
Drug-drug. *CYP450 inducers (such as
phenobarbital, rifampin):* decreased
montelukast effects
Drug-diagnostic tests. *Alanine aminotransferase, aspartate aminotransferase:*
increased levels

Precautions
Use cautiously in:
• acute asthma attacks, hepatic impairment, phenylketonuria
• pregnant or breastfeeding patients
• children younger than age 2 (safety
not established).

Patient monitoring
• Assess eosinophil count.
• Monitor temperature; watch for fever
and other signs and symptoms of infection.

Patient teaching
• Advise patient to take drug once a
day in evening.
• Tell patient he may sprinkle granules
onto soft food before taking.
• Inform patient that drug is for pre-
ventive use only and not for treatment
of acute asthma attacks.
• Caution patient to avoid driving and
other hazardous activities because drug
causes dizziness.
• Teach patient to minimize GI upset
by eating small, frequent servings of
healthy food and drinking plenty of
fluids.
• As appropriate, review all other significant adverse reactions and interactions, especially those related to the
drugs and tests mentioned above.

m

---

moricizine hydrochloride
Ethmozine

Pharmacologic class: Sodium channel blocker

Therapeutic class: Antiarrhythmic (class IA)

Pregnancy risk category B

Action
Suppresses abnormal automaticity and prolongs PR interval and QRS duration by blocking fast sodium channel in myocardial tissue; stabilizes membranes. Also has local anesthetic properties.

Availability
Tablets: 200 mg, 250 mg, 300 mg

🕧 Indications and dosages
➤ Life-threatening ventricular arrhythmias, including sustained ventricular tachycardia
Adults: 600 to 900 mg/day P.O. q 8 hours in divided doses; adjust dosage by 150 mg/day q 3 days as required and tolerated.
Dosage adjustment
• Hepatic or renal impairment

Contraindications
• Hypersensitivity to drug
• Cardiogenic shock
• Heart block
• Breastfeeding

Administration
• Administer drug with meals.
• Some patients may tolerate q-12-hour dosing. Assess these patients closely for increased dizziness and nausea.

Route	Onset	Peak	Duration
P.O.	1 hr	0.5-2 hr	10-24 hr

Adverse reactions
CNS: dizziness, fatigue, headache, nervousness, sleep disorders, weakness, paresthesia, **cerebrovascular events**
CV: chest pain, palpitations, hypotension, hypertension, thrombophlebitis, **arrhythmias, heart failure**
EENT: blurred vision
GI: nausea, vomiting, diarrhea, dyspepsia, dry mouth
Musculoskeletal: pain
Respiratory: dyspnea
Skin: sweating
Other: drug fever

Interactions
Drug-drug. *Cimetidine:* increased moricizine blood level
Digoxin: prolonged PR interval
Theophylline: decreased theophylline blood level

Precautions
Use cautiously in:
• electrolyte disturbances, severe renal or hepatic impairment, heart failure, coronary artery disease, sick sinus syndrome
• pregnant patients
• children (safety not established).

Patient monitoring
• Assess baseline ECG; monitor periodically thereafter.
• Monitor vital signs. Watch for drug-induced fever as well as hypotension and rebound hypertension (may occur 1 to 2 hours after administration).
• Monitor patient's weight and fluid intake and output.
• Assess cardiovascular and neurologic status carefully.

Patient teaching
• Instruct patient to take drug with meals to minimize GI upset.
• Advise patient to take drug exactly as prescribed and not to double the dose.

Tell him he may take a missed dose up to 6 hours after previous dose.

• Instruct patient not to stop taking drug suddenly; dosage must be tapered gradually.

◀╏ Teach patient to recognize and immediately report signs and symptoms of heart failure and cerebrovascular events.

• Caution patient to avoid driving and other hazardous activities until he knows how drug affects concentration and alertness.

• As appropriate, review all other significant and life-threatening adverse reactions and interactions, especially those related to the drugs mentioned above.

morphine hydrochloride
Dolora✤, Morphitec✤, MOS Syr

morphine sulfate
Astramorph PF, Avinza, Duramorph, Epimorph✤, Infumorph, Kadian, Morphine H.P.✤, MS Contin, MSIR, MS/S Suppositories, OMS Concentrate, Oramorph SR, RMS Uniserts, Roxanol, Roxanol 100, Roxanol Rescudose, Roxanol Suppositories, Statex✤

Pharmacologic class: Opioid agonist
Therapeutic class: Opioid analgesic
Controlled substance schedule II
Pregnancy risk category C

Action
Interacts with opiate receptor sites, primarily in the limbic system, thalamus, and spinal cord of the CNS, blocking neurotransmitters, which ultimately alters the perception of and relieves pain

Availability
morphine hydrochloride
Rectal suppositories: 20 mg, 30 mg
Syrup: 1 mg/ml, 5 mg/ml, 10 mg/ml, 20 mg/ml, 50 mg/ml
Tablets: 10 mg, 20 mg, 40 mg, 60 mg
morphine sulfate
Capsules: 15 mg, 30 mg
Capsules (sustained-release): 10 mg, 20 mg, 30 mg, 50 mg, 60 mg, 100 mg
Oral solution: 2 mg/ml, 4 mg/ml, 20 mg/ml (concentrate), 10 mg/5 ml, 20 mg/5 ml, 100 mg/5 ml
Rectal suppositories: 5 mg, 10 mg, 20 mg, 30 mg
Solution for epidural or I.V. injection (preservative-free): 0.5 mg/ml, 1 mg/ml
Solution for I.M., S.C., or I.V. injection: 1 mg/ml, 2 mg/ml, 4 mg/ml, 5 mg/ml, 8 mg/ml, 10 mg/ml, 15 mg/ml, 25 mg/ml, 50 mg/ml
Solution for epidural or intrathecal use (for continuous microinfusion device, preservative-free): 10 mg/ml and 25 mg/ml in 20-ml vials
Solution for I.V. injection (for patient-controlled analgesia [PCA] device): 1 mg/ml, 2 mg/ml, 3 mg/ml, 5 mg/ml
Tablets: 15 mg, 30 mg
Tablets (controlled-release, sustained-release): 15 mg, 30 mg, 60 mg, 100 mg, 200 mg
Tablets (soluble): 10 mg, 15 mg, 30 mg

🕐 Indications and dosages
➤ Severe to moderate pain
Adults: 5 to 30 mg P.O. (immediate-release) q 4 hours p.r.n. Or 20 mg P.O. (controlled-release, Kadian) once or twice daily p.r.n. Or 200 mg P.O. (MS Contin) only in opioid-tolerant patients who require daily morphine-equivalent dosages above 400 mg. Or 5 to 20 mg/70 kg S.C. or I.M. q 4 hours p.r.n. Or 2 to 10 mg/70 kg I.V. p.r.n. administered slowly over 4 to 5 minutes. As a continuous I.V. infusion, 0.1 to 1 mg/ml in dextrose 5% in water delivered by controlled-infusion device. For rectal use, 10 to 30 mg P.R. q 4 hours

m

p.r.n. As an epidural injection (Astramorph PF, Duramorph), initially 5 mg injected in lumbar region (may provide pain relief for up to 24 hours); if response isn't adequate within 1 hour, carefully give incremental doses of 1 to 2 mg as needed, up to 10 mg/24 hours. For continuous epidural infusion, 2 to 4 mg/24 hours. As an intrathecal injection, usual dosage is one-tenth of epidural dosage; 0.2 to 1 mg as a single injection in lumbar area may provide relief for up to 24 hours.

Dosage adjustment
• Adults weighing less than 50 kg (110 lb)
• Children

Contraindications
• Hypersensitivity to drug, tartrazine, bisulfites, or alcohol
• Acute bronchial asthma
• Upper airway obstruction
• GI obstruction

Administration
• Administer at onset of pain for best response.
• Give oral form with food or milk to minimize GI upset.
• Know that immediate-release form may be crushed and mixed with food or fluids.
• Don't crush or break extended-release form; remind patient to swallow it whole.
• When giving by direct I.V., dilute with at least 5 ml of sterile water for injection or normal saline solution; administer 2.5 to 10 mg over 4 to 5 minutes.
• For continuous I.V. infusion, use infusion pump or PCA pump; titrate dosage to provide adequate pain relief.
• Don't use parenteral form if it's cloudy or contains visible particulate matter.

Route	Onset	Peak	Duration
P.O.	Unknown	60-120 min	4-5 hr
P.O. (extended)	Unknown	Unknown	8-24 hr
I.V.	Rapid	20 min	4-5 hr
I.M.	10-30 min	30-60 min	4-5 hr
S.C.	20 min	50-90 min	4-5 hr
Epidural	6-30 min	Unknown	Up to 24 hr
Intrathecal	Rapid (min)	Unknown	Up to 24 hr
Rectal	Unknown	20-60 min	4-5 hr

Adverse reactions
CNS: confusion, sedation, dizziness, dysphoria, euphoria, floating feeling, hallucinations, headache, nightmares
CV: hypotension, bradycardia
EENT: blurred vision, diplopia, miosis
GI: nausea, vomiting, constipation, dry mouth
GU: urinary retention
Respiratory: apnea, respiratory depression, respiratory arrest
Skin: flushing, itching, sweating
Other: physical or psychological drug dependence, drug tolerance

Interactions
Drug-drug. *Antihistamines, barbiturates, clomipramine, sedative-hypnotics, tricyclic antidepressants:* additive CNS depression
Buprenorphine, butorphanol, dezocine, nalbuphine, pentazocine: decreased analgesia
Cimetidine: decreased morphine metabolism and increased effects
Mixed opioid agonist-antagonists: precipitation of withdrawal symptoms in physically dependent patients
Monoamine oxidase inhibitors: severe, unpredictable reactions
Warfarin: increased anticoagulant effect
Drug-diagnostic tests. *Amylase, lipase:* increased levels

Drug-herb. *Chamomile, hops, kava, skullcap, valerian:* increased CNS depression

Drug-behaviors. *Alcohol use:* increased CNS depression

Precautions
Use cautiously in:
• head trauma; increased intracranial pressure; severe renal, hepatic, or pulmonary disease; hypothyroidism; adrenal insufficiency; prostatic hypertrophy
• elderly or debilitated patients
• pregnant or breastfeeding patients.

Patient monitoring
• Monitor vital signs; contact prescriber if respiratory rate drops to 10 breaths/minutes or less.
• Assess pain location, character, and intensity.
• Monitor fluid intake and output; stay alert for urinary retention.
• Monitor bowel evacuation pattern; if constipation occurs, implement appropriate measures.
• Assess neurologic status; implement safety measures as needed to prevent injury.
• Evaluate patient for signs and symptoms of physical or psychological dependence; watch for drug hoarding.

Patient teaching
• Advise patient to take drug at first sign of pain, because continuous dosing is more effective than as-needed dosing.
• Tell patient and caregiver that drug may cause respiratory depression; instruct them to immediately report a respiratory rate of 10 breaths/minute or less.
• Teach patient that drug may cause constipation or urinary retention; encourage high-fiber diet and high fluid intake.
• Emphasize importance of taking drug only as prescribed; point out that

drug may cause psychological or physical dependence.
• Instruct patient to avoid driving and other hazardous activities until he knows how drug affects concentration, vision, and alertness.
• Teach patient and caregivers about appropriate home safety measures to prevent injury.
• Caution patient to avoid alcohol and other CNS depressants during therapy and for 24 hours afterward.
• Teach patient to avoid herbs, which may worsen adverse CNS effects.
• As appropriate, review all other significant and life-threatening adverse reactions and interactions, especially those related to the drugs, tests, herbs, and behaviors mentioned above.

moxifloxacin hydrochloride
Avelox

m

Pharmacologic class: Fluoroquinolone
Therapeutic class: Anti-infective
Pregnancy risk category C

Action
Selectively inhibits DNA synthesis by disrupting DNA replication and transcription and suppressing protein synthesis, causing bacterial cell death

Availability
Injection (premixed): 400 mg/250-ml bags
Tablets: 400 mg

⬤ Indications and dosages
➤ Acute bacterial sinusitis caused by *Haemophilus influenzae, Moraxella catarrhalis,* and *Staphylococcus pneumoniae*
Adults: 400 mg P.O. or I.V. q 24 hours for 10 days

➤ Acute bacterial exacerbation of chronic bronchitis

Adults: 400 mg P.O. or I.V. q 24 hours for 5 days

➤ Community-acquired pneumonia

Adults: 400 mg P.O. or I.V. q 24 hours for 7 to 14 days

➤ Uncomplicated skin and skin-structure infections

Adults: 400 mg P.O. or I.V. q 24 hours for 7 days

Contraindications

• Hypersensitivity to drug or other fluoroquinolones

• Children younger than age 18 (except in postexposure inhalation anthrax)

Administration

• Give premixed I.V. dose over 60 minutes; don't mix with other drugs in same I.V. line.

• Know that although milk or yogurt may impair drug absorption, drug may be given with other calcium products.

Route	Onset	Peak	Duration
P.O.	Within 1 hr	1-3 hr	24 hr
I.V.	Rapid	End of infusion	24 hr

Adverse reactions

CNS: dizziness, drowsiness, headache, insomnia, acute psychoses, agitation, confusion, light-headedness, hallucinations, tremor, **seizures**

CV: prolonged QT interval, vasodilation, tachycardia, hypertension, **arrhythmias**

GI: nausea, diarrhea, abdominal pain, altered taste, **pseudomembranous colitis**

GU: vaginitis

Hematologic: eosinophilia, **thrombocytopenia, leukopenia**

Musculoskeletal: joint pain, tendinitis, tendon rupture

Skin: rash, photosensitivity, phototoxicity

Other: phlebitis at I.V. site, superinfection, hypersensitivity reactions including **anaphylaxis, Stevens-Johnson syndrome**

Interactions

Drug-drug. *Amiodarone, bepridil, disopyramide, erythromycin, pentamidine, phenothiazines, pimozide, procainamide, quinidine, sotalol, tricyclic antidepressants:* increased risk of serious adverse cardiovascular reactions

Antacids, iron salts, bismuth subsalicylate, sucralfate, zinc salts: decreased moxifloxacin absorption

Theophylline: increased theophylline blood level, possible toxicity

Drug-diagnostic tests. *Alanine aminotransferase, alkaline phosphatase, aspartate aminotransferase, bilirubin, lactate dehydrogenase, platelets:* increased values

Drug-food. *Concurrent tube feedings, milk, yogurt:* impaired drug absorption

Drug-herb. *Dong quai, St. John's wort:* phototoxicity

Fennel: decreased moxifloxacin absorption

Drug-behaviors. *Sun exposure:* phototoxicity

Precautions

Use cautiously in:

• underlying CNS diseases and disorders, renal impairment, cirrhosis, bradycardia, acute myocardial ischemia, prolonged QTc interval, uncorrected hypokalemia, dialysis

• elderly patients

• pregnant or breastfeeding patients (safety not established except in postexposure inhalation anthrax).

Patient monitoring

• Watch for hypersensitivity reaction, anaphylaxis, and other allergic reactions; be aware that these may occur after initial dose.

• Monitor cardiovascular and neurologic status closely.

• Watch for tendinitis and Achilles tendon rupture.
• Monitor complete blood count and liver function tests.
• Assess GI status; report signs or symptoms of pseudomembranous colitis.
• Watch closely for superinfection.

Patient teaching
• Advise patient to take drug once a day with or without food.
• Tell patient to take oral form 4 hours before or 8 hours after antacids, multivitamins, sucralfate, or preparations containing aluminum, magnesium, iron, or zinc.
• Inform patient that drug may cause serious allergic reactions even several days after therapy begins; advise him to report these immediately.
• Teach patient to promptly report tendon pain, diarrhea with blood or pus, and signs and symptoms of superinfection.
• Instruct patient to avoid driving and other hazardous activities until he knows how drug affects concentration and alertness.
• As appropriate, review all other significant and life-threatening adverse reactions and interactions, especially those related to the drugs, tests, foods, herbs, and behaviors mentioned above.

muromonab-CD3
Orthoclone OKT3

Pharmacologic class: Murine monoclonal antibody

Therapeutic class: Immunosuppressant

Pregnancy risk category C

Action
Binds to and blocks the function of T lymphocytes responsible for antigen recognition, thereby reversing graft rejection

Availability
Injection: 1 mg/1 ml in 5-ml ampules

Indications and dosages
➤ Acute allograft rejection in kidney transplant patients; steroid-resistant acute allograft rejection in heart and liver transplant patients
Adults: 5 mg/day I.V. for 10 to 14 days
Dosage adjustment
• Children

Contraindications
• Hypersensitivity to drug or other products of murine origin
• Uncompensated heart failure
• Predisposition to or history of seizures
• Pregnancy or breastfeeding

Administration
• In kidney transplant patients, start therapy as soon as acute renal rejection is diagnosed. In heart and liver transplant patients, start therapy when physician determines that steroid therapy hasn't reversed allograft rejection.
• Be aware that drug must be given in facility equipped and staffed to treat cardiopulmonary arrest.
• For I.V. bolus injection, draw solution into syringe through low protein-binding 0.2- or 0.22-micron filter. Discard filter and attach needle-free adapter.
• Administer bolus over less than 1 minute.
• Give antipyretics to decrease fever and corticosteroids to reduce allergic response, as prescribed.

Route	Onset	Peak	Duration
I.V.	Immediate	Unknown	1 wk

Adverse reactions

CNS: tremors, hallucinations, fatigue, headache, weakness, **aseptic meningitis, cerebral edema, seizures, encephalopathy**

CV: chest pain, hypertension, hypotension, **heart failure, tachycardia, cardiac arrest, shock**

EENT: blindness, blurred vision, conjunctivitis, photophobia, tinnitus, otitis media

GI: nausea, vomiting, diarrhea

GU: oliguria, **anuria**

Respiratory: dyspnea, wheezing, **severe pulmonary edema, adult respiratory distress syndrome (ARDS)**

Skin: flushing

Other: fever, chills, flulike symptoms, infection, **anaphylaxis, cytokine release syndrome**

Interactions

Drug-drug. *Indomethacin:* increased muromonab blood level, encephalopathy, and other adverse CNS effects

Live-virus vaccines: increased vaccine replication and effects

Other immunosuppressants: increased risk of infection

Drug-diagnostic tests. *Blood urea nitrogen, creatinine:* increased levels

Drug-herb. *Astragalus, echinacea, melatonin:* interference with immunosuppressant effect

Precautions

Use cautiously in:
• fever
• children younger than age 2.

Patient monitoring

• Evaluate vital signs and cardiovascular status; monitor ECG closely.

• Stay alert for signs and symptoms of cytokine release syndrome, including fever up to 41.6° C (107° F), chills, rigor, nausea, vomiting, abdominal pain, diarrhea, malaise, joint and muscle pain, headache, and tremors.

◀╟ Be aware that most adverse reactions occur within 30 minutes to 6 hours of first dose.

• Monitor temperature closely; stay alert for fever and other signs and symptoms of infection.

• Assess neurologic status and respiratory status closely; evaluate for signs and symptoms of aseptic meningitis, encephalopathy, cerebral edema, pulmonary edema, and ARDS.

Patient teaching

• Inform patient that drug can cause serious adverse reactions; reassure him that he'll be monitored closely and will receive nursing and medical interventions to relieve these reactions. Teach him to recognize and immediately report adverse reactions.

• Reassure patient that adverse reactions will subside as treatment progresses.

• Advise female patients to avoid becoming pregnant during therapy.

• As appropriate, review all other significant and life-threatening adverse reactions and interactions, especially those related to the drugs, tests, and herbs mentioned above.

mycophenolate mofetil
CellCept

mycophenolate mofetil hydrochloride
CellCept Intravenous

Pharmacologic class: Mycophenolic acid derivative

Therapeutic class: Immunosuppressant

Pregnancy risk category C

Action
Inhibits binding of interleukin (IL)-1 with IL-1 receptors, preventing proliferation and differentiation of activated B and T cells; binds to intracellular proteins to prevent T-cell activation, thereby suppressing immune responses

Availability
Capsules: 250 mg
Injection: 500 mg/vial
Tablets: 500 mg

Indications and dosages
➣ To prevent organ rejection in patients receiving allogeneic kidney transplants
Adults: 1 g P.O. or I.V. b.i.d., given with corticosteroids and cyclosporine
➣ To prevent organ rejection in patients receiving allogeneic heart transplants
Adults: 1.5 g P.O. or I.V. b.i.d. given with corticosteroids and cyclosporine. May start I.V. administration less than 24 hours after transplantation; switch to P.O. dosing when tolerated.
➣ To prevent organ rejection in patients receiving allogeneic liver transplants
Adults: 1.5 g b.i.d P.O. or I.V. over 2 hours; usually given with corticosteroids and cyclosporine.
Dosage adjustment
• Severe chronic renal impairment
• Neutropenia

Contraindications
• Hypersensitivity to drug or its components, mycophenolic acid, or polysorbate 80 (I.V. form)
• Pregnancy or breastfeeding

Administration
• Give P.O. form at least 1 hour before or 2 hours after meals. To enhance absorption, don't administer with other drugs.

• Don't open or crush tablets or capsules, and don't allow patient to chew them.
• Drug is teratogenic. Avoid inhaling powder in capsules or letting it contact skin or mucous membranes. If contact occurs, wash skin thoroughly with soap and water or irrigate eyes with water.
• For I.V. use, reconstitute with dextrose 5% in water and dilute to 6 mg/ml; administer over 2 hours. Don't give by rapid I.V. push or bolus.

Route	Onset	Peak	Duration
P.O.	Unknown	30-75 min	7.5-18 hr
I.V.	Unknown	Unknown	10-17 hr

Adverse reactions
CNS: tremor, insomnia, dizziness, headache, asthenia
CV: chest pain, hypertension, peripheral edema
EENT: pharyngitis, oral moniliasis
GI: nausea, vomiting, diarrhea, constipation, dyspepsia, abdominal pain, **hemorrhage**
GU: urinary tract infection, hematuria, renal tubular necrosis
Hematologic: anemia, hypochromic anemia, leukocytosis, **leukopenia, thrombocytopenia**
Metabolic: hypercholesterolemia, hypophosphatemia, hypokalemia, hyperkalemia, hyperglycemia
Musculoskeletal: back pain
Respiratory: dyspnea, cough, bronchitis, pneumonia
Skin: acne, rash
Other: pain, fever, infection, lymphoma, **sepsis**

Interactions
Drug-drug. *Acyclovir, ganciclovir, other drugs that undergo renal tubular secretion:* increased risk of toxicity from either drug

m

Antacids containing aluminum or magnesium: decreased mycophenolate absorption
Cholestyramine: reduced mycophenolate bioavailability
Hormonal contraceptives: reduced contraceptive efficacy
Phenytoin, theophylline: increased blood levels of both drugs
Probenecid, salicylates: increased mycophenolate blood level
Drug-herb. *Astragalus, echinacea, melatonin:* interference with immunosuppressant effect

Precautions

Use cautiously in:
• lymphoma, cancer, neutropenia, renal disease, or GI disorders.

Patient monitoring

• Monitor complete blood count with white cell differential, electrolyte levels, lipid panel, blood chemistry, and liver function tests.
• Evaluate vital signs; assess cardiovascular and respiratory status carefully. Watch for signs and symptoms of bronchitis and pneumonia.
• Assess all body systems carefully for signs and symptoms of infection.
• Monitor patient for bleeding tendency.

Patient teaching

• Advise patient to take oral drug at least 1 hour before or 2 hours after meals. Tell him not to crush, break, or chew it or take it with other drugs.
• Instruct patient to take his temperature and promptly report fever or other signs or symptoms of infection.
• Teach patient to report unusual bleeding or bruising.
• Instruct patient to avoid driving and other hazardous activities until he knows how drug affects concentration and alertness.
• Instruct patient to avoid crowds and people with known infections.

• Teach female patient to use abstinence or two other contraceptive methods during therapy and for 6 weeks afterward (even if she has a history of infertility). Tell her to immediately report suspected pregnancy.
• As appropriate, review all other significant and life-threatening adverse reactions and interactions, especially those related to the drugs and herbs mentioned above.

nabumetone
Gen-Nabumetone✽, Relafen

Pharmacologic class: Nonsteroidal anti-inflammatory drug (NSAID)
Therapeutic class: Antiarthritic
Pregnancy risk category C, D (third trimester)

Action

Unknown; inhibits cyclooxygenase, an enzyme needed for prostaglandin synthesis, resulting in stimulation of anti-inflammatory response and blocking of pain impulses

Availability

Tablets: 500 mg, 750 mg

Indications and dosages

➤ Rheumatoid arthritis, osteoarthritis
Adults: 1,000 mg/day P.O. as a single dose or in two divided doses; may increase up to 2,000 mg/day

Contraindications

• Hypersensitivity to drug
• Active GI bleeding or ulcer disease

• History of aspirin- or NSAID-induced asthma, urticaria, or other allergic-type reactions
• Concurrent use of other NSAIDs
• Pregnancy (third trimester)

Administration
• Give drug with food or milk to increase absorption.
• In chronic therapy, use lowest effective dosage.

Route	Onset	Peak	Duration
P.O.	1-2 hr	5 hr	12-24 hr

Adverse reactions
CNS: dizziness, drowsiness, fatigue, headache, insomnia, malaise, nervousness
CV: vasculitis
EENT: abnormal vision, tinnitus
GI: nausea, vomiting, diarrhea, constipation, abdominal pain, dyspepsia, flatulence, stomatitis, dry mouth, **GI bleeding**
Skin: pruritus, rash, angioedema
Other: edema, fluid retention, allergic reactions including **anaphylaxis**

Interactions
Drug-drug. *Acetaminophen:* increased risk of adverse renal reactions (with chronic nabumetone use)
Anticoagulants, cefamandole, cefoperazone, cefotetan, clopidogrel, eptifibatide, plicamycin, thrombolytics, ticlopidine, tirofiban, valproic acid: increased risk of bleeding
Antihypertensives, diuretics: decreased nabumetone efficacy
Antineoplastics: increased risk of adverse hematologic reactions
Aspirin, corticosteroids, other NSAIDs, potassium supplements: additive adverse GI effects
Cyclosporine: increased risk of renal toxicity
Insulins, oral hypoglycemics: increased hypoglycemic effect

Methotrexate: increased risk of methotrexate toxicity

Precautions
Use cautiously in:
• severe cardiovascular, renal, or hepatic disease
• history of ulcer disease.

Patient monitoring
• Watch closely for signs and symptoms of hypersensitivity reaction, anaphylaxis, and angioedema, including hives, swelling, shortness of breath, and abdominal pain.
• Monitor GI status; report nutritional deficiencies.
• Assess vital signs.
• Monitor fluid intake and output.

Patient teaching
• Tell patient he may crush tablet if he can't swallow it whole.
• To minimize GI upset, teach patient to take drug with food; eat small, frequent servings of healthy food; and drink plenty of fluids.
• Inform patient that for drug to be effective, he must take it for entire length of therapy as prescribed.
◀ Teach patient to recognize and immediately report signs and symptoms of hypersensitivity reaction and angioedema (hives, swelling, shortness of breath, abdominal pain).
• Caution patient to avoid driving and other hazardous activities until he knows how drug affects concentration, vision, strength, and alertness.
• Instruct patient to avoid aspirin, ibuprofen, and over-the-counter preparations (unless prescribed). Also teach him to avoid alcohol.
• As appropriate, review all other significant and life-threatening adverse reactions and interactions, especially those related to the drugs mentioned above.

n

nadolol
Apo-Nadolol✚, Corgard,
Novo-Nadolol✚, Syn-Nadolol✚

Pharmacologic class: Beta-adrenergic
blocker (nonselective)

Therapeutic class: Antianginal, antihypertensive

Pregnancy risk category C

Action
Blocks stimulation of beta$_1$ and beta$_2$
receptor sites, decreasing cardiac output, thereby slowing heart rate and reducing blood pressure

Availability
Tablets: 20 mg, 40 mg, 80 mg, 120 mg,
160 mg

💊 Indications and dosages
➤ Angina pectoris

Adults: Initially, 40 mg P.O. once daily;
may increase by 40 to 80 mg q 3 to 7
days p.r.n., up to a maximum daily
dosage of 240 mg

➤ Hypertension

Adults: Initially, 40 mg P.O. once daily;
may increase by 40 to 80 mg q 7 days
p.r.n., up to 320 mg/day

Dosage adjustment
• Renal impairment

Off-label uses
• Hyperthyroidism
• Migraine headache
• Parkinson's tremor

Contraindications
• Hypersensitivity to drug or other
beta-adrenergic blockers
• Pulmonary edema or cardiogenic
shock
• Sinus bradycardia or heart block
• Chronic obstructive pulmonary dis-
ease

Administration
• Give drug with or without food.

Route	Onset	Peak	Duration
P.O.	5 days	3-4 hr	24 hr

Adverse reactions
CNS: dizziness, fatigue, paresthesia, behavior changes, sedation

CV: bradycardia, peripheral vascular
insufficiency (Raynaud's phenomenon), **heart failure**

EENT: blurred vision, dry eyes, nasal
congestion

GI: nausea, constipation, diarrhea, abdominal discomfort or bloating, indigestion, anorexia

Respiratory: bronchospasm

Skin: rash

Interactions
Drug-drug. *Amphetamines, ephedrine,
epinephrine, norepinephrine, phenylephrine, pseudoephedrine:* severe vasoconstriction and bradycardia

Antihypertensives, nitrates: additive hypotension

Clonidine: increased hypotension and
bradycardia

Digoxin: additive bradycardia

*Diltiazem, general anesthetics, pheny-
toin (I.V.), verapamil:* additive myocardial depression

Insulins, oral hypoglycemics: altered
glycemic control

Nonsteroidal anti-inflammatory drugs:
decreased antihypertensive action

Thyroid hormones: decreased nadolol
efficacy

Drug-behaviors. *Acute alcohol ingestion:* additive hypotension

Cocaine use: severe vasoconstriction
and bradycardia

Precautions
Use cautiously in:
• renal or hepatic impairment, pulmonary disease, diabetes mellitus, thyrotoxicosis

---

- history of severe allergic reactions
- elderly patients
- pregnant or breastfeeding patients
- children (safety not established).

Patient monitoring
- Monitor vital signs and peripheral circulation. Notify prescriber if heart rate is below 55 beats/minute.
- Assess for signs and symptoms of heart failure.

Patient teaching
- Advise patient to take drug with meals and bedtime snack to minimize GI upset.
- Teach patient how to measure pulse and blood pressure at home and when to notify prescriber.
- Instruct patient to avoid over-the-counter products containing stimulants, such as some cold and flu remedies and nasal decongestants.
- Tell diabetic patients and their families that drug may mask symptoms of low blood glucose; advise patient to monitor urine or blood glucose regularly.
- Caution patient to avoid driving and other hazardous activities until he knows how drug affects concentration and alertness.
- As appropriate, review all other significant and life-threatening adverse reactions and interactions, especially those related to the drugs and behaviors mentioned above.

nafarelin acetate
Synarel

Pharmacologic class: Gonadotropin-releasing hormone (GnRH)
Therapeutic class: Hormone
Pregnancy risk category X

Action
Inhibits secretion of gonadotropin, a luteinizing hormone (LH)-releasing hormone; increases pituitary production of LH and follicle-stimulating hormone (FSH) initially, ultimately deactivating testicular and ovarian functions.

Availability
Nasal spray: 2 mg/ml in 10-ml bottle (200 mcg/spray)

🖊 Indications and dosages
➤ Endometriosis
Adults: One spray (200 mcg) intranasally in one nostril in morning and one spray in other nostril in evening (400 mcg/day); may increase to one spray in each nostril in morning and evening (800 mcg/day)
➤ Central precocious puberty
Children: Two sprays in each nostril in morning and evening (1,600 mcg/day); may increase up to 1,800 mcg/day (three sprays in alternating nostrils t.i.d.)

Contraindications
- Hypersensitivity to GnRH, its analogs, or sorbitol
- Pregnancy or breastfeeding

Administration
- Make sure patient isn't pregnant before starting therapy.
- For endometriosis, begin therapy during second to fourth day of menstrual period.
- If patient needs topical decongestant, wait at least 2 hours after nafarelin dose before administering it.

Route	Onset	Peak	Duration
Intranasal	Within 4 wk	3-4 wk	3-6 mo

Adverse reactions
CNS: emotional lability, headache, depression, insomnia
CV: chest pain

n

EENT: nasal irritation, rhinitis
GU: vaginal dryness, bleeding, or discharge; menses cessation; decreased libido; transient breast enlargement
Musculoskeletal: decreased bone density, myalgia
Respiratory: dyspnea
Skin: urticaria, rash, pruritus, acne, oily skin, hirsutism, transient increase in pubic hair
Other: weight changes, hot flashes, edema, body odor, hypersensitivity reaction

Interactions
Drug-drug. *Topical nasal decongestants:* reduced nafarelin absorption

Precautions
Use cautiously in:
• rhinitis.

Patient monitoring
• Monitor patient for emotional lability or depression.
• Assess nasal mucosa for signs of nasal erosion.
• Monitor vital signs. Weigh patient regularly; report edema.
• Stay alert for adverse hormonal effects, including hot flashes, menses cessation followed by breakthrough bleeding, hirsutism, acne, decreased libido, and vaginal dryness.

Patient teaching
• Instruct patient to complete entire course of therapy. Advise her to keep enough drug on hand to prevent interruption.
• Inform patient that regular menstruation should cease after 4 to 6 weeks of therapy but that breakthrough bleeding may still occur.
• Caution patient that ovulation may still occur. Instruct her to use barrier birth-control method during therapy and to report suspected pregnancy.

• Teach patient about adverse hormonal effects; identify which signs and symptoms to report to prescriber.
• Inform patient that drug may cause emotional changes or depression; advise her to report these to prescriber.
• As appropriate, review all other significant adverse reactions and interactions, especially those related to the drugs mentioned above.

nafcillin sodium
Nafcil, Nallpen, Unipen

Pharmacologic class: Penicillinase-resistant penicillin
Therapeutic class: Anti-infective
Pregnancy risk category B

Action
Inhibits cell wall synthesis during microorganism multiplication; resists inactivation by staphylococcal penicillinase; bactericidal

Availability
Injection: 500 mg, 1 g, 2 g, 10 g
I.V. infusion (piggyback): 1 g, 2 g

⚠️ Indications and dosages
➤ Systemic infection caused by penicillinase-producing staphylococci
Adults: 500 mg I.M. q 4 to 6 hours or I.V. q 4 hours; for more severe infections, 1 g I.M. or I.V. q 4 hours, to a maximum daily dosage of 6 g
Dosage adjustment
• Children

Contraindications
• Hypersensitivity to drug or other penicillins

Administration
• For I.M. use, reconstitute 500 mg with sterile water or bacteriostatic water for final concentration of 250 mg/

♣ Canada   ◀€ Clinical alert   Reactions in **bold** are life-threatening

ml. Inject deep into large muscle mass, such as ventral gluteal or vastus lateralis.

• For I.V. use, reconstitute with normal saline solution, dextrose 5% in water (D_5W), dextrose 10% in water, half D_5W/normal saline solution, or half D_5W/lactated Ringer's solution. Administer over 30 to 60 minutes. Don't mix with other drugs in same solution.

Route	Onset	Peak	Duration
I.V.	Immediate	15 min	4 hr
I.M.	Rapid	30-90 min	4-6 hr

Adverse reactions
CNS: lethargy, hallucinations, anxiety, depression, twitching, **coma, seizures**
CV: thrombophlebitis
GI: nausea, vomiting, diarrhea
Hematologic: anemia, **bone marrow depression, granulocytopenia**
Skin: angioedema
Other: superinfection, vein irritation (with I.V. use), hypersensitivity reactions including serum sickness and **anaphylaxis**

Interactions
Drug-drug. *Aminoglycosides:* synergistic effects
Cyclosporine: subtherapeutic cyclosporine blood level
Hormonal contraceptives: decreased contraceptive efficacy
Probenecid: increased nafcillin blood level
Rifampin: antagonism (dose-dependent)
Warfarin: increased risk of bleeding
Drug-diagnostic tests. *Granulocytes, neutrophils, platelets:* decreased counts
Drug-herb. *Khat:* delayed and reduced nafcillin absorption

Precautions
Use cautiously in:
• hypersensitivity to cephalosporins
• renal disorders, GI distress

• pregnant or breastfeeding patients
• neonates.

Patient monitoring
• Assess for signs and symptoms of hypersensitivity, serum sickness, and angioedema; know that these reactions may occur several days after therapy begins.
• Monitor neurologic status. Stay alert for seizures, and assess for depression and hallucinations.
• Evaluate complete blood count with white cell differential.
• In prolonged therapy, assess for superinfection.

Patient teaching
• Instruct patient to complete entire course of therapy even if symptoms disappear.
◀€ Teach patient to recognize and immediately report signs and symptoms of hypersensitivity reaction, serum sickness, or angioedema, as well as bleeding and easy bruising.
• Teach patient about signs and symptoms of superinfection; instruct him to report these promptly.
• Caution patient to avoid driving and other hazardous activities until he knows how drug affects alertness and motor function.
• As appropriate, review all other significant and life-threatening adverse reactions and interactions, especially those related to the drugs, tests, and herbs mentioned above.

nalbuphine hydrochloride
Nubain

Pharmacologic class: Opioid agonist-antagonist

Therapeutic class: Analgesic, adjunct to anesthesia

Pregnancy risk category C

Action
Binds with opiate receptors in CNS, altering perception of and response to painful stimuli

Availability
Injection: 10 mg/ml, 20 mg/ml

🖊 Indications and dosages
➤ Moderate to severe pain
Adults: 10 mg/70 kg I.V., I.M., or S.C. q 3 to 6 hours p.r.n., up to 160 mg/day. Maximum of 20 mg as a single dose.
➤ Adjunct to balanced anesthesia
Adults: 0.3 mg to 3 mg/kg I.V. over 10 to 15 minutes, followed by maintenance doses of 0.25 mg to 0.50 mg/kg I.V. in single doses p.r.n.

Contraindications
• Hypersensitivity to drug
• Physical drug dependence

Administration
• Ensure that emergency resuscitation equipment and naloxone (antidote) are available before starting therapy.
• For I.M. use, inject deep into large muscle mass; rotate injection sites.
• For I.V. use, infuse undiluted over 2 to 3 minutes into a vein or I.V. line with compatible solution (such as dextrose 5% in water, normal saline solution, or lactated Ringer's solution).

Route	Onset	Peak	Duration
I.V.	2-3 min	30 min	3-6 hr
I.M.	15 min	1 hr	3-6 hr
S.C.	15 min	Unknown	3-6 hr

Adverse reactions
CNS: dizziness, sedation, headache, vertigo
CV: hypertension, hypotension, tachycardia, bradycardia
EENT: miosis
GI: nausea, vomiting, dry mouth
Respiratory: dyspnea, respiratory depression

Skin: sweating, clamminess
Other: hypersensitivity reactions including **anaphylaxis**

Interactions
Drug-drug. *CNS depressants (such as general anesthetics, monoamine oxidase inhibitors, sedative-hypnotics, tranquilizers, tricyclic antidepressants):* additive CNS effects
Drug-diagnostic tests. *Amylase, lipase:* increased levels
Drug-herb. *Chamomile, hops, kava, skullcap, valerian:* increased CNS depression
Drug-behaviors. *Alcohol use:* additive CNS and respiratory depression

Precautions
Use cautiously in:
• increased intracranial pressure, head trauma, myocardial infarction, severe heart disease, respiratory depression, renal or hepatic disease, impaired ventilation, hypothyroidism, adrenal insufficiency, prostatic hypertrophy, emotional instability, alcoholism
• history of substance abuse
• pregnant or breastfeeding patients
• children.

Patient monitoring
• Monitor vital signs; watch for respiratory depression and heart rate changes.
• Evaluate patient for CNS changes; institute safety measures as needed to prevent injury.
• Watch for hypersensitivity reactions, such as anaphylaxis.

Patient teaching
• Instruct patient to change position slowly and carefully to avoid dizziness or light-headedness from sudden blood pressure decrease.
• Teach patient to avoid CNS depressants (including alcohol, sedative-hypnotics, and some herbs) for at least 24 hours after taking nalbuphine.

• Caution patient to avoid driving and other hazardous activities until he knows how drug affects concentration, vision, and alertness.

• As appropriate, review all other significant and life-threatening adverse reactions and interactions, especially those related to the drugs, tests, herbs, and behaviors mentioned above.

nalidixic acid
NegGram

Pharmacologic class: Quinolone antibiotic

Therapeutic class: Urinary tract anti-infective

Pregnancy risk category B

Action
Interferes with DNA and RNA synthesis in susceptible gram-negative bacteria; bactericidal

Availability
Oral suspension: 250 mg/5 ml
Tablets: 250 mg, 500 mg, 1 g

Indications and dosages
➤ Urinary tract infections (UTIs) caused by susceptible gram-negative bacteria, including *Proteus* strains, *Klebsiella* and *Enterobacter* species, and *Escherichia coli*
Adults: Initially, 1 g P.O. q.i.d. for 1 to 2 weeks. In prolonged therapy, dosage may be reduced to 2 g/day.
Dosage adjustment
• Children

Contraindications
• Hypersensitivity to drug
• Seizure disorder
• Infants younger than 3 months

Administration
• Give drug with food or milk to avoid GI upset.

Route	Onset	Peak	Duration
P.O.	Variable	1-2 hr	Unknown

Adverse reactions
CNS: drowsiness, weakness, headache, dizziness, malaise, vertigo, syncope, excitement, hallucinations, confusion, depression, insomnia, **seizures**
EENT: blurred vision, light sensitivity, decreased visual acuity, diplopia, altered color perception
GI: nausea, vomiting, diarrhea, abdominal pain
Hematologic: eosinophilia
Skin: rash, urticaria, pruritus, photosensitivity, angioedema
Other: fever, chills, **anaphylaxis, Stevens-Johnson syndrome**

Interactions
Drug-drug. *Antacids:* decreased nalidixic acid absorption
Nitrofurantoin: decreased nalidixic acid effects
Oral anticoagulant: increased anticoagulant effects
Drug-diagnostic tests. *Urinary vanillylmandelic acid, urine 17-ketogenic steroids, urine 17-ketosteroids:* false increases
Urine glucose tests using cupric sulfate reagents (such as Benedict's test): false-positive reaction
Drug-food. *Caffeine-containing foods and beverages:* increased stimulation
Drug-herb. *Dong quai, St. John's wort:* photosensitivity

Precautions
Use cautiously in:
• renal or hepatic disease, glucose-6-phosphate dehydrogenase deficiency, cerebral arteriosclerosis, CNS damage
• elderly patients
• pregnant or breastfeeding patients
• prepubertal children.

Patient monitoring

• Monitor clinical response; if no improvement occurs, repeat culture and sensitivity tests.

• Assess neurologic and nutritional status carefully.

• Watch for GI signs and symptoms.

• Monitor for hypersensitivity reactions, including anaphylaxis and angioedema.

Patient teaching

• Instruct patient to take drug with food to minimize GI upset.

◀€ Teach patient to recognize and immediately report serious adverse effects, including CNS changes and angioedema.

• Advise patient to minimize GI upset by eating small, frequent servings of healthy food and ensuring adequate fluid intake.

• Instruct patient to avoid driving and other hazardous activities until he knows how drug affects concentration and alertness.

• As appropriate, review all other significant and life-threatening adverse reactions and interactions, especially those related to the drugs, tests, foods, and herbs mentioned above.

naloxone hydrochloride
Narcan

Pharmacologic class: Opioid antagonist

Therapeutic class: Opioid antidote

Pregnancy risk category B

Action

Unclear; thought to compete with opioids for the same receptor sites in brain. Prevents or reverses opioid effects, including respiratory depression, sedation, and hypotension; also reverses dysphoric effects of opioid agonists-antagonists.

Availability

Injection: 0.4 mg/ml, 1 mg/ml (with preservatives); 0.02 mg/ml, 0.4 mg/ml (paraben-free)

⚠ Indications and dosages

➢ Opioid overdose

Adults: 0.4 to 2 mg I.V., S.C., or I.M.; repeat q 2 to 3 minutes p.r.n., up to 10 mg

➢ Postoperative opioid-induced respiratory depression

Adults: 0.1 to 0.2 mg I.V. q 2 to 3 minutes p.r.n.

Dosage adjustment

• Children and neonates

Off-label uses

• Dementia associated with Alzheimer's disease or schizophrenia

• Reversal of alcoholic coma

Contraindications

• Hypersensitivity to drug or other opioid antagonists

Administration

• Administer only if resuscitation equipment is available.

• If ordered, give initial dose of 0.1 mg I.V. to assess patient's response. Give subsequent doses of 0.4 mg or less (undiluted) by direct injection over 15 seconds, or titrate based on response.

• As needed, give continuous I.V. infusion, further diluting drug with normal saline solution or dextrose 5% in water; titrate based on patient's response.

Route	Onset	Peak	Duration
I.V.	1-2 min	5-15 min	Variable
I.M., S.C.	2-5 min	5-15 min	Variable

Adverse reactions
CNS: tremors, **seizures**
CV: tachycardia, hypotension, hypertension (with higher doses), **ventricular tachycardia, ventricular fibrillation, cardiac arrest**
GI: nausea, vomiting
Respiratory: hyperpnea, **pulmonary edema**
Skin: diaphoresis
Other: withdrawal syndrome

Interactions
None significant

Precautions
Use cautiously in:
• cardiovascular disease, opioid dependency
• pregnant or breastfeeding patients
• children.

Patient monitoring
• Monitor vital signs every 3 to 5 minutes until opioid effects are reversed.
• Assess arterial blood gas results and oxygen saturation.
• Evaluate cardiac status with continuous ECG monitoring.
• If patient doesn't respond to 10-mg doses given in opioid overdose, reevaluate cause of underlying clinical condition.
• Evaluate neurologic status, including level of consciousness; stay alert for seizures.
• Once naloxone is effective (up to 2 hours after administration), watch for signs and symptoms of acute withdrawal syndrome in opioid-dependent patients.
• Follow facility guidelines regarding follow-up treatment of drug overdose.

Patient teaching
• Reassure patient that environment is safe.

naltrexone hydrochloride
Depade, ReVia

Pharmacologic class: Opioid antagonist
Therapeutic class: Opioid antidote
Pregnancy risk category C

Action
Unknown; thought to block opioid effects through competitive binding at opioid receptor sites in brain

Availability
Tablets: 50 mg

Indications and dosages
➤ Alcoholism
Adults: 50 mg P.O. once daily
➤ Opioid dependence
Adults: Initially, 25 mg P.O.; give an additional dose of 25 mg if no withdrawal symptoms occur within 1 hour. When patient is receiving 50 mg q 24 hours, a maintenance schedule (such as 50 to 150 mg/day P.O.) may be used.

Off-label uses
• Eating disorders
• Postconcussion syndrome unresponsive to other treatments

Contraindications
• Hypersensitivity to drug
• Acute hepatitis or hepatic failure
• Acute opioid withdrawal
• Concurrent opioid analgesic use

Administration
• Don't initiate therapy until patient has been opiate-free for 7 to 10 days.
• Know that naloxone challenge test should be performed.

Route	Onset	Peak	Duration
P.O.	15-30 min	60 min	24-72 hr

Adverse reactions
CNS: headache, lassitude, fatigue, insomnia, nervousness, anxiety, irritability, dizziness, depression, increased energy, **suicidal ideation**
GI: nausea, vomiting, constipation, abdominal pain and cramps, anorexia
Hepatic: hepatocellular injury
Musculoskeletal: joint and muscle pain
Skin: rash
Other: chills

Interactions
Drug-drug. *Opioid-containing preparations (such as some cough and cold remedies, analgesics, and antidiarrheal products):* lack of therapeutic benefit from these drugs
Drug-diagnostic tests. *Alanine aminotransferase, aspartate aminotransferase, lactate dehydrogenase, lymphocytes:* increased values

Precautions
Use cautiously in:
• mild hepatic disease, depression, suicidal tendencies
• pregnant or breastfeeding patients
• children.

Patient monitoring
• Monitor respiratory status; stay alert for respiratory depression and dysfunction.
• Evaluate neurologic status for change in level of consciousness, seizures, depression, and suicidal ideation.
• Watch for onset of nausea and vomiting; institute measures to prevent aspiration.
• In opioid-dependent patients, assess for signs and symptoms of opioid withdrawal, which may occur up to 2 hours after administration.
• In drug overdose, follow facility guidelines regarding follow-up treatment.

Patient teaching
• Explain all interventions to patient once he is alert and oriented.
• Reassure patient that environment is safe.
• As appropriate, review all significant and life-threatening adverse reactions and interactions, especially those related to the drugs and tests mentioned above.

nandrolone decanoate
Deca-Durabolin, Hybolin Decanoate

Pharmacologic class: Anabolic steroid
Therapeutic class: Erythropoietic
Controlled substance schedule III
Pregnancy risk category X

Action
Stimulates erythropoietin production in kidney, increasing red blood cells (RBCs); also promotes tissue development and reverses catabolism

Availability
Injection: 50 mg/ml, 100 mg/ml, 200 mg/ml

Indications and dosages
➤ Anemia associated with renal insufficiency
Adults and children older than age 14: In females, 50 to 100 mg I.M. q week at 1- to 4-week intervals; in males, 100 to 200 mg I.M. q week at 1- to 4-week intervals
Dosage adjustment
• Children younger than age 14

Contraindications
• Hypersensitivity to anabolic steroids or sesame oil
• Breast cancer
• Hypercalcemia
• Nephritis

- Prostate cancer
- Hepatic disorders
- Enhancement of physical appearance or athletic performance
- Pregnancy or breastfeeding

Administration
- Verify that female patients aren't pregnant before giving drug.
- Inject I.M. deep into upper outer quadrant of gluteal muscle.

Route	Onset	Peak	Duration
I.M.	Unknown	3-6 days	Unknown

Adverse reactions
CNS: insomnia, excitation, habituation, depression
GI: nausea, vomiting, diarrhea
GU: bladder irritability, increased creatinine level
Hematologic: suppression of clotting factors
Hepatic: reversible jaundice, hepatic dysfunction, elevated hepatic enzyme levels, **peliosis hepatitis**
Metabolic: virilism in women and prepubertal boys; premature epiphyseal closure in children; hypercalcemia; decreased high-density lipoprotein (HDL) and protein-bound iodine (PBI) levels; increased sodium, potassium, phosphate, and low-density lipoprotein (LDL) levels; increased triiodothyronine (T_3) uptake, thyroid-binding capacity, and radioactive iodine uptake; altered glucose tolerance (in diabetic patients)
Skin: acne, hirsutism
Other: chills, edema

Interactions
Drug-drug. *Hepatotoxic drugs:* increased risk of hepatotoxicity
Insulin, oral hypoglycemics: altered requirements for these drugs
Nonsteroidal anti-inflammatory drugs, salicylates, warfarin: increased risk of bleeding

Drug-diagnostic tests. *Alkaline phosphatase, aspartate aminotransferase, bilirubin, calcium, creatinine, prothrombin time, LDLs, phosphate, potassium, sodium, T_3 uptake:* increased values
Clotting factors II, V, VII, and X: suppressed levels
Glucose tolerance: altered test results
HDLs, PBI: decreased levels
Radioactive iodine uptake, thyroid-binding capacity: decreased

Precautions
Use cautiously in:
- cardiac or hepatic impairment, coronary artery disease, diabetes mellitus, benign prostatic hyperplasia
- elderly patients
- children.

Patient monitoring
- Assess skin color and character and body hair growth.
- Monitor electrolyte levels, lipid panels, thyroid function tests, liver function studies, coagulation studies, and long bone X-rays in children.
- Monitor diabetic patients carefully; anticipate adjusting insulin or oral hypoglycemic dosages.
- Assess fluid intake and output; evaluate patient for edema.

Patient teaching
- Teach patient to mark next injection date on calendar.
- Advise female patients to avoid pregnancy during therapy and to use barrier contraceptives.
- Instruct diabetic patients to monitor blood glucose levels closely.
- As appropriate, review all other significant and life-threatening adverse reactions and interactions, especially those related to the drugs and tests mentioned above.

n

naproxen

Apo-Naproxen✤, EC-Naprosyn,
Naprosyn, Naprosyn-E✤,
Naprosyn SR✤, Novo-Naprox✤

naproxen sodium

Aleve, Anaprox, Anaprox DS, Apo-
Napro-Na✤, Apo-Napro-Na DS✤,
Naprelan, Novo-Naprox Sodium✤,
Novo-Naprox Sodium DS✤, Synflex✤

Pharmacologic class: Nonsteroidal
anti-inflammatory drug (NSAID)
Therapeutic class: Nonopioid analgesic, antipyretic, anti-inflammatory
Pregnancy risk category B

Action

Unknown; thought to inhibit prostaglandin synthesis

Availability

naproxen
Oral suspension: 125 mg/5 ml
Suppositories: 500 mg
Tablets: 125 mg, 250 mg, 375 mg,
500 mg
Tablets (controlled-release): 375 mg,
500 mg
Tablets (delayed-release): 250 mg,
375 mg, 500 mg
Tablets (extended-release): 750 mg
naproxen sodium
Caplets, tablets: 220 mg, 275 mg,
550 mg

🕛 Indications and dosages

➣ Pain, osteoarthritis, ankylosing
spondylitis, dysmenorrhea, bursitis,
acute tendinitis
Adults: 250 to 500 mg (naproxen) P.O.
b.i.d. (up to 1.5 g/day); 375 to 500 mg
(naproxen delayed-release) P.O. t.i.d.;
250 mg, 375 mg or 500 mg (naproxen
oral suspension) P.O. b.i.d.; 275 to 550

mg P.O. (naproxen sodium) b.i.d. (up
to 1.65 g/day); or 750 or 1,000 mg/day
P.O. (naproxen controlled-release), not
to exceed 1,500 mg/day
➣ Mild to moderate pain, primary
dysmenorrhea
Adults: Initially, 500 mg (naproxen)
P.O., followed by 250 mg q 6 to 8 hours
p.r.n., to a maximum of 1.25 g/day. Or
initially, 550 mg (naproxen sodium)
P.O., followed by 275 mg q 6 to 8 hours
p.r.n., to a maximum of 1,375 mg/day.
Or 1,000 mg/day (naproxen controlled-
release) P.O., to a maximum of 1,500
mg/day for a limited time; then no
more than 1,000 mg/day.
➣ Gout
Adults: Initially, 750 mg (naproxen)
P.O., followed by 250 mg q 8 hours; or
initially, 825 mg (naproxen sodium)
P.O., followed by 275 mg q 8 hours.
Or 1,000 to 1,500 mg (naproxen
controlled-release) P.O. once on day 1,
followed by 1,000 mg daily.
Dosage adjustment
• Children

Contraindications

• Hypersensitivity to drug or other
NSAIDs
• Active GI bleeding or ulcer disease
• Asthma

Administration

• Give with food or milk to avoid GI
upset.

Route	Onset	Peak	Duration
P.O. (analgesia)	1 hr	2-4 hr	8-12 hr
P.O. (anti-inflam- matory)	14 days	2-4 wk	Unknown

Adverse reactions

CNS: dizziness, drowsiness, headache,
vertigo, light-headedness
CV: palpitations, tachycardia
EENT: visual disturbances, tinnitus,
auditory disturbances, stomatitis

GI: nausea, diarrhea, constipation, heartburn, abdominal pain, **GI bleeding**

Skin: rash, pruritus, skin eruptions, sweating, photosensitivity

Other: thirst, edema, allergic reactions including **anaphylaxis**

Interactions

Drug-drug. *Acetaminophen (chronic use), cyclosporine:* increased risk of adverse renal effects

Anticoagulants, thrombolytics: increased anticoagulant effects

Antihypertensives, cefamandole, cefoperazone, cefotetan, diuretics, eptifibatide: decreased response

Antineoplastics, methotrexate: increased risk of nephrotoxicity

Aspirin: decreased naproxen efficacy

Aspirin, corticosteroids, other NSAIDs: additive adverse GI effects

Clopidogrel, plicamycin, ticlopidine, valproic acid: increased risk of bleeding

Insulin, oral hypoglycemics: increased risk of hypoglycemia

Lithium: increased lithium blood level and risk of nephrotoxicity

Other photosensitizing agents: increased risk of photosensitivity

Probenecid: increased naproxen blood level, increased risk of toxicity

Drug-diagnostic tests. *Creatinine clearance, glucose, hematocrit, hemoglobin, leukocytes, platelets:* decreased values

Bleeding time: prolonged (for up to 4 days after therapy ends)

Alanine aminotransferase, alkaline phosphatase, aspartate aminotransferase, blood urea nitrogen, creatinine, lactate dehydrogenase, potassium: increased levels

Urine 5-hydroxy-indoleacetic acid, urine steroids: test interference

Drug-herb. *Anise, arnica, chamomile, clove, dong quai, fenugreek, feverfew, garlic, ginger, ginkgo, ginseng, licorice:* increased anticoagulant effect, increased risk of bleeding

Precautions

Use cautiously in:
• severe cardiovascular, renal, or hepatic disease
• history of ulcer disease
• chronic alcohol use or abuse
• breastfeeding patients
• children younger than age 2 (safety not established).

Patient monitoring

• Monitor GI status; stay alert for signs and symptoms of GI bleeding.
• In long-term use, assess complete blood count with white cell differential and coagulation studies; monitor for visual and hearing impairment.
• Monitor cardiovascular status for tachycardia, palpitations, and edema.
• Evaluate blood glucose levels closely in diabetic patients.

Patient teaching

• Instruct patient to take drug with food or milk followed by 8 oz of water, and to stay upright for 30 minutes afterward.
• Tell patient he may crush or break regular tablets but not extended-, delayed-, or controlled-release forms; he must swallow these whole.
• Inform patient that drug's full therapeutic effect may take up to 2 weeks.
• Caution patient not to exceed recommended dosage.
• Teach patient to use sunscreen to prevent photosensitivity reaction.
• Instruct patient not to take over-the-counter medications unless prescribed.
• As appropriate, review all other significant and life-threatening adverse reactions and interactions, especially those related to the drugs, tests, and herbs mentioned above.

naratriptan hydrochloride
Amerge

Pharmacologic class: Selective 5-hydroxytryptamine$_1$ (5-HT$_1$) agonist

Therapeutic class: Vascular headache suppressant, antimigraine drug

Pregnancy risk category C

Action
Binds with specific 5-HT$_1$ receptors in intracranial blood vessels and sensory trigeminal nerves, leading to vasoconstriction and migraine relief

Availability
Tablets: 1 mg, 2.5 mg

🕊 Indications and dosages
➣ Migraine headache with or without aura

Adults: 1 or 2.5 mg P.O. as a single dose; may repeat in 4 hours. Don't exceed 5 mg in 24 hours and don't use to treat more than four headaches per month.

Dosage adjustment
• Mild to moderate renal or hepatic impairment

Contraindications
• Hypersensitivity to drug or its components
• Severe renal, cardiovascular or hepatic impairment
• Ischemic bowel disease
• History of cerebrovascular or peripheral vascular conditions
• Monoamine oxidase (MAO) inhibitor use within 14 days
• Elderly patients

Administration
• Know that drug does not prevent migraine.

• Give drug only if cardiovascular status has been evaluated and determined to be safe and if first dose is given under supervision.

Route	Onset	Peak	Duration
P.O.	30-60 min	2-3 hr	Up to 24 hr

Adverse reactions
CNS: dizziness, drowsiness, malaise, fatigue, paresthesia

CV: coronary artery vasospasm, **myocardial infarction, ventricular fibrillation or tachycardia**

GI: nausea, vomiting

Other: pain or pressure sensation in throat or neck

Interactions
Drug-drug. *Ergot-type compounds (dihydroergotamine, methysergide):* prolonged vasospastic reactions

Hormonal contraceptives: increased naratriptan blood level and effects

MAO inhibitors: increased systemic exposure to naratriptan, increased risk of adverse reactions

Selective serotonin reuptake inhibitors: weakness, hyperreflexia, incoordination

Sibutramine: serotonin syndrome

Drug-herb. *S-adenosylmethionine (SAM-e), St. John's wort:* increased risk of adverse serotonergic effects

Drug-behaviors. *Cigarette smoking:* increased naratriptan metabolism

Precautions
Use cautiously in:
• mild to moderate renal or hepatic impairment, cardiovascular risk factors
• pregnant or breastfeeding patients
• children (safety not established).

Patient monitoring
• Perform especially close monitoring in patients with cardiovascular risk factors (such as hypertension, hypercholesterolemia, obesity, diabetes mellitus, cigarette smoking, strong family histo-

ry), postmenopausal women, and men over age 40.
• Assess vital signs and ECG.
• Monitor neurologic status closely; institute safety measures as needed to prevent injury.

Patient teaching
• Teach patient to take dose at first sign of headache.
• If prescriber has approved a second dose, advise patient to take it at least 4 hours after first dose if headache hasn't gone away completely or if it has returned.
• Caution patient not to take more than two tablets in a 24-hour period.
• Instruct patient to avoid driving and other hazardous activities until he knows how drug affects concentration and alertness.
• Teach patient to minimize GI upset by eating small, frequent servings of healthy food and ensuring adequate fluid intake.
• As appropriate, review all other significant and life-threatening adverse reactions and interactions, especially those related to the drugs, herbs, and behaviors mentioned above.

nateglinide
Starlix

Pharmacologic class: Amino acid derivative
Therapeutic class: Antidiabetic
Pregnancy risk category C

Action
Decreases blood glucose level by stimulating insulin secretion from pancreatic beta cells; interacts with calcium and potassium channels in pancreas

Availability
Tablets: 60 mg, 120 mg

Indications and dosages
➤ To decrease glucose levels in patients with type 2 diabetes mellitus not adequately controlled by diet and exercise (given alone or with metformin)
Adults: 120 mg P.O. t.i.d. up to 30 minutes before meals, or 60 mg P.O. t.i.d. if patient is near hemoglobin A1c (HbA1c) goal

Contraindications
• Hypersensitivity to drug or its components
• Diabetic ketoacidosis
• Type 1 diabetes mellitus

Administration
• Give 30 minutes before meals; if meal is missed, don't give dose.

Route	Onset	Peak	Duration
P.O.	Rapid	Within 1 hr	4 hr

Adverse reactions
CNS: dizziness
GI: diarrhea
Metabolic: hypoglycemia
Musculoskeletal: back pain, joint pain
Respiratory: upper respiratory tract infection, bronchitis, coughing
Other: flulike symptoms, trauma

Interactions
Drug-drug. *Beta-adrenergic blockers, monoamine oxidase inhibitors, nonsteroidal anti-inflammatory drugs, salicylates:* increased hypoglycemic effect
Corticosteroids, sympathomimetics, thiazides, thyroid products: reduced hypoglycemic effect
Drug-diagnostic tests. *Glucose:* decreased level

Precautions
Use cautiously in:
• renal or hepatic impairment, adrenal or pituitary insufficiency
• elderly or malnourished patients
• pregnant or breastfeeding patients.

Patient monitoring
• Monitor blood glucose and HbA1c levels.
• Assess pulmonary status for bronchitis, upper respiratory infection, and flulike signs and symptoms.
• Monitor musculoskeletal status; check for back pain and arthropathy.
• Note GI complaints; identify nutritional deficiencies.

Patient teaching
• Instruct patient to take doses up to 30 minutes before each of three main meals.
• Advise patient not to skip a meal; if he does, he should also skip accompanying nateglinide dose to prevent hypoglycemia.
• Teach patient how to monitor blood and urine for glucose and ketones, as prescribed.
• Instruct patient to report adverse CNS effects and signs and symptoms of respiratory infections.
• Caution patient to avoid driving and other hazardous activities until he knows how drug affects sensation and balance.
• As appropriate, review all other significant adverse reactions and interactions, especially those related to the drugs and tests mentioned above.

nedocromil sodium
Tilade

Pharmacologic class: Mast cell stabilizer
Therapeutic class: Antiasthmatic
Pregnancy risk category B

Action
Blocks allergen-triggered release of histamine and slow-releasing substance of anaphylaxis from mast cells, decreasing overall allergic response and inflammatory reaction

Availability
Aerosol for inhalation: 1.75 mg/spray in 16.2-g canister

Indications and dosages
➤ Maintenance therapy in mild to moderate bronchial asthma
Adults and children older than age 12: Two inhalations (1.75 mg/spray) two to four times daily

Contraindications
• Hypersensitivity to drug or its components
• Acute asthma attack, acute bronchospasm

Administration
• Know that therapeutic response may take up to 4 weeks.

Route	Onset	Peak	Duration
Inhalation	Unknown	30 min	3.5 hr

Adverse reactions
CNS: headache
CV: chest pain
EENT: conjunctivitis, rhinitis, sinusitis, pharyngitis
GI: nausea, diarrhea, abdominal pain, unpleasant taste
Respiratory: coughing, upper respiratory tract infection, increased sputum, bronchitis, dyspnea, worsening of bronchial asthma, **bronchospasm**
Other: viral infection, allergic reactions including **anaphylaxis**

Interactions
None significant

Precautions
Use cautiously in:
• pregnant or breastfeeding patients
• children younger than age 12 (safety not established).

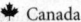

Patient monitoring
• Monitor pulmonary function tests.
• Assess respiratory status.

Patient teaching
• Teach patient to expectorate mucus from airway before using inhaler.
• Provide instructions on proper inhalation technique.
• Encourage patient to use spacer as needed to achieve therapeutic dosage.
• Teach patient to gargle and sip water after inhalation to reduce mouth irritation.
• Tell patient that therapeutic effect may take up to 4 weeks.
• Inform patient that drug should be used for asthma prevention only and not as rescue inhaler in emergencies.
• As appropriate, review all other significant and life-threatening adverse reactions.

nefazodone hydrochloride
Serzone

Pharmacologic class: Phenylpiperazine
Therapeutic class: Antidepressant
Pregnancy risk category C

Action
Potentiates effects of norepinephrine and serotonin by blocking synapse reuptake in nerve cells and disrupting alpha$_1$-adrenergic receptors

Availability
Tablets: 50 mg, 100 mg, 150 mg, 200 mg, 250 mg

⚕ Indications and dosages
➤ Major depression
Adults: Initially, 100 mg P.O. b.i.d.; may increase weekly up to 600 mg/day in two divided doses.

Dosage adjustment
• Elderly patients

Contraindications
• Hypersensitivity to drug or other phenylpiperazines
• Active hepatic disease or baseline transaminase elevations
• Monoamine oxidase (MAO) inhibitor use within 14 days
• Concurrent cisapride, pimozide, carbamazepine, or triazolam therapy

Administration
• Give with food or milk if GI upset occurs.
• Know that tablets may be crushed.

Route	Onset	Peak	Duration
P.O.	Days-wks	Few wks	Unknown

Adverse reactions
CNS: dizziness, asthenia, agitation, light-headedness, insomnia, drowsiness, confusion, weakness, headache, memory impairment, paresthesia, poor concentration, psychomotor retardation, tremor
CV: hypotension, orthostatic hypotension, peripheral edema
EENT: abnormal or blurred vision, eye pain, tinnitus, pharyngitis
GI: nausea, vomiting, diarrhea, constipation, dyspepsia, dry mouth
GU: urinary frequency or retention, urinary tract infection
Hematologic: decreased hematocrit
Respiratory: increased cough
Skin: rash, pruritus
Other: increased appetite, thirst, infection, chills, fever, flulike symptoms

Interactions
Drug-drug. *Alprazolam, triazolam:* increased blood level and effects of these drugs
Antihypertensives, nitrates: additive hypotension

Carbamazepine, cisapride, pimozide: increased nefazodone blood level, leading to toxicity

CNS depressants (including antihistamines, opioids, sedative-hypnotics): additive CNS depression

Digoxin: increased digoxin blood level

HMG-CoA reductase inhibitors: increased risk of myopathy

MAO inhibitors: potentially fatal reactions (such as hyperpyrexia, excitation, seizures, delirium, coma)

Drug-diagnostic tests. *Cholesterol, complete blood count, glucose, hematocrit:* decreased levels

Drug-herb. *Chamomile, hops, kava, skullcap, valerian:* increased CNS depression

S-adenosylmethionine (SAM-e), St. John's wort: increased risk of serotonergic effects, including serotonin syndrome

Drug-behaviors. *Acute alcohol ingestion:* additive hypotension

Alcohol use: increased CNS depression

Precautions

Use cautiously in:
• cardiovascular or cerebrovascular disease
• history of suicide attempt, drug abuse, or mania
• elderly patients
• pregnant or breastfeeding patients
• children younger than age 18 (safety not established).

Patient monitoring

• Monitor vital signs with patient lying down, sitting, and standing. Notify prescriber if blood pressure drops 20 mm Hg.
• Assess complete blood count.
• Closely monitor neurologic status.
• Evaluate patient for withdrawal symptoms (which may occur if therapy is stopped abruptly).

Patient teaching

• Tell patient to crush drug if he can't swallow it whole.
• Advise patient to take drug with food or milk to minimize GI upset.
• Inform patient that therapeutic effect may take up to 4 weeks; encourage him to keep taking drug as prescribed.
• Teach patient that drug may cause adverse CNS effects; advise him to report significant mood changes (especially depression or suicidal thoughts).
• Instruct patient to rise slowly and carefully to avoid dizziness and lightheadedness from temporary blood pressure drop.
• Instruct patient not to stop taking drug abruptly; dosage must be tapered.
• As appropriate, review all other significant adverse reactions and interactions, especially those related to the drugs, tests, herbs, and behaviors mentioned above.

nelfinavir mesylate
Viracept

Pharmacologic class: Protease inhibitor
Therapeutic class: Antiretroviral
Pregnancy risk category B

Action

Inhibits action of human immunodeficiency virus (HIV) protease and prevents cleavage of viral polyproteins, resulting in production of immature, noninfectious virus

Availability

Oral powder: 50 mg/1g powder (1 g powder/level scoopful)
Tablets: 250 mg, 625 mg

⏀ Indications and dosages
➤ Management of HIV infection
Adults and children over age 13: 750 mg P.O. t.i.d. or 1,250 mg b.i.d., given with other antiretrovirals
Dosage adjustment
• Children younger than age 13

Contraindications
• Hypersensitivity to drug or its components
• Concurrent use of amiodarone, astemizole, cisapride, dihydroergotamine, ergotamine, midazolam, quinidine, rifampin, terfenadine, or triazolam
• Breastfeeding (should be avoided by HIV-infected patients)

Administration
• Give tablets with food.
• Know that oral powder may be mixed with food or milk.

Route	Onset	Peak	Duration
P.O.	Rapid	2-4 hr	8 hr

Adverse reactions
CNS: anxiety, depression, dizziness, drowsiness, emotional lability, headache, hyperkinesia, insomnia, malaise, migraine headache, sleep disorders, weakness, myasthenia, paresthesia, **suicidal ideation, seizures**
EENT: acute iritis, rhinitis, sinusitis, pharyngitis
GI: nausea, diarrhea, abdominal pain, flatulence
GU: nephrolithiasis, sexual dysfunction
Hematologic: anemia, **leukopenia, thrombocytopenia**
Metabolic: dehydration, hyperlipidemia, hyperuricemia, hypoglycemia
Musculoskeletal: joint pain, arthritis, back pain, myalgia, myopathy
Respiratory: dyspnea, **bronchospasm**
Skin: pruritus, rash, sweating, fungal dermatitis, folliculitis, urticaria

Other: fever, body fat redistribution, allergic reactions

Interactions
Drug-drug. *Amiodarone, dihydroergotamine, ergotamine, midazolam, quinidine, triazolam:* excessive sedation, vasoconstriction, serious arrhythmias
Carbamazepine, phenobarbital, phenytoin, rifampin: decreased nelfinavir blood level and efficacy
Hormonal contraceptives: decreased contraceptive blood level and efficacy
Rifabutin: decreased rifabutin metabolism and effects
Drug-food. *Most foods:* enhanced drug absorption
Drug-herb. *St. John's wort:* decreased nelfinavir blood level and efficacy

Precautions
Use cautiously in:
• hemophilia, diabetes mellitus, hepatic impairment.

Patient monitoring
• Monitor patient for signs and symptoms of depression; assess for suicidal ideation.
• Evaluate neurologic status closely, particularly for seizures and sensorimotor dysfunction.
• Assess complete blood count, lipid panel, uric acid level, and HIV-specific tests.
• Watch for secondary infections, particularly fungal and EENT infections.

Patient teaching
• Teach patient to take drug with meals or snacks. Tell him he may mix oral powder with nonacidic fluids.
• Inform patient that he may take missed dose up to 1 hour before next scheduled dose.
• Instruct patient to report depression or suicidal thoughts.
• Tell patient that drug may predispose him to other infections, especially fungal and EENT infections. Advise him

to avoid crowds and to wash hands often and thoroughly.

• Instruct female patients to use reliable barrier contraception.

• Teach patient to avoid driving and other hazardous activities until he knows how drug affects concentration, vision, strength, and alertness.

• As appropriate, review all other significant and life-threatening adverse reactions and interactions, especially those related to the drugs, foods, and herbs mentioned above.

neomycin sulfate
Mycifradin, Myciguent, Neo-Biotec, Neo-fradin, Neo-Tabs

Pharmacologic class: Aminoglycoside
Therapeutic class: Anti-infective
Pregnancy risk category D

Action
Interferes with bacterial protein synthesis by binding to 30S ribosomal subunit, causing misreading of genetic code. Inaccurate peptide sequence then forms in protein chain, leading to bacterial death.

Availability
Cream: 0.5%
Ointment: 0.5%
Oral solution: 125 mg/5 ml
Otic suspension: 5 mg/ml (with polymyxin B sulfate 10,000 units/ml and hydrocortisone 1%)
Tablets: 350, 500 mg

Indications and dosages
➣ Preoperative intestinal antisepsis
Adults: 1 g P.O. q hour for four doses, then 1 g q 4 hours for 24 hours or 1 g at 19 hours, 18 hours, and 9 hours before surgery

➣ Hepatic encephalopathy
Adults: 4 to 12 g/day P.O. in divided doses
➣ Superficial bacterial infections
Adults and children: Apply cream or ointment topically one to five times daily.
Dosage adjustment
• Children

Contraindications
• Hypersensitivity to drug or other aminoglycosides
• Intestinal obstruction

Administration
• Give preoperative dose before bowel surgery, after cathartic administration.

Route	Onset	Peak	Duration
P.O.	Variable	1-4 hr	Unknown
Topical	Unknown	Unknown	Unknown

Adverse reactions
CNS: neuromuscular blockade
EENT: ototoxicity
GI: nausea, vomiting, diarrhea, malabsorption syndrome
GU: nephrotoxicity

Interactions
Drug-drug. *Acyclovir, amphotericin B, cephalosporin, cisplatin, other aminoglycosides, vancomycin:* increased risk of ototoxicity and nephrotoxicity
Digoxin: decreased digoxin absorption
Dimenhydrinate: masking of ototoxicity symptoms
Oral anticoagulants: increased anticoagulant effect
Potent loop diuretics: increased risk of ototoxicity

Precautions
Use cautiously in:
• renal impairment, hearing impairment, neuromuscular diseases (such as myasthenia gravis)
• obese patients

- elderly patients
- pregnant or breastfeeding patients
- infants (safety not established).

Patient monitoring
- Assess for neuromuscular blockade.
- Evaluate patient for ototoxicity.
- Monitor kidney function test results.

Patient teaching
- Inform patient that drug may cause muscular weakness.
- Instruct patient to report hearing problems.
- Advise patient to avoid driving and other hazardous activities until he knows how drug affects neuromuscular status.
- Tell patient he'll undergo frequent blood testing during therapy.
- As appropriate, review all other significant and life-threatening adverse reactions and interactions, especially those related to the drugs mentioned above.

neostigmine bromide
Prostigmin

neostigmine methylsulfate
PMS-Neostigmine Methylsulfate✤, Prostigmin

Pharmacologic class: Anticholinesterase

Therapeutic class: Muscle stimulant
Pregnancy risk category C

Action
Inhibits enzyme acetylcholinesterase, leading to increased acetylcholine concentration at synapse and prolonged acetylcholine effects. Exerts direct cholinomimetic effect on skeletal muscle.

Availability
Injection (methylsulfate): 2 mg/ml, 1 mg/ml, 0.5 mg/ml, 0.25 mg/ml
Tablets (bromide): 15 mg

Indications and dosages
➣ Myasthenia gravis
Adults: 15 mg/day P.O.; may increase p.r.n. up to 375 mg/day; average dosage is 150 mg/day. Or, 1 ml of 1:2,000 solution (0.5 mg) S.C. or I.M. based on response and tolerance.
➣ Postoperative abdominal distention and bladder atony
Adults: 0.5 to 1 mg I.M. or S.C.; if given for urinary retention and no response occurs within 1 hour after dose, catheterize patient and repeat dose q 3 hours for five doses.
➣ Antidote for nondepolarizing neuromuscular blockers
Adults: 0.5 to 2.5 mg I.V.; repeat p.r.n. up to 5 mg. Precede initial dose with 0.6 to 1.2 mg atropine sulfate I.V.
Dosage adjustment
- Children and neonates

n

Contraindications
- Hypersensitivity to cholinergics or bromide
- Peritonitis
- Mechanical obstruction of GI or urinary tract

Administration
◀℈ Before giving, ensure that atropine sulfate is available to treat cholinergic crisis.
- Know that atropine may be combined with usual dose to decrease risk of adverse reactions.
- Give oral form 1 hour before or 2 hours after a meal.
- Administer I.V. dose undiluted directly into vein or I.V. line; give doses of 0.5 mg slowly over 1 minute.
- Keep resuscitation equipment on hand.

Route	Onset	Peak	Duration
P.O.	45-75 min	1-2 hr	2-4 hr
I.V.	4-8 min	1-2 hr	2-4 hr
I.M., S.C.	20-30 min	1-2 hr	2-4 hr

Adverse reactions

CNS: dizziness, headache, drowsiness, asthenia, **loss of consciousness**
CV: hypotension, tachycardia, bradycardia, **atrioventricular (AV) block, cardiac arrest**
EENT: vision changes, lacrimation, miosis
GI: nausea, vomiting, diarrhea, abdominal cramping, flatulence, increased peristalsis
GU: urinary frequency
Musculoskeletal: muscle cramps, spasms, and fasciculations; joint pain
Respiratory: dyspnea, **bronchospasm, respiratory depression, respiratory arrest, laryngospasm**
Skin: rash, urticaria, flushing
Other: anaphylaxis

Interactions

Drug-drug. *Aminoglycosides, anticholinergics, atropine, corticosteroids, local and general anesthetics:* reversal of anticholinergic effects
Cholinergics: additive toxicity
Kanamycin, neomycin, streptomycin: increased neuromuscular blockade
Succinylcholine: potentiation of neuromuscular blockade, prolonged respiratory depression

Precautions

Use cautiously in:
• asthma, peptic ulcer, bradycardia, arrhythmias, recent coronary occlusion, vagotonia, hyperthyroidism, seizure disorder
• pregnant or breastfeeding patients.

Patient monitoring

◀≣ Monitor vital signs; assess patient for hypotension, bradycardia or tachycardia, AV block, and signs and symptoms of impending cardiac arrest.
• Evaluate respiratory and neurologic status.

Patient teaching

• Instruct patient to take tablets 1 hour before or 2 hours after meals.
• Tell patient that drug may alter his respiratory and cardiac status; teach him to recognize and report warning signs.
• Caution patient to avoid driving and other hazardous activities until he knows how drug affects concentration, vision, muscle function, and alertness.
• As appropriate, review all other significant and life-threatening adverse reactions and interactions, especially those related to the drugs mentioned above.

nesiritide
Natrecor

Pharmacologic class: Human B-type natriuretic peptide
Therapeutic class: Vasodilator
Pregnancy risk category C

Action

Binds to receptors on vascular smooth muscle and endothelial cells, causing smooth muscle relaxation and vasodilation. As a result, systemic and pulmonary pressures decrease and diuresis occurs.

Availability

Injection: 1.5 mg in single-use vials

⏩ Indications and dosages

➤ Acutely decompensated heart failure in patients who have dyspnea at rest or with minimal activity
Adults: 2 mcg/kg I.V. bolus, followed

by continuous I.V. infusion of 0.01 mcg/kg/minute

Contraindications
- Hypersensitivity to drug or its components
- Systolic blood pressure less than 90 mm Hg
- Primary therapy for cardiogenic shock

Administration
- For I.V. use, prime tubing before connecting to patient. Withdraw bolus and infuse over 60 seconds into I.V. port of tubing. Follow immediately with a constant infusion delivering 0.01 mcg/kg/minute. Drug should be mixed and infused in dextrose 5% in water, normal saline solution, or dextrose in half-normal saline solution.

◀€ Don't mix with other drug solutions. Always administer through a separate line.

- Know that nesiritide therapy exceeding 48 hours hasn't been studied.

Route	Onset	Peak	Duration
I.V.	Immediate	15 min	Unknown

Adverse reactions
CNS: dizziness, headache, insomnia, anxiety
CV: hypotension, angina pectoris, bradycardia, ventricular extrasystole, **ventricular tachycardia**
GI: nausea, vomiting, abdominal pain
Musculoskeletal: leg cramps, back pain
Respiratory: cough, hemoptysis, **apnea**
Other: injection site reactions

Interactions
Drug-drug. *Angiotensin-converting enzyme inhibitors, nitrates:* increased hypotension
Bumetanide, enalaprilat, ethacrynate sodium, furosemide, heparin, hydral-

azine, insulin: physical and chemical incompatibility with nesiritide
Drug-diagnostic tests. *Hematocrit, hemoglobin:* decreased values

Precautions
Use cautiously in:
- restrictive or obstructive cardiomyopathy, constrictive pericarditis, pericardial tamponade, renal dysfunction, hypotension
- pregnant or breastfeeding patients.

Patient monitoring
- Monitor vital signs and pulmonary artery wedge pressure continuously during infusion and for several hours afterward.
- Assess cardiovascular status closely.

Patient teaching
- Tell patient he'll be monitored closely during infusion and for several hours afterward.
- Inform patient that drug may cause serious adverse effects; reassure him that he'll receive appropriate interventions to relieve symptoms.
- Instruct patient to report chest pain, dizziness, palpitations, and other uncomfortable symptoms.
- As appropriate, review all other significant and life-threatening adverse reactions and interactions, especially those related to the drugs and tests mentioned above.

n

nevirapine
Viramune

Pharmacologic class: Nonnucleoside reverse transcriptase inhibitor
Therapeutic class: Antiretroviral
Pregnancy risk category C

Action
Inhibits human immunodeficiency virus (HIV) non-nucleoside reverse transcriptase by binding directly to reverse transcriptase and blocking RNA-dependent and DNA-dependent polymerase activity.

Availability
Oral suspension: 50 mg/5 ml
Tablets: 200 mg

⚠ Indications and dosages
➤ Adjunctive treatment in patients with HIV-1 infection who show clinical or immunologic deterioration
Adults: 200 mg P.O. daily for 14 days, then 200 mg P.O. b.i.d., given in conjunction with a nucleoside analogue
Dosage adjustment
• Hepatic impairment
• Chronic hemodialysis
• Children

Off-label uses
• Prophylaxis of maternal-fetal HIV transmission

Contraindications
• Hypersensitivity to drug

Administration
• Give with or without food.

Route	Onset	Peak	Duration
P.O.	Unknown	4 hr	Unknown

Adverse reactions
CNS: paresthesia, headache, malaise, fatigue
GI: nausea, diarrhea, abdominal pain
Hematologic: agranulocytosis
Hepatic: hepatitis, hepatotoxicity, hepatic failure
Musculoskeletal: myalgia, pain
Skin: rash, toxic epidermal necrolysis, blistering
Other: fever, **Stevens-Johnson syndrome**

Interactions
Drug-drug. *Drugs extensively metabolized by CYP3A-P450, hormonal contraceptives, protease inhibitors:* decreased blood levels of these drugs
Prednisone: increased risk of rash
Rifabutin, rifamycin: decreased nevirapine blood level
Drug-diagnostic tests. *Alanine aminotransferase, aspartate aminotransferase, bilirubin, gamma-glutamyltransferase:* increased levels
Hemoglobin, neutrophils: decreased levels
Drug-herb. *St. John's wort:* decreased nevirapine blood level

Precautions
Use cautiously in:
• impaired renal or hepatic function
• pregnant or breastfeeding patients
• children.

Patient monitoring
• Check closely for rash, especially during first 6 months of therapy.
• Monitor patient's weight, temperature, and chest X-ray periodically.
• Assess patient's appetite and energy and physical activity levels.
• Monitor liver function test results.

Patient teaching
• Tell patient he may take drug with or without food.
• Teach patient to take missed dose as soon as he remembers; however, if time for next dose is near, instruct him to skip previous dose. Caution him not to double the dose.
• Inform female patient that hormonal contraceptives, implants, or shots may be ineffective during nevirapine therapy. Urge her to use alternative birth-control method.
◄€ Teach patient to recognize and immediately report signs and symptoms of hepatotoxicity. Also tell patient to immediately report rash.

• Inform patient that nevirapine won't cure HIV or prevent its transmission.
• As appropriate, review all other significant and life-threatening adverse reactions and interactions, especially those related to the drugs, tests, and herbs mentioned above.

niacin (nicotinic acid, vitamin B₃)

Edur-Acin, Nia-Bid, Niac, Niacels, Niacor, Niaspan, Nicobid, Nico-400, Nicolar, Nicotinex, Novo-Niacin♣

niacinamide (nicotinamide)

Pharmacologic class: Water-soluble vitamin
Therapeutic class: Lipid-lowering drug, vitamin
Pregnancy risk category C

Action

Stimulates glycogenolysis, lipid metabolism, and tissue perfusion; decreases lipoprotein and triglyceride synthesis by inhibiting free fatty acid release from adipose tissue. Also causes peripheral vasodilation.

Availability

Capsules (extended-release): 125 mg, 250 mg, 300 mg, 400 mg, 500 mg
Elixir: 50 mg/5 ml
Tablets: 25 mg, 50 mg, 100 mg, 125 mg, 250 mg, 400 mg, 500 mg
Tablets (extended-release): 125 mg, 250 mg, 400 mg, 500 mg, 750 mg, 1,000 mg

🖊 Indications and dosages

➤ Treatment and prevention of niacin deficiency (pellagra)
Adults: As a dietary supplement, 10 to 20 mg/day P.O. For treatment of niacin deficiency, 300 to 500 mg/day P.O. in divided doses.

➤ Adjunctive therapy in certain hyperlipidemias (niacin only)
Adults: Initially, 100 to 500 mg/day P.O., increased slowly to 1 or 2 g t.i.d., up to a maximum daily dosage of 6 g
Dosage adjustment
• Children

Contraindications

• Hypersensitivity to niacin or tartrazine (with some products)
• Peptic ulcer
• Hepatic disease
• Hemorrhage
• Severe hypotension
• Breastfeeding

Administration

• Give with food or meals to minimize GI upset.
• Avoid crushing, breaking, or chewing extended-release tablets and capsules; make sure patient swallows them whole.
• When giving elixir, use calibrated measuring device to ensure accurate dosage.

Route	Onset	Peak	Duration
P.O.	Unknown	45 min	Unknown

Adverse reactions

CNS: anxiety, panic, paresthesia, headache, dizziness
CV: orthostatic hypotension, vasovagal attacks, arrhythmias, vasodilation, syncope
EENT: blurred vision, central vision loss, proptosis, toxic amblyopia
GI: nausea, vomiting, diarrhea, GI upset, bloating, flatulence, heartburn, hunger pains, peptic ulcers, dry mouth, anorexia
GU: dark urine
Hepatic: jaundice, **hepatotoxicity**
Metabolic: glycosuria, hyperglycemia, hyperuricemia
Respiratory: wheezing

n

♣ Canada　　◀€ Clinical alert　　Reactions in **bold** are life-threatening

Skin: facial and neck flushing, pruritus, burning, dry skin, hyperpigmentation, increased sebaceous gland activity, rash, skin stinging or tingling

Interactions

Drug-drug. *Ganglionic blockers (guanadrel, guanethidine):* additive hypotension

HMG-CoA reductase inhibitors: increased risk of myopathy

Probenecid, sulfinpyrazone: decreased uricosuric effects (with high doses)

Drug-diagnostic tests. *Alkaline phosphatase, bilirubin, hepatic enzymes, prothrombin time, lactate dehydrogenase, uric acid:* increased values

Cholesterol, serum albumin: decreased levels

Urinary catecholamines: false increase

Urine glucose: false-positive result

Drug-herb. *Chapparal, comfrey, germander, jin bu huan, kava, pennyroyal:* increased risk of hepatotoxicity

Precautions

Use cautiously in:

• arterial bleeding, gout, glaucoma, diabetes mellitus, schizophrenia

• history of peptic ulcer disease

• heavy alcohol consumption

• pregnant patients.

Patient monitoring

• Monitor liver function tests; watch for signs and symptoms of hepatotoxicity.

• Check vital signs; stay alert for orthostatic hypotension.

• Assess vision.

• Monitor blood glucose levels carefully in diabetic patients.

Patient teaching

• Tell patient to swallow extended-release form whole and not to crush, break, or chew it.

• Advise patient to take drug with food to minimize GI upset.

• If patient is taking elixir, teach him how to use calibrated measuring device to measure accurate dosage.

• Tell patient that transient flushing and warm sensation (especially in face, neck, and ears) may occur within 2 hours of taking drug.

◄€ Instruct patient to immediately report signs and symptoms of hepatotoxicity (such as flulike symptoms, dark urine, and gray stools).

◄€ Caution patient not to substitute extended-release for immediate-release nicotinic acid because of risk of severe liver problems.

• Caution patient to change positions slowly to minimize dizziness from orthostatic hypotension.

• Instruct patient to avoid driving and other hazardous activities until he knows how drug affects concentration and alertness.

• As appropriate, review all other significant and life-threatening adverse reactions and interactions, especially those related to the drugs, tests, and herbs mentioned above.

nicardipine
Cardene, Cardene IV, Cardene SR

Pharmacologic class: Calcium channel blocker

Therapeutic class: Antianginal, antihypertensive

Pregnancy risk category C

Action

Inhibits calcium transport into myocardial and vascular smooth muscle cells, causing a decrease in cardiac output and a reduction in myocardial contractions

Availability

Capsules: 20 mg, 30 mg
Capsules (sustained-release): 30 mg, 45 mg, 60 mg
Injection: 2.5 mg/ml in 10-ml ampules

✿ Indications and dosages

➤ Hypertension, angina pectoris, vasospastic (Prinzmetal's) angina, heart failure
Adults: 20 mg P.O. (immediate-release) t.i.d.; may increase q 3 days. Or 30 mg P.O. (sustained-release) b.i.d., to a maximum dosage of 60 mg b.i.d. To switch from P.O. to parenteral use, give 0.5 to 2.2 mg/hour I.V. by continuous infusion.

➤ Acute hypertensive episodes
Adults: 5 mg/hour I.V., titrated as needed up to 15 mg/hour

Contraindications

• Hypersensitivity to drug
• Sick sinus syndrome
• Second- or third-degree atrioventricular block (unless artificial pacemaker is in place)
• Systolic blood pressure less than 90 mm Hg
• Advanced aortic stenosis

Administration

• Give without regard to meals; if GI upset occurs, give with meal. Don't give with grapefruit juice.
• Don't open, crush, break, or let patient chew sustained-release capsules.
• For I.V. use, dilute each 25-mg ampule with 240 ml of dextrose 5% in water, normal saline solution, dextrose 5% with normal saline solution, or half-normal saline solution, to a concentration of 0.1 mg/ml.
• Don't mix with furosemide, heparin, or thiopental.
◀€ Give by slow I.V. infusion; titrate dosage according to blood pressure response.

Route	Onset	Peak	Duration
P.O.	20 min	0.5-2 hr	8 hr
P.O. (sustained)	Unknown	Unknown	12 hr
I.V.	Few min	45 min	Unknown

Adverse reactions

CNS: dizziness, headache, asthenia, drowsiness, paresthesia
CV: peripheral edema, chest pain, hypotension, palpitations, tachycardia
EENT: dry mouth
GI: nausea, dyspepsia
Musculoskeletal: myalgia
Respiratory: dyspnea
Skin: rash, flushing

Interactions

Drug-drug. *Beta blockers, digoxin, disopyramide, phenytoin:* bradycardia, conduction defects, heart failure
Carbamazepine, cimetidine, cyclosporine, prazosin, propranolol, quinidine: decreased nicardipine metabolism, greater risk of toxicity
Corticosteroids, diuretics, hypoglycemics: increased risk of hypokalemia
Fentanyl, nitrates, other antihypertensives, quinidine: additive hypotension
Nonsteroidal anti-inflammatory drugs: reduced antihypertensive effect of nicardipine, increased risk of GI bleeding
Theophylline: increased theophylline effects
Drug-food. *Grapefruit juice:* increased drug blood levels and effects
Drug-herb. *Ephedra, yohimbine:* antagonism of drug's antihypertensive effect
St. John's wort: decreased nifedipine blood level
Drug-behaviors. *Alcohol use:* additive hypotension

n

Precautions

Use cautiously in:

- severe hepatic or renal impairment, hypotension
- history of serious ventricular arrhythmias or heart failure
- elderly patients
- pregnant or breastfeeding patients (safety not established)
- children (safety not established).

Patient monitoring

- Assess vital signs and cardiovascular status.
- Monitor fluid intake and output; assess for signs and symptoms of heart failure.
- Watch closely for rash.

Patient teaching

- Tell patient he may take drug without regard to meals. If GI upset occurs, advise him to take it with food.
- Instruct patient not to drink grapefruit juice during therapy.
- Teach patient to monitor blood pressure and report abnormal findings.
- ◀﴾ Advise patient to immediately report chest pain or rash.
- Instruct patient to consult prescriber before drinking alcohol or taking over-the-counter drugs (especially cold remedies).
- As appropriate, review all other significant and life-threatening adverse reactions and interactions, especially those related to the drugs, foods, herbs, and behaviors mentioned above.

nicotine

nicotine polacrilex
Nicorette

nicotine inhaler
Nicotrol Inhaler

nicotine nasal spray
Nicotrol NS

nicotine transdermal system
Clear Nicoderm CQ, Habitrol, Nicoderm CQ, Nicotrol

Pharmacologic class: Cholinergic
Therapeutic class: Smoking deterrent
Pregnancy risk category C (gum), ***D*** (inhalation, nasal, transdermal)

Action

Supplies nicotine during controlled withdrawal from cigarette smoking. Binds selectively to nicotinic-cholinergic receptors in the peripheral and central nervous systems, autonomic ganglia, adrenal medulla, and neuromuscular junction. At low doses, exerts a stimulating effect; at high doses, a reward effect.

Availability

Chewing gum: 2 mg, 4 mg
Inhalation: 42 cartridges/system, each containing 10 mg nicotine (delivering 4 mg)
Nasal spray: 10 mg/ml (0.5 mg/spray) in 10-ml bottles (100 doses)
Transdermal patch: 7 mg/day, 11 mg/day, 14 mg/day, 15 mg/day, 21 mg/day, 22 mg/day

🖊 Indications and dosages

➤ Adjunctive therapy (with behavior modification) for nicotine withdrawal
Transdermal—
Adults: 21 mg/day transdermally (Habitrol) for 4 to 8 weeks, then 14 mg/day for 2 to 4 weeks, and then 7 mg/day for 2 to 4 weeks, for a total of 8 to 16 weeks; patient must wear system 24 hours/day. Or 21 mg/day transdermally (Nicoderm CQ) for 6 weeks, then 14 mg/day for 2 weeks, and then 7 mg/day for 2 weeks, for a total of 10 weeks; patient must wear system 24 hours/day. Or 15 mg/day transdermally (one Nicotrol patch) for 6 weeks; patient must wear system 16 hours/day and remove it at bedtime.
Adults, adolescents, and children weighing less than 45 kg (100 lb) who smoke fewer than 10 cigarettes daily or have underlying cardiovascular disease: 14 mg/day transdermally (Habitrol) for 4 to 8 weeks, then 7 mg/day for 2 to 4 weeks, for a total of 6 to 8 weeks; patient must wear system 24 hours/day. Or 14 mg/day transdermally (Nicoderm CQ) for 6 weeks, then 7 mg/day for 2 weeks, for a total of 8 weeks; patient must wear system 24 hours/day.
Nasal spray—
Adults: One spray intranasally in each nostril once or twice per hour, up to five times per hour or 40 times per day, for no longer than 3 months
Inhalation—
Adults: Initially for optimal response, at least six cartridges inhaled daily for first 3 to 6 weeks, to a maximum of 16 cartridges daily for 12 weeks. Patient self-titrates dosage to required nicotine level (usually, 6 to 16 cartridges daily), followed by gradual withdrawal over 6 to 12 weeks.
Chewing gum—
Adults: Use as needed depending on smoking urge or chewing rate, or use on fixed schedule q 1 to 2 hours. Usual initial requirement is 20 mg/day, not to exceed 60 mg/day.

Contraindications

• Hypersensitivity to menthol (inhaler only)
• Allergy to adhesive (transdermal forms only)
• Severe cardiovascular disease
• Gastric ulcer
• Immediately after myocardial infarction
• Children

Administration

• Apply patch (when patient awakens) and remove patch (as prescribed) at same time each day.
• Administer nasal spray regularly during first week to help patient get used to its irritant effects.
• With inhalation forms, give at least six cartridges daily for first 3 to 6 weeks.
• Encourage patient to titrate dosage to level required, followed by gradual withdrawal.

Route	Onset	Peak	Duration
Gum	Rapid	15-30 min	Unknown
Inhalation	Rapid	15 min	Unknown
Nasal spray	Rapid	4-15 min	Unknown
Transdermal (Habitrol)	Rapid	6-12 hr	Unknown
Transdermal (Nicoderm CQ)	Rapid	2-4 hr	Unknown

Adverse reactions

CNS: headache, insomnia, abnormal dreams, dizziness, drowsiness, poor concentration, nervousness, weakness, paresthesia
CV: atrial fibrillation, chest pain, hypertension, tachycardia
EENT: sinusitis; pharyngitis (with gum); nasopharyngeal irritation, rhinitis, sneezing, watering eyes, eye irritation (with nasal spray); mouth and

throat irritation (with inhaler)**GI:** nausea, vomiting, diarrhea, constipation, abdominal pain, abnormal taste, dry mouth, dyspepsia; increased salivation, sore mouth (with gum)
GU: dysmenorrhea
Musculoskeletal: joint pain, back pain, myalgia; jaw muscle ache (with gum)
Respiratory: increased cough (with nasal spray or inhaler), **bronchospasm**
Skin: burning at patch site, erythema, pruritus, cutaneous hypersensitivity, rash, sweating (all with transdermal patch)
Other: increased appetite (with gum), allergy, hiccups

Interactions

Drug-drug. *Acetaminophen, adrenergic antagonists (such as prazosin, labetalol), clozapine, furosemide, imipramine, oxazepam, pentazocine, propranolol and other beta blockers, theophylline:* increased effects of these drugs
Bupropion: treatment-emergent hypertension
Insulin: decreased insulin requirement
Isoproterenol, phenylephrine: increased requirements for these drugs
Propoxyphene: decreased nicotine metabolism
Drug-food. *Caffeine-containing foods and beverages:* increased nicotine effects
Drug-behaviors. *Cigarette smoking:* increased nicotine metabolism and effects

Precautions

Use cautiously in:
• cardiovascular disease, hypertension, diabetes mellitus, pheochromocytoma, peripheral vascular disease, hyperthyroidism, peptic ulcer disease, hepatic disease
• skin disorders (transdermal form only)
• dental disorders, esophagitis, pharyngitis, stomatitis (gum only)
• women of childbearing age
• pregnant or breastfeeding patients.

Patient monitoring

• Assess for signs and symptoms of nicotine withdrawal (irritability, drowsiness, fatigue, headache).
• Watch for evidence of nicotine toxicity (nausea, vomiting, diarrhea, increased salivation, headache, dizziness, visual disturbances).

Patient teaching

• Caution patient against any type of smoking during therapy.
• If patient is using gum, teach him to chew one piece whenever nicotine craving occurs. Advise him to chew it slowly until he feels tingling sensation, store it between cheek and gum until tingling disappears.
• Instruct patient to apply transdermal patch to clean, dry skin of upper arm or torso when he awakens; to keep it in place when showering, bathing, or swimming; and to remove it at same time each day.
• If patient is using nasal spray, instruct him to tilt head back slightly when spraying; remind him not to sniff, swallow, or inhale through nose.
• If patient is using inhalation form, teach him to puff continuously for 20 minutes and to use at least six cartridges daily for first 3 to 6 weeks.
• As appropriate, review all significant and life-threatening adverse reactions and interactions, especially those related to the drugs, foods, and behaviors mentioned above.

nifedipine
Adalat, Adalat CC, Adalat P.A.♣,
Adalat XL♣, Apo-Nifed♣,
Gen-Nifedical♣, Nifedical XL,
Novo-Nifedin♣, Nu-Nifed,
Procardia, Procardia XL

Pharmacologic class: Calcium channel blocker
Therapeutic class: Antianginal, antihypertensive
Pregnancy risk category C

Action
Inhibits calcium transport into myocardial and vascular smooth muscle cells, suppressing contractions. Dilates main coronary arteries and arterioles and inhibits coronary artery spasm, thus increasing oxygen delivery to the heart and decreasing frequency and severity of angina attacks.

Availability
Capsules: 5 mg, 10 mg, 20 mg
Tablets: 10 mg
Tablets (extended-release): 10 mg, 20 mg, 30 mg, 60 mg, 90 mg

🕖 Indications and dosages
➤ Hypertension, angina pectoris, vasospastic (Prinzmetal's) angina, heart failure, migraine
Adults: 10 to 30 mg P.O. t.i.d., not to exceed 180 mg daily; or 10 to 20 mg b.i.d. (Adalat P.A. extended-release) or 30 to 90 mg once daily (Adalat CC, P.A., XL extended-release), not to exceed 90 to 120 mg daily

Off-label uses
• Autonomic dysreflexia
• Preeclampsia
• Raynaud's disease
• Hypertrophic cardiomyopathy

Contraindications
• Hypersensitivity to drug or other calcium channel blockers
• Sick sinus syndrome
• Second- or third-degree atrioventricular block (unless artificial pacemaker is in place)
• Systolic blood pressure less than 90 mm Hg

Administration
• Give with or without food. If GI upset occurs, administer with meals—but never with grapefruit juice.
• Don't crush or break extended-release tablets; make sure patient swallows them whole.
• Know that Procardia XL and Adalat CC are not equivalent because of their pharmacokinetic differences.
• Be aware that extended-release tablets only are used for treatment of hypertension.

Route	Onset	Peak	Duration
P.O.	20 min	Unknown	6-8 hr
P.O. (PA)	Unknown	4 hr	12 hr
P.O. (CC, PA, XL)	Unknown	6 hr	24 hr

Adverse reactions
CNS: headache, dizziness, fatigue, asthenia, headache, paresthesia, vertigo
CV: peripheral edema, chest pain, hypotension, **arrhythmias, heart failure, myocardial infarction**
EENT: epistaxis, rhinitis
GI: nausea, constipation
GU: urinary frequency, impotence
Musculoskeletal: leg cramps
Skin: flushing, rash
Other: **Stevens-Johnson syndrome**

Interactions
Drug-drug. *Beta blockers, digoxin, disopyramide, phenytoin:* bradycardia, conduction defects, heart failure

Carbamazepine, cimetidine, cyclosporine, prazosin, propranolol, quinidine: decreased nifedipine metabolism, greater risk of toxicity
Corticosteroids, diuretics, hypoglycemics: increased risk of hypokalemia
Digoxin: increased digoxin blood level, greater risk of digoxin toxicity
Fentanyl, nitrates, other antihypertensives, quinidine: additive hypotension
Nonsteroidal anti-inflammatory drugs: decreased antihypertensive effect
Drug-diagnostic tests. *Antinuclear antibody, direct Coombs' test:* false-positive results
Drug-food. *Grapefruit juice:* increased nifedipine blood level and effects
Drug-herb. *Ginkgo, ginseng:* increased nifedipine blood level
Ephedra, yohimbine: antagonism of nifedipine effect
St. John's wort: decreased nifedipine blood level
Drug-behaviors. *Alcohol use:* additive hypotension

Precautions
Use cautiously in:
- severe hepatic or renal impairment, hypotension
- history of porphyria, serious ventricular arrhythmias, or heart failure
- elderly patients
- pregnant or breastfeeding patients (safety not established)
- children (safety not established).

Patient monitoring
- Monitor vital signs and cardiovascular status; stay alert for chest pain and edema.
- Watch for rash.

Patient teaching
- Advise patient that he may take drug with or without meals. If GI upset occurs, tell him to take it with meals—but never with grapefruit juice.
- Caution patient not to crush or break extended-release tablets; tell him to swallow them whole.
- Inform patient that angina attacks may occur 30 minutes after administration. Explain that these attacks are usually temporary and don't mean that drug should be withdrawn.

[Clinical alert] Teach patient to report rash immediately.
- Instruct patient to avoid driving and other hazardous activities until he knows how drug affects concentration, balance, and alertness.
- As appropriate, review all other significant and life-threatening adverse reactions and interactions, especially those related to the drugs, tests, foods, herbs, and behaviors mentioned above.

nilutamide
Anandron✦, Nilandron

Pharmacologic class: Antiandrogen
Therapeutic class: Antineoplastic
Pregnancy risk category C

Action
Inhibits testosterone uptake in target tissue, preventing normal androgenic response and arresting tumor growth in androgen-sensitive tissue

Availability
Tablets: 50 mg, 150 mg, 100 mg

Indications and dosages
➢ Metastatic prostate cancer, used in combination with surgical castration
Adults: 300 mg/day P.O. for 30 days, starting on day of or day after surgery; then 150 mg/day P.O.

Contraindications
- Hypersensitivity to drug
- Severe hepatic or respiratory insufficiency

Administration
- Give with or without food.
- Start therapy on same day as or day after surgical castration.

Route	Onset	Peak	Duration
P.O.	Rapid	Days	Wks

Adverse reactions
CNS: dizziness, depression, hyperesthesia, insomnia
CV: hypertension, peripheral edema, **heart failure**
EENT: impaired dark and light adaptation, abnormal vision, chromatopsia
GI: nausea, vomiting, dyspepsia, constipation, anorexia
GU: urinary tract infection, hematuria, nocturia, gynecomastia, testicular atrophy, decreased libido, impotence
Hepatic: increased alanine aminotransferase and aspartate aminotransferase levels, **hepatitis**
Hematologic: anemia, **aplastic anemia**
Respiratory: dyspnea, upper respiratory infection, **interstitial pneumonia**
Other: flulike symptoms, pain, fever

Interactions
Drug-drug. *Phenytoin, theophylline, vitamin K, warfarin:* increased risk of toxicity from these drugs
Drug-behaviors. *Alcohol use:* disulfiram-like reaction

Precautions
Use cautiously in:
- renal impairment.

Patient monitoring
- Check for signs and symptoms of hepatitis; monitor liver function tests.
- Monitor complete blood count.
- Assess fluid intake and output and weight; watch for signs and symptoms of heart failure.
- Monitor respiratory status, including chest X-rays.

Patient teaching
- Tell patient he may take drug with or without food.
- Inform patient that therapy will start on day of or day after surgical castration.
- Instruct patient to weigh himself daily and report sudden increases.
- 🔊 Teach patient to report new onset or worsening of dyspnea or signs and symptoms of hepatotoxicity.
- Tell patient that drug may impair his adaptation to darkness and light, which may cause difficulty driving at night or through tunnels.
- As appropriate, review all other significant and life-threatening adverse reactions and interactions, especially those related to the drugs and behaviors mentioned above.

nimodipine
Nimotop

n

Pharmacologic class: Calcium channel blocker
Therapeutic class: Cerebral vasodilator
Pregnancy risk category C

Action
Inhibits calcium transport into vascular smooth muscle cells, suppressing contractions; also dilates coronary and cerebral arteries

Availability
Capsules: 30 mg

💊 Indications and dosages
➤ Subarachnoid hemorrhage
Adults: 60 mg P.O. q 4 hours for 21 days. Therapy starts within 96 hours of subarachnoid hemorrhage.
Dosage adjustment
- Hepatic impairment

Contraindications
None known

Administration
• If patient can't swallow capsule, puncture it with sterile needle and empty contents into syringe; administer through nasogastric tube followed by a flush of normal saline solution (30 ml).

Route	Onset	Peak	Duration
P.O.	Unknown	1 hr	4 hr

Adverse reactions
CNS: headache, depression
CV: hypotension, peripheral edema, ECG abnormalities, bradycardia, tachycardia
GI: nausea, diarrhea, abdominal discomfort
Hepatic: abnormal liver function tests
Musculoskeletal: muscle cramps
Respiratory: dyspnea
Skin: acne, flushing, rash

Interactions
Drug-drug. *Nitrates, other antihypertensives, quinidine:* additive hypotension
Drug-diagnostic tests. *Alanine aminotransferase, alkaline phosphatase, lactate dehydrogenase:* increased levels
Platelets: decreased count
Drug-food. *Grapefruit juice:* increased drug blood level and effects
Drug-herb. *Ephedra, yohimbine:* antagonism of nimodipine effects
St. John's wort: decreased drug blood level
Drug-behaviors. *Alcohol use:* increased hypotension

Precautions
Use cautiously in:
• severe hepatic or renal impairment, hypotension
• history of serious ventricular arrhythmias or heart failure
• elderly patients
• pregnant or breastfeeding patients (safety not established)
• children (safety not established).

Patient monitoring
• Monitor weight and fluid intake and output; stay alert for fluid retention.
• Assess neurologic status and mood, watching for signs of depression.
• Check vital signs and ECG.

Patient teaching
• Tell patient to take drug for full course of therapy (21 days).
• Tell patient to take drug on empty stomach 1 hour before or 2 hours after a meal and to avoid grapefruit juice 1 hour before or 2 hours after taking drug.
• Instruct patient to report irregular heartbeat, shortness of breath, rash, or swollen hands or feet.
• Teach patient to minimize GI upset by eating small, frequent meals.
• Advise patient to weigh himself daily and report sudden weight gain.
• As appropriate, review all other significant and life-threatening adverse reactions and interactions, especially those related to the drugs, tests, foods, herbs, and behaviors mentioned above.

nisoldipine
Sular

Pharmacologic class: Calcium channel blocker
Therapeutic class: Antihypertensive
Pregnancy risk category C

Action
Suppresses calcium transport into vascular smooth muscle cells, inhibiting vasoconstriction and dilating coronary arteries, thereby improving myocardial oxygen uptake

Availability
Tablets (extended-release): 10 mg, 20 mg, 30 mg, 40 mg

Indications and dosages
➤ Hypertension
Adults: Initially, 20 mg daily as a single dose; may increase by 10 mg daily q 7 days, up to 60 mg daily (usual range is 20 to 40 mg daily).

Contraindications
• Hypersensitivity to drug or other calcium channel blockers

Administration
• Give without regard to meals; if GI upset occurs, give with food.
• Don't crush or break extended-release tablets; make sure patient swallows them whole.

Route	Onset	Peak	Duration
P.O.	Unknown	6-12 hr	24 hr

Adverse reactions
CNS: headache, dizziness
CV: peripheral edema, chest pain, vasodilation, hypotension, palpitations, **myocardial infarction**
EENT: pharyngitis, sinusitis
GI: nausea
Skin: rash

Interactions
Drug-drug. *Azole antifungals, cimetidine, ranitidine:* increased nisoldipine blood level
Hydantoin: decreased nisoldipine effects
Nitrates, other antihypertensives: additive hypotension
Phenytoin, other CYP3A4 inducers: decreased nisoldipine blood level and efficacy
Drug-food. *Grapefruit juice:* significantly increased drug blood level and effects
High-fat meal: increased drug blood level

Drug-herb. *Ephedra, yohimbine:* antagonism of nimodipine effects
St. John's wort: decreased nimodipine blood level
Drug-behaviors. *Alcohol use:* increased hypotensive effects

Precautions
Use cautiously in:
• heart failure and left ventricular dysfunction, hepatic impairment, renal disease, coronary artery disease, hypotension
• concurrent phenytoin use
• elderly patients
• pregnant or breastfeeding patients
• children (safety not established).

Patient monitoring
• Check vital signs and ECG.
• Monitor fluid intake and output; watch for peripheral edema.

Patient teaching
• Tell patient to swallow extended-release tablets whole and not to crush or break them.
• If GI upset occurs, teach patient to take drug with food and to eat small, frequent meals.
• Advise patient to avoid high-fat meals, alcohol, and grapefruit juice.
• Teach patient to immediately report irregular heart beat, shortness of breath, swelling, pronounced dizziness, rash, or chest pain.
• As appropriate, review all other significant and life-threatening adverse reactions and interactions, especially those related to the drugs, foods, herbs, and behaviors mentioned above.

n

nitrofurantoin
Macrobid, Macrodantin

nitrofurantoin macrocrystals
Apo-Nitrofurantoin✥, Furadantin

Pharmacologic class: 5-nitrofuran derivative

Therapeutic class: Anti-infective, urinary tract anti-infective

Pregnancy risk category B

Action
Inhibits bacterial enzymes required for normal cell activity (at low concentrations); inhibits normal cell wall synthesis (at high concentrations)

Availability
Capsules: 25 mg, 50 mg, 100 mg
Capsules (extended-release): 100 mg
Oral suspension: 25 mg/5 ml
Tablets: 50 mg, 100 mg

⃠ Indications and dosages
➤ Active urinary tract infections (UTIs) caused by susceptible organisms
Adults: 50 to 100 mg P.O. q.i.d. or 100 mg q 12 hours (extended-release)
➤ Chronic suppression of UTIs
Adults: 50 to 100 mg P.O. at bedtime
Dosage adjustment
• Children

Contraindications
• Hypersensitivity to drug or parabens (oral suspension only)
• Severe renal disease
• Oliguria or anuria
• Glucose-6-phosphate dehydrogenase deficiency
• Infants younger than 1 month
• Pregnancy near term

Administration
• Give with food or milk to avoid GI upset.

Route	Onset	Peak	Duration
P.O.	Unknown	30 min	6-12 hr

Adverse reactions
CNS: dizziness, drowsiness, headache, peripheral neuropathy, nystagmus, vertigo
CV: chest pain
GI: nausea, vomiting, diarrhea, abdominal pain, anorexia, **pseudomembranous colitis**
Hematologic: agranulocytosis, thrombocytopenia
Hepatic: hepatitis, hepatic necrosis
Respiratory: asthma attacks, **pulmonary hypersensitivity reactions**
Skin: photosensitivity, exfoliative dermatitis, alopecia, pruritus, urticaria, angioedema
Other: drug fever, hypersensitivity reactions including **anaphylaxis, Stevens-Johnson syndrome**

Interactions
Drug-drug. *Anticholinergics:* increased nitrofurantoin absorption and bioavailability
Drugs that can cause pulmonary toxicity: increased risk of pneumonitis
Hepatotoxic drugs: increased risk of hepatotoxicity
Magnesium salts: decreased nitrofurantoin absorption
Neurotoxic drugs: increased risk of neurotoxicity
Uricosurics (such as probenecid): decreased renal clearance of nitrofurantoin and increased blood level
Drug-diagnostic tests. *Alkaline phosphatase, bilirubin, blood urea nitrogen, creatinine:* increased levels
Granulocytes, platelets: decreased levels
Urine glucose tests using Benedict's reagent or Fehling's solution: false-positive results

Precautions
Use cautiously in:
- diabetes mellitus, renal impairment
- elderly or debilitated patients
- pregnant or breastfeeding patients.

Patient monitoring
- Monitor patient's response to therapy; obtain specimens for repeat urine culture and sensitivity tests if no improvement occurs.
- Assess respiratory status; watch for signs and symptoms of pulmonary hypersensitivity reaction.
- Monitor complete blood count and liver function tests; stay alert for indications of hepatic involvement.
- Evaluate patient for rash.

Patient teaching
- Tell patient to take drug with food or milk at regular intervals around the clock.
- Advise patient to complete entire course of therapy.
- Instruct patient to use caution when driving and performing other hazardous activities until he knows how drug affects vision, concentration, and alertness.
- ◀ℰ Teach patient to immediately report fever, chills, cough, chest pain, difficulty breathing, rash, severe diarrhea, bleeding or easy bruising, dark urine, yellowing of skin or eyes, numbness or tingling of fingers or toes, or intolerable GI upset.
- As appropriate, review all other significant and life-threatening adverse reactions and interactions, especially those related to the drugs and tests mentioned above.

nitroglycerin
Deponit, Minitran, Nitrek, Nitro-Bid, Nitro-Bid IV, Nitrocot, Nitrodisc, Nitro-Dur, Nitrogard, Nitrogard SR, Nitroglyn E-R, Nitrong, Nitro-par, Nitro-Time, Notroject✤, Nitrolingual, Nitrol, NitroQuick, Nitrostat, Transderm-Nitro, Tridil

Pharmacologic class: Nitrate
Therapeutic class: Antianginal
Pregnancy risk category C

Action
Inhibits calcium transport into myocardial and vascular smooth muscle cells, suppressing contractions. Dilates main coronary arteries and arterioles and inhibits coronary artery spasm, thus increasing oxygen delivery to the heart and decreasing frequency and severity of angina attacks.

n

Availability
Capsules (extended-release): 2.5 mg, 6.5 mg, 9 mg
Injection: 0.5 mg/ml, 5 mg/ml
Ointment (transdermal): 2%
Solution for injection: 25 mg/250 ml, 50 mg/250 ml, 50 mg/500 ml, 100 mg/250 ml, 200 mg/500 ml
Spray (translingual): 0.4 mg/spray in 14.5-g canister (200 doses)
Tablets (buccal, extended-release): 1 mg, 2 mg, 3 mg, 5 mg
Tablets (extended-release): 2.6 mg, 6.5 mg, 9 mg
Tablets (sublingual): 0.3 mg, 0.4 mg, 0.6 mg
Transdermal system (patch): 0.1 mg/hour, 0.2 mg/hour, 0.3 mg/hour, 0.4 mg/hour, 0.6 mg/hour, 0.8 mg/ hour

⚡ Indications and dosages
➣ Prophylactic management of angina pectoris

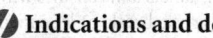

Adults: For acute angina attack, 0.3 to 0.6 mg S.L., repeated q 5 minutes for 15 minutes p.r.n.; or one to two translingual sprays, repeated q 5 minutes for 15 minutes p.r.n. For long-term or prophylactic use in angina, 1-mg extended-release buccal tablet q 5 hours, with dosage and frequency increased p.r.n.; or 2.5 to 9 mg (extended-release tablets) P.O. q 8 to 12 hours; or 1.3 to 6.5 mg (extended-release capsules) P.O. q 8 to 12 hours.

➤ Hypertension during surgical procedures; adjunct in heart failure
Adults: 5 mcg/minute I.V., increased by 5 mcg/minute q 3 to 5 minutes up to 20 mcg/minute, then increased by 10 to 20 mcg/minute q 3 to 5 minutes (dosage determined by hemodynamic parameters)

➤ Acute myocardial infarction
Adults: 12.5 to 25 mcg I.V., then a continuous infusion of 10 to 20 mcg/minute q 5 to 10 minutes; increase by 5 to 10 mcg/minute q 5 to 10 minutes as needed to a maximum of 200 mcg/minute

Off-label uses
• Pulmonary edema

Contraindications
• Hypersensitivity to drug or adhesives (transdermal)
• Closed-angle galucoma
• Orthostatic hypotension
• Hypotension or uncorrected hypovolemia (I.V.)
• Early myocardial infarction (S.L.)
• Head trauma or cerebral hemorrhage
• Severe anemia
• Pericardial tamponade or constrictive pericarditis
• Concurrent sildenafil therapy

Administration
• Administer tablets and capsules with water. Don't crush, break, or let patient chew them.

• For sublingual use, administer under tongue or in buccal pouch; instruct patient not to swallow the tablet. For acute angina, give at pain onset. For angina prophylaxis, give before activities that may cause anginal pain. Make sure tablet fizzles or burns under patient's tongue.
• For translingual use, spray directly onto oral mucosa. Don't let patient inhale spray. Give at pain onset and administer as needed prophylactically before activities that trigger angina.
• For transdermal use, apply system to skin site with little hair and movement. Don't apply to distal extremities. Rotate application sites to avoid irritation and sensitization.
• Apply transdermal ointment to skin by spreading prescribed amount over a 6″ x 6″ area (using an applicator, not your fingers). Cover area with plastic wrap and tape. Rotate sites to reduce risk of irritation and inflammation.
• For I.V. use, administer with infusion pump. Increase dosage in increments of 5 mcg/minute every 3 to 5 minutes, as needed, to achieve desired blood pressure response; once achieved, reduce dosage and lengthen dosage adjustment intervals.

Route	Onset	Peak	Duration
P.O. (extended)	40-60 min	Unknown	8-12 hr
I.V.	Immediate	Unknown	Several min
Buccal (extended)	Unknown	Unknown	5 hr
S.L.	1-3 min	Unknown	30-60 min
Transdermal (ointment)	20-60 min	Unknown	4-8 hr
Transdermal (patch)	40-60 min	Unknown	8-24 hr
Translingual	2-4 min	Unknown	30-60 min

Adverse reactions
CNS: dizziness, headache, apprehension, restlessness, weakness
CV: hypotension, syncope, **tachycardia**
EENT: blurred vision, dry eyes
GI: nausea, vomiting, abdominal pain
Hematologic: methemoglobinemia
Skin: contact dermatitis (with transdermal or ointment use), rash, exfoliative dermatitis, flushing

Interactions
Drug-drug. *Antihypertensives, beta blockers, calcium channel blockers, haloperidol, phenothiazines:* additive hypotension
Drugs with anticholinergic properties (antihistamines, phenothiazines, tricyclic antidepressants): decreased absorption of lingual, sublingual, or buccal nitroglycerin
Sildenafil: increased risk of potentially fatal hypotension
Drug-diagnostic tests. *Cholesterol:* false elevations
Methemoglobin: increased level (with excessive doses)
Urine catecholamines, urine vanillylmandelic acid: increased levels
Drug-behaviors. *Alcohol use or acute alcohol ingestion:* increased risk of potentially fatal hypotension

Precautions
Use cautiously in:
• renal or severe hepatic impairment, glaucoma, hypertrophic cardiomyopathy
• hypovolemia or normal or decreased pulmonary capillary wedge pressure (with I.V. use)
• alcohol intolerance (with large I.V. doses)
• pregnant or breastfeeding patients
• children (safety not established).

Patient monitoring
◀｜≶ With I.V. use, frequently monitor blood pressure; titrate dosage to obtain desired results.

• With transdermal use, check for rash or skin irritation.
• Monitor patient for angina relief.

Patient teaching
• Instruct patient to place S.L. tablet directly under tongue and hold it there as it dissolves. Caution him not to chew or swallow tablet.
• Teach patient to use drug before physical activities that may cause angina.
• Instruct patient to take drug at pain onset and repeat every 5 minutes for three doses. If pain doesn't subside, advise him to seek medical attention.
• Tell patient not to chew or crush sustained-release tablets.
• Teach patient to apply correct amount of ointment using applicator. Caution him to avoiding rubbing site; instruct him to cover ointment with plastic wrap and tape it, to wash hands after placement, and to rotate sites.
• Advise patient to consult prescriber or pharmacist before changing brands of transdermal system; different brands may have different drug concentrations.
• As appropriate, review all significant and life-threatening adverse reactions and interactions, especially those related to the drugs, tests, and behaviors mentioned above.

n

nitroprusside sodium
Nipride✤, Nitropress

Pharmacologic class: Vasodilator
Therapeutic class: Antihypertensive
Pregnancy risk category C

Action
Interferes with calcium influx and intracellular activation of calcium, causing peripheral vasodilation and a direct decrease in blood pressure

---

✤ Canada   ◀｜≶ Clinical alert   Reactions in **bold** are life-threatening

Availability

Injection: 50 mg/vial in 2 ml- and 5-ml vials

💋 Indications and dosages

➤ Hypertensive emergencies; controlled hypotension during anesthesia; cardiac pump failure or cardiogenic shock

Adults: 0.5 to 10 mcg/kg/ minute I.V.
Children: 0.3 to 0.5 mcg/kg/minute I.V., titrated to patient's response

Dosage adjustment
- Hepatic insufficiency
- Renal impairment
- Elderly patients

Contraindications

- Hypersensitivity to drug
- Hypertension caused by aortic coarctation or atrioventricular shunting
- Acute heart failure caused by reduced peripheral vascular resistance

Administration

◀≶ Give only in settings with trained personnel and continuous blood pressure monitoring equipment.
- Dilute 50 mg in 2 to 3 ml of dextrose 5% in water (D_5W); then dilute in 250 to 1,000 ml of D_5W.
- Administer only with microdrip regulator, infusion pump, or another device that allows precise flow rate measurement.
- Wrap infusion solution in aluminum foil or other opaque material to protect it from light.

Route	Onset	Peak	Duration
I.V.	1-2 min	1-10 min	10 min

Adverse reactions

CNS: dizziness, headache, agitation, twitching, decreased reflexes, ataxia, restlessness, **loss of consciousness, increased intracranial pressure**
CV: ECG changes, hypotension, bradycardia, tachycardia

GI: nausea, vomiting, abdominal pain, ileus
Hematologic: decreased platelet aggregation, **methemoglobinemia**
Musculoskeletal: muscle twitching
Metabolic: acidosis, hypothyroidism
Respiratory: dyspnea
Skin: pinkish skin, rash, pruritus, diaphoresis, flushing
Other: pain, irritation at injection site, **thiocynate or cyanide toxicity**

Interactions

Drug-drug. *Enflurane, ganglionic blockers, halothane, negative inotropic drugs, volatile liquid anesthetics:* severe hypotension
Drug-diagnostic tests. *Creatinine:* increased level

Precautions

Use cautiously in:
- fluid and electrolyte imbalances, hepatic or renal disease, hypothyroidism
- elderly patients
- pregnant or breastfeeding patients
- children.

Patient monitoring

◀≶ Measure blood pressure frequently (preferably with continuous arterial line) to detect rapid drop.
- Monitor injection site for extravasation. Use central line whenever possible.
- Obtain baseline ECG and monitor for changes.
◀≶ Watch for signs and symptoms of cyanide toxicity (acidosis, dyspnea, headache, vomiting, dizziness, ataxia, loss of consciousness).

Patient teaching

- Tell patient he'll be closely monitored during therapy.
◀≶ Instruct patient to immediately report pain in chest or at injection site.
- As appropriate, review all other significant and life-threatening adverse reactions and interactions, especially

---

those related to the drugs and tests mentioned above.

nizatidine
Axid, Axid AR

Pharmacologic class: Histamine$_2$ (H$_2$)-receptor antagonist
Therapeutic class: Antiulcer drug
Pregnancy risk category B

Action
Inhibits histamine action at H$_2$-receptor sites in gastric parietal cells, reducing gastric acid secretion and pepsin production

Availability
Capsules: 150 mg, 300 mg
Tablets: 75 mg

⚡ Indications and dosages
➤ Active duodenal ulcer
Adults: 300 mg once daily at bedtime or 150 mg b.i.d.
➤ To prevent duodenal ulcers
Adults: 150 mg once daily at bedtime
➤ Gastroesophageal reflux disease (GERD)
Adults: 150 mg b.i.d.
➤ To prevent and treat heartburn, acid indigestion, and sour stomach
Adults: 75 mg P.O. immediately to 60 minutes before consuming foods or beverages expected to cause symptoms
Dosage adjustment
• Renal impairment
• Elderly patients

Contraindications
• Hypersensitivity to drug or other H$_2$-receptor antagonists

Administration
• Give with or without food.

• If patient is to take drug twice a day, give one dose in morning and one at bedtime.

Route	Onset	Peak	Duration
P.O.	Unknown	0.5-3 hr	8-12 hr

Adverse reactions
CNS: dizziness, insomnia, abnormal dreams, drowsiness, anxiety, nervousness, headache
CV: chest pain, **arrhythmias**
EENT: amblyopia, pharyngitis, sinusitis, rhinitis, tooth disorder
GI: nausea, vomiting, diarrhea, constipation, flatulence, dyspepsia, abdominal pain, anorexia, dry mouth
Hematologic: anemia
Hepatic: elevated liver enzyme levels
Musculoskeletal: back pain, myalgia
Respiratory: cough
Skin: rash, pruritus
Other: infection, fever

Interactions
Drug-drug. *Salicylates (high doses):* increased salicylate blood level
Drug-diagnostic tests. *Alanine aminotransferase, alkaline phosphatase, aspartate aminotransferase:* elevated levels
Skin tests using allergenic extracts: false-negative results
Urobilinogen determination using Multistix: false-positive result
Drug-herb. *Pennyroyal:* altered rate of herbal metabolite formation

Precautions
Use cautiously in:
• renal impairment
• elderly patients
• pregnancy or breastfeeding patients.

Patient monitoring
• Monitor liver function tests.
• Check temperature; watch for fever and other signs and symptoms of infection.

n

Patient teaching

• Advise patient to take once-daily doses at bedtime with or without food, and twice-daily doses in the morning and at bedtime.

• Instruct patient to take drug exactly as prescribed and not to take other OTC drugs (especially aspirin).

• Tell patient to promptly report signs and symptoms of infection.

• Instruct patient to avoid driving and other hazardous activities until he knows how drug affects concentration and alertness.

• As appropriate, review all other significant and life-threatening adverse reactions and interactions, especially those related to the drugs, tests, and herbs mentioned above.

norelgestromin/ethinyl estradiol

Ortho Evra

Pharmacologic class: Estrogen
Therapeutic class: Hormone
Pregnancy risk category X

Action

Suppresses gonadotropin and inhibits ovulation by causing changes in cervical mucus and endometrium, preventing implantation of egg

Availability

Transdermal patch: 6 mg norelgestromin and 0.75 mg ethinyl estradiol; releases 150 mcg norelgestromin and 20 mcg ethinyl estradiol q 24 hours

🕛 Indications and dosages

➤ To prevent pregnancy
Adults: Apply patch on day 1 of menstrual cycle (or first Sunday after period begins); change patch weekly thereafter for 3 weeks (on same day each

week), and then remove patch for fourth week. Repeat q month.

Contraindications

• Thromboembolism
• Undiagnosed vaginal bleeding
• Breast or reproductive system cancer
• Cerebrovascular disease
• Coronary artery disease
• Severe hypertension or diabetes with vascular involvement
• Cholestatic jaundice
• Pregnancy or breastfeeding

Administration

• Apply patch to clean, dry, intact skin on buttocks, abdomen, upper torso, or upper outer arm.
• Change patch on same day each week, except for fourth week, when patch is removed.

Route	Onset	Peak	Duration
Transdermal	Rapid	2 days	Unknown

Adverse reactions

CNS: headache, dizziness, lethargy, depression, emotional lability, **increased risk of cerebrovascular accident**
CV: edema, hypertension, **myocardial infarction, thromboembolism**
EENT: contact lens intolerance, worsening of myopia or astigmatism
GI: nausea, vomiting, jaundice, abdominal cramps, bloating, gallbladder disease, anorexia, **pancreatitis**
GU: amenorrhea, dysmenorrhea, breakthrough bleeding, cervical erosion, vaginal candidiasis, breast tenderness, breast enlargement or secretion, menstrual cramps, loss of libido, **increased risk of breast or endometrial cancer**
Hepatic: cholestatic jaundice, **hepatic adenoma**
Metabolic: hyperglycemia, hypercalcemia, sodium and water retention
Musculoskeletal: leg cramps
Respiratory: upper respiratory infection, **pulmonary embolism**

Skin: acne, oily skin, increased pigmentation, urticaria, reaction at patch site
Other: increased appetite, weight changes

Interactions
Drug-drug. *Acetaminophen:* decreased acetaminophen blood level
Antibiotics, barbiturates, carbamazepine, fosphenytoin, phenobarbital, phenytoin, rifampin: decreased contraceptive efficacy
Corticosteroids: enhanced corticosteroid effects
Cyclosporine: increased risk of cyclosporine toxicity
CYP3A4 inhibitors (such as ketoconazole, itraconazole): increased hormone level
Dantrolene, other hepatotoxic drugs: increased risk of hepatotoxicity
Miconazole (vaginal capsules): increased ethinyl estradiol blood level
Insulin, oral hypoglycemics, warfarin: altered requirements for these drugs
Protease inhibitors: increased contraceptive metabolism
Tamoxifen: interference with tamoxifen effects
Drug-diagnostic tests. *Antithrombin III, folate, low-density lipoproteins, pyridoxine, total cholesterol, urine pregnanediol:* decreased values
Cortisol; factors VII, VIII, IX, and X; glucose; high-density lipoproteins; phospholipids; prolactin; prothrombin; sodium; triglycerides: increased levels
Metyrapone test: false decrease
Thyroid function tests: false interpretation
Drug-food. *Caffeine:* increased blood caffeine level
Drug-herb. *Black cohosh:* increased adverse drug effects
Red clover: interference with hormonal therapy
Saw palmetto: antiestrogenic effects
St. John's wort: decreased drug blood level and effects

Drug-behaviors. *Smoking (15 or more cigarettes daily):* increased risk of adverse cardiovascular reactions

Precautions
Use cautiously in:
• cardiovascular disease, severe hepatic or renal disease, asthma, bone disease, migraine, lipid disorders, fibrocystic breasts, increased risk for endometrial cancer, sexually transmitted diseases
• family history of breast or genital tract cancer
• abnormal mammogram.

Patient monitoring
• Evaluate menstrual pattern.
◀€ Monitor blood pressure; watch for signs and symptoms of thromboembolic disease (swelling or warmth in calves, sudden chest pain, shortness of breath).
• Check blood glucose level in diabetic patients.

Patient teaching
• Instruct patient to start using patch on first day of menstrual period or on first Sunday after period starts. Advise her to use calendar to keep track of which day each week to change patch.
• Teach patient to remove patch during week 4 of each cycle; tell her she should expect to have bleeding that week.
• Tell patient to check daily that patch is firmly attached to skin. Explain that if patch was detached for 1 day or less, she should try to reattach it more firmly. But if patch was detached for more than 1 day or for an unknown length of time, she should start with a new patch and a new calendar.
• Instruct patient to use alternative contraception during first week of patch use.
◀€ Inform patient that smoking while using patch increases risk of thromboembolic disease. Tell her to immediately report swelling or warmth in

calves, chest pain, or shortness of breath.

• As appropriate, review all other significant and life-threatening adverse reactions and interactions, especially those related to the drugs, tests, foods, herbs, and behaviors mentioned above.

norepinephrine bitartrate
Levophed

Pharmacologic class: Sympathomimetic

Therapeutic class: Alpha-adrenergic agonist, beta$_1$-adrenergic agonist, cardiac stimulant, vasopressor

Pregnancy risk category C

Action
Stimulates beta$_1$ and alpha$_1$ receptors in sympathetic nervous system, causing vasoconstriction, increased blood pressure, enhanced contractility, and decreased heart rate

Availability
Injection: 1 mg/ml

Indications and dosages
➢ Severe hypotension
Adults: 8 to 12 mcg/minute I.V.; then titrate based on blood pressure response. Maintenance dosage is 2 to 4 mcg/minute.

Contraindications
• Hypersensitivity to drug
• Ventricular fibrillation
• Tachyarrhythmias
• Pheochromocytoma
• Concurrent cyclopropane or halothane anesthesia

Administration
• Mix with dextrose 5% in water or dextrose 5% in normal saline solution.

• Inspect solution to make sure it's clear and colorless; don't infuse if it's brown or pink.
• Administer through infusion pump; titrate infusion rate to achieve and maintain low-normal systolic blood pressure (80 to 100 mmHg).
• Continue infusion until adequate blood pressure and tissue perfusion persist without drug therapy.
• Gradually titrate dosage downward.
• To avoid extravasation, administer only into large vein (antecubital) or through central line. Don't use femoral vein in patients who are elderly or have occlusive vascular disorders.
• Avoid line stasis or flushing to prevent delivery of large drug concentrations.

Route	Onset	Peak	Duration
I.V.	Immediate	Immediate	1-2 min after infusion ends

Adverse reactions
CNS: headache, anxiety, weakness, dizziness, tremor, restlessness, insomnia
CV: bradycardia, **severe hypertension, arrhythmias, cardiac arrest**
Respiratory: respiratory difficulty, **asthmatic episodes**
Skin: irritation with extravasation, necrosis
Other: anaphylaxis

Interactions
Drug-drug. *Alpha-adrenergic blockers:* antagonism of norepinephrine effects
Antihistamines, ergot alkaloids, guanethidine, monoamine oxidase inhibitors, oxytocin, tricyclic antidepressants: severe hypertension
Bretylium, inhalation anesthetics: increased risk of arrhythmias

Precautions
Use cautiously in:
• arterial embolism, peripheral vascular disease, hypertension, hyperthyroidism, cardiac disease

- elderly patients
- pregnant or breastfeeding patients.

Patient monitoring

◀€ Check blood pressure every 2 minutes until desired pressure is achieved; recheck every 5 minutes for duration of infusion.

- Use continuous ECG monitoring as well as blood pressure monitoring.
- Monitor infusion site for extravasation.

◀€ Watch for signs and symptoms of peripheral vascular insufficiency (decreased capillary refill, pale to cyanotic to black skin color).

Patient teaching

- When patient is alert, explain why he's receiving drug.
- Reassure patient he'll be monitored continuously until he's stable.

norethindrone acetate
Aygestin

Pharmacologic class: Progesterone, hormone

Therapeutic class: Progestin

Pregnancy risk category X

Action

Inhibits secretion of pituitary gonadotropins, suppressing follicular maturation and ovulation and stimulating mammary tissue growth

Availability

Tablets: 5 mg

⚕ Indications and dosages

➢ Endometriosis

Adults: 5 mg P.O. daily for 2 weeks, increased in increments of 2.5 mg/day q 2 weeks until 15 mg daily is reached.

➢ Amenorrhea, abnormal uterine bleeding

Adults: 2.5 to 10 mg P.O. daily starting on day 5 of menstrual cycle

Contraindications

- Hypersensitivity to drug
- Severe hepatic disease
- Thromboembolic disorders
- Cancer of breast or genital organs
- Undiagnosed vaginal bleeding
- Missed abortion
- Pregnancy

Administration

- Give with or without food.
- Therapy may be maintained for 6 to 9 months or until breakthrough bleeding necessitates temporary halt.

Route	Onset	Peak	Duration
P.O.	Variable	Unknown	24 hr

Adverse reactions

CNS: migraine, depression, insomnia, drowsiness, headache, precipitation of acute intermittent porphyria, **cerebrovascular accident**

CV: hypotension, hypertension, thrombophlebitis, **thromboembolism, myocardial infarction**

EENT: sudden partial or complete vision loss, proptosis, diplopia

GI: nausea, cholestatic jaundice

GU: breakthrough bleeding, menstrual flow changes, amenorrhea, changes in cervical erosion and secretions, breast tenderness and secretion

Metabolic: hyperglycemia, fluid retention, decreased glucose tolerance

Respiratory: pulmonary embolism

Skin: rash, urticaria, acne, hirsutism, alopecia, chloasma, oily skin, seborrhea, purpura, melasma, photosensitivity

Other: edema, weight gain, fever

n

Interactions
Drug-drug. *Hepatic enzyme-inducing drugs (such as carbamazepine, phenobarbital, phenytoin, rifampin):* decreased norethindrone efficacy
Drug-diagnostic tests. *Alkaline phosphatase; amino acids; factors VII, VIII, IX, and X; nitrogen; pregnanediol:* increased levels
Gamma-glutamyltransferase, high-density lipoproteins: decreased levels
Drug-herb. *Cola nut, guarana, yerba maté:* increased CNS stimulation
St. John's wort: decreased contraceptive efficacy

Precautions
Use cautiously in:
• hypertension, blood dyscrasias, bone marrow disease, gallbladder disease, heart failure, diabetes mellitus, depression, migraine, asthma, seizure disorders, hepatic or renal disease
• family history of breast or reproductive tract cancer
• breastfeeding patients.

Patient monitoring
• Monitor pretreatment and annual physical exams to check blood pressure, breasts, abdomen, pelvic organs, and Pap smear results.
◀€ Assess for signs and symptoms of thromboembolic disease (calf swelling or warmth, sudden chest pain, or shortness of breath).
• Check blood glucose level in diabetic patients.

Patient teaching
◀€ Teach patient to recognize and immediately report signs or symptoms of thromboembolic disease.
• Instruct patient to avoid pregnancy or to discontinue drug if she gets pregnant; drug may cause serious fetal anomalies or fetal death.
◀€ Instruct patient to discontinue drug and consult prescriber if she has sudden partial or complete vision loss.

• If patient is using drug to treat amenorrhea, tell her to mark administration days on calendar.
• Teach diabetic patients to monitor blood glucose level closely and to watch for hyperglycemia.
• Instruct patient to report breakthrough bleeding, spotting, change in menstrual flow, or amenorrhea.
• As appropriate, review all other significant and life-threatening adverse reactions and interactions, especially those related to the drugs, tests, and herbs mentioned above.

norfloxacin
Noroxin

Pharmacologic class: Fluoroquinolone
Therapeutic class: Anti-infective
Pregnancy risk category C

Action
Inhibits bacterial DNA synthesis by blocking DNA gyrase in susceptible gram-negative and gram-positive aerobic and anaerobic bacteria

Availability
Tablets: 400 mg

Indications and dosages
➤ Urinary tract infections (UTIs) caused by *Escherichia coli, Klebsiella pneumoniae,* and *Proteus mirabilis*
Adults: 400 mg P.O. q 12 hours for 3 days
➤ UTIs caused by all other organisms
Adults: 400 mg q 12 hours for 7 to 10 days
➤ Gonorrhea
Adults: 800 mg P.O. as a single dose
➤ Prostatitis due to *E. coli*
Adults: 400 mg P.O. q 12 hours for 28 days
Dosage adjustment
• Renal impairment

Contraindications
• Hypersensitivity to drug
• History of tendinitis or tendon rupture with fluoroquinolone use
• Pregnancy
• Children younger than age 18

Administration
• Give with a glass of water 1 hour before or 2 hours after a meal.
• Don't give antacids within 2 hours of norfloxacin.

Route	Onset	Peak	Duration
P.O.	Rapid	2-3 hr	12 hr

Adverse reactions
CNS: dizziness, drowsiness, headache, insomnia, acute psychoses, agitation, confusion, hallucinations, increased intracranial pressure, light-headedness, tremors, asthenia, **seizures**
CV: QT prolongation, vasodilation, **arrhythmias**
GI: nausea, diarrhea, abdominal pain, altered taste, **pancreatitis, pseudomembranous colitis**
GU: interstitial cystitis, vaginitis
Hematologic: eosinophilia, **leukopenia**
Hepatic: elevated hepatic enzyme levels, **hepatitis**
Metabolic: hyperglycemia, hypoglycemia
Musculoskeletal: tendinitis, tendon rupture
Skin: photosensitivity, phototoxicity, rash
Other: hyperhidrosis, hypersensitivity reactions including **anaphylaxis, Stevens-Johnson syndrome**

Interactions
Drug-drug. *Antacids, bismuth, iron salts, subsalicylate, sucralfate, zinc salts:* decreased norfloxacin absorption
Antineoplastics: decreased norfloxacin blood level
Cimetidine: interference with norfloxacin elimination
Corticosteroids: increased risk of tendon rupture
Nitrofurantoin: antagonism of norfloxacin's antibacterial effects in GU tract
Other fluoroquinolones: increased risk of nephrotoxicity
Probenecid: decreased renal elimination of norfloxacin
Theophylline: increased theophylline blood level, greater risk of toxicity
Warfarin: increased anticoagulant effect
Drug-diagnostic tests. *Alanine aminotransferase, alkaline phosphatase, aspartate aminotransferase, bilirubin, lactate dehydrogenase, platelets:* increased levels
Hemoglobin, hematocrit: decreased values
Drug-food. *Caffeine:* decreased hepatic metabolism of caffeine
Milk or yogurt (consumed alone): impaired drug absorption
Tube feedings: impaired drug absorption
Drug-herb. *Dong quai, St. John's wort:* phototoxicity
Fennel: decreased drug absorption
Drug-behaviors. *Sun exposure:* phototoxicity

Precautions
Use cautiously in:
• CNS diseases or disorders, renal impairment, cirrhosis, bradycardia, acute myocardial ischemia
• elderly patients
• breastfeeding (safety not established except in post-exposure inhalation or cutaneous anthrax).

Patient monitoring
• Monitor vital signs and cardiovascular status.
• Check fluid intake and output; keep patient well-hydrated.
• Assess patient's response to therapy; obtain specimens for repeat culture and sensitivity tests if he relapses or doesn't improve.

n

• Monitor renal function; as necessary, adjust dosage for renal dysfunction.

Patient teaching

• Teach patient to take drug on empty stomach with a glass of water 1 hour before or 2 hours after a meal.

• If patient requires antacids for GI upset, instruct him not to take them within 2 hours of norfloxacin.

◀€ Advise patient to report rash, severe GI problems, or weakness.

• Caution patient to avoid driving and other hazardous activities until he knows how drug affects concentration and alertness.

• Teach patient ways to counteract photosensitivity.

• As appropriate, review all other significant and life-threatening adverse reactions and interactions, especially those related to the drugs, tests, foods, herbs, and behaviors mentioned above.

norgestrel
Ovrette

Pharmacologic class: Estrogen
Therapeutic class: Contraceptive
Pregnancy risk category X

Action
Suppresses gonadotropin and inhibits ovulation by causing changes in endometrium, preventing implantation of egg

Availability
Tablets: 0.075 mg

🕖 Indications and dosages
➤ To prevent pregnancy
Adults: 1 tablet P.O. daily

Contraindications
• Thromboembolism
• Undiagnosed vaginal bleeding

• Breast or reproductive organ cancer
• Cerebrovascular or coronary artery disease
• Cholestatic jaundice or hepatic disease
• Pregnancy or breastfeeding

Administration
• Give daily starting on first day of menstrual period.
• Administer tablet at same time each day.

Route	Onset	Peak	Duration
P.O.	Unknown	Unknown	24 hr

Adverse reactions
CNS: headache, dizziness, lethargy, depression, emotional lability, **increased risk of cerebrovascular accident, seizures**
CV: edema, hypertension, **myocardial infarction, thromboembolism**
EENT: contact lens intolerance, worsening of myopia or astigmatism
GI: nausea, vomiting, jaundice, abdominal cramps, bloating, gallbladder disease, anorexia, **pancreatitis**
GU: amenorrhea, breakthrough bleeding, dysmenorrhea, cervical erosion, vaginal candidiasis, breast tenderness, breast enlargement or secretion, loss of libido, **increased risk of breast and endometrial cancer**
Hepatic: cholestatic jaundice, **hepatic adenoma**
Metabolic: hyperglycemia, hypercalcemia, sodium and water retention
Musculoskeletal: leg cramps
Respiratory: pulmonary embolism
Skin: acne, oily skin, increased pigmentation, urticaria
Other: increased appetite, weight changes

Interactions
Drug-drug. *Acetaminophen:* decreased acetaminophen blood level

---

Antibiotics, barbiturates, carbamazepine, fosphenytoin, phenobarbital, phenytoin, rifampin: decreased norgestrel efficacy

Corticosteroids: enhanced corticosteroid effects

Cyclosporine: increased risk of cyclosporine toxicity

Dantrolene, other hepatotoxic drugs: increased risk of hepatotoxicity

Insulin, oral hypoglycemics, warfarin: altered requirement for these drugs

Miconazole (vaginal capsules): increased norgestrel blood level

Protease inhibitors: increased norgestrel metabolism

Tamoxifen: interference with tamoxifen effects

Drug-diagnostic tests. *Antithrombin III, pyridoxine, folate, low-density lipoproteins, total cholesterol, urine pregnanediol:* decreased values

Cortisol; factors VII, VIII, IX, and X; glucose; high-density lipoproteins; phospholipids; prolactin; prothrombin; sodium; triglycerides: increased levels

Metyrapone tests: false decrease

Thyroid function tests: false interpretation

Drug-food. *Caffeine:* increased caffeine blood level

Drug-herb. *Black cohosh:* increased adverse reactions to norgestrel

Red clover: interference with norgestrel therapy

Saw palmetto: antiestrogenic effects

St. John's wort: decreased drug blood level and effects

Drug-behaviors. *Smoking:* increased risk of adverse cardiovascular reactions

Precautions

Use cautiously in:
• underlying cardiovascular disease, severe hepatic or renal disease, asthma, bone disease, migraine, seizures, lipid disorders, diabetes, fibrocystic breasts, sexually transmitted disease
• increased risk of endometrial cancer

• family history of breast or genital tract cancer
• cigarette smokers.

Patient monitoring

• Check vital signs and cardiovascular status.

◀€ Watch for signs and symptoms of thromboembolic disease (leg pain, swelling, shortness of breath).

Patient teaching

• Teach patient to take drug at bedtime or with a meal to establish a daily routine.

• Inform patient that taking drug during pregnancy can cause serious fetal anomalies.

◀€ Instruct patient to immediately report calf swelling or warmth, chest pain, shortness of breath, sudden severe headache, and bleeding or spotting.

• Advise patient to avoid driving and other hazardous activities until she knows how drug affects concentration and alertness.

• As appropriate, review all other significant and life-threatening adverse reactions and interactions, especially those related to the drugs, tests, foods, herbs, and behaviors mentioned above.

n

nortriptyline hydrochloride
Aventyl, Norventyl✦, Pamelor, PMS-Nortriptyline✦

Pharmacologic class: Tricyclic compound

Therapeutic class: Antidepressant

Pregnancy risk category D

Action

Increases serotonin and norepinephrine release by blocking reuptake by presynaptic neurons; also possesses anticholinergic properties

---

Availability
Capsules: 10 mg, 25 mg, 50 mg, 75 mg
Oral solution: 10 mg/5 ml

🔘 Indications and dosages
➤ Depression, chronic neurogenic pain
Adults: 25 mg P.O. t.i.d. or q.i.d., up to a maximum of 150 mg daily
Dosage adjustment
• Elderly patients
• Children

Off-label uses
• Postherpetic neuralgia
• Neurologic pain

Contraindications
• Hypersensitivity to drug
• Acute recovery phase of myocardial infarction
• Monoamine oxidase inhibitor use within 14 days
• Children younger than age 12

Administration
• Give drug as prescribed, either in divided doses three or four times a day or as a single dose at bedtime.
• Administer with meals or snack to minimize stomach upset.

Route	Onset	Peak	Duration
P.O.	2-3 wk	6 wk	Unknown

Adverse reactions
CNS: drowsiness, fatigue, lethargy, agitation, confusion, extrapyramidal reactions, hallucinations, headache, insomnia, dizziness, **seizures**
CV: hypotension, ECG changes, heart block, palpitations, **arrhythmias, myocardial infarction, cerebrovascular accident**
EENT: blurred vision, dry eyes
GI: nausea, constipation, unpleasant taste, anorexia, dry mouth, **paralytic ileus**
GU: urinary retention, gynecomastia
Hematologic: blood dyscrasias

Hepatic: jaundice, **hepatotoxicity**
Metabolic: weight gain, altered glucose level
Skin: photosensitivity

Interactions
Drug-drug. *Anticholinergics and anticholinergic-like drugs (including antidepressants, antihistamines, atropine, disopyramide, haloperidol, phenothiazines, quinidine):* additive anticholinergic effects
Antihypertensives: lack of therapeutic response to antihypertensives
Antithyroid drugs: increased risk of agranulocytosis
Cimetidine, fluoxetine, hormonal contraceptives: increased nortriptyline blood level and possible toxicity
Clonidine: hypertensive crisis
CNS depressants (including antihistamines, opioid analgesics, sedative-hypnotics): additive CNS depression
Decongestants, vasoconstrictors: additive adrenergic effects
MAO inhibitors: hypertension, hyperpyrexia, seizures, death
Drug-diagnostic tests. *Alkaline phosphatase, bilirubin:* increased levels
Glucose: increased or decreased level
Drug-herb. *Angel's trumpet, belladonna, henbane, jimson weed, scopolia:* increased anticholinergic effects
Chamomile, hops, kava, skullcap, scopolia, valerian: increased CNS depression
St. John's wort: decreased drug blood level and efficacy
Drug-behaviors. *Alcohol use:* increased drowsiness, impaired motor skills

Precautions
Use cautiously in:
• asthma, cardiovascular disease, severe depression, increased intraocular pressure, narrow-angle glaucoma, urinary retention, cardiac or hepatic disease, hyperthyroidism
• history of seizures
• elderly patients (especially elderly men with prostatic hyperplasia)

- pregnant or breastfeeding patients
- children.

Patient monitoring
- Check vital signs and ECG.
- Monitor bowel and bladder function; stay alert for urine retention and constipation.
- Assess neurologic status; document mood swings.
◀ Watch for suicidal tendencies.

Patient teaching
- Tell patient that full effect of drug may not occur for 4 weeks.
- Teach patient that drug may cause drowsiness or dizziness, but that these effects should subside within a few weeks.
◀ Advise patient (and family, as appropriate) to immediately report worsening depression or suicidal ideation.
- Caution patient to avoid driving and other hazardous activities until he knows how drug affects him.
- Instruct patient to notify prescriber immediately if she's planning or suspects pregnancy.
- As appropriate, review all other significant and life-threatening adverse reactions and interactions, especially those related to the drugs, tests, herbs, and behaviors mentioned above.

nystatin
Mycostatin, Nadostine✤, Nilstat, Nyaderm, Nystex, Pedi-Dri, PMS-Nystatin✤

Pharmacologic class: Antifungal
Therapeutic class: Anti-infective
Pregnancy risk category A

Action
Interferes with fungal cell wall synthesis, inhibiting formation of ergo sterols and increasing cell wall permeability, which causes osmotic instability

Availability
Cream: 100,000 units/g
Ointment: 100,000 units/g
Powder: 100,000 units/g
Suspension: 100,000 units/ml
Tablets: 500,000 units
Troches: 200,000 units
Vaginal tablets: 100,000 units

🔰 Indications and dosages
➤ Candidiasis (topical use)
Adults and children: Apply cream, ointment, or powder two or three times daily until healing is complete.
➤ Oral candidiasis
Adults: 400,000 to 600,000 units suspension q.i.d. Have patient gargle and then swallow half of dose in each side of mouth.
Infants: 200,000 units suspension q.i.d. Use half of dose in each side of mouth.
Newborn and premature infants: 100,000 units suspension q.i.d. Use half of dose in each side of mouth.
➤ GI infections
Adults: 500,000 to 1 million units (1 to 2 tablets) P.O. t.i.d.; continue for 48 hours after desired response occurs.
➤ Vaginal candidiasis
Adults: One vaginal tablet (100,000 units) daily for 2 weeks

Contraindications
- Hypersensitivity to drug or its components

Administration
- Give oral suspension by placing half of dose in each side of patient's mouth. Instruct patient to hold suspension in mouth, swish it around, or gargle for several minutes before swallowing it.
- To prepare oral solution from powder, add one-eighth teaspoon to 120 ml of water and stir well. Give immediately after preparing.

• Advise patient to let troche dissolve slowly and completely in mouth; teach him not to chew or swallow it whole.
• Know that nystatin vaginal tablets can be given orally to treat oral candidiasis.
• Apply cream, ointment, or powder two to three times daily until healing is complete.
• Consult prescriber for proper cleaning technique before applying vaginal form. Use applicator provided for vaginal administration.

Route	Onset	Peak	Duration
P.O., topical, vaginal	Unknown	Unknown	Unknown

Adverse reactions
GI: nausea, vomiting, diarrhea, GI distress, oral irritation
GU: vulvovaginal irritation (with vaginal form)
Skin: pruritus, rash

Interactions
Drug-drug. *Topical corticosteroids:* increased corticosteroid absorption
Drug-behaviors. *Latex contraceptive use:* damage to contraceptive (with intravaginal nystatin)

Precautions
Use cautiously in:
• renal or hepatic disease, achlorhydria
• pregnant or breastfeeding patients
• children under age 2.

Patient monitoring
• If patient is taking oral tablets, inspect oral mucous membranes for irritation.
• With topical use, monitor affected area for increase in redness, swelling, or irritation.

Patient teaching
• Advise patient to continue taking drug for at least 48 hours after symptoms resolve.

• Instruct patient to let lozenge dissolve slowly in mouth; teach him not to chew or swallow it.
• If patient misses a dose, tell her to apply or take it as soon as possible and then resume her regular dosing schedule.
• Advise patient that diabetes mellitus, reinfection by sexual partner, tight-fitting pantyhose, and use of antibiotics, hormonal contraceptives, or corticosteroids predispose her to vaginal infection. Urge her to wear cotton underwear.
• Teach female patients to practice careful hygiene in affected areas.
• Teach patient using vaginal tablets to wash applicator thoroughly after each use.
• Tell patient to continue therapy during menstruation.
• As appropriate, review all significant adverse reactions and interactions, especially those related to the drugs and behaviors mentioned above.

octreotide acetate
Sandostatin, Sandostatin LAR Depot

Pharmacologic class: Somatostatin analog
Therapeutic class: Antidiarrheal
Pregnancy risk category B

Action
Suppresses secretion of serotonin, serotonin metabolites, and gastrohepatic peptides, increasing absorption of fluids and electrolytes from the GI tract. Also suppresses growth hormone, insulin, and glucagon.

Availability
Depot injection: 10 mg, 20 mg, 30 mg
Injection: 0.05 mg/ml, 0.1 mg/ml, and
0.5 mg/ml in 1-ml ampules, 0.2 mg/ml
and 1 mg/ml in 5-ml vials

💊 Indications and dosages
➢ Diarrhea
Adults: 100 to 600 mcg (Sandostatin)
daily S.C. or I.V. in two to four divided
doses during first 2 weeks of therapy.
Then, depending on response, 20 mg
(LAR Depot) I.M. q 4 weeks for 2
months.
➢ Diarrhea caused by vasoactive in-
testinal peptide tumors (VIPomas)
Adults: 200 to 300 mcg (Sandostatin)
daily S.C. or I.V. in two to four divided
doses during first 2 weeks of therapy.
Then, depending on response, 20 mg
(LAR Depot) I.M. q 2 weeks for 2
months.
➢ Acromegaly
Adults: 50 to 100 mcg (Sandostatin)
S.C. or I.V. two or three times daily.
Then, depending on response, 20 mg
(LAR Depot) I.M. q 4 weeks for 3
months. Then adjust on basis of
growth hormone levels.
Dosage adjustment
• Renal impairment

Off-label uses
• Dumping syndrome (postprandial
hypotension)
• GI and pancreatic fistulas
• Variceal bleeding

Contraindications
• Hypersensitivity to drug or its components

Administration
• When giving S.C., rotate administration sites with each injection.
◀€ Don't give LAR Depot I.V.
• Mix I.M. solution and inject deep
into gluteal muscle over 3 minutes;
don't use deltoid muscle.

• For I.V. administration, dilute in 50
to 200 ml of dextrose 5% in water or
normal saline solution; infuse over 15
to 30 minutes.
• Know that octreotide suppression
test and octreotide scintigraphy may be
done to determine if drug will aid carcinoid tumor treatment.
• Drug may be kept at room temperature for 2 weeks; refrigerate ampules.

Route	Onset	Peak	Duration
S.C., I.V.	Unknown	0.4 hr	Up to 12 hr
I.M.	Unknown	2 wk	Up to 4 wk

Adverse reactions
CNS: dizziness, drowsiness, fatigue,
headache, weakness
CV: edema, bradycardia, conduction
abnormalities, **arrhythmias**
EENT: vision disturbances
GI: nausea, vomiting, diarrhea, abdom-
inal pain, cholelithiasis, fat malabsorp-
tion
Skin: flushing
Metabolic: hyperglycemia, hypogly-
cemia, hypothyroidism
Other: injection site pain

Interactions
Drug-drug. *Cyclosporine:* reduced cy-
closporine blood level
Insulin, oral hypoglycemics: altered re-
quirements for these drugs
Oral drugs: altered absorption of these
drugs
Drug-diagnostic tests. *Glucose:* in-
creased or decreased level
Hepatic enzymes: slightly increased
levels
Schilling's test: abnormal results
Thyroxine, vitamin B$_{12}$: decreased
levels
Drug-food. *Fats:* altered octreotide
absorption

Precautions
Use cautiously in:
• gallbladder disease, renal impair-

ment, hyperglycemia or hypoglycemia, fat malabsorption

• pregnant or breastfeeding patients
• children.

Patient monitoring

• Assess bowel sounds and stool frequency and consistency.
• Monitor vital signs.
• Monitor fluid intake and output; stay alert for dehydration or edema.
• Evaluate diabetic patients for hypoglycemia or hyperglycemia.

Patient teaching

• If patient is being treated for carcinoid tumor, teach him to keep track of number of daily stools or flushing episodes (reflects drug efficacy in suppressing amine-induced symptoms).
• Instruct patient to weigh himself daily and report significant changes.
• If patient will use drug at home, teach correct methods for injection, storage, and needle disposal.
• Instruct patient to avoid driving and other hazardous activities until he knows how drug affects concentration, vision, and alertness.
• As appropriate, review all other significant and life-threatening adverse reactions and interactions, especially those related to the drugs, tests, and foods mentioned above.

ofloxacin
Floxin

Pharmacologic class: Fluoroquinolone
Therapeutic class: Anti-infective
Pregnancy risk category C

Action

Inhibits bacterial DNA synthesis by inhibiting DNA gyrase in susceptible gram-negative and gram-positive aerobic and anaerobic bacteria

Availability

Injection: 20 mg/ml, 40 mg/ml
Ophthalmic solution: 3 mg/ml (0.3%)
Otic solution: 0.3%
Premixed injection: 200 mg/50 ml, 400 mg/100 ml
Tablets: 200 mg, 300 mg, 400 mg

Indications and dosages

➣ **Prostatitis,** *Escherichia coli*
Adults: 300 mg P.O. or I.V. q 12 hours for 6 weeks
➣ **Urinary tract infections**
Adults: 200 mg P.O. or I.V. q 12 hours for 3 to 10 days
➣ **Gonorrhea**
Adults: 400 mg P.O. or I.V. as a single dose
➣ **Bacterial conjunctivitis**
Adults and children ages 1 and older: One to two drops of ophthalmic solution in affected eye q 2 to 4 hours on days 1 and 2; then one to two drops q.i.d. on days 3 through 7
➣ **Corneal ulcers**
Adults: One to two drops of ophthalmic solution in affected eye q 30 minutes while awake on days 1 and 2; then one to two drops q hour while awake on days 3 to 7; and then one to two drops q.i.d. while awake on days 7 to 9
➣ **Otitis externa**
Adults and children ages 12 older: 10 drops of otic solution into affected ear b.i.d. for 10 days
➣ **Chronic suppurative otitis media with perforated tympanic membrane**
Adults and children ages 12 and older: 10 drops of otic solution into affected ear b.i.d. for 14 days
Dosage adjustment
• Renal impairment
• Severe hepatic impairment

Contraindications

• Hypersensitivity to drug or other fluoroquinolones
• Uncorrected hypokalemia
• Pregnancy

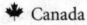 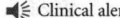

• Children under age 18 (except in postexposure inhalation or cutaneous anthrax and in ophthalmic and otic use)

Administration

• For intermittent I.V. infusion, dilute to a concentration of 4 mg/ml using normal saline solution, dextrose 5% in water (D_5W), dextrose 5% in normal saline solution, or dextrose 5% in lactated Ringer's solution. Infuse over at least 60 minutes.
• Don't give zinc- or iron-containing drugs within 2 hours of ofloxacin.

Route	Onset	Peak	Duration
P.O.	Rapid	1-2 hr	12 hr
I.V.	Rapid	End of infusion	12 hr
Ophthalmic, otic	Unknown	Unknown	Unknown

Adverse reactions

CNS: dizziness, drowsiness, headache, insomnia, acute psychoses, agitation, confusion, light-headedness, tremors, hallucinations, **increased intracranial pressure, seizures**
CV: chest pain, vasodilation
GI: nausea, diarrhea, constipation, abdominal pain, altered taste, **pseudomembranous colitis**
GU: interstitial cystitis, vaginitis
Hematologic: eosinophilia, **leukopenia**
Musculoskeletal: tendinitis, tendon rupture, joint pain, back pain
Skin: photosensitivity, phototoxicity, rash
Other: superinfection, phlebitis at I.V. site, hypersensitivity reactions including **anaphylaxis, Stevens-Johnson syndrome**

Interactions

Drug-drug. *Amiodarone, bepridil, disopyramide, erythromycin, pentamidine, phenothiazines, pimozide, procainamide, quinidine, sotalol, tricyclic antidepressants:* increased risk of serious adverse cardiovascular reactions
Antacids, bismuth subsalicylate, iron salts, sucralfate, zinc salts: decreased ofloxacin absorption
Corticosteroids: increased risk of tendon rupture
Probenecid: decreased renal elimination of ofloxacin
Theophylline: increased theophylline blood level and possible toxicity
Warfarin: increased warfarin effects
Drug-diagnostic tests. *Alanine aminotransferase, aspartate aminotransferase, platelets:* increased levels
Hemoglobin, hematocrit: decreased values
Drug-food. *Milk or yogurt (consumed alone), tube feedings:* impaired drug absorption
Drug-herb. *Fennel:* decreased drug absorption
Dong quai, St. John's wort: phototoxicity
Drug-behaviors. *Sun exposure:* phototoxicity

Precautions

Use cautiously in:
• underlying CNS disease, renal impairment, cirrhosis, bradycardia, acute myocardial ischemia
• dialysis patients
• elderly patients
• breastfeeding patients (safety not established except in postexposure inhalation or cutaneous anthrax).

Patient monitoring

• Assess patient for signs and symptoms of superinfection.
• Inspect for rash; check for signs and symptoms of hypersensitivity reaction.
• Monitor patient for fever with diarrhea; severe, persistent diarrhea; or diarrhea containing pus.
• Evaluate neurologic status closely.

Patient teaching

• Encourage patient to maintain fluid intake of at least 1,500 ml daily to prevent crystalluria.

• Inform patient being treated for gonorrhea that partners must be treated.

• Tell patient to report fever and diarrhea, especially if stool contains blood, pus, or mucus. Caution him not to treat diarrhea without consulting prescriber.

◀€ Instruct patient to immediately report rash or tendon pain or inflammation.

• Instruct patient not to take zinc- or iron-containing drugs or antacids within 2 hours of ofloxacin.

• As appropriate, review all other significant and life-threatening adverse reactions and interactions, especially those related to the drugs, tests, foods, herbs, and behaviors mentioned above.

---

olanzapine
Zyprexa, Zyprexa Zydis

Pharmacologic class: Thienobenzodiazepine
Therapeutic class: Antipsychotic
Pregnancy risk category C

Action

Unknown; thought to antagonize dopamine and serotonin type 2 in CNS. Also antagonizes muscarinic receptors in the respiratory tract, providing cholinergic activation.

Availability

Tablets: 2.5 mg, 5 mg, 7.5 mg, 10 mg, 15 mg
Tablets (orally disintegrating): 5 mg, 10 mg, 15 mg, 20 mg

🕖 Indications and dosages

➤ Long-term treatment or maintenance of schizophrenia
Adults: Initially, 5 to 10 mg P.O. daily; may increase q week by 5 mg/day (not to exceed 20 mg/day)
➤ Psychotic disorders, including acute manic episodes linked to bipolar disorder
Adults: Initially, 10 to 15 mg P.O. daily; may increase q 24 hours by 5 mg/day (not to exceed 20 mg/day)
Dosage adjustment
• Elderly patients

Off-label uses

• Borderline personality disorder

Contraindications

• Hypersensitivity to drug
• Phenylketonuria (with orally disintegrating tablets)
• Breastfeeding

Administration

• Administer without regard to meals.
• To remove orally disintegrating tablet from package, peel back foil; don't push tablet through foil.

Route	Onset	Peak	Duration
P.O.	Unknown	6 hr	Unknown

Adverse reactions

CNS: agitation, dizziness, headache, restlessness, sedation, weakness, dystonia, insomnia, mood changes, personality disorder, speech impairment, tardive dyskinesia, tremor, extrapyramidal effects, **neuroleptic malignant syndrome**
CV: orthostatic hypotension, chest pain, tachycardia
EENT: amblyopia, rhinitis, increased salivation, pharyngitis
GI: nausea, constipation, abdominal pain, dry mouth
GU: urinary incontinence, urinary tract infection
Hematologic: leukopenia

Metabolic: diabetes mellitus, goiter, increased thirst
Musculoskeletal: hypertonia, joint pain
Respiratory: cough, dyspnea
Skin: photosensitivity, ecchymosis
Other: increased appetite, weight gain or loss, fever, flulike symptoms, impaired body temperature regulation

Interactions
Drug-drug. *Antihypertensives:* additive hypotension
Carbamazepine, omeprazole, rifampin: decreased olanzapine effects
CNS depressants: additive CNS depression
Dopamine agonists, levodopa: antagonism of these drugs' effects
Drug-diagnostic tests. *Alanine aminotransferase, alkaline phosphatase, aspartate aminotransferase, bilirubin, creatinine phosphokinase, gamma-glutamyltransferase:* elevated levels
Platelets: decreased count
Drug-behaviors. *Alcohol use:* additive CNS depression
Smoking: increased drug clearance
Sun exposure: increased risk of photosensitivity

Precautions
Use cautiously in:
• hepatic impairment, cardiovascular or cerebrovascular disease, prostatic hypertrophy, narrow-angle glaucoma
• history of seizures, paralytic ileus, or attempted suicide
• elderly patients
• pregnant patients
• children under age 18 (safety not established).

Patient monitoring
• Assess mental status throughout therapy.
• Check vital signs during dosage adjustment periods.
• Watch patient to ensure that he takes drug and doesn't hoard it.

◀€ Monitor patient for signs and symptoms of neuroleptic malignant syndrome (fever, respiratory distress, tachycardia, seizures, diaphoresis, hypertension or hypotension, tiredness, severe muscle stiffness, loss of bladder control).
• Evaluate patient for onset of akathisia, tardive dyskinesia, and extrapyramidal effects.

Patient teaching
• Tell patient he may take drug without regard to meals.
• Teach patient to remove orally disintegrating tablet from package by peeling back foil, not by pushing tablet through foil. Instruct him to remove tablet from foil (using dry hands) and place entire tablet in mouth. Tell him tablet will disintegrate with or without liquid.
• Inform patient that drug may cause extrapyramidal symptoms, akathisia, and tardive dyskinesia leading to involuntary movements, tremors, rigidity, muscle contractions, and restlessness.
• Advise patient to avoid alcohol and other CNS depressants.
• Tell patient to exercise in moderation and to avoid overly hot baths and showers, because drug impairs body temperature regulation.
• Instruct patient to avoid driving and other hazardous activities until he knows how drug affects concentration and alertness.
• As appropriate, review all other significant and life-threatening adverse reactions and interactions, especially those related to the drugs, tests, and behaviors mentioned above.

O

olmesartan medoxomil
Benicar

Pharmacologic class: Angiotensin II type 1-receptor antagonist

Therapeutic class: Antihypertensive

Pregnancy risk category C (first trimester), *D* (second and third trimesters)

Action
Selectively blocks binding of angiotensin II to specific tissue receptors found in vascular smooth muscle and adrenal gland. This action blocks vasoconstrictive effects of the renin-angiotensin system as well as release of aldosterone, reducing blood pressure and possibly preventing vascular remodeling related to arteriosclerosis.

Availability
Tablets: 5 mg, 20 mg, 40 mg

Indications and dosages
➢ Hypertension

Adults: 20 mg P.O. once daily; may titrate to 40 mg daily after 2 weeks, if needed.

Dosage adjustment
• Volume depletion

Contraindications
• Hypersensitivity to drug
• Pregnancy

Administration
• Give with or without food.
• Know that drug may be used alone or with other antihypertensives.

Route	Onset	Peak	Duration
P.O.	Variable	1-2 hr	Unknown

Adverse reactions
CNS: fatigue, dizziness, headache, insomnia

CV: orthostatic hypotension, chest pain, peripheral edema, syncope, tachycardia

EENT: sinusitis, rhinitis, pharyngitis, dental pain

GI: nausea, diarrhea, constipation, abdominal pain, dry mouth

GU: hematuria

Hematologic: hyperglycemia, hypertriglyceridemia

Musculoskeletal: back pain, arthritis, muscle weakness

Respiratory: upper respiratory infection symptoms, bronchitis, cough

Skin: rash, inflammation, pruritus, alopecia, dry skin, angioedema

Other: flulike symptoms

Interactions
Drug-herb. *Ephedra:* antagonism of antihypertensive effect

Precautions
Use cautiously in:
• hypersensitivity to drug
• hepatic disease, renal dysfunction, hypovolemia, sodium depletion
• elderly patients
• pregnant or breastfeeding patients
• children.

Patient monitoring
• Monitor vital signs and cardiovascular status; stay alert for orthostatic hypotension, syncope, and peripheral edema.
• Check temperature and watch for flulike symptoms and signs and symptoms of infections, especially respiratory and EENT infections.
• Watch for angioedema.
• Monitor blood pressure carefully after initial dose in volume-depleted patients; drug may cause transient blood pressure drop.

Patient teaching
• Teach patient to take drug at same time each day, with or without food.

• Advise patient to promptly report signs and symptoms of infection, particularly respiratory symptoms.

• Caution patient that when he begins therapy, inadequate fluid intake, excessive perspiration, vomiting, or diarrhea may cause blood pressure to drop. Teach him to change position slowly to avoid dizziness and fainting.

• Instruct patient to avoid driving and other hazardous activities until he knows how drug affects concentration and alertness.

◀≋ Tell female patient to notify prescriber immediately if she suspects pregnancy.

• As appropriate, review all other significant adverse reactions and interactions, especially those related to the herb mentioned above.

olsalazine sodium
Dipentum

Pharmacologic class: Salicylate
Therapeutic class: Anti-inflammatory
Pregnancy risk category C

Action
Unknown; converts to active form, mesalamine, which blocks cyclooxygenase and inhibits prostaglandin production in colon

Availability
Capsules: 250 mg

Indications and dosages
➣ Remission of ulcerative colitis in patients who can't tolerate sulfasalazine
Adults: 500 mg P.O. b.i.d

Contraindications
• Hypersensitivity to drug or other salicylates

Administration
• Give with meals to reduce GI irritation.

Route	Onset	Peak	Duration
P.O.	Variable	60 min	Unknown

Adverse reactions
CNS: headache, fatigue, depression, vertigo
EENT: stomatitis
GI: nausea, vomiting, diarrhea, abdominal pain, cramps, dyspepsia, bloating
Musculoskeletal: joint pain
Respiratory: upper respiratory infection
Skin: rash, itching

Interactions
Drug-drug. *Anticoagulants, coumarin derivatives:* prolonged prothrombin time, increased International Normalized Ratio
Drug-food. *Any food:* decreased GI irritation

Precautions
Use cautiously in:
• hepatic or renal impairment, severe allergy, bronchial asthma
• pregnant or breastfeeding patients
• children under age 14.

Patient monitoring
• Monitor neurologic status; stay alert for depression.
• Assess GI symptoms; encourage adequate fluid intake to avoid dehydration.
• Monitor urinalysis, blood urea nitrogen, and creatinine in patients with renal impairment.

Patient teaching
• Instruct patient to take drug with food and to continue taking it even after symptoms improve.
• Teach patient to eat appropriate foods in small frequent servings to minimize GI upset.

- Advise patient to notify prescriber if symptoms worsen or don't improve after 1 to 2 months of therapy.
- Inform patient that he may require periodic proctoscopy and sigmoidoscopy to determine his response to drug.
- Caution patient to avoid driving and other hazardous activities until he knows how drug affects mood and wakefulness.
- As appropriate, review all significant adverse reactions and interactions, especially those related to the drugs and foods mentioned above.

omeprazole
Losec✸, Prilosec

Pharmacologic class: Proton pump inhibitor
Therapeutic class: Antiulcer drug
Pregnancy risk category C

Action
Reduces gastric acid secretion and increases gastric mucus and bicarbonate production, creating a protective coating on the gastric mucosa; relieves discomfort from excessive gastric acid.

Availability
Capsules (delayed-release): 10 mg, 20 mg, 40 mg

Indications and dosages
➤ Gastroesophageal reflux disease
Adults: 20 mg P.O. once daily
➤ Duodenal ulcers associated with *Helicobacter pylori*
Adults: 40 mg P.O. once daily in morning, with clarithromycin 500 mg P.O. b.i.d. for 2 weeks, then 20 mg once daily for 2 weeks; or 20 mg b.i.d. with

clarithromycin 500 mg P.O. b.i.d. and amoxicillin 1,000 mg b.i.d. for 10 days.
➤ Gastric ulcers
Adults: 40 mg once daily for 4 to 6 weeks
➤ Pathologic hypersecretory conditions, including Zollinger-Ellison syndrome
Adults: Initially, 60 mg once daily; may increase up to 120 mg t.i.d. Divide daily dosages above 80 mg.

Off-label uses
- Posterior laryngitis
- To enhance pancreatin efficacy in treating steatorrhea in cystic fibrosis patients

Contraindications
- Hypersensitivity to drug or its components

Administration
- Give dose 30 to 60 minutes before a meal, preferably in morning.
- If desired, administer concurrently with antacids.
- Know that if patient has ulcer at beginning of therapy, treatment may be extended.
- When giving through nasogastric tube, separate capsule and mix pellets with water. Agitate syringe while injecting drug. After administration, flush with 30 to 60 ml of water.
- Don't crush capsules.
- Be aware that symptomatic response to omeprazole doesn't rule out gastric cancer.

Route	Onset	Peak	Duration
P.O.	Within 1 hr	Within 2 hr	72-96 hr

Adverse reactions
CNS: dizziness, drowsiness, headache, weakness, asthenia, vertigo, insomnia, apathy, anxiety, paresthesia, abnormal dreams

GI: nausea, vomiting, diarrhea, constipation, abdominal pain, acid regurgitation, flatulence

Hepatic: increased hepatic enzyme levels

Musculoskeletal: back pain

Respiratory: cough, upper respiratory tract infection

Skin: itching, rash

Other: allergic reactions, weight gain

Interactions

Drug-drug. *Ampicillin, cyanocobalamine, digoxin, iron salts, ketoconazole:* interference with absorption of these drugs

Clarithromycin: increased omeprazole blood level

Cyclosporine, diazepam, disulfiram, flurazepam, phenytoin, triazolam, warfarin: prolonged elimination and increased effects of these drugs

Drugs metabolized by CYP450 system: competition for metabolism

Drug-diagnostic tests. *Alanine phosphatase, alkaline aminotransferase, aspartate aminotransferase, bilirubin:* increased levels

Gastrin: increased level during first 1 to 2 weeks of therapy

Precautions

Use cautiously in:
• hepatic disease
• pregnant or breastfeeding patients
• children (safety not established).

Patient monitoring

• Assess vital signs.
• Check for abdominal pain, emesis, diarrhea, or constipation.
• Evaluate fluid intake and output.
• Monitor liver function test; evaluate patient for signs and symptoms of hepatotoxicity.

Patient teaching

• Teach patient to take drug 30 to 60 minutes before a meal, preferably in morning.
• Instruct patient to swallow capsules whole and not to open them.
◀€ Teach patient to recognize and immediately report signs and symptoms of hepatotoxicity, such as flulike symptoms, dark urine, or yellowing of skin or eyes.
• Instruct patient to avoid driving and other hazardous activities until he knows how drug affects concentration and alertness.
• As appropriate, review all other significant and life-threatening adverse reactions and interactions, especially those related to the drugs and tests mentioned above.

ondansetron hydrochloride
Zofran, Zofran ODT

Pharmacologic class: Serotonin (5HT$_3$) antagonist
Therapeutic class: Antiemetic
Pregnancy risk category B

Action

Blocks serotonin at 5HT$_3$ receptor sites in vagal nerve terminals by disrupting the chemoreceptor trigger zone in CNS

Availability

Injection: 2 mg/ml in 2- and 20-ml vials
Injection (premixed): 32 mg/50 ml single-dose containers
Oral solution: 4 mg/5 ml
Tablets: 4 mg, 8 mg, 24 mg
Tablets (orally disintegrating): 4 mg, 8 mg

⚡ Indications and dosages

➤ To prevent nausea and vomiting caused by chemotherapy

Adults and children over age 12: 8 mg P.O. 30 minutes before chemotherapy, repeated 8 hours later (may give 8 mg P.O. q 12 hours for 1 to 2 days after chemotherapy); or 0.15 mg/kg I.V. over 15 minutes, starting 30 minutes before chemotherapy, repeated 4 hours and 8 hours later; or 32 mg I.V. as a single dose 30 minutes before chemotherapy.

➤ To prevent nausea and vomiting caused by radiation

Adults and children over age 12: 8 mg P.O. 1 to 2 hours before radiation; may repeat q 8 hours, depending on type, location, and extent of radiation.

➤ Prevention and treatment of post-operative nausea and vomiting

Adults and children over age 12: 16 mg P.O. 1 hour before anesthesia induction, or 4 mg I.V. or I.M. before anesthesia or postoperatively

Dosage adjustment
• Hepatic impairment
• Children younger than age 12

Contraindications

• Hypersensitivity to drug
• Phenylketonuria (with orally disintegrating tablets)

Administration

• Give first dose before emetogenic event.
• Don't remove orally disintegrating tablets by pushing them through foil backing. Instead, peel back foil with dry hands and remove tablet. Place tablet on patient's tongue, where it will dissolve in seconds. Tell patient to swallow saliva.
• Give undiluted drug by direct I.V. route immediately before anesthesia induction, or postoperatively if nausea and vomiting occur. Administer over at least 30 seconds—preferably 2 to 5 minutes.

• For intermittent I.V. infusion, dilute in 50 ml of dextrose 5% in water (D_5W) and normal saline solution or D_5W and half-normal saline solution; infuse over 15 minutes.

Route	Onset	Peak	Duration
P.O., I.V.	Rapid	15-30 min	4-8 hr
I.M.	Rapid	40 min	Unknown

Adverse reactions

CNS: headache, dizziness, malaise, drowsiness, fatigue, weakness, extrapyramidal reactions
CV: chest pain, hypotension
GI: constipation, diarrhea, abdominal pain, dry mouth
GU: urinary retention
Hepatic: increased hepatic enzyme levels
Respiratory: bronchospasm
Other: pain at injection site, shivering, **anaphylaxis**

Interactions

Drug-drug. *Drugs that alter hepatic enzyme activity:* altered pharmacokinetics of ondansetron
Drug-diagnostic tests. *Alanine aminotransferase, aspartate aminotransferase, bilirubin:* transient elevations

Precautions

Use cautiously in:
• hepatic disease
• pregnancy or breastfeeding patients
• children younger than age 12.

Patient monitoring

• Monitor GI status.
• Assess for extrapyramidal reactions.
• Check vital signs; watch for hypotension or bronchospasm.
• Monitor fluid intake and output; watch for urinary retention.

Patient teaching

• Teach patient taking orally disintegrating tablets to remove tablet by peeling back foil (with dry hands) rather than pushing tablet through foil backing. Instruct him to place tablet on tongue, where it will dissolve in seconds, and then to swallow saliva.

◀€ Advise patient to immediately report extrapyramidal symptoms.

• Instruct patient to avoid driving and other hazardous activities until he knows how drug affects concentration and alertness.

• As appropriate, review all other significant and life-threatening adverse reactions and interactions, especially those related to the drugs and tests mentioned above.

orlistat
Xenical

Pharmacologic class: GI lipase inhibitor
Therapeutic class: Weight control drug
Pregnancy risk category B

Action
Inhibits absorption of dietary fats in stomach and small intestines

Availability
Capsules: 120 mg

Indications and dosages
➤ Obesity management used in conjunction with reduced-calorie diet; to reduce risk of regain after weight loss
Adults: 120 mg P.O. t.i.d. with each meal containing fat

Contraindications
• Hypersensitivity to drug or its components
• Chronic malabsorption syndrome or cholestasis

Administration
• Know that organic causes of obesity should be ruled out before therapy begins.
• Give three times daily with meals, or up to 1 hour after a meal.
• If patient misses a meal or eats a fat-free meal, omit dose.
• Know that orlistat therapy is frequently combined with psychotherapy.

Route	Onset	Peak	Duration
P.O.	Unknown	8 hr	48-72 hr

Adverse reactions
CNS: insomnia, depression, anxiety, dizziness, headache, fatigue
EENT: ear, nose, and throat symptoms; dental pain; tooth disorder
GI: fecal urgency, flatus with discharge, oily or increased bowel movements, oily spotting, fecal incontinence
GU: urinary tract infection (UTI), vaginitis, menstrual irregularities
Musculoskeletal: back pain, arthritis, myalgia, tendinitis
Respiratory: upper or lower respiratory infection
Skin: dry skin, rash
Other: influenza

O

Interactions
Drug-drug. *Beta-carotene, fat-soluble vitamins:* reduced vitamin absorption
Cyclosporine: reduced cyclosporine blood level
Pravastatin: increased lipid-lowering effects

Precautions
Use cautiously in:
• hypothyroidism, diabetes mellitus, clinically significant GI disease, fat-soluble vitamin deficiencies
• history of bulimia or anorexia nervosa
• nephrolithiasis
• pregnant or breastfeeding patients
• children.

Patient monitoring

• Watch for signs and symptoms of UTI, respiratory infection, and ear, nose, and throat disorders.
• Monitor patient for weight loss.
• Evaluate patient's diet for appropriate caloric intake.

Patient teaching

• Instruct patient to take drug with meals as directed. Tell him he may omit a dose if he misses a meal or eats a fat-free meal.
• Teach patient to consume reduced-calorie diet and to spread daily fat intake over three main meals.
• Inform patient that drug predisposes him to ear, nose, throat, respiratory, and urinary infections; instruct him to promptly report signs and symptoms.
• Tell patient about common adverse GI effects, including problems controlling bowel movements. If significant GI upset occurs, encourage him to consult prescriber about taking psyllium at bedtime or with each dose.
• Encourage patient to ask prescriber if he should take supplemental daily multivitamin containing vitamins D, E, K, and beta-carotene at least 2 hours before or after orlistat.
• Advise patient to notify prescriber if pregnancy is planned or suspected.
• As appropriate, review all other significant adverse reactions and interactions, especially those related to the drugs mentioned above.

oseltamivir phosphate
Tamiflu

Pharmacologic class: Viral neuraminidase inhibitor
Therapeutic class: Antiviral
Pregnancy risk category C

Action

Inhibits influenza virus neuraminidase, causing alteration of viral particle aggregation and decreased viral release from infected cells

Availability

Capsules: 75 mg
Powder for oral suspension: 12 mg/ml

Indications and dosages

➤ To prevent influenza type A virus infection
Adults and children over age 13: 75 mg P.O. daily for more than 7 days, starting within 2 days of exposure
➤ Treatment of influenza type A virus infection
Adults and children over age 13: 75 mg P.O. b.i.d for 5 days, starting within 2 days of symptom onset
Dosage adjustment
• Renal impairment

Contraindications

• Hypersensitivity to drug

Administration

• For treatment, give first dose at onset of flu symptoms; for prevention, give within 2 days of exposure.

Route	Onset	Peak	Duration
P.O.	Variable	2.5	6 hr

Adverse reactions

CNS: headache, dizziness, fatigue, insomnia
GI: nausea, vomiting, diarrhea
Respiratory: cough, rhinitis, bronchitis

Interactions

None significant

Precautions

Use cautiously in:
• chronic cardiac or renal disease, respiratory disorders

- elderly patients
- pregnant or breastfeeding patients.

Patient monitoring

- Monitor respiratory status; watch for signs and symptoms of secondary infection.

Patient teaching

- Instruct patient to take drug as soon as flu symptoms occur and to complete entire course of therapy.
- Teach patient to prepare oral solution by adding water to powder and shaking well.
- Advise patient to take drug with food or milk to minimize GI irritation.
- Caution patient not to share drug with others, even if they have similar symptoms.
- Advise patient to consult prescriber before taking other drugs.
- As appropriate, review all other significant adverse reactions.

---

oxacillin sodium
Bactocil, Prostaphlin

Pharmacologic class: Penicillinase-resistant penicillin

Therapeutic class: Broad-spectrum anti-infective

Pregnancy risk category B

Action

Interferes with bacterial cell wall synthesis during multiplication of susceptible organisms; overall, exhibits minimal immunosuppressive activity

Availability

Capsules: 250 mg, 500 mg
Injection: 250 mg, 500 mg, 1 g, 2 g, 4 g
I.V. infusion: 1 g, 2 g
Oral solution: 250 mg/5 ml

⚕ Indications and dosages

➢ Systemic infections caused by penicillinase-producing staphylococci
Adults and children weighing more than 40 kg (88 lb): 500 mg to 1 g P.O. q 4 to 6 hours, or 250 mg to 1g I.M. or I.V. q 4 to 6 hours
Dosage adjustment
- Children and neonates

Contraindications

- Hypersensitivity to drug, other penicillins, cephalosporins, imipenem, or beta-lactamase inhibitors (piperacillin/tazobactam)

Administration

- Give oral forms on empty stomach 1 hour before or 2 hours after meals.
- For I.M. use, reconstitute to a dilution of 250 mg/1.5 ml sterile water; inject deep into muscle.
- For I.V. use, infuse slowly to prevent vein irritation.

Route	Onset	Peak	Duration
P.O.	Unknown	0.5-2 hr	Unknown
I.V.	Immediate	Immediate	Unknown
I.M.	Unknown	0.5 hr	Unknown

Adverse reactions

CNS: neuropathy, depression, agitation, confusion, anxiety, hallucinations, lethargy, twitching, neuromuscular irritability, **seizures, coma**
CV: thrombophlebitis
EENT: oral lesions
GI: nausea, vomiting, diarrhea, enterocolitis, abdominal pain, **pseudomembranous colitis**
GU: oliguria, proteinuria, hematuria, vaginitis, moniliasis, **glomerulonephritis**
Hematologic: anemia, increased bleeding, eosinophilia, hemolytic anemia, **bone marrow depression, granulocytopenia, thrombocytopenia, neutropenia**
Hepatic: hepatotoxicity

Other: overgrowth of nonsusceptible organisms, hypersensitivity reaction, **anaphylaxis, serum sickness**

Interactions
Drug-drug. *Aminoglycosides:* aminoglycoside inactivation
Aspirin, disulfiram, probenecid: increased oxacillin blood level, increased bone marrow depression
Hormonal contraceptives: decreased contraceptive efficacy
Rifampin, tetracyclines: decreased antimicrobial activity
Drug-diagnostic tests. *Alanine aminotransferase, alkaline phosphatase, aspartate aminotransferase, eosinophils, low-density lipoproteins:* increased levels
Granulocytes, hemoglobin, neutrophils, platelets: decreased levels
Drug-herb. *Khat:* delayed drug absorption

Precautions
Use cautiously in:
• renal disorders
• pregnant or breastfeeding patients
• neonates.

Patient monitoring
◀≀ Stay alert for severe anaphylaxis.
• Watch for signs and symptoms of infection; obtain specimen for repeat culture test if therapeutic effects don't occur.
• Monitor complete blood count with white cell differential; watch for signs and symptoms of blood dyscrasias.
• Monitor neurologic status carefully; stay alert for seizures or impending coma.
• Check bowel movements for severe persistent diarrhea (with or without fever) and pus in stool.

Patient teaching
• Advise patient to take oral form 1 hour before or 2 hours after meals on an empty stomach.

• Teach patient to complete entire course of therapy even if he feels better.
• Instruct patient to report rash, severe diarrhea, or black or furry tongue.
• Teach patient to avoid driving and other hazardous activities until he knows how drug affects concentration and alertness.
• As appropriate, review all other significant and life-threatening adverse reactions and interactions, especially those related to the drugs, tests, and herbs mentioned above.

oxaliplatin
Eloxitan

Pharmacologic class: Alkylator
Therapeutic class: Antineoplastic
Pregnancy risk category D

Action
Thought to interfere with bacterial cell wall synthesis by cross-linking strands of DNA and disrupting RNA transcription, causing bacterial cell to rupture and die. Overall, exhibits minimal immunosuppressive activity.

Availability
Powder for injection: 50 mg, 100 mg in single-use vials

🖊 Indications and dosages
➤ Metastatic cancer of colon or rectum, given in combination with 5-fluorouracil (5-FU) and leucovorin
Adults: On day one, 85 mg/m² oxaliplatin I.V. infusion and 200 mg/m² leucovorin; give both drugs simultaneously over 2 hours, followed by 400 mg/m² I.V. bolus of 5-FU over 2 to 4 minutes, and then 600 mg/m² 5-FU I.V. infusion as a 22-hour continuous infusion. On day two, 200 mg/m² leucovorin I.V. infusion over 2 hours, followed by 400 mg/m² 5-FU I.V. bolus

over 2 to 4 minutes, and then 600 mg/m² 5-FU I.V. infusion as a 22-hour continuous infusion.

Contraindications
• Hypersensitivity to drug or platinum products
• Thrombocytopenia
• Radiation therapy
• Smallpox vaccination
• Pregnancy

Administration
◀€ Follow facility policy for preparing and administering mutagenic, teratogenic, and carcinogenic drugs.
• Premedicate patient with antiemetics, as prescribed.
• Reconstitute with sterile water or D₅W, but never with normal saline solution or other solutions containing chloride.
• Further dilute reconstituted drug in 250 to 500 ml of D₅W.
• Infuse over 2 hours simultaneously with leucovorin but in a separate I.V. bag.
• Don't use administration sets or needles that contain aluminum.
◀€ Be aware of importance of using leucovorin rescue with this drug.
• Know that cycles are usually repeated every 2 weeks

Route	Onset	Peak	Duration
I.V.	Unknown	Unknown	Unknown

Adverse reactions
CNS: peripheral neuropathy, fatigue, headache, dizziness, insomnia
CV: cardiac abnormalities
EENT: decreased visual acuity, tinnitus, hearing loss, rhinitis, pharyngitis
GI: severe nausea, vomiting, diarrhea, weight loss, stomatitis, anorexia, gastroesophageal reflux, constipation, dyspepsia, mucositis, flatulence
GU: hematuria, dysuria
Hematologic: anemia, **thrombocytopenia, leukopenia, pancytopenia,**

neutropenia, hemolytic uremic syndrome
Metabolic: hypokalemia
Respiratory: dyspnea, cough, upper respiratory infection, **fibrosis**
Skin: alopecia, rash, flushing, extravasation, redness, swelling, angioedema
Other: increased sensitivity to cold, pain at injection site, **anaphylaxis**

Interactions
Drug-drug. *Aminoglycosides, loop diuretics:* increased risk of nephrotoxicity
Aspirin, nonsteroidal anti-inflammatory drugs: increased risk of bleeding
Live-virus vaccines: decreased antibody response to vaccine
Myelosuppressants: increased bone marrow depression
Drug-diagnostic tests. *Alanine aminotransferase, aspartate aminotransferase, bilirubin, creatinine:* increased levels
Hemoglobin, neutrophils, platelets, white blood cells: decreased levels
Drug-behaviors. *Alcohol use:* increased risk of bleeding

Precautions
Use cautiously in:
• recent pneumococcal vaccination
• elderly patients
• breastfeeding patients
• children.

Patient monitoring
• Monitor complete blood count, blood chemistry, and kidney and liver function tests before each treatment cycle.
◀€ Watch closely for blood dyscrasias, hemolytic uremic syndrome, and anaphylaxis.
• Conduct complete neurologic examination before and after each dose.
• Monitor vital signs and ECG; assess cardiovascular and respiratory status closely.
• Assess patient's comfort level; keep him warm during infusion to minimize neurologic effects.

• Monitor patient for signs and symptoms of toxicity (paresthesia, nausea, vomiting).

Patient teaching
• Inform patient that chemotherapy drugs can cause many adverse effects.
• Tell patient that he'll receive drug from trained healthcare professional in hospital setting.
• Instruct patient to inform nurse immediately if drug contacts his skin, eyes, or mouth.
• Advise patient to stay warm and avoid iced drinks, to minimize neurologic symptoms.
◀€ Tell patient to report itching, hives, swelling of hands or face, chest tightness, difficulty breathing, unsteadiness, severe diarrhea or vomiting, or tingling sensation in hands, arms, legs, or feet.
• As appropriate, review all other significant and life-threatening adverse reactions and interactions, especially those related to the drugs, tests, and behaviors mentioned above.

oxandrolone
Oxandrin

Pharmacologic class: Hormone
Therapeutic class: Anabolic steroid
Controlled substance schedule III
Pregnancy risk category X

Action
Promotes body tissue building process, reverses catabolic or tissue-depleting processes, and increases hemoglobin and red cell mass. Also has androgenic and anabolic properties.

Availability
Tablets: 2.5 mg

Indications and dosages
➢ Adjunctive therapy to promote weight gain; to promote weight gain after weight loss; to relieve bone pain accompanying osteoporosis
Adults: 2.5 mg P.O. two to four times daily, to a maximum of 20 mg/day, usually for 2 to 4 weeks; repeat intermittently p.r.n.
Children: Total daily dosage of less than 0.1 mg/kg P.O.

Off-label uses
• Alcoholic hepatitis

Contraindications
• Hypersensitivity to anabolic steroids
• Nephrotic phase of nephritis
• Women with breast cancer and hypercalcemia
• Men with prostate or breast cancer
• Pregnancy or breastfeeding

Administration
• Verify that patient isn't pregnant before giving.
• Administer with food or meals if GI upset occurs.

Route	Onset	Peak	Duration
P.O.	Slow	Unknown	Unknown

Adverse reactions
CNS: excitation, insomnia, toxic confusion
GI: nausea, vomiting, diarrhea, abdominal fullness, burning sensation of tongue, anorexia, **intra-abdominal hemorrhage**
GU: increased risk of prostatic hypertrophy, virilization, phallic enlargement in prepubertal boys, inhibited testicular function in postpubertal males, gynecomastia, priapism, epididymitis, changes in libido, clitoral enlargement, menstrual irregularities
Hematologic: iron deficiencies
Hepatic: hepatotoxicity, peliosis hepatitis, hepatic cell tumor

Metabolic: blood lipid changes, hypercalcemia; altered cholesterol levels; decreased glucose tolerance; fluid retention

Musculoskeletal: premature epiphyseal closure in children

Skin: acne, increased skin pigmentation, baldness

Other: chills, ankle swelling, hoarseness, hirsutism and deepening of voice in women

Interactions

Drug-drug. *Anticoagulants:* potentiation of anticoagulant action

Insulin, oral hypoglycemics: decreased requirements for these drugs

Drug-diagnostic tests. *Creatinine, creatinine clearance:* increased values

Glucose tolerance tests: altered results

Thyroid function: decreased values

Precautions

Use cautiously in:

• renal, hepatic, or cardiac impairment; benign prostatic hypertrophy; pituitary insufficiency; myocardial infarction

• pregnant or breastfeeding patients.

Patient monitoring

• Assess patient for edema and need for diuretic therapy.

• Monitor periodic liver function tests and electrolyte levels.

• Assess periodic cholesterol levels in patients with increased risk for coronary artery disease.

• Monitor diabetic patients carefully; drug may alter glucose tolerance.

Patient teaching

• Teach patient to take drug with food or meals.

• Caution patient that drug shouldn't be taken to increase muscle strength; it doesn't enhance athletic ability and can cause serious side effects.

• Advise diabetic patients to monitor urine or blood glucose carefully and report abnormal levels.

• Instruct patient to report ankle swelling, skin color changes, severe nausea or vomiting, body hair growth, acne, and menstrual changes.

• As appropriate, review all other significant and life-threatening adverse reactions and interactions, especially those related to the drugs and tests mentioned above.

oxaprozin
Daypro

Pharmacologic class: Propionic acid derivative, nonsteroidal anti-inflammatory drug (NSAID)

Therapeutic class: Anti-inflammatory, analgesic

Pregnancy risk category C (first and second trimesters), *D* (third trimester)

Action

Unclear; thought to inhibit prostaglandin synthesis by blocking cyclooxygenase (COX-2), reducing inflammation

Availability

Tablets: 600 mg

Indications and dosages

➤ Rheumatoid arthritis, osteoarthritis

Adults: 1,200 mg once daily in two to three divided doses. (Onset may be more rapid if an initial dose of 1,800 mg is given.) Maximum dosage is 1,800 mg daily.

Dosage adjustment

• Mild disease

• Renal impairment

• Low body weight

Contraindications
- Hypersensitivity to drug
- Concurrent use of other NSAIDs, including aspirin
- Active GI bleeding or ulcer disease

Administration
- Give with food or after meals if GI upset occurs.
- Use lowest effective dosage to minimize adverse reactions.

Route	Onset	Peak	Duration
P.O.	Unknown	3-5 hr	Unknown

Adverse reactions
CNS: agitation, anxiety, confusion, depression, dizziness, fatigue, headache, insomnia, malaise, paresthesia, tremor
CV: edema, vasculitis, blood pressure changes
EENT: abnormal vision, tinnitus
GI: nausea, vomiting, diarrhea, constipation, abdominal pain, dyspepsia, anorexia, duodenal ulcer, flatulence, gastritis, stomatitis, dry mouth, **GI bleeding**
GU: albuminuria, azotemia, interstitial nephritis, **acute renal failure**
Hematologic: prolonged bleeding time, anemia
Hepatic: abnormal liver function studies, cholestatic jaundice, **hepatitis**
Respiratory: dyspnea, hypersensitivity pneumonitis
Skin: diaphoresis, photosensitivity, pruritus, rash, angioedema
Other: increased appetite, weight gain, allergic reactions including **anaphylaxis, Stevens-Johnson syndrome**

Interactions
Drug-drug. *Alcohol, aspirin and other NSAIDs, corticosteroids, potassium supplements:* additive adverse GI effects and toxicity
Anticoagulants, cefamandole, cefoperazone, cefotetan, clopidogrel, eptifibatide, plicamycin, thrombolytics, ticlopidine,

tirofiban, vitamin A: increased risk of bleeding
Antineoplastics: increased risk of adverse hematologic reactions
Insulin, hypoglycemics: increased hypoglycemic effects of these drugs
Methotrexate: increased risk of methotrexate toxicity
Drug-diagnostic tests. *Alanine aminotransferase, alkaline phosphatase, aspartate aminotransferase, blood urea nitrogen, creatinine, lactate dehydrogenase, potassium:* increased levels
Bleeding time: prolonged (for up to 2 weeks after drug discontinuation)
Creatinine clearance, glucose, hemoglobin, hematocrit, platelets, white blood cells: decreased levels
Drug-herb. *Alfalfa, anise, arnica, astragalus, bilberry, black currant seed oil, bladderwrack, bogbean, boldo (with fenugreek), borage oil, buchu, capsaicin, cat's claw, celery, chamomile, chapparal, chincona bark, clove, clove oil, dandelion, dong quai, evening primrose oil, fenugreek, feverfew, garlic, ginger, ginkgo, ginseng, guggul, licorice, papaya extract, red clover, rhubarb, safflower oil, skullcap, tan-shen:* increased anticoagulant effect and bleeding risk

Precautions
Use cautiously in:
- severe cardiovascular or hepatic disease, renal impairment
- history of ulcer disease
- pregnant or breastfeeding patients
- children (safety not established).

Patient monitoring
- Monitor kidney and liver function studies, coagulation studies, and complete blood count.
- Watch for signs and symptoms of acute renal failure, nephritis, hepatitis, bleeding tendencies, and anemia.
- Monitor hearing and vision, including results of eye exams.
- Watch for and promptly report rash or swelling.

• Assess respiratory status closely; stay alert for dyspnea and pneumonitis.

Patient teaching

• Instruct patient to take drug with food or meals.
• Inform patient that many common over-the-counter drugs (including acetaminophen, aspirin, and other NSAIDs) and many herbal preparations increase drug's adverse effects. Tell him to consult prescriber before taking these products.
• Instruct patient to report weight gain, swelling in extremities, vision changes, and black or tarry stools.
• Advise patient to minimize GI upset by eating small, frequent servings of healthy food and drinking plenty of fluids.
• Instruct patient to avoid driving and other hazardous activities until he knows how drug affects concentration and alertness.
• Teach patient on long-term therapy to have periodic eye examinations.
• As appropriate, review all other significant and life-threatening adverse reactions and interactions, especially those related to the drugs, tests, and herbs mentioned above.

oxazepam
Apo-Oxazepam✤, Novoxapam✤, Serax

Pharmacologic class: Benzodiazepine
Therapeutic class: Anxiolytic, sedative-hypnotic
Controlled substance schedule IV
Pregnancy risk category D

Action
Suppresses CNS stimulation at the limbic and subcortical levels by potentiating the effects of gamma-aminobutyrate, an inhibitory neurotransmitter, thereby reducing anxiety and diminishing alcohol withdrawal symptoms

Availability
Capsules: 10 mg, 15 mg, 30 mg
Tablets: 15 mg

Indications and dosages
➤ Mild to moderate anxiety
Adults: 10 to 15 mg P.O. three to four times daily
➤ Severe anxiety, alcohol withdrawal symptoms
Adults: 15 to 30 mg P.O. three to four times daily
Dosage adjustment
• Elderly patients

Off-label uses
• Insomnia

Contraindications
• Hypersensitivity to drug or tartrazine (with some products)
• CNS depression
• Uncontrolled severe pain
• Concurrent use of other benzodiazepines
• Pregnancy or breastfeeding

Administration
• Administer with or without food.
• Taper dosage after long-term therapy.

Route	Onset	Peak	Duration
P.O.	45-90 min	3 hr	6-12 hr

Adverse reactions
CNS: dizziness, drowsiness, confusion, hangover, headache, poor memory, depression, paradoxical stimulation, slurred speech
CV: orthostatic hypotension, hypotension, ECG changes, tachycardia
EENT: blurred vision, mydriasis, tinnitus
GI: nausea, vomiting, constipation, diarrhea

O

GU: urinary retention, urinary incontinence
Hematologic: leukopenia
Hepatic: hepatitis
Respiratory: respiratory depression
Skin: rash, dermatitis, itching
Other: physical and psychological drug dependence, drug tolerance, withdrawal symptoms

Interactions

Drug-drug. *Azole antifungals:* increased oxazepam blood level, greater risk of toxicity
Hormonal contraceptives, phenytoin: decreased oxazepam efficacy
Levodopa: decreased levodopa efficacy
Other CNS depressants (including antidepressants, antihistamines, other benzodiazepines, sedative-hypnotics, opioids): additive CNS depression
Theophylline: decreased sedative effect of oxazepam
Drug-diagnostic tests. *Thyroid uptake of sodium iodide ^{123}I and ^{131}I:* decreased
Drug-food. *Cabbage:* decreased drug blood level
Drug-herb. *Chamomile, hops, kava, valerian, skullcap:* increased CNS depression
Drug-behaviors. *Alcohol use:* increased CNS depression

Precautions

Use cautiously in:
• hepatic dysfunction, severe chronic obstructive pulmonary disease, myasthenia gravis
• history of suicide attempt or drug abuse
• elderly or debilitated patients.

Patient monitoring

• Monitor liver function studies; watch for signs and symptoms of hepatitis.
• Check vital signs; stay alert for respiratory depression, orthostatic hypotension, and tachycardia.

• Monitor neurologic status; as needed, protect patient from injury.
• Watch for signs and symptoms of psychological or physical dependence; when dosage is tapered, watch for withdrawal symptoms.

Patient teaching

• Teach patient he may take drug with or without meals but should avoid cabbage.
• Instruct patient to take drug exactly as prescribed. Tell him it can cause dependence, and emphasize importance of following prescriber's tapering instructions to avoid withdrawal symptoms.
• Teach patient to change position slowly to avoid blood pressure decrease.
• Instruct patient to report severe dizziness, weakness, persistent drowsiness, palpitations, or visual changes.
• Advise patient not to drink alcohol.
• Caution patient not to drive or perform hazardous activities until he knows how drug affects vision, cognition, and balance.
• As appropriate, review all other significant and life-threatening adverse reactions and interactions, especially those related to the drugs, tests, foods, herbs, and behaviors mentioned above.

oxcarbazepine
Trileptal

Pharmacologic class: Carboxamide derivative
Therapeutic class: Anticonvulsant
Pregnancy risk category C

Action

Blocks sodium channels in neural membranes, stabilizing hyperexcitable states and inhibiting neuronal firing and transmission of impulses in the brain

♦ Canada   ◀€ Clinical alert   Reactions in **bold** are life-threatening

Availability
Oral suspension: 60 ml/ml in 250-ml bottle
Tablets: 150 mg, 300 mg, 600 mg

Indications and dosages
➤ Adjunctive therapy for partial seizures in adults; adjunctive therapy for partial seizures in children ages 4 to 16
Adults: 300 mg P.O. b.i.d.; may increase by up to 600 mg/day weekly, to a maximum of 1,200 mg daily.
Children ages 4 to 16: Initially, 8 to 10 mg/kg/day P.O. to a maximum of 600 mg daily
➤ Conversion to monotherapy for partial seizures in adults
Adults: 300 mg P.O. b.i.d.; may increase by 600 mg/day at weekly intervals over 2 to 4 weeks, to a maximum of 2,400 mg/day
➤ Initiation of monotherapy
Adults: 300 mg P.O. b.i.d.; increased by 300 mg/day P.O. q 3 days up to 1,200 mg/daily
Dosage adjustment
• Renal impairment
• Children under age 16

Contraindications
• Hypersensitivity to drug
• Breastfeeding

Administration
• Administer twice daily with or without food.
• Shake oral suspension well; if desired, mix in small glass of water.

Route	Onset	Peak	Duration
P.O.	Unknown	Unknown	Unknown

Adverse reactions
CNS: dizziness, vertigo, drowsiness, fatigue, headache, ataxia, tremor, emotional lability
EENT: abnormal vision, diplopia, nystagmus, rhinitis

GI: nausea, vomiting, diarrhea, constipation, abdominal pain, dyspepsia
Metabolic: hyponatremia
Skin: acne, rash
Other: thirst, allergic reactions, edema, lymphadenopathy

Interactions
Drug-drug. *Carbamazepine, valproic acid, verapamil:* decreased oxcarbazepine blood level
CNS depressants (including antidepressants, antihistamines, opioids, sedative-hypnotics): additive CNS depression
Felodipine, hormonal contraceptives: decreased blood levels of these drugs
Phenobarbital: decreased oxcarbazepine and increased phenobarbital blood levels
Phenytoin: increased phenytoin blood level
Drug-diagnostic tests. *Sodium:* decreased level (usually during first 3 months of therapy)
Drug-behaviors. *Alcohol use:* additive CNS depression

Precautions
Use cautiously in:
• renal impairment
• pregnant patients
• children under age 4 (safety not established).

Patient monitoring
• Monitor neurologic status closely for changes in cognition, mood, wakefulness, balance, and gait.
• Check sodium level; watch for signs and symptoms of hyponatremia.

Patient teaching
• Instruct patient to take drug at same time each day and to take it with or without food.
• Inform women that drug makes hormonal contraceptives less effective.

- Teach patient to report vision changes and significant neurologic changes.
- Advise patient to have periodic eye examinations.
- Teach patient not to drink alcohol.
- Tell patient he may need frequent blood tests to check drug blood levels.
- Teach patient to avoid driving and other hazardous activities until he knows how drug affects him.
- As appropriate, review all significant adverse reactions and interactions, especially those related to the drugs, tests, and behaviors mentioned above.

oxybutynin
Oxytrol

oxybutynin chloride
Ditropan, Ditropan XL

Pharmacologic class: Anticholinergic
Therapeutic class: Urinary tract antispasmodic
Pregnancy risk category B

Action
Inhibits acetylcholine action at postganglionic receptors, relaxing smooth muscle lining of the gentourinary tract, thereby preventing bladder irritability

Availability
Syrup: 5 mg/5 ml
Tablets: 5 mg
Tablets (extended-release): 5 mg, 10 mg, 15 mg
Transdermal system (patch): 39 cm^2/ 36 mg

⧸ Indications and dosages
➤ Frequent urination, urinary urgency or incontinence, and nocturia secondary to neurogenic bladder; overactive bladder

Adults: 5 mg P.O. two to three times daily (not to exceed 5 mg q.i.d.); or 5 to 15 mg P.O. once daily (extended-release); or one 3.9 mg/day transdermal system applied twice weekly (q 3 to 4 days)
Dosage adjustment
- Elderly patients
- Children

Contraindications
- Hypersensitivity to drug
- Glaucoma
- Intestinal obstruction, atony, or hemorrhage
- Severe colitis
- Myasthenia gravis
- Acute hemorrhage with shock

Administration
- Give without regard to food.
- Don't crush or break tablets.

Route	Onset	Peak	Duration
P.O.	30-60 min	3-6 hr	6-10 hr
P.O. (extended)	30-60 min	3-6 hr	Up to 24 hr
Transdermal	24-48 hr	48-96 hr	96 hr after removal

Adverse reactions
CNS: dizziness, drowsiness, hallucinations, insomnia, weakness, anxiety, restlessness, headache
CV: palpitations, hypotension, tachycardia
EENT: blurred vision, cycloplegia, increased intraocular pressure, mydriasis, photophobia
GI: nausea, vomiting, diarrhea, constipation, bloating, dry mouth
GU: urinary hesitancy, urinary retention, impotence
Metabolic: hyperthermia, suppressed lactation
Skin: decreased sweating, urticaria
Other: allergic reactions, fever, hot flashes

Interactions
Drug-drug. *Anticholinergics and anticholinergic-like drugs (including amantadine, antidepressants, disopyramide, haloperidol, phenothiazines):* additive anticholinergic effects
Atenolol: increased atenolol absorption
CNS depressants (including antidepressants, antihistamines, opioids, sedative-hypnotics): additive CNS depression
Digoxin: increased digoxin blood level (with extended-release oxybutynin)
Haloperidol: decreased haloperidol blood level, tardive dyskinesia, worsening of schizophrenia
Levodopa: decreased levodopa efficacy
Nitrofurantoin: increased nitrofurantoin blood level, greater risk of toxicity
Drug-herb. *Angel's trumpet, jimsonweed, scopolia:* increased anticholinergic effects
Drug-behaviors. *Alcohol use:* additive CNS depression

Precautions
Use cautiously in:
• cardiovascular disease, hyperthyroidism, GI disease
• elderly patients
• pregnant or breastfeeding patients
• children under age 5 (safety not established).

Patient monitoring
• Monitor vital signs and temperature; watch for hypotension, fever, and tachycardia.
• Evaluate patient's vision.
• Assess results of cystometric studies; stay alert for urinary retention.

Patient teaching
• Teach patient he may take drug with or without food; remind him not to crush, break, or chew extended-release tablets.
• Tell patient to apply transdermal patch to dry, intact skin on abdomen, hip, or buttock. Teach him to choose a new skin area with each new system

and not to reapply new patch to same site within 7 days. Instruct him not to cut or puncture patch.
• Teach patient to report blurred vision, fever, skin rash, nausea, or vomiting.
• Advise patient he'll need to undergo periodic bladder exams.
• Caution patient to avoid driving and other hazardous activities if drug causes drowsiness or blurred vision.
• As appropriate, review all other significant and life-threatening adverse reactions and interactions, especially those related to the drugs, herbs, and behaviors mentioned above.

oxycodone hydrochloride
Endocodone, OxyContin, OxyIR, Roxicodone, Roxicodone Intensol, Supeudol✚

Pharmacologic class: Opioid agonist
Therapeutic class: Narcotic analgesic
Controlled substance schedule II
Pregnancy risk category B

Action
Unknown; interacts with opiate receptor sites primarily in the limbic system, thalamus, and spinal cord of the CNS, blocking neurotransmission of pain impulses

Availability
Capsules (immediate-release): 5 mg
Solution (oral): 5 mg/5 ml
Solution (oral concentrate): 20 mg/ml
Tablets: 5 mg
Tablets (controlled-release): 10 mg, 20 mg, 40 mg, 80 mg, 160 mg
Tablets (immediate-release): 15 mg, 30 mg

🖊 Indications and dosages
➤ Moderate to severe pain
Adults: 5 mg P.O. q 6 hours p.r.n., in-

creased gradually to 10 to 30 mg q 6 hours p.r.n.

➤ Moderate or severe pain when continuous around-the-clock analgesia is needed

Adults: 10 mg P.O. (controlled-release) q 12 hours. For patients already taking opioids, use total oral oxycodone daily equianalgesic dose and then round down to closest tablet strength. For breakthrough pain, give supplemental immediate-release doses.

Dosage adjustment
• Hepatic disease
• Renal impairment
• Debilitated or opioid-naive patients

Off-label uses
• Postherpetic neuralgia (controlled-release form)

Contraindications
• Hypersensitivity to drug
• Paralytic ileus
• When opioids are contraindicated (as in respiratory depression, severe bronchial asthma, hypercarbia)
• Labor and delivery
• Breastfeeding
• Children younger than age 18

Administration
• Be aware that drug has high abuse potential.
• Know that controlled-release Oxy-Contin isn't indicated for p.r.n. pain control but is reserved for patients who need continuous, around-the-clock analgesia.
• Be aware that 80-mg and 160-mg controlled-release tablets are for opioid-tolerant patients only.
◀︎ Never break, crush, or let patient chew controlled-release forms; otherwise, controlled delivery mechanism is eliminated, causing rapid release and absorption of potentially fatal dose.
• Add concentrated solution to juice, applesauce, pudding, or other semisolid food immediately before giving.

• When discontinuing drug, taper dosage gradually to prevent withdrawal symptoms.

Route	Onset	Peak	Duration
P.O.	15-30 min	1 hr	4-6 hr
P.O. (controlled)	Unknown	24-36 hr	>12 hr

Adverse reactions
CNS: dizziness, asthenia, drowsiness, euphoria, light-headedness, insomnia, confusion, anxiety, twitching, abnormal dreams and thoughts
CV: orthostatic hypotension, **circulatory depression, bradycardia, shock**
GI: nausea, vomiting, constipation, diarrhea, ileus, abdominal pain, dyspepsia, gastritis, anorexia
GU: urinary retention
Respiratory: apnea, respiratory depression, respiratory arrest
Skin: pruritus, sweating
Other: chills, fever, hiccups, physical and psychological drug dependence

Interactions
Drug-drug. *Antihistamines, sedative-hypnotics:* additive CNS depression
Barbiturates, protease inhibitors: increased respiratory and CNS depression
Opioid agonist-antagonists: precipitation of opioid withdrawal in physically dependent patients
Drug-diagnostic tests. *Amylase, lipase:* increased levels
Drug-behaviors. *Alcohol use:* additive CNS depression

Precautions
Use cautiously in:
• head trauma; increased intracranial pressure; severe renal, hepatic, or pulmonary disease; hypothyroidism; adrenal insufficiency; urethral stricture; undiagnosed abdominal pain or prostatic hyperplasia; extensive burns; alcoholism
• history of substance abuse

- prolonged or high-dose therapy
- elderly or debilitated patients
- pregnant patients.

Patient monitoring

◀≋ Monitor vital signs and respiratory status; withhold drug if patient has significant respiratory or CNS depression.
- Assess patient's pain level frequently.
- Monitor bowel and bladder function.
- Assess patient for anxiety, twitching, and other CNS symptoms.
- Closely monitor head-trauma patients; drug may increase intracranial pressure while masking signs and symptoms.
- Carefully assess patients with acute abdominal pain; drug may obscure diagnosis.
- Stay alert for drug hoarding, dependence, and tolerance.

Patient teaching

◀≋ Caution patient not to break, crush, chew, or dissolve controlled-release tablets; warn him that rapid drug release and absorption may be fatal.
- Teach patient taking controlled-release form not to drive for 3 to 4 days after dosage increase, after consuming even a single alcoholic beverage, or if also taking antihistamines or other drugs that cause drowsiness.

◀≋ Instruct patient to promptly report adverse reactions, especially difficulty breathing or slow pulse.
- Advise patient not to drink alcohol.
- Teach patient to notify prescriber if she's pregnant or breastfeeding.
- Tell patient not to be alarmed if tablets appear in stools; drug has already been absorbed.
- Advise ambulatory patients to change position slowly to avoid dizziness from orthostatic hypotension.
- Instruct patient to consult prescriber before taking other drugs.

- Teach patient to avoid driving and other hazardous activities because drug may cause drowsiness or dizziness.
- As appropriate, review all other significant and life-threatening adverse reactions and interactions, especially those related to the drugs, tests, and behaviors mentioned above.

oxymorphone hydrochloride
Numorphan

Pharmacologic class: Opioid agonist
Therapeutic class: Narcotic analgesic
Controlled substance schedule II
Pregnancy risk category C

Action

Unknown; interacts with opiate receptor sites primarily in the limbic system, thalamus, and spinal cord of the CNS, blocking neurotransmission of pain impulses

Availability

Injection: 1 mg/ml, 1.5 mg/ml
Suppositories: 5 mg

⟋ Indications and dosages

➤ Moderate to severe pain
Adults: 1 to 1.5 mg I.M. or S.C. q 4 to 6 hours p.r.n.; or initially, 0.5 mg I.V., increased cautiously until pain relief is satisfactory; or 5 mg P.R. q 4 to 6 hours p.r.n., increased cautiously until pain relief is satisfactory
➤ To reduce labor pain
Adults: 0.5 to 1 mg I.M.

Contraindications

- Hypersensitivity to drug
- Respiratory disease
- Labor and delivery
- Breastfeeding
- Children younger than age 18

Administration

◀€ Keep naloxone available to reverse respiratory depression, if necessary.

• Give I.V. dose by direct injection over 2 to 3 minutes.

Route	Onset	Peak	Duration
I.V.	5-10 min	30-60 min	3-6 hr
I.M., S.C.	10-15 min	30-60 min	3-6 hr
P.R.	15-30 min	1-2 hr	3-6 hr

Adverse reactions

CNS: headache, drowsiness, confusion, dysphoria, euphoria, dizziness, hallucinations, lethargy, impaired mental and physical performance, depression, restlessness, insomnia, paradoxical stimulation, **seizures**

CV: hypotension, orthostatic hypotension, palpitations, **bradycardia, tachycardia**

EENT: blurred vision, miosis, diplopia, visual disturbances, tinnitus

GI: nausea, vomiting, constipation, biliary tract spasm, cramps, dry mouth, anorexia, **paralytic ileus, toxic megacolon**

GU: urethral spasm, urinary hesitancy or retention, antidiuretic effect

Respiratory: suppression of cough reflex, atelectasis, **respiratory depression, allergic bronchospastic reaction, allergic laryngeal edema or laryngospasm, apnea**

Skin: rash, urticaria, pruritus, facial flushing, diaphoresis

Other: physical or psychological drug dependence, drug tolerance, allergic reaction, injection site reaction

Interactions

Drug-drug. *Antihistamines (first-generation), antipsychotics, barbiturates, general anesthetics, monoamine oxidase inhibitors, sedative-hypnotics, skeletal muscle relaxants, tricyclic antidepressants:* increased risk of respiratory depression

Drug-diagnostic tests. *Amylase, lipase:* increased levels

Drug-behaviors. *Alcohol use or abuse, opiate abuse:* increased risk of respiratory depression

Precautions

Use cautiously in:

• head trauma; increased intracranial pressure; severe renal, hepatic, or pulmonary disease; hypothyroidism; adrenal insufficiency; urethral stricture; undiagnosed abdominal pain or prostatic hyperplasia; extensive burns; alcoholism

• history of substance abuse

• prolonged or high-dose therapy

• elderly or debilitated patients

• pregnant patients.

Patient monitoring

◀€ Closely monitor respiratory status; stay alert for respiratory depression and allergic responses affecting the bronchi and larynx.

• Monitor vital signs and ECG.

• With prolonged use, watch for signs and symptoms of drug dependence.

• Assess neurologic status carefully; institute protective measures as needed.

Patient teaching

◀€ Instruct patient to immediately report seizures or difficulty breathing.

• Caution patient to rise slowly when changing position to avoid dizziness from blood pressure decrease.

• Advise patient to avoid alcohol; caution him not to drive or perform other hazardous activities.

• Caution patient not to stop taking drug suddenly after several weeks because withdrawal symptoms may occur.

• As appropriate, review all other significant and life-threatening adverse reactions and interactions, especially those related to the drugs, tests, and behaviors mentioned above.

oxytocin
Pitocin, Syntocinon

Pharmacologic class: Posterior
pituitary hormone
Therapeutic class: Uterine-active agent
Pregnancy risk category NR

Action
Unknown; thought to directly stimulate smooth muscle contractions in the uterus and cervix

Availability
Injection: 10 units/ml ampule or vial

Indications and dosages
➤ To induce or stimulate labor
Adults: Initially, 1-ml ampule (10 units) in compatible I.V. solution infused at 1 to 2 milliunits/minute (0.001 to 0.002 units/minute). Increase rate in increments of 1 to 2 milliunits/minute q 15 to 30 minutes until an acceptable contraction pattern is established.
➤ To control postpartum bleeding
Adults: 10 to 40 units in compatible I.V. solution infused at an adequate rate needed to control bleeding; or 10 units I.M. after placenta delivery
➤ Incomplete abortion
Adults: 10 units in compatible I.V. solution infused at 10 to 20 milliunits/ minute (0.01 to 0.02 units/minute)

Off-label uses
• Antepartal fetal heart rate testing
• Breast enlargement

Contraindications
• Hypersensitivity to drug
• Cephalopelvic disproportion
• Fetal distress when delivery is not imminent
• Prolonged use in uterine inertia or severe toxemia

• Hypertonic or hyperactive uterine pattern
• Unfavorable fetal position or presentation that's undeliverable without conversion
• Labor induction or augmentation when vaginal delivery is contraindicated (as in invasive cervical cancer, active genital herpes, or total placenta previa)
• Children

Administration
• Reconstitute by adding 1 ml (10 units) to 1,000 ml of normal saline solution, lactated Ringer's solution, or dextrose 5% in water.
◀€ Don't give by I.V. bolus injection.
• Infuse I.V. using controlled-infusion device.
• Be aware that drug isn't routinely given I.M.
• Know that drug should be used only with inpatients at critical care facility and when prescriber is immediately available.

Route	Onset	Peak	Duration
I.V.	Immediate	40 min	1 hr
I.M.	3-5 min	40 min	2-3 hr

Adverse reactions
CNS: seizures or coma from water intoxication, neonatal brain damage, subarachnoid hemorrhage
CV: premature ventricular contractions, **arrhythmias, neonatal bradycardia**
GI: nausea, vomiting
GU: postpartal hemorrhage; pelvic hematoma; uterine hypertonicity, spasm, or tetanic contraction; abruptio placentae; uterine rupture (with excessive doses)
Hematologic: afibrinogenemia
Hepatic: neonatal jaundice
Other: hypersensitivity reactions including **anaphylaxis, low 5-minute Apgar score (neonate)**

♣ Canada   ◀€ Clinical alert   Reactions in **bold** are life-threatening

Interactions
Drug-drug. *Sympathomimetics:* postpartum hypertension
Thiopental anesthetics: delayed anesthesia induction
Vasoconstrictors: severe hypertension (when given within 3 to 4 hours of oxytocin)
Drug-herb. *Ephedra:* increased hypertension

Precautions
Use cautiously in:
• previous cervical or uterine surgery, history of uterine sepsis
• breastfeeding patients.

Patient monitoring
◀▓ Continuously monitor contractions, fetal and maternal heart rate, and maternal blood pressure and ECG; discontinue infusion if uterine hyperactivity occurs.
◀▓ Monitor patient extremely carefully during first and second stages of labor because of risk of cervical laceration, uterine rupture, and maternal and fetal death.
• When giving drug to control postpartum bleeding, monitor and record vaginal bleeding.
• Assess fluid intake and output; watch for signs and symptoms of water intoxication.

Patient teaching
• Inform patient about risks and benefits of oxytocin-induced labor.
• Teach patient to recognize and immediately report adverse drug effects.

paclitaxel
Onxol, Taxol

Pharmacologic class: Antimicrotubule
Therapeutic class: Antineoplastic
Pregnancy risk category D

Action
Stabilizes cellular microtubules to prevent depolymerization; this action inhibits microtubule network (essential for vital interphase and mitotic cellular functions) and induces abnormal microtubule arrays or bundles throughout cell cycle and during mitosis

Availability
Concentrate for injection: 30 mg/5-ml vial, 100 mg/16.7-ml vial, 300 mg/50-ml vial

🖊 Indications and dosages
➤ Advanced ovarian cancer
Adults: As first-line therapy, 175 mg/m^2 I.V. over 3 hours q 3 weeks, or 135 mg/m^2 I.V. over 24 hours q 3 weeks, followed by cisplatin. After failure of first-line therapy, 135 mg/m^2 I.V. or 175 mg/m^2 I.V. over 3 hours q 3 weeks.
➤ Breast cancer after failure of combination chemotherapy
Adults: As adjuvant treatment for node-positive breast cancer, 175 mg/m^2 I.V. over 3 hours q 3 weeks for four courses sequentially with doxorubicin combination chemotherapy. After chemotherapy failure for metastatic disease or relapse within 6 months of adjuvant therapy, 175 mg/m^2 I.V. over 3 hours q 3 weeks.
➤ Non-small-cell lung cancer
Adults: 135 mg/m^2 I.V. over 24 hours q 3 weeks, followed by cisplatin

> AIDS-related Kaposi's sarcoma
Adults: 135 mg/m² I.V. over 3 hours q 3 weeks, or 100 mg/m² I.V. over 3 hours q 2 weeks
Dosage adjustment
• Advanced HIV infection (when used for Kaposi's sarcoma)

Off-label uses
• Advanced head and neck cancer
• Small-cell lung cancer
• Upper GI tract adenocarcinoma
• Non-Hodgkin's lymphoma
• Pancreatic cancer
• Polycystic kidney disease

Contraindications
• Hypersensitivity to drug or castor oil
• Solid tumors in patients with baseline neutrophil counts below 1,500 cells/mm³
• AIDS-related Kaposi's sarcoma in patients with baseline neutrophil counts below 1,000 cells/mm³

Administration
◀≶ Follow facility protocol for handling chemotherapeutic drugs and preparing solutions.
• Dilute in dextrose 5% in water, normal saline solution, or dextrose 5% in lactated Ringer's solution, according to manufacturer's guidelines.
• Inspect solution for particles; administer through polyethylene-lined administration set attached to 0.22 micron in-line filter.
• To prevent severe hypersensitivity reaction, premedicate with dexamethasone 20 mg, as prescribed, 12 and 6 hours before infusion; also give diphenhydramine 50 mg I.V., plus either cimetidine 300 mg or ranitidine 50 mg I.V. 30 to 60 minutes before paclitaxel dose.
◀≶ Keep epinephrine available. If severe hypersensitivity reaction occurs, stop infusion immediately and administer epinephrine, I.V. fluids, and additional antihistamine and corticosteroid doses, as indicated and prescribed.

Route	Onset	Peak	Duration
I.V.	Unknown	Unknown	Unknown

Adverse reactions
CNS: abnormal ECG, peripheral neuropathy
CV: hypotension, syncope, hypertension, bradycardia, **venous thrombosis**
GI: nausea, vomiting, diarrhea, stomatitis, mucositis
Hematologic: anemia, bleeding, **leukopenia, neutropenia, thrombocytopenia**
Hepatic: abnormal liver function studies
Musculoskeletal: joint pain, myalgia
Skin: alopecia, radiation reactions
Other: infection, injection site reaction, hypersensitivity reactions including **anaphylaxis**

Interactions
Drug-drug. *Carbamazepine, phenobarbital:* decreased paclitaxel blood level and efficacy
Cisplatin: increased bone marrow depression (when paclitaxel dose follows cisplatin dose)
Cyclosporine, diazepam, doxorubicin, felodipine, ketoconazole, midazolam: inhibited paclitaxel metabolism and greater risk of toxicity
Doxorubicin: increased doxorubicin blood level and toxicity
Live-virus vaccines: decreased antibody response to vaccine, increased risk of adverse reactions
Other antineoplastics: increased risk of bone marrow depression
Drug-diagnostic tests. *Triglycerides:* increased levels

Precautions
Use cautiously in:
• severe hepatic impairment, active infection, decreased bone marrow reserve, chronic debilitating illnesses

P

• patients with childbearing potential
• children (safety not established).

Patient monitoring
◀€ Watch closely for hypersensitivity reaction.
• Monitor heart rate and blood pressure.
• Assess infusion site for local effects and extravasation, especially during prolonged infusions.
• Monitor complete blood count, including platelet count. If neutropenia develops, monitor patient for infection; if thrombocytopenia develops, watch for signs and symptoms of bleeding.
• If patient has preexisting conduction abnormality, maintain continuous cardiac monitoring.

Patient teaching
• Instruct neutropenic patient to minimize infection risk by avoiding crowds, plants, and fresh fruits and vegetables.
• Teach thrombocytopenic patient to avoid activities that can cause injury; advise him to use soft toothbrush and electric razor.
• Advise patient to promptly report signs and symptoms of infection, bleeding, or peripheral neuropathy (such as numbness and tingling of feet and hands).
• Tell patient to promptly report pain or burning at injection site.
• Explain that temporary hair loss is likely to occur.
• As appropriate, review all other significant and life-threatening adverse reactions and interactions, especially those related to the drugs and tests mentioned above.

palivizumab
Synagis

Pharmacologic class: Monoclonal antibody
Therapeutic class: Immunologic agent
Pregnancy risk category C

Action
Neutralizes and suppresses activity of syncytial virus in respiratory tract, inhibiting respiratory syncytial virus (RSV) replication

Availability
Injection: 50 mg, 100-mg vial

Indications and dosages
➤ Prevention of serious lower respiratory tract disease caused by RSV in high-risk children
Children: 15 mg/kg I.M. q month throughout RSV season

Contraindications
• Hypersensitivity to drug or its components
• Adults

Administration
◀€ Keep epinephrine 1:1,000 available in case anaphylaxis occurs. (However, drug isn't known to cause anaphylaxis.)
• Dilute in sterile water for injection; gently swirl for 30 seconds to avoid foaming.
• Keep reconstituted solution at room temperature for at least 20 minutes before administering. Give within 6 hours of reconstitution.
• Inject I.M. into anterolateral thigh. Avoid gluteal injection, which may damage sciatic nerve.

Route	Onset	Peak	Duration
I.M.	Unknown	Unknown	Unknown

Adverse reactions

CNS: nervousness, pain

EENT: otitis media, rhinitis, pharyngitis, sinusitis, conjunctivitis, oral monilia

GI: vomiting, diarrhea, gastroenteritis

Hematologic: anemia

Hepatic: increased alanine aminotransferase (ALT) and aspartate aminotransferase (AST) levels

Respiratory: upper respiratory tract infection, cough, wheezing, bronchiolitis, bronchitis, pneumonia, asthma, croup, dyspnea, **apnea**

Skin: rash, fungal dermatitis, eczema

Other: failure to thrive, hernia, pain, fever, injection site reaction, viral infection, flulike symptoms

Interactions

Drug-diagnostic tests. *ALT, AST:* increased levels

Hemoglobin: decreased level

Precautions

Use cautiously in:
• thrombocytopenia, coagulation disorders, established RSV.

Patient monitoring

◀€ Watch closely for signs and symptoms of anaphylaxis immediately after administration.
• Assess for signs and symptoms of infection, particularly EENT and respiratory infection.
• Monitor liver function studies and complete blood count.
• Assess patient's weight and hydration status.

Patient teaching

• Teach parent that monthly injections are necessary during RSV season (November through April).
• Inform parent that drug may cause GI symptoms and failure to thrive; provide dietary counsultation as needed.
• Caution parent that EENT and respiratory infections may occur after administration; advise parent to contact prescriber immediately if child has fever or other signs or symptoms of infection.
• As appropriate, review all other significant and life-threatening adverse reactions and interactions, especially those related to the tests mentioned above.

palonosetron hydrochloride
Aloxi

Pharmacologic class: Selective serotonin subtype 3 (5-HT$_3$) receptor antagonist

Therapeutic class: Antiemetic

Pregnancy risk category B

Action

Selectively binds to and antagonizes 5-HT$_3$ receptor

Availability

Solution: 0.25 mg (free base) in 5-ml vial

⟋ Indications and dosages

➤ To prevent nausea and vomiting associated with emetogenic cancer chemotherapy

Adults: 0.25 mg I.V. as a single dose 30 minutes before chemotherapy begins; repeated doses within 7 days are not recommended.

Contraindications

• Hypersensitivity to drug or its components

Administration

• Flush I.V. line with normal saline solution before and after giving drug.
• Give 30 minutes before start of chemotherapy.

• Administer directly into I.V. line over 30 seconds; don't mix with other drugs.

Route	Onset	Peak	Duration
I.V.	Unknown	Unknown	Unknown

Adverse reactions
CNS: headache, fatigue, insomnia, dizziness, anxiety
CV: hypotension, vein discoloration and distention, nonsustained tachycardia, bradycardia
GI: constipation, diarrhea, abdominal pain, anorexia
GU: glycosuria
Hepatic: transient asymptomatic increases in alanine aminotransferase (ALT), aspartate aminotransferase (AST), and bilirubin levels
Metabolic: hyperkalemia, fluctuating electrolyte levels, hyperglycemia, metabolic acidosis
Musculoskeletal: joint pain
Other: fever, flulike symptoms

Interactions
Drug-diagnostic tests: *ALT, AST, bilirubin, blood and urine glucose, potassium:* increased levels

Precautions
Use cautiously in:
• hypersensitivity to other $5HT_3$ receptor antagonists
• diabetes mellitus, hepatic dysfunction
• pregnant or breastfeeding patients
• children.

Patient monitoring
• Assess vital signs and ECG; watch closely for tachycardia, bradycardia, and hypotension.
• Monitor electrolyte levels for fluctuations (especially hyperkalemia and metabolic acidosis).
• Evaluate temperature; watch for flulike symptoms.

• Closely monitor blood and urine glucose levels in diabetic patients; stay alert for hyperglycemia.

Patient teaching
• Describe drug's antiemetic effect; reassure patient that prevention of nausea and vomiting counterbalance drug's transient adverse reactions.
• Teach patient to recognize and promptly report signs and symptoms of hyperkalemia and metabolic acidosis.
• Advise patient to report flulike symptoms.
• Instruct diabetic patients to closely watch blood and urine glucose levels.
• As appropriate, review all other significant and life-threatening adverse reactions and interactions, especially those related to the tests mentioned above.

pamidronate disodium
Aredia

Pharmacologic class: Bisphosphonate, hypocalcemic

Therapeutic class: Bone resorption inhibitor

Pregnancy risk category C

Action
Inhibits normal and abnormal bone resorption and decreases calcium levels

Availability
Injection: 30 mg/vial, 90 mg/vial

⚠ Indications and dosages
➢ Hypercalcemia associated with cancer
Adults: For moderate hypercalcemia, 60 to 90 mg as a single-dose I.V. infusion over 4 to 24 hours. For severe hypercalcemia, 90 mg as a single-dose I.V. infusion over 2 to 24 hours.

➤ Osteolytic lesions caused by multiple myeloma
Adults: 90 mg I.V. every month infused over 4 hours
➤ Osteolytic bone metastases of breast cancer
Adults: 90 mg I.V. as a 2-hour infusion q 3 to 4 weeks
➤ Paget's disease
Adults: 30 mg I.V. daily as a 4-hour infusion for 3 days

Contraindications
• Hypersensitivity to drug, its components, or other bisphosphonates

Administration
• Hydrate patient, as needed, with saline solution before starting therapy.
• Because of risk of renal failure, don't give single doses exceeding 90 mg.
◀ℰ Reconstitute vial using 10 ml of sterile water for injection. When completely dissolved, further dilute in 250 to 1,000 ml of half-normal or normal saline solution or dextrose 5% in water.
◀ℰ Don't mix with solutions containing calcium, such as lactated Ringer's solution.
• Administer in separate I.V. line from all other drugs and fluids.

Route	Onset	Peak	Duration
I.V.	Unknown	Unknown	Unknown

Adverse reactions
CNS: anxiety, headache, insomnia, psychosis, drowsiness, weakness
CV: hypertension, syncope, atrial flutter, tachycardia, **arrhythmias, heart failure**
EENT: stomatitis, sinusitis
GI: nausea, vomiting, diarrhea, abdominal pain, constipation, dyspepsia, anorexia, **GI hemorrhage**
GU: urinary tract infection
Hematologic: anemia, **neutropenia, leukopenia, granulocytopenia, thrombocytopenia**

Metabolic: hypothyroidism, reduced electrolyte levels, elevated creatinine level
Musculoskeletal: bone pain, joint pain, myalgia
Respiratory: crackles, coughing, dyspnea, pleural effusion, upper respiratory infection
Other: fever, generalized pain, injection site reaction

Interactions
Drug-diagnostic tests. *Calcium, hemoglobin, magnesium, phosphorus, platelets, potassium, red blood cells, white blood cells:* decreased levels
Creatinine: increased level

Precautions
Use cautiously in:
• renal impairment
• pregnant or breastfeeding patients
• children (safety not established).

Patient monitoring
• Monitor hydration status carefully.
• Assess vital signs and ECG; evaluate cardiovascular and respiratory status closely.
• Monitor hematologic studies and creatinine level before each treatment.
• Assess electrolyte levels, especially calcium, magnesium, and phosphorus.
• Closely monitor fluid intake and output; watch for signs and symptoms of urinary tract infection.

Patient teaching
• Instruct patient to weigh himself regularly and report sudden gain.
• Advise patient to promptly report significant respiratory problems, peripheral edema, or GI bleeding.
• Inform patient that drug lowers resistance to some infections; advise him to immediately report fever and other signs and symptoms of infection.
• Explain importance of laboratory tests before, during, and after therapy.

p

• Caution patient to avoid driving and other hazardous activities until he knows how drug affects concentration, cognition, and alertness.

• Teach patient to minimize GI upset by eating small, frequent servings of healthy food and drinking plenty of fluids.

• As appropriate, review all other significant and life-threatening adverse reactions and interactions, especially those related to the tests mentioned above.

pancreatin
Donnazyme, Hi-Vegi-Lip,
4X Pancreatin, 8X Pancreatin,
Pancrezyme 4X

pancrelipase
Cotazym, Cotazym-65B✢, Cotazym
ECS 8, Cotazym ECS 20, Cotazym-S,
Creon 5, Creon 10, Creon 20,
Ilozyme, Ku-Zyme HP, Lipram-CR20,
Lipram-PN 10, Lipram-PN 16,
Lipram-UL 12, Pancrease Capsules,
Pancrease MT4, Pancrease MT10,
Pancrease MT16, Pancrease MT20,
Protilase, Ultrase MT12, Ultrase
MT18, Ultrase MT20, Viokase,
Zymase

Pharmacologic class: Pancreatic enzyme
Therapeutic class: Digestant
Pregnancy risk category C

Action
Promotes fat absorption by increasing digestion in the duodenum

Availability
Cotazym
Capsules: 8,000 units lipase, 30,000
units protease, 30,000 units amylase, 25 mg calcium carbonate
Cotazym-S
Capsules (enteric-coated): 5,000 units lipase, 20,000 units protease, 20,000 units amylase
Creon 5
Capsules (delayed-release): 5,000 units lipase, 18,750 units protease, 16,600 units amylase
Creon 10
Capsules (delayed-release): 20,000 units lipase, 75,000 units protease, 33,200 units amylase
Creon 20, Lipram-CR20
Capsules (delayed-release): 20,000 units lipase, 75,000 units protease, 66,400 units amylase
Donnazyme
Tablets: 500 mg pancreatin, 1,000 units lipase, 12,500 units protease, 12,500 units amylase
Hi-Vegi-Lip
Tablets (enteric-coated): 2,400 mg pancreatin, 4,800 units lipase, 60,000 units protease, 60,000 units amylase
Ilozyme
Tablets: 11,000 units lipase, 30,000 units protease, 30,000 units amylase
Ku-Zyme HP
Capsules: 8,000 units lipase, 30,000 units protease, 30,000 units amylase
Lipram-PN 10, Pancrease MT10
Capsules (enteric-coated microtablets): 10,000 units lipase, 30,000 units protease, 30,000 units amylase
Lipram-PN 16, Pancrease MT16
Capsules (enteric-coated microtablets): 16,000 units lipase, 48,000 units protease, 48,000 units amylase
Lipram-UL12, Ultrase MT12
Capsules (delayed-release): 12,000 units lipase, 39,000 units protease, 39,000 units amylase
Pancrease
Capsules (enteric-coated microspheres): 4,000 units lipase, 12,000 units protease, 12,000 units amylase
Pancrease MT4
Capsules (enteric-coated microtablets):

4,500 units lipase, 30,000 units protease, 30,000 units amylase

Pancrease MT20
Capsules (enteric-coated microtablets): 20,000 units lipase, 60,000 units protease, 60,000 units amylase

4X Pancreatin
Tablets (600 mg, enteric-coated): 2,400 mg pancreatin, 12,000 units lipase, 60,000 units protease, 60,000 units amylase

8X Pancreatin
Tablets (900 mg, enteric-coated): 7,200 mg pancreatin, 22,500 units lipase, 180,000 units protease, 180,000 units amylase

Pancrelipase
Capsules (enteric-coated pellets): 4,000 units lipase, 25,000 units protease, 20,000 units amylase

Pancrezyme 4X
Tablets (enteric-coated): 2,400 mg pancreatin, 12,000 units lipase, 60,000 units protease, 60,000 units amylase

Protilase
Capsules (enteric-coated spheres): 4,000 units lipase, 25,000 units protease, 20,000 units amylase

Ultrase MT18
Capsules (delayed-release): 18,000 units lipase, 58,500 units protease, 58,000 units amylase

Ultrase MT20
Capsules (delayed-release): 20,000 units lipase, 65,000 units protease, 65,000 units amylase

Viokase
Powder: 16,800 units lipase, 70,000 units protease, 70,000 units amylase per 0.7 g powder
Tablets: 8,000 units lipase, 30,000 units protease, 30,000 units amylase

Zymase
Capsules (enteric-coated sphere): 12,000 units lipase, 24,000 units protease, 24,000 units amylase

✒ Indications and dosages

➤ Replacement therapy in exocrine pancreatic secretion insufficiency; digestive aid in diseases associated with pancreatic enzyme deficiency (such as cystic fibrosis)

Adults: Dosage varies with patient's condition and digestive requirements. For pancreatin, usual initial dosage is 8,000 to 24,000 USP units of lipase activity P.O. before or with each meal or snack; may increase as needed to reduce steatorrhea if nausea, vomiting, or diarrhea doesn't occur. For pancrelipase, usual initial dosage is 4,000 to 33,000 units of lipase activity P.O. before or with each meal or snack; may increase as needed or decrease as symptoms improve.

Dosage adjustment
• Children

Contraindications

• Hypersensitivity to drug or pork
• Acute pancreatitis, acute exacerbation of chronic pancreatic disease

Administration

• Give before or with each meal or snack.
• Make sure patient doesn't crush or chew pancreatin tablets or hold tablet in mouth before swallowing; drug may irritate oral mucosa.
• If desired, open pancrelipase delayed-release capsule and give contents with liquid or mixed with soft food with pH above 5.5; don't let patient chew or crush capsule contents.
• If desired, give pancrelipase powder with liquids or mixed with soft food; make sure powder isn't inhaled.

Route	Onset	Peak	Duration
P.O.	Unknown	Unknown	1-2 hr

Adverse reactions

GI: nausea, vomiting, diarrhea (with high doses), cramping, anorexia
Metabolic: hyperuricemia
Skin: perianal irritation
Other: allergic reaction

P

Interactions

Drug-drug. *Antacids (calcium carbonate, magnesium hydroxide):* negation of digestive enzyme's beneficial effects
Iron salts: decreased effects of oral iron
Drug-diagnostic tests. *Uric acid:* increased level

Precautions

Use cautiously in:
• pregnant or breastfeeding patients.

Patient monitoring

• Assess patient's stools; if steatorrhea doesn't improve, dosage may need to be increased.
• When giving high doses, monitor patient for nausea, vomiting, and diarrhea.
• Evaluate dietary intake and nutritional status.
• Assess uric acid level.

Patient teaching

• Teach patient to take drug with plenty of fluids before or with each meal or snack.
• Instruct patient not to crush or chew pancreatin tablets or hold them in mouth before swallowing.
• Tell patient he may open pancrelipase delayed-release capsules and take contents with liquids or mix them with soft food; caution him not to chew or crush capsule contents.
• Instruct patient not to take antacids or iron salts within 2 hours of pancreatic enzymes.
• Teach patient to report perianal irritation or joint pain.
• Advise patient to minimize GI upset by eating small, frequent servings of healthy food and drinking plenty of fluids.
• As appropriate, review all other significant adverse reactions and interactions, especially those related to the drugs and tests mentioned above.

pancuronium bromide
Pavulon

Pharmacologic class: Nondepolarizing neuromuscular blocker

Therapeutic class: Muscle relaxant, adjunct to anesthesia

Pregnancy risk category C

Action

Inhibits action of acetylcholine at motor endplate receptor sites, blocking neuromuscular transmission

Availability

Injection: 1 mg/ml, 2 mg/ml

Indications and dosages

➤ Adjunct to balanced anesthesia to relax skeletal muscles for intubation
Adults and children age 1 month and older: Initially, 0.04 to 0.1 mg/kg I.V.; may follow with 0.01 mg/kg q 25 to 60 minutes if needed. (*Note:* Dosage is individualized according to type of anesthesia used, patient needs, and patient response. Dosages given above are typical representations.)

Contraindications

• Hypersensitivity to drug

Administration

◀€ Know that drug should be given only by specially trained personnel in settings where respiratory support is available.
• Administer through established I.V. line containing normal saline solution, lactated Ringer's solution, or dextrose 5% in water.
• Know that neostigmine can reverse drug's effects.
• Be aware that dosages are highly individualized.

◀€ Make sure patient's analgesic and sedative needs are met; drug doesn't relieve pain or provide sedation.

Route	Onset	Peak	Duration
I.V.	2-3 min	Unknown	22-65 min

Adverse reactions

CV: increased mean arterial pressure, increased cardiac output, tachycardia
GI: salivation
Musculoskeletal: prolonged weakness, prolonged skeletal muscle relaxation
Respiratory: cyanosis, **prolonged apnea, bronchospasm, respiratory insufficiency**
Skin: rash
Other: altered neuromuscular blockade in patients with electrolyte imbalances, hypersensitivity reaction

Interactions

Drug-drug. *Aminoglycosides (such as gentamicin, kanamycin, dihydrostreptomycin, neomycin, streptomycin), colistin, magnesium salts, polymyxin B, potassium-depleting drugs, sodium colistimethate, tetracyclines:* prolonged neuromuscular blockade
Enflurane, haloflurane, isoflurane, succinylcholine: enhanced neuromuscular blockade
Opioid analgesics: additive respiratory depression
Quinidine: recurrent paralysis
Tricyclic antidepressants (given with both halothane and pancuronium): severe ventricular arrhythmias

Precautions

Use cautiously in:
• cardiac, hepatic, neuromuscular, renal, or respiratory disease; electrolyte imbalances; severe obesity
• concurrent use of tricyclic antidepressants
• pregnant or breastfeeding patients
• neonates.

Patient monitoring

• Monitor heart rhythm, vital signs, and pulse oximetry during and after administration.
• Assess patient's sedation level.
• Evaluate fluid intake and output and potassium level.
• Assess muscle recovery using peripheral nerve stimulator and train-of-four monitoring.

Patient teaching

• Explain all procedures to patient as appropriate.

pantoprazole sodium
Protonix, Protonix IV

Pharmacologic class: Proton pump inhibitor
Therapeutic class: GI agent
Pregnancy risk category B

Action

Reduces gastric acid secretion and increases gastric mucus and bicarbonate production, creating a protective coating on the gastric mucosa

Availability

Powder for injection (freeze-dried): 40 mg/vial
Tablets (delayed-release): 20 mg, 40 mg

🖊 Indications and dosages

➤ Erosive esophagitis associated with gastroesophageal reflux disease
Adults: 40 mg I.V. daily for 7 to 10 days or 40 mg P.O. daily for 8 weeks; may repeat P.O. course
➤ Pathologic hypersecretory conditions
Adults: 80 mg I.V. q 12 hours, up to a maximum of 240 mg/day (80 mg q 8 hours); then 40 mg P.O. b.i.d as needed

p

Contraindications
• Hypersensitivity to drug

Administration
• For I.V. administration, use in-line filter provided. If Y-site is used, place filter below Y-site closest to patient.
• Dilute I.V. form with 10 ml of normal saline solution; further dilute in dextrose 5% in water, normal saline solution, or lactated Ringer's solution, as directed. Give over 15 minutes no faster than 3 mg/minute.
• Don't give I.V. form with other I.V. solutions.

Route	Onset	Peak	Duration
P.O.	Rapid	2.5 hr	>24 hr
I.V.	Rapid	Unknown	>24 hr

Adverse reactions
CNS: dizziness, headache
CV: chest pain
EENT: rhinitis
GI: vomiting, diarrhea, abdominal pain, dyspepsia
Hepatic: increased aspartate aminotransferase (AST) level
Metabolic: hyperglycemia
Skin: rash, pruritus
Other: injection site reaction

Interactions
Drug-drug. *Ampicillin, cyanocobalamin, digoxin, iron salts, ketoconazole:* delayed absorption of these drugs
Clarithromycin, diazepam, flurazepam, phenytoin, triazolam: increased pantoprazole blood level
Sucralfate: delayed pantoprazole absorption
Warfarin: increased bleeding
Drug-diagnostic tests. *AST, glucose:* increased levels
Tetrahydrocannabinol test: false-positive result

Precautions
Use cautiously in:
• severe hepatic disease
• pregnant or breastfeeding patients
• children.

Patient monitoring
• Assess patient for symptomatic improvement.
• Monitor blood glucose level in diabetic patients.

Patient teaching
• Teach patient to swallow delayed-release tablets whole without crushing, chewing, or splitting them.
• Tell patient he may take tablets with or without food.
• Explain that antacids don't affect absorption of delayed-release tablets.
• Instruct diabetic patients to monitor blood glucose level carefully and stay alert for signs and symptoms of hyperglycemia.
• As appropriate, review all other significant adverse reactions and interactions, especially those related to the drugs and tests mentioned above.

paroxetine hydrochloride
Paxil, Paxil CR

Pharmacologic class: Selective serotonin reuptake inhibitor (SSRI)
Therapeutic class: Antidepressant, anxiolytic
Pregnancy risk category C

Action
Unknown; thought to inhibit neuronal reuptake of serotonin in CNS

Availability
Oral suspension: 10 mg/5 ml
Tablets: 10 mg, 20 mg, 30 mg, 40 mg

Tablets (controlled-release): 12.5 mg, 25 mg, 37.5 mg

🕖 Indications and dosages
➤ Depression
Adults: Initially, 20 mg/daily P.O. (immediate-release) as a single dose; may increase by 10 mg/day at weekly intervals (dosage range is 20 to 50 mg). Or initially, 25 mg P.O. (controlled-release) once daily; may increase by 12.5 mg/day at weekly intervals, up to 62.5 mg/day P.O.
➤ Obsessive-compulsive disorder
Adults: Initially, 20 mg/day P.O. (immediate-release); increase by 10 mg/day at weekly intervals, up to 60 mg P.O. (dosage range is 20 to 60 mg/day). Or initially, 25 mg/day P.O. (controlled-release); may be titrated upward by 10 mg/day at weekly intervals, to a maximum of 60 mg/day.
➤ Panic disorder
Adults: Initially, 10 mg/day P.O. (immediate-release); may increase by 10 mg/day at weekly intervals, up to 40 mg P.O. (range 10 to 60 mg/day). Or initially, 12.5 mg/day P.O. (controlled-release); may be titrated upward by 10 mg/day at weekly intervals, to a maximum of 75 mg/day.
➤ Social anxiety disorder
Adults: 20 to 60 mg P.O. (immediate-release) daily
Dosage adjustment
• Hepatic impairment, severe renal impairment
• Elderly or debilitated patients

Off-label uses
• Premenstrual dysphoric disorder

Contraindications
• Hypersensitivity to drug
• Monoamine oxidase (MAO) inhibitor use within 14 days
• Concurrent thioridazine use

Administration
• Give with or without food.

• Don't administer to patients taking MAO inhibitors.

Route	Onset	Peak	Duration
P.O.	Unknown	2-8 hr	Unknown
P.O. (controlled)	Unknown	6-10 hr	Unknown

Adverse reactions
CNS: anxiety, agitation, dizziness, drowsiness, vascular headache, insomnia, confusion, hangover, depression, paresthesia, tremor, twitching, myoclonus, amnesia, abnormal dreams, cerebral ischemia, asthenia
CV: chest pain, hypertension, hypotension, palpitations, postural hypotension, angina pectoris, myocardial ischemia, supraventricular extrasystoles, thrombophlebitis, ventricular extrasystole, tachycardia, bradycardia
EENT: blurred vision, rhinitis, dry mouth
GI: nausea, vomiting, diarrhea, constipation, abdominal pain, dyspepsia, flatulence
GU: urinary disorders, urinary frequency, urinary tract infection, ejaculatory disturbance, decreased libido, genital disorders
Musculoskeletal: back pain, myalgia, myasthenia, myopathy, joint pain
Respiratory: cough, bronchitis, respiratory disorders, yawning
Skin: sweating, pruritus, pallor, rash, photosensitivity
Other: chills, appetite and weight changes, accidental injury, edema

Interactions
Drug-drug. *Cimetidine:* increased paroxetine blood level
Digoxin: decreased digoxin efficacy
Drugs metabolized by liver (such as amitriptyline, class IC antiarrhythmics, desipramine, fluoxetine, imipramine, nortriptyline, phenothiazines, procyclidine, quinidine): decreased metabolism and increased effects of these drugs

5-hydroxytryptamine receptor agonists (such as frovatriptan, naratriptan, rizatriptan, sumatriptan, zolmitriptan): weakness, hyperreflexia, incoordination

MAO inhibitors: potentially fatal reactions (hyperthermia, rigidity, myoclonus, autonomic instability, fluctuating vital signs, extreme agitation, delirium, coma)

Phenobarbital, phenytoin: decreased paroxetine efficacy

Theophylline: increased risk of theophylline toxicity

Tryptophan: headache, nausea, sweating, dizziness

Warfarin: increased risk of bleeding (without altering prothrombin time)

Drug-diagnostic tests. *Alkaline phosphatase, bilirubin, glucose:* increased levels

Urinary catecholamines: false increases

VMA, 5-hydroxyindole acetic acid: decreased level

Drug-herb. *S-adenosylmethionine (SAM-e), St. John's wort:* increased risk of adverse serotonergic effects, including serotonin syndrome

Precautions

Use cautiously in:
• severe renal or hepatic impairment
• history of seizures or mania, history or risk of suicide attempt
• patients at increased risk for hyponatremia or abnormal bleeding
• elderly or debilitated patients
• pregnant or breastfeeding patients
• children (safety not established).

Patient monitoring

• Check for signs and symptoms of toxicity, including drowsiness, nausea, tremor, tachycardia, confusion, and dizziness.
• Assess vital signs and cardiovascular status.
• Monitor neurologic status, especially for depression and suicidal ideation.

• Evaluate respiratory status; stay alert for infection and pulmonary embolism.

Patient teaching

• Teach patient to recognize and immediately report signs and symptoms of toxicity.
• Tell patient to swallow controlled-release tablets whole without chewing or crushing them.
• Tell patient that he should continue to take drug even if he feels better. Caution him not to stop therapy abruptly.
• Advise patient to consult prescriber before taking other prescription or over-the-counter drugs.
• Caution patient to avoid driving and other hazardous activities until he know how drug affects him.
• As appropriate, review all other significant adverse reactions and interactions, especially those related to the drugs, tests, and herbs mentioned above.

pegaspargase
Oncaspar, PEG-L-Asparaginase

Pharmacologic class: Enzyme
Therapeutic class: Antineoplastic
Pregnancy risk category C

Action

Stimulates production of effector proteins, such as serum neopterin and 2,5 oligodenylate synthetase; raises body temperature and reversibly lowers white blood cell and platelet counts

Availability

Injection: 750 IU/ml, 5-ml vial in phosphate buffered saline solution

---

Indications and dosages

> Acute lymphoblastic leukemia in patients hypersensitive to native forms of L-asparaginase

Adults and children with body surface area (BSA) above 0.6 m²: 2,500 IU/m² I.M. or I.V. q 14 days

Adults and children with BSA below 0.6 m²: 82.5 IU/m² I.M. or I.V. q 14 days

Contraindications

• Hypersensitivity to drug
• Pancreatitis or history of pancreatitis
• Previous hemorrhagic events related to L-asparaginase therapy

Administration

◀≋ Follow facility protocol for handling, preparing, and disposal of chemotherapeutic drugs.

◀≋ Keep resuscitation equipment, epinephrine, oxygen, steroids, and antihistamines readily available.

• Know that I.M. route is preferred because it's less likely to cause hepatotoxicity, coagulopathy, and GI or renal disorders. For single I.M. injection, volume shouldn't exceed 2 ml.

• For I.V. use, dilute in 100 ml of normal saline solution or dextrose 5% in water; infuse over 1 to 2 hours.

◀≋ Don't freeze. Freezing inactivates drug.

Route	Onset	Peak	Duration
I.V.	Unknown	72-96 hr	2 wk
I.M.	Unknown	Unknown	Unknown

Adverse reactions

CNS: neuritis, dizziness, headache, confusion, hallucinations, emotional lability, drowsiness, Parkinson-like syndrome, malaise, **coma, seizures**
CV: hypertension, hypotension, chest pain, endocarditis, peripheral edema, tachycardia

GI: nausea, vomiting, diarrhea, constipation, abdominal pain, flatulence, anorexia, **pancreatitis**
GU: glycosuria, polyuria, urinary frequency, hematuria, increased blood urea nitrogen (BUN) and creatinine levels
Hematologic: hemolytic anemia, **leukopenia, pancytopenia, thrombocytopenia, disseminated intravascular coagulation, decreased clotting factors**
Hepatic: fatty liver deposits, jaundice, abnormal liver function tests, **hepatotoxicity, hepatomegaly**
Metabolic: hyperglycemia, hypoproteinemia, hypoglycemia, hyperuricemia, hyperammonemia, hyponatremia
Respiratory: dyspnea, cough, **bronchospasm**
Skin: alopecia, rash, urticaria, pruritus, night sweats
Other: increased appetite and thirst, weight loss, chills, fever, injection site reaction, facial or lip edema, hypersensitivity reactions including **anaphylaxis, septic shock**

Interactions

Drug-drug. *Aspirin, dipyridamole, heparin, nonsteroidal anti-inflammatory drugs (NSAIDs), warfarin:* increased risk of bleeding or thrombosis (from coagulatory imbalances)
Methotrexate: decreased methotrexate action
Drug-diagnostic tests. *Amylase, lipase:* increased levels
Glucose: increased or decreased level
Lymphoblasts: decreased count
Plasma proteins: altered levels
Uric acid: increased level

Precautions

Use cautiously in:
• renal, hepatic disease; CNS disorders
• concurrent use of anticoagulants, aspirin or other NSAIDs, or hepatotoxic agents
• pregnant or breastfeeding patients.

Patient monitoring

🔊 Watch for anaphylaxis and other hypersensitivity reactions, especially during first hour of therapy.

• Monitor complete blood count (including platelet count); fibrinogen; prothrombin and partial thromboplastin times; International Normalized Ratio; and serum amylase, lipase, and uric acid levels.

• Assess neurologic status; stay alert for decreased level of consciousness and signs of impending seizures.

• Check for signs and symptoms of bleeding, infection, and hyperglycemia.

• Monitor heart rate, blood pressure, respiratory rate, temperature, and fluid intake and output.

Patient teaching

🔊 Teach patient to recognize and immediately report signs and symptoms of hypersensitivity reactions, bleeding, infection, and other adverse reactions.

• Tell patient that drug is likely to cause reversible hair loss.

• Teach patient about importance of follow-up laboratory tests.

• Advise patient to avoid situations that increase risk for infection.

• Instruct patient to consult prescriber before taking other prescription drugs or over-the-counter preparations.

• As appropriate, review all other significant and life-threatening adverse reactions and interactions, especially those related to the drugs and tests mentioned above.

pegfilgrastim
Neulasta

Pharmacologic class: Granulocytic colony stimulating factor
Therapeutic class: Hematopoietic drug
Pregnancy risk category C

Action

Binds to specific cell-surface receptors on hematopoietic cells, stimulating proliferation and differentiation in bone marrow

Availability

Injection: 6 mg/0.6 ml in prefilled syringes

Indications and dosages

➤ To decrease risk of infection in patients who are receiving myelosuppressive drugs associated with severe febrile neutropenia
Adults: 6 mg S.C. as a single dose once per chemotherapy cycle

Contraindications

• Hypersensitivity to drug, *Escherichia coli*-derived proteins, filgrastim, or other drug components

Administration

• Inspect solution for particles. Discard solution if it contains particles or is discolored.

• Don't administer 14 days before to 24 hours after administration of cytotoxic chemotherapy.

Route	Onset	Peak	Duration
S.C.	Variable	Variable	Variable

Adverse reactions

CNS: headache, generalized weakness, fatigue, dizziness, insomnia
CV: peripheral edema
EENT: stomatitis, taste perversion
GI: nausea, vomiting, diarrhea, abdominal pain, dyspepsia, **splenic rupture**
Hematologic: leukocytosis, **granulocytopenia**
Hepatic: increased alkaline phosphatase (ALP) and lactate dehydrogenase (LD) levels
Metabolic: increased uric acid level
Musculoskeletal: bone pain, myalgia, joint pain

Respiratory: adult respiratory distress syndrome (ARDS) in septic patients
Skin: alopecia, mucositis
Other: allergic reaction, increased pain, fever, neutropenic fever, **aggravation of sickle cell disease**

Interactions
Drug-drug. *Lithium:* potentiation of neutrophil release
Drug-diagnostic tests. *ALP, LD, uric acid:* increased levels

Precautions
Use cautiously in:
• myeloid cancers, sickle cell disease
• patients undergoing chemotherapy or radiation
• pregnant or breastfeeding patients
• children.

Patient monitoring
◀╪ Assess for signs and symptoms of impending splenic rupture, such as left upper quadrant or shoulder pain and splenic enlargement.
• Monitor vital signs and temperature.
• Watch for signs and symptoms of sepsis, ARDS, and neutropenic fever.
• Monitor complete blood count, liver function tests, and uric acid level.

Patient teaching
• Teach patient or caregiver how to administer injection and dispose of syringes at home, if appropriate.
◀╪ Teach patient to recognize and immediately report signs and symptoms of splenic rupture.
• Caution patient to avoid driving and other hazardous activities until he knows how drug affects concentration and alertness.
• Advise patient to minimize GI upset by eating small, frequent servings of healthy food and drinking plenty of fluids.
• Instruct patient to have follow-up laboratory tests as needed.

• Tell patient to notify prescriber if she becomes pregnant.
• As appropriate, review all other significant and life-threatening adverse reactions and interactions, especially those related to the drugs and tests mentioned above.

peginterferon alfa-2a
Pegasys

Pharmacologic class: Interferon
Therapeutic class: Biological response modifier
Pregnancy risk category C

Action
Unclear; thought to bind to specific receptors on cell surface, suppressing cell proliferation and virus replication. Also increases level of effector proteins and decreases leukocyte and platelet counts

Availability
Injection: 180-mcg/ml vial

Indications and dosages
➤ Chronic hepatitis C infection in adults who haven't previously received interferon alfa
Adults: 180 mcg S.C. in abdomen or thigh q week for 48 weeks. If drug is poorly tolerated, reduce dosage to 135 mcg weekly; some patients may need a reduction to 90 mcg.
Dosage adjustment
• Neutrophil count below 750 cells/mm^3 or platelet count below 50,000 cells/mm^3
• Hepatic disease
• End-stage renal disease requiring dialysis

Off-label uses
• Renal cell carcinoma

p

Contraindications

- Hypersensitivity to drug
- Autoimmune hepatitis
- Decompensated hepatic disease
- Infants and neonates

Administration

- Keep drug refrigerated. Before giving, roll vial between palms for 1 minute to warm; don't shake. Protect solution from light.
- Don't use solution that is cloudy or contains visible particles.
- Administer S.C. in abdomen or thigh.

Route	Onset	Peak	Duration
S.C.	Gradual	72-96 hr	Unknown

Adverse reactions

CNS: dizziness, insomnia, fatigue, rigors, poor memory and concentration, asthenia, depression, irritability, anxiety, peripheral neuropathy, **coma, suicidal ideation, cerebral hemorrhage**
CV: endocarditis, pulmonary embolism
EENT: corneal ulcer, retinopathy
GI: bleeding, colitis, peptic ulcer, **pancreatitis**
Hematologic: anemia, slight hematocrit decrease, **leukopenia, thrombocytopenia, neutropenia**
Hepatic: hepatic dysfunction
Metabolic: diabetes mellitus
Musculoskeletal: myalgia, back pain, joint pain, myositis
Respiratory: pneumonia, **interstitial pneumonitis**
Skin: alopecia, pruritus, diaphoresis, rash, dermatitis
Other: fever, injection site reaction, pain, hypersensitivity reactions, **autoimmune phenomena**

Interactions

Drug-diagnostic tests. *Absolute neutrophil count, platelets, white blood cells:* decreased counts

Precautions

Use cautiously in:

- thyroid disorders; bone marrow depression; hepatic, renal, or cardiac disease; depression; ophthalmic disorders; pancreatitis; autoimmune disorders; pulmonary disorders; colitis
- elderly patients
- pregnant or breastfeeding patients
- children younger than age 18.

Patient monitoring

- Assess cardiac and pulmonary status.
- Before therapy begins, assess complete blood count (including platelet count), blood glucose level, and thyroid, kidney, and liver function tests. Continue to monitor these tests at 1, 2, 4, 6, and 8 weeks and then every 4 weeks during therapy (or more often if abnormalities occur).

◀€ Monitor neurologic status; watch for signs and symptoms of cerebral hemorrhage or behavioral changes (such as irritability, hopelessness, depression, and suicidal ideation).

Patient teaching

- Teach patient how to administer injection S.C. in thigh or abdomen, if appropriate.

◀€ Advise patient to promptly report bleeding, infection symptoms, chest pain, shortness of breath, depression, or suicidal thoughts.

- Tell patient that drug should be administered exactly as prescribed on same day, and approximately same time of day, each week. If he misses a dose but remembers it within 2 days, he should take dose as soon as possible; if more than 2 days have elapsed, tell him to contact prescriber.
- Caution patient not to switch brands without prescriber's approval.
- Instruct patient to have periodic eye exams.
- Advise females of childbearing age to avoid pregnancy and use two birth control methods before, during, and

up to 6 months after therapy. Instruct male patients to use condoms.

• As appropriate, review all significant and life-threatening adverse reactions and interactions, especially those related to the tests mentioned above.

pegvisomant
Somavert

Pharmacologic class: Growth hormone receptor antagonist

Therapeutic class: Growth hormone analog

Pregnancy risk category B

Action
Selectively binds to growth hormone (GH) receptors on cell surfaces, where it blocks binding of endogenous GH and interferes with GH signal transduction. This action decreases blood levels of insulin-like growth factor-I (IGF-1) and other GH-responsive serum proteins.

Availability
Solution: 10-mg, 15-mg, and 20-mg vials

⚕ Indications and dosages
➤ Acromegaly in patients who haven't responded adequately to surgery, radiation, and other medical therapies
Adults: Initial loading dose of 40 mg S.C., followed by 10 mg S.C. daily; may adjust dosage in 5-mg increments after serum IGF-1 measurement q 4 to 6 weeks, not to exceed a maximum daily maintenance dosage of 30 mg

Contraindications
• Hypersensitivity to drug or its components

Administration
• Reconstitute in vial with 1 ml of sterile water for injection.
• Roll vial gently between palms to mix; don't shake.
• Withdraw prescribed dose and administer S.C.

Route	Onset	Peak	Duration
S.C.	Unknown	Unknown	24 hr

Adverse reactions
CNS: dizziness, paresthesia
CV: chest pain, hypertension, peripheral edema
EENT: sinusitis
GI: diarrhea, nausea, abdominal pain
Hepatic: abnormal liver function tests
Musculoskeletal: back pain
Other: infection, pain, injection site reaction, accidental injury, flulike symptoms

Interactions
Drug-drug. *Insulin, oral hypoglycemics:* decreased insulin sensitivity, reduced requirements for these drugs
Opioids: increased pegvisomant requirement
Drug-diagnostic tests. *Growth-hormone assays:* interference with growth hormone measurement
Drug-behaviors. *Opioid addiction:* increased pegvisomant requirement

Precautions
Use cautiously in:
• growth hormone-excreting tumors, diabetes mellitus, hepatic dysfunction
• pregnant or breastfeeding patients
• children.

Patient monitoring
• Assess liver function test results; watch for signs and symptoms of hepatic dysfunction.
• Monitor serum IGF-1 level; as appropriate, discuss dosage adjustments with prescriber.

P

• Monitor vital signs; check for hypertension, chest pain, and peripheral edema.
• Measure temperature and watch for signs and symptoms of infection, especially sinusitis or flulike symptoms.
• Assess blood glucose levels closely in diabetic patients; notify prescriber of significant decrease.

Patient teaching

• Teach patient proper technique for reconstituting and administering drug S.C.
◀€ Instruct patient to immediately report chest pain, peripheral edema, or signs or symptoms of infection.
• Caution patient to avoid driving and other hazardous activities until he knows how drug affects him.
• Teach diabetic patients to monitor blood glucose level closely and report significant decrease.
• Advise patient that he'll undergo frequent liver function tests; teach him to report yellowing of skin or eyes and other signs of hepatic dysfunction.
• As appropriate, review all other significant adverse reactions and interactions, especially those related to the drugs, tests, and behaviors mentioned above.

pemoline
Cylert, PemADD, PemADD CT

Pharmacologic class: CNS stimulant
Therapeutic class: Analeptic
Controlled substance schedule IV
Pregnancy risk category B

Action
Unknown; may act through dopaminergic mechanisms

Availability
Tablets: 18.75 mg, 37.5 mg, 75 mg
Tablets (chewable): 37.5 mg

⚕ Indications and dosages
➤ Attention deficit hyperactivity disorder
Children ages 6 and older: Initially, 37.5 mg/day as a single morning dose; may increase by 18.75 mg at weekly intervals until optimum response occurs. Dosage range is 56.25 to 75 mg/day, not to exceed 112.5 mg/day.

Off-label uses
• Narcolepsy
• Fatigue
• Excessive daytime sleepiness

Contraindications
• Hypersensitivity to drug
• Hepatic impairment

Administration
• Administer in morning to minimize insomnia.
• Give with food if GI upset occurs.

Route	Onset	Peak	Duration
P.O.	Unknown	2-4 hr	Unknown

Adverse reactions
CNS: headache, irritability, Tourette syndrome, insomnia, dyskinetic movements, depression, nervousness, drowsiness, hallucinations, **seizures**
CV: tachycardia
EENT: abnormal oculomotor function, nystagmus, oculogyric crisis
GI: nausea, diarrhea, abdominal pain, anorexia
GU: elevated acid phosphatase level
Hematologic: aplastic anemia
Hepatic: increased hepatic enzyme levels, jaundice, **hepatic failure, hepatitis**
Metabolic: growth suppression
Skin: rash, sweating
Other: fever, weight loss

Interactions
Drug-drug. *Anticonvulsants:* lowered seizure threshold
Other CNS stimulants: additive CNS stimulation
Drug-diagnostic tests. *Alanine aminotransferase, alkaline phosphatase, aspartate aminotransferase, lactate dehydrogenase:* increased levels

Precautions
Use cautiously in:
• renal impairment, tics, psychosis, emotional instability, drug abuse
• history of seizure disorders
• pregnant or breastfeeding patients (safety not established)
• children younger than age 6.

Patient monitoring
• Assess neurologic function; watch for seizures, tics, depression, and dyskinetic movements.
• Monitor complete blood count and liver function tests; watch for signs and symptoms of hepatic dysfunction.
• Check for symptomatic improvement, which should occur by third week.
• Assess height and weight (long-term therapy may cause growth abnormalities).

Patient teaching
• Teach patient and parents that drug should be taken in morning to minimize insomnia; recommend taking it with food if it causes GI upset.
◀ Inform patient and parents about drug's risks and benefits; emphasize importance of immediately reporting signs or symptoms of hepatic dysfunction (such as yellowing of skin or eyes, anorexia, malaise, and GI complaints).
• Teach patient and parents to recognize and promptly report adverse CNS effects.
• Advise patient and parents of need for periodic eye exams.

• Explain that patient should have follow-up laboratory tests to monitor hepatic function.
• As appropriate, review all other significant and life-threatening adverse reactions and interactions, especially those related to the drugs and tests mentioned above.

penicillin G benzathine
Bicillin L-A, Megacillin✚, Permapen

Pharmacologic class: Penicillin
Therapeutic class: Anti-infective
Pregnancy risk category B

Action
Inhibits biosynthesis of cell wall mucopeptide; kills penicillin-susceptible bacteria during active multiplication stage

Availability
Suspension for I.M. injection: 600,000 units/ml in 1-, 2-, and 4-ml prefilled syringes

Indications and dosages
➤ Streptococcal (group A) upper respiratory tract infections
Adults: 1.2 million units I.M. as a single dose
➤ Early syphilis (primary, secondary, or latent)
Adults: 2.4 million units I.M. as a single dose
Children: 50,000 units/kg I.M. as a single dose, increased as necessary up to adult dosage
➤ Congenital syphilis
Children under age 2: 50,000 units/kg I.M. as a single dose
➤ Neurosyphilis
Adults: 2.4 million units I.M. q week for up to 3 weeks, after aqueous penicillin G or procaine penicillin regimen

➤ Gummas and cardiovascular syphilis (latent)
Adults: 2.4 million units I.M. q week for 3 weeks
➤ Yaws, bejel, and pinta
Adults: 1.2 million units I.M. as a single dose
➤ Prophylaxis of rheumatic fever and glomerulonephritis
Adults: 1.2 million units I.M. q month or 600,000 units q 2 weeks after acute attack

Contraindications

• Hypersensitivity to penicillins, cephalosporins, imipenem, beta-lactamase inhibitors (piperacillin/tazobactam), or benzathine

Administration

• Inject deep I.M. at a slow, steady rate; administer in upper outer quadrant of buttock in adults or in midlateral thigh in infants and small children. Rotate injection sites with repeated doses.
• If using prefilled syringes, carefully follow manufacturer's instructions.
◀€ Keep epinephrine and emergency equipment readily available in case of anaphylaxis.
• Be aware that Hoigne's syndrome (transient bizarre behavior and neurologic reactions) may immediately follow I.M. injection.
• Know that in syphilis treatment, Jarisch-Hersheimer reaction (fever, chills, headache, sweating, malaise, hypotension or hypertension) may occur 2 to 12 hours after therapy begins but usually subsides within 24 hours.

Route	Onset	Peak	Duration
I.M.	Delayed	Dose dependent	Dose dependent

Adverse reactions

CNS: lethargy, hallucinations, anxiety, neuropathy, fatigue, headache, nervousness, tremors, euphoria, asthenia, Hoigne's syndrome, **cerebrovascular accident, seizures, coma**
CV: hypotension, palpitations, pulmonary hypertension, vasodilation, vasovagal reaction, syncope, tachycardia, **cardiac arrest, pulmonary embolism**
EENT: blurred vision, vision loss, laryngeal edema
GI: nausea, vomiting, diarrhea, epigastric distress, abdominal pain, glossitis, colitis, blood in stool, **pseudomembranous colitis**
GU: nephropathy, urogenic bladder, hematuria, proteinuria, impotence, priapism, **renal failure**
Hematologic: eosinophilia, hemolytic anemia, **leukopenia, thrombocytopenia**
Hepatic: increased alanine aminotransferase (ALT) level
Metabolic: hyperkalemia, hypernatremia, increased blood urea nitrogen and creatinine levels
Respiratory: dyspnea, hypoxia, **apnea, pulmonary embolism**
Skin: rash, urticaria, sweating
Other: fever, pain at I.M. site, superinfection, injection site reactions, Jarisch-Hersheimer reaction, **anaphylaxis, serum sickness**

Interactions

Drug-drug. *Aspirin, probenecid:* increased penicillin blood level
Erythromycins, tetracyclines: decreased antimicrobial activity of penicillin
Hormonal contraceptives: decreased contraceptive efficacy
Drug-diagnostic tests. *ALT, eosinophils, granulocytes, hemoglobin, platelets, potassium, white blood cells:* increased levels
Direct Coombs' test: positive result
Sodium: decreased level
Urine glucose, urine protein: false-positive results

Precautions
Use cautiously in:
• severe renal insufficiency, significant allergies or asthma
• pregnant or breastfeeding patients.

Patient monitoring
◀€ Watch closely for anaphylaxis and serum sickness.
• In long-term therapy, monitor complete blood count with white cell differential, as well as electrolyte levels; watch for blood dyscrasias and electrolyte imbalances.
• Assess neurologic status, especially for seizures and decreasing level of consciousness.
• Stay alert for evidence of superinfection and pseudomembranous colitis.

Patient teaching
◀€ Teach patient to recognize anaphylaxis symptoms and to contact emergency medical services immediately if these occur.
• Instruct patient to report signs and symptoms of superinfection.
• Tell patient that drug may cause diarrhea; instruct him to report severe, persistent diarrhea (with or without pus) and fever.
• Teach patient to complete entire course of therapy as prescribed, even after symptoms improve.
• Advise patient to contact prescriber if signs and symptoms of infection get worse.
• Tell female patient that drug may make hormonal contraceptives ineffective; encourage use of barrier birth control methods if she wishes to avoid pregnancy.
• As appropriate, review all other significant and life-threatening adverse reactions and interactions, especially those related to the drugs and tests mentioned above.

penicillin G potassium
Pfizerpen

Pharmacologic class: Penicillin
Therapeutic class: Anti-infective
Pregnancy risk category B

Action
Inhibits the biosynthesis of cell wall mucopeptide; bactericidal against penicillin-susceptible microorganisms during active multiplication stage

Availability
Powder for injection: 1 million, 5 million, and 20 million units/vial
Premixed (frozen) solution for injection: 1 million, 2 million, and 3 million units/50 ml

Indications and dosages
➤ Meningococcal meningitis
Adults: 1 to 2 million units I.M. q 2 hours or 20 to 30 million units/day by continuous I.V. infusion for 14 days or until afebrile for 7 days
➤ Meningitis caused by susceptible strains of pneumococcus or meningococcus
Children: 250,000 units/kg/day in equally divided doses I.M. or by continuous I.V. infusion q 4 hours for 7 to 14 days (depending on infecting organism)
Infants older than 7 days: 200,000 to 300,000 units/kg/day I.V. in divided doses q 6 hours
Neonates less than 7 days old: 100,000 to 150,000 units/kg/day I.V. in divided doses q 6 hours
➤ Actinomycosis
Adults: 1 to 6 million units/day I.M. or I.V. for cervicofacial infections; 10 to 20 million units/day I.V. q 4 to 6 hours for 6 weeks for thoracic and abdominal infections

P

➤ Clostridial infections
Adults: 20 million units/day I.M. or I.V. infusion q 4 to 6 hours, given with antitoxin therapy

➤ Fusospirochetal infections
Adults: 5 to 10 million units/day I.M. or 200,000 to 500,000 units I.V. infusion q 4 to 6 hours

➤ Rat bite fever, Haverhill fever
Adults: 12 to 20 million units/day I.M. or I.V. infusion q 4 to 6 hours for 3 or 4 weeks

➤ *Pasteurella* infections
Adults: 4 to 6 million units/day I.M. or I.V. infusion q 4 to 6 hours for 2 weeks

➤ Erysipeloid endocarditis
Adults: 12 to 20 million units/day I.M. or I.V. infusion q 4 to 6 hours for 4 to 6 weeks

➤ Diphtheria (as adjunctive therapy with antitoxin to prevent carrier state)
Adults: 2 to 3 million units/day I.M. or I.V. infusion in divided doses q 4 to 6 hours for 10 to 12 days

➤ Anthrax
Adults: At least 5 million units/day I.M. or I.V. infusion

➤ Serious streptococcal infections
Adults: 5 to 24 million units/day I.M. or I.V. infusion in divided doses q 4 to 6 hours

➤ Neurosyphilis
Adults: 18 to 24 million units/day I.V. (given in doses of 3 to 4 million units q 4 hours) for 10 to 14 days

➤ *Listeria* infections
Adults: 15 to 20 million units/day I.M. or I.V. infusion q 4 to 6 hours for 2 weeks (for meningitis); 15 to 20 million units/day I.M. or I.V. infusion q 4 to 6 hours for 4 weeks (for endocarditis)

➤ Disseminated gonococcal infections
Adults: 10 million units/day I.V. (3 to 4 million units q 4 hours) for 10 to 14 days

Off-label uses
• Lyme disease

• Predental prophylaxis against bacterial endocarditis

Contraindications
• Hypersensitivity to penicillins, imipenem, beta-lactamase inhibitors (piperacillin/tazobactam), or cephalosporins

Administration
◀⟨ Keep epinephrine and emergency equipment available in case anaphylaxis occurs.

• For I.V. use, dilute in sterile water for injection, normal saline solution, or dextrose 5% in water (D_5W). Shake vigorously. For continuous infusion, further dilute in 1 to 2 L of compatible solution and infuse over 24 hours. For intermittent infusion, further dilute in 50 or 100 ml of normal saline solution or D_5W; administer over 1 to 2 hours in adults or 15 to 30 minutes in children and infants.

• Know that drug also may be given by intrapleural or intrathecal route.

• Be aware that in syphilis treatment, Jarisch-Hersheimer reaction (fever, chills, headache, sweating, malaise, hypotension or hypertension) may occur 2 to 12 hours after therapy starts, but usually subsides within 24 hours.

Route	Onset	Peak	Duration
I.M.	Rapid	15-30 min	4-6 hr
I.V.	Rapid	End of infusion	4-6 hr

Adverse reactions
CNS: hyperreflexia, neuropathy, **coma, seizures**
CV: arrhythmias, cardiac arrest, heart failure (with high I.V. doses)
GI: nausea, vomiting, diarrhea, epigastric distress, abdominal pain, glossitis, colitis, blood in stool, **pseudomembranous colitis**
GU: nephropathy
Hematologic: hemolytic anemia, **leukopenia, thrombocytopenia**

Metabolic: hyperkalemia (with continuous high-dose I.V. infusion)
Skin: rash, urticaria, exfoliative dermatitis
Other: pain at I.M. site, phlebitis at I.V. site, Jarisch-Hersheimer reaction, superinfection, **anaphylaxis, serum sickness**

Interactions
Drug-drug. *Aspirin, probenecid:* increased penicillin blood level
Erythromycins, tetracyclines: decreased antimicrobial activity of penicillin
Hormonal contraceptives: decreased contraceptive efficacy
Drug-diagnostic tests. *Alanine aminotransferase, eosinophils, granulocytes, hemoglobin, platelets, potassium, white blood cells:* increased levels
Direct Coombs' test: positive results
Sodium: decreased level
Urine glucose, urine protein: false-positive results

Precautions
Use cautiously in:
• severe renal insufficiency, significant allergies or asthma
• pregnant or breastfeeding patients.

Patient monitoring
◀≣ Watch closely for anaphylaxis and serum sickness.
• In long-term therapy, monitor complete blood count with white cell differential, as well as electrolyte levels; watch for blood dyscrasias and electrolyte imbalances.
• Closely monitor neurologic status, especially for seizures and decreasing level of consciousness.
• Stay alert for signs and symptoms of superinfection.

Patient teaching
◀≣ Teach patient to recognize signs and symptoms of anaphylaxis and to contact emergency medical services immediately if these occur.

• Instruct patient to report signs and symptoms of superinfection.
• Tell patient that drug may cause diarrhea; instruct him to report severe, persistent diarrhea and fever.
• Advise patient to complete entire course of therapy as prescribed, even after symptoms improve.
• Teach patient to contact prescriber if signs and symptoms of infection worsen.
• Tell female patient that drug may make hormonal contraceptives ineffective; encourage use of barrier birth-control methods if she wishes to avoid pregnancy.
• As appropriate, review all other significant and life-threatening adverse reactions and interactions, especially those related to the drugs and tests mentioned above.

penicillin G procaine
Ayercillin✤, Crysticillin-AS✤, Wycillin

Pharmacologic class: Penicillin
Therapeutic class: Anti-infective
Pregnancy risk category B

P

Action
Inhibits the biosynthesis of cell wall mucopeptide; bactericidal against penicillin-susceptible microorganisms during active multiplication stage

Availability
Suspension for I.M. injection: 600,000 units/vial, 1.2 million units/vial

🛈 Indications and dosages
➤ Anthrax, bacterial endocarditis, erysipeloid and fusospirochetal infections, rat bite fever, group A streptococcal infections
Adults: 600,000 to 1 million units/day I.M.

---

818 penicillin G procaine

➤ Diphtheria
Adults: 300,000 to 600,000 units/day I.M. with antitoxin for 14 days; for carrier state, 300,000 units/day I.M. for 10 days
➤ Syphilis, yaws, bejel, and pinta
Adults: 600,000 units/day I.M. for 8 days; for late infections, continue for 10 to 15 days. For neurosyphilis, 2.4 million units/day I.M. with probenecid for 10 to 14 days.

Off-label uses
• Lyme disease
• Predental prophylaxis against bacterial endocarditis

Contraindications
• Hypersensitivity to penicillins, imipenem, beta-lactamase inhibitors (piperacillin/tazobactam), cephalosporins, or procaine

Administration
◀€ Keep epinephrine and emergency equipment available in case anaphylaxis occurs.
• In adults, inject deep I.M. into upper outer aspect of buttock.
• In infants and small children, inject at a slow, steady rate into midlateral aspect of thigh.
• Be aware that Hoigne's syndrome (transient bizarre behavior and neurologic reactions) may immediately follow I.M. injection.
• Know that in syphilis treatment, Jarisch-Hersheimer reaction (fever, chills, headache, sweating, malaise, hypotension or hypertension) may occur 2 to 12 hours after therapy starts, but usually subsides within 24 hours.

Route	Onset	Peak	Duration
I.M.	Delayed	1-3 hr	24 hr

Adverse reactions
CNS: lethargy, hallucinations, anxiety, depression, twitching, Hoigne's syndrome, **seizures, coma**

EENT: laryngeal edema
GU: interstitial nephritis
Hematologic: increased bleeding, eosinophilia, hemolytic anemia, **bone marrow depression, leukopenia, thrombocytopenia, granulocytopenia**
Skin: rash, urticaria
Other: pain at I.M. site, fever, superinfection, Jarisch-Hersheimer reaction, sterile abscess, **anaphylaxis, serum sickness**

Interactions
Drug-drug. *Aspirin, probenecid:* increased penicillin blood level
Erythromycins, tetracyclines: decreased penicillin antimicrobial activity
Hormonal contraceptives: decreased contraceptive efficacy
Drug-diagnostic tests. *Alanine aminotransferase, eosinophils, granulocytes, hemoglobin, platelets, potassium, white blood cells:* increased levels
Direct Coombs' test: positive result
Sodium: decreased level
Urine glucose, urine protein: false-positive results

Precautions
Use cautiously in:
• severe renal insufficiency, significant allergies or asthma
• pregnant or breastfeeding patients
• neonates.

Patient monitoring
◀€ Watch closely for anaphylaxis and serum sickness.
• In long-term therapy, monitor complete blood count with white cell differential, as well as electrolyte levels; stay alert for blood dyscrasias and electrolyte imbalances.
• Assess neurologic status, especially for seizures and decreasing level of consciousness.
• Monitor patient for signs and symptoms of superinfection.

♣ Canada   ◀€ Clinical alert   Reactions in **bold** are life-threatening

Patient teaching

◀€ Teach patient to recognize anaphylaxis signs and symptoms and to contact emergency medical services if these occur.

• Instruct patient to report signs and symptoms of superinfection.

• Advise patient that drug may cause diarrhea; teach him to report severe, persistent diarrhea and fever.

• Emphasize the importance of completing the entire course of therapy as prescribed, even after symptoms improve.

• Advise patient to contact prescriber if signs and symptoms of infection worsen.

• Tell female patient that drug may make hormonal contraceptives ineffective; encourage use of barrier birth-control methods if she wishes to avoid pregnancy.

• As appropriate, review all other significant and life-threatening adverse reactions and interactions, especially those related to the drugs and tests mentioned above.

penicillin V potassium

Apo-Pen VK✤, Beepen-VK, Nadopen-V✤, Novo-Pen-VK✤, Pen-Vee, Pen-Vee K✤, PVF K✤, Veetids

Pharmacologic class: Penicillin
Therapeutic class: Anti-infective
Pregnancy risk category B

Action

Inhibits the biosynthesis of cell wall mucopeptide; bactericidal against penicillin-susceptible microorganisms during active multiplication stage

Availability

Oral solution: 200,000 units (125 mg)/ 5 ml, 400,000 units (250 mg)/5 ml
Tablets: 400,000 units (250 mg), 800,000 units (500 mg)

💋 Indications and dosages

➤ Mild to moderately severe streptococcal infections of upper respiratory tract, including scarlet fever and mild erysipelas
Adults and children age 12 and older: 125 to 250 mg P.O. q 6 to 8 hours for 10 days
Children younger than age 12: 25 to 50 mg/kg/day P.O. daily in divided doses q 6 hours for 10 days
➤ Mild to moderately severe pneumococcal respiratory infections, including otitis media
Adults and children age 12 and older: 250 to 500 mg P.O. q 6 hours until afebrile for at least 2 days
➤ Mild staphylococcal infections of skin and soft tissue, mild to moderately severe fusospirochetosis (Vincent's infection) of oropharynx
Adults and children age 12 and older: 250 to 500 mg P.O. q 6 to 8 hours
➤ To prevent recurrence of rheumatic fever or chorea
Adults and children age 12 and older: 125 to 250 mg P.O. b.i.d. on a continuing basis

Off-label uses

• Prophylaxis of *Streptococcus pneumoniae* septicemia in children with sickle cell anemia or splenectomy
• Early Lyme disease
• Actinomycosis
• Anthrax preexposure prophylaxis
• Prophylaxis of bacterial endocarditis after dental procedures

Contraindications

• Hypersensitivity to penicillins, imipenem, beta-lactamase inhibitors (piperacillin/tazobactam), or cephalosporins

P

Administration

🔊 Have epinephrine and emergency equipment available in case anaphylaxis is occurs.

• Give with water 1 hour before or 2 hours after meals. Don't give with fruit juice or carbonated beverages.

Route	Onset	Peak	Duration
P.O.	Unknown	1 hr	6 hr

Adverse reactions

CNS: lethargy, hallucinations, anxiety, depression, twitching, **seizures, coma**
EENT: stomatitis, glossitis, sore mouth or tongue, black or furry tongue
GI: nausea, vomiting, diarrhea, bloody diarrhea, epigastric distress, enterocolitis, rectal bleeding, flatulence, abdominal pain, dry mouth, **pseudomembranous colitis**
GU: interstitial nephritis
Hematologic: increased bleeding, anemia, eosinophilia, hemolytic anemia, **leukopenia, granulocytopenia, bone marrow depression, thrombocytopenia, thrombocytopenic purpura**
Metabolic: hyperkalemia, alkalosis, hypokalemia
Skin: rash, urticaria
Other: fever, superinfection, **anaphylaxis, serum sickness**

Interactions

Drug-drug. *Aspirin, probenecid:* increased penicillin blood level
Erythromycins, tetracyclines: decreased penicillin antimicrobial activity
Hormonal contraceptives: decreased contraceptive efficacy
Drug-diagnostic tests. *Alanine aminotransferase (ALT), eosinophils, granulocytes, hemoglobin, platelets:* increased levels
Albumin, lymphocytes, protein, uric acid, white blood cells: decreased levels
Direct Coombs' test: positive result
Potassium: increased or decreased level
Sodium: decreased level

Urine glucose, urine protein: false-positive results
Drug-herb. *Khat:* delayed and reduced penicillin absorption

Precautions

Use cautiously in:
• severe renal insufficiency
• pregnant or breastfeeding patients.

Patient monitoring

🔊 Watch for anaphylaxis and serum sickness.

• In long-term therapy, monitor complete blood count with white cell differential, as well as electrolyte levels; watch for blood dyscrasias and electrolyte imbalances.

• Assess neurologic status, especially for seizures and decreasing level of consciousness.

• Monitor patient closely for signs and symptoms of superinfection and pseudomembranous colitis.

Patient teaching

• Instruct patient to take drug with water 1 hour before or 2 hours after meals. Tell him not to take it with fruit juice or carbonated beverages.

🔊 Teach patient to recognize anaphylaxis symptoms; instruct him to contact emergency medical services if these occur.

• Instruct patient to report signs and symptoms of superinfection.

• Advise patient to contact prescriber if infection symptoms get worse.

• Tell patient that drug may cause diarrhea; instruct him to report severe, persistent diarrhea and fever.

• Teach patient to complete entire course of therapy as prescribed, even after symptoms improve.

• Tell female patient that drug may make hormonal contraceptives ineffective; encourage use of barrier birth-control methods if she wishes to avoid pregnancy.

• As appropriate, review all other significant and life-threatening adverse reactions and interactions, especially those related to the drugs, tests, and herbs mentioned above.

pentamidine isethionate
NebuPent, Pentacarinat✤,
Pentam 300, Pneumopent✤

Pharmacologic class: Antiprotozoal
Therapeutic class: Anti-infective
Pregnancy risk category C

Action
Unknown; may interfere with nuclear metabolism and synthesis of DNA, RNA, and proteins

Availability
Aerosol: 300 mg
Injection: 300 mg/vial

⟩ Indications and dosages
➤ *Pneumocystis jiroveci* (formerly *Pneumocystis carinii*) pneumonia
Adults and children: 4 mg/kg I.V. or deep I.M. daily for 14 days
➤ To prevent *P. jiroveci* pneumonia in high-risk patients with human immunodeficiency virus
Adults: 300 mg by inhalation once q 4 weeks using Respigard II nebulizer

Off-label uses
• Trypanosomiasis
• Visceral leishmaniasis

Contraindications
• History of anaphylaxis from pentamidine

Administration
• For I.V. infusion, dilute 300 mg-vial with sterile water for injection; withdraw prescribed dose, then dilute further in 50 to 250 ml of dextrose 5% in water and infuse over 60 to 120 minutes.
• For I.M. use, dilute 300 mg-vial with 3 ml of sterile water for injection; withdraw prescribed dose and administer deep I.M. using Z-track method.
• Keep patient supine during I.M. or I.V. administration to minimize hypotension.
• For inhalation, dilute in 6 ml of sterile water and administer through nebulizer with flow rate of 6 L/minute from 50-p.s.i. compressed air source.

Route	Onset	Peak	Duration
I.V.	Unknown	1 hr	Unknown
I.M., Inhalation	Unknown	0.5 hr	Unknown

Adverse reactions
CNS: disorientation, hallucinations, dizziness, confusion, fatigue, headache, neuralgia, **cerebrovascular accident**
CV: chest pain, ECG abnormalities, vasodilation, vasculitis, phlebitis, hypertension, palpitations, syncope, **arrhythmias, hypotension, ventricular tachycardia**
EENT: pharyngitis
GI: nausea, vomiting, diarrhea, abdominal pain, anorexia, metallic or bad taste, **pancreatitis**
GU: increased creatinine level, **acute renal failure, renal toxicity**
Hematologic: anemia, **leukopenia, thrombocytopenia**
Hepatic: increased liver function test results
Metabolic: hypoglycemia, hyperglycemia, hypocalcemia, hyperkalemia
Musculoskeletal: myalgia
Respiratory: cough, dyspnea, congestion, **pneumothorax, bronchospasm**
Skin: rash, night sweats, sterile abscess, urticaria, induration at injection site
Other: fever, chills, pain at injection site or elsewhere, edema, **Stevens-Johnson syndrome**

P

Interactions
Drug-diagnostic tests. *Blood urea nitrogen, creatinine, potassium:* increased levels
Calcium: decreased level
ECG: alterations
Glucose: increased or decreased level
Hemoglobin, hematocrit, platelets, white blood cells: decreased levels

Precautions
Use cautiously in:
• blood dyscrasias, hepatic or renal disease, diabetes mellitus, ventricular tachycardia, hypocalcemia, hypertension, hypotension, hypoglycemia, pancreatitis
• pregnant or breastfeeding patients
• children.

Patient monitoring
• Monitor blood pressure closely during and after I.M. or I.V. administration until patient is stable.
• Assess I.V. site closely during and after I.V. administration; extravasation may cause tissue necrosis.
• Evaluate neurologic status; watch for signs and symptoms of cerebrovascular accident.
• Monitor complete blood count (including platelet count); calcium, potassium, and glucose levels; and kidney and liver function test results.

Patient teaching
• Explain purpose of therapy; stress importance of completing entire course.
• Teach patient to recognize and immediately report serious adverse cardiovascular and neurologic effects.
• Teach patient how to use aerosol.
• Tell patient to notify prescriber if infection worsens.
• Teach patient to minimize GI upset by eating small, frequent servings of healthy food and drinking plenty of fluids.

• Instruct patient to avoid driving and other hazardous activities until he knows how drug affects concentration and alertness.
• As appropriate, review all other significant and life-threatening adverse reactions and interactions, especially those related to the tests mentioned above.

pentazocine hydrochloride
Talwin, Talwin 50

pentazocine hydrochloride and naloxone hydrochloride
Talwin NX

Pharmacologic class: Opioid agonist-antagonist
Therapeutic class: Opioid analgesic, adjunct to anesthesia
Controlled substance schedule IV
Pregnancy risk category C

Action
Unknown; interacts with opiate receptor sites primarily in the limbic system, thalamus, and spinal cord of the CNS, blocking neurotransmission of pain impulses.

Availability
Injection: 30 mg/ml
Tablets: 50 mg

Indications and dosages
➤ Moderate to severe pain, preoperative or preanesthetic medication, or as an adjunct to surgical anesthesia
Adults: 50 to 100 mg P.O. q 3 to 4 hours (not to exceed 600 mg/day) or 30 mg S.C., I.M., or I.V. q 3 to 4 hours (not to exceed 30 mg/dose I.V. or 60 mg/dose I.M. or S.C.) When given S.C., I.V., or I.M., maximum daily dosage is 360 mg.

➤ Labor
Adults: 20 mg I.V. for two or three doses at 2- to 3-hour intervals, or 30 mg I.M. as a single dose

Contraindications
• Hypersensitivity to drug or naloxone (with oral form)

Administration
• Inject I.V. slowly by direct infusion with patient lying supine.
• Use S.C. route only when necessary (may cause tissue damage).

Route	Onset	Peak	Duration
P.O.	15-30 min	60-180 min	3 hr
I.V.	12-30 min	Unknown	3 hr
I.M., S.C.	15-20 min	15-60 min	3 hr

Adverse reactions
CNS: dizziness, drowsiness, euphoria, hallucinations, headache, sedation, dysphoria, unusual dreams, weakness, depression, insomnia, irritability, excitement, tremor, paresthesia
CV: hypertension, hypotension, syncope, tachycardia, **circulatory depression, shock**
EENT: blurred vision, diplopia, nystagmus, miosis (with high doses), tinnitus, taste alteration
GI: nausea, vomiting, constipation, diarrhea, dry mouth, ileus, cramps, abdominal distress, anorexia
GU: urinary retention, altered rate and strength of labor contractions
Hematologic: decreased white blood cell (WBC) count
Respiratory: dyspnea, transient apnea in neonates whose mothers received pentazocine during labor, **respiratory depression**
Skin: clamminess, diaphoresis, rash, urticaria, nodules, cutaneous depression, sclerosis of skin and S.C. tissues, dermatitis, pruritus, flushing
Other: chills, physical or psychological drug dependence, drug tolerance, soft-tissue induration, facial edema, stinging on injection, **anaphylaxis**

Interactions
Drug-drug. *Barbiturates, first-generation (sedating) antihistamines, other sedating drugs:* additive CNS depression
Monoamine oxidase inhibitors: unpredictable reactions
Opioids: decreased analgesic effects
Drug-diagnostic tests. *Amylase, lipase:* increased levels
Granulocytes, WBCs: reduced counts
Drug-herb. *Chamomile, hops, kava, skullcap, valerian:* increased CNS depression
Drug-behaviors. *Alcohol use:* increased CNS depression

Precautions
Use cautiously in:
• head trauma, increased intracranial pressure, respiratory conditions, adrenal insufficiency, seizure disorder, acute CNS manifestations, hepatic impairment, acute myocardial infarction, alcohol or narcotic use
• history of drug abuse
• pregnant or breastfeeding patients
• children (safety not established).

Patient monitoring
• Monitor vital signs, especially for shock, dyspnea, and circulatory or respiratory depression.
• Monitor drug efficacy.
• In prolonged use, assess for signs and symptoms of dependence.

Patient teaching
◀€ Teach patient that Talwin NX is for oral use only; life-threatening reactions may result from misusing drug by injection.
• Inform patient that withdrawal symptoms may occur if drug is stopped suddenly after prolonged use.
• Teach patient to avoid alcohol.

P

• Advise patient to consult prescriber before taking other prescription drugs or over-the-counter preparations.
• Caution patient to avoid driving and other hazardous activities until he knows how drug affects him.
• Advise patient to have periodic eye exams.
• As appropriate, review all significant and life-threatening adverse reactions and interactions, especially those related to the drugs, tests, herbs, and behaviors mentioned above.

pentobarbital
Nembutal

pentobarbital sodium
Nembutal Sodium

Pharmacologic class: Barbiturate
Therapeutic class: Sedative-hypnotic, anticonvulsant
Controlled substance schedule II
Pregnancy risk category D

Action
Depresses sensory cortex, decreases motor activity, and alters cerebellar function; may interfere with nerve impulse transmission in brain

Availability
Capsules: 100 mg
Elixir: 20 mg/5 ml
Injection: 50 mg/ml in 2-ml prefilled syringes

⚕ Indications and dosages
➤ Sedation
Adults: 20 to 30 mg P.O. three to four times daily
Children: 2 to 6 mg/kg P.O. daily in divided doses, with a maximum of 100 mg/dose

➤ Preoperative sedation
Adults: Initially 100 mg P.O., 150 to 200 mg I.M., or 100 mg I.V.
➤ Seizures
Adults: Initially, 100 mg. I.V.; may give additional doses after 1 minute. Maximum dosage is 500 mg.
Children: Initially, 50 mg. I.V.; may give additional doses until desired response occurs. Don't exceed 100 mg/dose.

Contraindications
• Hypersensitivity to drug or other barbiturates
• Nephritis
• Severe hepatic impairment
• Severe respiratory disease with dyspnea or obstruction
• History of sedative-hypnotic abuse
• S.C. or intra-arterial administration

Administration
◀€ When giving drug I.V., make sure resuscitation equipment is available.
• Give I.V. by direct injection no faster than 50 mg/minute.
• Inject I.M. deep into large muscle mass.

Route	Onset	Peak	Duration
P.O.	15-60 min	3-4 hr	3-4 hr
I.V.	Immediate	1 min	3-4 hr
I.M.	10-25 min	Unknown	3-4 hr

Adverse reactions
CNS: drowsiness, agitation, confusion, hyperkinesia, ataxia, nightmares, nervousness, hallucinations, insomnia, anxiety, abnormal thinking
CV: hypotension, syncope, **bradycardia** (all with I.V. use)
GI: nausea, vomiting, constipation, diarrhea
Hepatic: hepatic damage
Musculoskeletal: joint pain, myalgia, neuralgia
Respiratory: laryngospasm (with I.V.

use), **bronchospasm, respiratory depression**

Skin: rash, urticaria, exfoliative dermatitis

Other: phlebitis at I.V. site, physical or psychological drug dependence, fever, hypersensitivity reactions including angioedema, **serum sickness**

Interactions

Drug-drug. *Acetaminophen:* increased risk of hepatotoxicity

Activated charcoal: decreased pentobarbital absorption

Anticoagulants, beta-blockers (except timolol), carbamazepine, clonazepam, corticosteroids, digoxin, doxorubicin, doxycycline, felodipine, fenoprofen, griseofulvin, hormonal contraceptives, metronidazole, quinidine, theophylline, verapamil: decreased efficacy of these drugs

Antihistamines (first-generation), opioids, other sedative-hypnotics: additive CNS depression

Chloramphenicol, hydantoins, narcotics: increased or decreased effects of these drugs or pentobarbital

Divalproex, monoamine oxidase (MAO) inhibitors, valproic acid: decreased pentobarbital metabolism, increased sedation

Rifampin: increased pentobarbital metabolism, decreased effects

Drug-diagnostic tests. *Sulfobromophthalein:* false increase

Drug-herb. *Chamomile, hops, kava, valerian, or skullcap:* increased CNS depression

St. John's wort: decreased pentobarbital effects

Drug-behaviors. *Alcohol use:* increased sedation, additive CNS depression

Precautions

Use cautiously in:
• hepatic impairment
• patients who may be suicidal or who have a history of drug addiction
• alcohol use

• labor and delivery
• elderly or debilitated patients.

Patient monitoring

◀€ Closely monitor blood pressure and heart and respiratory rates; watch for signs and symptoms of respiratory depression.
• Monitor neurologic status before and during therapy.
• Assess complete blood count and kidney and liver function test results.
• In long-term therapy, monitor patient for signs of drug dependence.

Patient teaching

• Instruct patient to take drug exactly as prescribed.
• Inform patient that increasing dosage without prescriber's approval may lead to dependence.
• Advise patient to avoid St. John's wort, alcohol, and other CNS depressants.
• Caution patient to avoid driving and other hazardous activities.
• Advise patients taking hormonal contraceptives to use alternate birth-control method.
• As appropriate, review all significant and life-threatening adverse reactions and interactions, especially those related to the drugs, tests, herbs, and behaviors mentioned above.

pentostatin
Nipent

Pharmacologic class: Antimetabolite
Therapeutic class: Antineoplastic
Pregnancy risk category D

Action

Unknown; inhibits adenosine deaminase, thus increasing levels of deoxyadenosine triphosphate in the cells;

blocking DNA synthesis and inhibiting ribonucleotide reductase.

Availability
Powder for injection: 10 mg vial

🕖 Indications and dosages
➤ Hairy cell leukemia refractory to alpha-interferon therapy
Adults: 4 mg/m^2 I.V. every other week; may be given by bolus or diluted to a larger volume and given over 20 to 30 minutes

Contraindications
• Hypersensitivity to drug

Administration
• Before giving drug, hydrate patient with 500 to 1,000 ml of dextrose 5% and normal saline solution (or its equivalent). After administering drug, give 500 ml of dextrose 5% in water (D$_5$W) or its equivalent.
◀€ Follow facility protocol for handling and preparing chemotherapeutic drugs.
• Give by direct I.V. injection or dilute with 25 to 50 ml of D$_5$W or normal saline solution; infuse over 20 to 30 minutes.

Route	Onset	Peak	Duration
I.V.	Unknown	Unknown	Unknown

Adverse reactions
CNS: headache, malaise, anxiety, confusion, depression, dizziness, insomnia, nervousness, paresthesia, drowsiness, abnormal thinking, fatigue, asthenia, hallucinations, hostility, amnesia
CV: peripheral edema, cellulitis, vasculitis, hypotension, angina, phlebitis, thrombophlebitis, tachycardia, bradycardia, **cardiac arrest, heart failure, hemorrhage, ventricular asystole, pericardial effusion, sinus arrest**
EENT: abnormal vision, nonreactive pupils, photophobia, retinopathy, eye pain, conjunctivitis, dry or watery eyes, hearing loss, tinnitus, ear pain, epistaxis, pharyngitis, rhinitis, gingivitis
GI: nausea, vomiting, diarrhea, constipation, dyspepsia, abdominal pain, ileus, flatulence, stomatitis, glossitis, unusual taste, anorexia
GU: abnormal renal function, renal insufficiency, renal calculi, decreased libido, amenorrhea, breast lump, impotence, **renal failure**
Hematologic: ecchymosis, anemia, hemolytic anemia, **agranulocytosis, aplastic anemia, leukopenia, thrombocytopenia**
Hepatic: elevated liver function test results
Metabolic: hyperuricemia, hypercalcemia, hyponatremia
Musculoskeletal: myalgia, joint pain
Respiratory: cough, dyspnea, respiratory tract infection, **pulmonary embolus**
Skin: rash, eczema, petechiae, dry skin, pruritus, skin disorder, furunculosis, acne, alopecia, diaphoresis, photosensitivity
Other: fever, chills, pain, facial edema, lymphadenopathy, herpes simplex, herpes zoster, flulike symptoms, viral or bacterial infection, allergic reaction, infection, **sepsis, neoplasm**

Interactions
Drug-drug. *Allopurinol:* hypersensitivity vasculitis
Carmustine, cyclophosphamide, etoposide: potentially fatal acute pulmonary edema and hypotension
Fludarabine: severe or fatal pulmonary toxicity
Vidarabine: increased risk and severity of adverse reactions
Drug-diagnostic tests. *Calcium, serum uric acid:* increased levels
Granulocytes, platelets, sodium, white blood cells: decreased levels

---

Precautions
Use cautiously in:
- renal disease, bone marrow depression
- pregnant or breastfeeding patients
- children.

Patient monitoring
- Monitor complete blood count (including platelet count); watch for signs and symptoms of blood dyscrasias.
- Assess kidney and liver function tests; watch for signs and symptoms of organ dysfunction.
- Monitor temperature; stay alert for signs and symptoms of bacterial and viral infections.
- Closely monitor vital signs and ECG, particularly for life-threatening arrhythmias, heart failure, and pulmonary edema.

Patient teaching
◀፪ Teach patient that drug lowers resistance to infection. Instruct him to avoid crowds and to immediately report fever, cough, breathing problems, sore throat, and other signs and symptoms of infection.
- Teach patient to minimize GI upset by eating small, frequent servings of healthy food and drinking plenty of fluids.
- Advise female patients of childbearing age to avoid pregnancy while taking drug and to seek medical advice before becoming pregnant.
- Instruct patient to avoid driving and other hazardous activities until he knows how drug affects concentration and alertness.
- As appropriate, review all other significant and life-threatening adverse reactions and interactions, especially those related to the drugs and tests mentioned above.

pentoxifylline
Trental

Pharmacologic class: Hemorrheologic, xanthine derivative
Therapeutic class: Hematologic agent
Pregnancy risk category C

Action
Unknown; thought to increase blood flow to circulatory system by increasing vasoconstriction and oxygen concentrations

Availability
Tablets (controlled-release): 400 mg
Tablets (extended-release): 400 mg

🕖 Indications and dosages
➤ Intermittent claudication
Adults: 400 mg t.i.d.; if adverse effects occur, decrease to 400 mg b.i.d.
Dosage adjustment
- Renal impairment

Off-label uses
- Diabetic angiopathies and neuropathies
- Transient ischemic attacks
- Severe idiopathic recurrent aphthous stomatitis
- Raynaud's phenomenon

Contraindications
- Hypersensitivity to drug or methylxanthines
- Breastfeeding

Administration
- Give drug with meals to minimize GI distress.
- Make sure patient swallows tablets whole without crushing, breaking, or chewing them.

Route	Onset	Peak	Duration
P.O.	Variable	2-4 hr	8 hr

Adverse reactions
CNS: agitation, dizziness, drowsiness, headache, insomnia, nervousness, tremor, anxiety, confusion, malaise
CV: angina, edema, hypotension, **arrhythmias**
EENT: blurred vision, epistaxis, laryngitis, nasal congestion, sore throat, bad taste
GI: nausea, vomiting, constipation, diarrhea, abdominal discomfort, belching, bloating, dyspepsia, flatus, cholecystitis, dry mouth, excessive salivation, anorexia
Hematologic: leukopenia
Respiratory: dyspnea
Skin: brittle fingernails, pruritus, rash, urticaria, flushing, angioedema
Other: weight changes, thirst, flulike symptoms, lymphadenopathy

Interactions
Drug-drug. *Anticoagulants, nonsteroidal anti-inflammatory drugs (NSAIDs):* increased risk of bleeding
Antihypertensives: additive hypotension
Theobromide, theophylline: increased risk of theophylline toxicity
Drug-herb. *Anise, arnica, asafetida, chamomile, clove, dong quai, fenugreek, feverfew, garlic, ginger, ginkgo, ginseng, licorice:* increased risk of bleeding
Drug-behaviors. *Smoking:* decreased pentoxifylline efficacy

Precautions
Use cautiously in:
• patients at risk for bleeding
• pregnant patients
• children (safety not established).

Patient monitoring
• Monitor vital signs and cardiovascular status; watch for angina, edema, and hypotension.
• Frequently monitor prothrombin time and International Normalized Ratio in patients receiving warfarin concurrently.

• Assess theophylline levels in patients receiving theophylline-containing drugs concurrently.

Patient teaching
• Teach patient to take tablets with meals and to swallow them whole without crushing, breaking, or chewing them.
• Advise patient to contact prescriber if adverse reactions occur.
◀€ Caution patient that drug can cause serious adverse effects; instruct him to immediately report chest pain, swelling, and flulike symptoms.
• Tell patient that smoking may make drug less effective and that many over-the-counter preparations (including aspirin, NSAIDs, and herbs) increase risk of bleeding. Discourage use of these products.
• As appropriate, review all other significant and life-threatening adverse reactions and interactions, especially those related to the drugs, herbs, and behaviors mentioned above.

perindopril erbumine
Aceon

Pharmacologic class: Angiotensin-converting enzyme (ACE) inhibitor

Therapeutic class: Antihypertensive

Pregnancy risk category C (first trimester), ***D*** (second and third trimesters)

Action
Inhibits conversion of angiotensin I to angiotensin II (a potent vasoconstrictor); this effect leads to decreased plasma angiotensin II, reduced vasoconstriction, enhanced plasma renin activity, and decreased aldosterone activity

---

Availability
Tablets: 2 mg, 4 mg, 8 mg

🔋 Indications and dosages
➤ Essential hypertension
Adults: 4 mg P.O. daily; may be titrated upward to 16 mg/day, given as a single dose or in two divided doses (start with 2 to 4 mg/day in patients receiving diuretics). May be given alone or with other agents.
Dosage adjustment
• Renal impairment
• Elderly patients

Off-label uses
• Heart failure
• To prevent renal damage secondary to diabetes mellitus

Contraindications
• Hypersensitivity to drug or other ACE inhibitors
• Angioedema during previous ACE inhibitor use
• Pregnancy

Administration
• Give drug without regard to food.
◀ᕍ Know that drug (especially first dose) may cause angioedema. Keep epinephrine and antihistamines available in case angioedema causes airway obstruction.
• For elderly patients, titrate dosage upward very slowly.

Route	Onset	Peak	Duration
P.O.	1 hr	3-7 hr	12-24 hr

Adverse reactions
CNS: dizziness, fatigue, headache, insomnia, weakness, asthenia, drowsiness, vertigo, sleep disorder, depression, paresthesia
CV: hypotension, angina pectoris, palpitations, chest pain, abnormal ECG, tachycardia
EENT: ear infection, sinusitis, rhinitis, pharyngitis

GI: nausea, vomiting, diarrhea, abdominal pain, flatulence
GU: proteinuria, urinary tract infection, impotence, decreased libido, male sexual dysfunction, menstrual disorder, **renal failure**
Metabolic: hyperkalemia
Musculoskeletal: back, arm, leg pain, neck, or joint pain; hypertonia; myalgia; arthritis
Respiratory: cough, upper respiratory infection
Skin: rash, angioedema
Other: fever, viral infection, edema

Interactions
Drug-drug. *Antacids:* decreased perindopril absorption
Antihypertensives, general anesthetics, nitrates, phenothiazines: additive hypotension
Cyclosporine, heparin, indomethacin, potassium-sparing diuretics, potassium supplements: hyperkalemia
Diuretics: excessive hypotension
Lithium: increased lithium toxicity
Nonsteroidal anti-inflammatory drugs: blunted antihypertensive response
Drug-diagnostic tests. *Alanine aminotransferase, aspartate aminotransferase, blood urea nitrogen, creatinine, potassium, triglycerides:* increased levels
Hematocrit, hemoglobin: decreased values
Drug-food. *Salt substitutes containing potassium:* hyperkalemia
Drug-herb. *Capsaicin:* cough
Drug-behaviors. *Acute alcohol ingestion:* additive hypotension

Precautions
Use cautiously in:
• renal impairment, hepatic failure, renal artery stenosis, hyperkalemia, cough
• black patients with hypertension
• pregnant or breastfeeding patients
• children (safety not established).

P

Patient monitoring

• Assess blood pressure; dosage adjustments or concomitant diuretic use may cause severe hypotension.

• Monitor for angioedema, especially after first dose.

• Watch for signs and symptoms of infection, particularly EENT and respiratory infections.

• Monitor potassium level; watch for signs and symptoms of hyperkalemia.

• Monitor liver and kidney function tests before and during therapy.

• In black patients, watch closely for angioedema and monitor drug efficacy; monotherapy may be less effective in these patients.

Patient teaching

• Teach patient to take drug at same time each day, with or without food.

◀❧ Instruct patient to stop using drug and immediately report difficulty swallowing or breathing or hoarseness.

• Tell patient to avoid excessive perspiration or decreased fluid intake, which may cause symptomatic blood pressure drop. Inform him that vomiting or diarrhea may also decrease blood pressure.

• Teach patient to report signs and symptoms of infection.

• Advise patient not to use potassium-containing salt substitutes.

◀❧ Caution female patients of childbearing age to contact prescriber immediately if they suspect pregnancy.

• As appropriate, review all significant and life-threatening adverse reactions and interactions, especially those related to the drugs, tests, foods, herbs, and behaviors mentioned above.

perphenazine
Apo-Perphenazine✹, Phenazine✹, Trilafon

Pharmacologic class: Phenothiazine, dopaminergic antagonist
Therapeutic class: Antipsychotic, antiemetic
Pregnancy risk category NR

Action
Unknown; thought to antagonize dopamine and serotonin type 2 in CNS. Also antagonizes muscarinic receptors in the respiratory tract, providing cholinergic activation.

Availability
Injection: 5 mg/ml
Oral concentrate: 16 mg/5 ml
Tablets: 2 mg, 4 mg, 8 mg, 16 mg

⬆ Indications and dosages
➤ Psychosis in moderately disturbed nonhospitalized patients
Adults and children over age 12: Initially, 4 to 8 mg P.O. t.i.d.
➤ Psychosis in hospitalized patients
Adults and children over age 12: Initially, 8 to 16 mg P.O. two to four times daily, increased p.r.n.; avoid dosages above 64 mg daily. Or 5 to 10 mg deep I.M. injection q 6 hours p.r.n.
➤ Severe nausea and vomiting
Adults: 8 to 16 mg P.O. daily in divided doses, to a maximum of 24 mg; or 5 to 10 mg by deep I.M. injection p.r.n.; or up to 5 mg I.V. by slow injection or infusion.

Off-label uses
• Intractable hiccups

Contraindications
• Hypersensitivity to drug
• Blood dyscrasias

- Bone marrow depression
- Hepatic damage
- Subcortical damage
- Coma
- Concurrent use of high-dose CNS depressants

Administration
- Give oral forms with food to avoid GI upset.
- Dilute oral solution in water or fruit juice just before giving; use at least 60 ml of diluent for each 5 ml of oral solution.
- Avoid contact with oral or injection solution; contact dermatitis may occur.
- Give I.M injection deep into upper outer aspect of buttocks; massage site to prevent abscess.
- Know that I.V. route is rarely indicated and should be used only in recumbent hospitalized patients. For I.V. use, dilute with normal saline solution to a concentration of 0.5 mg/ml; give slowly at no more than 1 mg q 2 minutes.
- Replace parenteral therapy with oral therapy as soon as possible.

Route	Onset	Peak	Duration
P.O.	Variable	1-3 hours	Unknown
I.M., I.V.	5-10 min	1-2 hr	6 hr

Adverse reactions
CNS: drowsiness, insomnia, vertigo, headache, tremor, ataxia, slurring, exacerbation of psychotic symptoms, Parkinsonism, dystonias, akathisia, tardive dyskinesia, numbness and aching of arms and legs, hyperreflexia, cerebrospinal fluid abnormality, catatonic-like state, paranoid reactions, paradoxical stimulation, hyperactivity, nocturnal confusion, bizarre dreams, **seizures, neuroleptic malignant syndrome**
CV: hypotension, orthostatic hypotension, hypertension, dizziness, peripheral edema, ECG changes, tachycardia, bradycardia, **cardiac arrest, heart failure**

EENT: glaucoma, photophobia, blurred vision, miosis, mydriasis, corneal and lens deposits, pigmentary retinopathy, oculogyric crisis, nasal congestion, abnormal tongue color or movement, dysphagia
GI: nausea, vomiting, diarrhea, constipation, obstipation, anorexia, dry mouth, **adynamic ileus**
GU: urine retention, polyuria, dark urine, urinary frequency, urinary incontinence, bladder paralysis, galactorrhea, lactation, breast enlargement, menstrual irregularities, inhibited ejaculation, changes in libido, false-positive pregnancy test
Hematologic: eosinophilia, hemolytic anemia, **leukopenia, agranulocytosis, thrombocytopenic purpura**
Hepatic: jaundice, biliary stasis
Metabolic: hyperglycemia, hypoglycemia, hyponatremia, glycosuria, pituitary tumor, **syndrome of inappropriate antidiuretic hormone secretion**
Respiratory: dyspnea, suppressed cough reflex, asthma, **bronchospasm, laryngospasm, laryngeal edema**
Skin: urticaria, photosensitivity, pallor, erythema, eczema, pruritus, perspiration, pigmentation changes, angioedema, exfoliative dermatitis
Other: increased appetite, weight gain, fever, systemic lupus erythematosus-like syndrome, pain at I.M. site, hypersensitivity reactions including **anaphylactoid reaction**

Interactions
Drug-drug. *Anticholinergic drugs:* increased risk of anticholinergic adverse effects
CNS depressants: increased perphenazine effects, increased adverse CNS reactions
Tricyclic antidepressants: increased perphenazine blood level, greater risk of adverse effects
Drug-diagnostic tests. *Eosinophils, liver function tests:* increased values
Glucose: increased or decreased level

P

Granulocytes, hemoglobin, platelets, sodium, white blood cells: decreased levels
Pregnancy tests: false-positive result
Drug-herb. *Kava:* dystonic reactions
St. John's wort: photosensitivity
Yohimbe: yohimbe toxicity
Drug-behaviors. *Alcohol use:* increased CNS depression
Sun exposure: increased risk of photosensitivity reaction

Precautions

Use cautiously in:
• respiratory disorders, hepatic or renal dysfunction, breast cancer, alcohol withdrawal symptoms, suicidal tendencies, surgery
• patients taking CNS depressants or anticholinergics
• elderly patients
• pregnant or breastfeeding patients
• children younger than age 12.

Patient monitoring

◀€ Watch for anaphylactoid reaction and angioedema. Monitor neurologic status; stay alert for signs and symptoms of neuroleptic malignant syndrome (high fever, sweating, unstable blood pressure, stupor, muscle rigidity, and autonomic dysfunction), Parkinson-like symptoms, and catatonic-like state.
• Assess blood pressure and heart rate continuously during I.V. use; monitor cardiovascular status and vital signs periodically.
• Evaluate respiratory status, especially for dyspnea and airway spasms.
• Monitor complete blood count, glucose level, and liver function tests; watch for signs and symptoms of blood dyscrasias.

Patient teaching

• Explain importance of combining drug therapy with psychotherapy.
• Teach patient to take drug exactly as prescribed and to report adverse reactions promptly.

• Instruct patient to avoid sun exposure and to wear sunscreen outdoors to prevent photosensitivity reactions.
• Advise patient to consult prescriber before taking other prescription drugs or over-the-counter preparations.
• Caution patient to avoid driving and other hazardous activities until he knows how drug affects him.
• Advise patient to avoid alcohol, smoking, caffeine, and herbs.
• As appropriate, review all other significant and life-threatening adverse reactions and interactions, especially those related to the drugs, tests, herbs, and behaviors mentioned above.

phenazopyridine hydrochloride

Azo-Standard, Baridium, Geridium, Phenazo✣, Prodium, Pyridiate, Pyridium, Urogesic, UTI Relief

Pharmacologic class: Nonopioid analgesic
Therapeutic class: Urinary analgesic
Pregnancy risk category B

Action

Unknown; thought to act locally on urinary tract mucosa to produce analgesic or anesthetic effects, relieving burning, urgency, and frequency

Availability

Tablets: 95 mg, 97.2 mg, 100 mg, 150 mg, 200 mg

🔘 Indications and dosages

➤ Pain caused by irritation of lower urinary tract mucosa
Adults: 200 mg P.O. t.i.d.

Contraindications

• Hypersensitivity to drug
• Renal insufficiency

Administration
- Give with or after meals.
- Discontinue drug after 2 days, as prescribed, when given in combination with antibiotics.

Route	Onset	Peak	Duration
P.O.	Unknown	Unknown	6-8 hr

Adverse reactions
CNS: headache, vertigo
EENT: staining of contact lenses
GI: GI disturbances
GU: bright orange urine, **renal toxicity**
Hepatic: hepatotoxicity
Hematologic: hemolytic anemia, **methemoglobinemia**
Skin: rash
Other: anaphylactoid reaction

Interactions
Drug-diagnostic tests. *Bilirubin, glucose, ketones, protein, steroids:* interference with urine tests based on spectrophotometry or color reactions

Precautions
Use cautiously in:
- hepatitis
- pregnant or breastfeeding patients
- children younger than age 12.

Patient monitoring
- Monitor patient for symptomatic improvement of urinary tract infection (UTI).
- Assess follow-up urine culture after antibiotic therapy ends.

Patient teaching
- Explain drug therapy and measures to help prevent repeat UTIs.
- Inform patient that drug may discolor urine and tears and may stain clothing and contact lenses.
- ◄ Advise patient to promptly contact prescriber if symptoms don't improve or if skin or eyes become yellow.
- As appropriate, review all other significant and life-threatening adverse

reactions and interactions, especially those related to the tests mentioned above.

phenelzine sulfate
Nardil

Pharmacologic class: Monoamine oxidase (MAO) inhibitor
Therapeutic class: Antidepressant
Pregnancy risk category C

Action
Nonselectively inhibits metabolism of monoamine oxidase, an enzyme that increases accumulation of endogenous epinephrine, norepinephrine, and serotonin in CNS storage sites

Availability
Tablets: 15 mg

⚠ Indications and dosages
➤ Neurotic and atypical depression (usually used in conjunction with psychotherapy in patients who don't respond to more commonly prescribed drugs)
Adults: Initially, 15 mg P.O. t.i.d.; may increase rapidly to at least 60 mg/day, then 90 mg/day if needed based on patient tolerance. After adequate response occurs, reduce dosage slowly to a maintenance dosage of 15 mg daily.

Contraindications
- Hypersensitivity to drug
- Renal impairment
- Pheochromocytoma
- Heart failure or other cardiovascular disease
- Abnormal liver function tests
- History of headache
- Concurrent use of sympathomimetic drugs, guanethidine, dextromethor-

phan, CNS depressants, buspirone, or serotonergic drugs
• Consumption of tyramine-rich foods

Administration

◀€ If hypertensive crisis occurs, discontinue drug immediately and give phentolamine 5 mg I.V. slowly as ordered.

◀€ Ask patient about other drugs he's using; MAO inhibitors can cause dangerous interactions with many drugs.

Route	Onset	Peak	Duration
P.O.	Unknown	2-6 hr	Variable

Adverse reactions

CNS: dizziness, headache, drowsiness, hyperreflexia, hypersomnia, tremors, muscle twitching, fatigue, insomnia, palilalia, euphoria, paresthesia, ataxia, toxic delirium, manic reaction, acute anxiety reaction, precipitation of schizophrenia, **shock-like coma, seizures**
CV: orthostatic hypotension, edema, **hypertensive crisis, arrhythmias**
GI: nausea, vomiting, diarrhea, constipation, GI disturbances, epigastric or abdominal pain, dry mouth
GU: urinary retention, sexual disturbances
Hematologic: leukopenia
Hepatic: elevated serum transaminase levels, jaundice, **fatal progressive necrotizing hepatocellular disease**
Metabolic: hypernatremia, hypermetabolic syndrome
Skin: pruritus, rash, sweating
Other: weight changes, fever, lupuslike syndrome, edema

Interactions

Drug-drug. *Amphetamines, dextromethorphan, CNS depressants, dibenzazepine derivatives, other MAO inhibitors, serotonergic agents (such as fluoxetine, fluvoxamine, paroxetine, sertraline):* hypertensive crisis, seizures, fever, diaphoresis, excitation, delirium, tremor, coma, circulatory collapse

Antidepressants, buspirone: hypertension
Antihypertensives, beta blockers, thiazide diuretics: increased hypotensive effects
Dextromethorphan, tryptophan: hypertension, excitation, hyperpyrexia
Epinephrine, guanadrel, guanethidine, norepinephrine, reserpine, vasoconstrictors: hypertensive crisis
Insulin, oral hypoglycemics: additive hypoglycemia
Drug-diagnostic tests. *Sodium, transaminases:* increased levels
White blood cells: decreased count
Drug-food. *Aged, pickled, fermented, or smoked foods; wine; alcohol-free wine and beer; broad bean pods; cheese (except cottage and cream cheese); excessive amounts of chocolate and caffeine; dry sausage (including hard salami, pepperoni, and Lebanon bologna); foods containing L-tryptophan (such as dairy foods, soy, poultry, and meat); liver; spoiled, improperly refrigerated, handled, or stored protein-rich foods; yeast extract; yogurt:* hypertensive crisis
Drug-herb. *Ephedra, L-tryptophan:* hypertensive crisis
Drug-behaviors. *Alcohol use:* hypertensive crisis

Precautions

Use cautiously in:
• hyperthyroidism, seizure disorders, hypotension, hypomania, diabetes mellitus, hepatic complications, myocardial ischemia
• patients who are switching MAO inhibitors
• suicidal or drug-dependent patients
• elderly patients
• pregnant or breastfeeding patients
• children younger than age 16.

Patient monitoring

• Monitor blood pressure; drug may cause hypertensive crisis.
• Assess patient for symptomatic improvement.

• Monitor complete blood count, liver function studies, and blood glucose level before and during therapy.

Patient teaching
• Explain importance of taking drug exactly as prescribed.
• Teach patient to discontinue drug at least 10 days before elective surgery.
• Emphasize importance of avoiding certain foods, beverages, prescription drugs, and over-the-counter preparations during therapy and for 14 days afterward. Ask pharmacist to provide patient with complete list.
◀€ Instruct patient to immediately report occipital headache, palpitations, stiff neck, nausea, sweating, dilated pupils, and photophobia (indications of hypertensive crisis).
• Advise patient to rise slowly from a lying or sitting position to avoid dizziness.
• Caution patient to avoid driving and other hazardous activities until he knows how drug affects concentration, vision, and alertness.
• As appropriate, review all other significant and life-threatening adverse reactions and interactions, especially those related to the drugs, tests, foods, herbs, and behaviors mentioned above.

phenobarbital
Luminal, Solfoton

phenobarbital sodium
Luminal Sodium

Pharmacologic class: Barbiturate
Therapeutic class: Anticonvulsant, sedative-hypnotic, anxiolytic
Controlled substance schedule IV
Pregnancy risk category D

Action
Interferes with gamma-aminobutyric acid receptors, blocking nerve impulse transmission in the CNS, depressing the sensory cortex, thereby reducing motor activity and raising seizure threshold

Availability
Capsules: 16 mg
Elixir: 15 mg/5 ml, 20 mg/5 ml
Injection: 30 mg/ml and 60 mg/ml in 1-ml prefilled syringes; 65 mg/ml in 1-ml vials; 130 mg/ml in 1-ml prefilled syringes, 1-ml vials, and 1-ml ampules
Tablets: 15 mg, 16 mg, 30 mg, 60 mg, 100 mg

🖊 Indications and dosages
➤ Tonic-clonic (grand mal) and partial seizures; febrile seizures in children
Adults: 60 to 100 mg/day P.O. as a single dose or in two or three divided doses; or initially, 100 to 320 mg I.V. p.r.n. (a total of 600 mg I.V. in a 24-hour period).
➤ Sedation or hypnotic effect
Adults: For sedation, 30 to 120 mg/day P.O. in two or three divided doses or 30 to 120 mg/day I.M. or I.V. in two or three divided doses. As a hypnotic, 100 to 200 mg P.O. at bedtime or 100 to 320 mg I.M. or I.V. at bedtime.
➤ Preoperative sedative
Adults: 100 to 200 mg I.M. 60 to 90 minutes before surgery
Dosage adjustment
• Impaired hepatic or renal function
• Elderly or debilitated patients
• Children

Off-label uses
• Prevention and treatment of hyperbilirubinemia

Contraindications
• Hypersensitivity to drug or other barbiturates
• Marked hepatic impairment
• Nephritis

- Severe respiratory disease with dyspnea or obstruction
- History of sedative-hypnotic abuse

Administration

- Inject I.M. deep into large muscle mass.
- Give I.V. at a maximum rate of 60 mg/minute; make sure resuscitation equipment is available.

◀️ Stop injection immediately if patient complains of pain or if circulation at injection site diminishes; inadvertent intra-arterial injection may have occurred.

Route	Onset	Peak	Duration
P.O.	30-60 min	Unknown	10-16 hr
I.V.	5 min	30 min	10-16 hr
I.M., S.C.	10-30 min	Unknown	10-16 hr

Adverse reactions

CNS: delirium, depression, drowsiness, excitation, lethargy, agitation, confusion, hyperkinesia, ataxia, vertigo, CNS depression, nightmares, nervousness, paradoxical stimulation, abnormal thinking, hallucinations, insomnia, anxiety, dizziness, headache
CV: hypotension, syncope, **bradycardia** (with I.V. use)
GI: nausea, vomiting, constipation
Hematologic: megaloblastic anemia
Hepatic: hepatic damage
Musculoskeletal: joint pain, myalgia
Respiratory: hypoventilation, **laryngospasm, bronchospasm, apnea** (with I.V. use); **respiratory depression**
Skin: photosensitivity, rash, urticaria
Other: physical or psychological drug dependence, phlebitis at I.V. site, hypersensitivity reactions including **angioedema, serum sickness, Stevens-Johnson syndrome**

Interactions

Drug-drug. *Acetaminophen:* increased risk of hepatotoxicity

Activated charcoal: decreased phenobarbital absorption
Anticoagulants, beta blockers (except timolol), carbamazepine, clonazepam, corticosteroids, digoxin, doxorubicin, doxycycline, felodipine, fenoprofen, griseofulvin, hormonal contraceptives, metronidazole, quinidine, theophylline, verapamil: decreased efficacy of these drugs
Chloramphenicol, hydantoins, narcotics: increased or decreased effects of these drugs or phenobarbital
Cyclophosphamide: increased risk of hematologic toxicity
Divalproex, monoamine oxidase inhibitors, valproic acid: decreased phenobarbital metabolism, increased sedative effect
Other CNS depressants (including first-generation antihistamines, opioids, other sedative-hypnotics): additive CNS depression
Rifampin: increased phenobarbital metabolism and decreased effects
Drug-diagnostic tests. *Bilirubin:* decreased level in neonates and patients with seizure disorders or congenital nonhemolytic unconjugated hyperbilirubinemia
Drug-herb. *Chamomile, hops, kava, skullcap, valerian:* increased CNS depression
St. John's wort: decreased drug effects
Drug-behaviors. *Alcohol use:* additive CNS effects, death
Sun exposure: photophobia

Precautions

Use cautiously in:
- hepatic dysfunction, renal impairment, seizure disorder, fever, hyperthyroidism, diabetes mellitus, severe anemia, pulmonary or cardiac disease
- history of suicide attempt or drug abuse

- chronic use
- elderly and debilitated patients
- pregnant or breastfeeding patients
- children under age 6.

Patient monitoring

- Monitor vital signs; watch for bradycardia and hypotension.

◀≣ In patients with seizure disorder, be aware that drug withdrawal may cause status epilepticus.

- Assess neurologic status; institute safety measures as needed.
- Closely monitor respiratory status, especially for respiratory depression and airway spasms.
- Monitor phenobarbital blood level and liver function tests.
- Watch for signs of drug dependence.

Patient teaching

◀≣ Instruct patient to promptly report rash, facial and lip edema, syncope, dyspnea, or depression.

◀≣ Stress importance of taking drug exactly as prescribed, with or without food; caution patient not to stop therapy abruptly, especially if he's taking drug to treat seizures.

- Caution patient that prolonged use may lead to dependence.
- Instruct patient to seek medical advice before taking other prescription or over-the-counter drugs.
- Caution patient to avoid driving and other hazardous activities until he knows how drug affect him.
- Advise patient to avoid alcohol.
- As appropriate, review all other significant and life-threatening adverse reactions and interactions, especially those related to the drugs, tests, herbs, and behaviors mentioned above.

phentolamine mesylate
Regitine, Rogitine ♣

Pharmacologic class: Alpha-adrenergic blocker

Therapeutic class: Diagnostic agent, antihypertensive agent in pheochromocytoma

Pregnancy risk category C

Action
Competively blocks postsynaptic (alpha$_1$) and presynaptic (alpha$_2$) adrenergic receptors; acts on arterial tree and venous bed, reducing total peripheral resistance and lowering venous return to heart

Availability
Injection: 5 mg/vial
Powder for injection: 5 mg

🕭 Indications and dosages
➤ To prevent or control hypertensive episodes before or during pheochromocytomectomy
Adults: Inject 5 mg I.V. or I.M. 1 to 2 hours before surgery; then 5 mg I.V. during surgery as indicated.
➤ To aid diagnosis of pheochromocytoma
Adults: 2.5 or 5 mg (in 1 ml of sterile water) by I.V. injection; record blood pressure q 30 seconds for 3 minutes, then q minute for the next 7 minutes. Or 5 mg (in 1 ml sterile water) I.M.; record blood pressure q 5 minutes for 30 to 45 minutes.
➤ Prevention and treatment of dermal necrosis after extravasation of norepinephrine
Adults: For prevention, add 10 mg to each liter of I.V. solution containing norepinephrine. For treatment, inject 5 to 10 mg in 10 ml of normal saline so-

P

lution into area of extravasation within 12 hours.

Off-label uses
• Hypertensive crisis caused by monoamine oxidase inhibitor use
• Rebound hypertension caused by withdrawal of clonidine, propranolol, or other antihypertensives
• Impotence (given with papaverine)

Contraindications
• Hypersensitivity to drug
• Coronary artery disease
• Myocardial infarction
• Coronary insufficiency
• Angina

Administration
• Reconstitute powder by diluting with 1 ml of sterile water for injection.
• When treating extravasation, infiltrate area with solution. Make sure treatment occurs within 12 hours of extravasation.
• For pheochromocytoma diagnosis, withhold sedatives, analgesics, and nonessential drugs for 24 to 72 hours before test (until blood pressure returns to hypertensive level). Keep patient supine until blood pressure stabilizes; then rapidly inject drug I.V. Maximum effect usually occurs within 2 minutes of administration.

Route	Onset	Peak	Duration
I.V., I.M.	Immediate	Unknown	Brief

Adverse reactions
CNS: weakness, dizziness
CV: tachycardia, acute and prolonged hypotension, **arrhythmias**
EENT: nasal congestion
GI: nausea, vomiting, diarrhea
Skin: flushing

Interactions
Drug-drug. *Ephedrine, epinephrine:* antagonism of these drugs' effects

Drug-herb. *Ephedra:* antagonism of vasoconstrictive effects

Precautions
Use cautiously in:
• patients receiving cardiac glycosides concurrently
• pregnant and breastfeeding patients.

Patient monitoring
• When using for norepinephrine extravasation, monitor injection site closely and assess blood pressure, heart rate, and respiratory rate.
• For pheochromocytoma diagnosis, monitor blood pressure; patients with pheochromocytoma show an immediate, steep drop in systolic and diastolic pressures. Monitor and record blood pressure immediately after injection, at 30-second intervals for first 3 minutes, and at 1-minute intervals for next 7 minutes. Systolic decrease of 60 mmHg and diastolic decrease of 25 mmHg within 2 minutes after I.V. administration indicates a positive reaction for pheochromocytoma.

Patient teaching
• Explain drug administration procedure.
◀€ Instruct patient to promptly report adverse reactions; assure him he'll be monitored closely.
• Tell patient to withhold other medications (especially sedatives and analgesics) for at least 24 hours before pheochromocytoma testing, if appropriate.
• Advise patient to avoid ephedra (ma huang).
• As appropriate, review all other significant adverse reactions and interactions, especially those related to the drugs and herbs mentioned above.

phenylephrine hydrochloride

Afrin Children's Pump Mist, AH-Chew D, Coricidin, Dioephrine✤, Neo-Synephrine, Rhinall, Vicks Sinex Ultra Fine Mist

Pharmacologic class: Sympatho-mimetic, alpha-adrenergic agonist

Therapeutic class: Vasopressor, nasal decongestant, ophthalmic vasoconstrictor

Pregnancy risk category C

Action

Stimulates alpha-adrenergic receptors, producing pronounced vasoconstriction and increasing blood pressure. Produces vasoconstriction in skin, mucous membranes, and mucosa; produces mydriasis by contracting pupillary dilator muscle.

Availability

Injection: 10 mg/ml
Nasal solution: 0.125%, 0.25%, 0.5%, 1%
Tablets (chewable): 10 mg

💊 Indications and dosages

➤ Mild to moderate hypotension
Adults: 1 to 10 mg S.C. or I.M., not to exceed an initial dosage of 5 mg
➤ Severe hypotension and shock
Adults: 0.1 to 0.18 mg/minute I.V. infusion. Maintainance infusion is 40 to 60 mcg/minute.
➤ To prevent hypotension during spinal anesthesia
Adults: 2 to 3 mg S.C. or I.M. 3 to 4 minutes before injection of spinal anesthetic
➤ Hypotensive emergency during spinal anesthesia
Adults: 0.2 mg I.V., up to a maximum of 0.5 mg/dose

➤ To prolong spinal anesthesia
Adults: 2 to 5 mg added to anesthetic solution (increases duration of spinal block up to 50%)
➤ Vasoconstrictor for regional anesthesia
Adults: 1 mg of phenylephrine added to every 20 ml of local anesthetic solution
➤ Paroxysmal supraventricular tachycardia
Adults: 0.5 mg by rapid I.V. injection, not to exceed an initial dosage of 0.5 mg. Subsequent dosages (determined by blood pressure) shouldn't exceed preceding dosage by more than 0.1 to 0.2 mg; maximum dosage is 1 mg.
➤ Nasal congestion
Adults: One or two sprays of 0.25% or 0.5% solution in each nostril q 3 to 4 hours p.r.n.; in severe cases, 1% solution may be needed. Or 10 mg to 20 mg (chewable tablets) P.O. q 4 hours.

Dosage adjustment
• Elderly patients

Contraindications

• Hypersensitivity to drug
• Severe hypertension
• Ventricular tachycardia

p

Administration

• In emergencies, drug may be given by direct I.V. injection; dilute 1 ml of solution containing 10 mg/ml with 9 ml of sterile water for injection.
◀€ For I.V. infusion, dilute 10 mg in 500 ml of dextrose 5% in water or normal saline solution; titrate dosage until blood pressure is slightly below patient's normal blood pressure or until maximum dosage is reached. Infuse I.V. in large vein (preferably through central venous catheter) using an infusion pump. After condition stabilizes, taper dosage gradually; do not withdraw abruptly. Avoid extravasation.

Route	Onset	Peak	Duration
P.O.	Unknown	Unknown	Unknown
I.V.	Immediate	Unknown	15-20 min
I.M., S.C.	10-15 min	Unknown	0.5-2 hr
Nasal	15-20 min	Unknown	0.5-4 hr

Adverse reactions

CNS: anxiety, restlessness, tremor, headache, light-headedness, dizziness, drowsiness, insomnia, hallucinations, nervousness, restlessness, giddiness, prolonged psychosis, weakness, photophobia, orofacial dystonia
CV: hypertension, palpitations, tachycardia, bradycardia, **arrhythmias**
GI: nausea, vomiting, gastric irritation, anorexia
GU: urinary retention (in males with prostatitis)
Hematologic: leukopenia, agranulocytosis, thrombocytopenia
Respiratory: asthmatic episodes
Skin: sweating, rash, urticaria, contact dermatitis, necrosis and sloughing (with extravasation at I.V. site)

Interactions

Drug-drug. *Beta blockers:* blocked cardiostimulatory effects of phenylephrine
Bretylium, sympathomimetics: serious arrhythmias
Furazolidone: excessive hypertension
Guanethidine, methyldopa: decreased antihypertensive effects
Halogenated hydrocarbon anesthetics: serious arrhythmias
Monoamine oxidase inhibitors: severe headache, hypertension, hyperpyrexia
Oxytocics, tricyclic antidepressants: increased pressor response
Drug-behaviors. *Sun exposure:* photophobia

Precautions

Use cautiously in:
• hyperthyroidism, partial heart block, bradycardia, hypertension, cardiac dis-ease, arteriosclerosis, unstable vasomotor syndrome
• elderly patients
• pregnant or breastfeeding patients.

Patient monitoring

• Monitor ECG continuously during I.V. administration; monitor blood pressure every 5 to 15 minutes until it stabilizes, and then every 30 to 60 minutes.
• Monitor central venous pressure and fluid intake and output; keep in mind that drug doesn't eliminate need for fluid resuscitation.
• Assess complete blood count; watch for signs and symptoms of blood dyscrasias.
• Monitor I.V. site; extravasation can cause tissue damage.
• Assess for symptomatic improvement in patients using nasal preparations.
◀€ Monitor patient for adverse reactions, particularly life-threatening asthmatic episodes.

Patient teaching

• Teach patient to take drug exactly as directed and not to exceed recommended dosage.
• Tell patient using nasal solution that dropper, inhaler, or spray dispenser shouldn't be used by more than one person. Teach proper instillation technique: Instill nasal solution into dependent nostril with head down in a lateral position; stay in this position for 5 minutes, and then instill solution in other nostril in same manner. Advise patient to rinse container tip with hot water after each use. Instruct him to discontinue use and contact prescriber if symptoms don't improve after 3 days.
• As appropriate, review all significant and life-threatening adverse reactions and interactions, especially those related to the drugs and behaviors mentioned above.

phenytoin
(diphenylhydantoin)
Dilantin-125, Dilantin Infatabs

phenytoin sodium
(diphenylhydantoin
sodium)
Dilantin Kapseals, Diphenylan♣,
Phenytek♣

Pharmacologic class: Hydantoin
derivative
Therapeutic class: Anticonvulsant
Pregnancy risk category D

Action
Unknown; limits seizure activity, possibly by promoting sodium efflux from
neurons in motor cortex during nerve
impulse generation; reduces activity in
brain stem centers responsible for tonic phase of tonic-clonic seizures

Availability
Capsules (prompt-release): 30 mg,
100 mg
Capsules (extended-release): 30 mg,
100 mg
Injection: 50 mg/ml in 2- and 5-ml
ampules
Oral suspension: 30 mg/5 ml, 125 mg/
5 ml
Tablets (chewable): 50 mg

💊 Indications and dosages
➤ Status epilepticus
Adults: Loading dose of 10 to 15 mg/
kg by slow I.V., followed by maintenance dosage of 100 mg P.O. or I.V. q 6
to 8 hours
Neonates and children: Loading dose
of 15 to 20 mg/kg I.V. in divided doses
of 5 to 10 mg/kg

➤ To control generalized tonic-clonic
(grand mal) and complex partial (psychomotor, temporal lobe) seizures
Adults: Loading dose of 1 g P.O.
(extended-release) in three divided
doses at 2-hour intervals, or 1 g P.O.
(extended-release) daily in three divided doses; usual maintenance dosage is
600 mg/day starting 24 hours after
loading dose.
Children: Initially, 5 mg/kg/day P.O. in
two or three equally divided doses;
maintenance dosage is individualized
and given in two to three divided doses
(not to exceed 300 mg/day).
➤ To prevent seizures during neurosurgery
Adults: 100 to 200 mg I.M. at 4-hour
intervals during surgery and postoperatively

Off-label uses
- Arrhythmias
- Severe preeclampsia
- Trigeminal neuralgia
- Recessive dystrophic epidermolysis
bullosa, junctional epidermolysis bul-
losa

Contraindications
- Hypersensitivity to drug
- Sinus bradycardia, sinoatrial block,
second- or third-degree atrioventricular (AV) block, Adams-Stokes syndrome

Administration
- Before I.V. use, check designated line
for patency and flush with normal
saline solution. Administer no faster
than 50 mg/minute; afterward, flush
with normal saline solution. Avoid extravasation, which can cause severe tissue damage.
🔊 Don't administer I.V. into dorsal
hand veins; purple glove syndrome
may occur.
- If giving oral solution through nasogastric (NG) tube, dilute dose with
sterile water or normal saline solution;

after administration, flush tube with at least 20 ml of diluent.
- Withhold enteral feedings for at least 1 hour before and 1 hour after oral administration.
- Administer I.M. only as a last resort (may cause pain and is poorly absorbed).
- If rash occurs, withhold drug and notify prescriber.

Route	Onset	Peak	Duration
P.O.	Unknown	3 hr	6-12 hr
P.O. (extended)	Unknown	4-12 hr	12-36 hr
I.V.	Unknown	Rapid	12-24 hr
I.M.	Unknown	Erratic	12-24 hr

Adverse reactions

CNS: ataxia, slurred speech, confusion, agitation, depression, dizziness, drowsiness, dysarthria, dyskinesia, extrapyramidal symptoms, fatigue, headache, insomnia, irritability, twitching, nervousness, numbness, psychotic disturbances, tremor, weakness, CNS depression (with I.V. use), **coma**
CV: vasodilation, edema, chest pain, **tachycardia, hypotension** (increased with I.V. use), **cardiovascular collapse** (with I.V. use)
EENT: diplopia, amblyopia, nystagmus, visual field defect, eye pain, conjunctivitis, photophobia, mydriasis, hearing loss, tinnitus, ear pain, sinusitis, rhinitis, epistaxis, lip enlargement, altered taste
GI: nausea, vomiting, diarrhea, constipation, gingival hyperplasia, dry mouth
GU: pink, red, or reddish-brown urine; gynecomastia; Peyronie's disease
Hepatic: jaundice, **toxic hepatitis, liver damage**
Hematologic: macrocytosis, megaloblastic anemia, eosinophilia, monocytosis, leukocytosis, simple anemia, hemolytic anemia, **thrombocytopenia,**

agranulocytosis, granulocytopenia, leukopenia, pancytopenia
Metabolic: hypocalcemia, diabetes insipidus, hyperglycemia, decreased serum thyroxine and free thyroxine levels
Musculoskeletal: back pain, osteomalacia, pelvic pain
Respiratory: pneumonia, pharyngitis, hyperventilation, apnea, aspiration pneumonia, asthma, dyspnea, increased cough and sputum, hypoxia, hemoptysis, bronchitis, chest pain, **pulmonary fibrosis, atelectasis, pneumothorax**
Skin: hypertrichosis, rash, pruritus, hirsutism, alopecia, bruising, exfoliative dermatitis
Other: fever, lymphadenopathy, weight gain or loss, injection site reaction, coarsened facial features, lupus erythematosus syndrome, allergic reactions, **Stevens-Johnson syndrome**

Interactions

Drug-drug. *Acetaminophen, amiodarone, carbamazepine, cardiac glycosides, corticosteroids, dicumarol, disopyramide, doxycycline, estrogens, haloperidol, hormonal contraceptives, methadone, metapyrone, mexiletine, quinidine, theophylline, valproic acid:* increased metabolism and decreased effects of these drugs
Activated charcoal, antacids, sucralfate: decreased phenytoin absorption
Allopurinol, amiodarone, benzodiazepines, chloramphenicol, cimetidine, disulfiram, fluconazole, isoniazid, metronidazole, miconazole, omeprazole, phenacemide, phenylbutazone, succinimides, sulfonamides, trimethoprim, valproic acid: inhibited phenytoin metabolism and increased effects
Antineoplastics, folic acid, influenza vaccine, loxapine, nitrofurantoin, pyridoxine: decreased phenytoin effects
Barbiturates, carbamazepine, diazoxide, rifampin, theophylline: increased

phenytoin metabolism and decreased effects

Chlorpheniramine, ibuprofen, phenothiazines: increased phenytoin effects
Cyclosporine, dopamine, furosemide, levodopa, levonorgestrel, mebendazole, muscle relaxants, nondepolarizing phenothiazines, sulfonylureas: decreased effects of these drugs
Salicylates, tricyclic antidepressants, valproic acid: phenytoin displacement, increased phenytoin effects
Drug-diagnostic tests. *Alkaline phosphatase, gamma-glutamyltransferase, glucose:* increased levels
Dexamethasone (1-mg) suppression test, metyrapone test: interference with test results
Free thyroxine, serum thyroxine: decreased levels
Drug-food. *Enteral tube feedings:* decreased phenytoin absorption
Folic acid: decreased folic acid absorption
Drug-behaviors. *Acute alcohol ingestion:* increased phenytoin blood level
Chronic alcohol ingestion: decreased phenytoin blood level

Precautions
Use cautiously in:
• hepatic disease, skin rash, diabetes mellitus
• pregnant or breastfeeding patients (safety not established).

Patient monitoring
• Assess blood pressure, ECG, and heart rate, especially during I.V. loading dose; watch for adverse reactions.
• Monitor phenytoin blood level; therapeutic range is 10 to 20 mcg/ml.
• Evaluate complete blood count and kidney and liver function tests.
• Closely monitor prothrombin time and Internationalized Normal Ratio in patients receiving warfarin concurrently.
• Monitor drug efficacy.

Patient teaching
• Explain drug therapy, need for follow-up tests, and importance of taking drug exactly as prescribed.
• Caution patient not to stop therapy abruptly.
• Advise patient to refrain from alcohol use.
◀╢ Instruct patient to report rash immediately.
• Inform patient that drug may discolor urine.
• Caution female patient that drug may make hormonal contraceptives ineffective.
• Teach patient to practice good dental hygiene to minimize gingival hyperplasia.
• Encourage patient to seek medical advice before taking over-the-counter preparations.
• As appropriate, review all other significant and life-threatening adverse reactions and interactions, especially those related to the drugs, tests, foods, and behaviors mentioned above.

pimozide
Orap

Pharmacologic class: Diphenylbutylpiperidine
Therapeutic class: Antipsychotic
Pregnancy risk category C

Action
Unknown; thought to dopaminergic receptors on neurons in CNS, relieving tics

Availability
Tablets: 1 mg, 2 mg

Indications and dosages
➤ Suppression of motor and phonic tics in patients with Tourette syndrome

who are unresponsive to first-line therapy

Adults: Initially, 1 to 2 mg P.O. daily in divided doses, increased every other day p.r.n. Maintenance dosage is less than 0.2 mg/kg/day or 10 mg/day (whichever is smaller).

Contraindications
- Hypersensitivity to drug
- Severe toxic CNS depression
- Congenital long-QT syndrome
- History of arrhythmias
- Concurrent use of itraconazole, ketoconazole, macrolide antibiotics, protease inhibitors, nefazodone, other drugs that prolong the QT interval, or other drugs known to cause motor and phonic tics

Administration
- Give with or without food.
- To minimize daytime sedation, entire daily dose may be given at bedtime.

Route	Onset	Peak	Duration
P.O.	Unknown	6-8 hr	Unknown

Adverse reactions
CNS: Parkinsonian-like symptoms, drowsiness, headache, insomnia, dizziness, akathisia, rigidity, speech disorder, handwriting changes, tardive dyskinesia, sedation, depression, excitement, nervousness, abnormal dreams, hyperkinesia, torticollis, tremor, **neuroleptic malignant syndrome**
CV: abnormal ECG, hypotension, orthostatic hypotension, hypertension, palpitations, chest pain, tachycardia, **prolonged QT interval**
EENT: visual disturbance, perception of spots before eyes, photosensitivity, decreased visual accommodation, excessive salivation, taste changes
GI: nausea, vomiting, diarrhea, constipation, eructation, dysphagia, dry mouth

GU: urinary frequency, menstrual disorder, breast secretions, impotence, loss of libido
Musculoskeletal: muscle cramps, muscle tightness, stooped posture
Skin: rash, skin irritation, sweating
Other: thirst, weight gain or loss, increased appetite

Interactions
Drug-drug. *Amphetamines, methylphenidate, pemoline:* tics
Antiarrhythmics, azole antifungals, macrolide antibiotics, phenothiazines, protease inhibitors, tricyclic antidepressants: ECG abnormalities
Anticholinergics: increased anticholinergic effects
CNS depressants: additive CNS depression
Drug-diagnostic tests. *ECG:* abnormalities
Drug-food. *Grapefruit juice:* inhibited pimozide metabolism
Drug-behaviors. *Alcohol use:* increased CNS depression

Precautions
Use cautiously in:
- history of seizures, cardiovascular disorders, hepatic or renal dysfunction, ECG abnormalities
- disorders that could be worsened by adverse anticholinergic effects
- pregnant or breastfeeding patients
- children younger than age 12.

Patient monitoring
◀€ Assess neurologic status, especially for signs and symptoms of neuroleptic malignant syndrome (high fever, sweating, unstable blood pressure, stupor, muscle rigidity, and autonomic dysfunction) and Parkinsonian-like symptoms.
- Monitor for tardive dyskinesia, even after drug therapy ends.
- Assess vital signs and ECG; stay alert for prolonged QT interval, hypertension, or orthostatic hypotension.

Patient teaching

• Tell patient he can take drug with or without food, but shouldn't take it grapefruit juice.

• Caution patient not to stop taking drug suddenly; dosage must be tapered.

◀╪ Teach patient to recognize and immediately report signs and symptoms of neuroleptic malignant syndrome and tardive dyskinesia. Tell patient that tardive dyskinesia may develop long after drug therapy ends.

• Instruct patient to rise slowly and carefully because drug may cause a temporary blood pressure drop if he stands up suddenly.

• Advise patient that drug may cause impotence and loss of libido; encourage him to discuss these problems with prescriber.

• Tell patient that drug may cause appetite changes; encourage good dietary practices.

• Caution patient that drug may cause vision changes and photosensitivity, which he should report.

• Instruct patient not to drink alcohol or grapefruit juice while taking drug.

• Caution patient to avoid driving and other hazardous activities until he knows how drug affects concentration, vision, and alertness.

• As appropriate, review all other significant and life-threatening adverse reactions and interactions, especially those related to the drugs, tests, foods, and behaviors mentioned above.

pindolol
Apo-Pindol✦, Novo-Pindol✦, Nu-Pindol✦, Visken

Pharmacologic class: Beta-adrenergic blocker (nonselective)
Therapeutic class: Antihypertensive
Pregnancy risk category B

Action

Competes with beta-adrenergic agonists for available receptor sites, inhibiting both beta$_1$ (myocardial) and beta$_2$ (respiratory) sites. Inhibits chronotropic, inotropic, and vasodilator responses to beta-adrenergic stimulation.

Availability

Tablets: 5 mg, 10 mg

⧉ Indications and dosages

➤ Hypertension

Adults: Initially, 5 mg b.i.d.; may increase by 10 mg/day q 3 to 4 weeks p.r.n., up to a maximum of 60 mg/day.

Contraindications

• Overt heart failure
• Cardiogenic shock
• Severe bradycardia
• Second- or third-degree heart block
• Bronchial asthma

Administration

• Give with or without food.
• Know that drug may be used alone or with other antihypertensives.

Route	Onset	Peak	Duration
P.O.	Rapid	1 hr	8-15 hr

Adverse reactions

CNS: lethargy, weakness, anxiety, depression, dizziness, drowsiness, insomnia, nervousness, paresthesia
CV: orthostatic hypotension, peripheral vasoconstriction, chest pain, palpitations, tachycardia, bradycardia, **heart failure**
EENT: blurred vision, dry eyes
GI: nausea, vomiting, constipation, diarrhea
GU: impotence, decreased libido
Musculoskeletal: joint pain, back pain, muscle cramps
Metabolic: hyperglycemia, hypoglycemia

P

Respiratory: wheezing, dyspnea, **bronchospasm**
Skin: itching, rash
Other: drug-induced lupus syndrome, edema, cold extremities

Interactions
Drug-drug. *Amphetamines, ephedrine, epinephrine, norepinephrine, phenylephrine, pseudoephedrine:* unopposed alpha-adrenergic stimulation, causing excessive hypertension and bradycardia
Beta-adrenergic bronchodilators, theophylline: decreased theophylline antagonism or antagonism of both drugs
Catecholamine-depleting drugs (such as reserpine): additive beta blockade
Insulin, oral hypoglycemics: altered efficacy of these drugs
Nonsteroidal anti-inflammatory drugs: decreased antihypertensive action
Other antihypertensives, nitrates: additive hypotension
Thyroid preparations: decreased pindolol efficacy
Drug-diagnostic tests. *Alanine aminotransferase, alkaline phosphatase, aspartate aminotransferase, lactate dehydrogenase, uric acid:* increased levels
Glucose: increased or decreased level
Drug-herb. *Cocaine, ephedra:* unopposed alpha-adrenergic stimulation

Precautions
Use cautiously in:
• renal or hepatic impairment, pulmonary disease, diabetes mellitus, thyrotoxicosis, severe allergic reactions, major surgery
• elderly patients
• pregnant or breastfeeding patients
• children (safety not established).

Patient monitoring
• Monitor apical heart rate; withhold drug and notify prescriber if rate is below 60 beats/minute.
• Closely monitor ECG, vital signs, and cardiovascular status; stay alert for signs and symptoms of heart failure.

• Assess respiratory status, especially for wheezing and dyspnea.
• Monitor blood glucose level in patients with diabetes; drug may mask signs and symptoms of hypoglycemia.

Patient teaching
• Instruct patient to take drug at same time each day, with or without food.
• Caution patient that stopping drug abruptly may worsen angina or cause severe cardiac problems.
• Advise patient to rise slowly from a lying or sitting position to avoid dizziness from orthostatic hypotension.
• Instruct patient to report signs and symptoms of heart failure or breathing difficulty.
• Advise diabetic patients to monitor blood glucose levels closely.
• As appropriate, review all other significant and life-threatening adverse reactions and interactions, especially those related to the drugs, tests, and herbs mentioned above.

pioglitazone hydrochloride
Actos

Pharmacologic class: Thiazolidinedione
Therapeutic class: Hypoglycemic
Pregnancy risk category C

Action
Enhances insulin sensitivity in muscle and adipose tissue; inhibits hepatic gluconeogenesis

Availability
Tablets: 15 mg, 30 mg, 45 mg

🖊 Indications and dosages
➤ Adjunct to diet and exercise to improve glycemic control in patients with type 2 diabetes mellitus

Adults: 15 to 30 mg once daily; may be increased to 45 mg/day if needed

Contraindications
• Hypersensitivity to drug, its components, or rosiglitazone

Administration
• Give with or without food.
• Know that drug may be used with sulfonylureas, metformin, or insulin when combination of diet, exercise, and monotherapy doesn't achieve adequate glycemic control.

Route	Onset	Peak	Duration
P.O.	30 min	2 hr	24 hr

Adverse reactions
CNS: headache
EENT: tooth disorders, sinusitis, pharyngitis
Hematologic: anemia
Metabolic: aggravation of diabetes mellitus, **hypoglycemia, hyperglycemia**
Musculoskeletal: myalgia
Respiratory: upper respiratory infection
Other: pain, edema

Interactions
Drug-drug. *Hormonal contraceptives:* decreased contraceptive efficacy
Ketoconazole: increased pioglitazone effects
Drug-diagnostic tests. *Creatinine kinase:* transient increase
Hematocrit, hemoglobin: decreased values (usually during first 4 to 12 weeks of therapy)
Drug-herb. *Chromium, coenzyme Q10, fenugreek:* additive hypoglycemic effects
Glucosamine: poor glycemic control

Precautions
Use cautiously in:
• edema, hepatic impairment

• female patients of childbearing age
• pregnant or breastfeeding patients
• children.

Patient monitoring
• Assess patient's weight and compliance with diet and exercise program.
• Monitor liver function tests before and during therapy.
• Monitor hemoglobin A1c, hemoglobin, hematocrit, and blood glucose levels.
• Assess for signs and symptoms of hypoglycemia or hyperglycemia.

Patient teaching
• Explain drug therapy and need for follow-up tests.
• Instruct patient to take drug exactly as prescribed; tell him he may take it without regard to food.
• Caution patient not to double the dosage if he misses a dose.
• Tell patient that drug may increase his risk for EENT and respiratory infections; instruct him to contact prescriber if these occur.
◀᭣ Advise patient to immediately report unexplained nausea, vomiting, abdominal pain, fatigue, anorexia, dark urine, fever, trauma, infection, rapid weight gain, edema, or shortness of breath.
• Explain to premenopausal anovulatory women that drug may cause ovulation; recommend reliable contraception.
• Tell females of childbearing age to contact prescriber immediately if pregnancy occurs.
• As appropriate, review all other significant and life-threatening adverse reactions and interactions, especially those related to the drugs, tests, and herbs mentioned above.

p

piperacillin sodium
Pipracil, Zosyn

Pharmacologic class: Penicillin
(extended-spectrum)
Therapeutic class: Anti-infective
Pregnancy risk category B

Action
Inhibits biosynthesis of bacterial cell
wall during active multiplication stage,
resulting in cell death

Availability
Injection: 2 g, 3 g, 4 g, 40 g

🖊 Indications and dosages
➤ Prophylaxis of infection during abdominal and vaginal surgery
Adults: For intra-abdominal surgery,
2 g I.V. just before surgery, followed by
2 g during surgery, and then 2 g q 6
hours for no more than 24 hours. For
vaginal hysterectomy, 2 g I.V. just before surgery, followed by 2 g at 6 hours
and 2 g at 12 hours. In cesarean delivery, 2 g I.V. after cord is clamped, followed by 2 g at 4 hours and 2 g at 8
hours. In abdominal hysterectomy, 2 g
I.V. just before surgery, followed by 2 g
on return to in recovery room and 2 g
6 hours later.
➤ Serious infections, such as septicemia, nosocomial pneumonia, intra-
abdominal infections, aerobic and
anaerobic gynecologic infections, and
skin and soft-tissue infections
Adults: 12 to 18 g/day I.V. in divided
doses q 4 to 6 hours
➤ Complicated urinary tract infection (UTI)
Adults: 8 to 16 g/day I.V. in divided
doses q 6 to 8 hours
➤ Uncomplicated UTI or community-acquired pneumonia

Adults: 6 to 8 g/day I.M. or I.V. in di-
vided doses q 6 to 12 hours
➤ Uncomplicated gonorrhea
Adults: 2 g I.M. as a single dose, with 1
g probenecid given P.O. 30 minutes be-
fore piperacillin injection
Dosage adjustment
• Renal impairment
• Elderly patients
• Children

Contraindications
• Hypersensitivity to penicillin or
cephalosporins

Administration
◀🖊 Keep epinephrine and emergency
equipment available.
• For I.M. injection, dilute in sterile
water for injection or normal saline solution to yield a final concentration of
400 mg/ml. Limit I.M. injection dosage
to 2 g. Preferably, inject into upper outer buttock area.
• For intermittent I.V. infusion, dilute
reconstituted solution in 50 ml of dextrose 5% in water (D_5W), normal
saline solution, dextrose 5% in normal
saline solution, or lactated Ringer's solution; infuse over 30 minutes.
• When giving I.V. bolus, inject reconstituted solution over 3 to 5 minutes.
• Don't mix with aminoglycosides in
syringe or infusion container; doing so
inactivates aminoglycoside.

Route	Onset	Peak	Duration
I.V.	Immediate	Immediate	Dose dependent
I.M.	Unknown	30-50 min	Dose dependent

Adverse reactions
CNS: headache, dizziness, fatigue,
seizures
CV: thrombophlebitis, hematoma,
deep vein thrombosis
GI: nausea, vomiting, diarrhea, bloody
diarrhea, constipation, **pseudomem-**
branous colitis

GU: increased creatinine and blood urea nitrogen levels

Hematologic: eosinophilia, **neutropenia, leukopenia, thrombocytopenia**

Hepatic: increased hepatic enzyme levels, hyperbilirubinemia, **cholestatic hepatitis**

Metabolic: hypokalemia, hypernatremia, sodium overload

Musculoskeletal: prolonged muscle relaxation

Skin: rash, erythema, induration, bruising, erythema multiforme

Other: pain, superinfection, **Stevens-Johnson syndrome, anaphylaxis**

Interactions

Drug-drug. *Aminoglycosides:* aminoglycoside inactivation

Aspirin, probenecid: increased piperacillin blood level

Hormonal contraceptives: decreased contraceptive efficacy

Methotrexate: increased risk of methotrexate toxicity

Tetracyclines: decreased piperacillin efficacy

Vecuronium: prolonged neuromuscular blockade

Drug-diagnostic tests. *Coombs' test (with I.V. piperacillin):* false-positive results

Eosinophils: increased count

Granulocytes, hemoglobin, platelets, white blood cells: decreased levels

Precautions

Use cautiously in:
• uremia, hypokalemia, cystic fibrosis, bleeding tendencies, drug allergies, sodium restriction
• pregnant or breastfeeding patients
• children.

Patient monitoring

◀€ Monitor for signs and symptoms of anaphylaxis or superinfection.

◀€ Be aware that high doses may cause seizures.

• Watch for signs and symptoms of thrombophlebitis and deep-vein thrombosis.

• Assess drug efficacy; obtain repeat cultures after therapy ends.

• Monitor complete blood count with white cell differential, as well as potassium level; check for blood dyscrasias and hypokalemia.

• Assess for signs and symptoms of erythema multiforme (sore throat, rash, cough, iris lesions, mouth sores, cough, fever). Report early signs before condition can progress to Stevens-Johnson syndrome.

Patient teaching

• Teach patient about importance of completing entire course of therapy.

◀€ Instruct patient to immediately report allergic reactions, rash, severe diarrhea with pus (with or without fever), or extremity pain.

• Instruct patient to contact prescriber if signs and symptoms of infection worsen or if new symptoms develop.

• Advise female patient taking hormonal contraceptives to use alternate birth-control method.

• As appropriate, review all other significant and life-threatening adverse reactions and interactions, especially those related to the drugs and tests mentioned above.

p

piperacillin sodium and tazobactam sodium
Zosyn

Pharmacologic class: Penicillin (extended-spectrum), beta-lactamase inhibitor

Therapeutic class: Anti-infective

Pregnancy risk category B

Action
Inhibits bacterial cell wall synthesis, resulting in cell death; tazobactam increases piperacillin efficacy by inhibiting penicillinases that can inactivate penicillin.

Availability
Powder for injection: 2 g piperacillin and 0.25 g tazobactam/vial, 3 g piperacillin and 0.375 g tazobactam/vial, 4 g piperacillin and 0.5 g tazobactam/vial

🕖 Indications and dosages
➤ Ruptured appendix, peritonitis, pelvic inflammatory disease, moderately severe community-acquired pneumonia, skin and skin-structure infections
Adults and children older than age 12: 3.375 g (3 g piperacillin and 0.375 g tazobactam) I.V. q 6 hours for 7 to 10 days
➤ Moderate to severe nosocomial pneumonia
Adults and children age 12 and older: 3.375 g (3 g piperacillin and 0.375 g tazobactam) I.V. over 30 minutes q 4 hours for 7 to 14, days given with an aminoglycoside
Dosage adjustment
• Renal impairment

Contraindications
• Hypersensitivity to penicillins, cephalosporins, or beta-lactamase inhibitors
• Neonates

Administration
• Dilute each gram with 5 ml of diluent, such as sterile or bacteriostatic water for injection, normal saline solution for injection, dextrose 5% in water, dextrose 5% in normal saline solution for injection, or 6% dextran in normal saline solution. Don't use lactated Ringer's solution.

• Shake vial until drug dissolves. Dilute again to a final volume of 50 ml; infuse over 30 minutes.
• Don't mix with other drugs; if possible, stop primary infusion while piperacillin is infusing.
• Don't mix in same container with aminoglycosides, which are chemically incompatible with piperacillin.

Route	Onset	Peak	Duration
I.V.	Immediate	Immediate	Unknown

Adverse reactions
CNS: headache, insomnia, agitation, dizziness, anxiety, lethargy, hallucinations, depression, twitching, **coma, seizures**
CV: hypertension, chest pain, tachycardia
EENT: rhinitis, glossitis
GI: nausea, vomiting, diarrhea, constipation, dyspepsia, abdominal pain, **pseudomembranous colitis**
GU: vaginal candidiasis, vaginitis, interstitial nephritis, oliguria, proteinuria, hematuria, glomerulonephritis
Hematologic: anemia, eosinophilia, increased bleeding, **bone marrow depression, leukopenia, thrombocytopenia**
Metabolic: hypokalemia, hypernatremia
Respiratory: dyspnea
Skin: rash, pruritus
Other: fever; pain, edema, inflammation, or phlebitis at I.V. site; superinfection; hypersensitivity reactions including serum sickness and **anaphylaxis**

Interactions
Drug-drug. *Aminoglycosides:* aminoglycoside inactivation
Aspirin, probenecid: increased piperacillin blood level
Hormonal contraceptives: decreased contraceptive efficacy
Methotrexate: increased risk of methotrexate toxicity

Tetracyclines: decreased piperacillin efficacy
Vecuronium: prolonged neuromuscular blockade
Drug-diagnostic tests. *Coombs' test, urine glucose tests using copper reduction method (Clinitest, Benedict's solution, or Fehling's solution): urine protein: false-positive results*
Eosinophils: increased count
Granulocytes, hemoglobin, platelets, white blood cells: decreased levels

Precautions

Use cautiously in:
• heart failure, renal insufficiency (in children), seizures, bleeding disorders, uremia, hypokalemia, cystic fibrosis
• patients with dietary sodium restrictions
• pregnant or breastfeeding patients.

Patient monitoring

• Assess neurologic status, especially for seizures.
• Monitor vital signs and fluid intake and output.
• Evaluate electrolyte levels, complete blood count with white cell differential, and culture and sensitivity test results.
• In patients receiving high doses or prolonged therapy, monitor for signs and symptoms of bacterial or fungal superinfection and pseudomembranous colitis.
• Monitor patient's dietary sodium intake (drug has high sodium content).
◀≋ Immediately report rash, hives, severe diarrhea, black tongue, sore throat, fever, unusual bleeding, or bruising.

Patient teaching

• Teach patient to monitor urinary output and report significant changes.
• Instruct patient to report unusual pain, redness, swelling, or other changes at infusion site.

• As appropriate, review all other significant and life-threatening adverse reactions and interactions, especially those related to the drugs and tests mentioned above.

pirbuterol acetate
Maxair Autohaler

Pharmacologic class: Beta-adrenergic agonist
Therapeutic class: Bronchodilator
Pregnancy risk category C

Action

Increases production of cyclic adenosine monophosphate at beta-adrenergic receptors, producing bronchodilation and inhibiting histamine release. Primarily selective for beta$_2$-adrenergic (pulmonary) receptor sites, with minimal effect on beta$_1$-adrenergic (cardiac) receptors.

Availability

Inhalation aerosol: 200 mcg/spray (up to 400 inhalations/14.0-g canister)

◢ Indications and dosages

➤ Reversible airway disease caused by intermittent asthma or chronic obstructive pulmonary disease
Adults and children over age 12: One or two inhalations q 4 to 6 hours (not to exceed 12 inhalations/day)

Contraindications

• Hypersensitivity to drug, adrenergic amines, or fluorocarbons

Administration

• If patient also uses a corticosteroid inhaler, give pirbuterol first, then wait 5 minutes before giving steroid.

Route	Onset	Peak	Duration
Inhalation	Within 5 min	1.5 hr	6-8 hr

Adverse reactions

CNS: nervousness, restlessness, tremor, headache, insomnia

CV: angina, hypertension, tachycardia, **arrhythmias**

GI: nausea, vomiting

Metabolic: hyperglycemia

Respiratory: paradoxical broncho-spasm

Interactions

Drug-drug. *Beta-adrenergic blockers:* negation of pirbuterol's therapeutic effects

Diuretics: hypokalemia, exacerbation of ECG changes

Monoamine oxidase inhibitors: hypertensive crisis

Other adrenergics: additive adverse adrenergic effects

Drug-diagnostic tests. *Glucose:* increased level

Drug-food. *Caffeine-containing foods and beverages:* increased stimulant effects

Drug-herb. *Caffeine-containing herbs (such as cola nut, guarana, yerba maté), ephedra:* increased stimulant effects

Precautions

Use cautiously in:
• cardiac disease, hypertension, hyperthyroidism, diabetes mellitus, glaucoma, hypokalemia
• elderly patients
• pregnant (near term) or breastfeeding patients
• children under age 12 (safety not established).

Patient monitoring

◀€ Be aware that excessive use may lead to tolerance and paradoxical bronchospasm.
• Monitor respiratory status before and after administering drug; note improvements.
• Assess dosage (number of inhalations) and dosing frequency needed to control symptoms.

• Notify prescriber if patient needs higher dosage to control symptoms.
• Assess vital signs and cardiovascular status; stay alert for angina, hypertension, and arrhythmias.
• Monitor patient for worsening bronchospasm after administration.

Patient teaching

• Teach patient how to use metered-dose inhaler or autoinhaler.
• Instruct patient to wait at least 2 minutes between inhalations.
• If patient is also using an inhaled corticosteroid, teach him to use pirbuterol first and then wait 5 minutes before using the steroid.
• Advise patient to contact prescriber if he needs higher or more frequent doses to control symptoms.
• Teach patient to recognize signs and symptoms of bronchospasm; advise him to notify prescriber if these worsen after he takes drug.
• Inform patient that herbs containing ephedra or caffeine may worsen stimulant effects, such as nervousness and tremors.
• As appropriate, review all other significant and life-threatening adverse reactions and interactions, especially those related to the drugs, tests, foods, and herbs mentioned above.

piroxicam

Apo-Piroxicam✦, Feldene, Novo-Pirocam✦, Nu-Pirox✦

Pharmacologic class: Oxicam derivative, nonsteroidal anti-inflammatory drug (NSAID)

Therapeutic class: Analgesic, anti-inflammatory, antipyretic

Pregnancy risk category C (first and second trimesters), *D* (third trimester)

Action
Inhibits cyclooxygenase, an enzyme needed for prostaglandin synthesis, thereby stimulating anti-inflammatory response and blocking pain impulses

Availability
Capsules: 10 mg, 20 mg

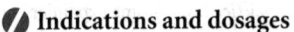 Indications and dosages
➤ Inflammatory disorders (including rheumatoid arthritis, osteoarthritis)
Adults: 20 mg P.O. daily as a single dose or in two divided doses
Dosage adjustment
- Hepatic or renal impairment
- Elderly patients

Off-label uses
- Dysmenorrhea
- Ankylosing spondylitis
- Gout

Contraindications
- Hypersensitivity to drug or other NSAIDs, including aspirin
- Active GI bleeding or ulcer disease
- Third trimester of pregnancy, breast-feeding

Administration
- Give with milk, antacids, or food to minimize GI upset.

Route	Onset	Peak	Duration
P.O. (analgesia)	1 hr	Unknown	48-72 hr
P.O. (anti-inflam.)	7-12 days	2-3 wk	Unknown

Adverse reactions
CNS: drowsiness, headache, dizziness
CV: edema, hypertension, vasculitis, tachycardia, **arrhythmias**
EENT: blurred vision, tinnitus
GI: nausea, vomiting, diarrhea, constipation, abdominal pain, flatulence, dyspepsia, anorexia, **severe GI bleeding**
GU: proteinuria, **renal failure**

Hematologic: prolonged bleeding time, anemia, **blood dyscrasias**
Hepatic: abnormal liver function studies, jaundice, **hepatitis**
Skin: rash
Other: allergic reactions including **anaphylaxis**

Interactions
Drug-drug. *Acetaminophen (chronic use), cyclosporine, gold compounds:* increased risk of adverse renal effects
Anticoagulants, cefamandole, cefoperazone, cefotetan, clopidogrel, eptifibatide, heparin, plicamycin, thrombolytics, ticlopidine, tirofiban, valproic acid, vitamin A: increased risk of bleeding
Antineoplastics: increased risk of hematologic toxicity
Aspirin: decreased piroxicam blood level and efficacy
Corticosteroids, other NSAIDs: additive adverse GI effects
Diuretics, other antihypertensives: decreased response to these drugs
Insulin, oral hypoglycemics: increased risk of hypoglycemia
Lithium: increased lithium blood level and risk of toxicity
Probenecid: increased piroxicam blood level and risk of toxicity
Drug-diagnostic tests. *Alanine aminotransferase, alkaline phosphatase, aspartate aminotransferase, blood urea nitrogen, creatinine, electrolytes, lactate dehydrogenase:* increased levels
Hematocrit, hemoglobin, platelets, white blood cells: decreased levels
Drug-herb. *Alfalfa, anise, arnica, astragalus, bilberry, black currant seed oil, bladderwrack, bogbean, boldo, borage oil, buchu, capsaicin, cat's claw, celery, chaparral, cinchona bark, clove oil, coenzyme Q10, dandelion, danshen, dong quai, evening primrose oil, fenugreek, feverfew, garlic, ginger, ginkgo, guggul, papaya extract, red clover, rhubarb, safflower oil, skullcap, St. John's wort:* increased anticoagulant effect and bleeding risk

P

Precautions

Use cautiously in:

- renal impairment, severe cardiovascular or hepatic disease
- history of ulcer disease
- pregnant patients (first or second trimester)
- children (safety not established).

Patient monitoring

- Monitor vital signs and cardiovascular status; stay alert for hypertension and arrhythmias.
- Monitor kidney and liver function studies, hearing, and complete blood cell count.
- Watch for signs and symptoms of drug-induced hepatitis and GI toxicity, including ulcers and bleeding.
- Monitor for signs and symptoms of infection, which drug may mask.

Patient teaching

- Advise patient to take drug with milk, antacids, or food to minimize GI upset.
- Teach patient that drug may mask signs and symptoms of infection; instruct him to contact prescriber if he suspects an infection.
- Teach patient to recognize and report signs and symptoms of allergic reaction or GI bleeding.
- Inform patient that many herbs increase the risk of GI bleeding; caution him not to use herbs without prescriber's approval.
- Instruct patient to drink plenty of fluids and to report decreased urination.
- Advise patient to avoid driving and other hazardous activities until he knows how drug affects concentration and alertness.
- As appropriate, review all other significant and life-threatening adverse reactions and interactions, especially those related to the drugs, tests, and herbs mentioned above.

plasma protein fraction
Plasmanate, Plasma-Plex, Plasmatein, Protenate

Pharmacologic class: Human plasma protein
Therapeutic class: Plasma expander
Pregnancy risk category C

Action

Maintains plasma colloid osmotic pressure, enhancing movement of fluid from interstitial tissues into circulatory system, thereby regulating blood volume

Availability

Solution for injection: 5% in 50-ml, 250-ml, and 500-ml vials

⚕ Indications and dosages

➢ Hypovolemic shock
Adults: Initially, 250 to 500 ml by I.V. infusion, up to a maximum of 10 ml/minute
➢ Hypoproteinemia
Adults: 1,000 to 1,500 ml daily by I.V. infusion, up to a maximum of 8 ml/minute

Contraindications

- Hypersensitivity to drug or albumin
- Heart failure
- Severe anemia
- Normal or increased intravascular volume
- During cardiopulmonary bypass

Administration

- Ensure that patient is adequately hydrated before administering drug.
- Know that dosage and infusion rate depend on patient's condition and response to drug.

- Don't infuse through same I.V. line with solutions containing amino acids or alcohol.
- Don't use infusion that has been frozen or contains visible sediment.
- Infuse at a site distant from infection or trauma, usually at a rate no faster than 10 ml/minute.
- Be aware that rapid infusion (especially in normovolemic patients) may cause vascular overload, dyspnea, and pulmonary edema.
- Monitor blood pressure; slow infusion rate if hypotension occurs.

Route	Onset	Peak	Duration
I.V.	Immediate	Immediate	Unknown

Adverse reactions
CNS: headache, paresthesia
CV: hypotension, tachycardia, **vascular overload and heart failure** (with rapid I.V. infusion)
GI: nausea, vomiting, increased salivation
Respiratory: dyspnea, **pulmonary edema** (with rapid I.V. infusion)
Skin: rash, flushing
Other: fever, chills

Interactions
Drug-diagnostic tests. *Alkaline phosphatase:* false increase

Precautions
Use cautiously in:
- hepatic or renal impairment, reduced cardiac reserve, decreased sodium intake
- pregnant patients.

Patient monitoring
◀▒ Assess for signs and symptoms of vascular overload, including heart failure and pulmonary edema.
- Monitor vital signs hourly; expect a gradual return to normal during and after drug therapy.
- Monitor fluid intake and output.

Patient teaching
- Instruct patient to report difficulty breathing.
- Tell patient that drug may cause headache, nausea, and vomiting; advise him to report these problems.
- Inform patient that he'll undergo regular blood tests.
- As appropriate, review all other significant and life-threatening adverse reactions and interactions, especially those related to the tests mentioned above.

plicamycin (mithramycin)
Mithracin

Pharmacologic class: Crystalline compound produced by *Streptomyces plicatus*
Therapeutic class: Antibiotic antineoplastic
Pregnancy risk category X

Action
Unknown; antitumor activity may stem from drug's formation of a complex, which causes cross-linking of DNA strands, inhibiting cellular RNA and enzymatic RNA synthesis.

Availability
Injection: 2.5-mg vials

⚕ Indications and dosages
➤ Testicular cancer
Adults: 25 to 30 mcg/kg/day I.V. over 4 to 6 hours for 8 to 10 days
➤ Hypercalcemia and hypercalciuria associated with advanced cancer
Adults: 25 mcg/kg/day I.V. over 4 to 6 hours for 3 to 4 days; may repeat weekly until adequate response occurs.
Dosage adjustment
- Renal failure

P

Contraindications

- Hypersensitivity to drug
- Thrombocytopenia, thrombocytopathy
- Bone marrow depression
- Coagulation disorders or increased risk of bleeding
- Pregnancy or breastfeeding

Administration

◀꒐ Follow facility policy for preparing, handling, and administering carcinogenic, mutagenic, or teratogenic drugs. Don't let drug touch skin or mucous membranes.

- Administer antiemetic before plicamycin, as prescribed, to reduce nausea and vomiting.
- Dilute with 4.9 ml of sterile water for injection; shake vial to dissolve.
- Further dilute in 1,000 ml of dextrose 5% in water or normal saline solution.
- Infuse I.V. over 4 to 6 hours; discard unused portion.

Route	Onset	Peak	Duration
I.V.	1-2 days	3 days	3-15 days

Adverse reactions

CNS: drowsiness, asthenia, lethargy, depression, headache, malaise
CV: phlebitis
GI: nausea, vomiting, diarrhea, stomatitis, anorexia
GU: proteinuria, increased creatinine and blood urea nitrogen levels
Hematologic: leukopenia, thrombocytopenia, bleeding syndrome
Hepatic: increased hepatic enzyme levels, mild and reversible hepatotoxicity
Metabolic: hypokalemia, hypocalcemia, hypophosphatemia
Skin: facial flushing; rash; pain, redness, or swelling at injection site; cellulitis with extravasation
Other: fever

Interactions

Drug-drug. *Other antineoplastics:* increased plicamycin toxicity

Drug-diagnostic tests. *Blood urea nitrogen, creatinine, hepatic enzymes:* increased levels
Calcium, phosphate, potassium, platelets, white blood cells (WBCs): decreased levels

Drug-herb. *Anise, arnica, chamomile, clove, dong quai, fenugreek, garlic, ginger, ginkgo, ginseng, licorice:* increased risk of bleeding
Chaparral, comfrey, eucalyptus, germander, jin bu huan, kava, pennyroyal, skullcap, valerian: increased risk of hepatotoxicity

Precautions

Use cautiously in:
- renal or hepatic disease, electrolyte imbalances.

Patient monitoring

◀꒐ Watch closely for bleeding syndrome, which usually starts with epistaxis and progresses quickly.

- Monitor liver function test results, electrolyte levels, platelet and WBC counts, and prothrombin time. Notify prescriber if platelet count falls below 150,000/mm³, WBC count falls below 4,000/mm³, or prothrombin time is more than 4 seconds longer than control.

◀꒐ Assess for indications of sudden drop in calcium level, such as Chvostek's sign, muscle cramps, carpopedal spasm, or tetany.

- Monitor I.V. site closely to avoid extravasation.

Patient teaching

◀꒐ Teach patient to recognize and immediately report easy bruising, bleeding, and hypocalcemia. Inform patient that nosebleed may be first sign of a bleeding problem.

- Instruct patient to report unusual pain, redness, swelling, or other changes at infusion site.
- Caution females of childbearing age to avoid pregnancy during therapy; ad-

vise them to report suspected pregnancy right away.

• Advise patient to avoid herbs because many herbs increase the risk of liver damage.

• As appropriate, review all other significant and life-threatening adverse reactions and interactions, especially those related to the drugs, tests, and herbs mentioned above.

poractant alfa
Curosurf

Pharmacologic class: Porcine lung extract

Therapeutic class: Exogenous pulmonary agent

Pregnancy risk category NR

Action
Stabilizes and expands alveoli by reducing their surface tension and replenishing surfactant, preventing alveolar collapse

Availability
Suspension for endotracheal instillation: 120 mg (1.5 ml), 240 mg (3 ml)

⚠ Indications and dosages
➤ Respiratory distress syndrome (RDS) in premature infants
Infants: Administer 2.5 ml/kg birth weight endotracheally, instilling half of dose into each bronchus; up to two subsequent doses of 1.25 ml/kg birth weight at 12-hour intervals may be needed. Maximum dosage is 5 ml/kg (initial dose plus two subsequent doses).

Off-label uses
• Adult RDS caused by viral pneumonia or near-drowning

• HIV-infected infants with *Pneumocystis jiroveci* (formerly *Pneumocystis carinii*) pneumonia

Contraindications
None

Administration
• Give first dose as soon as possible after RDS diagnosis and when patient is on ventilator.

• Know that drug is meant for endotracheal use only.

◀◊ Be aware that drug should be given only by clinicians experienced in intubation, ventilatory management, and resuscitation of neonates because it can rapidly affect oxygenation and pulmonary function.

• Before use, slowly warm vial to room temperature and gently turn upside-down to ensure uniform suspension. Don't shake.

• Using a large-gauge needle, slowly withdraw entire contents of vial into 3-ml or 5-ml plastic syringe. Attach precut, 8-cm 5 French catheter to syringe. Fill catheter with drug; discard excess drug through catheter so that only prescribed dose remains in syringe.

• Before giving, verify proper placement and patency of endotracheal tube. Make sure catheter doesn't extend beyond endotracheal tube.

Route	Onset	Peak	Duration
Intratracheal	Immediate	3 hr	Unknown

Adverse reactions
CV: transient hypotension and bradycardia
Respiratory: transient endotracheal tube blockage, decreased oxygen saturation, airway obstruction

Interactions
None significant

Precautions

Use cautiously in:
• bradycardia, crackles, infection
• family history of allergy to pork products.

Patient monitoring

• Monitor vital signs and ECG; watch for hypotension and bradycardia.
◀€ Assess closely for endotracheal tube blockage and proper ventilation.

Patient teaching

• Reassure parents that infant will be monitored closely.

porfimer sodium
Photofrin

Pharmacologic class: Photosensitizing agent
Therapeutic class: Antineoplastic
Pregnancy risk category C

Action

Exerts photosensitizing action by damaging cancer cells through propagation of radical reactions; subsequent laser light photoactivation produces cytotoxic reaction in affected tissues

Availability

Injection (cake or freeze-dried powder): 75 mg/vial

⃠ Indications and dosages

➤ Esophageal cancer, microinvasive endobronchial non-small-cell lung cancer

Adults: 2 mg/kg I.V. for 3 to 5 minutes, followed 40 to 50 hours later by illumination with laser light. A second laser light application may be given 96 to 120 hours after injection; a total of three courses may be given, separated by at least 30 days.

Contraindications

• Hypersensitivity to porphyrins
• Porphyria
• Bronchoesophageal or tracheoesophageal fistula, tumor erosion into major blood vessels, and other conditions that rule out photodynamic therapy

Administration

• Be aware that drug should be given by slow I.V. push over 3 to 5 minutes only by clinicians trained in photodynamic therapy.
• Reconstitute with 31.8 ml of 5% dextrose injection or normal saline solution injection. Shake well until dissolved. Use immediately after reconstitution.
• Don't mix with other drugs in same syringe.
• Take care to prevent extravasation; if extravasation occurs, protect area from light.
• Don't let drug contact skin or eyes. Wear rubber gloves and eye protection. If contact occurs, avoid bright light; otherwise, photosensitivity reaction may occur.

Route	Onset	Peak	Duration
I.V.	30-40 hr	Unknown	Up to 90 days

Adverse reactions

CNS: anxiety, confusion, insomnia, asthenia
CV: hypotension, hypertension, chest pain, sick sinus syndrome, tachycardia, **heart failure, atrial fibrillation, myocardial infarction**
EENT: diplopia, photophobia, pharyngitis
GI: nausea, vomiting, diarrhea, constipation, abdominal pain, gastric ulcer, dyspepsia, melena, hematemesis, dysphagia, eructation, esophagitis, anorexia, **esophageal edema, esophageal tumor bleeding, esophageal stricture, esophageal perforation, peritonitis**
GU: urinary tract infection, candidiasis

Hematologic: anemia
Hepatic: jaundice
Metabolic: dehydration
Musculoskeletal: back pain
Respiratory: cough, dyspnea, bronchitis, pneumonia, stridor, **respiratory insufficiency or failure, bronchospasm, tracheoesophageal fistula, laryngotracheal edema, pleural effusion, pulmonary edema**
Skin: photosensitivity, local inflammatory response
Other: substernal or general pain, weight loss, fever, surgical complications, edema

Interactions

Drug-drug. *Glucocorticoids:* decreased efficacy of photodynamic therapy
Other photosensitizing drugs (fluoroquinolones, griseofulvin, phenothiazines, sulfonamides, sulfonylureas, tetracyclines, thiazide diuretics): increased photosensitivity
Drug-diagnostic tests. *Hemoglobin:* decreased level
Drug-behaviors. *Sun exposure:* increased risk of photosensitivity

Precautions

Use cautiously in:
• esophageal varices, endobronchial tumors in sites where treatment-induced inflammation could block main airway
• elderly patients
• pregnant or breastfeeding patients
• children (safety not established).

Patient monitoring

◄€ Monitor for signs and symptoms of esophageal obstruction.
◄€ Assess vital signs and cardiovascular status; watch for signs and symptoms of cardiac complications.
◄€ Monitor respiratory status, especially for difficulty breathing.
• Evaluate nutritional and hydration status.

• Watch for photosensitivity reaction; protect patient's skin and eyes from direct sunlight and bright indoor light.

Patient teaching

◄€ Teach patient to immediately report difficulty breathing or swallowing.
• Emphasize importance of avoiding sun exposure for at least 30 days (and even up to 90 or more days) after therapy ends. Instruct patient to wear dark sunglasses with average white light transmittance less than 4%.
• Inform patient that conventional ultraviolet sunscreens don't prevent photosensitivity reactions caused by this drug.
• As appropriate, review all other significant and life-threatening adverse reactions and interactions, especially those related to the drugs, tests, and behaviors mentioned above.

potassium acetate

Pharmacologic class: Mineral, electrolyte
Therapeutic class: Electrolyte replacement, nutritional supplement
Pregnancy risk category C

Action

Maintains acid-base balance, isotonicity, and electrophysiologic balance throughout body tissues; crucial to nerve impulse transmission and contraction of cardiac, skeletal, and smooth muscle. Also essential for normal renal function and carbohydrate metabolism.

Availability

Concentrate for injection: 2 mEq/ml in 20-, 50-, and 100-ml vials; 4 mEq/ml in 50-ml vials

✒ Indications and dosages

➤ Prevention or treatment of potassium depletion

Adults: Dosage highly individualized. If potassium level exceeds 2.5 mEq/L, give 40 mEq/L as additive to I.V. infusion at a maximum rate of 10 mEq/hour; maximum daily dosage is 200 mEq. If potassium level is below 2 mEq/L, give 80 mEq/L as additive to I.V. infusion at a maximum rate of 40 mEq/hour; maximum daily dosage is 400 mEq.

Children: Dosage highly individualized; up to 3 mEq/kg or 40 mEq/m^2/day as additive to I.V. infusion.

Contraindications

- Acute dehydration
- Heat cramps
- Hyperkalemia
- Hyperkalemic familial periodic paralysis
- Severe renal impairment
- Severe hemolytic reactions
- Untreated Addison's disease
- Severe tissue trauma
- Concurrent use of potassium-sparing diuretics, angiotensin-converting enzyme (ACE) inhibitors, or salt substitutes containing potassium

Administration

◀🎧 Give as additive to I.V. infusion only. Never give by I.V. push or I.M. route or undiluted. Use peripheral line with maximum rate of 40 mEq/hour.

◀🎧 To ensure that potassium is well mixed in compatible solution, don't add potassium to I.V. bottle in hanging position.

◀🎧 Dilute in compatible I.V. solution; administer slowly to reduce risk of fatal hyperkalemia.

- If patient complains of burning with I.V. administration, decrease flow rate.
- Ensure that patient is well hydrated and urinating before starting therapy.

- Be aware that potassium preparations are not interchangeable.
- Know that dosages are expressed in milliequivalents (mEq) of potassium and that potassium acetate contains 10.2 mEq/g.

Route	Onset	Peak	Duration
I.V.	Rapid	End of infusion	Unknown

Adverse reactions

CNS: confusion, unusual fatigue, restlessness, asthenia, flaccid paralysis, paresthesia, absence of reflexes

CV: ECG changes, hypotension, **arrhythmias, heart block, cardiac arrest**

GI: nausea, vomiting, diarrhea, abdominal discomfort, flatulence

Metabolic: hyperkalemia

Musculoskeletal: weakness and heaviness of legs

Respiratory: respiratory paralysis

Other: irritation at I.V. site

Interactions

Drug-drug. *ACE inhibitors, potassium-sparing diuretics, other potassium-containing preparations:* increased risk of hyperkalemia

Drug-diagnostic tests. *Potassium:* increased level

Drug-food. *Salt substitutes containing potassium:* increased risk of hyperkalemia

Drug-herb. *Dandelion:* increased risk of hyperkalemia

Licorice: decreased response to potassium

Precautions

Use cautiously in:

- cardiac disease, renal impairment, diabetes mellitus, hypomagnesemia
- pregnant or breastfeeding patients
- children (safety and efficacy not established).

Patient monitoring

• Monitor renal function; fluid intake and output; and potassium, creatinine, and blood urea nitrogen levels.

◀ℰ Know that potassium is contraindicated in severe renal impairment and must be used with extreme caution (if at all) in patients with any degree of renal impairment because of risk of life-threatening hyperkalemia.

• Assess vital signs and ECG; watch for arrhythmias.

• Evaluate patient's neurologic status; watch for neurologic complications.

• Monitor I.V. site for signs of irritation.

Patient teaching

• Instruct patient to report unusual pain, redness, swelling, or other reactions at infusion site.

• Advise patient to report nausea, vomiting, confusion, numbness and tingling, unusual tiredness or weakness, or a heavy feeling in legs.

• Instruct patient to avoid salt substitutes.

• As appropriate, review all other significant and life-threatening adverse reactions and interactions, especially those related to the drugs, tests, foods, and herbs mentioned above.

potassium bicarbonate
K+Care ET

Pharmacologic class: Mineral, electrolyte

Therapeutic class: Electrolyte replacement, nutritional supplement

Pregnancy risk category C

Action

Maintains acid-base balance, isotonicity, and electrophysiologic balance throughout body tissues; crucial to nerve impulse transmission and contraction of cardiac, skeletal, and smooth muscle. Also essential for normal renal function and carbohydrate metabolism.

Availability

Tablets for effervescent oral solution: 25 mEq

⚫ Indications and dosages

➤ Prevention of potassium depletion

Adults: Dosage highly individualized. Usual dosage is 25 mEq/day P.O. in divided doses.

➤ Treatment of potassium depletion

Adults: 50 to 100 mEq/day P.O. in divided doses, not to exceed a maximum daily dosage of 150 mEq

Contraindications

• Hypersensitivity to tartrazine or alcohol (with some products)

• Acute dehydration

• Heat cramps

• Hyperkalemia

• Hyperkalemic familial periodic paralysis

• Severe renal impairment

• Severe hemolytic reaction

• Untreated Addison's disease

• Severe tissue trauma

• Concurrent use of potassium-sparing diuretics, angiotensin-converting enzyme (ACE) inhibitors, or salt substitutes containing potassium

Administration

• Ensure that patient is adequately hydrated and urinating before starting therapy.

• Give with meals and a full glass of water or juice to minimize GI upset.

• Be aware that potassium preparations are not interchangeable.

• Know that dosages are expressed in milliequivalents (mEq) of potassium and that potassium bicarbonate contains 10 mEq potassium/g.

p

Route	Onset	Peak	Duration
P.O.	Unknown	1-2 hr	Unknown

Adverse reactions

CNS: confusion, unusual fatigue, restlessness, asthenia, flaccid paralysis, paresthesia

CV: ECG changes, hypotension, **heart block, arrhythmias, cardiac arrest**

GI: nausea, vomiting, diarrhea, abdominal discomfort, flatulence

Metabolic: hyperkalemia

Musculoskeletal: weakness and heaviness of legs

Interactions

Drug-drug. *ACE inhibitors, potassium-sparing diuretics, other potassium-containing preparations:* increased risk of hyperkalemia

Drug-diagnostic tests. *Potassium:* increased level

Drug-food. *Salt substitutes containing potassium:* increased risk of hyperkalemia

Drug-herb. *Dandelion:* increased risk of hyperkalemia

Licorice: decreased response to potassium

Precautions

Use cautiously in:
• cardiac disease, renal impairment, diabetes mellitus, hypomagnesemia
• pregnant or breastfeeding patients
• children (safety and efficacy not established).

Patient monitoring

• Monitor renal function; fluid intake and output; and potassium, creatinine, and blood urea nitrogen levels.

◀€ Be aware that potassium is contraindicated in patients with severe renal impairment and must be used with extreme caution (if at all) in patients with any degree of renal impairment because of risk of life-threatening hyperkalemia.

• Assess vital signs; check ECG for arrhythmias.

• Monitor neurologic status; stay alert for neurologic complications.

Patient teaching

• Instruct patient to dissolve tablets thoroughly in 4 to 8 oz of cold water or juice, to add flavor packet, and to sip solution over 5 to 10 minutes with a meal.

• Teach patient to minimize GI upset by eating small, frequent servings of healthy food and drinking plenty of fluids.

• Advise patient to report nausea, vomiting, confusion, numbness and tingling, unusual tiredness or weakness, or a heavy feeling in legs.

• Instruct patient to avoid salt substitutes.

• As appropriate, review all other significant and life-threatening adverse reactions and interactions, especially those related to the drugs, tests, foods, and herbs mentioned above.

potassium chloride

Apo-K✤, Cena-K, Gen-K, K+ Care, K+ 10, Kaochlor, Kaochlor S-F, Kaon-Cl, Kay Ciel, K-Dur, K-Lease, K-Lor, Klor-Con, Klorvess Liquid, Klotrix, K-Lyte/Cl Powder, K-Med✤, K-Norm, K-Sol, K-Tab, Micro-K, Micro-K Extencaps, Micro-LS, Potasalan, Roychlor, Rum-K, Slow-K, Ten-K

Pharmacologic class: Mineral, electrolyte

Therapeutic class: Electrolyte replacement, nutritional supplement

Pregnancy risk category C

Action
Maintains acid-base balance, isotonicity, and electrophysiologic balance throughout body tissues; crucial to nerve impulse transmission and contraction of cardiac, skeletal, and smooth muscle. Also essential for normal renal function and carbohydrate metabolism.

Availability
Capsules (extended-release): 8 mEq, 10 mEq
Powder for oral solution: 20 mEq, 25 mEq
Parenteral injection (concentrate): 1.5 mEq/ml, 2 mEq/ml
Parenteral injection (concentrate for I.V. infusion): 0.1 mEq/ml, 0.2 mEq/ml, 0.3 mEq/ml, 0.4 mEq/ml
Potassium chloride in 5% dextrose injection: 10 mEq/L, 20 mEq/L, 30 mEq/L, 40 mEq/L
Potassium chloride in 0.9% sodium chloride injection: 20 mEq/L, 40 mEq/L
Potassium chloride in dextrose and lactated Ringer's injection: various strengths
Potassium chloride in dextrose and sodium chloride injection: various strengths
Solution, oral: 6.7 mEq, 10 mEq, 13.3 mEq, 15 mEq, 20 mEq, 30 mEq, 40 mEq
Tablets: 500 mg, 595 mg
Tablets (effervescent): 25 mEq, 50 mEq
Tablets (extended-release): 8 mEq, 10 mEq
Tablets (extended-release crystals): 10 mEq, 20 mEq
Tablets (extended-release, film coated): 8 mEq, 10 mEq
Tablets (film-coated): 2.5 mEq, 10 mEq

⚕ Indications and dosages
➣ Prevention of potassium depletion
Adults: Dosage highly individualized. Usual single dosage is 20 mEq/day P.O. in divided doses.
➣ Treatment of potassium depletion
Adults: Dosage highly individualized. 40 to 100 mEq/day P.O. in divided doses, not to exceed 20 mEq in a single dose. Or for a serum potassium level above 2.5 mEq/L, give 40 mEq/L as additive to I.V. infusion at a maximum rate of 10 mEq/hour; maximum daily dosage is 200 mEq. For a potassium level below 2 mEq/L, give 80 mEq/L as additive to I.V. infusion at a maximum rate of 40 mEq/hour; maximum daily dosage is 400 mEq.
Children: Dosage highly individualized; give up to 3 mEq/kg or 40 mEq/m^2/day as additive to I.V. infusion.

Contraindications
• Hypersensitivity to tartrazine or alcohol (with some products)
• Acute dehydration
• Heat cramps
• Hyperkalemia
• Hyperkalemic familial periodic paralysis
• Severe renal impairment
• Severe hemolytic reactions
• Untreated Addison's disease
• Severe tissue trauma
• Concurrent use of potassium-sparing diuretics, angiotensin-enzyme converting (ACE) inhibitors, or salt substitutes containing potassium
• Esophageal compression caused by enlarged left atrium (with wax matrix forms)

Administration
◀€ Give I.V. form as an additive by infusion only; never give undiluted or by I.V. push or I.M. route. Use peripheral line and infuse at a maximum rate of 40 mEq/hour.
◀€ Dilute in compatible I.V. solution following manufacturer's instructions; administer slowly to reduce risk of fatal hyperkalemia.
◀€ To ensure that potassium is well mixed in compatible solution, don't add potassium to I.V. bottle in hanging position.

p

• Make sure patient is well-hydrated and urinating before starting therapy.
• If patient complains of burning with I.V. administration, decrease flow rate.
• Give oral form with meals and a full glass of water or juice to minimize GI upset.
• Ensure that patient swallows wax-matrix tablets completely to avoid serious esophageal problems.
• Don't give wax matrix tablets to patients with swallowing problems or who might have esophageal compression.
• Be aware that potassium preparations aren't interchangeable.
• Know that dosages are expressed in milliequivalents (mEq) of potassium and that potassium chloride contains 13.4 mEq potassium/g.

Route	Onset	Peak	Duration
P.O.	Unknown	1-2 hr	Unknown
I.V.	Rapid	End of infusion	Unknown

Adverse reactions

CNS: confusion, unusual fatigue, restlessness, asthenia, flaccid paralysis, paresthesia, absence of reflexes
CV: ECG changes, hypotension, **arrhythmias, heart block, cardiac arrest**
GI: nausea, vomiting, diarrhea, abdominal discomfort, flatulence
Metabolic: hyperkalemia
Musculoskeletal: weakness and heaviness of legs
Respiratory: respiratory paralysis
Other: irritation at I.V. site

Interactions

Drug-drug. *ACE inhibitors, potassium-sparing diuretics, other potassium-containing preparations:* increased risk of hyperkalemia
Drug-diagnostic tests. *Potassium:* increased level
Drug-food. *Salt substitutes containing potassium:* increased risk of hyperkalemia

Drug-herb. *Dandelion:* increased risk of hyperkalemia
Licorice: decreased response to potassium

Precautions

Use cautiously in:
• cardiac disease, renal impairment, diabetes mellitus, hypomagnesemia
• pregnant or breastfeeding patients
• children (safety and efficacy not established).

Patient monitoring

• Monitor renal function; fluid intake and output; and potassium, creatinine, and blood urea nitrogen levels.
• Assess vital signs and ECG; stay alert for arrhythmias.
• Monitor neurologic status; watch for neurologic complications.
• Monitor I.V. site for signs of irritation.
◀€ Know that potassium is contraindicated in patients with severe renal impairment and must be used with extreme caution (if at all) in patients with any degree of renal impairment because of risk of life-threatening hyperkalemia.

Patient teaching

• Instruct patient to mix and dissolve powder completely in 3 to 8 oz of water or juice.
• Teach patient to swallow extended-release capsules whole without crushing or chewing them.
• Instruct patient to take oral form with or just after a meal, with a glass of water or fruit juice to minimize GI upset.
• Teach patient to sip diluted liquid form over 5 to 10 minutes.
• Advise patient to report nausea, vomiting, confusion, numbness and tingling, unusual fatigue or weakness, or a heavy feeling in legs.
• Teach patient to minimize GI upset by eating frequent, small servings of

healthy food and drinking plenty of fluids.

• Tell patient that although wax matrix form may appear in stool, drug has already been absorbed.

• Advise patient not to use salt substitutes.

• As appropriate, review all other significant and life-threatening adverse reactions and interactions, especially those related to the drugs, tests, foods, and herbs mentioned above.

potassium gluconate
Kaon, Kaylixir, K-G Elixir, Potassium-Rougier♣

Pharmacologic class: Mineral, electrolyte

Therapeutic class: Electrolyte replacement, nutritional supplement

Pregnancy risk category C

Action
Maintains acid-base balance, isotonicity, and electrophysiologic balance throughout body tissues; crucial to nerve impulse transmission and contraction of cardiac, skeletal, and smooth muscle. Also essential for norma renal function and carbohydrate metabolism.

Availability
Elixir: 20 mEq/15 ml
Tablets: 2 mEq, 5 mEq

🖊 Indications and dosages
➤ Prevention of potassium depletion
Adults: Dosage highly individualized. Usual daily dosage is 20 mEq P.O. in divided doses.
➤ Treatment of potassium depletion
Adults: 40 to 100 mEq/day P.O. in divided doses, not to exceed 20 mEq in a single dose

Contraindications
• Hypersensitivity to tartrazine or alcohol (some products)
• Acute dehydration
• Heat cramps
• Hyperkalemia
• Hyperkalemic familial periodic paralysis
• Severe renal impairment
• Severe hemolytic reactions
• Untreated Addison's disease
• Severe tissue trauma
• Concurrent use of potassium-sparing diuretics, angiotensin-converting enzyme (ACE) inhibitors, or salt substitutes containing potassium

Administration
• Make sure patient is adequately hydrated and urinating before starting therapy.
• Give with food or meals and a full glass of water or juice to minimize GI upset.
• Be aware that potassium preparations are not interchangeable.
• Know that dosages are expressed in milliequivalents (mEq) of potassium and that potassium gluconate contains 4.3 mEq/g.

Route	Onset	Peak	Duration
P.O.	Unknown	1-2 hr	Unknown

Adverse reactions
CNS: confusion, unusual tiredness restlessness, asthenia, flaccid paralysis, paresthesia
CV: ECG changes, hypotension, **arrhythmias, heart block, cardiac arrest**
GI: nausea, vomiting, diarrhea, abdominal discomfort, flatulence
Metabolic: hyperkalemia
Musculoskeletal: weakness and heaviness of legs

P

Interactions

Drug-drug. *ACE inhibitors, potassium-sparing diuretics, other potassium preparations:* increased risk of hyperkalemia

Drug-diagnostic tests. *Potassium:* increased level

Drug-food. *Salt substitutes containing potassium:* increased risk of hyperkalemia

Drug-herb. *Dandelion:* increased risk of hyperkalemia

Licorice: decreased response to potassium

Precautions

Use cautiously in:

• cardiac disease, renal impairment, diabetes mellitus, hypomagnesemia

• pregnant or breastfeeding patients

• children (safety and efficacy not established).

Patient monitoring

• Monitor renal function; fluid intake and output; and potassium, creatinine, and blood urea nitrogen levels.

◀€ Know that potassium is contraindicated in patients with severe renal impairment and must be used with extreme caution (if at all) in patients with any degree of renal impairment because of risk of life-threatening hyperkalemia.

• Monitor vital signs; check ECG for arrhythmias.

• Monitor patient's neurologic status; watch for neurologic complications.

Patient teaching

• Teach patient to take oral form with or just after meals, with a glass of water or fruit juice.

• Instruct patient to dilute liquid form in water or juice and to sip it over 5 to 10 minutes.

• Advise patient to report nausea, vomiting, confusion, numbness and tingling, unusual tiredness or weakness, or a heavy feeling in legs.

• Teach patient to minimize GI upset by eating small, frequent servings of healthy food and drinking plenty of fluids.

• Advise patient not to use salt substitutes.

• As appropriate, review all other significant and life-threatening adverse reactions and interactions, especially those related to the drugs, tests, foods, and herbs mentioned above.

potassium iodide
Pima, Thyro-Block

Pharmacologic class: Iodine, iodide

Therapeutic class: Antithyroid agent, expectorant

Pregnancy risk category D

Action

Rapidly inhibits release and synthesis of thyroid hormones, reduces thyroid vascularity, and decreases thyroid uptake of radioactive iodine after radiation emergencies or administration of radioactive iodine isotopes. Thought to act as expectorant by increasing respiratory tract secretions, thus decreasing mucus viscosity.

Availability

Saturated solution (SSKI): 1 g potassium iodide/ml in 30- and 240-ml bottles

Solution (strong iodine solution, Lugol's solution): 5% iodine and 10% potassium iodide in 120-ml bottle

Syrup: 325 mg potassium iodide/5 ml

Tablets: 130 mg (available only through state and federal agencies)

🕖 Indications and dosages

➢ Preparation for thyroidectomy

Adults and children: One to five drops SSKI P.O. t.i.d. or three to six drops

---

strong iodine solution P.O. t.i.d. for 10 days before surgery

➤ Thyrotoxic crisis

Adults and children: 500 mg P.O. (approximately 10 drops SSKI) q 4 hours or 1 ml P.O. (strong iodine solution) t.i.d., given at least 1 hour after initial dose of propylthiouracil or methimazole

➤ Radiation protectant in emergencies

Adults over age 40 with predicted thyroid exposure of 500 centigrays (cGy) or more, adults ages 18 to 40 with predicted thyroid exposure of 10 cGy or more, pregnant or breastfeeding women with predicted thyroid exposure of 5 cGy or more, and adolescents weighing 70 kg (154 lb) or more with predicted thyroid exposure of 5 cGy or more: 130 mg P.O. (tablet)

Children ages 3 to 18 (except adolescents weighing 70 kg [154 lb] or more) with predicted thyroid exposure of 5 cGy or more: 65 mg P.O. (tablet)

Children ages 1 month to 3 years with predicted thyroid exposure of 5 cGy or more: 32 mg P.O. (tablet)

Infants from birth to age 1 month with predicted thyroid exposure of 5 cGy or more: 16 mg P.O. (tablet)

➤ Expectorant

Adults: 300 to 650 mg P.O. (SSKI) three or four times daily given with at least 6 oz of fluid

Children: 60 to 250 mg P.O. (SSKI) q.i.d. given with at least 6 oz of fluid

Off-label uses
• Lymphocutaneous sporotrichosis

Contraindications
• Hypersensitivity to iodine, shellfish, or bisulfites (with some products)
• Hypothyroidism
• Renal impairment
• Acute bronchitis
• Addison's disease
• Acute dehydration

• Heat cramps
• Hyperkalemia
• Tuberculosis
• Iodism
• Concurrent use of potassium-containing drugs, potassium-sparing diuretics, or salt substitutes containing potassium

Administration
• Dilute saturated solution with at least 6 oz of water.

◀€ Don't give concurrently with other potassium-containing drugs or potassium-sparing diuretics because of increased risk of hyperkalemia, arrhythmias, and cardiac arrest.

• Know that U.S. government stockpiles potassium iodide 130-mg tablets for emergency use.

• When giving to very young children or patients who can't swallow tablets, crush tablet and dissolve in 20 ml of water; then add 20 ml of selected beverage (such as orange juice).

• Be aware that use of potassium iodide as an expectorant has been largely replaced by safer and more effective drugs.

Route	Onset	Peak	Duration
P.O.	24 hr	10-15 days	Variable

p

Adverse reactions
CNS: confusion; paresthesia, pain, or weakness in hands or feet; weakness or heaviness in legs; unusual fatigue

EENT: tooth discoloration (with strong iodide solution)

Metabolic: hyperkalemia, severe hypothyroidism, thyroid hyperplasia, thyroid adenoma, goiter (with prolonged use), **iodism** with large dosages or prolonged use

Other: hypersensitivity reactions (angioneurotic edema, fever, cutaneous and mucosal hemorrhage, serum sickness–like reaction)

Interactions
Drug-drug. *Lithium, other thyroid drugs:* additive hypothyroidism
Potassium-sparing diuretics, other potassium preparations: increased risk of hyperkalemia, arrhythmias, and cardiac arrest
Drug-diagnostic tests. *Radionuclide thyroid imaging:* altered test results
Thyroid uptake of ^{131}I, ^{123}I, sodium pertechnetate Tc 99m: decreased uptake
Drug-food. *Salt substitutes containing potassium:* increased risk of hyperkalemia

Precautions
Use cautiously in:
• cystic fibrosis, adolescent acne, hypocomplementemic vasculitis, goiter, autoimmune thyroid disease
• pregnant or breastfeeding patients
• children.

Patient monitoring
◀€ In long-term use, check for signs and symptoms of iodism (including metallic taste, sore teeth and gums, sore throat, burning of mouth and throat, coldlike symptoms, severe headache, productive cough, GI irritation, diarrhea, angioneurotic edema, rash, fever, and cutaneous or mucosal hemorrhage). Discontinue drug immediately if these occur.
• Monitor potassium level; watch for signs and symptoms of potassium toxicity.
• Assess ECG, renal function, fluid intake and output, and creatinine and blood urea nitrogen levels.
• Monitor thyroid function test results; watch for signs and symptoms of hypothyroidism or hyperthyroidism.

Patient teaching
• Teach patient to dilute drug in at least 6 oz of water or juice and to take it with meals.
• Advise patient to sip strong iodine

solution through a straw to help prevent tooth discoloration.
◀€ Teach patient to recognize and immediately report signs and symptoms of iodism and potassium toxicity.
• Instruct patient to minimize GI upset by eating small, frequent servings of healthy food and drinking plenty of fluids.
• Inform patient that many salt substitutes are high in potassium; advise him not to use these without prescriber's approval.
• As appropriate, review all other significant and life-threatening adverse reactions and interactions, especially those related to the drugs, tests, and foods mentioned above.

pramipexole dihydrochloride
Mirapex

Pharmacologic class: Non-ergot dopamine agonist
Therapeutic class: Antidyskinetic
Pregnancy risk category C

Action
Unknown; thought to directly stimulate postsynaptic dopamine receptors in corpus striatum (unlike levodopa, which may increase brain's dopamine concentration)

Availability
Tablets: 0.125 mg, 0.25 mg, 0.5 mg, 1 mg, 1.5 mg

Ⓘ Indications and dosages
➤ Idiopathic Parkinson's disease
Adults: Initially, 0.125 mg P.O. t.i.d.; may increase by 0.125 mg q 5 to 7 days over 6 to 7 weeks. Maintenance range is 1.5 to 4.5 mg/day in three divided doses.

Dosage adjustment
• Renal impairment

Contraindications
• Hypersensitivity to drug or its components

Administration
• Don't give drug at same time as other CNS depressants.
• Don't stop therapy abruptly; dosage should be tapered over 1 week.

Route	Onset	Peak	Duration
P.O.	Unknown	2 hr	8 hr

Adverse reactions
CNS: amnesia, dizziness, drowsiness, hallucinations, asthenia, abnormal dreams, confusion, dyskinesia, extrapyramidal symptoms, headache, insomnia, hypertonia, unsteadiness, sleep attacks
CV: orthostatic hypotension
GI: nausea, constipation, dyspepsia, dry mouth
GU: urinary frequency, impotence
Musculoskeletal: leg cramps
Respiratory: fibrotic complications (such as retroperitoneal fibrosis, pulmonary infiltrates, pleural effusion or thickening)
Other: accidental injury, edema

Interactions
Drug-drug. *Cimetidine:* increased pramipexole blood level
Dopamine antagonists (such as butyrophenones, metoclopramide, phenothiazines, thioxanthenes): decreased pramipexole efficacy
Levodopa: increased risk of hallucinations and dyskinesia

Precautions
Use cautiously in:
• renal impairment
• elderly patients
• pregnant or breastfeeding patients
• children (safety not established).

Patient monitoring
• Evaluate patient for therapeutic and adverse effects.
• Assess blood pressure; watch for orthostatic hypotension.
• Monitor neurologic status, especially for sleep attacks and extrapyramidal symptoms.

Patient teaching
• Instruct patient to take drug with food if it causes nausea and not to take it at same time as other CNS depressants.
• Advise patient to report dyskinesia, hallucinations, or sleep attacks.
• Inform patient that drug may cause impotence; encourage him to discuss this effect with prescriber.
• Tell patient and significant other that drug's neurologic and motor effects increase risk of accidental injury; teach them how to prevent injury.
• Teach patient to move slowly when sitting up or standing to avoid dizziness or light-headedness from sudden blood pressure decrease.
• As appropriate, review all other significant and life-threatening adverse reactions and interactions, especially those related to the drugs mentioned above.

p

pravastatin sodium
Pravachol

Pharmacologic class: HMG-CoA reductase inhibitor
Therapeutic class: Antilipemic
Pregnancy risk category X

Action
Inhibits HMG-CoA reductase, an enzyme that catalyzes cholesterol synthesis pathway; this action decreases cholesterol, triglyceride, apolipoprotein B,

and low-density lipoprotein (LDL) levels and increases high-density lipoprotein levels

Availability

Tablets: 10 mg, 20 mg, 40 mg, 80 mg

⏀ Indications and dosages

➤ Adjunct to diet to control levels of LDL, total cholesterol, apolipoprotein B, and triglycerides in patients with primary hypercholesterolemia, mixed dyslipidemia (including Fredrickson types IIa and IIb), primary dysbeta-lipoproteinemia (Fredrickson type III), hypertriglyceridemia (including Fredrickson type IV), and primary and secondary prevention of cardiovascular events

Adults: 10 to 80 mg P.O. once daily

Contraindications

• Hypersensitivity to drug or other HMG-CoA reductase inhibitors
• Active hepatic disease or unexplained, persistent transaminase elevations
• Pregnancy, breastfeeding, females of childbearing age

Administration

• If patient is also receiving a bile-acid resin, give pravastatin at bedtime, at least 4 hours after resin.

Route	Onset	Peak	Duration
P.O.	Unknown	Unknown	Unknown

Adverse reactions

CNS: amnesia, abnormal dreams, emotional lability, facial paresis, headache, hyperkinesia, poor coordination, malaise, paresthesia, peripheral neuropathy, drowsiness, syncope, asthenia
CV: orthostatic hypotension, palpitations, phlebitis, vasodilation, **arrhythmias**
EENT: amblyopia, glaucoma, eye hemorrhage, altered refraction, dry eyes, hearing loss, tinnitus, epistaxis, gingi-val hemorrhage, glossitis, sinusitis, pharyngitis
GI: nausea, vomiting, diarrhea, constipation, abdominal or biliary pain, colitis, gastric ulcer, dysphagia, esophagitis, flatulence, dyspepsia, heartburn, gastroenteritis, melena, tenesmus, abdominal cramps, stomatitis, dry mouth, taste loss, **pancreatitis, rectal hemorrhage**
GU: dysuria, hematuria, nocturia, urinary frequency or urgency, urinary retention, renal calculi, nephritis, abnormal ejaculation, cystitis, epididymitis, decreased libido, impotence
Hematologic: anemia, **thrombocytopenia**
Hepatic: jaundice, **hepatic failure, hepatitis**
Metabolic: hyperglycemia, hypoglycemia
Musculoskeletal: joint pain, bursitis, back pain, gout, leg cramps, myalgia, myositis, neck rigidity, torticollis, myasthenia gravis, rhabdomyolysis, increased creatine kinase level
Respiratory: dyspnea, pneumonia, bronchitis
Skin: diaphoresis, acne, alopecia, contact dermatitis, eczema, dry skin, pruritus, rash, urticaria, skin ulcers, seborrhea, photosensitivity
Other: increased or decreased appetite, weight gain, facial or generalized edema, fever, flulike symptoms, infection, allergic reaction

Interactions

Drug-drug. *Antacids, colestipol:* decreased pravastatin blood level
Azole antifungals, cyclosporine, erythromycin, niacin, gemfibrozil, other HMG-CoA reductase inhibitors: increased risk of myopathy
Digoxin: increased pravastatin blood level and risk of toxicity
Hormonal contraceptives: increased hormone levels

Drug-diagnostic tests. *Alanine aminotransferase, aspartate aminotransferase:* increased levels

Drug-food. *Grapefruit juice:* increased drug blood level

Drug-herb. *Chaparral, comfrey, eucalyptus, germander, jin bu huan, kava, pennyroyal, skullcap, valerian:* increased risk of hepatotoxicity

Red yeast rice: increased risk of adverse drug reactions

Precautions
Use cautiously in:
• renal impairment; severe hypotension or hypertension; severe acute infection; severe metabolic, endocrine, or electrolyte disorders; uncontrolled seizures; visual disturbances; myopathy; major surgery; trauma; alcoholism
• history of hepatic disease
• concurrent use of gemfibrozil or azole antifungals
• children under age 18 (safety not established).

Patient monitoring
• Monitor for signs and symptoms of allergic reaction.
• Monitor vital signs and cardiovascular status.
• Evaluate liver function test results before starting therapy, 6 to 12 weeks later, and at least semiannually thereafter; also monitor lipid levels.
• Assess creatine kinase levels of patients experiencing muscle pain or receiving other drugs associated with myopathy.

Patient teaching
• Caution patient not to take drug with grapefruit juice or antacids.
• Teach patient to recognize and immediately report signs and symptoms of allergic response and other adverse reactions, especially myositis.
• Inform patient that drug may cause headache, musculoskeletal pain, and leg cramps. Encourage him to discuss activity recommendations and pain management with prescriber.
• Advise females of childbearing age to notify prescriber of possible pregnancy.
• Tell male patient that drug may cause erectile dysfunction (impotence) and abnormal ejaculation. Recommend that he discuss these issues with prescriber.
• Instruct patient to avoid driving and other hazardous activities until he knows how drug affects concentration, alertness, and vision.
• Instruct patient not to take herbs unless prescriber approves.
• As appropriate, review all other significant and life-threatening adverse reactions and interactions, especially those related to the drugs, tests, foods, and herbs mentioned above.

prazosin hydrochloride
Minipress

Pharmacologic class: Alpha$_1$-adrenergic blocker (peripherally acting)
Therapeutic class: Antihypertensive
Pregnancy risk category C

Action
Induces peripheral vasodilation by blocking postsynaptic alpha$_1$-adrenergic receptors, thereby lowering blood pressure; decreases smooth muscle contractions of prostatic capsule and relaxes smooth muscles by alpha$_1$-adrenoceptor blockade in bladder neck and prostate

Availability
Capsules: 1 mg, 2 mg, 5 mg

p

💊 Indications and dosages

➤ Hypertension

Adults: Initially, 1 mg P.O. two or three times daily for 3 days, with first dose given at bedtime; increase gradually to a maintenance dosage of 6 to 15 mg/day in two or three divided doses (not to exceed 40 mg/day).

Off-label uses

• Benign prostatic hypertrophy

Contraindications

• Hypersensitivity to drug or other alpha$_1$-adrenergic blockers

Administration

• Give test dose of 1 mg at bedtime to prevent first-dose syncope.
• Don't stop therapy suddenly; dosage must be tapered.

Route	Onset	Peak	Duration
P.O.	2 hr	2-4 hr	10 hr

Adverse reactions

CNS: dizziness, headache, asthenia, drowsiness, depression, syncope
CV: first-dose orthostatic hypotension, palpitations, angina, edema
EENT: blurred vision, nasal congestion, epistaxis
GI: nausea, vomiting, diarrhea, abdominal cramps, dry mouth
GU: impotence, priapism
Musculoskeletal: joint and bone pain, myalgia

Interactions

Drug-drug. *Antihypertensives, nitrates:* additive hypotension
Nonsteroidal anti-inflammatory drugs: decreased antihypertensive effect
Drug-diagnostic tests. *Sodium, urinary vanillylmandelic acid:* increased levels
Pheochromocytoma screening test: false-positive result
Drug-herb. *Ephedra (ma huang):* acute hypertension

Precautions

Use cautiously in:
• renal insufficiency, angina pectoris, hepatic impairment
• patients receiving diuretics concurrently
• pregnant or breastfeeding patients
• children (safety not established).

Patient monitoring

• After first dose, observe closely for hypotension and syncope.
• Monitor blood pressure and pulse; watch for orthostatic hypotension.

Patient teaching

• Caution patient not to stop therapy suddenly; dosage must be tapered.
• Teach patient that drug may cause headache, muscle aches, or bone pain. Encourage him to discuss activity recommendations and pain management with prescriber.
• Tell patient that drug may cause sexual dysfunction; advise him to discuss these issues with prescriber.
• Instruct patient to move slowly when sitting up or standing to avoid dizziness or light-headedness from sudden blood pressure decrease.
• Caution patient not to take the herb ephedra (ma huang).
• As appropriate, review all other significant and life-threatening adverse reactions and interactions, especially those related to the drugs, tests, and herbs mentioned above.

---

prednisolone
Delta-Cortef, Prelone

prednisolone acetate
Econopred Ophthalmic, Econopred
Plus Ophthalmic, Key-Pred-25,
Key-Pred-50, Predalone 50,
Predcor-50, Pred Forte Ophthalmic,
Pred Mild Ophthalmic

prednisolone sodium phosphate
AK-Pred Ophthalmic, Hydeltrasol,
Inflamase Mild Ophthalmic,
Key-Pred-SP, Orapred, Pediapred

prednisolone tebutate
Predate TBA, Prednisol TBA

Pharmacologic class: Corticosteroid
(intermediate-acting)
Therapeutic class: Anti-inflammatory,
immunosuppressant
Pregnancy risk category C

Action
Shows potent anti-inflammatory (glucocorticoid) and weak sodium-retaining (mineralocorticoid) activity. Glucocorticoid activity causes profound
and varied metabolic effects.

Availability
Oral solution: 3 mg/ml, 5 mg/ml
Suspension for injection (acetate): 25
mg/ml, 50 mg/ml
Suspension for injection (tebutate): 20
mg/ml
Suspension (ophthalmic): 0.12%,
0.125%, 1%
Syrup: 15 mg/5 ml
Tablets: 4 mg, 5 mg, 8 mg, 16 mg,
24 mg, 32 mg

Indications and dosages
➤ Severe inflammation, immunosuppression
Adults: Individualized according to diagnosis, severity of condition, and response. 5 to 60 mg P.O. (prednisolone)
daily in two to four divided doses; or 4
to 60 mg I.M. (acetate) daily in divided
doses q 12 hours; or 5 to 50 mg P.O.
(sodium phosphate) daily in divided
doses.
➤ Short-term adjunctive therapy for
severe inflammation
Adults: 20 to 30 mg (tebutate) injected
into large joints or bursae, 8 to 10 mg
injected into small joints, 4 to 10 mg
injected into tendon sheaths, or 10 to
20 mg injected into ganglia
➤ Acute exacerbation of multiple
sclerosis
Adults: 200 mg P.O. daily for 1 week,
followed by 80 mg every other day for
1 month
➤ Refractory bronchial asthma
Children: 1 to 2 mg/kg/day (sodium
phosphate) in single or divided doses;
may continue for 3 to 10 days or until
symptoms resolve or until patient
achieves peak expiratory flow rate of
80% of his personal best.
➤ Nephrotic syndrome in children
Children: 60 mg/m^2 P.O. (sodium
phosphate solution) daily in three divided doses for 4 weeks, followed by 4
weeks of alternate-day therapy at single
doses of 40 mg/m^2
➤ Steroid-responsive inflammatory
eye conditions
Adults: For initial therapy in severe
cases, one to two drops (acetate or sodium phosphate) instilled into conjunctival sac q hour during day and q 2
hours at night. In mild or moderate inflammation or in severe cases when fa-
vorable response occurs, dosage may
be reduced to one to two drops q 3 to
12 hours.

p

Contraindications

- Hypersensitivity to drug, other corticosteroids, alcohol, bisulfite, or tartrazine (with some products)
- Systemic fungal infections
- Idiopathic thrombocytopenic purpura (with I.M. use)
- Live virus vaccines (with immunosuppressive steroid dosages)
- Active untreated infections (except in selected patients with certain types of meningitis)

Administration

◀€ Be aware that prednisolone has many different formulations that may be given by various routes: P.O., I.M., intralesional, intra-articular, soft tissue, or ophthalmic. Before administering, make sure formulation can be given by prescribed route.

- Inject I.M. form deep into gluteal muscle; rotate injection sites.
- Avoid S.C. injection.
- In systemic therapy, don't discontinue drug abruptly—even if inhaled steroid is added.
- Know that additional corticosteroids are needed during stress or trauma.

Route	Onset	Peak	Duration
P.O. (prednisolone, sod. phos.)	Unknown	1-2 hr	1.25-1.5 days
I.M. (acetate)	Slow	Unknown	Unknown
Intralesional, soft tissue, intra-artic.	Slow	Unknown	Prolonged
Ophthalmic (acetate, sod. phos.)	Unknown	Unknown	Unknown

Adverse reactions

CNS: headache, nervousness, depression, euphoria, personality changes, psychosis, vertigo, paresthesia, insomnia, restlessness, **increased intracranial pressure, seizures, meningitis**

CV: hypotension, vasculitis, thrombophlebitis, hypertension, **shock, heart failure, thromboembolism, fat embolism, arrhythmias**

EENT: cataracts, glaucoma, visual disturbances, exacerbation of infection, secondary ocular infections, perforation of globe at site of corneal or scleral thinning, transient stinging or burning of eyes, dry eyes, corneal ulcers, mydriasis (with ophthalmic use); posterior subcapsular cataracts (especially in children), glaucoma, nasal irritation and congestion, rebound congestion, sneezing, epistaxis, nasopharyngeal and oropharyngeal fungal infections, perforated nasal septum, anosmia, dysphonia, hoarseness, throat irritation (with long-term use)

GI: nausea, vomiting, abdominal distention, rectal bleeding, dry mouth, bad taste, esophageal candidiasis, esophageal ulcer, **pancreatitis, peptic ulcer**

GU: amenorrhea, irregular menses

Hematologic: purpura

Metabolic: sodium and fluid retention, hypokalemia, hypocalcemia, hyperglycemia, increased cholesterol level, decreased triiodothyronine (T_3) and thyroxine (T_4) levels, growth retardation (in children), decreased carbohydrate tolerance, diabetes mellitus, cushingoid effects (with long-term use), hypothalamic-pituitary-adrenal suppression (with systemic use longer than 5 days), **adrenal suppression** (with high-dose, long-term use)

Musculoskeletal: muscle weakness or atrophy, myalgia, myopathy, osteoporosis, aseptic joint necrosis, spontaneous fractures (with long-term use), osteonecrosis, tendon rupture

Respiratory: cough, wheezing, **bronchospasm**

Skin: rash, pruritus, contact dermatitis, acne, striae, poor wound healing, thin fragile skin, bruising, hirsutism, petechiae, subcutaneous fat atrophy, urticaria, angioedema

---

Other: increased or decreased appetite; aggravation or masking of infections; weight gain (with long-term use); facial edema; pain, burning, and atrophy at injection site; hypersensitivity reaction

Interactions

Drug-drug. *Amphotericin B, mezlocillin, piperacillin, thiazide and loop diuretics, ticarcillin:* additive hypokalemia
Anticholinesterase drugs: decreased anticholinesterase effect (when prednisolone is used for myasthenia gravis)
Aspirin, other nonsteroidal anti-inflammatory drugs: increased risk of GI discomfort and bleeding
Cardiac glycosides: increased risk of digitalis toxicity associated with hypokalemia
Cyclosporine: therapeutic benefits in organ transplant recipients, but with increased risk of toxicity
Erythromycin, indinavir, itraconazole, ketoconazole, ritonavir, saquinavir: increased prednisolone blood level and effects
Hormonal contraceptives: impaired metabolism and increased effects of prednisolone
Isoniazid: decreased isoniazid blood level
Live-virus vaccines: decreased antibody response to vaccine, increased risk of adverse effects
Oral anticoagulants: reduced anticoagulant requirement, opposition to anticoagulant action
Phenobarbital, phenytoin, rifampin: decreased prednisolone efficacy
Salicylates: reduced salicylate blood level
Somatrem: inhibition of somatrem's growth-promoting effects
Theophylline: altered pharmacologic effects of either drug
Drug-diagnostic tests. *Calcium, potassium, T_3, T_4, thyroid ^{131}I uptake:* decreased levels

Cholesterol, glucose: increased levels
Nitroblue tetrazolium test for bacterial infection: false-negative result
Drug-herb. *Alfalfa:* activation of quiescent systemic lupus erythematosus
Echinacea: increased immune-stimulating effects
Ephedra (ma huang): decreased drug blood level
Ginseng: potentiation of immunomodulating effect
Licorice: prolonged drug activity
Drug-behaviors. *Alcohol use:* increased risk of gastric irritation and GI ulcers

Precautions

Use cautiously in:
• diabetes mellitus, glaucoma, renal or hepatic disease, hypothyroidism, cirrhosis, diverticulitis, nonspecific ulcerative colitis, recent intestinal anastomoses, inflammatory bowel disease, thromboembolic disorders, seizures, myasthenia gravis, heart failure, hypertension, osteoporosis, ocular herpes simplex, immunosuppression, emotional instability
• pregnant or breastfeeding patients
• children under age 6.

Patient monitoring

• Monitor weight, blood pressure, and electrolyte levels.
• Watch for cushingoid effects (moon face, central obesity, buffalo hump, hair thinning, high blood pressure, frequent infections).
• Assess patient for depression and psychosis.
• Monitor blood glucose levels carefully in diabetic patients.
• Evaluate for signs and symptoms of infection, which drug may mask or exacerbate.
• Monitor for signs and symptoms of early adrenal insufficiency (fatigue, weakness, joint pain, fever, anorexia, shortness of breath, dizziness, syncope).

p

• Assess musculoskeletal status for joint, tendon, and muscle pain.

Patient teaching

• Tell patient to take oral dose with food or milk to reduce GI upset.

🔈 Teach patient to recognize and immediately report cushingoid effects and signs and symptoms of early adrenal insufficiency.

🔈 Advise patient and significant other to immediately report depression or psychosis.

• Explain that drug increases risk of infection; instruct patient to contact prescriber at first sign of infection.

• Caution patient not to stop therapy (including ophthalmic forms) suddenly and to discuss any changes in drug use with prescriber.

• Tell patient to report joint, muscle, or tendon pain.

• Inform patient that he may need increased dosage during periods of stress; encourage him to wear or carry medical identification stating this.

• Advise patient to avoid vaccinations during therapy. Tell him that others living in same household shouldn't receive oral polio vaccine because they could pass poliovirus to him.

• Caution patient not to take over-the-counter drugs or herbs.

• As appropriate, review all other significant and life-threatening adverse reactions and interactions, especially those related to the drugs, tests, herbs, and behaviors mentioned above.

prednisone

Apo-Prednisone✱, Cordrol, Deltasone, Liquid Pred, Meticorten, Orasone 1, Orasone 5, Orasone 10, Orasone 20, Orasone 50, Panasol-S, Prednicen-M, Prednicot, Sterapred, Winpred✱

Pharmacologic class: Corticosteroid (intermediate acting)

Therapeutic class: Anti-inflammatory, immunosuppressant

Pregnancy risk category C

Action

Shows potent anti-inflammatory (glucocorticoid) and weak sodium-retaining (mineralocorticoid) activity. Glucocorticoid activity causes profound and varied metabolic effects.

Availability

Oral solution: 5 mg/ml, 5 mg/5 ml
Syrup: 5 mg/5 ml
Tablets: 1 mg, 2.5 mg, 5 mg, 10 mg, 20 mg, 50 mg

Indications and dosages

➢ Severe inflammation, immunosuppression

Adults: Individualized according to diagnosis, severity of condition, and response For most uses, 5 to 60 mg P.O. daily as a single dose or in divided doses

➢ Acute exacerbation of multiple sclerosis

Adults: 200 mg P.O. daily for 1 week, then 80 mg every other day for 1 month

➢ Adjunctive therapy in *Pneumocystis jiroveci* (formerly *Pneumocystis carinii*) pneumonia in AIDS patients

Adults: 40 mg P.O. b.i.d. for 5 days, then 40 mg once daily for 5 days, then 20 mg once daily for 11 days

Contraindications

• Hypersensitivity to drug, other corticosteroids, alcohol, bisulfite, or tartrazine (with some products)
• Systemic fungal infections
• Live-virus vaccines (with immunosuppressive doses)
• Active untreated infections (except in selected patients with some types of meningitis)

Administration

• Give drug with food or milk to reduce GI upset.
• Administer once-daily dose early in morning.

Route	Onset	Peak	Duration
P.O.	Unknown	1-2 hr	1.25-1.5 days

Adverse reactions

CNS: headache, nervousness, depression, euphoria, personality changes, psychosis, vertigo, paresthesia, insomnia, restlessness, **seizures, meningitis, increased intracranial pressure**
CV: hypotension, vasculitis, thrombophlebitis, hypertension, **heart failure, thromboembolism, fat embolism, arrhythmias, shock**
EENT: posterior subcapsular cataracts (especially in children), glaucoma, nasal irritation and congestion, rebound congestion, sneezing, epistaxis, nasopharyngeal and oropharyngeal fungal infections, perforated nasal septum, anosmia, dysphonia, hoarseness, throat irritation (with long-term use)
GI: nausea, vomiting, abdominal distention, rectal bleeding, esophageal candidiasis, bad taste, dry mouth, esophageal ulcer, **pancreatitis, peptic ulcer**
GU: amenorrhea, irregular menses
Hematologic: purpura
Metabolic: sodium and fluid retention, hypokalemia, hypocalcemia, hyperglycemia, increased cholesterol level, decreased triiodothyronine (T_3) and thyroxine (T_4) levels, growth retardation (in children), decreased carbohydrate tolerance, diabetes mellitus, cushingoid effects (with long-term use), hypothalamic-pituitary-adrenal suppression (with systemic use exceeding 5 days), **adrenal suppression** (with high-dose, long-term use)
Musculoskeletal: muscle weakness or atrophy, myalgia, myopathy, osteoporosis, aseptic joint necrosis, spontaneous fractures (with long-term use), osteonecrosis, tendon rupture
Respiratory: cough, wheezing, **bronchospasm**
Skin: rash, pruritus, contact dermatitis, acne, striae, poor wound healing, hirsutism, thin fragile skin, petechiae, bruising, subcutaneous fat atrophy, urticaria, angioedema
Other: aggravation or masking of infections, increased or decreased appetite, weight gain (with long-term use), facial edema, hypersensitivity reaction

Interactions

Drug-drug. *Amphotericin B, mezlocillin, piperacillin, thiazide and loop diuretics, ticarcillin:* additive hypokalemia
Aspirin, other nonsteroidal anti-inflammatory drugs: increased risk of GI discomfort and bleeding
Cardiac glycosides: increased risk of digitalis toxicity associated with hypokalemia
Cyclosporine: therapeutic benefits in organ transplant recipients, but with increased risk of toxicity
Erythromycin, indinavir, itraconazole, ketoconazole, ritonavir, saquinavir: increased prednisone blood level and effects
Hormonal contraceptives: impaired metabolism and increased effects of prednisone
Isoniazid: decreased isoniazid blood level

p

Live-virus vaccines: decreased antibody response to vaccine, increase risk of adverse effects

Oral anticoagulants: reduced anticoagulant requirements, opposition to anticoagulant action

Phenobarbital, phenytoin, rifampin: decreased prednisone efficacy

Salicylates: reduced salicylate blood level

Somatrem: inhibition of somatrem's growth-promoting effects

Theophylline: altered pharmacologic effects of either drug

Drug-diagnostic tests. *Calcium, potassium, T_3, T_4, thyroid ^{131}I uptake:* decreased levels

Cholesterol, glucose: increased levels

Nitroblue tetrazolium test for bacterial infection: false-negative result

Drug-herb. *Alfalfa:* activation of quiescent systemic lupus erythematosus

Echinacea: increased immune-stimulating effects

Ephedra (ma huang): decreased drug blood level

Ginseng: potentiation of immunomodulating effect

Licorice: prolonged drug activity

Drug-behaviors. *Alcohol use:* increased risk of gastric irritation and GI ulcers

Precautions

Use cautiously in:
• diabetes mellitus, glaucoma, renal or hepatic disease, hypothyroidism, cirrhosis, diverticulitis, nonspecific ulcerative colitis, recent intestinal anastomoses, inflammatory bowel disease, thromboembolic disorders, seizures, myasthenia gravis, heart failure, hypertension, osteoporosis, hypothyroidism, ocular herpes simplex, immunosuppression, emotional instability
• pregnant or breastfeeding patients
• children under age 6.

Patient monitoring

• Monitor weight, blood pressure, and electrolyte levels.

• Watch for cushingoid effects (moon face, central obesity, buffalo hump, hair thinning, high blood pressure, and more frequent infections).
• Check for signs and symptoms of depression and psychosis.
• Assess blood glucose level carefully in diabetic patients.
• Monitor patient for signs and symptoms of infection, which drug may mask or exacerbate.
• Assess for early indications of adrenal insufficiency (fatigue, weakness, joint pain, fever, appetite loss, shortness of breath, dizziness, syncope).
• Monitor musculoskeletal status for joint, tendon, and muscle pain.

Patient teaching

• Tell patient to take drug with food or milk to reduce GI upset.
◀€ Teach patient to recognize and immediately report signs and symptoms of early adrenal insufficiency and cushingoid effects.
• Inform patient that drug increases his risk of infection; instruct him to contact prescriber at first sign or symptom of infection.
• Caution patient not to discontinue therapy suddenly; advise him to discuss any changes in drug use with prescriber.
• Teach patient to report joint, muscle, or tendon pain.
◀€ Advise patient or significant other to immediately report depression or psychosis.
• Advise patient not to take herbs or over-the-counter drugs during therapy.
• Caution patient to avoid vaccinations during therapy. Tell him that others in household shouldn't receive oral polio vaccine because they could pass poliovirus to him.
• Tell patient he may need higher dosage during periods of stress; encourage him to wear or carry medical identification stating this.

• As appropriate, review all other significant and life-threatening adverse reactions and interactions, especially those related to the drugs, tests, herbs, and behaviors mentioned above.

primaquine phosphate

Pharmacologic class: 8-aminoquinoline compound
Therapeutic class: Antimalarial
Pregnancy risk category C

Action
Unknown; thought to disrupt parasitic mitochondria and bind to native DNA, leading to structural changes that disrupt metabolic processes and to inhibition of gametocyte and erythrocyte forms; destroys some gametocytes and makes other incapable of undergoing maturation division.

Availability
Tablets: 26.3 mg (15 mg base)

Indications and dosages
➤ Treatment or prevention of relapse of malaria caused by *Plasmodium vivax*
Adults: 15 mg base P.O. daily for 14 days
Children: 0.3 mg base/kg/day P.O. for 14 days, increased to a maximum of 15 mg base

Off-label uses
• *Pneumocystis jiroveci* (formerly *Pneumocystis carinii*) pneumonia

Contraindications
• Hypersensitivity to drug
• Concurrent use of quinacrine, other hemolytic drugs, or myelosuppressants
• Bone marrow depression
• Systemic disease with history of or tendency to granulocytopenia (such as lupus erythematosus or rheumatoid arthritis)

Administration
◀€ Before giving, check prescription to see if dosage is written as mg or mg base.
• Start therapy during last 2 weeks of suppression course with chloroquine or comparable drugs, or after suppression course ends.

Route	Onset	Peak	Duration
P.O.	Unknown	1-3 hr	Unknown

Adverse reactions
CNS: headache, dizziness, asthenia
CV: hypertension
EENT: blurred vision, difficulty focusing
GI: nausea, vomiting, diarrhea, constipation, abdominal pain, epigastric distress
Hematologic: mild anemia, hemolytic anemia, and leukocytosis; **methemoglobinemia**
Skin: pruritus, skin eruptions, pallor

Interactions
Drug-drug. *Aluminum and magnesium salts:* decreased GI absorption of primaquine
Quinacrine: increased risk of primaquine toxicity
Drug-diagnostic tests. *Hemoglobin, red blood cells:* decreased levels
White blood cells: increased or decreased count

Precautions
Use cautiously in:
• porphyria, methemoglobinemia, methemoglobin reductase deficiency, glucose-6-phosphate dehydrogenase deficiency, iodine deficiency, anemia
• pregnant patients.

p

Patient monitoring

◀€ Monitor complete blood count; watch for signs and symptoms of blood dyscrasias or hemolytic reaction (dark urine, chills, fever, chest pain, bluish skin). Stop drug and notify prescriber at once if these occur.

• Monitor blood pressure.

Patient teaching

• Advise patient to take drug with food to minimize GI upset.

◀€ Teach patient to recognize and immediately report signs and symptoms of hemolytic reactions.

• Instruct patient to avoid driving and other hazardous activities until he knows how drug affects concentration, vision, and alertness.

• Teach patient to complete entire course of therapy as prescribed, even after symptoms improve.

• As appropriate, review all other significant and life-threatening adverse reactions and interactions, especially those related to the drugs and tests mentioned above.

primidone
Apo-Primidone✦, Mysoline, PMS-Primidone✦, Sertan✦

Pharmacologic class: Barbiturate
Therapeutic class: Anticonvulsant
Pregnancy risk category NR

Action
Unknown; may raise seizure threshold by its conversion to phenobarbital, which decreases neuronal firing

Availability
Suspension: 250 mg/5 ml
Tablets: 50 mg, 250 mg

⚡ Indications and dosages
➤ Tonic-clonic and simple partial seizures

Adults and children ages 8 and older: Initially, 100 to 125 mg P.O. at bedtime on days 1 to 3, followed by 100 to 125 mg P.O. b.i.d. on days 4 to 6, then 100 to 125 mg P.O. t.i.d. on days 7 to 9, followed by a maintenance dosage of 250 mg P.O. three or four times daily.

Children younger than age 8: Initially, 50 mg P.O. at bedtime on days 1 to 3, followed by 50 mg P.O. b.i.d. on days 4 to 6, then 100 mg P.O. b.i.d. on days 7 to 9. Daily maintenance dosage is 125 to 250 mg t.i.d. or 10 to 25 mg/kg/day in divided doses.

Dosage adjustment
• Renal impairment

Off-label uses
• Benign familial (essential) tremor

Contraindications
• Hypersensitivity to drug or phenobarbital
• Porphyria

Administration
• Don't change brands; bioequivalency problems have occurred.
• Don't stop therapy suddenly; dosage must be tapered.

Route	Onset	Peak	Duration
P.O.	Unknown	3-4 hr	Unknown

Adverse reactions
CNS: headache, dizziness, stimulation, drowsiness, sedation, confusion, hallucinations, psychosis, ataxia, vertigo, hyperirritability, emotional disturbances, paranoid symptoms, **coma**
EENT: diplopia, nystagmus, eyelid edema
GI: nausea, vomiting, anorexia
GU: impotence
Hematologic: megaloblastic anemia, **thrombocytopenia**

Hepatic: altered liver function test results
Skin: flushing, rash

Interactions
Drug-drug. *Acetazolamide, succinimide:* decreased primidone blood level
Carbamazepine: decreased primidone blood level, increased carbamazepine blood level
Hydantoins, isoniazid, nicotinamide: increased primidone blood level
Drug-diagnostic tests. *Hemoglobin, platelets:* decreased levels
Liver function tests: altered results

Precautions
Use cautiously in:
• hepatic, renal, or chronic obstructive pulmonary disease
• pregnant or breastfeeding patients
• hyperactive children.

Patient monitoring
• Monitor primidone and phenobarbital blood levels.
• Monitor complete blood count and blood chemistry; watch for signs and symptoms of blood dyscrasias.
• Assess neurologic status regularly; stay alert for excessive drowsiness and emotional status changes.

Patient teaching
• Caution patient not to discontinue therapy suddenly. Advise him to discuss any dosage changes with prescriber.
• Instruct patient to report unusual bleeding, bruising, or rash.
• Inform patient that drug may cause sexual dysfunction; advise him to discuss this issue with prescriber.
• Caution patient to avoid driving and other hazardous activities until he knows how drug affects concentration, vision, and alertness.
• As appropriate, review all other significant and life-threatening adverse reactions and interactions, especially those related to the drugs and tests mentioned above.

probenecid
Benemid, Benuryl✦, Probalan

Pharmacologic class: Sulfonamide-derived uricosuric
Therapeutic class: Antigout drug, tubular blocking agent
Pregnancy risk category B

Action
Promotes excretion of uric acid from the kidneys by blocking tubular reabsorption; also inhibits tubular secretion of weak organic acids (most penicillins and cephalosporins and some beta-lactam anti-infectives)

Availability
Tablets: 0.5 g

🕡 Indications and dosages
➤ Hyperuricemia associated with gout
Adults and children weighing more than 50 kg (110 lb): After acute gout attack subsides, 250 mg P.O. b.i.d. for 1 week, followed by 500 mg b.i.d.; may increase by 500 mg/day q 4 weeks (not to exceed 3 g/day)
➤ To prolong action or increase blood level of penicillins
Adults: 500 mg P.O. q.i.d.
Children ages 2 to 14: Initially, 25 mg/kg or 0.7 g/m² $, then a maintenance dosage of 40 mg/kg/day or 1.2 g/m² $ in four divided doses
➤ Gonorrhea
Adults: 1 g P.O. as a single dose immediately before or with prescribed amoxicillin dose
Dosage adjustment
• Renal impairment

p

Off-label uses

• Hyperuricemia secondary to thiazide therapy

Contraindications

• Hypersensitivity to drug
• Acute gout attack
• Uric acid calculi
• Blood dyscrasias
• Concurrent salicylate use
• Concurrent penicillin use in patients with renal impairment
• Children under age 2

Administration

• Don't give drug until acute gout attack subsides.
• Ensure high fluid intake and alkaline urine during therapy.

Route	Onset	Peak	Duration
P.O.	30 min	2-4 hr	8 hr

Adverse reactions

CNS: headache, dizziness
GI: nausea, vomiting, diarrhea, anorexia, abdominal pain, sore gums
GU: urinary frequency, uric acid calculi, renal colic, nephrotic syndrome
Hematologic: anemia, hemolytic anemia, **aplastic anemia**
Hepatic: hepatitis, hepatic necrosis
Musculoskeletal: costovertebral pain
Skin: flushing, rash, pruritus
Other: fever, gout exacerbation, hypersensitivity reactions including **anaphylaxis**

Interactions

Drug-drug. *Acyclovir, allopurinol, barbiturates, cephalosporins, pantothenic acid, penicillins:* increased blood levels of these drugs, increased uric acid–reducing effect of probenecid
Benzodiazepines: faster onset and prolonged effect of benzodiazepines
Clofibrate: increased clofibrate blood level
Dapsone: accumulation of dapsone and its metabolites

Dyphylline: increased half-life and decreased clearance of dyphylline
Methotrexate, nonsteroidal anti-inflammatory drugs, rifampin, sulfonamides: increased blood level, therapeutic effect, and toxicity of these drugs
Oral hypoglycemics: increased half-life and hypoglycemic effect of these drugs
Penicillamine: increased pharmacologic effects of penicillamine
Salicylates: decreased probenecid or salicylate activity
Thiopental: extended anesthetic effect of thiopental
Zidovudine: increased risk of zidovudine toxicity
Drug-diagnostic tests. *Urine glucose tests using copper reduction method (Clinitest, Benedict's solution, Fehling's solution):* false-positive result

Precautions

Use cautiously in:
• peptic ulcer, renal impairment
• pregnant or breastfeeding patients.

Patient monitoring

• Monitor kidney and liver function test results, complete blood count, and blood urea nitrogen level.
• Assess fluid intake and output to ensure good hydration and reduce urinary side effects.
• Monitor pattern and severity of acute gout attacks to assess need for additional anti-inflammatory drugs during first 6 to 12 months of therapy.

Patient teaching

• Advise patient to take drug with food or milk to minimize GI upset.
• Teach patient about causes of gout and proper use of drug. Emphasize that he must wait until acute attack has subsided and should then take drug regularly to prevent further attacks.
• Tell patient that drug may exacerbate acute gout attacks for first 6 to 12 months and that he'll need to take

colchicine or other anti-inflammatory drug for 3 to 6 months.

• Instruct patient to drink 2 to 3 liters of fluids daily.

• Tell patient with gout to limit foods high in purine (such as anchovies, organ meats, and legumes) because purine breakdown leads to uric acid formation.

• Instruct diabetic patients to test urine with Clinistix or Tes-Tape during therapy.

• As appropriate, review all other significant and life-threatening adverse reactions and interactions, especially those related to the drugs and tests mentioned above.

procainamide hydrochloride
Apo-Procainamide✦, Procanbid, Procan SR, Promine, Pronestyl, Pronestyl-SR✦

Pharmacologic class: Membrane stabilizer

Therapeutic class: Antiarrhythmic (class IA)

Pregnancy risk category C

Action
Decreases myocardial excitability by inhibiting conduction velocity. Also depresses myocardial contractility.

Availability
Capsules: 250 mg, 375 mg, 500 mg
Injection: 100 mg/ml, 500 mg/ml
Tablets: 250 mg, 375 mg, 500 mg
Tablets (extended-release): 250 mg, 500 mg, 750 mg, 1,000 mg

⚕ Indications and dosages
➢ Life-threatening ventricular arrhythmias
Adults: 50 to 100 mg by slow I.V. push

at a rate of 50 mg/minute, repeated q 5 minutes until arrhythmias subside. Alternatively, give loading dose of 500 to 600 mg by I.V. infusion over 25 to 30 minutes. Maximum loading dose by either I.V. administration method is 1 g. When arrhythmia subsides, give continuous I.V. infusion of 2 to 6 mg/minute.

Or give 50 mg/kg I.M. in divided doses q 3 to 6 hours until oral therapy is tolerated.

For long-term maintenance, usual dosage is 50 mg/kg (extended-release) P.O. daily in equally divided doses q 6 hours.

Dosage adjustment
• Renal impairment

Contraindications
• Hypersensitivity to drug, tartrazine, or sulfites
• Asymptomatic premature ventricular contractions
• Complete heart block
• Lupus erythematosus
• Torsades de pointes
• Breastfeeding
• Children under age 18

Administration
• Don't crush tablets including extended-release.
• Ask patient about procaine sensitivity before giving drug (cross-sensitivity may occur).
• For I.V. use, dilute with dextrose 5% in water.
• Administer I.V. doses with patient in supine position to avoid hypotensive effects.
• When giving by I.V. infusion, use infusion pump to ensure that drug infuses at 50 mg/minute or less.
◀ᴇ Don't leave patient's bedside during I.V. administration.

p

Route	Onset	Peak	Duration
P.O.	Unknown	90-120 min	Unknown
I.V.	Immediate	Immediate	Unknown
I.M.	10-30 min	15-60 min	Unknown

Adverse reactions

CNS: headache, dizziness, confusion, psychosis, restlessness, asthenia, depression, neuropathy, **seizures**

CV: hypotension, bradycardia, atrioventricular block, **ventricular fibrillation, ventricular asystole, cardiovascular collapse, cardiac arrest**

EENT: bitter taste

GI: nausea, vomiting, diarrhea, anorexia

Hematologic: hemolytic anemia, **agranulocytosis, thrombocytopenia, neutropenia**

Skin: rash, urticaria, pruritus, flushing

Other: lupuslike syndrome, edema

Interactions

Drug-drug. *Amiodarone:* increased procainamide blood level and risk of toxicity

Anticholinesterase drugs: decreased anticholinesterase effects

Antihypertensives: additive hypotension

Beta-adrenergic blockers, cimetidine, ranitidine, trimethoprim: increased procainamide blood level

Lidocaine: additive cardiodepressant action, conduction abnormalities

Neuromuscular blockers: increased skeletal muscle relaxation

Other antiarrhythmics: additive or antagonistic effects, additive toxicity

Trimethoprim: increased pharmacologic effects of procainamide

Drug-herb. *Henbane:* increased anticholinergic activity

Jimsonweed: adverse cardiovascular effects

Licorice: prolonged QT interval

Drug-behaviors. *Alcohol use:* altered drug blood level

Precautions

Use cautiously in:

• procaine hypersensitivity, renal impairment, ischemic heart disease, heart failure, first-degree heart block, atypical ventricular tachycardia, myasthenia gravis, systemic lupus erythematosus, cytopenia

• patients receiving other antiarrhythmics concurrently

• pregnant patients

• children.

Patient monitoring

◀❧ When giving drug I.V., stay at patient's bedside and monitor blood pressure and ECG continuously.

◀❧ If ECG shows prolonged QT intervals and QRS complexes, heart block, or worsening arrhythmia, stop drug administration, run rhythm strip, and contact prescriber immediately.

• Assess blood levels of procainamide and *N*-acetylprocainamide (drug's active metabolite).

• Monitor electrolyte levels, complete blood count, and antinuclear antibody titer; watch for signs and symptoms of blood dyscrasias.

• Evaluate patient for signs and symptoms of lupuslike syndrome.

Patient teaching

• Teach patient not to crush extended-released tablets.

◀❧ Advise patient to immediately report cardiovascular symptoms or bleeding tendency.

• Emphasize importance of taking drug exactly as prescribed; advise patient to use alarm clock to help him remember to take nighttime doses.

• Advise patient to avoid alcohol intake.

• Instruct patient not to take herbal remedies unless prescriber approves.

• As appropriate, review all other significant and life-threatening adverse reactions and interactions, especially those related to the drugs, herbs, and behaviors mentioned above.

---

procaine hydrochloride
Novocain

Pharmacologic class: Benzoic acid
Therapeutic class: Ester-type local anesthetic (short-acting)
Pregnancy risk category C

Action
Blocks generation and conduction of impulses through sensory, motor, and autonomic nerve fibers by making nerve cell membrane less permeable to sodium ions; reversibly blocks nerve conduction near injection site, causing temporary loss of feeling or sensation in limited area

Availability
Injection: 1% solution in ampules and multidose vials, 2% and 10% solution in multidose vials

Indications and dosages
➤ Infiltration anesthesia
Adults: 350 to 600 mg of 0.25% to 0.5% diluted solution injected into area to be anesthetized as a single dose
➤ Peripheral nerve block
Adults: 100 ml of 1% diluted solution or 50 ml of 2% solution injected into area where peripheral nerve block is needed
➤ Spinal anesthesia
Adults: 0.5, 1, or 2 ml of 10% solution injected into spinal area, depending on area of anesthesia needed, diluted in 0.5, 1, or 2 ml of normal saline solution, sterile distilled water, or spinal fluid (respectively); administer at 1.5 ml/5 seconds.

Contraindications
• Hypersensitivity to drug, its components (including sodium sulfite with some products), or para-aminobenzoic acid

Administration
• Know that drug should be given only by personnel with expertise in administering it (and in avoiding intravascular injections) and in assessing and managing dose-related toxicities and other acute emergencies that may arise.
• Follow label directions to reconstitute drug for selected route.
• Make sure emergency resuscitation equipment is available before drug is given.
• Know that if necessary, epinephrine may be added to slow procaine absorption, prolong action, or maintain hemostasis.

Route	Onset	Peak	Duration
All routes discussed above	2-5 min	Unknown	1 hr

Adverse reactions
CNS: anxiety, restlessness, shivering, drowsiness, disorientation, tremor, **seizures, loss of consciousness**
CV: hypotension, hypertension, bradycardia, **fetal bradycardia, myocardial depression, cardiac arrest, arrhythmias**
EENT: blurred vision, miosis, tinnitus
GI: nausea, vomiting, diarrhea, abdominal pain
Respiratory: status asthmaticus, respiratory arrest
Skin: flushing, rash, urticaria, burning, skin discoloration at injection site, tissue necrosis
Other: hypersensitivity reactions including **anaphylaxis**

Interactions
Drug-drug. *Diuretics:* prolonged procaine half-life and effect
Enflurane, epinephrine, halothane: arrhythmias

P

Monoamine oxidase inhibitors, pheno-thiazines, tricyclic antidepressants: hypertension
Sulfonamides: inhibition of sulfonamide action

Precautions
Use cautiously in:
- severe drug allergies
- elderly patients
- pregnant patients
- children.

Patient monitoring
◀€ Monitor patient's vital signs and ECG closely, especially when drug is given as spinal anesthestic; stay alert for signs of impending cardiac arrest.
◀€ Stay alert for signs and symptoms of status asthmaticus and anaphylaxis.
◀€ Monitor patient's position carefully, especially after spinal anesthesia, to help prevent damage to nerves and other body tissues.
- Inspect infusion site for extravasation.

Patient teaching
- Explain use of drug to patient; reassure him that he'll be closely monitored during anesthesia.
- Inform patient that infiltration causes temporary numbness.
- As appropriate, review all other significant and life-threatening adverse reactions and interactions, especially those related to the drugs mentioned above.

procarbazine hydrochloride
Matulane, Natulan♣

Pharmacologic class: Alkylating agent
Therapeutic class: Antineoplastic
Pregnancy risk category D

Action
Thought to inhibit DNA, RNA, and protein synthesis, resulting in death of rapidly dividing cells; also inhibits monoamine oxidase

Availability
Capsules: 50 mg

⏀ Indications and dosages
➤ Hodgkin's disease
Adults: 2 to 4 mg/kg P.O. daily as a single dose or in divided doses for 1 week, followed by 4 to 6 mg/kg P.O. daily until white blood cell (WBC) count falls below 4,000/mm³ or platelets fall below 100,000/mm³, or until desired response occurs. With desired response, give maintenance dose of 1 to 2 mg/kg P.O. daily (round off dosage to nearest 50 mg). As a component of MOPP (mechlorethamine, vincristine, procarbazine, prednisone) regimen for advanced Hodgkin's disease, usual dosage is 100 mg/m² P.O. daily on days 1 to 14 of 28-day cycle.
Children: Dosage highly individualized. Usual dosage is 50 mg/m² P.O. daily for first week, followed by 100 mg/m² P.O. daily until leukopenia, thrombocytopenia, or desired response occurs. With desired response, maintenance dosage is 50 mg/m² P.O. daily.

Off-label uses
- Brain tumor
- Lymphoma

Contraindications
- Hypersensitivity to drug
- Inadequate bone marrow reserve
- Pregnancy or breastfeeding

Administration
- Weigh patient. Know that dosages are based on patient's weight; however, use caution in patients with edema or ascites.

Route	Onset	Peak	Duration
P.O.	Rapid	1 hr	Unknown

Adverse reactions

CNS: confusion, dizziness, drowsiness, hallucinations, headache, mania, depression, nightmares, psychosis, syncope, tremor, neuropathy, paresthesia, **seizures**

CV: edema, hypotension, tachycardia

EENT: nystagmus, photophobia, retinal hemorrhage

GI: nausea, vomiting, diarrhea, dysphagia, ascites, stomatitis, dry mouth, anorexia

GU: gonadal suppression, gynecomastia

Hematologic: anemia, **leukopenia, thrombocytopenia**

Hepatic: hepatic dysfunction

Respiratory: cough, pleural effusion

Skin: alopecia, photosensitivity, pruritus, rash

Interactions

Drug-drug. *Digoxin:* decreased digoxin blood level

Levodopa: flushing, hypertension

Opioid analgesics: deep coma, death

Sympathomimetics (indirect-acting): abrupt, life-threatening hypertension

Tricyclic antidepressants: severe toxicity and fatal reactions (including blood pressure fluctuations, seizures, and coma)

Drug-diagnostic tests. *Hematocrit, hemoglobin, platelets, reticulocytes, WBCs:* decreased levels

Drug-food. *Caffeine-containing foods and beverages:* hypertension, arrhythmias

Tyramine-containing foods and beverages: life-threatening hypertension

Drug-behaviors. *Alcohol use:* disulfiram-like reaction

Precautions

Use cautiously in:
• infection, chronic debilitating illness, headache, hepatic or renal impairment, cardiovascular disease, heart failure, diarrhea, stomatitis, pheochromocytoma, psychiatric illness, alcoholism
• patients who have had radiation therapy or received other chemotherapy agents within previous month
• elderly patients
• women of childbearing age.

Patient monitoring

• Monitor vital signs and nutritional status.
• Assess fluid intake and output; watch for signs and symptoms of fluid overload.
◄€ Monitor neurologic status, especially for seizures, paresthesia, neuropathy, and confusion. Discontinue drug and notify prescriber if these occur.
◄€ Monitor complete blood count and platelet count; discontinue drug and contact prescriber if WBC count falls below 4,000/mm³ or platelet count falls below 100,000/mm³.
◄€ Evaluate patient's concurrent drug use to ensure that he isn't receiving other drugs that could cause potentially fatal interactions.
◄€ Check for diarrhea; discontinue therapy and contact prescriber if patient has frequent bowel movements or watery stools.
• Monitor blood urea nitrogen level, liver and kidney function test results, and urinalysis.
◄€ Discontinue therapy at first sign of hypersensitivity, stomatitis, diarrhea, or bleeding.

Patient teaching

• Instruct patient to avoid caffeine-containing foods and beverages.
◄€ Teach patient to avoid foods and beverages containing tyramine (such as cheese, Chianti wine, tea, coffee, cola, and bananas).

• Advise patient to avoid alcohol.
• As appropriate, review all other significant and life-threatening adverse reactions and interactions, especially those related to the drugs, tests, foods, and behaviors mentioned above.

prochlorperazine
Compazine, Stemetil❧

prochlorperazine edisylate
Compazine

prochlorperazine maleate
Compazine, Compazine Spansule, Stemetil❧

Pharmacologic class: Phenothiazine
Therapeutic class: Antiemetic, antipsychotic, anxiolytic
Pregnancy risk category C

Action
Possesses anticholinergic, CNS depressant, and antihistaminic effects; decreases sensitivity of middle-ear labyrinth and depresses conduction in vestibular-cerebellar pathways

Availability
Capsules (extended-release): 10 mg, 15 mg, 30 mg (all maleate)
Oral solution: 5 mg/5 ml (edisylate)
Injection: 5 mg/ml (edisylate)
Suppositories: 2.5 mg, 5 mg, 25 mg
Tablets: 5 mg, 10 mg, 25 mg

🝝 Indications and dosages
➤ Nausea
Adults: 5 to 10 mg P.O. three to four times daily or 15 mg P.O. once daily or 10 mg P.O. (extended-release) b.i.d., up to 40 mg/day. Or 2.5 to 10 mg I.V., not to exceed 40 mg/day.

Children weighing 40 to 85 lb: 2.5 mg P.O. or P.R. t.i.d. or 5 mg P.O. or P.R. b.i.d., not to exceed 15 mg/day
Children weighing 30 to 39 lb: 2.5 mg P.O. or P.R. two or three times daily, not to exceed 10 mg/day
Children weighing 20 to 29 lb: 2.5 mg P.O. or P.R. daily to b.i.d., not to exceed 7.5 mg/day
➤ Nausea and vomiting associated with surgery
Adults: 5 to 10 mg I.V. 15 to 30 minutes before anesthesia induction, repeated once if necessary; or 5 to 10 mg I.M. 1 to 2 hours before anesthesia induction, repeated once in 30 minutes if necessary
➤ Management of psychotic symptoms
Adults and children older than age 12: 5 to 10 mg P.O. three to four times daily; may be increased q 2 to 3 days up to 150 mg/day. Or 10 to 20 mg I.M.; may repeat q 2 to 4 hours for up to four doses if necessary.
➤ Anxiety
Adults and children older than age 12: 5 mg P.O. three to four times daily; or 15 mg P.O. (sustained-release) once daily or 10 mg P.O. (sustained-release) q 12 hours; up to 20 mg/day for a maximum of 12 weeks

Off-label uses
• Migraine

Contraindications
• Hypersensitivity to drug or other phenothiazines
• Coma
• Concurrent use of large amounts of CNS depressants
• Pediatric surgery
• Children younger than age 2 or weighing less than 9 kg (20 lb)

Administration
• For I.V. infusion, dilute 20 mg in 1 L of compatible I.V. solution, such as normal saline solution.

• Don't mix in same syringe with other drugs.

• Know that injection solution may cause contact dermatitis; don't get it on hands or clothing.

◀€ Give I.V. by slow infusion only; don't give as bolus.

• Know that I.M. injection isn't preferred because it can cause local irritation. However, if I.M. route is prescribed, inject deep into upper outer quadrant of gluteal area.

• Don't give by S.C. route.

• After desired response is attained, switch to oral form at same or higher dosage.

Route	Onset	Peak	Duration
P.O.	30-40 min	Unknown	3-4 hr
P.O. (extended)	30-40 min	Unknown	10-12 hr
I.V.	Rapid (min)	10-30 min	3-4 hr
I.M.	10-20 min	10-30 min	3-4 hr
P.R.	60 min	Unknown	3-4 hr

Adverse reactions

CNS: extrapyramidal reactions, sedation, tardive dyskinesia, **neuroleptic malignant syndrome**

CV: ECG changes, orthostatic hypotension, tachycardia

EENT: blurred vision, lens opacities, pigmentary retinopathy, dry eyes

GI: constipation, ileus, dry mouth, anorexia

GU: pink or reddish brown urine, urinary retention

Hematologic: agranulocytosis, leukopenia

Hepatic: cholestatic jaundice, **hepatitis**

Metabolic: hyperthermia

Skin: photosensitivity, pigmentation changes, rash

Other: galactorrhea, allergic reactions

Interactions

Drug-drug. *Anticonvulsants:* reduced seizure threshold

Antineoplastics: masking of toxicity caused by antineoplastics

CNS depressants (including antihistamines, anticholinergics, opioid analgesics, other phenothiazines, sedative-hypnotics): additive CNS depression

Guanethidine: inhibition of antihypertensive effects

Oral anticoagulants: decreased anticoagulant effect

Phenytoin: increased or decreased phenytoin blood level

Propranolol: increased blood levels of both drugs

Thiazide diuretics: increased risk of orthostatic hypotension

Drug-diagnostic tests. *Liver function tests:* abnormal results

Phenylketonuria test: false-positive result

Drug-herb. *Betel nut:* increased risk of extrapyramidal reactions

Evening primrose oil: increased risk of seizures

Kava: increased risk of drug-related adverse reactions

Drug-behaviors. *Alcohol use:* additive CNS depression

Precautions

Use cautiously in:

• cardiovascular or hepatic disease, glaucoma, seizures

• patients who expect to be exposed to extreme heat

• children with acute illness.

Patient monitoring

◀€ Monitor neurologic status, especially for signs and symptoms of neuroleptic malignant syndrome (high fever, sweating, unstable blood pressure, stupor, muscle rigidity, and autonomic dysfunction).

• In long-term therapy, assess for other adverse CNS effects, including extrapyramidal symptoms and tardive dyskinesia.

• When giving by I.V. infusion, watch for hypotension; keep patient supine for 30 minutes after infusion.
• Monitor patient closely if he's receiving prochlorperazine for nausea and vomiting associated with chemotherapy, because drug may mask symptoms of chemotherapy toxicity.
• Evaluate complete blood count and liver function test results.

Patient teaching

• Instruct patient to dilute oral solution with tomato or fruit juice, milk, coffee, soda, tea, water, or soup.
◀♬ Teach patient to recognize and immediately report signs and symptoms of an allergic reaction or neuroleptic malignant syndrome.
• Inform patient about drug's other CNS effects; instruct him to contact prescriber if these occur.
• Advise patient to avoid driving and other hazardous activities until he knows how drug affects concentration, vision, alertness, and motor skills.
• Caution patient to avoid alcohol and herbal products.
• Tell patient that drug may turn urine pink or reddish brown.
• As appropriate, review all other significant and life-threatening adverse reactions and interactions, especially those related to the drugs, tests, herbs, and behaviors mentioned above.

progesterone
Crinone, Progesterone Injection, Prometrium

Pharmacologic class: Progestin
Therapeutic class: Hormone
Pregnancy risk category B (oral), *D* (injection), *NR* (vaginal)

Action
Suppresses ovulation by causing changes in vaginal epithelium, relaxing smooth muscle of the uterus, and promoting mammary alveolar tissue growth. Also inhibits pituitary activity and causes withdrawal bleeding in presence of estrogen.

Availability
Injection (in sesame or peanut oil with benzyl alcohol): 50 mg/ml in 10-ml vials
Micronized capsules (oral): 100 mg, 200 mg
Micronized vaginal gel: 4%, 8%

🕖 Indications and dosages
➤ Secondary amenorrhea
Adults: 400 mg/day P.O. in evening for 10 days, or 5 to 10 mg/day I.M. for 6 to 8 days given 8 to 10 days before expected menstrual period. Or 45 mg (one applicatorful of 4% gel) vaginally once every other day for up to six doses; may increase to 90 mg (one applicatorful of 8% gel) once every other day for up to six doses.
➤ Dysfunctional uterine bleeding
Adults: 5 to 10 mg I.M. daily for 6 days
➤ To prevent postmenopausal estrogen-induced endometrial hyperplasia
Adults: 200 mg/day P.O. at bedtime for 14 days on days 8 to 21 of 28-day cycle or on days 12 to 25 of 30-day cycle. If patient currently receives estrogen 1.25 mg/day, give 300 mg progesterone divided in two doses (100 mg 2 hours after breakfast and 200 mg at bedtime); further adjustment may be required.
➤ Corpus luteum insufficiency or assisted reproduction technology
Adults: For luteal phase support, 90 mg (one applicatorful of 8% gel) vaginally once daily. For in vitro fertilization, 90 mg (one applicatorful of 8% gel) vaginally once daily, starting within 24 hours of embryo transfer and continued through day 30 after trans-

fer; if pregnancy occurs, treatment may continue for up to 12 weeks. For partial or complete ovarian failure, 90 mg (one applicatorful of 8% gel) vaginally b.i.d. while patient undergoes donor oocyte transfer; if pregnancy occurs, treatment may last up to 12 weeks.

Contraindications
- Hypersensitivity to drug, peanuts, or sesame
- Thromboembolic disease
- Cerebrovascular disease
- Severe hepatic disease
- Breast or genital cancer
- Porphyria
- Missed abortion
- Undiagnosed vaginal bleeding
- Pregnancy (except in corpus luteum dysfunction)

Administration
- Before first dose, ensure that patient has read package insert regarding adverse effects. Reinforce written information with an oral review.
- Before first I.M. dose, ask if patient has allergy to peanuts or sesame.
- Inject I.M. dose deep into muscle; rotate injection sites.

Route	Onset	Peak	Duration
P.O.	Unknown	2-4 hr	Unknown
I.M., vaginal	Unknown	Unknown	Unknown

Adverse reactions
CNS: depression, emotional lability, **cerebrovascular accident**
CV: thrombophlebitis, **thromboembolism**
EENT: retinal thrombosis, gingival bleeding
GI: abdominal cramps
GU: amenorrhea, breakthrough bleeding, spotting, cervical erosions, breast tenderness, changes in menstrual flow, galactorrhea
Hepatic: elevated hepatic enzyme levels, **hepatitis**

Metabolic: altered thyroid function tests
Respiratory: pulmonary embolism
Skin: melasma, rash, angioedema
Other: weight gain or loss, hypersensitivity reactions including **anaphylaxis**

Interactions
Drug-drug. *Conjugated estrogens:* increased levels of both drugs
Drug-diagnostic tests. *Alkaline phosphatase, amino acids, low-density lipoproteins:* increased levels
Chloride and sodium excretion: decreased (with high doses)
High-density lipoproteins: decreased level
Pregnanediol excretion: decreased
Thyroid function tests: altered results
Drug-herb. *Red clover:* interference with drug effects
Drug-behaviors. *Smoking:* increased risk of thromboembolic effects

Precautions
Use cautiously in:
- renal or cardiovascular disease, seizure disorders, fluid retention, diabetes mellitus, asthma, migraine, depression
- history of hepatic disease
- breastfeeding patients.

Patient monitoring
◀ Watch for evidence of thromboembolic disorders, including cerebrovascular accident, pulmonary embolism, diplopia, proptosis, or sudden partial or complete vision loss (may signal retinal thrombosis). If these occur, discontinue therapy and notify prescriber immediately.
◀ Assess for emotional lability and depression.

Patient teaching
◀ Teach patient to recognize and immediately report signs and symptoms of thromboembolic disorders.

◀≶ Instruct patient and significant other to stay alert for and immediately report depression.

• Advise women that drug may cause menstrual abnormalities.

◀≶ Instruct patient to immediately report possible pregnancy.

• Advise patient to monitor weight regularly and report significant changes.

• Tell patient that smoking increases risk of thromboembolism; encourage her to stop smoking if she smokes.

• As appropriate, review all other significant and life-threatening adverse reactions and interactions, especially those related to the drugs, tests, herbs, and behaviors mentioned above.

promethazine

Antinaus 50, Histanil, Pentazine, Phenazine 50, Phencen-50, Phenergan, Phenergan Fortis, Phenergan Plain, Phenerzine, Pro-50, Promacot, Promet, Prothazine, Shogan

Pharmacologic class: Phenothiazine (nonselective)

Therapeutic class: Antihistamine, antiemetic, sedative-hypnotic

Pregnancy risk category C

Action

Blocks effects of histamine and inhibits chemoreceptor trigger zone in medulla. Alters dopamine effects in CNS, possesses significant anticholinergic activity, and produces CNS depression by indirectly reducing reticular stimulation.

Availability

Injection: 25 mg/ml and 50 mg/ml in 1-ml ampules and 1- and 10-ml vials
Suppositories: 2.5 mg, 5 mg, 25 mg

Syrup: 3.25 mg/5 ml, 6.25 mg/5 ml, 10 mg/5 ml, 25 mg/5 ml
Tablets: 12.5 mg, 25 mg, 50 mg

✔ Indications and dosages

➤ Type 1 hypersensitivity reaction
Adults: 25 mg P.O. or P.R. at bedtime or 12.5 mg P.O. before meals and at bedtime. Or 25 mg I.M. or I.V.; may repeat in 2 hours.

Children older than age 2: 25 mg P.O. or P.R. at bedtime or 6.25 to 12.5 mg P.O. t.i.d.

➤ Motion sickness
Adults: Initially, 25 mg P.O. or P.R. 30 to 60 minutes before traveling; may repeat 8 to 12 hours later if needed. On successive travel days, 25 mg P.O. or P.R. b.i.d. (on arising and before evening meal).

Children older than age 2: 12.5 to 25 mg P.O. or P.R. b.i.d.

➤ Sedation
Adults: 25 to 50 mg P.O., I.M., I.V., or P.R. at bedtime

Children older than age 2: 12.5 to 25 mg P.O. or P.R. at bedtime

➤ Adjunct to preoperative or postoperative analgesia
Adults: 25 to 50 mg P.O., P.R., I.M., or I.V. given with appropriately reduced dosage of a narcotic or barbiturate and required amount of belladonna alkaloid

Children older than age 2: 0.5 mg/lb P.O., P.R., I.M., or I.V., given with appropriately reduced dosage of a narcotic or barbiturate and required amount of belladonna alkaloid. Parenteral dosages shouldn't exceed half of adult dosage.

➤ Nausea
Adults: 25 mg P.O. or P.R.; may repeat doses of 12.5 to 25 mg P.O. or P.R. q 4 to 6 hours p.r.n. Or 12.5 to 25 mg I.M. or I.V.; may repeat q 4 hours p.r.n.

Children older than age 2: 25 mg or 0.5 mg/lb P.O. or P.R.; may repeat doses of 12.5 to 25 mg P.O. or P.R. q 4 to 6 hours p.r.n. May give I.M. or I.V. in dosages not exceeding half of adult dosage. Don't administer if cause of vomiting is unknown.

Contraindications
• Hypersensitivity to drug
• Previous idiosyncratic reaction to phenothiazines
• Coma
• CNS depression related to barbiturates, general anesthesia, tranquilizers, alcohol, or narcotics
• Asthma, chronic obstructive pulmonary disease, sleep apnea
• Acutely ill or dehydrated children

Administration
• Don't give I.V. at concentrations above 25 mg/ml or faster than 25 mg/minute.
• Use light-resistant covering for I.V. drug.
◀€ Inject I.M. deep into large muscle. Don't give by S.C. route.

Route	Onset	Peak	Duration
P.O., I.M. P.R.	20 min	Unknown	4-12 hr
I.V.	3-5 min	Unknown	4-12 hr

Adverse reactions
CNS: confusion, disorientation, marked drowsiness, sedation, dizziness, extrapyramidal reactions, fatigue, insomnia, nervousness, **neuroleptic malignant syndrome**
CV: hypertension, hypotension, bradycardia, tachycardia
EENT: blurred vision, diplopia, tinnitus, dry mouth
GI: constipation
Hematologic: blood dyscrasias
Hepatic: cholestatic jaundice
Respiratory: respiratory depression
Skin: photosensitivity, rash
Other: hypersensitivity reaction

Interactions
Drug-drug. *Anticholinergics:* additive anticholinergic effects

CNS depressants: additive CNS depression
Epinephrine: reversal of epinephrine's vasopressor effects
Monoamine oxidase inhibitors: increased extrapyramidal effects
Drug-diagnostic tests. *Glucose:* increased level
Granulocytes, platelets, white blood cells: decreased counts
Pregnancy test: false-positive or false-negative results
Skin tests using allergen extracts: false-negative results
Drug-herb. *Betel nut:* increased risk of extrapyramidal effects
Evening primrose oil: increased risk of seizures
Kava: increased risk of adverse drug effects
Drug-behaviors. *Alcohol use:* additive CNS depression
Sun exposure: increased risk of photosensitivity

Precautions
Use cautiously in:
• cardiovascular or hepatic disease, seizures, bone marrow depression, narrow-angle glaucoma, prostatic hypertrophy, stenosing peptic ulcer, pyloroduodenal or bladder neck obstruction
• pregnant or breastfeeding patients
• children.

Patient monitoring
◀€ Monitor neurologic status; stay alert for signs and symptoms of neuroleptic malignant syndrome (high fever, sweating, unstable blood pressure, stupor, muscle rigidity, and autonomic dysfunction).
• In long-term therapy, assess for other adverse CNS effects, including extrapyramidal reactions.
• Monitor complete blood count and liver function test results.

Patient teaching

🔊 Teach patient to recognize and immediately report signs and symptoms of hypersensitivity reaction or neuroleptic malignant syndrome.

• Teach patient about drug's other significant neurologic effects; instruct him to contact prescriber if these occur.

• Instruct patient to avoid driving and other hazardous activities until he knows how drug affects concentration, vision, alertness, and motor skills.

• Tell patient to avoid alcohol and herbal products during therapy.

• As appropriate, review all other significant and life-threatening adverse reactions and interactions, especially those related to the drugs, tests, herbs, and behaviors mentioned above.

propafenone hydrochloride
Rythmol

Pharmacologic class: Direct membrane stabilizer

Therapeutic class: Antiarrhythmic (class IC)

Pregnancy risk category C

Action

Slows conduction velocity in the atrioventricular node, decreases automaticity, and increases ratio of effective refractory period to action potential duration; also possesses mild beta-adrenergic blocking properties

Availability

Tablets: 150 mg, 225 mg, 300 mg

💋 Indications and dosages

➤ Life-threatening ventricular arrhythmias, including sustained ventricular tachycardia

Adults: Dosage highly individualized based on patient response and tolerance. Initially, 150 mg P.O. q 8 hours (450 mg/day); may be increased after 3 to 4 days to 225 mg P.O. q 8 hours (675 mg/day) or, if necessary, up to 300 mg P.O. q 8 hours (900 mg/day). Dosage shouldn't exceed 900 mg/day P.O.

Dosage adjustment

• Hepatic disease

• Supraventricular tachycardia, arrhythmias associated with Wolff-Parkinson-White syndrome

• Elderly patients

Contraindications

• Hypersensitivity to drug

• Sick-sinus syndrome, sinoatrial or atrioventricular (AV) block (unless artificial pacemaker is in place)

• Cardiogenic shock

• Bradycardia

• Uncontrolled heart failure

• Marked hypotension

• Bronchospastic disorders

• Electrolyte imbalances

• Breastfeeding

Administration

• Give drug with food (but not with grapefruit juice) in three divided doses daily, once every 8 hours.

Route	Onset	Peak	Duration
P.O.	Variable	3.5 hr	Unknown

Adverse reactions

CNS: headache, dizziness, drowsiness, syncope, vertigo, confusion, asthenia, speech disturbances, memory loss, ataxia, paresthesia, anxiety, abnormal dreams, insomnia, tremor

CV: palpitations, angina, chest pain, hypotension, bradycardia, premature ventricular contractions, first-degree AV block, proarrhythmias, **supraventricular or ventricular arrhythmias, heart failure, atrial fibrillation, intraventricular conduction delay**

EENT: blurred vision, tinnitus

GI: nausea, vomiting, diarrhea, constipation, dyspepsia, cholestasis, abdominal pain or cramps, flatulence, altered taste, dry mouth, anorexia

GU: reversible disorders of spermatogenesis

Hematologic: purpura, hemolytic anemia, **leukopenia, agranulocytosis, thrombocytopenia, neutropenia**

Hepatic: abnormal liver function

Musculoskeletal: muscle weakness, myalgia, leg cramps

Respiratory: dyspnea

Skin: rash, alopecia, diaphoresis

Other: myasthenia gravis exacerbation, edema

Interactions

Drug-drug. *Beta-adrenergic blockers:* increased blood level and effects of beta-adrenergic blockers metabolized by liver

Cimetidine: increased propafenone blood level

Cyclosporine, desipramine, digoxin, theophylline, warfarin: increased blood levels of these drugs

Quinidine: delayed propafenone metabolism

Rifampin: decreased blood level and antiarrhythmic efficacy of propafenone

Drug-diagnostic tests. *Antinuclear antibody:* positive titer

Bleeding time: prolonged

Creatine kinase, glucose: increased levels

Granulocytes, white blood cells: decreased counts

Drug-herb. *Aloe, buckthorn, cascara sagrada, senna pod or leaf:* increased antiarrhythmic action, decreased potassium level

Precautions

Use cautiously in:
• hepatic or renal impairment, myasthenia gravis
• pregnant patients
• children.

Patient monitoring

• Monitor ECG and vital signs.
• Evaluate neurologic status; stay alert for decreasing level of consciousness.
• Monitor complete blood count and liver function test results; watch for blood dyscrasias and abnormal liver function.
• Monitor respiratory status for dyspnea.

Patient teaching

◀€ Teach patient which cardiac, neurologic, and respiratory adverse effects to report immediately.

◀€ Instruct patient to immediately report unusual bleeding or bruising.

• Caution patient to avoid driving and other hazardous activities until he knows how drug affects concentration, vision, and alertness.

• As appropriate, review all other significant and life-threatening adverse reactions and interactions, especially those related to the drugs, tests, and herbs mentioned above.

propantheline bromide
Pro-Banthine, Propanthel✦

Pharmacologic class: Parasympatholytic

Therapeutic class: Anticholinergic, antimuscarinic, antispasmodic

Pregnancy risk category C

Action

Prevents muscarinic action of acetylcholine at postganglionic parasympathetic neuroeffector sites, thus relaxing GI tract and blocking gastric acid secretion

Availability

Tablets: 7.5 mg, 15 mg

ⓘ Indications and dosages
➤ Peptic ulcer
Adults: 15 mg P.O. 30 minutes before each meal and 30 mg at bedtime, for a total of four daily doses
➤ Mild spasmodic conditions
Adults of normal stature: 15 mg P.O. t.i.d. before each meal and 30 mg at bedtime, for a total of four daily doses
Adults of small stature: 7.5 mg P.O. t.i.d. before each meal
Dosage adjustment
• Mild peptic ulcer symptoms
• Elderly patients

Off-label uses
• Neurogenic bladder
• Urinary incontinence
• Antisecretory and antispasmodic effects

Contraindications
• Hypersensitivity to drug or other anticholinergics
• Narrow-angle glaucoma
• Tachycardia
• Arrhythmias
• Myocardial ischemia
• Acute hemorrhage
• GI obstruction
• Paralytic ileus
• GI atony in elderly or debilitated patients
• Toxic megacolon
• Stenosing peptic ulcer
• Prostatic hypertrophy
• Bladder neck obstruction
• Renal disease
• Myasthenia gravis
• Breastfeeding

Administration
• Give 30 minutes before meals and at bedtime—except in adults of small stature, who should receive drug three times a day before meals.

Route	Onset	Peak	Duration
P.O.	30-60 min	2-6 hr	6 hr

Adverse reactions
CNS: confusion, stimulation, headache, insomnia, dizziness, anxiety, asthenia, hallucinations
CV: palpitations, orthostatic hypotension, tachycardia
EENT: blurred vision, photophobia, mydriasis, cycloplegia, increased intraocular pressure, nasal congestion
GI: nausea, vomiting, constipation, heartburn, dysphagia, bloating, gastroesophageal reflux disease (GERD), dry mouth, taste loss, **paralytic ileus**
GU: urinary hesitancy or retention, impotence, suppressed lactation
Skin: rash, urticaria, pruritus, anhidrosis
Other: fever, heat prostration, allergic reaction

Interactions
Drug-drug. *Amantadine:* increased propantheline effects
Atenolol: increased pharmacologic effects of atenolol
Phenothiazines: decreased antipsychotic efficacy of phenothiazines, increased adverse effects of propantheline
Tricyclic antidepressants: increased anticholinergic effects
Drug-herb. *Henbane, jimsonweed, scopolia:* increased anticholinergic effects

Precautions
Use cautiously in:
• heart failure, hypertension, arrhythmias, coronary artery disease, hepatic disease, hiatal hernia, prostatic hypertrophy, glaucoma, chronic lung disease in debilitated patients, hyperthyroidism, autonomic neuropathy
• elderly patients
• pregnant patients
• children.

Patient monitoring
• Monitor vital signs; watch for orthostatic hypotension.

• Assess patient for sensory and neuro-logic impairment.

Patient teaching
• Inform patient that drug may inhibit sweating and make him susceptible to heat prostration. Teach him effective ways to maintain normal body temperature.
• Describe drug's adverse anticholinergic effects; recommend appropriate measures to minimize these.
• Advise patient to report GERD symptoms to prescriber.
• Tell male patient that drug may cause impotence; encourage him to discuss this problem with prescriber.
• Instruct patient to avoid driving and other hazardous activities until he knows how drug affects concentration, vision, and alertness.
• Teach patient to move slowly when sitting up or standing to avoid dizziness or light-headedness from sudden blood pressure decrease.
• As appropriate, review all other significant adverse reactions and interactions, especially those related to the drugs and herbs mentioned above.

propofol
Diprivan

Pharmacologic class: General anesthetic

Therapeutic class: Sedative-hypnotic
Pregnancy risk category B

Action
Unknown; thought to inhibit sympathetic nerve impulse transmission, causing CNS depression

Availability
Injection: 10 mg/ml in 20-ml ampules; 50-ml prefilled syringes; 50-ml and 100-ml infusion vials

⚠ Indications and dosages
➤ General anesthesia induction
Adults younger than age 55: 40 mg or 2 to 2.5 mg/kg I.V. q 10 seconds until induction onset. In neurosurgical patients, 20 mg or 1 to 2 mg/kg q 10 seconds until induction onset. In patients receiving cardiac anesthesia, 20 mg or 0.5 to 1.5 mg/kg q 10 seconds until induction onset.
➤ General anesthesia maintenance
Adults younger than age 55: 100 to 200 mcg/kg/minute by I.V. infusion, given with nitrous oxide and oxygen; or 25 to 50 mg (2.5 to 5 ml) by intermittent I.V. bolus, given with nitrous oxide
➤ To initiate monitored anesthesia care sedation
Adults younger than age 55: 100 to 150 mcg/kg/minute by I.V. infusion for 3 to 5 minutes, titrated to desired effect; or approximately 0.5 mg/kg by slow I.V. injection over 3 to 5 minutes, titrated to desired effect
➤ To maintain monitored anesthesia care sedation
Adults younger than age 55: 25 to 75 mcg/kg/minute by slow I.V. infusion for 10 to 15 minutes, decreased to 25 to 50 mcg/kg/minute
➤ To initiate and maintain sedation in mechanically ventilated patients in intensive care unit (ICU)
Adults younger than age 55: Initially, I.V. infusion of 5 mcg/kg/minute for 5 minutes with highly individualized dosage; may be increased at 5- to 10-minute intervals in increments of 5 to 10 mcg/kg/minute until desired sedation level is reached.
Dosage adjustment
• Adults older than age 55
• American Society of Anesthesiologists Class III or IV patients
• Debilitated patients
• Children

p

Contraindications

• Hypersensitivity to drug, its components, eggs, soybean oil, or glycerol
• When general anesthesia or sedation is contraindicated
• Breastfeeding

Administration

• Be aware that drug usually doesn't require dilution. However, if prescribed, use only dextrose 5% in water and dilute to a concentration of no less than 2 mg/ml; then infuse at prescribed rate.
• Don't use drug if emulsion phases have separated.
• Don't use filter with pores smaller than 5 microns.
• Don't mix with other drugs before infusing; don't deliver through same I.V. line as blood or plasma.
• After 12 hours, discard unused portion along with tubing.
• Don't stop administering drug suddenly; dosage must be tapered.
• Shield drug from light.

Route	Onset	Peak	Duration
I.V.	<40 sec	Unknown	10-15 min

Adverse reactions

CNS: headache, abnormal movements, dizziness, shivering, tremor, confusion, drowsiness, paresthesia, agitation, abnormal dreams, euphoria, fatigue
CV: hypotension, hypertension, premature ventricular or atrial contractions, abnormal ECG, ST-segment depression, tachycardia, bradycardia, **asystole**
EENT: blurred vision, eye pain, tinnitus, sneezing, strange taste, dry mouth
GI: nausea, vomiting, abdominal pain
GU: urinary retention, green urine
Musculoskeletal: myalgia
Respiratory: cough, hiccups, dyspnea, hypoventilation, wheezing, tachypnea, hypoxia, **apnea**
Skin: flushing, phlebitis, urticaria

Other: fever, burning or stinging sensation at injection site, hypersensitivity reaction

Interactions

Drug-drug. *Inhalation anesthetics, opioids, sedative-hypnotics, skeletal muscle relaxants:* increased CNS depression
Drug-behaviors. *Alcohol use:* increased CNS depression

Precautions

Use cautiously in:
• renal or hepatic disease, heart failure, arrhythmias, hypertension, respiratory disorders, hyperlipidemia
• elderly patients
• pregnant patients
• patients in labor and delivery
• children.

Patient monitoring

• Monitor vital signs and ECG continuously.
• Monitor arterial blood gas results and respiratory status.
• When giving drug in ICU, evaluate patient's neurologic status frequently to help determine minimal dosage required.
• Assess blood lipid levels.

Patient teaching

• Inform patient that drug may impair mental alertness briefly after therapy ends.
• Assure patient that he'll be monitored continuously.
• Tell patient that drug normally turns urine green.

---

propoxyphene hydrochloride
Darvon

propoxyphene napsylate
Darvon-N

Pharmacologic class: Opioid-like agonist

Therapeutic class: Nonopioid analgesic

Controlled substance schedule IV

Pregnancy risk category C

Action
Alters perception of and emotional response to pain by binding with opiate receptors in brain, causing depression of CNS

Availability
propoxyphene hydrochloride
Capsules: 65 mg
propoxyphene napsylate
Tablets: 100 mg

⬤ Indications and dosages
➤ Mild to moderate pain
Adults: 65 mg (hydrochloride) P.O. q 4 hours or 100 mg (napsylate) P.O. q 4 hours as needed. Don't exceed 390 mg/ day hydrochloride or 600 mg/day napsylate.
Dosage adjustment
• Hepatic or renal impairment
• Elderly or debilitated patients

Contraindications
• Hypersensitivity to drug or its components
• Suicidal or substance abuse–prone patients

Administration
• Give with milk or food to reduce GI upset.

• Be aware that 100 mg of propoxyphene napsylate is equivalent to 65 mg of propoxyphene hydrochloride.

Route	Onset	Peak	Duration
P.O.	15-60 min	2-3 hr	4-6 hr

Adverse reactions
CNS: dizziness, headache, dysphoria, euphoria, insomnia, paradoxical excitement, asthenia, sedation
CV: hypotension
EENT: blurred vision
GI: nausea, vomiting, constipation, abdominal pain
Hepatic: altered liver function test results
Skin: rash
Other: physical or psychological drug dependence, drug tolerance

Interactions
Drug-drug. *Antidepressants, sedative-hypnotics:* additive CNS depression
Buprenorphine, dezocine, nalbuphine, pentazocine: decreased analgesic effect
Monoamine oxidase (MAO) inhibitors: unpredictable and potentially fatal effects
Partial-antagonist opioid analgesics: precipitation of withdrawal in physically dependent patients
Drug-diagnostic tests. *Alanine aminotransferase, alkaline phosphatase, aspartate aminotransferase:* altered levels
Drug-herb. *Chamomile, hops, kava, skullcap, valerian:* increased CNS depression
Drug-behaviors. *Alcohol use:* increased CNS depression
Smoking: increased metabolism and decreased analgesic efficacy of propoxyphene

Precautions
Use cautiously in:
• head trauma; increased intracranial pressure; severe renal, hepatic, or pulmonary disease; hypothyroidism; adre-

P

nal insufficiency; undiagnosed abdominal pain; prostatic hypertrophy; alcoholism
- patients receiving MAO inhibitors
- elderly or debilitated patients
- pregnant or breastfeeding patients
- children.

Patient monitoring
- Advise patient to take drug with milk or food to minimize GI upset.
- Assess patient's pain level 30 minutes after administering drug.
- Evaluate drug's CNS effects; implement protective measures, as needed, to prevent injury.
- In long-term therapy, monitor liver function studies and evaluate patient regularly for signs of physical or psychological drug dependence.

Patient teaching
- Inform patient that drug may cause physical or psychological dependence; stress that he should take it only as prescribed and only when needed.
- Teach patient that alcohol and smoking affect drug blood level; discourage these habits.
- Instruct patient to avoid driving and other hazardous activities until he knows how drug affects concentration, vision, and alertness.
- As appropriate, review all other significant adverse reactions and interactions, especially those related to the drugs, tests, herbs, and behaviors mentioned above.

propranolol hydrochloride
Apo-Propranolol✤, Betachron E-R, Inderal, Inderal LA, Novopranol✤, PMS Propranolol✤

Pharmacologic class: Beta-adrenergic blocker (nonselective)

Therapeutic class: Antianginal, antiarrhythmic (class II), antihypertensive, vascular headache suppressant

Pregnancy risk category C

Action
Blocks stimulation of beta$_1$-adrenergic (myocardial) and beta$_2$-adrenergic (pulmonary, vascular, and uterine) receptor sites, decreasing cardiac output, thereby slowing heart rate and reducing blood pressure

Availability
Capsules (extended-release, sustained-release): 60 mg, 80 mg, 120 mg, 160 mg
Injection: 1 mg/ml
Oral solution: 4 mg/ml, 8 mg/ml, 80 mg/ml
Tablets: 10 mg, 20 mg, 40 mg, 60 mg, 90 mg, 120 mg

Indications and dosages
➤ Angina pectoris
Adults: 80 to 320 mg P.O. in divided doses three to four times daily or 80 mg (extended- or sustained-release) P.O. daily; maximum daily dosage is 320 mg.
➤ Hypertension
Adults: 40 mg P.O. b.i.d. or 80 mg (extended- or sustained-release) P.O. daily; maximum daily dosage is 640 mg.
➤ Prophylaxis after myocardial infarction
Adults: 180 to 240 mg P.O. in divided doses three to four times daily; maximum daily dosage is 240 mg.

➤ Hypertrophic subaortic stenosis
Adults: 20 to 40 mg P.O. three to four times daily (before meals and at bedtime) or 80 to 160 mg (extended- or sustained-release) P.O. daily
➤ Adjunctive therapy in pheochromocytoma
Adults: 60 mg P.O. daily in divided doses for 3 days, given after primary treatment with alpha-adrenergic blocker
➤ To prevent migraine or vascular headache
Adults: 80 mg P.O. (extended- or sustained-release) daily; may increase as needed up to 240 mg/day
➤ Essential tremor
Adults: 40 mg P.O. b.i.d., adjusted as needed up to 120 mg/day; maximum daily dosage is 320 mg.
➤ Arrhythmias
Adults: 10 to 30 mg P.O. (tablets or oral solution) three or four times daily
➤ Life-threatening arrhythmias, arrhythmias that occur during anesthesia
Adults: 1 to 3 mg slow I.V. injection under careful monitoring; if necessary, give second dose after 2 minutes and additional doses at intervals of no less than 4 hours until desired response occurs.

Contraindications
• Uncompensated heart failure
• Pulmonary edema
• Cardiogenic shock
• Sinus bradycardia, heart block greater than first degree
• Bronchospastic disease
• Raynaud's syndrome
• Hypertensive emergencies
• Myasthenia gravis
• Concurrent thioridazine use

Administration
◀€ Take apical pulse for 1 full minute; withhold dose and notify prescriber if patient has bradycardia or tachycardia.

• Be aware that I.V. use is usually reserved for arrhythmias that are life-threatening or occur during anesthesia.
• Inject I.V. dose directly into large vein or into tubing of compatible I.V. solution (dextrose 5% in water, normal or half-normal saline solution, or lactated Ringer's solution).
• Don't administer as continuous I.V. infusion.
• For intermittent I.V. infusion, dilute with normal saline solution and infuse in 0.1- to 0.2-mg increments over 10 to 15 minutes.
◀€ Have I.V. isoproterenol, atropine, or glucagon available in case of emergency.
◀€ Don't stop giving drug suddenly. Dosage must be tapered.

Route	Onset	Peak	Duration
P.O.	30 min	60-90 min	6-12 hr
P.O. (extended, sustained)	Unknown	6 hr	24 hr
I.V.	Immediate	1 min	4-6 hr

Adverse reactions
CNS: fatigue, asthenia, anxiety, dizziness, drowsiness, insomnia, memory loss, depression, mental status changes, nervousness, paresthesia, nightmares
CV: peripheral vasoconstriction, orthostatic hypotension, bradycardia, **arrhythmias, heart failure, myocardial infarction and sudden death** (with abrupt withdrawal in angina therapy)
EENT: blurred vision, dry eyes, nasal congestion, rhinitis, sore throat
GI: nausea, vomiting, diarrhea, constipation, dry mouth
GU: elevated blood urea nitrogen (BUN), impotence, decreased libido
Hematologic: transient eosinophilia, purpura, **thrombocytopenic purpura**
Metabolic: fluid retention; hyperglycemia; hypoglycemia (increased in children); increased transaminase, alkaline phosphatase (ALP), lactate de-

hydrogenase (LD), and triiodothyronine (T_4) levels; decreased thyroxine (T_3) level; **thyrotoxicosis** (with abrupt withdrawal in hypertension therapy)
Musculoskeletal: joint pain, back pain, myalgia, muscle cramps
Respiratory: wheezing, **bronchospasm, pulmonary edema**
Skin: pruritus, rash
Other: fever

Interactions

Drug-drug. *Antacids (aluminum-based):* decreased propranolol absorption
Anticholinergics, tricyclic antidepressants: antagonism of cardiac beta-adrenergic blocking effect
Chlorpromazine: additive hypotension
Cimetidine: increased propranolol blood level and risk of toxicity
Digoxin: additive bradycardia
Diuretics, other antihypertensives: increased hypotensive effect
Glucagon, isoproterenol: antagonism of propranolol's effects
Insulin, oral hypoglycemics: impaired glucose tolerance, increased risk of hypoglycemia
Neuromuscular blockers: increased neuromuscular blockade (with high propranolol doses)
Nonsteroidal anti-inflammatory drugs: decreased hypotensive effect
Theophylline: decreased theophylline clearance, antagonism of theophylline's bronchodilating effect
Thioridazine: increased thioridazine blood level, leading to prolonged QT interval
Drug-diagnostic tests. *ALP, BUN, eosinophils, LD, serum transaminases, T_4:* increased levels
Glucose: decreased or increased level
Platelets: decreased count
T_3: decreased level
Drug-behaviors. *Acute alcohol ingestion:* additive hypotension

Precautions

Use cautiously in:
• renal or hepatic impairment, sinus node dysfunction, pulmonary disease, diabetes mellitus, hyperthyroidism
• history of severe allergic reactions
• elderly patients
• pregnant or breastfeeding patients
• children (safety not established).

Patient monitoring

• Monitor vital signs, ECG, and central venous pressure.
• Assess fluid balance; check for signs and symptoms of heart failure.
• Monitor complete blood count and liver and thyroid function test results.
• Watch closely for signs and symptoms of hypoglycemia (drug may mask these).
• Monitor blood glucose levels in diabetic patients to identify need for altered insulin or oral hypoglycemic dosage. Be aware that in labile diabetes, hypoglycemia may be accompanied by steep blood pressure rise.

Patient teaching

• Advise patient to take drug with meals at same time every day to minimize GI upset.
◀﹦ Caution patient not to stop taking drug suddenly. Tell him that dosage must be tapered.
• Teach patient to monitor pulse and to report promptly bradycardia or tachycardia.
• Tell patient that drug may cause muscle aches or bone pain. Advise him to discuss activity recommendations and pain management with prescriber.
• Instruct patient to avoid driving and other hazardous activities until he knows how drug affects concentration, vision, and alertness.
• As appropriate, review all other significant and life-threatening adverse

---

reactions and interactions, especially those related to the drugs, tests, and behaviors mentioned above.

propylthiouracil (PTU)
Propyl-Thyracil ♣

Pharmacologic class: Thioamide derivative

Therapeutic class: Antithyroid agent
Pregnancy risk category D

Action
Directly interferes with thyroid synthesis by preventing iodine from combining with thyroglobulin, leading to decreased thyroid hormone levels

Availability
Tablets: 50 mg

Indications and dosages
➤ Hyperthyroidism
Adults: Initially, 300 to 450 mg P.O. daily in equally divided doses q 8 hours; maintenance dosage is 100 to 150 mg P.O. daily.
➤ Thyrotoxic crisis
Adults: 200 mg P.O. q 4 to 6 hours during first 24 hours, followed by a maintenance dosage of 100 to 150 mg P.O. daily

Contraindications
• Hypersensitivity to drug
• Breastfeeding

Administration
• Give with meals to reduce GI upset.

Route	Onset	Peak	Duration
P.O.	Unknown	1-1.5 hr	Unknown

Adverse reactions
CNS: drowsiness, headache, vertigo, neuritis, paresthesia

GI: nausea, vomiting, diarrhea, epigastric distress, taste loss
Hematologic: agranulocytosis, leukopenia, thrombocytopenia
Hepatic: jaundice, **hepatic necrosis**
Metabolic: hypothyroidism
Musculoskeletal: joint pain, myalgia
Skin: rash, urticaria, pruritus, alopecia, skin discoloration, cutaneous vasculitis
Other: fever, lymphadenopathy, parotitis, edema

Interactions
Drug-drug. *Anticoagulants:* potentiation of anticoagulant effect
Drug-diagnostic tests. *Alanine aminotransferase, alkaline phosphatase, aspartate aminotransferase, bilirubin, lactate dehydrogenase:* increased levels
Granulocytes, platelets: decreased levels
Prothrombin time: prolonged

Precautions
Use cautiously in:
• decreased bone marrow reserve
• pregnant patients.

Patient monitoring
• Monitor complete blood count and liver and thyroid function test results.
• Assess for signs and symptoms of hypothyroidism (cold intolerance, nonpitting edema, fatigue, weight gain, and depression).
• Monitor for severe rash, fever, or enlarged cervical lymph nodes. If these effects occur, stop therapy and notify prescriber.

Patient teaching
• Instruct patient to take drug with meals to reduce GI upset.
• Teach patient to recognize and report signs and symptoms of hypothyroidism and jaundice.
• Advise patient to discuss iodine intake (as in iodized salt and shellfish) with prescriber.
• Tell patient to avoid over-the-counter cold remedies that contain iodine.

P

- Instruct patient to avoid driving and other hazardous activities until he knows how drug affects concentration and alertness.
- As appropriate, review all other significant and life-threatening adverse reactions and interactions, especially those related to the drugs and tests mentioned above.

protamine sulfate

Pharmacologic class: Low-molecular-weight protein
Therapeutic class: Heparin antagonist
Pregnancy risk category C

Action
Binds with heparin, causing immediate neutralization of anticoagulant activity

Availability
Injection: 10 mg/ml

⚡ Indications and dosages
➤ Heparin overdose
Adults and children: 1 mg slow I.V. over 10 minutes

Contraindications
- Hypersensitivity to drug

Administration
- One milligram of protamine neutralizes approximately 90 USP units of heparin activity derived from lung tissue or 115 USP units of heparin activity derived from intestinal mucosa.
- Before giving drug, ask patient about fish allergies; patient may develop hypersensitivity reaction (however, no true relationship has been established).
- Ensure that emergency equipment is available in case of anaphylaxis or sudden hypotension.
- ◀⧉ Give slowly by direct I.V. injection. Rapid administration exacerbates adverse cardiovascular and respiratory effects.

Route	Onset	Peak	Duration
I.V.	5 min	Unknown	2 hr

Adverse reactions
CNS: lassitude
CV: hypotension, bradycardia, **circulatory collapse**
GI: nausea, vomiting, anorexia
Hematologic: bleeding
Respiratory: dyspnea, **pulmonary edema, severe respiratory distress**
Skin: rash, dermatitis, angioedema
Other: anaphylaxis

Interactions
None significant

Precautions
Use cautiously in:
- fish allergy
- pregnant or breastfeeding patients
- children.

Patient monitoring
- Monitor vital signs and ECG continuously.
- Watch closely for signs and symptoms of hypersensitivity reaction.
- Check for spontaneous bleeding from heparin rebound, particularly after cardiac surgery or dialysis.
- Monitor activated partial thromboplastin time 15 minutes after drug administration.

Patient teaching
- Teach patient about drug's purpose; advise him of common adverse effects.
- ◀⧉ Instruct patient to notify nurse immediately of adverse effects, especially respiratory distress or abnormal bleeding or bruising.

pseudoephedrine hydrochloride

Allermed, Cenafed, Children's Congestion Relief, Decofed, DeFed-60, Dimetapp Decongestant Pediatric Drops, Dorcol Children's Decongestant Liquid, Efidac/24, Genaphed, Halofed, PediaCare Infants' Oral Decongestant Drops, Pedia Relief, Pseudo, Pseudo-Gest, Robidrine♣, Seudotabs, Simply Stuffy, Sudafed, Sudafed Children's Nasal Decongestant, Sudafed 12 Hour, Suphedrin, Triaminic AM Decongestant Formula, Triaminic Infant Oral Decongestant Drops♣

pseudoephedrine sulfate

Drixoral Nasal Decongestant, Drixoral Non-Drowsy Formula

Pharmacologic class: Sympathomimetic

Therapeutic class: Decongestant (systemic)

Pregnancy risk category C

Action

Stimulates alpha-adrenergic receptors, causing vasoconstriction of respiratory tract; relaxes bronchial smooth muscle through beta$_2$-adrenergic stimulation

Availability
pseudoephedrine hydrochloride
Capsules: 60 mg
Capsules (extended-release): 120 mg, 240 mg
Drops: 7.5 mg/0.8 ml (0.8 ml = 1 dropperful)
Oral solution: 15 mg/5 ml, 30 mg/5 ml
Syrup: 30 mg/5 ml
Tablets: 30 mg, 60 mg

Tablets (extended-release): 120 mg, 240 mg
pseudoephedrine sulfate
Tablets (extended-release, film-coated): 120 mg

🖉 Indications and dosages
➤ Nasal, sinus, and eustachian tube congestion
Adults and children ages 12 and older: 60 mg P.O. q 4 to 6 hours p.r.n. (not to exceed 240 mg/day); or 120 mg (extended-release) q 12 hours or 240 mg (extended-release) q 24 hours

Contraindications
• Hypersensitivity to drug or other sympathomimetics
• Alcohol intolerance (with some liquid products)
• Hypertension
• Severe coronary artery disease
• Monoamine oxidase (MAO) inhibitor use within 14 days
• Breastfeeding
• Children under age 12 (extended-release forms)

Administration
• Give at least 2 hours before bedtime to minimize insomnia.

Route	Onset	Peak	Duration
P.O.	30 min	Unknown	4-8 hr
P.O. (extended)	60 min	Unknown	12 hr

Adverse reactions
CNS: anxiety, nervousness, dizziness, drowsiness, excitability, fear, hallucinations, headache, insomnia, restlessness, asthenia, **seizures**
CV: palpitations, hypertension, tachycardia, **cardiovascular collapse**
GI: anorexia, dry mouth
GU: dysuria
Respiratory: respiratory difficulty

p

Interactions
Drug-drug. *Beta-adrenergic blockers:* increased pressor effects of pseudo-ephedrine
MAO inhibitors: hypertensive crisis
Mecamylamine, methyldopa, reserpine: decreased antihypertensive effect of these drugs
Other sympathomimetics: additive effects and greater risk of toxicity
Drug-food. *Foods that acidify urine:* decreased drug efficacy
Foods that alkalinize urine: increased drug efficacy

Precautions
Use cautiously in:
• hyperthyroidism, diabetes mellitus, prostatic hypertrophy, ischemic heart disease, glaucoma
• elderly patients who are sensitive to drug's CNS effects
• pregnant patients.

Patient monitoring
• Monitor vital signs.
• Assess neurologic and cardiovascular status regularly.

Patient teaching
• Advise patient to take drug at least 2 hours before bedtime to reduce insomnia.
• Instruct patient not to crush or break extended-release tablets or capsules.
• Advise patient to discontinue use and consult prescriber if he experiences nervousness, dizziness, or insomnia.
• Tell patient to consult prescriber before taking other over-the-counter products.
• Instruct patient to avoid driving and other hazardous activities until he knows how drug affects concentration and alertness.
• As appropriate, review all other significant and life-threatening adverse reactions and interactions, especially those related to the drugs and foods mentioned above.

psyllium
Alramucil, Fiberall, Genfiber, Hydrocil Instant, Karacil❦, Konsyl, Maalox Daily Fiber Therapy, Metamucil, Metamucil Orange Flavor, Metamucil Sugar Free, Modane Bulk, Mylanta Natural Fiber Supplement, Perdiem, Prodiem Plain❦, Reguloid Natural, Reguloid Natural Sugar Free, Reguloid Orange, Reguloid Orange Sugar Free, Restore, Restore Sugar Free, Serutan, Syllact, V-Lax

Pharmacologic class: Psyllium colloid
Therapeutic class: Bulk-forming laxative
Pregnancy risk category B

Action
Stimulates lining of colon, increasing peristalsis and water absorption of stool, thereby promoting evacuation

Availability
Chewable pieces: 1.7 g/piece, 3.4 g/piece
Granules: 2.5 g/tsp, 4.03 g/tsp
Powder: 3.3 g/tsp, 3.4 g/tsp, 3.5 g/tsp, 4.94 g/tsp
Powder (effervescent): 3.4 g/packet, 3.7 g/packet
Wafers: 3.4 g/wafer

⚠ Indications and dosages
➤ Chronic constipation, ulcerative colitis, irritable bowel syndrome
Adults and children ages 12 and older: 30 g daily in divided doses of 2.5 to 7.5 g/dose P.O. in 8 oz of water or juice

Contraindications
• Hypersensitivity to drug
• Intestinal obstruction
• Abdominal pain or other appendicitis symptoms
• Fecal impaction

Administration
• Mix powder with 8 oz of cold liquid (such as orange juice) to mask taste.
• Give diluted drug immediately after mixing, before it congeals; then give another glass of fluid.

Route	Onset	Peak	Duration
P.O.	12-24 hr	3 days	Variable

Adverse reactions
GI: nausea; vomiting; diarrhea (with excessive use); abdominal cramps with severe constipation; anorexia; **esophageal, gastric, small intestinal, or rectal obstruction** (with dry form)
Respiratory: asthma (rare)
Other: severe allergic reactions including **anaphylaxis**

Interactions
None significant

Precautions
Use cautiously in:
• phenylketonuria
• pregnant patients.

Patient monitoring
• Monitor patient's bowel movements.
• Check for signs and symptoms of rare but severe allergic reactions, such as anaphylaxis or asthma.

Patient teaching
• Teach patient to dissolve drug in 8 oz of a cold beverage and drink it immediately, followed by another glass of liquid.
• Caution patient not to take drug without dissolving it in liquid.
• Instruct patient to take drug after meals if it decreases his appetite.
• Tell patient that drug usually causes bowel movement within 12 to 24 hours but may take as long as 3 days.
◀€ Instruct patient to immediately stop taking drug and notify prescriber if signs and symptoms of allergic reaction occur.

• Advise diabetic patients to use sugar-free form.
• Instruct patients with phenylketonuria to avoid forms containing phenylalanine.
• As appropriate, review all other significant and life-threatening adverse reactions.

pyrantel pamoate
Antiminth, Combantrin♣, Pin-Rid, Pin-X, Reese's Pinworm

Pharmacologic class: Pyrimidine derivative
Therapeutic class: Anthelmintic
Pregnancy risk category C

Action
Stimulates ganglionic receptors in worm, causing it to become paralyzed; worm is then expelled through normal peristalsis.

Availability
Capsules: 180 mg
Liquid: 50 mg/ml
Oral suspension: 50 mg/ml, 144 mg/ml
Tablets: 360 mg

🍷 Indications and dosages
➤ Pinworm (enterobiasis), roundworm (ascariasis)
Adults and children older than age 2: 11 mg/kg P.O. as a single dose (maximum dosage of 1 g/day), repeated in 2 weeks

Contraindications
• Hypersensitivity to drug

Administration
• Shake suspension well. Give all forms without regard to food, milk, or juice.

p

Route	Onset	Peak	Duration
P.O.	Slow	1-3 hr	Unknown

Adverse reactions
CNS: dizziness, headache, drowsiness, insomnia, asthenia
GI: nausea, vomiting, diarrhea, abdominal cramps, gastralgia, anorexia
Hepatic: transiently elevated aspartate aminotransferase level
Skin: rash
Other: fever

Interactions
Drug-drug. *Piperazine:* antagonism of both drugs' effects

Precautions
Use cautiously in:
• malnutrition, dehydration, hepatic disease, seizure disorder
• *Trichostrongylus* infection
• pregnant or breastfeeding patients
• children under age 2.

Patient monitoring
• Monitor for rash and fever.

Patient teaching
• Teach patient to shake suspension well; tell him that he may take it with or without food, juice, or milk.
• Instruct patient to report rash or fever.
• If pinworm is suspected, tell patient that everyone in household should be treated.
• Teach patient to practice strict hygiene to prevent reinfection.
• Instruct patient to avoid driving and other hazardous activities until he knows how drug affects concentration and alertness.
• As appropriate, review all other significant adverse reactions and interactions, especially those related to the drugs mentioned above.

pyrazinamide
PMS Pyrazinamide♣, Tebrazid♣

Pharmacologic class: Niacinamide derivative
Therapeutic class: Antitubercular
Pregnancy risk category C

Action
Unknown; thought to exhibit bacteriostatic action

Availability
Tablets: 500 mg

🔓 Indications and dosages
➤ Tuberculosis (usually used as adjunct)
Adults and children: 15 to 30 mg/kg/day P.O., not to exceed 2 g/day; or 50 to 70 mg/kg P.O. twice weekly, up to a maximum of 4 g/dose; or 50 to 70 mg/kg/dose P.O. three times weekly, up to a maximum of 3 g/dose
Dosage adjustment
• Renal impairment

Contraindications
• Hypersensitivity to drug
• Severe hepatic disease
• Acute gout

Administration
• Give with other antituberculars, as prescribed, to reduce risk of resistant organisms.
• Be aware that drug therapy may last 6 months or longer.

Route	Onset	Peak	Duration
P.O.	Rapid	2 hr	Unknown

Adverse reactions
CNS: headache
GI: nausea, vomiting, diarrhea, peptic ulcer, abdominal cramps, anorexia

GU: dysuria, increased uric acid secretion

Hematologic: hemolytic anemia

Hepatic: abnormal liver function test results, **hepatotoxicity**

Metabolic: hyperuricemia

Musculoskeletal: gout, joint pain

Skin: urticaria, photosensitivity

Interactions

Drug-drug. *Ethionamide:* increased risk of hepatotoxicity

Probenecid: decreased probenecid efficacy (possibly precipitating gout)

Drug-diagnostic tests. *Acetest or Ketostix urine test:* false interpretation

Uric acid: increased level

Precautions

Use cautiously in:
• renal failure, diabetes mellitus, porphyria, chronic gout, history of gout
• pregnant or breastfeeding patients
• children under age 13.

Patient monitoring

• Monitor complete blood count, uric acid level, and liver and kidney function test results.

• Assess for signs and symptoms of gout, hepatic failure, and hemolytic anemia.

◀ Discontinue drug at first sign of hepatic impairment or hyperuricemia accompanied by acute gouty arthritis.

Patient teaching

• Advise patient to take drug regularly, as prescribed, in combination with other antituberculars so that resistant organisms don't proliferate.

◀ Teach patient to recognize and immediately report signs and symptoms of gout and liver impairment.

• As appropriate, review all other significant and life-threatening adverse reactions and interactions, especially those related to the drugs and tests mentioned above.

pyridostigmine bromide

Mestinon, Mestinon-SR✤, Mestinon Timespans, Regonol

Pharmacologic class: Anticholinesterase

Therapeutic class: Muscle stimulant, antimyasthenic

Pregnancy risk category C

Action

Prevents acetylcholine destruction, resulting in stronger contractions of muscles weakened by myasthenia gravis or curare-like neuromuscular blockers

Availability

Injection: 5 mg/ml
Syrup: 60 mg/5 ml
Tablets: 60 mg
Tablets (extended-release): 180 mg

⃠ Indications and dosages

➤ Myasthenia gravis

Adults: 600 mg P.O. given over 24 hours, spaced for maximum symptom relief; dosage range is 60 to 1,500 mg. For myasthenic crisis, 2 mg or 1/30 of oral dose I.M. or very slow I.V. q 2 to 3 hours.

➤ Reversal of nondepolarizing neuromuscular blockers after surgery

Adults: 10 to 20 mg slow I.V. injection (range is 0.1 to 0.25 mg/kg) with or immediately after 0.6 to 1.2 mg atropine sulfate I.V.

Dosage adjustment
• Renal impairment
• Seizure disorders

Off-label uses

• Myasthenia gravis in children
• Constipation in patients with Parkinson's disease
• Nerve agent prophylaxis

p

Contraindications
• Hypersensitivity to drug or bromides
• Mechanical intestinal or urinary tract obstruction

Administration
🔊 Don't exceed I.V. injection rate of 1 mg/minute.
🔊 Don't give concurrently with other anticholinesterase drugs.
• Have atropine available for use in emergencies.

Route	Onset	Peak	Duration
P.O.	20-30 min	Unknown	Unknown
P.O. (extended)	30-60 min	Unknown	6-12 hr
I.V.	2-5 min	Unknown	2-4 hr
I.M.	<15 min	Unknown	2-4 hr

Adverse reactions
CNS: headache, dysarthria, dysphoria, drowsiness, dizziness, headache, syncope, **loss of consciousness, seizures**
CV: nodal rhythm, decreased cardiac output leading to hypotension, bradycardia, **atrioventricular block, cardiac arrest, arrhythmias**
EENT: diplopia, lacrimation, miosis, spasm of accommodation, conjunctival hyperemia, increased salivation
GI: nausea, vomiting, diarrhea, abdominal cramps, flatulence, increased peristalsis, dysphagia
GU: urinary frequency, urgency, or incontinence
Musculoskeletal: muscle weakness, fasciculations, and cramps; joint pain
Respiratory: increased pharyngeal and tracheobronchial secretions, dyspnea, **central respiratory paralysis, respiratory muscle paralysis, laryngospasm, bronchospasm, bronchiolar constriction**
Skin: diaphoresis, flushing, rash, urticaria
Other: thrombophlebitis at I.V. site, **cholinergic crisis, anaphylaxis**

Interactions
Drug-drug. *Aminoglycosides:* potentiation of neuromuscular blockade
Anesthetics (general and local), antiarrhythmics: decreased anticholinesterase effects
Atropine, belladonna derivatives: suppression of parasympathomimetic GI symptoms (leaving only fasciculation and voluntary muscle paralysis as signs of anticholinesterase overdose)
Corticosteroids: decreased anticholinesterase effects; after corticosteroid withdrawal, increased anticholinesterase effects
Ganglionic blockers (mecamylamine): increased anticholinesterase effects
Magnesium: antagonism of beneficial anticholinesterase effects
Nondepolarizing neuromuscular blockers (atropine, pancuronium, tubocurarine): antagonism of neuromuscular blockade and reversal of muscle relaxation after surgery (with parenteral pyridostigmine)
Other anticholinesterase drugs: in patient with myasthenia gravis, symptoms of anticholinesterase overdose that mimic underdose, causing patient's condition to worsen
Succinylcholine: increased and prolonged neuromuscular blockade (including respiratory depression)

Precautions
Use cautiously in:
• seizure disorders, bronchial asthma, coronary occlusion, hyperthyroidism, arrhythmias, peptic ulcer, vagotonia, cholinergic crisis, bradycardia
• pregnant or breastfeeding patients
• children (safety and efficacy not established).

Patient monitoring
• Assess patient's response to each dose.
• Monitor vital signs, ECG, and cardiovascular and respiratory status.

◀€ Assess for signs and symptoms of overdose, which indicate cholinergic crisis.

Patient teaching

• If patient is using syrup, teach him to pour it over ice.

• Instruct patient using extended-release tablets not to crush them.

◀€ Teach patient to recognize and promptly report signs and symptoms of overdose, including muscle fasciculations, sweating, excessive salivation, and constricted pupils.

• Tell patient that drug may cause headache and muscle cramps. Encourage him to discuss activity recommendations and pain management with prescriber.

• Advise patient to monitor and report his response to ongoing therapy so that optimal dosage can be determined.

• As appropriate, review all other significant and life-threatening adverse reactions and interactions, especially those related to the drugs mentioned above.

pyrimethamine
Daraprim

Pharmacologic class: Folic acid antagonist

Therapeutic class: Antiprotozoal, antimalarial

Pregnancy risk category C

Action

Inhibits reduction of dihydrofolic acid to tetrahydrofolic acid (folinic acid) by binding to and reversibly inhibiting dihydrofolate reductase

Availability

Tablets: 25 mg

⚫ Indications and dosages

➤ To suppress and control transmission of susceptible *Plasmodium* strains in semi-immune patients

Adults and children ages 10 and older: 25 mg P.O. daily for 2 days, given with a sulfonamide

➤ Toxoplasmosis

Adults: Initially, 50 to 75 mg P.O. daily for 1 to 3 weeks, given with a sulfonamide. Depending on patient's response and tolerance, dosages of both drugs should then be reduced by 50% and continued for 4 to 5 more weeks. Alternatively, 25 to 100 mg P.O. daily with leucovorin for 3 to 4 weeks, given in conjunction with a sulfonamide q.i.d. for 3 to 4 weeks.

Children: 1 mg/kg P.O. daily in two equally divided doses for 2 to 4 days, then reduced to 0.5 mg/kg daily for approximately 1 month. Alternatively, 2 mg/kg (up to 100 mg) P.O. daily in two equally divided doses for 3 days, followed by 1 mg/kg (up to 25 mg) in two equally divided doses for 4 weeks, given with sulfadiazine for 4 weeks.

➤ To prevent toxoplasmosis in AIDS patients

Adults and adolescents: 50 mg P.O. once weekly with oral leucovorin once weekly and dapsone daily. Alternatively, 75 mg P.O. daily with oral leucovorin, and dapsone once weekly; or 25 mg P.O. daily with oral leucovorin daily and atovaquone daily; or 25 to 50 mg P.O. daily with oral leucovorin daily and sulfadiazine daily or clindamycin q 6 to 8 hours. Any of these regimens may be continued in various dosages lifelong.

Children and infants: 1 mg/kg P.O. daily with oral leucovorin q 3 days and dapsone daily. Lifelong regimen is a combination of pyrimethamine, oral leucovorin, and either sulfadiazine or clindamycin in various dosages.

P

Off-label uses
• Isosporiasis
• Prophylaxis for *Pneumocystis jiroveci* (formerly *Pneumocystis carinii*) pneumonia

Contraindications
• Hypersensitivity to drug
• Megaloblastic anemia caused by folate deficiency
• Concurrent folate antagonist therapy
• Breastfeeding

Administration
• Administer with meals.
• When giving tablets to young children, crush them and administer as an oral suspension in water, cherry syrup, or sweetened solution.
• Be aware that because of worldwide resistance to pyrimethamine, its use alone to prevent or treat acute malaria is no longer recommended.
• Know that fixed combination of pyrimethamine and sulfadoxine is available and has been used for uncomplicated mild to moderate malaria caused by chloroquine-resistant *Plasmodium falciparum* and for presumptive self-treatment by travelers.

Route	Onset	Peak	Duration
P.O.	Unknown	2-6 hr	2 wk

Adverse reactions
CNS: headache, light-headedness, insomnia, malaise, depression, **seizures**
CV: arrhythmias
EENT: dry throat, atrophic glossitis
GI: nausea, vomiting, diarrhea, anorexia
GU: hematuria
Hematologic: megaloblastic anemia, **leukopenia, pancytopenia, thrombocytopenia**
Metabolic: hyperphenylalaninemia
Respiratory: pulmonary eosinophilia
Skin: pigmentation changes, dermatitis, erythema multiforme, **toxic epidermal necrolysis**

Other: fever, **anaphylaxis, Stevens-Johnson syndrome**

Interactions
Drug-drug. *Lorazepam:* hepatotoxicity
Myelosuppressants (including antineoplastics): increased risk of bone marrow depression
Drug-diagnostic tests. *Platelets, white blood cells:* decreased counts

Precautions
Use cautiously in:
• anemia, bone marrow depression, hepatic or renal impairment, glucose-6-phosphate dehydrogenase deficiency
• history of seizures
• patients more than 16 weeks pregnant.

Patient monitoring
• Monitor complete blood count; watch for signs and symptoms of blood dyscrasias.
• Assess for signs and symptoms of folic acid deficiency.
• Closely monitor neurologic and cardiovascular status; watch for seizures and arrhythmias.
• Watch for evidence of erythema multiforme, including sore throat, cough, mouth sores, rash, iritic lesions, and fever. Report early signs before condition can progress to Stevens-Johnson syndrome.

Patient teaching
• Advise patient to take drug with meals.
◀€ Caution patient to discontinue drug and contact prescriber at first sign of rash.
• Instruct patient to avoid driving and other hazardous activities until he knows how drug affects concentration and alertness.
• As appropriate, review all other significant and life-threatening adverse reactions and interactions, especially those related to the drugs and tests mentioned above.

quetiapine fumarate
Seroquel

Pharmacologic class: Dibenzothiazepine derivative

Therapeutic class: Atypical antipsychotic

Pregnancy risk category C

Action
Unknown; thought to achieve antipsychotic effects by antagonizing dopamine type 2 and serotonin type 2 receptors. Other effects may result partly from antagonizing other receptors, such as histamine H_1 receptors and adrenergic alpha$_1$ receptors.

Availability
Tablets: 25 mg, 100 mg, 200 mg, 300 mg

Indications and dosages
➤ Schizophrenia
Adults: Initially, 25 mg P.O. b.i.d., increased by 25 to 50 mg two to three times daily over 3 days, up to 300 to 400 mg/day in two to three divided doses by day 4 (not to exceed 800 mg/day)

Dosage adjustment
- Hepatic impairment
- History of hypotensive reactions
- Elderly or debilitated patients

Off-label uses
- Bipolar disorder
- Mania
- Obsessive-compulsive disorder
- Posttraumatic stress disorder
- Psychosis related to Parkinson's disease

Contraindications
- Hypersensitivity to drug or its components

Administration
- Give with or without food.
- Don't confuse Seroquel with Serzone (an antidepressant).

Route	Onset	Peak	Duration
P.O.	Rapid	1.5 hr	8-12 hr

Adverse reactions
CNS: dizziness, cognitive impairment, extrapyramidal symptoms, sedation, tardive dyskinesia, **neuroleptic malignant syndrome, seizures**
CV: palpitations, peripheral edema, orthostatic hypotension
EENT: ear pain, rhinitis, pharyngitis
GI: constipation, dyspepsia, dry mouth, anorexia
Hematologic: leukopenia
Respiratory: cough, dyspnea
Skin: diaphoresis
Other: weight gain, flulike symptoms

Interactions
Drug-drug. *Antihistamines, opioid analgesics, sedative-hypnotics, other CNS depressants:* additive CNS depression
Antihypertensives: increased risk of hypotension
Barbiturates, carbamazepine, corticosteroids, phenytoin, rifampin, thioridazine: increased clearance and decreased efficacy of quetiapine
Dopamine agonists, levodopa: antagonism of these drugs' effects
Erythromycin, fluconazole, itraconazole, ketoconazole, other CYP450-3A4 inhibitors: increased quetiapine effects
Drug-diagnostic tests. *Alanine aminotransferase, aspartate aminotransferase:* asymptomatic elevations
Total cholesterol, triglycerides: increased levels
Urine tricyclic antidepressant assay: false-positive screen

q

White blood cells: decreased count
Drug-behaviors. *Alcohol use:* increased CNS effects

Precautions

Use cautiously in:
- hepatic impairment, cardiovascular or cerebrovascular disease, dehydration, hypovolemia, Alzheimer's dementia, hypothyroidism
- history of seizures, suicide attempt, or hypotensive reactions
- elderly or debilitated patients
- pregnant patients
- children (safety not established).

Patient monitoring

◀€ Monitor neurologic status, especially for signs and symptoms of tardive dyskinesia or neuroleptic malignant syndrome.
- Watch blood pressure for orthostatic hypertension.

Patient teaching

- Tell patient he can take drug with or without food.
◀€ Teach patient to recognize and immediately report signs and symptoms of neuroleptic malignant syndrome, such as high fever, sweating, unstable blood pressure, stupor, muscle rigidity, and tardive dyskinesia.
- Instruct patient to move slowly when sitting up or standing to avoid dizziness or light-headedness from sudden blood pressure decrease.
- Advise female patients to notify prescriber of possible pregnancy.
- Teach patient not to stop taking drug abruptly; tell him dosage must be tapered.
- Caution patient not to drink alcohol.
- Instruct patient to avoid driving and other hazardous activities until he knows how drug affects concentration and alertness.

- As appropriate, review all other significant and life-threatening adverse reactions and interactions, especially those related to the drugs, tests, and behaviors mentioned above.

quinapril hydrochloride
Accupril

Pharmacologic class: Angiotensin-converting enzyme (ACE) inhibitor
Therapeutic class: Antihypertensive
Pregnancy risk category C (first trimester), *D* (second and third trimesters)

Action

Inhibits conversion of angiotensin I to angiotensin II, a potent vasoconstrictor; decreases cardiac output. Increases plasma renin levels and reduces aldosterone levels, causing systemic vasodilation.

Availability

Tablets: 5 mg, 10 mg, 20 mg, 40 mg

⨂ Indications and dosages

➤ Hypertension
Adults: Initially, 10 to 20 mg P.O. daily for patients not receiving diuretics, with subsequent dosages adjusted at 2-week intervals according to blood pressure response at peak (2 to 6 hours) and trough (predose) blood levels; maintenance dosage is 20 to 80 mg/day as a single dose or in two divided doses. If quinapril alone doesn't adequately control blood pressure, diuretic may be added. In patients receiving diuretics, discontinue diuretic 2 to 3 days before starting quinapril; if blood pressure is not controlled, resume diuretic. If diuretic can't be discontinued, initiate therapy with 5 mg quinapril daily.

➤ Adjunct in heart failure

Adults: Initially, 5 mg P.O. b.i.d., titrated weekly until effective dosage is determined. Maintenance dosage is 20 to 40 mg/day in two evenly divided doses.

Dosage adjustment

• Renal impairment
• Elderly patients

Off-label uses

• Aortic insufficiency
• Atherosclerosis
• Postoperative hypertension
• Myocardial infarction
• Diabetic or nondiabetic neuropathy

Contraindications

• Hypersensitivity to drug or other ACE inhibitors
• Angioedema caused by other ACE inhibitors
• Pregnancy (second and third trimesters)

Administration

• Administer with or without food, but not with a high-fat meal.

Route	Onset	Peak	Duration
P.O.	0.5-1 hr	2-6 hr	Up to 24 hr

Adverse reactions

CNS: dizziness, drowsiness, fatigue, headache, insomnia, depression, vertigo, paresthesia, asthenia, malaise, nervousness, syncope

CV: hypotension, angina pectoris, palpitations, chest pain, tachycardia, **arrhythmias**

EENT: amblyopia, sinusitis, pharyngitis

GI: nausea, vomiting, diarrhea, constipation, abdominal pain, anorexia, taste disturbances, dry mouth

GU: impotence

Metabolic: hyperkalemia

Musculoskeletal: back pain

Respiratory: cough, dyspnea

Skin: rash, pruritus, alopecia, flushing, diaphoresis, photosensitivity

Other: fever, viral infections, hypersensitivity reactions including **anaphylaxis**

Interactions

Drug-drug. *Allopurinol:* increased risk of hypersensitivity reactions

Antacids: decreased quinapril absorption

Digoxin, lithium: increased blood levels and risk of toxicity of these drugs

Diuretics, other antihypertensives: increased hypotension

Indomethacin: decreased hypotensive effect of quinapril

Phenothiazines: increased pharmacologic effect of quinapril

Potassium-sparing diuretics, potassium supplements: increased risk of hyperkalemia

Tetracyclines: decreased tetracycline absorption

Drug-diagnostic tests. *Alanine aminotransferase, alkaline phosphatase, aspartate aminotransferase, bilirubin, blood urea nitrogen, creatinine, potassium:* increased levels

Drug-food. *High-fat foods:* decreased rate and extent of drug absorption

Salt substitutes containing potassium: increased risk of hyperkalemia

Drug-herb. *Capsaicin:* increased incidence of cough

Ephedra (ma huang): decreased drug efficacy, exacerbation of hypertension

Yohimbe: interference with drug's antihypertensive effect

Drug-behaviors. *Alcohol use:* increased hypotension

Precautions

Use cautiously in:

• autoimmune diseases, aortic stenosis, hypertrophic cardiomyopathy, cerebrovascular or cardiac insufficiency, collagen vascular disease, febrile illness, hepatic or renal impairment, hypovolemia, hyponatremia, hypotension, neutropenia, chronic cough, proteinuria, renal artery stenosis

q

- family history of angioedema
- concurrent immunosuppressant or diuretic therapy
- black patients
- elderly patients
- pregnant (first trimester) or breast-feeding patients
- children (safety not established).

Patient monitoring
- Monitor vital signs and cardiovascular status; be sure to ask patient if he's experiencing angina.
- Assess complete blood count and liver function tests.
- Monitor potassium level; watch for signs and symptoms of hyperkalemia.
- Watch closely for signs and symptoms of angioedema, especially in black patients after first dose.
- Assess for dry, nonproductive cough and signs and symptoms of infection.

Patient teaching
- Tell patient he may take drug with or without food, but not with a high-fat meal.
- ◀ Teach patient to immediately report facial or tongue swelling or difficulty breathing.
- Instruct patient to monitor and record his blood pressure.
- Teach patient to promptly report dry, nonproductive cough or signs and symptoms of infection.
- Instruct patient to move slowly when sitting up or standing to avoid dizziness or light-headedness from sudden blood pressure decrease.
- Inform patient that excessive fluid loss, as from sweating, vomiting, or diarrhea, and inadequate intake increase the risk of light-headedness (especially in hot weather).
- Advise patient to avoid driving and other hazardous activities until he knows how drug affects concentration and alertness.

- Caution patient to avoid herbal products and salt substitutes containing potassium.
- As appropriate, review all other significant and life-threatening adverse reactions and interactions, especially those related to the drugs, tests, foods, herbs, and behaviors mentioned above.

quinidine gluconate
Quinaglute Dura-tabs, Quinate❖

quinidine sulfate
Apo-Quinidine❖, Novoquinidin❖, Quinidex Extentabs, Quinora

Pharmacologic class: Cinchona alkaloid
Therapeutic class: Antiarrhythmic (class IA), antimalarial
Pregnancy risk category C

Action
Slows conduction and prolongs refractory period, reducing myocardial irritability, thereby interrupting or preventing certain arrhythmias. As an antimalarial, acts primarily as an intra-erythrocytic schizonticide.

Availability
quinidine gluconate
Injection: 80 mg/ml
Tablets (extended-release): 324 mg
quinidine sulfate
Tablets: 200 mg, 300 mg
Tablets (extended-release): 300 mg

⚕ Indications and dosages
➤ Test dose
Adults: 200 mg quinidine sulfate P.O. as a single dose or 200 mg quinidine gluconate I.M. to determine if patient has idiosyncratic reaction
➤ Premature atrial and ventricular contractions

Adults: 200 to 300 mg quinidine sulfate P.O. three to four times daily, or quinidine gluconate (extended-release) given as 324 to 660 mg P.O. q 8 to 12 hours

➤ Paroxysmal supraventricular tachycardia (PSVT)

Adults: 400 to 600 mg quinidine sulfate P.O. q 2 or 3 hours until arrhythmia is terminated; or 324 to 660 mg (extended-release) P.O. q 8 to 12 hours. For parenteral use, 400 mg quinidine gluconate I.M., repeated q 2 hours if necessary; or 330 mg quinidine gluconate I.V. (up to 750 mg) in diluted solution, infused no faster than 1 ml/minute.

➤ Conversion of atrial fibrillation

Adults: 200 mg quinidine sulfate P.O. q 2 or 3 hours for five to eight doses, increased daily until sinus rhythm returns or toxic effects occur; maximum daily dosage is 4 g. Or 300 mg quinidine sulfate (extended-release) P.O. q 8 to 12 hours, increased cautiously if necessary. Or 324 to 660 mg quinidine gluconate (extended-release) P.O. q 8 to 12 hours. For parenteral use, 800 mg quinidine gluconate I.V. in diluted solution, infused no faster than 0.25 mg/kg/minute.

➤ Severe, life-threatening *Plasmodium falciparum* malaria

Adults: Loading dose of 10 mg/kg quinidine gluconate I.V. diluted in 5 ml/kg of normal saline solution (or 250 ml of normal saline solution in an otherwise healthy, 50-kg [110-lb] patient) by continuous infusion over 1 to 2 hours, followed by continuous maintenance infusion of 0.02 mg/kg/minute for 72 hours or until parasitemia is reduced to less than 1% or oral therapy can begin. Or alternate loading dose of 24 mg/kg quinidine gluconate I.V. diluted in 250 ml of 0.9% sodium chloride injection given by intermittent infusion over 4 hours, followed by a maintenance dosage of 12 mg/kg quinidine gluconate I.V. at 8-hour in-

tervals, starting 8 hours after loading dose, infused over 4 hours for 7 days or until patient can tolerate oral therapy.

Dosage adjustment
• Hepatic insufficiency

Off-label uses
• Myocardial infarction

Contraindications
• Hypersensitivity to drug or related cinchona derivatives
• Thrombocytopenia with previous quinidine therapy
• Myasthenia gravis
• Complete heart block
• Left bundle-branch block or other severe intraventricular conduction defects
• Aberrant ectopic impulses and abnormal rhythm
• History of prolonged QT interval or drug-induced torsades de pointes
• When cardiac rhythm depends on pacemaker
• Digoxin toxicity

Administration
◀€ Before first dose, assess apical pulse and blood pressure. If patient has bradycardia or tachycardia, withhold dose and contact prescriber.
• If patient has atrial fibrillation, expect to give digoxin, a calcium channel blocker, a beta-adrenergic blocker, and possibly an anticoagulant before administering quinidine.
• If sinus rhythm isn't restored after a total of 10 mg/kg quinidine gluconate has been given, other means of cardioversion may be considered.
• Monitor blood pressure and ECG; titrate flow rate to correct arrhythmia.
• Be aware that quinidine gluconate may be given I.M.; however, I.V. route is preferred in life-threatening situations.
• When giving large doses, monitor blood pressure and ECG continuously.

q

• Know that quinidine gluconate is the only parenteral cinchona alkaloid antimalarial commercially available in the United States. Because newer antiarrhythmics have replaced quinidine for many cardiac uses, it may not be readily available and prescribers may not be familiar with its use. For information about availability or use, contact manufacturer at 800-821-0538.

Route	Onset	Peak	Duration
P.O. (extended)	Unknown	3-5 hr	Unknown
P.O. (sulfate)	Unknown	1-3 hr	Unknown
I.V.	Immediate	Immediate	Unknown
I.M.	30-90 sec	Unknown	Unknown

Adverse reactions

CNS: vertigo, headache, ataxia, apprehension, excitement, delirium, syncope, confusion, depression, dementia
CV: ECG changes, hypotension, vasculitis, increased creatine kinase level, tachycardia, premature ventricular contractions, paradoxical tachycardia, **ventricular tachycardia, ventricular fibrillation, ventricular flutter, ventricular ectopy, torsades de pointes, complete atrioventricular (AV) block, widened QRS complex, prolonged QT interval, asystole, aggravated heart failure, arterial embolism, vascular collapse**
EENT: diplopia, blurred vision, mydriasis, abnormal color perception, scotoma, photophobia, night blindness, optic neuritis, decreased hearing, tinnitus
GI: nausea, vomiting, diarrhea, abdominal pain, increased salivation, anorexia
GU: lupus nephritis
Hematologic: purpura, hemolytic anemia, **hypothrombinemia, leukocytosis, shift to left in white blood cell differential, neutropenia, thrombocytopenia, thrombocytopenic purpura, agranulocytosis**

Hepatic: increased hepatic enzyme levels, **hepatotoxicity**
Respiratory: acute asthma attack, respiratory arrest
Skin: rash, pruritus, urticaria, photosensitivity, angioedema
Other: fever, cinchonism, lupuslike syndrome, hypersensitivity reaction

Interactions

Drug-drug. *Amiodarone:* increased quinidine blood level, causing potentially fatal arrhythmias
Antacids, cimetidine: increased quinidine blood level
Anticholinergics: additive vagolytic effect
Anticoagulants, beta-adrenergic blockers (such as metoprolol, propranolol), procainamide, propafenone, tricyclic antidepressants: increased effects of these drugs
Barbiturates, hydantoins, nifedipine, rifampin, sucralfate: decreased therapeutic effect of quinidine
Cardiac glycosides: increased cardiac glycoside blood level, greater risk of toxicity
Cholinergics: decreased quinidine effect (may lead to failure to terminate PSVT)
Depolarizing (decamethonium, succinylcholine) and nondepolarizing (tubocurarine, pancuronium) neuromuscular blockers: potentiation of neuromuscular blockade
Diltiazem, verapamil: decreased quinidine clearance, resulting in hypotension, bradycardia, ventricular tachycardia, AV block, or pulmonary edema
Disopyramide: increased disopyramide or decreased quinidine blood level
Potassium, urinary alkalinizers: increased blood level and effects of quinidine
Drug-diagnostic tests. *Granulocytes, hemoglobin, platelets:* decreased levels
Hepatic enzymes: increased levels
Renal function tests: altered results

Drug-food. *Grapefruit juice:* inhibited drug metabolism
Reduced sodium intake: increased quinidine blood level
Drug-herb. *Jimsonweed:* adverse cardiovascular effects
Licorice: additive effects

Precautions

Use cautiously in:
• potassium imbalance, renal or hepatic disease, heart failure, respiratory depression
• elderly patients
• pregnant or breastfeeding patients
• children.

Patient monitoring

◀≤ Monitor ECG and vital signs closely; assess for worsening heart failure, especially with I.V. use.
• Assess kidney and liver function test results, complete blood count, and quinidine blood level.
• Watch for signs and symptoms of blood dyscrasias.
◀≤ Closely monitor respiratory status; stay alert for asthma attacks or impending respiratory arrest.
• Monitor for adverse GI effects, which may signify drug toxicity.

Patient teaching

• Advise patient to take drug with food to reduce GI upset.
• Instruct patient not to crush or chew extended-release tablets.
◀≤ Teach patient to recognize and immediately report signs and symptoms of toxicity, including tinnitus, nausea, headache, dizziness, and visual disturbances.
• Caution patient to avoid potassium supplements, licorice, and grapefruit juice and to maintain a constant level of sodium intake.
• Advise patient to discuss herbal use with prescriber.
• As appropriate, review all other significant and life-threatening adverse

reactions and interactions, especially those related to the drugs, tests, foods, and herbs mentioned above.

quinine sulfate

Pharmacologic class: Cinchona alkaloid
Therapeutic class: Antimalarial
Pregnancy risk category X

Action

Unknown; interferes with DNA synthesis by increasing pH in intracellular organelles of susceptible parasites

Availability

Capsules: 200 mg, 300 mg, 325 mg
Tablets: 260 mg

Indications and dosages

➤ Uncomplicated, chloroquine-resistant *Plasmodium falciparum* malaria
Adults: 650 mg P.O. q 8 hours for 3 to 7 days, given with another oral antimalarial (sulfadoxine and pyrimethamine, clindamycin, doxycycline, or tetracycline)
Children: 25 mg/kg P.O. daily in three evenly divided doses for 3 to 7 days, given with another oral antimalarial (sulfadoxine and pyrimethamine, clindamycin, doxycycline, or tetracycline)

Off-label uses

• Nocturnal recumbency leg cramps

Contraindications

• Hypersensitivity to drug or other cinchona alkaloids
• Glucose-6-phosphate dehydrogenase deficiency
• Optic neuritis
• Tinnitus

q

• History of blackwater fever or thrombocytopenic purpura
• Pregnancy

Administration
• Give with or without food.

Route	Onset	Peak	Duration
P.O.	Unknown	1-3 hr	4-11 hr

Adverse reactions
CNS: headache, vertigo, syncope, apprehension, restlessness, excitement, confusion, delirium, dizziness, **seizures**
CV: angina, vasculitis
EENT: diplopia, blurred vision, scotoma, abnormal color perception, photophobia, night blindness, amblyopia, mydriasis, optic atrophy, hearing loss, tinnitus
GI: nausea, vomiting, diarrhea, abdominal cramps, epigastric pain, dysphagia
Hematologic: hemolytic anemia, **hypoprothrombinemia, acute hemolysis, thrombocytopenic purpura, agranulocytosis**
Hepatic: hepatotoxicity
Metabolic: hypoglycemia, hypothermia
Respiratory: asthma symptoms
Skin: rash, pruritus, photosensitivity, flushing, diaphoresis
Other: cinchonism, facial edema, hypersensitivity reactions including fever and **hemolytic uremic syndrome**

Interactions
Drug-drug. *Aluminum-containing antacids:* delayed or decreased quinine absorption
Cimetidine: decreased metabolism and increased effects of quinine
Digoxin: increased digoxin blood level
Mefloquine: increased risk of seizures, ECG abnormalities, and cardiac arrest
Neuromuscular blockers: increased effects of these drugs, resulting in respiratory difficulty
Rifabutin, rifampin: increased metabolism and decreased effects of quinine

Succinylcholine: delayed succinylcholine metabolism
Urinary alkalinizers (such as acetazolamide, sodium bicarbonate): increased quinine blood level and risk of toxicity
Warfarin: increased warfarin effects, increased risk of bleeding
Drug-diagnostic tests. *Urinary 17-ketogenic steroids:* elevated levels

Precautions
Use cautiously in:
• myasthenia gravis, recurrent or interrupted malaria therapy
• history of arrhythmias (especially prolonged QT interval), asthma, or heart disease
• breastfeeding patients.

Patient monitoring
◀€ Monitor for signs and symptoms of hypersensitivity reaction, including fever and hemolytic uremic syndrome.
• Stay alert for signs and symptoms of cinchonism, including tinnitus, headache, nausea, and visual disturbances.
• Assess for bleeding tendency and hepatotoxicity.
• Monitor complete blood count, liver function tests, and quinine and glucose levels.

Patient teaching
• Tell patient he may take drug with or without food.
◀€ Teach patient to recognize and immediately report signs and symptoms of cinchonism and hepatotoxicity.
• Instruct patient to report unusual bleeding or bruising.
• As appropriate, review all other significant and life-threatening adverse reactions and interactions, especially those related to the drugs and tests mentioned above.

quinupristin and dalfopristin
Synercid

Pharmacologic class: Streptogramin
Therapeutic class: Anti-infective
Pregnancy risk category B

Action
Synergistic effects of drug combination interfere with bacterial cell wall synthesis by disrupting DNA and RNA transcription

Availability
Injection: 500 mg/10 ml (150 mg quinupristin and 350 mg dalfopristin)

Indications and dosages
➤ Serious or life-threatening infections associated with vancomycin-resistant *Enterococcus faecium*
Adults and adolescents ages 16 and older: 7.5 mg/kg by I.V. infusion over 1 hour q 8 hours
➤ Complicated skin and skin-structure infections caused by *Staphylococcus aureus* (methicillin-susceptible) and *Streptococcus pyogenes*
Adults and adolescents ages 16 and older: 7.5 mg/kg by I.V. infusion over 1 hour q 12 hours for at least 7 days
Dosage adjustment
• Hepatic impairment

Contraindications
• Hypersensitivity to drug or other streptogramins

Administration
◄€ Don't mix with other drugs or saline solution.
• For intermittent infusion through a common I.V. line, flush line with dextrose 5% in water (D_5W) before and after giving this drug.

• Add 5 ml of sterile water or D_5W to powdered drug in vial, and swirl gently by hand until powder dissolves; don't shake vial. Solution should be clear.
• Within 30 minutes of first dilution, draw up prescribed dose and dilute further in D_5W to a final concentration of 2 mg/ml or less.
• If patient has a central venous catheter and is fluid-restricted, drug may be given in 100 ml of D_5W.
• Administer by infusion pump over 60 minutes.
• If significant peripheral vein irritation occurs, dilute in 500 to 750 ml of D_5W.
• Know that duration of therapy depends on infection site and severity.

Route	Onset	Peak	Duration
I.V.	Unknown	Unknown	Unknown

Adverse reactions
CNS: headache
CV: thrombophlebitis
GI: nausea, vomiting
Hepatic: hyperbilirubinemia, increased hepatic enzyme levels
Musculoskeletal: joint pain, myalgia
Skin: rash, pruritus
Other: inflammation, pain, or edema at infusion site

Interactions
Drug-drug. *Cyclosporine:* reduced metabolism and increased blood level of cyclosporine
Drugs metabolized by CYP450-3A4 (antiretrovirals; antineoplastics, such as vinca alkaloids, docetaxel, and paclitaxel; benzodiazepines; calcium channel blockers; HMG-CoA reductase inhibitors; immunosuppressants; corticosteroids; carbamazepine; cisapride; disopyramide; lidocaine; quinidine): increased therapeutic and adverse effects of these drugs
Drug-diagnostic tests. *Alanine aminotransferase, aspartate aminotransferase, bilirubin:* increased levels

q

Precautions

Use cautiously in:
- hepatic impairment
- breastfeeding patients.

Patient monitoring

- Monitor closely for infusion site reaction and thrombophlebitis. If these problems occur, consider increasing infusion volume, changing infusion site, or infusing through peripherally inserted central catheter or central venous catheter.
- Assess weight and fluid intake and output to help detect edema.
- Monitor bilirubin level.

Patient teaching

◀€ Instruct patient to immediately report pain or redness at infusion site.
- Tell patient to report muscle aches and pains.
- Advise patient to minimize GI upset by eating small, frequent servings of healthy food and drinking plenty of fluids.
- As appropriate, review all other significant adverse reactions and interactions, especially those related to the drugs and tests mentioned above.

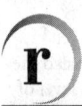

rabeprazole sodium

AcipHex

Pharmacologic class: Proton pump inhibitor

Therapeutic class: Gastric antisecretory agent

Pregnancy risk category B

Action

Reduces gastric acid secretion and increases gastric mucus and bicarbonate production, creating a protective coating on the gastric mucosa

Availability

Tablets (delayed-release): 20 mg

🖊 Indications and dosages

➤ Healing of erosive or ulcerative gastroesophageal reflux disease (GERD)
Adults: 20 mg P.O. daily for 4 to 8 weeks. If healing doesn't occur within 8 weeks, another 8 weeks of therapy may be considered. Maintenance dosage is 20 mg P.O. daily.
➤ GERD
Adults: 20 mg P.O. daily for 4 weeks. If symptoms don't resolve after 4 weeks, another course of therapy may be considered.
➤ Hypersecretory conditions, including Zollinger-Ellison syndrome
Adults: Initially, 60 mg P.O. daily; dosage adjusted as needed up to 100 mg P.O. daily as a single dose or 60 mg P.O. b.i.d.; maximum daily dosage is 120 mg.
➤ Duodenal ulcer
Adults: 20 mg P.O. daily for up to 4 weeks
➤ *Helicobacter pylori* eradication
Adults: 20 mg P.O. b.i.d. for 7 days (given with amoxicillin and clarithromycin)

Off-label uses

- Dyspepsia
- Benign gastric ulcer

Contraindications

- Hypersensitivity to drug, its components, or benzimidazoles
- Breastfeeding

Administration

- Don't crush or split tablet.
- Give single daily dose after morning meal.

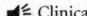

Route	Onset	Peak	Duration
P.O.	Within 1 hr	Unknown	24 hr

Adverse reactions
CNS: headache

Interactions
Drug-drug. *Gastric pH–dependent drugs (such as digoxin, ketoconazole):* increased or decreased absorption
Warfarin: increased risk of bleeding

Precautions
Use cautiously in:
• severe hepatic impairment
• pregnant patients
• children (safety not established).

Patient monitoring
• Stay alert for symptomatic response; however, be aware that a positive response doesn't rule out gastric cancer.

Patient teaching
• Tell patient he may take drug with or without food; teach him not to crush, chew, or split tablets.
• As appropriate, review all significant adverse reactions and interactions, especially those related to the drugs mentioned above.

raloxifene
Evista

Pharmacologic class: Nonsteroidal benzothiophene derivative

Therapeutic class: Selective estrogen receptor modulator, bone resorption inhibitor

Pregnancy risk category X

Action
Binds to estrogen receptors, activating its pathways and increasing bone mineral density, thereby decreasing bone resorption and turnover

Availability
Tablets: 60 mg

🕖 Indications and dosages
➤ Prevention and treatment of osteoporosis in postmenopausal women
Adults: 60 mg P.O. daily

Off-label uses
• Prophylaxis of cardiovascular disease

Contraindications
• Hypersensitivity to drug or its components
• History of thromboembolic events
• Concurrent estrogen therapy
• Premenopausal women
• Females of childbearing age
• Pregnancy or breastfeeding
• Children

Administration
• Give with or without food.

Route	Onset	Peak	Duration
P.O.	Unknown	6 hr	Unknown

Adverse reactions
CNS: depression, insomnia, vertigo, syncope, hypoesthesia, migraine, neuralgia
CV: varicose veins, thrombophlebitis, chest pain, peripheral edema, deep-vein thrombosis
EENT: conjunctivitis, sinusitis, rhinitis, pharyngitis, laryngitis
GI: nausea, vomiting, diarrhea, dyspepsia, flatulence, gastroenteritis, abdominal pain
GU: urinary tract infection or disorder, cystitis, vaginitis, leukorrhea, endometrial disorder, **vaginal hemorrhage**
Metabolic: decreased total cholesterol and low-density lipoprotein (LDL) levels
Musculoskeletal: leg cramps, joint pain, myalgia, arthritis, tendon disorder

r

Respiratory: cough, pneumonia, bronchitis, **pulmonary embolism**
Skin: rash, diaphoresis
Other: weight gain, hot flashes, infection, pain, flulike symptoms

Interactions
Drug-drug. *Cholestyramine:* reduced raloxifene absorption
Highly protein-bound drugs (such as diazepam, diazoxide, lidocaine): interference with binding of these drugs
Warfarin: decreased prothrombin time
Drug-diagnostic tests. *Albumin, calcium, inorganic phosphate, platelets, protein:* decreased levels
Apolipoprotein A1: increased level
Apolipoprotein B, fibrinogen, LDLs, total cholesterol: decreased levels
Corticosteroid-binding, sex steroid–binding, and thyroid-binding globulin: increased levels

Precautions
Use cautiously in:
• altered lipid metabolism, hepatic dysfunction
• immobilized patients and others at increased risk for thromboembolic events.

Patient monitoring
• Watch for thromboembolic events, especially during first 4 months of therapy.
• Stay alert for other adverse effects, particularly leg cramps, other musculoskeletal complaints, and respiratory disorders.
• Assess bone mineral density results.
• Monitor for unexplained vaginal bleeding.

Patient teaching
• Tell patient she may take drug with or without food.
• Instruct patient to read package insert before starting drug and to review it periodically.

◀€ Teach patient to recognize and immediately report symptoms of blood clots.
• Instruct patient to stop taking drug 3 days before expected period of prolonged immobility and to restart it only after she regains normal mobility.
• Inform patient that drug may cause hot flashes; assure her that these are normal effects.
• Instruct patient to report unexplained vaginal bleeding or leg cramps.
• As appropriate, review all other significant and life-threatening adverse reactions and interactions, especially those related to the drugs and tests mentioned above.

ramipril
Altace

Pharmacologic class: Angiotensin-converting enzyme (ACE) inhibitor
Therapeutic class: Antihypertensive
Pregnancy risk category C (first trimester), *D* (second and third trimesters)

Action
Inhibits conversion of angiotensin I to angiotensin II, a potent vasoconstrictor; decreases cardiac output. Increases plasma renin levels and reduces aldosterone levels, causing systemic vasodilation.

Availability
Capsules: 1.25 mg, 2.5 mg, 5 mg, 10 mg

⌀ Indications and dosages
➢ Hypertension (used alone or with other agents)
Adults: Initially, 2.5 mg P.O. daily in patients not receiving diuretics; may increase dosage slowly p.r.n. according to blood pressure response. Mainte-

nance dosage is 2.5 to 20 mg/day P.O. as a single dose or in two equally divided doses. If ramipril alone doesn't control blood pressure, thiazide diuretic may be added.

➤ To reduce the risk of myocardial infarction (MI), cerebrovascular accident, or death from cardiovascular causes

Adults: Initially, 2.5 mg P.O. daily for 1 week, followed by 5 mg P.O. daily for the next 3 weeks, then increased as tolerated to a maintenance dosage of 10 mg P.O. daily. In hypertensive patients and those who've had a recent MI, divide maintenance dose.

➤ Heart failure after MI

Adults: Initially, 2.5 mg P.O. b.i.d.; may decrease to 1.25 mg b.i.d. if patient becomes hypotensive at higher dosage. Titrate toward target dosage of 5 mg b.i.d. at 3-week intervals.

Dosage adjustment
• Renal impairment
• Concurrent diuretic use

Off-label uses
• Angina associated with syndrome X
• Atherosclerosis
• Mitral insufficiency
• Renovascular hypertension
• Diabetic or nondiabetic nephropathy
• Erythrocytosis

Contraindications
• Hypersensitivity to drug or other ACE inhibitors
• Angioedema with previous ACE inhibitor therapy
• Pregnancy (second and third trimesters)

Administration
• Be aware that diuretics should be discontinued 2 to 3 days before ramipril therapy begins, if possible, to avoid severe hypotension.
• If patient can't swallow capsules, open them and mix in water or apple

juice, or sprinkle contents in small amount of applesauce.

Route	Onset	Peak	Duration
P.O.	1-2 hr	2-4 hr	24 hr

Adverse reactions
CNS: dizziness, fatigue, headache, vertigo, asthenia
CV: hypotension, orthostatic hypotension, angina pectoris, tachycardia, **MI, heart failure**
EENT: blurred vision, sinusitis
GI: nausea, vomiting, diarrhea
Hematologic: purpura, **agranulocytosis**
Metabolic: hyperkalemia
Musculoskeletal: muscle cramps
Respiratory: cough, asthma, upper respiratory tract infection, **bronchospasm**
Skin: rash, pruritus, urticaria, photosensitivity, angioedema
Other: fever

Interactions
Drug-drug. *Allopurinol:* increased risk of hypersensitivity reaction
Antacids: decreased ramipril absorption
Digoxin, lithium: increased blood levels and risk of toxicity of these drugs
Diuretics, other antihypertensives: increased hypotension
Indomethacin: reduced hypotensive effect of ramipril
Phenothiazines: increased pharmacologic effects of ramipril
Potassium-sparing diuretics, potassium supplements: increased risk of hyperkalemia
Tetracyclines: decreased tetracycline absorption
Drug-diagnostic tests. *Alanine aminotransferase, alkaline phosphatase, aspartate aminotransferase, bilirubin, blood urea nitrogen, creatinine, potassium:* increased levels
Drug-food. *Any food:* decreased rate (but not extent) of drug absorption

r

Salt substitutes containing potassium: increased risk of hyperkalemia

Drug-herb. *Capsaicin:* increased incidence of cough

Ephedra (ma huang): decreased drug efficacy, exacerbation of hypertension

Yohimbe: interference with drug's antihypertensive effect

Drug-behaviors. *Alcohol use:* increased hypotension

Precautions

Use cautiously in:

• autoimmune diseases, aortic stenosis, hypertrophic cardiomyopathy, cerebrovascular or cardiac insufficiency, collagen vascular disease, febrile illness, hepatic or renal impairment, hypotension, neutropenia, chronic cough, proteinuria, renal artery stenosis

• family history of angioedema

• concurrent immunosuppressant or diuretic therapy

• black patients

• elderly patients

• pregnant (first trimester) or breastfeeding patients

• children (safety not established).

Patient monitoring

• Assess vital signs and cardiovascular status; be sure to ask patient if he's experiencing angina.

• Monitor complete blood count and liver function test results.

• Closely monitor potassium level; watch for signs and symptoms of hyperkalemia.

• Stay alert for signs and symptoms of angioedema, especially in black patients after first dose.

• Evaluate for dry, nonproductive cough.

Patient teaching

• Tell patient he may take drug with or without food.

◀€ Instruct patient to immediately report swelling of tongue or face or difficulty breathing.

• Teach patient to monitor and record his blood pressure.

• Inform patient that drug may cause dry, nonproductive cough. Instruct him to report this problem if it becomes bothersome.

• Instruct patient to avoid driving and other hazardous activities until he knows how drug affects concentration and alertness.

• Advise patient to move slowly when sitting up or standing to avoid dizziness or light-headedness from sudden blood pressure decrease.

• Caution patient that excessive fluid loss (as from sweating, vomiting, or diarrhea) and inadequate fluid intake increase risk of light-headedness (especially in hot weather).

• Tell patient to avoid salt substitutes containing potassium and herbs.

• As appropriate, review all other significant and life-threatening adverse reactions and interactions, especially those related to the drugs, tests, foods, herbs, and behaviors mentioned above.

ranitidine hydrochloride
Apo-Ranitidine✦, Zantac, Zantac 75, Zantac EFFERdose

Pharmacologic class: Histamine$_2$ (H$_2$)-receptor antagonist

Therapeutic class: Antiulcerative

Pregnancy risk category B

Action

Reduces gastric acid secretion and increases gastric mucus and bicarbonate production, creating a protective coating on the gastric mucosa

Availability

Capsules (liquid-filled): 150 mg, 300 mg

Granules (effervescent): 150 mg/packet

✦ Canada   ◀€ Clinical alert   Reactions in **bold** are life-threatening

Solution for injection: 25 mg/ml in 2-, 10-, and 40-ml vials
Solution for injection (pre-mixed): 50 mg/50 ml in 0.45% sodium chloride in single-dose plastic containers
Syrup: 15 mg/ml
Tablets: 75 mg, 150 mg, 300 mg
Tablets (effervescent): 150 mg

🟊 Indications and dosages

➤ Active duodenal ulcer
Adults: 150 mg or 10 ml P.O. b.i.d.; or 300 mg or 20 ml P.O. daily. Maintenance dosage is 150 mg or 10 ml P.O. at bedtime.
➤ Benign gastric ulcer
Adults: 150 mg or 10 ml P.O. b.i.d.; maintenance dosage is 150 mg or 10 ml P.O. at bedtime.
➤ Pathologic hypersecretory conditions, including Zollinger-Ellison syndrome; gastroesophageal reflux disease (GERD)
Adults: 150 mg or 10 ml P.O. b.i.d.
➤ Erosive esophagitis
Adults: 150 mg or 10 ml P.O. q.i.d.; maintenance dosage is 150 mg P.O. b.i.d.
➤ Duodenal and gastric ulcers
Children ages 1 month to 16 years: 2 to 4 mg/kg P.O. daily, up to a maximum of 300 mg/day. Maintenance dosage is 2 to 4 mg/kg P.O. daily, up to a maximum of 150 mg/day.
➤ GERD and erosive esophagitis
Children ages 1 month to 16 years: 5 to 10 mg/kg P.O. daily in two divided doses
➤ Hospitalized patients with pathologic hypersecretory conditions (including Zollinger-Ellison syndrome); intractable duodenal ulcers; patients who can't receive oral drugs
Adults: 50 mg I.M. q 6 to 8 hours or 50 mg intermittent I.V. bolus q 6 to 8 hours; or 50 mg intermittent I.V. infusion q 6 to 8 hours. For continuous I.V. infusion in patients with Zollinger-Ellison syndrome, add prescribed raniti-

dine dose to dextrose 5% in water (D_5W) or other compatible solution, dilute to a concentration of no more than 2.5 mg/ml, and start infusion at 1 mg/kg/hour; if, after 4 hours, measured gastric acid output exceeds 10 mEq/hour or patient becomes symptomatic, increase dosage
in increments of 0.5 mg/kg/hour and remeasure acid output. Some patients may need up to 2.5 mg/kg/hour with infusion rates as high as 220 mg/hour. For continuous I.V. infusion in other patients, add prescribed ranitidine dose to 250 ml D_5W or other compatible I.V. solution and administer at 6.25 mg/hour.
Children ages 1 month to 16 years: 2 to 4 mg/kg/day I.V. in divided doses q 6 to 8 hours, up to a maximum of 50 mg q 6 to 8 hours
Dosage adjustment
• Renal impairment
• Hepatic impairment
• Debilitaed patients

Off-label uses
• Asthma
• GI hemorrhage
• *Helicobacter pylori* infection
• Short bowel syndrome
• Immunosuppression reversal
• Psoriasis
• Aspiration pneumonitis prophylaxis

Contraindications
• Hypersensitivity to drug or its components
• Alcohol intolerance (with some oral products)
• History of acute porphyria

Administration
• For intermittent I.V. bolus injection, dilute prescribed dose in normal saline solution or other compatible solution to a concentration not exceeding 2.5 mg/ml, and inject no faster than 4 ml/minute (5 minutes).

r

• Give oral doses after meals and at bedtime.

• For intermittent I.V. infusion, dilute prescribed dose in D_5W or other compatible solution to a concentration not exceeding 0.5 mg/ml, and infuse no faster than 7 ml/minute (15 to 20 minutes).

• Note that premixed Zantac solution of 50 mg in half-normal saline solution (50 ml) doesn't require dilution and should be infused over 15 to 20 minutes.

• Know that I.V. form may be added to total parenteral nutrition solutions.

• Be aware that I.M. dose can be given undiluted deep into a large muscle.

Route	Onset	Peak	Duration
P.O.	Unknown	1-3 hr	8-12 hr
I.V., I.M.	Unknown	15 min	8-12 hr

Adverse reactions

CNS: headache, agitation, anxiety
GI: nausea, vomiting, diarrhea, constipation, abdominal discomfort or pain
GU: slightly increased creatinine level
Hematologic: reversible granulocytopenia and **thrombocytopenia**
Hepatic: increased hepatic enzyme levels, **hepatitis**
Skin: rash
Other: pain at I.M. injection site, burning or itching at I.V. site, hypersensitivity reaction

Interactions

Drug-drug. *Antacids:* decreased ranitidine absorption
Propantheline: delayed absorption and increased peak ranitidine level
Drug-diagnostic tests. *Urine protein tests using Multistix:* false-negative results
Drug-herb. *Yerba maté:* decreased drug clearance
Drug-behaviors. *Smoking:* decreased ranitidine effects

Precautions

Use cautiously in:
• renal or hepatic impairment, heart rhythm disturbances, phenylketonuria
• elderly patients
• pregnant or breastfeeding patients.

Patient monitoring

• Assess vital signs.
• Monitor complete blood count and liver function studies.

Patient teaching

• Tell patient he may take oral drug with or without food; advise him to take once-daily prescription drug at bedtime.

• Instruct patient to dissolve EFFERdose in 6 to 8 oz of water before taking.

• Caution patient to avoid driving and other hazardous activities until he knows how drug affects concentration and alertness.

• As appropriate, review all other significant and life-threatening adverse reactions and interactions, especially those related to the drugs, tests, herbs, and behaviors mentioned above.

rasburicase
Elitek

Pharmacologic class: Recombinant urate oxidase enzyme
Therapeutic class: Antineoplastic, antimetabolite
Pregnancy risk category C

Action

Catalyzes oxidation of uric acid into an inactive soluble metabolite

Availability

Powder for injection: 1.5 mg/vial

Indications and dosages
➤ Chemotherapy-induced hyper-uricemia in children with leukemia, lymphoma, or solid-tumor cancers
Children: 0.15 to 0.2 mg/kg by I.V. infusion over 30 minutes as a single daily dose for 5 days; chemotherapy should begin 4 to 24 hours after first dose.

Off-label uses
• Chemotherapy-induced hyper-uricemia in adults with leukemia, lymphoma, or solid-tumor cancers

Contraindications
• Hypersensitivity to drug or its components
• History of anaphylaxis, hemolytic anemia, or methemoglobinemia as a reaction to rasburicase
• Glucose-6-phosphate dehydrogenase (G6PD) deficiency

Administration
• Know that patients at high risk for G6PD deficiency (those of African or Mediterranean descent) should be screened for this disorder before starting therapy.
• Give drug 4 to 24 hours before first chemotherapy dose.
• Dilute by adding 1-ml vial of diluent provided with drug. Swirl gently; don't shake. Dilute further by injecting prescribed diluted dose into infusion bag containing appropriate volume of normal saline solution to achieve final volume of 50 ml.
• Administer by I.V. infusion over 30 minutes once daily.
◄€ Don't give as I.V. bolus.
• Don't use I.V. filters.
• Don't mix with other drugs. Use a separate I.V. line, or flush line with 15 ml of normal saline solution before and after infusing rasburicase.
• Know that administration of more than one course isn't recommended.

Route	Onset	Peak	Duration
I.V.	4 hr	96 hr	Unknown

Adverse reactions
CNS: headache
GI: nausea, vomiting, diarrhea, constipation, abdominal pain
Hematologic: neutropenia, methemoglobinemia, severe hemolysis (in patients with G6PD deficiency)
Respiratory: respiratory distress
Skin: rash
Other: fever, mucositis, hypersensitivity reactions including **anaphylaxis, sepsis**

Interactions
Drug-diagnostic tests. *Neutrophils:* decreased count
Uric acid: interference with measurement (if blood is at room temperature)

Precautions
Use cautiously in:
• pregnant or breastfeeding patients
• children under age 2.

Patient monitoring
• Monitor for signs and symptoms of hypersensitivity reaction.
• Assess for respiratory distress and signs and symptoms of infection.
• Monitor uric acid level and complete blood count.

Patient teaching
• Teach parents and patient (if appropriate) to recognize and immediately report adverse effects, including hypersensitivity reaction.
◄€ Caution parents that drug may cause sepsis. Instruct them to monitor child's temperature and immediately report fever and other signs and symptoms of infection.
• As appropriate, review all other significant and life-threatening adverse reactions and interactions, especially

r

those related to the tests mentioned above.

remifentanil hydrochloride
Ultiva

Pharmacologic class: Opioid agonist
Therapeutic class: Opioid analgesic
Controlled substance schedule II
Pregnancy risk category C

Action
Unknown; thought to bind to mu-opioid receptors in CNS, altering perception of and emotional response to pain. Also inhibits ascending pain pathways in limbic system, thalamus, midbrain, and hypothalamus.

Availability
Injection: 1 mg/ml in 3-, 5-, and 10-ml vials

Indications and dosages
➤ Induction of anesthesia through intubation
Adults: 0.5 to 1 mcg/kg/minute I.V. given with a hypnotic or volatile drug. May give 1 mcg/kg I.V. over 30 to 60 seconds if endotracheal intubation will occur less than 8 minutes after start of infusion.
➤ Maintenance of anesthesia
Adults: 0.25 to 0.4 mcg/kg/minute. Increase dosage by 25% to 100% or decrease by 25% to 50% q 2 to 5 minutes, as needed. If rate exceeds 1 mcg/kg/minute, anesthetic doses may be increased. A supplemental I.V. bolus dose of 1 mcg/kg may be given.
➤ To continue analgesic effect during immediate postoperative period
Adults: Initially, 0.1 mcg/kg/minute I.V.; adjust in increments of 0.025 mcg/kg/minute q 5 minutes p.r.n.
➤ Monitored anesthesia care

Adults: 0.5 to 1 mcg/kg I.V. over 30 to 60 seconds, 90 seconds before anesthetic is given. As a continuous infusion, 0.05 to 0.1 mcg/kg/minute I.V. 5 minutes before anesthetic is given; after anesthetic is given, titrate rate to 0.025 to 0.05 mcg/kg/minute. Then adjust rate by 0.025 mcg/kg/minute q 5 minutes p.r.n.
Dosage adjustment
• Elderly patients
• Obese patients

Off-label uses
• Peripartum anesthesia

Contraindications
• Hypersensitivity to drug or other opioid analgesics
• Acute or severe bronchial asthma
• Upper airway obstruction
• Significant respiratory depression
• Epidural or intrathecal administration
• During labor when delivery of premature neonate is anticipated

Administration
◀€ Have emergency resuscitation equipment and naloxone available in case of respiratory arrest.
• Add 1 ml of diluent per milligram of drug; shake well to create clear, colorless solution of 1 mg/ml.
• Further dilute drug in normal or half-normal saline solution, dextrose 5% in water, dextrose 5% in normal saline solution, or dextrose 5% in lactated Ringer's solution.
• Use infusion control pump for continuous infusion; choose site close to venous cannula. After administering, clear I.V. tubing by flushing.
• Know that rates over 0.2 mcg/kg/minute may cause respiratory depression.

Route	Onset	Peak	Duration
I.V.	Immediate	Unknown	5-10 min

Adverse reactions

CNS: headache, agitation, dizziness, confusion, sedation, euphoria, delirium, anxiety

CV: hypertension, hypotension, palpitations, tachycardia, bradycardia, **asystole**

EENT: blurred vision, miosis, diplopia, tinnitus

GI: nausea, vomiting, diarrhea, constipation, abdominal cramps, anorexia, dry mouth

GU: urinary retention, dysuria

Musculoskeletal: muscle rigidity

Respiratory: respiratory depression, apnea

Skin: flushing, rash, urticaria, bruising, pruritus, diaphoresis

Interactions

Drug-drug. *Benzodiazepines, hypnotics, inhalation anesthetics:* synergistic effects

Centrally acting muscle relaxants, other opioid analgesics: increased risk of respiratory depression

Drug-herb. *Kava:* increased CNS depression

Precautions

Use cautiously in:
• bradycardia, heart failure, pulmonary disease, hypothyroidism
• elderly patients
• pregnant patients.

Patient monitoring

◀≶ When giving high doses, assess for muscle rigidity and be prepared to stop therapy.

• Continuously monitor respiratory and cardiovascular function, oxygenation, and vital signs.

• Assess fluid intake and output; watch for urinary retention.

Patient teaching

• Tell patient he'll be monitored closely throughout anesthesia period.

• Reassure patient that he'll receive drugs to control pain before remifentanil is discontinued during perioperative period.

repaglinide
Prandin

Pharmacologic class: Meglitinide
Therapeutic class: Hypoglycemic
Pregnancy risk category C

Action

Inhibits alpha-glucosidases, enzymes that convert oligosaccharides and disaccharides to glucose; inhibition of these enzymes lowers blood glucose level, especially in postprandial hyperglycemia

Availability

Tablets: 0.5 mg, 1 mg, 2 mg

⦸ Indications and dosages

➤ Adjunct to diet and exercise in type 2 diabetes mellitus uncontrolled by diet and exercise alone

Adults: 0.5 to 4 mg P.O. before each meal; may adjust at 1-week intervals based on blood glucose response; maximum daily dosage is 16 mg.

Contraindications

• Hypersensitivity to drug or its components
• Diabetic ketoacidosis
• Type 1 diabetes mellitus

Administration

• Give 15 to 30 minutes before meals.

Route	Onset	Peak	Duration
P.O.	Within 30 min	60-90 min	<4 hr

Adverse reactions

CNS: headache, paresthesia
CV: angina, chest pain

r

EENT: sinusitis, rhinitis, tooth disorder
GI: nausea, vomiting, diarrhea, constipation, dyspepsia
GU: urinary tract infection
Metabolic: hypoglycemia, hyperglycemia
Musculoskeletal: joint pain, back pain
Respiratory: upper respiratory tract infection, bronchitis
Other: hypersensitivity reaction

Interactions

Drug-drug. *Barbiturates, carbamazepine, rifampin:* decreased repaglinide blood level
Beta-adrenergic blockers, chloramphenicol, monoamine oxidase inhibitors, nonsteroidal anti-inflammatory drugs, probenecid, sulfonamides, warfarin: potentiation of repaglinide effects
Calcium channel blockers, corticosteroids, estrogens, hormonal contraceptives, isoniazid, phenothiazines, phenytoin, nicotinic acid, sympathomimetics, thyroid preparations: hyperglycemia, loss of glycemic control
Erythromycin, ketoconazole, miconazole: decreased repaglinide metabolism, increased risk of hypoglycemia
Drug-food. *Any food:* decreased drug bioavailability
Drug-herb. *Aloe gel (oral), bitter melon, chromium, coenzyme Q10, fenugreek, gymnema sylvestre, psyllium, St. John's wort:* additive hypoglycemic effects
Glucosamine: poor glycemic control

Precautions

Use cautiously in:
• renal or hepatic impairment; adrenal or pituitary insufficiency; stress caused by infection, fever, trauma, or surgery
• elderly or malnourished patients
• pregnant or breastfeeding patients
• children.

Patient monitoring

• Monitor blood glucose and glycosylated hemoglobin levels.

• Monitor patient's meal pattern; consult prescriber about adjusting dosage if patient adds or misses a meal.
• Assess for angina, shortness of breath, or other discomforts.
• Watch for signs and symptoms of urinary or upper respiratory tract infection, bronchitis, and EENT infections.

Patient teaching

• Tell patient to take drug 15 to 30 minutes before each meal.
• Instruct patient to monitor blood glucose level carefully; teach him to recognize signs and symptoms of hypoglycemia and hyperglycemia.
• Advise patient to immediately report signs and symptoms of infection.
• As appropriate, review all other significant adverse reactions and interactions, especially those related to the drugs, foods, and herbs mentioned above.

reteplase, recombinant
Retavase

Pharmacologic class: Tissue plasminogen activator
Therapeutic class: Thrombolytic enzyme
Pregnancy risk category C

Action

Converts plasminogen to plasmin, which in turn breaks down fibrin and fibrinogen, thereby dissolving thrombus

Availability

Injection: 10.4 units (18.1 mg)/vial

⏷ Indications and dosages
➤ Acute myocardial infarction
Adults: 10 units by I.V. bolus over 2 minutes, repeated in 30 minutes

Off-label uses
• Pulmonary embolism

Contraindications
• Hypersensitivity to drug or alteplase
• Active internal bleeding
• Bleeding diathesis
• Recent intracranial or intraspinal surgery or trauma
• Intracranial neoplasm
• Arteriovenous malformation or aneurysm
• Severe uncontrolled hypertension
• History of cerebrovascular accident

Administration
◀€ If patient shows signs or symptoms of bleeding or anaphylaxis after first bolus dose, withhold second bolus and contact prescriber immediately.
• Use sterile water for injection (without preservatives) to reconstitute drug into colorless solution of 1 unit/ml.
• If drug foams, let it sit until foam subsides.
• Don't use solution that is discolored or contains visible precipitates.
• Don't give with other drugs in same I.V. line; know that drug is incompatible with heparin.

Route	Onset	Peak	Duration
I.V.	Immediate	End of infusion	Variable

Adverse reactions
CNS: intracranial hemorrhage
CV: arrhythmias, hemorrhage
GI: nausea, vomiting, **GI bleeding**
GU: hematuria
Hematologic: anemia, **bleeding tendency**
Other: bleeding at puncture sites, fever

Interactions
Drug-drug. *Anticoagulants, indomethacin, phenylbutazone, platelet aggregation inhibitors (such as abciximab, aspirin, dipyridamole):* increased risk of bleeding
Drug-diagnostic tests. *Hemoglobin:* decreased level
International Normalized Ratio, partial thromboplastin time, prothrombin time: increased
Drug-herb. *Ginkgo, many other herbs:* increased risk of bleeding

Precautions
Use cautiously in:
• previous puncture of noncompressible vessels, major surgery, obstetric delivery, organ biopsy, trauma, hypertension, conditions that may cause left-sided heart thrombus (including mitral stenosis), acute pericarditis, subacute bacterial endocarditis, hemostatic defects, diabetic hemorrhagic retinopathy, cerebrovascular disease, severe hepatic or renal dysfunction, septic thrombophlebitis or occluded AV cannula at a seriously infected site, other conditions in which bleeding poses a significant hazard
• concurrent use of oral anticoagulants (such as warfarin)
• patients older than age 75
• pregnant or breastfeeding patients.

Patient monitoring
◀€ Check closely for signs and symptoms of bleeding in all body systems; monitor coagulation studies and complete blood count.
• Monitor ECG for arrhythmias secondary to coronary thrombolysis.
• Assess neurologic status to detect early signs of intracranial hemorrhage.

Patient teaching
• Teach patient about drug's anticoagulant effect; instruct him in safety measures to avoid injury that can lead to uncontrolled bleeding.

r

◀€ Instruct patient to immediately report signs and symptoms of bleeding problems.

• Tell patient he'll undergo frequent blood testing during therapy.

ribavirin
Copegus, Rebetol, Virazole

Pharmacologic class: Synthetic nucleoside analog
Therapeutic class: Antiviral
Pregnancy risk category X

Action
Unknown; thought to inhibit RNA and DNA synthesis by depleting nucleotides and blocking replication and maturation of viral cells

Availability
Capsules: 200 mg
Powder to be reconstituted for inhalation (Virazole): 6 g in 100-ml glass vial
Tablets: 200 mg

⚕ Indications and dosages
➤ Chronic hepatitis C infection (*Note:* Dosage is calculated solely on body weight of patient.)
Adults and children weighing 75 kg (165 lb) or more: 600 mg P.O. q morning and evening, given with interferon alfa-2b
Adults and children weighing less than 75 kg (165 lb): 400 mg P.O. q morning and 600 mg P.O. q evening, given with interferon alfa-2b
➤ Hospitalized infants and young children with severe lower respiratory tract infection caused by respiratory syncytial virus
Infants and young children: 20 mg/ml by inhalation as a starting solution in Viratek Small Particle Aerosol Generator (SPAG-2) for 12 to 18 hours daily

for 3 to 7 days. Infants who aren't mechanically ventilated should receive drug by oxygen hood from SPAG-2 unit.
Dosage adjustment
• Cardiovascular disease
• Chronic obstructive pulmonary disease (COPD)
• Renal impairment
• Hemoglobin below 10 g/dl

Off-label uses
• Influenza A or B
• Pneumonia caused by adenovirus
• Severe lower respiratory tract infection in adults
• Herpes genitalis
• Hemorrhagic fever

Contraindications
• Hypersensitivity to drug or its components
• Autoimmune hepatitis (oral combination therapy)
• Creatinine clearance below 50 ml/minute
• Significant or unstable cardiac disease
• Hemoglobinopathies, such as sickle cell anemia and thalassemia major
• Females of childbearing age (inhalation form)
• Pregnancy or pregnant partner of male patient (oral drug)
• Breastfeeding

Administration
◀€ Be aware that oral form must be given in conjunction with interferon alfa-2b injection.
• Give aerosol by Viratek SPAG-2 only; don't use other aerosol-generating equipment.
• Dilute powder in sterile water for injection; don't use solutions with antimicrobial ingredients.
• Know that drug may be given by oral or nasal inhalation
• Discard solution in SPAG-2 every 24 hours before adding new solution.

◀≶ Avoid prolonged contact with aerosol, which can cause headache or eye irritation.

Route	Onset	Peak	Duration
Oral	Unknown	Unknown	Unknown
Inhalation	Slow	60-90 min	Unknown

Adverse reactions
CNS: fatigue, headache, nervousness, depression, **suicidal ideation**
CV: hypotension, bradycardia (with inhalation form), **cardiac arrest**
EENT: conjunctivitis, eyelid erythema or rash
GI: nausea, dyspepsia, anorexia, **pancreatitis**
Hematologic: hemolytic anemia, reticulocytosis
Hepatic: increased alanine aminotransferase (ALT), aspartate aminotransferase (AST), and bilirubin levels
Respiratory: bacterial pneumonia, **pneumothorax, bronchospasm, pulmonary edema, apnea, worsening respiratory status** (inhalation form)
Skin: rash, pruritus

Interactions
Drug-drug. *Abacavir, didanosine, lamivudine, stavudine, zalcitabine, zidovudine:* potentially fatal lactic acidosis
Stavudine, zidovudine: decreased antiviral activity
Drug-diagnostic tests. *ALT, AST, bilirubin:* increased levels
Hemoglobin: decreased level
Reticulocytes: increased count

Precautions
Use cautiously in:
• liver transplant and other transplant recipients
• decompensated hepatic disease or co-infection with hepatitis B or human immunodeficiency virus
• COPD
• patients who haven't responded to interferon.

Patient monitoring
◀≶ Carefully monitor respiratory status; check ventilator frequently to ensure that drug precipitates don't interfere with effective function.
◀≶ Monitor ECG and vital signs; watch for hypotension, bradycardia, and other evidence of impending cardiac arrest or worsening respiratory condition.
• Assess neurologic status; stay alert for depression and suicidal ideation.
• Monitor complete blood count with white cell differential as well as liver function test results.

Patient teaching
• Explain drug delivery system and precautions carefully to patient and parents of children receiving inhalation form.
◀≶ Caution patient or parents that drug may cause depression or suicidal thoughts, which should be reported immediately.
◀≶ Instruct patient or parents to immediately report new or worsening respiratory symptoms.
• Counsel sexually active patients (both males and females) about appropriate birth control methods, and tell them to use extreme care to avoid pregnancy. Emphasize importance of using two forms of effective contraception during treatment and for 6 months afterward (with oral therapy).
• As appropriate, review all other significant and life-threatening adverse reactions and interactions, especially those related to the drugs and tests mentioned above.

r

rifabutin
Mycobutin

Pharmacologic class: Rifamycin derivative

Therapeutic class: Antimycobacterial

Pregnancy risk category B

Action
Inhibits RNA synthesis by blocking RNA transcription in susceptible organisms (mycobacteria and some gram-positive and gram-negative bacteria)

Availability
Capsules: 150 mg

🕖 Indications and dosages
➤ To prevent disseminated *Mycobacterium avium intracellulare* complex in patients with advanced human immunodeficiency virus (HIV) infection
Adults: 300 mg P.O. daily as a single dose or in two divided doses

Off-label uses
- Tuberculosis
- HIV infection
- Prophylaxis and treatment of *M. avium intracellulare* in children

Contraindications
- Hypersensitivity to drug
- Active tuberculosis

Administration
- Give in divided doses twice daily with food to reduce GI upset.

Route	Onset	Peak	Duration
P.O.	Unknown	2-3 hr	>24 hr

Adverse reactions
CNS: headache, asthenia
CV: sensation of pressure in chest
EENT: uveitis; discolored tears, saliva, or sputum
GI: nausea, vomiting, diarrhea, dyspepsia, abdominal pain, eructation, flatulence, discolored feces, anorexia, abnormal taste
GU: discolored urine
Hematologic: eosinophilia, **neutropenia, leukopenia, thrombocytopenia**
Hepatic: slightly increased hepatic enzyme levels
Musculoskeletal: joint pain, myalgia
Respiratory: dyspnea
Skin: rash, discolored skin or sweat
Other: fever, flulike symptoms

Interactions
Drug-drug. *Clarithromycin, itraconazole, saquinavir:* reduced blood levels and efficacy of these drugs
Delavirdine: decreased delavirdine blood level, increased rifabutin blood level
Drugs metabolized by liver (such as zidovudine): altered blood levels of these drugs
Hormonal contraceptives: decreased contraceptive efficacy
Indinavir, nelfinavir, ritonavir: increased rifabutin blood level
Drug-diagnostic tests. *Alanine aminotransferase, aspartate aminotransferase, eosinophils:* increased levels
Neutrophils, platelets, white blood cells: decreased counts
Drug-food. *High-fat foods:* delayed drug absorption

Precautions
Use cautiously in:
- severe hepatic disease
- pregnant or breastfeeding patients.

Patient monitoring
- Monitor complete blood count with white cell differential; watch for signs and symptoms of blood dyscrasias.
- Assess nutritional status.

• Closely monitor vital signs and temperature; stay alert for dyspnea and flu-like symptoms.

Patient teaching
• Advise patient to take drug twice daily with food (but not high-fat foods) if GI upset occurs. To further minimize GI upset, teach him to eat small, frequent servings of healthy food and drink plenty of fluids.
• Teach patient to take drug exactly as prescribed, even when symptoms subside.
• Tell patient that drug may turn tears, urine, and other body fluids reddish or brownish orange. Instruct him not to wear contact lenses during therapy because drug may stain them permanently.
• Inform patient that drug occasionally causes eye inflammation; instruct him to promptly report symptoms to prescriber.
• Caution patient to avoid driving and other hazardous activities until effects of drug are known; drug may cause weakness.
• As appropriate, review all other significant and life-threatening adverse reactions and interactions, especially those related to the drugs, tests, and foods mentioned above.

rifampin (rifampicin)
Rifadin, Rimactane, Rofact✤

Pharmacologic class: Rifamycin derivative
Therapeutic class: Antitubercular
Pregnancy risk category C

Action
Inhibits RNA synthesis by blocking RNA transcription in susceptible organisms (mycobacteria and some gram-positive and gram-negative bacteria)

Availability
Capsules: 150 mg, 300 mg
Powder for injection: 600 mg/vial

Indications and dosages
➤ Tuberculosis
Adults: 10 mg/kg/day (up to 600 mg/day) P.O. or I.V. infusion as a single dose
Children: 10 to 20 mg/kg/day (up to 600 mg/day) P.O. or I.V. infusion as a single dose
➤ Asymptomatic *Neisseria meningitidis* carriers
Adults: 600 mg P.O. or I.V. infusion q 12 hours for 2 days
Children older than 1 month: 10 mg/kg/day P.O. or I.V. infusion (up to 600 mg/day) q 12 hours for 2 days

Off-label uses
• *Mycobacterium avium intracellulare* complex infection
• Brucellosis
• *Haemophilus influenzae* type B
• Severe staphylococcal bone and joint infections
• Prosthetic valve endocarditis caused by coagulase-negative staphylococci
• Leprosy
• Prophylaxis in high-risk close contacts of patients with *N. meningitidis* infections

Contraindications
• Hypersensitivity to drug or other rifamycin derivatives
• Breastfeeding

Administration
• Add 10 ml of sterile water to vial to yield a 60-mg/ml solution for I.V. infusion.
• Further dilute in 100 ml of dextrose 5% in water (D_5W) and infuse over 30 minutes, or add to 500 ml of D_5W and infuse over 3 hours.

r

• Give oral doses with a full glass of water 1 hour before or 2 hours after a meal.
• If patient can't receive dextrose, use normal saline solution for dilution; however, don't use other I.V. solutions.

Route	Onset	Peak	Duration
P.O.	Rapid	2-4 hr	12-24 hr
I.V.	Rapid	End of infusion	12-24 hr

Adverse reactions

CNS: ataxia, confusion, drowsiness, fatigue, headache, asthenia, psychosis, generalized numbness
EENT: conjunctivitis; discolored tears, saliva, and sputum
GI: nausea, vomiting, diarrhea, abdominal cramps, flatulence, discolored feces, heartburn, epigastric distress, anorexia, sore mouth and tongue, **pseudomembranous colitis**
GU: discolored urine
Hematologic: decreased hemoglobin, eosinophilia, transient leukopenia, hemolytic anemia, **hemolysis, disseminated intravascular coagulation (DIC), thrombocytopenia**
Hepatic: jaundice, transient abnormalities in liver function studies
Metabolic: hyperuricemia
Musculoskeletal: myalgia, joint pain
Respiratory: dyspnea, wheezing
Skin: flushing, rash, pruritus, discolored sweat, erythema multiforme, **toxic epidermal necrolysis**
Other: flulike symptoms, hypersensitivity reactions including vasculitis and **Stevens-Johnson syndrome**

Interactions

Drug-drug. *Barbiturates, beta-adrenergic blockers, cardiac glycosides, clarithromycin, clofibrate, cyclosporine, dapsone, diazepam, doxycycline, fluoroquinolones (such as ciprofloxacin), haloperidol, levothyroxine, methadone, progestins, quinine, tacrolimus, theophylline, tricyclic antidepressants (such as amitriptyline, nortriptyline), zidovudine:* increased metabolism of these drugs
Chloramphenicol, corticosteroids, disopyramide, efavirenz, estrogens, fluconazole, hormonal contraceptives, itraconazole, ketoconazole, nevirapine, quinidine, opioid analgesics, oral hypoglycemics, phenytoin, quinidine, ritonavir, theophylline, tocainide, verapamil, warfarin: decreased efficacy of these drugs
Delavirdine, indinavir, nelfinavir, saquinavir: decreased blood levels of these drugs
Hepatotoxic drugs (including isoniazid, ketoconazole, pyrazinamide): increased risk of hepatotoxicity
Drug-diagnostic tests. *Alanine aminotransferase, alkaline phosphatase, aspartate aminotransferase, bilirubin, blood urea nitrogen, uric acid:* increased levels
Dexamethasone suppression test: interference with results
Direct Coombs' test: false-positive result
Folate, vitamin B$_{12}$ assay: interference with standard assays
Sulfobromophthalein uptake and excretion test: delayed hepatic uptake and excretion
Drug-behaviors. *Alcohol use:* increased risk of hepatotoxicity

Precautions

Use cautiously in:
• porphyria
• history of hepatic disease
• concurrent use of other hepatotoxic drugs
• pregnant patients.

Patient monitoring

• Monitor kidney and liver function test results, complete blood count, and uric acid level.
◀╪ Watch for signs and symptoms of bleeding tendency, especially DIC.
• Assess for signs and symptoms of hepatic impairment.

• Monitor bowel movements for diarrhea, which may indicate pseudomembranous colitis.

Patient teaching

• Advise patient to take oral dose 1 hour before or 2 hours after meals. If drug causes significant GI upset, instruct him to take it with meals. To further minimize GI upset, teach him to eat small, frequent servings of healthy food and drink plenty of fluids.

◀€ Instruct patient to immediately report fever, malaise, appetite loss, nausea, vomiting, or yellowing of skin or eyes.

• Tell patient that drug may color his tears, urine, and other body fluids reddish or brownish orange. Instruct him not to wear contact lenses during therapy because drug may stain them permanently.

• Instruct patient not to drink alcohol.

• Caution patient to avoid driving and other hazardous activities until he knows how drug affects concentration and alertness.

• As appropriate, review all other significant and life-threatening adverse reactions and interactions, especially those related to the drugs, tests, and behaviors mentioned above.

rifapentine
Priftin

Pharmacologic class: Rifamycin derivative

Therapeutic class: Antitubercular
Pregnancy risk category C

Action

Inhibits RNA synthesis by blocking RNA transcription in susceptible organisms (mycobacteria and some gram-positive and gram-negative bacteria)

Availability

Tablets: 150 mg

Indications and dosages

➢ Pulmonary tuberculosis (given with at least one other antitubercular)
Adults: *Intensive-phase treatment*—600 mg P.O. twice weekly for 2 months, with doses given 72 hours apart; must be administered with at least one other antitubercular. *Continuation-phase treatment*—600 mg P.O. once weekly for 4 months, given with another appropriate antitubercular.

Off-label uses

• *Mycobacterium avium intracellulare* complex infection

Contraindications

• Hypersensitivity to drug or other rifamycin derivatives

Administration

• Expect to give drug with pyridoxine to adolescents, malnourished patients, and patients at risk for neuropathy.

Route	Onset	Peak	Duration
P.O.	Slow	5-6 hr	17-18 hr

Adverse reactions

CNS: headache, fatigue, anxiety, dizziness, aggressive behavior
CV: hypertension, peripheral edema
EENT: visual disturbances; discolored tears, sputum, and saliva
GI: nausea, vomiting, diarrhea, heartburn, esophagitis, gastritis, discolored feces, anorexia, **pancreatitis**
GU: hematuria, pyuria, proteinuria, urinary casts, discolored urine
Hematologic: anemia, thrombocytosis, hematoma, purpura, eosinophilia, **neutropenia, leukopenia**
Hepatic: increased alanine aminotransferase (ALT), alkaline phosphatase (ALP), aspartate aminotransferase (AST), bilirubin, and lactate dehydrogenase (LD) levels; **hepatitis**

r

Metabolic: hyperuricemia, hyperkalemia, hypovolemia
Musculoskeletal: gout, arthritis, joint pain
Skin: rash, pruritus, acne, urticaria, discolored skin and sweat
Other: edema

Interactions

Drug-drug. *Amitriptyline, anticoagulants, barbiturates, beta-adrenergic blockers, chloramphenicol, clofibrate, corticosteroids, cyclosporine, dapsone, delavirdine, diazepam, digoxin, diltiazem, disopyramide, doxycycline, fentanyl, fluconazole, fluoroquinolones, haloperidol, hormonal contraceptives, indinavir, itraconazole, ketoconazole, methadone, mexiletine, nelfinavir, nifedipine, nortriptyline, oral hypoglycemics, phenothiazines, progestin, quinidine, quinine, ritonavir, saquinavir, sildenafil, tacrolimus, theophylline, thyroid preparations, tocainide, verapamil, warfarin, zidovudine:* decreased actions of these drugs
Antiretroviral drugs: decreased efficacy of these drugs
Drug-diagnostic tests. *ALP, ALT, AST, bilirubin, eosinophils, LD, potassium, uric acid:* increased levels
Folate, vitamin B_{12} assays: interference with standard assays
Hemoglobin, neutrophils, platelets, white blood cells: decreased values

Precautions

Use cautiously in:
• hepatic disorders, porphyria
• concurrent use of protease inhibitors for human immunodeficiency virus infection
• elderly patients
• pregnant patients
• children under age 12.

Patient monitoring

• Monitor complete blood count, uric acid level, and liver function test re-

sults; watch for signs and symptoms of blood dyscrasias and hepatitis.
• Assess vital signs and fluid intake and output; stay alert for hypertension and edema.
• Closely monitor nutritional status and hydration.

Patient teaching

◀€ Instruct patient to immediately report fever, malaise, appetite loss, nausea, vomiting, or yellowing of skin or eyes.
• Emphasize importance of taking rifapentine with companion drugs as prescribed to prevent growth of resistant tuberculosis strains.
• Inform patient that drug may color his tears, urine, and other body fluids reddish or brownish orange. Instruct him not to wear contact lenses during therapy because drug may stain them permanently.
• Advise patient to minimize GI upset by eating small, frequent servings of healthy food and drinking plenty of fluids.
• Tell patient to monitor his weight and report sudden gains; also tell him to report swelling.
• Instruct patient to report unusual bleeding, bruising, or rash.
• Caution patient to avoid driving and other hazardous activities until he knows how drug affects concentration, vision, and alertness.
• As appropriate, review all other significant and life-threatening adverse reactions and interactions, especially those related to the drugs and tests mentioned above.

Safe drug administration

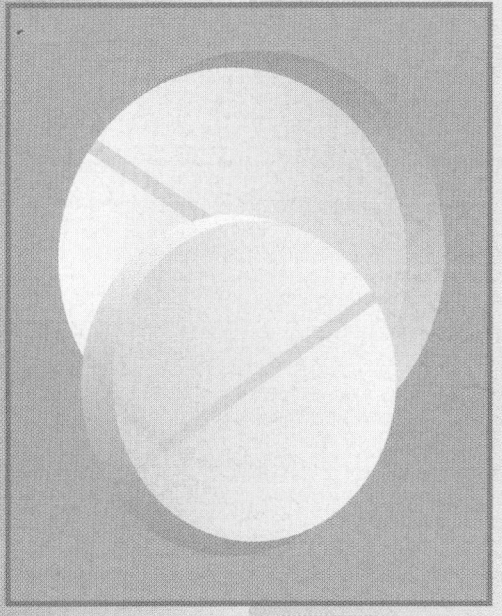

The following guidelines on preparing, administering, and monitoring drug therapy will help you ensure patient safety and drug effectiveness.

Body surface area in adults

SAFETY
GUIDELINES

To estimate an adult's body surface area (BSA) with the nomogram below, use a straightedge to connect the patient's weight in the right column with height in the left column. The point of intersection in the middle column is the BSA. For example, a patient who weighs 120 lb and is 62" tall has a BSA of 1.60 m².

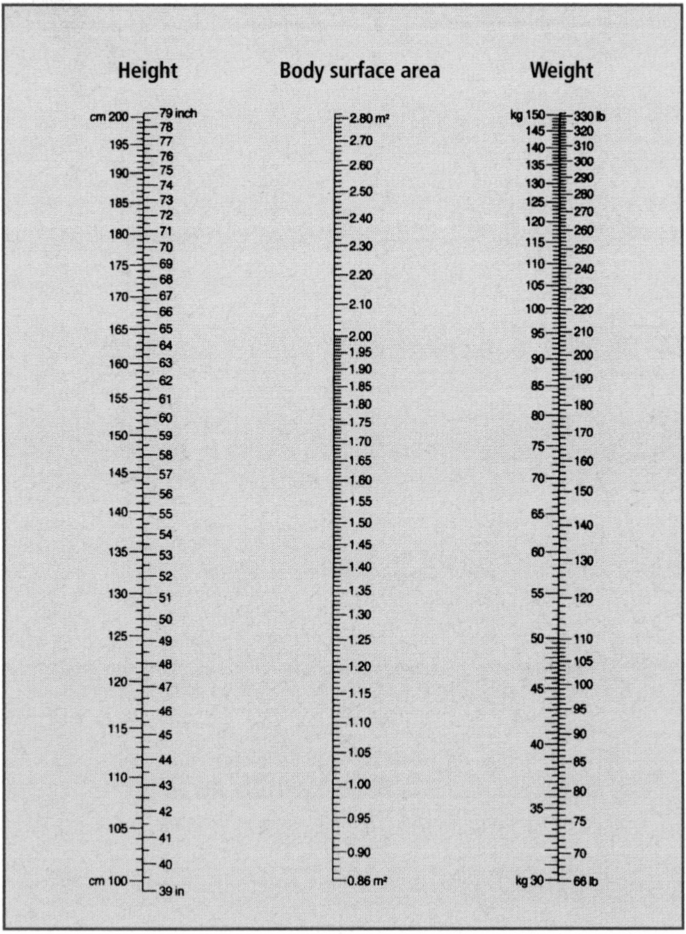

Height	Body surface area	Weight

Height

cm 200 — 79 inch
78
195 — 77
76
190 — 75
74
185 — 73
72
180 — 71
70
175 — 69
68
170 — 67
66
165 — 65
64
160 — 63
62
155 — 61
60
150 — 59
58
145 — 57
56
140 — 55
54
135 — 53
52
130 — 51
50
125 — 49
48
120 — 47
46
115 — 45
44
110 — 43
42
105 — 41
40
cm 100 — 39 in

Body surface area

2.80 m²
2.70
2.60
2.50
2.40
2.30
2.20
2.10
2.00
1.95
1.90
1.85
1.80
1.75
1.70
1.65
1.60
1.55
1.50
1.45
1.40
1.35
1.30
1.25
1.20
1.15
1.10
1.05
1.00
0.95
0.90
0.86 m²

Weight

kg 150 — 330 lb
145 — 320
140 — 310
135 — 300
130 — 290
125 — 280
120 — 270
115 — 260
250
110 — 240
105 — 230
100 — 220
95 — 210
90 — 200
85 — 190
80 — 180
75 — 170
70 — 160
150
65 — 140
60 — 130
55 — 120
50 — 110
105
45 — 100
95
40 — 90
85
35 — 80
75
70
kg 30 — 66 lb

From Lentner, C. (1981). *Geigy Scientific Tables: Units of Measurement, Body Fluid, Composition of Body, and Nutrition* (8th ed.). Basel, Switzerland: Novartis Medical Education. Used with permission from Icon Learning Systems, a division of MediMedia USA, Inc. All rights reserved.

Conversions and calculations

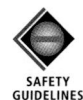

SAFETY
GUIDELINES

Accurate conversions and calculations are crucial to ensuring safe drug administration. Use the tables below when you need to convert one unit to another, find
equivalent measures, convert temperatures between Celsius and Fahrenheit, or
calculate dosages or administration rates.

Metric measures

Solids
1 milligram (mg) = 1,000 micrograms (mcg)
1 gram (g) = 1,000 mg
1 kilogram (kg) = 1,000 g

Liquids
1 milliliter (ml) = 1 cubic centimeter (cc)
1 ml = 1,000 microliters (mcl)
1 cc = 1,000 mcl
1 liter (L) = 1,000 ml
1 L = 1,000 cc

Household to metric equivalents
1 teaspoon (tsp) = 5 ml
1 tablespoon (tbs) = 15 ml
1 ounce (oz) = 30 ml
2 tbs = 30 ml
1 oz = 30 g
1 pound (lb) = 454 g
2.2 lb = 1 kg
1 inch = 2.54 centimeters (cm)

Temperature conversions

To convert Celsius (°C) to Fahrenheit (°F)
Use the following equation:
$(°C \times \frac{9}{5}) + 32 = °F$
Example: 38 °C times $\frac{9}{5}$ is 68.4; 68.4 plus 32 equals 100.4 °F.

To convert °F to °C
$(°F - 32) \times \frac{5}{9} = °C$
Example: 98.6 °F minus 32 is 66.6; 66.6 times $\frac{5}{9}$ equals 37 °C.

Calculating dosages and administration rates

Concentration of solution in mg/ml = $\dfrac{\text{mg of drug}}{\text{ml of solution}}$

Infusion rate in mg/minute = $\dfrac{\text{mg of drug}}{\text{ml of solution}} \times$ flow rate (ml/hour) $\div$ 60 minutes

Concentration of solution in mcg/ml = $\dfrac{\text{mg of drug} \times 1,000}{\text{ml of solution}}$

Infusion rate in mcg/minute =
$\dfrac{\text{mg of drug} \times 1,000}{\text{ml of solution}} \times$ flow rate (ml/hour) $\div$ 60 minutes

Infusion rate in mcg/kg/minute =
$\dfrac{\text{mg of drug} \times 1,000}{\text{ml of solution}} \times$ flow rate (ml/hour) $\div$ 60 minutes $\div$ weight in kg

Infusion rate in ml/hour = ml of solution $\div$ 60 minutes

Infusion rate in gtt/minutes = $\dfrac{\text{ml of solution}}{\text{time in minutes}} \times$ drip factor (gtt/ml)

Identifying injection sites

SAFETY
GUIDELINES

Drug injection sites vary with the administration route. The instructions below describe appropriate procedures and injection sites for I.M., S.C., and I.V. drugs.

To begin, wash your hands, put on gloves, and locate the appropriate site. Clean the site with an alcohol pad, and administer the injection as described here.

I.M. injections
You can administer an I.M. injection into the muscles shown below. In these illustrations, specific injection sites are shaded.

Deltoid site
• Locate the lower edge of the acromial process.
• Insert the needle 1" to 2" below the acromial process at a 90-degree angle.

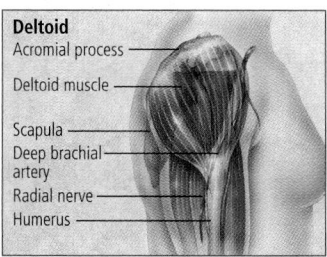

Deltoid
Acromial process
Deltoid muscle
Scapula
Deep brachial artery
Radial nerve
Humerus

Dorsogluteal site
• Draw an imaginary line from the posterior superior iliac spine to the greater trochanter.
• Insert the needle at a 90-degree angle above and outside the drawn line.
• You can administer a Z-track injection through this site. After drawing up the drug, change the needle, displace the skin lateral to the injection site, withdraw the needle, and then release the skin.

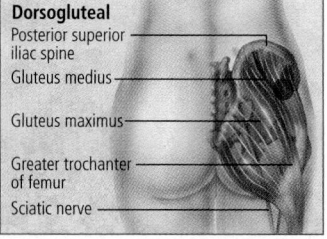

Dorsogluteal
Posterior superior iliac spine
Gluteus medius
Gluteus maximus
Greater trochanter of femur
Sciatic nerve

Ventrogluteal site
• With the palm of your hand, locate the greater trochanter of the femur.
• Spread your index and middle fingers posteriorly from the anterior superior iliac spine to the furthest area possible. This is the correct injection site.
• Remove your fingers and insert the needle at a 90-degree angle.

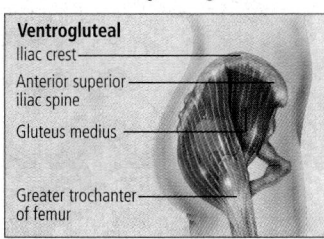

Ventrogluteal
Iliac crest
Anterior superior iliac spine
Gluteus medius
Greater trochanter of femur

Vastus lateralis and rectus femoris sites
• Find the lateral quadriceps muscle for the vastus lateralis, or the anterior thigh for the rectus femoris.
• Insert the needle at a 90-degree angle into the middle third of the muscle, parallel to the skin surface.

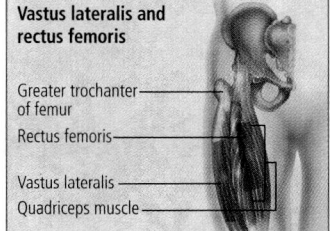

Vastus lateralis and rectus femoris
Greater trochanter of femur
Rectus femoris
Vastus lateralis
Quadriceps muscle

S.C. injections

S.C. drugs can be injected into the fat pads on the abdomen, buttocks, upper back, and lateral upper arms and thighs (shaded in the illustrations below). If your patient requires frequent S.C. injections, make sure to rotate injection sites.
• Gently gather and elevate or spread S.C. tissue.
• Insert the needle at a 45- or 90-degree angle, depending on the drug or the amount of S.C. tissue at the site.

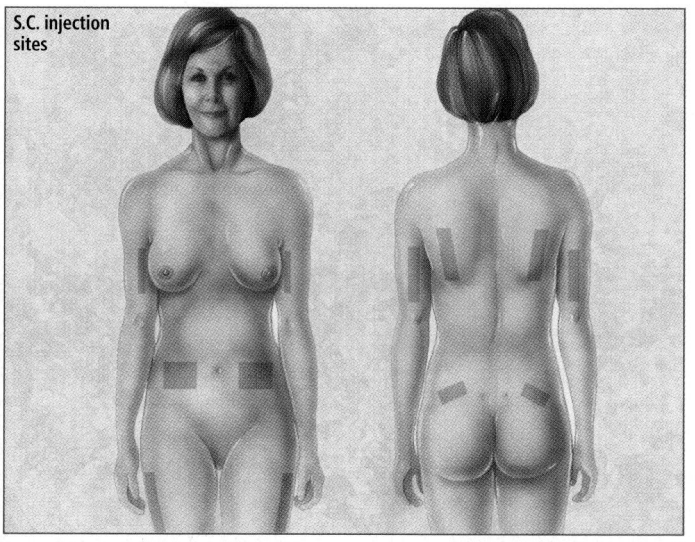

S.C. injection sites

I.V. injections

I.V. drugs can be injected into the veins of the arms and hands. The illustration at right shows commonly used sites.
• Locate the vein using a tourniquet.
• Insert the catheter at a slight angle (about 10 degrees).
• Release the tourniquet when blood appears in the syringe or tubing.
• Slowly inject the drug into the vein.

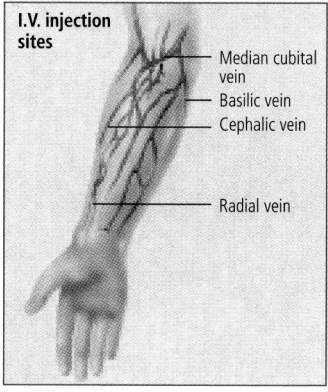

I.V. injection sites

Median cubital vein
Basilic vein
Cephalic vein
Radial vein

Drug compatibilities

Use the table below to determine if you can safely mix two drugs together in the same syringe or administer them together through the same I.V. line.

KEY
C: compatible
I: incompatible
∗: conflicting data exist
Blank space: no data available

	amikacin	amiodarone	amphotericin B	aztreonam	calcium chloride	calcium gluconate	cefazolin	ceftazidime	clindamycin	cyclosporine	dexamethasone	digoxin	diltiazem	diphenhydramine	dobutamine	dopamine	enalaprilat
amikacin		C	I	C	C	C	C	I	C	C	C	C	C	C			C
amiodarone	C		C		C	C	I	I	I		C	I			C	C	
amphotericin B	I	C		I									C	∗		I	I
aztreonam	C		I		C	C	C	C	C		C		C	C	C	C	C
calcium chloride	C	C													∗	C	
calcium gluconate	C	C		C			I		I		C			C	∗		C
cefazolin	C	I		C		I			∗	C	C		C				C
ceftazidime	I	I		C			∗		C				C				C
clindamycin	C	C		C		I	∗	C			C						C
cyclosporine	C						C	C								∗	
dexamethasone	C	C		C	C	C	C		C					∗			
digoxin		I													I		
diltiazem	C		C	C			C	C	C						C	C	C
diphenhydramine	C		∗	C		C					∗						
dobutamine		C		C	∗	∗						I	C			C	C
dopamine		C	I	C	C					∗			C		C		C
enalaprilat	C		I	C		C	C	C	C						C	C	
epinephrine	C	C			∗	∗									C		
esmolol	C	C		C			C	C	C		C				C	C	C
famotidine		C	C			C	C	C			C	C		C	C	C	C
furosemide	∗	∗											I	I	I		
heparin	I			I	C		C	∗	∗	C		C	C	∗	∗	∗	C
hydrocortisone	C		I	C	C	C			C		C		∗		C	C	C

SAFETY
GUIDELINES

	epinephrine	esmolol	famotidine	furosemide	heparin	hydrocortisone	imipenem and cilastatin sodium	insulin	labetalol	levofloxacin	lorazepam	magnesium	methylprednisolone	metoprolol	metronidazole	midazolam	milrinone	morphine	nitroglycerin	nitroprusside	norepinephrine	ondansetron	phenylephrine	potassium chloride	propofol	sodium bicarbonate	tobramycin	vancomycin	vecuronium
	C	C		*	I	C			C	C	C	C			C	C	C	C				C			C	I	C		C
	C	C	C	*				C	C		C	*	C		C	C	C	C	C	*			C	C		I	C	C	C
			C		I	I						*	C									I			I	I			
				C	C	C	C			I	C	C		I		C				C				C	C	C	*		
	*	C				C					I				C	C		C						I	I			
	*		C		C	C			C			*	C		C	C							C	C	C	I	C	C	
		C	C	*				C	C			C	C	*	C	C	C			C			C	C		C	*	C	
		C	C	*				C				C	I		C					C			C	C	I	*	*	
		C			C	C			C	C		I	C		C	C	C	C			C				C		*		
												*				C					*			C	C		C	C	
			C		C	C				C	*					*	C	C			*		C	C				I	
		C	C		C			I							C	C	C						C	C				
		C		*	*	C	*			C										C								
			C	I	*						I		I				C				C	C	*	C			C	
	C	C	C	I	*			*	C	C		*			*	C	C	C	C	C	C		C	*	C	I			C
		C	C		C	C		I	C	C			C	*	C	C	C	C	C	C	C	C		C	C	I			C
	C	C		*	C	C	C	C		C	C	C			C		C	C	C	C	C	C		C					C
	C	I	*		C	C				I	I	C				I	I	I	C	C		I		I	C	C	*		
	C	C	C	C		*	C	I	*	I	C	C	*		C	C	C	I	*	C		C	C	C	C	C	I	*	C
	C	C	C	C	*			C			C	*		C	I		C					C	C					C

Drug compatibilities (continued)

KEY
C: compatible
I: incompatible
∗: conflicting data exist
Blank space: no data available

	amikacin	amiodarone	amphotericin B	aztreonam	calcium chloride	calcium gluconate	cefazolin	ceftazidime	clindamycin	cyclosporine	dexamethasone	digoxin	diltiazem	diphenhydramine	dobutamine	dopamine	enalaprilat
imipenem and cilastatin sodium		I		C									C				
insulin		C		C			C					I	∗		∗	I	
labetalol	C	C				C	C	C	C						C	C	C
levofloxacin	C							C		C					C	C	
lorazepam	C	C		I							C		C	I			
magnesium	C	∗	∗	C	I	∗	C		I	C				∗			C
methylprednisolone		C	C	C		C			C				∗	I		C	C
metoprolol																	
metronidazole	C	C		I			∗	C	C	C						∗	C
midazolam	C	C				C	C	I	C		∗	C			∗	C	
milrinone	C	C			C	C	C	C	C		C	C	C		C	C	
morphine	C	C		C	C		C	C	C		C	C		C	C	C	C
nitroglycerin		C											C		C	C	
nitroprusside		∗			C										C	C	C
norepinephrine		C											C		C	C	
ondansetron	C		I	C			C	C	C	∗	∗			C		C	
phenylephrine		C				C							C	C			
potassium chloride	C	C		C		C	C	C			C	C		∗	∗	C	C
propofol	I		I	C	I	C	C	C	C	C	C	C	C		C	C	C
sodium bicarbonate	C	I		C	I	I		I					∗		I	I	
tobramycin		C		C		C	C	∗	∗	C			C				C
vancomycin	C	C		∗		C	∗	∗				I		C	C		C
vecuronium		C					C								C	C	

Drug compatibility chart (continued). Column headings (left to right): epinephrine, esmolol, famotidine, furosemide, heparin, hydrocortisone, imipenem and cilastatin sodium, insulin, labetalol, levofloxacin, lorazepam, magnesium, methylprednisolone, metoprolol, metronidazole, midazolam, milrinone, morphine, nitroglycerin, nitroprusside, norepinephrine, ondansetron, phenylephrine, potassium chloride, propofol, sodium bicarbonate, tobramycin, vancomycin, vecuronium. Cell symbols: C = compatible, I = incompatible, * = special consideration, ■ = diagonal (same drug).

	epinephrine	esmolol	famotidine	furosemide	heparin	hydrocortisone	imipenem and cilastatin sodium	insulin	labetalol	levofloxacin	lorazepam	magnesium	methylprednisolone	metoprolol	metronidazole	midazolam	milrinone	morphine	nitroglycerin	nitroprusside	norepinephrine	ondansetron	phenylephrine	potassium chloride	propofol	sodium bicarbonate	tobramycin	vancomycin	vecuronium
imipenem and cilastatin sodium			C		C		■	C			I					I	I					C							
insulin		C	C		I	C	C	■	I	I		C				C	C	C	C	C	I			C	C	*	C	C	
labetalol		C	C	I	*			I	■			C			C	C						C		C	C	*	C	C	
levofloxacin	C			I	I			I		■		C					C	I	I				C			C		C	
lorazepam			C	C	C	C	C	I		C	■				C		C				*			C	C			C	C
magnesium		C	C		C	*		C	C			■			C		C	C		C	*		C	C	I	I	C	C	
methylprednisolone			C		*								■	C	*	C	C			*				I	I	I			
metoprolol														■				C											
metronidazole		C			C	C			C		C	C	C		■	C	C	C								C			
midazolam		C	C	I	C	I	I	C	C				*		C	■	C	C	C	C	C	C		C	*	I	C	C	C
milrinone	C			I	C		I	C			C	C	C		C	C	■	C	C	C	C		C	C	C	C	C	C	C
morphine		C	C	I	I	C		C	C	C		C	C	C	C	C	■		C	C	C		C	C	I	C	C	C	C
nitroglycerin			C	C	C	*		C	C	C	I		C	C		C		■					C					C	
nitroprusside	C	C	C	C	C			C	C	I		C		C	C	C	C		■	C		C		C					C
norepinephrine			C					I	C			C	C	C		C			C	■		C						C	
ondansetron		C	I	C	C	C					*		*		C		C				■		C	C	I			C	
phenylephrine		C		C					C										C			■				I		C	
potassium chloride	C	C	C	I	C			C	C		C	C			C	C	C		C		C		■	C	C				
propofol	C	C	C	C	C	C		C	C		C	C	C		*	C	C	C		C	C	I		■	C	I	C	C	
sodium bicarbonate			C	C	C		*	*	C			I			I	C	I			I	■	C	C			I			
tobramycin		C		*	I		C	C			C					C	C	C	C					I	■	I			
vancomycin		C	C		*	I		C	C	C	C	C			C	C	C				C	C		C	I	■		C	
vecuronium		C		C	C			C				C	C	C	C	C				C	■							C	

Anaphylaxis: Treatment guidelines

SAFETY
GUIDELINES

A hypersensitivity reaction may occur when a patient comes in contact with a certain agent, such as a drug, food, or other foreign protein. In some patients, this reaction progresses to life-threatening anaphylaxis, marked by sudden development of urticaria and respiratory distress. If this reaction continues, it may precipitate vascular collapse, leading to shock and, occasionally, death.

Hypersensitivity reaction

Adults: Epinephrine 0.2 to 0.5 ml of 1:1,000 solution S.C.; repeat q 10 to 15 minutes to a maximum dosage of 1 mg.
Children: Epinephrine 10 mcg/kg of 1:1,000 solution S.C., to a maximum of 500 mcg/dose; may repeat dose q 15 minutes for 2 doses, then q 4 hours as needed

Adults or children: Diphenhydramine 1 to 2 mg/kg I.V.

Adults: Hydrocortisone 100 mg I.V. initially; then administer as indicated.
Children: Hydrocortisone 0.16 to 1 mg/kg I.V. given once or twice daily

If poor response, use anaphylaxis algorithm.

Anaphylaxis

Administer CPR if patient loses circulation or breathing; follow Advanced Cardiac Life Support guidelines.

If hypotension occurs, give vasopressors (such as dopamine, norepinephrine, or neosynephrine). Provide fluid resuscitation with large volumes of normal saline or lactated Ringer's solution.

Adults and children: If bronchospasm occurs, give 1 to 2 inhalations of inhaled bronchodilator and loading dose of 6 mg/kg theophylline I.V., followed by maintenance dose as indicated.

Adults: Epinephrine 0.2 to 0.5 ml of 1:1,000 solution S.C.; repeat q 10 to 15 minutes to maximum dosage of 1 mg.
Children: Epinephrine 10 mcg/kg of 1:1,000 solution S.C., to maximum of 500 mcg/dose; may repeat dose q 15 minutes for 2 doses, then q 4 hours as needed

If patient doesn't respond to S.C. epinephrine, dilute epinephrine to yield 1:10,000 solution. For adults, infuse at 1 mcg/minute; may titrate to 2 to 10 mcg/minute. For children, infuse at 0.1 mcg/kg/minute.

KEY:
CPR: cardiopulmonary resuscitation

Cardiac arrest: Treatment guidelines

SAFETY
GUIDELINES

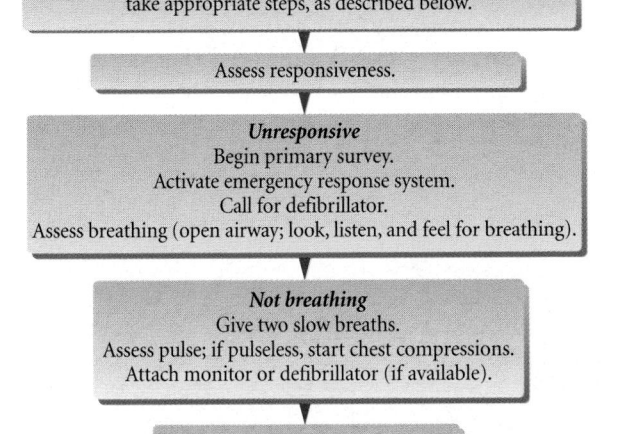

If you suspect your patient is in cardiac arrest, take appropriate steps, as described below.

Assess responsiveness.

Unresponsive
Begin primary survey.
Activate emergency response system.
Call for defibrillator.
Assess breathing (open airway; look, listen, and feel for breathing).

Not breathing
Give two slow breaths.
Assess pulse; if pulseless, start chest compressions.
Attach monitor or defibrillator (if available).

No pulse
Continue CPR.
Assess heart rhythm.

VF or VT on monitor
Attempt defibrillation (up to three shocks if VF/VT persists).

Asystole or PEA on monitor

Administer CPR for 1 minute.

Administer CPR for up to 3 minutes.

Conduct secondary ABCD survey

Airway: Attempt to insert airway device.

Breathing: Confirm and secure airway device; provide ventilation and oxygenation.

Circulation: Obtain I.V. access; administer adrenergic drug; consider antiarrhythmics, buffer agents, and pacing.
For asystole or PEA, give epinephrine 1 mg I.V.; repeat every 3 to 5 minutes.
For VF/VT, give vasopressin 40 units I.V. for one dose, or give epinephrine 1 mg I.V., repeated every 3 to 5 minutes.

Differential diagnosis: Search for and treat reversible causes.

KEY   ABCD: airway, breathing, circulation,   CPR: cardiopulmonary resuscitation   VF: ventricular fibrillation
         differential diagnosis   PEA: pulseless electrical activity   VT: ventricular tachycardia

Source: American Heart Association

Stroke: Treatment guidelines

SAFETY
GUIDELINES

This algorithm for the treatment of cerebrovascular accident (stroke) or suspected stroke is based on the one created by the American Heart Association.

Suspected stroke

Within 10 minutes of arrival at ED:
- Assess ABCs and vital signs.
- Give oxygen.
- Obtain I.V. access; draw blood.
- Check blood glucose level; treat accordingly.
- Obtain 12-lead ECG.
- Perform neurocheck.
- Alert stroke team.

Within 25 minutes of arrival at ED:
- Review patient history.
- Establish symptom onset (< 3 hours required for fibrinolytics).
- Perform physical exam.
- Obtain noncontrast CT scan; read CT scan (<45 minutes of arrival).
- Obtain lateral C-spine X-ray (if comatose or history of trauma).

CT scan shows intracerebral or subarachnoid hemorrhage (SAH)?

No

Yes

Probable ischemic stroke:
- CT scan exclusions?
- Improving neurologic deficits?
- Fibrinolytic exclusions?
- Symptom onset > 3 hours?

Consult neurosurgery.

Treat for acute hemorrhage:
- Reverse anticoagulants and bleeding disorder.
- Monitor neurologic status.
- Treat hypertension if patient is conscious.

No to above

Patient is candidate for fibrinolytic therapy?

No

Yes

Blood on LP

- Obtain informed consent.
- Begin fibrinolytic therapy within 1 hour of arrival at ED.
- Monitor neurologic status; obtain CT scan if condition deteriorates.
- Monitor BP; treat as indicated.
- Admit to CCU.
- Withhold anticoagulants and antiplatelet drugs for 24 hours.

If high suspicion of SAH despite negative CT, perform LP.

No blood on LP

Initiate supportive care.

ABCs: airway, breathing, and circulation
BP: blood pressure
CCU: critical care unit
CT: computed tomography

ECG: electrocardiogram
ED: emergency department
LP: lumbar puncture
SAH: subarachnoid hemorrhage

Source: American Heart Association

Hypertensive crisis: Treatment guidelines

SAFETY GUIDELINES

Hypertensive crisis is a severe blood pressure rise that can lead to irreversible heart, brain, and kidney damage—and even death—unless treated promptly. Suspect this condition if your patient has systemic blood pressure above 240/130 mm Hg without symptoms, or elevated blood pressure with chest pain, headache, or heart failure.

↓

Immediately reduce blood pressure.
Do not reduce blood pressure by more than 25% of mean arterial pressure over first 2 hours. Consider arterial line insertion for continuous blood pressure monitoring.

↓

Initial drug choices

Systemic blood pressure > 240/130 mm Hg without symptoms, or with headache	**Elevated blood pressure with chest pain or heart failure**	**Elevated blood pressure in pregnant woman with preeclampsia**
Nitroprusside I.V. at a rate of 0.25 to 10 mcg/kg/minute (drug of choice)	Nitroglycerin I.V. at a rate of 20 to 200 mcg/minute (drug of choice)	Hydralazine 5 to 10 mg I.V. q 20 minutes, to a maximum dosage of 20 mg (drug of choice)
or Fenoldopam I.V. at a rate of 0.05 to 1.6 mcg/kg/minute	**or** Nicardipine I.V. at a rate of 5 to 15 mg/hour	**or** Labetalol 20 mg I.V., followed by 40 mg I.V. 10 minutes later; then 80-mg doses at 10-minute intervals for 2 additional doses, to a maximum cumulative dosage of 220 mg
or Labetalol 20 mg I.V. initially; repeat injection q 10 minutes p.r.n., to maximum dosage of 300 mg	**or** Enalaprilat 1.25 to 5 mg I.V. q 6 hours	

Begin oral antihypertensives when blood pressure decreases to a satisfactory level.

Hyperglycemic crisis: Treatment guidelines

SAFETY GUIDELINES

If you suspect your patient has hyperglycemic crisis (also called diabetic ketoacidosis or DKA), complete the initial evaluation. DKA is present if the blood glucose level exceeds 250 mg/dl, arterial pH is below 7.3, bicarbonate level is below 15 mEq/L, and moderate ketonuria is present.

Give I.V. fluid.	Give insulin.
Give NSS I.V. at 15 to 20 ml/kg/hour.	Give regular insulin 0.15 units/kg as I.V. bolus.
When glucose level reaches 250 mg/dl, change to D₅ ½NSS at 150 to 250 ml/hour.	Start infusion of regular insulin at 0.1 unit/kg/hour. If glucose level doesn't fall by 50 to 70 mg/dl in first hour, double the infusion rate q hour until level falls by 50 to 70 mg/dl.

Monitor serum K+ level.	Assess need for NaHCO₃₋
K^+ < 3.3 mEq/L: Withhold insulin and give KCL or KPO₄ until level rises to 3.3 mEq/L or higher.	pH < 6.9: Dilute 100 mmol NaHCO₃₋ in 400 ml SWI; infuse at 200 ml/hour. Repeat dose until pH exceeds 7.0.
K^+ ≥ 5 mEq/L: Monitor K^+ level q 2 hours.	pH 6.9 to 7.0: Dilute 50 mmol NaHCO₃₋ in 200 ml SWI; infuse at 200 ml/hour. Repeat NaHCO₃₋ dose until pH exceeds 7.0.
K^+ ≥ 3.3 mEq/L but < 5 mEq/L: Give 20 to 30 mEq KCL in each liter of I.V. fluid to maintain K^+ at 4 to 5 mEq/L.	pH > 7.0: Don't give NaHCO₃₋.

Check electrolyte, BUN, creatinine, and glucose levels q 2 to 4 hours until stable. After DKA resolves, continue insulin infusion if patient is NPO status. When oral intake is tolerated, start S.C. insulin regimen. Continue I.V. infusion for 1 to 2 hours after S.C. insulin therapy begins.

KEY   BUN: blood urea nitrogen
D₅ ½NSS: dextrose 5% in
half-normal saline solution
K^+: potassium

KCL: potassium chloride
KPO₄: potassium phosphate
NaHCO₃₋: sodium bicarbonate

NPO: nothing by mouth
NSS: normal saline solution
SWI: sterile water for injection

Insulin shock: Treatment guidelines

SAFETY
GUIDELINES

If your patient has signs or symptoms of hypoglycemia, immediately obtain a fingerstick blood glucose level. If the level is 60 mg/dl or lower, have a STAT venous blood glucose level drawn. Then, as appropriate, take the actions described below.

Mild hypoglycemia (fingerstick blood glucose 50 to 60 mg/dl):

Give 4 oz of orange or apple juice, 8 oz of skim milk, or 3 packets of sugar in small amount of water. (Don't give orange juice if serum potassium level is 5 mEq/ml or more or if patient's on dialysis.)

Recheck fingerstick blood glucose level in 15 minutes. If it's 80 mg/dl or lower, repeat treatment.

Observe patient closely for further signs and symptoms of hypoglycemia.

Recheck fingerstick blood glucose level in 1 hour.

Moderate hypoglycemia (fingerstick blood glucose 40 to 50 mg/dl):

Give 4 oz of orange or apple juice, 8 oz of skim milk, or 3 packets of sugar in small amount of water. (Do not give orange juice if serum potassium level is 5 mEq/ml or more or if patient's on dialysis.)

Observe patient closely for further signs and symptoms of hypoglycemia.

Recheck fingerstick blood glucose level in 15 minutes.

Give 1 vial dextrose 50% in water (25 g) I.V. over 15 minutes if patient can't take oral carbohydrate.

Severe hypoglycemia (fingerstick blood glucose 40 mg/dl or lower with unconscious or symptomatic patient, or conscious but argumentative patient):

Establish I.V. access; give dextrose 50% in water I.V. over 15 minutes.

Monitor fingerstick blood glucose level q 15 minutes until it's 80 mg/dl or higher.

Provide diabetic meal or carbohydrate and protein snack as soon as patient's stable and can eat.

Follow-up care

Stay with the patient if he has moderate or severe hypoglycemia. Monitor blood pressure, heart rate, respiratory rate, and fingerstick blood glucose level every 15 minutes until it reaches 80 mg/dl or higher. Assess level of consciousness and institute safety precautions, as appropriate.

Preventing and treating extravasation

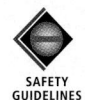

**SAFETY
GUIDELINES**

Extravasation—escape of a vesicant drug into surrounding tissues—can result
from a damaged vein or from leakage around a venipuncture site. Vesicant drugs
(such as daunorubicin and vincristine) can cause severe tissue damage if extravasation occurs.

To help prevent extravasation, make sure the existing I.V. line is patent before you
administer a drug by the I.V. route. Check patency by:
• inspecting the site for edema or pain
• flushing the I.V. line with 0.9% sodium chloride solution
• gently aspirating blood from the catheter.

   Alternatively, you may insert a new I.V. catheter to ensure correct catheter
placement. For vesicant drugs, consider using a central venous catheter.

If extravasation occurs, stop the infusion at once. Aspirate the remaining drug
from the catheter and remove the I.V. line (unless you need the catheter to administer an antidote). If the extravasated drug was daunorubicin or doxorubicin, apply a cold compress to the area; if it was vinblastine or vincristine, apply a warm
compress. Then instill the appropriate antidote according to facility policy.

Administering antidotes
Antidotes for extravasation typically are either given through the existing I.V. line
or injected S.C. around the infiltrated site using a 1-ml tuberculin syringe. Be sure
to use a new needle for each antidote injection.

Extravasated drug	Antidote and dosage
• aminophylline • calcium solutions • contrast media • dextrose solutions (concentrations of 10% or more) • etoposide • nafcillin • potassium solutions • teniposide • total parenteral nutrition solutions • vinblastine • vincristine • vindesine	**hyaluronidase:** 15 units/ml S.C., as 0.2 ml S.C. injection near extravasation site
• dactinomycin	**ascorbic acid injection:** 50 mg
• daunorubicin • doxorubicin	**hydrocortisone sodium succinate** 100 mg/ml: 50 to 200 mg
• dobutamine • dopamine • epinephrine • metaraminol • norepinephrine	**phentolamine:** 5 to 10 mg diluted in 10 to 15 ml of normal saline solution, administered within 12 hours of extravasation
• mechlorethamine	**sodium thiosulfate 10%:** 10 ml

riluzole
Rilutek

Pharmacologic class: Glutamate antagonist

Therapeutic class: Amyotrophic lateral sclerosis (ALS) agent

Pregnancy risk category C

Action
Unknown; thought to inhibit the accumulation of amino acids that build up on the motor neurons of the CNS, improving nerve impulse transmission

Availability
Tablets: 50 mg

Indications and dosages
➢ ALS
Adults: 50 mg P.O. q 12 hours

Off-label uses
- Cervical dystonia
- Huntington's disease

Contraindications
- Hypersensitivity to drug or its components

Administration
- Give at least 1 hour before or 2 hours after a meal to maximize absorption.

Route	Onset	Peak	Duration
P.O.	Unknown	Unknown	Unknown

Adverse reactions
CNS: headache, dizziness, drowsiness, asthenia, hypertonia, depression, insomnia, malaise, vertigo, circumoral paresthesia

CV: hypertension, orthostatic hypotension, tachycardia, phlebitis, palpitations, peripheral edema, **cardiac arrest**

EENT: rhinitis, sinusitis, tooth disorders, oral candidiasis

GI: nausea, vomiting, diarrhea, abdominal pain, dyspepsia, flatulence, stomatitis, dry mouth, anorexia

GU: urinary tract infection, dysuria

Hematologic: neutropenia

Hepatic: elevated alanine aminotransferase (ALT), aspartate aminotransferase (AST), bilirubin, and gamma-glutamyltransferase (GGT) levels

Musculoskeletal: back pain, joint pain

Respiratory: decreased lung function, increased cough, pneumonia

Skin: pruritus, eczema, alopecia, exfoliative dermatitis

Other: weight loss

Interactions
Drug-drug. *Allopurinol, methyldopa, sulfasalazine:* increased risk of hepatotoxicity

CYP450-1A2 inducers (such as omeprazole, rifampin): increased riluzole elimination

CYP450-1A2 inhibitors (such as amitriptyline, phenacetin, quinolones, theophylline): decreased riluzole elimination

Drug-diagnostic tests. *ALT, AST, bilirubin, GGT:* increased levels

Drug-food. *High-fat foods:* decreased riluzole absorption

Drug-behaviors. *Alcohol use:* increased risk of hepatotoxicity

Precautions
Use cautiously in:
- hepatic or renal insufficiency, neutropenia, febrile illness
- elderly patients
- female patients and Japanese patients (who may have decreased metabolic capacity to eliminate drug)
- pregnant or breastfeeding patients
- children.

Patient monitoring
- Monitor liver function studies and complete blood count.
- Assess vital signs and cardiovascular status, particularly for hypertension,

r

orthostatic hypotension, and peripheral edema.
• Closely monitor respiratory status for decreased lung function or pneumonia.
• Monitor weight, nutritional status, and hydration.

Patient teaching
• Teach patient to take drug 1 hour before or 2 hours after a meal, at same time each day.
• Instruct patient to take his temperature regularly and report fever.
◀⁚ Teach patient to immediately report arm or leg swelling as well as difficulty breathing and other signs of decreased lung function.
• Advise patient to minimize GI upset by eating small, frequent servings of healthy food and drinking plenty of fluids.
• Teach patient to avoid high-fat foods and alcohol.
• Instruct patient to move slowly when sitting up or standing to avoid dizziness or light-headedness from sudden blood pressure decrease.
• As appropriate, review all other significant and life-threatening adverse reactions and interactions, especially those related to the drugs, tests, foods, and behaviors mentioned above.

rimantadine hydrochloride
Flumadine

Pharmacologic class: Miscellaneous and anticholinergic-like agent
Therapeutic class: Antiviral
Pregnancy risk category C

Action
Prevents nucleic acid uncoating in viral cells, preventing penetration in host; also causes dopamine release from neurons

Availability
Syrup: 50 mg/5 ml
Tablets: 100 mg

🕭 Indications and dosages
➤ Treatment of influenza type A
Adults: 100 mg P.O. b.i.d.
➤ Prophylaxis of influenza type A
Adults and children older than age 10: 100 mg P.O. b.i.d.
Children younger than age 10: 5 mg/kg P.O. daily; maximum dosage is 150 mg daily.
Dosage adjustment
• Renal or hepatic disease
• Seizure disorders
• Elderly patients

Off-label uses
• Parkinson's disease

Contraindications
• Hypersensitivity to drug or amantadine

Administration
• Give several hours before bedtime.
• Know that therapy should start within 48 hours of symptom onset and continue for at least 1 week.

Route	Onset	Peak	Duration
P.O.	Slow	6 hr	Unknown

Adverse reactions
CNS: headache, dizziness, fatigue, depression, insomnia, poor concentration, asthenia, nervousness
CV: hypotension
EENT: tinnitus
GI: nausea, vomiting, diarrhea, abdominal pain, dyspepsia, dry mouth, anorexia
Respiratory: dyspnea
Skin: rash

Interactions
Drug-drug. *Acetaminophen, aspirin:* decreased rimantadine peak blood level

---

risedronate sodium   943

Cimetidine: increased rimantadine blood level

Precautions

Use cautiously in:
• history of seizures or renal or hepatic disease
• pregnant or breastfeeding patients
• children under age 1.

Patient monitoring

• Assess patient's flu symptoms; notify prescriber if symptoms don't improve over 2 to 3 days.
• Monitor vital signs, and watch for hypotension.
• Closely monitor nutritional status and hydration.

Patient teaching

• Teach patient to take drug several hours before bedtime.
• If patient is taking syrup, tell him to use specially marked oral syringe or measuring device to obtain accurate dose.
• Advise patient to contact prescriber if symptoms don't improve within 2 to 3 days.
• Instruct patient to avoid driving and other hazardous activities until he knows how drug affects concentration, motor function, and alertness.
• As appropriate, review all other significant adverse reactions and interactions, especially those related to the drugs mentioned above.

risedronate sodium
Actonel

Pharmacologic class: Bisphosphonate
Therapeutic class: Calcium regulator
Pregnancy risk category C

Action

Inhibits osteoclast-mediated bone resorption; also exerts antiresorptive effect, probably by directly inhibiting mature osteoclast activity or indirectly inhibiting osteoblasts

Availability

Tablets: 5 mg, 30 mg, 35 mg

💊 Indications and dosages

➤ Treatment and prevention of postmenopausal or glucocorticoid-induced osteoporosis
Adults: 5 mg P.O. daily taken in an upright position with 6 to 8 oz of water at least 30 minutes before any other beverage or food (other than water). Alternatively for postmenopausal osteoporosis only, 35 mg P.O. weekly.
➤ Paget's disease
Adults: 30 mg P.O. daily for 2 months taken in an upright position with 6 to 8 oz of water at least 30 minutes before any other beverage or food (other than water). If indicated, may retreat with same dosage after post-treatment observation period of at least 2 months.

Off-label uses

• Hypercalcemia of malignancy
• Primary hyperparathyroidism

Contraindications

• Hypersensitivity to drug or other bisphosphonates
• Hypocalcemia
• Inability to stand or sit upright for at least 30 minutes

Administration

• Give drug with 6 to 8 oz of water 30 minutes before first food or drink of the day (other than water); make sure patient stays upright for at least 30 minutes after taking drug.
• Be aware that patients with poor dietary intake may need calcium and vitamin D supplements.

r

♣ Canada   ◀€ Clinical alert   Reactions in **bold** are life-threatening

• Give calcium, magnesium, or aluminum supplements or antacids at a different time of day so they don't interfere with risedronate absorption.

Route	Onset	Peak	Duration
P.O.	Rapid	1 hr	Unknown

Adverse reactions

CNS: headache, anxiety, depression, dizziness, vertigo, syncope, asthenia
CV: angina, chest pain, cardiovascular disorder, hypertension, vasodilation, peripheral edema
EENT: cataract, conjunctivitis, dry eyes, otitis media, rhinitis, sinusitis, pharyngitis
GI: nausea, vomiting, diarrhea, constipation, abdominal pain, dyspepsia, dry mouth, flatulence, gastroenteritis, colitis, esophageal irritation, anorexia
GU: urinary tract infection
Hematologic: anemia
Musculoskeletal: bone, back, or joint pain; bone fracture; bursitis; myalgia; arthritis; leg and muscle cramps
Respiratory: bronchitis, cough, pneumonia, crackles
Skin: rash, pruritus, ecchymosis, **skin cancer**
Other: accidental injury, infection, neck pain, flulike symptoms, allergic reactions, **neoplasm**

Interactions

Drug-drug. *Antacids, aspirin, calcium or magnesium supplements:* decreased risedronate absorption
Nonsteroidal anti-inflammatory drugs, salicylates: increased GI irritation
Drug-diagnostic tests. *Bone-imaging agents used in diagnostic tests:* interference with test agents
Calcium, phosphorus: decreased levels
Drug-food. *Any food:* decreased drug absorption

Precautions

Use cautiously in:
• renal disease, hypotension, upper GI

disorders, difficulty swallowing
• pregnant or breastfeeding patients.

Patient monitoring

• Monitor patient for difficulty swallowing and signs and symptoms of esophageal irritation.
• Assess skin for unusual findings that may indicate skin cancer.

Patient teaching

• Advise patient to read patient information insert before starting therapy.
◀€ Emphasize importance of taking drug with a full glass (6 to 8 oz) of water at least 30 minutes before first food or drink of day and staying upright for at least 30 minutes afterward.
• Caution patient that chewing or sucking tablet may cause mouth irritation.
◀€ Instruct patient to stop taking drug and notify prescriber if she experiences difficulty or pain on swallowing, midline chest pain, or severe, persistent heartburn.
• Teach patient to report signs and symptoms of colitis.
• If patient must take calcium, magnesium, or aluminum supplements or antacids, tell her to take them at least 2 hours after risedronate.
• Tell patient that drug may cause leg cramps and bone or joint pain; advise her to discuss these problems with prescriber.
• As appropriate, review all other significant and life-threatening adverse reactions and interactions, especially those related to the drugs, tests, and foods mentioned above.

---

risperidone
Risperdal

Pharmacologic class: Benzisoxazole derivative

Therapeutic class: Antipsychotic

Pregnancy risk category C

Action
Antagonizes receptors for serotonin$_2$ and dopamine$_2$; also binds to alpha$_1$- and alpha$_2$-adrenergic receptors and histamine H$_1$ receptors

Availability
Oral solution: 1 mg/ml in 30- and 100-ml bottles
Tablets: 0.25 mg, 0.5 mg, 1 mg, 2 mg, 3 mg, 4 mg
Tablets (orally disintegrating): 0.5 mg, 1 mg, 2 mg

Indications and dosages
➤ Schizophrenia
Adults: 1 mg P.O. b.i.d., increased by 1 mg b.i.d. as tolerated on days 2 and 3, up to a target dosage of 3 mg b.i.d. by day 3. Further increments or decrements of 1 mg b.i.d. may be made at weekly intervals; usual dosage range is 4 to 8 mg/day. Alternatively, may be given as a single daily dose after initial titration.

Dosage adjustment
• Hepatic or renal impairment
• Elderly or debilitated patients

Off-label uses
• Tourette syndrome

Contraindications
• Hypersensitivity to drug
• Breastfeeding

Administration
• Record baseline blood pressure before starting therapy.

Route	Onset	Peak	Duration
P.O.	1-2 wk	Unknown	Up to 6 wk

Adverse reactions
CNS: aggressive behavior, dizziness, drowsiness, extrapyramidal reactions, headache, increased dreams, longer sleep periods, insomnia, sedation, fatigue, nervousness, tardive dyskinesia, hyperkinesia, agitation, anxiety, akathisia, **transient ischemic attack (TIA), cerebrovascular accident (CVA), neuroleptic malignant syndrome**
CV: orthostatic hypotension, chest pain, tachycardia, **arrhythmias**
EENT: vision disturbances, rhinitis, sinusitis, pharyngitis, toothache
GI: nausea, vomiting, diarrhea, constipation, abdominal pain, dyspepsia, dry mouth, increased salivation, anorexia
GU: difficulty urinating, polyuria, galactorrhea, decreased libido, dysmenorrhea, menorrhagia
Musculoskeletal: joint or back pain
Respiratory: cough, dyspnea, upper respiratory tract infection
Skin: pruritus, diaphoresis, rash, dry skin, seborrhea, increased pigmentation, photosensitivity
Other: fever, weight changes, impaired temperature regulation

Interactions
Drug-drug. *Antihistamines, opioids, sedative-hypnotics:* additive CNS depression
Carbamazepine: increased metabolism and decreased efficacy of risperidone
Clozapine: decreased metabolism and increased effects of risperidone
Levodopa, other dopamine agonists: decreased antiparkinsonian effects of these drugs
Drug-behaviors. *Alcohol use:* increased CNS depression

r

Sun exposure: increased risk of photosensitivity

Precautions

Use cautiously in:
• renal or hepatic impairment, cardiovascular disease, prolonged QT interval, dysphagia, hyperprolactinemia, hypothermia or hyperthermia, Parkinson's disease, phenylketonuria, tardive dyskinesia, previous diagnosis of breast cancer or prolactin-dependent tumors
• history of seizures, drug abuse, or suicide attempt
• elderly or debilitated patients
• pregnant patients
• children (safety not established).

Patient monitoring

◀ɛ Closely monitor neurologic status, especially for evidence of neuroleptic malignant syndrome (such as high fever, sweating, unstable blood pressure, stupor, muscle rigidity, and autonomic dysfunction), extrapyramidal reactions, TIA, CVA, and tardive dyskinesia.
• Monitor blood pressure, particularly for orthostatic hypotension.
• Assess body temperature; watch for fever and other signs and symptoms of infection.

Patient teaching

• Instruct patient to remove orally disintegrating tablet from blister pack, place it on tongue immediately, and swallow it with or without liquid as tablet dissolves.
• Teach patient to mix oral solution with water, coffee, orange juice, or low-fat milk; tell him solution isn't compatible with cola or tea.
• Advise patient to establish an effective bedtime routine to minimize sleep disorders.
◀ɛ Teach patient to recognize and immediately report serious adverse reactions, including tardive dyskinesia and neuroleptic malignant syndrome.

• Instruct patient to move slowly when sitting up or standing to avoid dizziness or light-headedness from sudden blood pressure decrease.
• Inform patient that excessive fluid loss (as from sweating, vomiting, or diarrhea) and inadequate fluid intake increase the risk of light-headedness (especially in hot weather).
• Caution patient to avoid driving and other hazardous activities until he knows how drug affects concentration and alertness.
• Advise patient not to drink alcohol.
• As appropriate, review all other significant and life-threatening adverse reactions and interactions, especially those related to the drugs and behaviors mentioned above.

ritonavir
Norvir

Pharmacologic class: Protease inhibitor
Therapeutic class: Antiretroviral
Pregnancy risk category B

Action

Inhibits human immunodeficiency virus (HIV) nonnucleoside reverse transcriptase by binding directly to reverse transcriptase and blocking RNA-dependent and DNA-dependent polymerase activity.

Availability

Capsules: 100 mg
Oral solution: 80 mg/ml

🕖 Indications and dosages
➤ HIV (in combination with other antiretrovirals)
Adults: Initially, 300 mg P.O. b.i.d., increased by 100 mg b.i.d. q 2 to 3 days, up to a usual maintenance dosage of 600 mg b.i.d.

Children ages 2 and older: 400 mg/m² b.i.d, not to exceed 600 mg b.i.d. To minimize nausea, start with 250 mg/m².

Off-label uses
• Chronic hepatitis B

Contraindications
• Hypersensitivity to drug or its components
• Concurrent use of amiodarone, bepridil, cisapride, dihydroergotamine, ergotamine, flecainide, midazolam, pimozide, propafenone, quinidine, or triazolam

Administration
• Give drug with meals to increase its absorption.
• Mix oral solution with chocolate milk or liquid nutritional supplement to mask taste.

Route	Onset	Peak	Duration
P.O.	Rapid	2-4 hr	Unknown

Adverse reactions
CNS: headache, dizziness, depression, insomnia, drowsiness, asthenia, paresthesia, syncope, malaise
CV: vasodilation
EENT: pharyngitis
GI: nausea, vomiting, diarrhea, constipation, dyspepsia, flatulence, abnormal taste, abdominal pain, anorexia
Hematologic: increased alanine aminotransferase (ALT), aspartate aminotransferase (AST), cholesterol, creatine kinase (CK), gamma-glutamyltransferase (GTT), and triglyceride levels
Musculoskeletal: myalgia
Skin: diaphoresis
Other: fever, pain

Interactions
Drug-drug. *Amiodarone, bepridil, cisapride, flecainide, midazolam, pimozide, propafenone, quinidine, triazolam:* inhibited metabolism of these drugs, leading to life-threatening reactions (such as arrhythmias, prolonged sedation, and respiratory depression)
Amitriptyline, anticoagulants, atovaquone, carbamazepine, clozapine, cyclosporine, desipramine, diltiazem, disopyramide, divalproex, dofetilide, dronabinol, ethinyl estradiol, lamotrigine, phenytoin, sulfamethoxazole, theophylline, zidovudine: increased risk of toxicity of these drugs
Amprenavir: increased amprenavir blood level
Astemizole, cisapride, encainide: increased risk of arrhythmias
Atorvastatin, cerivastatin, lovastatin, simvastatin: increased blood levels of these drugs, increased risk of rhabdomyolysis
Barbiturates, nevirapine, phenytoin, rifamycins: decreased ritonavir blood level
Bupropion: increased risk of seizures
Clarithromycin, efavirenz: increased blood levels of both drugs
Dihydroergotamine, ergotamine: ergot toxicity
Fluconazole: increased ritonavir blood level
Drug-diagnostic tests. *ALT, AST, cholesterol, CK, GGT, triglycerides, uric acid:* increased levels
Hematocrit, hemoglobin, neutrophils, red blood cells, white blood cells: decreased levels
Drug-herb. *St. John's wort:* decreased ritonavir blood level

Precautions
Use cautiously in:
• hepatic disease, diabetes mellitus, hemophilia types A and B
• pregnant or breastfeeding patients.

Patient monitoring
• Monitor complete blood count, liver function test results, electrolyte levels, and lipid panel.
• Assess neurologic status closely; stay alert for depression.

r

• Monitor vital signs and watch for syncope.
• Closely monitor nutritional and hydration status.

Patient teaching
• Teach patient to take drug with meals to increase its absorption.
• Encourage patient to mix oral solution with chocolate milk or liquid nutritional supplement to mask taste.
• Tell patient that drug may cause numbness, tingling, weakness, and other CNS effects that increase his risk of injury. Encourage him to use appropriate safety precautions.
• Instruct patient to report depression.
• As appropriate, review all other significant adverse reactions and interactions, especially those related to the drugs, tests, and herbs mentioned above.

rituximab
Rituxan

Pharmacologic class: Murine/human monoclonal antibody
Therapeutic class: Antineoplastic
Pregnancy risk category C

Action
Binds to CD20 antigen on malignant B lymphocytes and recruits immune effector functions to mediate B-cell lysis (possibly through complement-dependent cytotoxicity and antibody-dependent cell-mediated cytotoxicity)

Availability
Injection: 10 mg/ml in 10-ml (100-mg) and 50-ml (500-mg) vials

🕊 Indications and dosages
➤ Relapsed or refractory low-grade or follicular CD20-positive B-cell non-Hodgkin's lymphoma
Adults: 375 mg/m² by I.V. infusion once weekly for four or eight doses at 50 mg/hour; increase rate by 50 mg/hour q 30 minutes to a maximum of 400 mg/hour. Subsequent infusions may be started at 100 mg/hour, then increased by 100 mg/hour q 30 minutes to a maximum of 400 mg/hour as tolerated.

Off-label uses
• Waldenström's macroglobulinemia

Contraindications
• Hypersensitivity to drug, its components, or murine products

Administration
• Premedicate patient with diphenhydramine and acetaminophen, as prescribed.
• Give drug as I.V. infusion.
◀€ Never give as I.V. bolus or I.V. push.
• Dilute drug in dextrose 5% in water (D₅W) or normal saline solution to a concentration of 1 to 4 mg/ml.
• Invert bag gently to mix solution; infuse at prescribed rate.
• If hypersensitivity (non-IgE-mediated) reaction or infusion reaction occurs, interrupt or temporarily slow infusion; when symptoms improve, infusion can continue at half of previous rate.

Route	Onset	Peak	Duration
I.V.	Variable	Variable	6-12 mo

Adverse reactions
CNS: dizziness, headache, nervousness, hypertonia, hyperesthesia, insomnia, agitation, malaise, paresthesia, asthenia, fatigue, tremor, rigors
CV: hypotension, hypertension, peripheral edema, chest pain, tachycardia, bradycardia, angina, **arrhythmias**

EENT: conjunctivitis, lacrimation disorders, rhinitis, sinusitis, pharyngitis, altered taste

GI: nausea, vomiting, diarrhea, constipation, abdominal pain, dyspepsia, anorexia

GU: renal toxicity

Hematologic: anemia, **neutropenia, leukopenia, thrombocytopenia**

Metabolic: hyperglycemia, hypocalcemia

Musculoskeletal: myalgia, back pain

Respiratory: dyspnea, cough, bronchitis, **bronchospasm**

Skin: pruritus, rash, urticaria, flushing, dermatitis, angioedema, toxic epidermal necrolysis

Other: fever, chills, pain at injection site, hypersensitivity reactions including **Stevens-Johnson syndrome, sepsis**

Interactions

Drug-drug. *Cisplatin:* increased risk of renal failure

Live-virus vaccines: increased risk of infection from vaccine

Drug-diagnostic tests. *Calcium, hemoglobin, neutrophils, platelets, white blood cells:* decreased values

Glucose, lactate dehydrogenase: increased levels

Precautions

Use cautiously in:
• history of drug allergy or sensitivity
• prior exposure to murine-based monoclonal antibodies
• high level of circulating malignant cells
• cardiac or pulmonary conditions
• pregnant or breastfeeding patients
• children.

Patient monitoring

• Monitor closely for signs and symptoms of hypersensitivity reaction.

◀€ Stop drug and notify prescriber if patient develops signs or symptoms of Stevens-Johnson syndrome or other severe mucocutaneous reactions (including severe rash).

◀€ Monitor pulse and blood pressure throughout I.V. infusion; stop infusion if hypotension, bronchospasm, or angioedema occurs. Then consult prescriber about restarting infusion at half of previous rate.

◀€ Monitor ECG throughout infusion; stop infusion if serious arrhythmia develops.

• Monitor complete blood count as well as blood glucose and electrolyte levels.

• Assess for signs and symptoms of infection, including fever.

Patient teaching

◀€ Teach patient to immediately report signs and symptoms of hypersensitivity reaction or severe skin reactions.

◀€ Instruct patient to take his temperature every day and immediately report fever and other signs or symptoms of infection.

• Teach patient to minimize GI upset by eating small, frequent servings of healthy food and drinking plenty of fluids.

• Instruct patient to report unusual bleeding or bruising.

• As appropriate, review all other significant and life-threatening adverse reactions and interactions, especially those related to the drugs and tests mentioned above.

rivastigmine tartrate
Exelon

Pharmacologic class: Cholinesterase inhibitor

Therapeutic class: Anti-Alzheimer's drug

Pregnancy risk category B

Action
Unknown; thought to enhance cholinergic function by increasing acetylcholine concentration through reversible inhibition of its hydrolysis by cholinesterase

Availability
Capsules: 1.5 mg, 3 mg, 4.5 mg, 6 mg
Oral solution: 2 mg/ml

🚺 Indications and dosages
➣ Mild to moderate dementia of Alzheimer's disease
Adults: Initially, 1.5 mg P.O. b.i.d. with food. If tolerated, may increase to 3 mg b.i.d. after 2 weeks; may increase further to 4.5 mg b.i.d. and 6 mg b.i.d. if tolerated, after 2 weeks at previous dosage. Effective dosage range is 6 to 12 mg/day, up to a maximum of 12 mg/day.

Off-label uses
• Huntington's disease
• Parkinson's disease

Contraindications
• Hypersensitivity to drug, its components, or carbamate derivatives

Administration
• Give drug with food in morning and evening.

Route	Onset	Peak	Duration
P.O.	Unknown	1 hr	12 hr

Adverse reactions
CNS: depression, dizziness, headache, confusion, insomnia, psychosis, hallucinations, anxiety, tremor, drowsiness, fatigue, syncope, asthenia
CV: chest pain, hypertension, peripheral edema
EENT: rhinitis, pharyngitis
GI: nausea, vomiting, diarrhea, constipation, abdominal pain, flatulence, eructation, dyspepsia, anorexia
GU: urinary tract infection, urinary incontinence
Musculoskeletal: back pain, joint pain, bone fractures
Respiratory: upper respiratory tract infection, cough, bronchitis
Skin: rash, diaphoresis
Other: weight loss, pain, flulike symptoms

Interactions
Drug-drug. *Anticholinergics:* interference with anticholinergic effects
Cholinergic agonists (such as bethanechol), succinylcholine and similar neuromuscular blockers: synergistic effects
Drug-herb. *S-adenosylmethionine (SAM-e), St. John's wort:* increased risk of serotonin syndrome
Drug-behaviors. *Nicotine use:* increased drug clearance

Precautions
Use cautiously in:
• renal or hepatic impairment, diabetes mellitus, obstructive pulmonary disease, neurologic conditions that can cause seizures, peptic ulcers, GI bleeding, supraventricular conduction disorders
• patients older than age 85
• pregnant patients.

Patient monitoring
• Monitor patient's nutritional and hydration status, especially at start of therapy.
• Assess vital signs and cardiovascular status; stay alert for chest pain and peripheral edema.
• Closely monitor cognitive status, particularly memory; report significant decline or improvement.
• Assess temperature; watch for fever and other signs and symptoms of infections.

Patient teaching
• Instruct caregiver to give drug with food in morning and evening.

• Inform caregiver that drug initially may worsen CNS impairment; recommend appropriate safety measures.

• Teach caregiver that memory improvement generally is subtle and that drug usually works by preventing further memory loss.

• Inform caregiver that drug commonly causes nausea, vomiting, decreased appetite, and weight loss, especially at start of therapy.

• Advise caregiver to watch for and report weight loss, dehydration, and signs and symptoms of GI bleeding.

• Tell caregiver that drug interacts with many over-the-counter products and nicotine. Advise him to discuss such products with prescriber before giving to patient.

• As appropriate, review all other significant adverse reactions and interactions, especially those related to the drugs, herbs, and behaviors mentioned above.

rizatriptan benzoate
Maxalt, Maxalt-MLT

Pharmacologic class: Serotonin 5-hydroxytryptamine (5-HT$_1$) receptor agonist
Therapeutic class: Antimigraine drug
Pregnancy risk category C

Action
Thought to act as an agonist at specific 5-HT$_1$ receptor sites in intracranial blood vessels, causing vasoconstriction; may also act on sensory trigeminal nerves, reducing transmission along pain pathways

Availability
Tablets: 5 mg, 10 mg
Tablets (orally disintegrating): 5 mg, 10 mg

Indications and dosages
➤ Acute migraine with or without aura

Adults: 5 to 10 mg P.O.; may repeat in 2 hours, not to exceed three doses in 24 hours. For patients receiving propranolol concurrently, 5 mg P.O., up to a maximum of three doses in 24 hours.

Contraindications
• Hypersensitivity to drug or its components
• Ischemic heart disease or other significant cardiovascular disease
• Ischemic bowel disease
• Transient ischemic attacks
• Basilar or hemiplegic migraine
• Uncontrolled hypertension
• Use of other 5-HT$_1$ agonists or ergot-type compounds (dihydroergotamine, methysergide) within 24 hours
• Monoamine oxidase (MAO) inhibitor use within 14 days

Administration
• Place orally disintegrating tablet on patient's tongue to dissolve; encourage him to swallow it with saliva only.
• Don't give with beverages.

Route	Onset	Peak	Duration
P.O.	30 min	1-1.5 hr	Unknown

Adverse reactions
CNS: headache, dizziness, drowsiness, asthenia, fatigue, paresthesia, decreased mental acuity, euphoria, tremor
CV: chest pain, tightness, heaviness, or pressure
GI: nausea, vomiting, diarrhea, dry mouth
Respiratory: dyspnea
Skin: flushing
Other: neck, throat, or jaw pain, tightness, or pressure; hot flashes; warm or cold sensations

Interactions
Drug-drug. *Ergot or ergot-type compounds (such as dihydroergotamine,*

r

methysergide), other 5-HT₁ agonists:
additive vasoactive effects
MAO inhibitors, propranolol: increased
rizatriptan blood level, greater risk of
adverse effects
Selective serotonin reuptake inhibitors:
weakness, hyperreflexia, incoordination
tion
Drug-herb. *S-adenosylmethionine
(SAM-e), St. John's wort:* increased risk
of adverse serotonergic effects, including serotonin syndrome

Precautions
Use cautiously in:
• severe renal impairment (especially
in dialysis patients), moderate hepatic
impairment, cardiovascular risk factors
• phenylketonuria (PKU) in patients
receiving orally disintegrating tablets
• pregnant or breastfeeding patients
• children under age 18 (safety not established).

Patient monitoring
• Monitor patient's response to drug;
assess need for repeat doses.
• Assess vital signs and cardiovascular
status, especially in patients with cardiovascular risk factors.

Patient teaching
• Teach patient how to use drug; emphasize that it's effective only in treating diagnosed migraine—not in preventing migraine or treating other
types of headache.
• Advise patient to peel back blister
pack of Maxalt-MLT with dry hands
and place tablet on tongue. Tell him to
swallow drug with saliva only, not beverages.
• Tell patient he may repeat dose in 2
hours if headache recurs but should
take no more than 30 mg in 24 hours.
• Inform patients with PKU that orally
disintegrating tablets contain phenylalanine.
• Instruct female patients to immediately report possible pregnancy.

• As appropriate, review all other significant adverse reactions and interactions, especially those related to the
drugs and herbs mentioned above.

rocuronium bromide
Zemuron

Pharmacologic class: Nondepolarizing
neuromuscular blocker
Therapeutic class: Muscle relaxant,
adjunct to anesthesia
Pregnancy risk category B

Action
Competes for cholinergic receptors at
motor end-plate, interrupting nerve
impulse transmission, thereby causing
muscle relaxation

Availability
Injection: 10 mg/ml

🖋 Indications and dosages
➤ Adjunct to general anesthesia to allow endotracheal intubation and relax
skeletal muscles during mechanical
ventilation or surgery
Adults: Initial I.V. bolus of 0.6 mg/kg
usually allows endotracheal intubation
within 2 minutes and paralyzes muscles for 30 minutes. Start continuous
infusion at 0.01 to 0.012 mg/kg/minute
only after early evidence of recovery
from intubating dose.
Dosage adjustment
• Elderly patients

Contraindications
• Hypersensitivity to drug

Administration
◀€ Have emergency resuscitation
equipment available when giving drug.
• Ensure that patient has received a
sedative or general anesthetic before
starting drug.

• Give by rapid I.V. injection or continuous I.V. infusion in compatible solution (dextrose 5% in water, normal saline solution, dextrose 5% in normal saline solution, sterile water for injection, or lactated Ringer's solution).
• Know that an extra 12 minutes of muscle relaxation is produced by a maintenance dose of 0.1 mg/kg; an extra 17 minutes, by dose of 0.15 mg/kg; and an extra 24 minutes, by a dose of 0.2 mg/kg.

Route	Onset	Peak	Duration
I.V.	1 min	2 min	22-67 min

Adverse reactions

CV: transient hypotension or hypertension
Musculoskeletal: prolonged skeletal muscle relaxation

Interactions

Drug-drug. *Aminoglycosides (amikacin, gentamicin, kanamycin, neomycin, streptomycin), beta-adrenergic blockers, clindamycin, general anesthetics, lincomycin, lithium, magnesium sulfate, opioid analgesics, polymyxin antibiotics, quinidine, quinine:* enhanced neuromuscular blockade, causing increased skeletal muscle relaxation
Anticonvulsants (such as carbamazepine, phenytoin): shortened duration of neuromuscular blockade
Enflurane, isoflurane: prolonged rocuronium duration of action
Succinylcholine: increased intensity and duration of neuromuscular blockade

Precautions

Use cautiously in:
• cardiac disease, electrolyte imbalances, dehydration, neuromuscular disease (such as myasthenia gravis, Eaton-Lambert syndrome), respiratory or metabolic acidosis, significant hepatic disease
• pregnant or breastfeeding patients.

Patient monitoring

• Assess respiratory status frequently.
• Monitor vital signs and ECG continuously until patient recovers fully from neuromuscular blockade. Closely monitor recovery with nerve stimulator and train-of-four monitoring.

Patient teaching

• Unless patient is under general anesthesia, provide ongoing explanation of all procedures.
• Assure patient that he'll be monitored closely.

rofecoxib
Vioxx

Pharmacologic class: Nonsteroidal anti-inflammatory drug (NSAID), selective cyclooxygenase-2 (COX-2) inhibitor

Therapeutic class: Anti-inflammatory, nonopioid analgesic

Pregnancy risk category C, D (third trimester)

Action

Inhibits COX-2, an enzyme required for prostaglandin synthesis

Availability

Oral suspension: 12.5 mg/5 ml, 25 mg/5 ml
Tablets: 12.5 mg, 25 mg, 50 mg

Indications and dosages

➤ Osteoarthritis
Adults: Initially; 12.5 mg P.O. daily; may be increased to 25 mg daily if needed
➤ Rheumatoid arthritis
Adults: 25 mg P.O. daily
➤ Acute pain and primary dysmenorrhea
Adults: 50 mg P.O. daily for up to 5 days

r

Contraindications

• Hypersensitivity to drug or its components
• History of asthma, urticaria, or allergic reactions to aspirin or other NSAIDs
• Advanced renal disease
• Moderate or severe hepatic impairment
• Third trimester of pregnancy

Administration

• Give with or without food.

Route	Onset	Peak	Duration
P.O.	Within 45 min	2-3 hr	≥6 hr

Adverse reactions

CNS: fatigue, dizziness, headache, asthenia
CV: hypertension, lower extremity edema, angina pectoris, **myocardial infarction**
EENT: sinusitis
GI: nausea, diarrhea, dyspepsia, heartburn, epigastric or abdominal pain, **GI bleeding**
GU: urinary tract infection
Hematologic: anemia
Musculoskeletal: back pain
Respiratory: bronchitis, upper respiratory tract infection
Other: flulike symptoms

Interactions

Drug-drug. *Anticoagulants:* increased risk of bleeding
Aspirin, other NSAIDs: increased risk of GI bleeding
Diuretics, other antihypertensives: decreased efficacy of these drugs
Lithium, theophylline: increased blood levels of these drugs
Methotrexate: increased methotrexate blood level, greater risk of toxicity
Rifampin: decreased rofecoxib blood level
Drug-behaviors. *Chronic alcohol use:* increased risk of GI bleeding

Precautions

Use cautiously in:
• dehydration, asthma, anemia, hypertension, heart failure
• history of GI ulcer disease, bleeding, or perforation; hepatic or renal dysfunction; or coagulation defects
• elderly or debilitated patients
• breastfeeding patients
• children under age 18 (safety not established).

Patient monitoring

• Monitor closely for signs and symptoms of GI bleeding.
• Assess complete blood count; monitor patient for signs and symptoms of anemia.

Patient teaching

• Teach patient to take drug with food to reduce GI upset.
• Tell patient not to take drug with aspirin or other NSAIDs unless prescriber approves.
◀︎ Instruct patient to report GI bleeding immediately.
• Advise patient to avoid alcohol.
• Caution patient not to take drug during late pregnancy.
• As appropriate, review all other significant and life-threatening adverse reactions and interactions, especially those related to the drugs and behaviors mentioned above.

ropinirole hydrochloride
Requip

Pharmacologic class: Dopamine agonist
Therapeutic class: Antidyskinetic
Pregnancy risk category C

Action
Unknown; thought to stimulate dopamine receptors in brain

Availability
Tablets: 0.25 mg, 0.5 mg, 1 mg, 2 mg, 5 mg

⟋ Indications and dosages
➤ Idiopathic Parkinson's disease
Adults: Initially, 0.25 mg P.O. t.i.d. for 1 week, followed by 0.5 mg P.O. t.i.d. for 1 week, then 0.75 mg t.i.d. for 1 week, and then 1 mg t.i.d. for 1 week. After week 4, may increase by 1.5 mg/day q week, up to 9 mg/day; then may increase further by up to 3 mg/day q week, up to 24 mg/day.

Off-label uses
• Restless leg syndrome

Contraindications
• Hypersensitivity to drug or its components
• Breastfeeding

Administration
• Give drug with food if it causes nausea.

Route	Onset	Peak	Duration
P.O.	30-60 min	1-2 hr	16 hr

Adverse reactions
CNS: headache, dizziness, confusion, drowsiness, fatigue, increased dyskinesia, hyperkinesia, neuralgia, amnesia, hyperesthesia, yawning, dystonia, akathisia, hallucinations, abnormal thinking, poor concentration, syncope, vertigo, myoclonus, asthenia, malaise, sleep attacks
CV: orthostatic hypotension, hypertension, palpitations, extrasystole, peripheral edema, peripheral ischemia, chest pain, tachycardia, **atrial fibrillation**
EENT: abnormal vision, rhinitis, sinusitis, pharyngitis

GI: nausea, vomiting, flatulence, abdominal pain, dyspepsia, dry mouth, anorexia
GU: urinary tract infection, decreased libido, impotence
Hepatic: increased alkaline phosphatase (ALP) level
Metabolic: increased blood urea nitrogen (BUN)
Respiratory: bronchitis, dyspnea
Skin: diaphoresis, flushing
Other: viral infection, pain, edema

Interactions
Drug-drug. *Butyrophenones (such as haloperidol), metoclopramide, phenothiazines, thioxanthenes:* decreased ropinirole effects
Ciprofloxacin, estrogens: increased ropinirole effects
Drugs that alter activity of CYP450-1A2 enzyme system: altered ropinirole clearance
Levodopa: increased levodopa effects
Drug-diagnostic tests. *ALP, BUN:* increased levels
Drug-herb. *Kava:* decreased ropinirole efficacy

Precautions
Use cautiously in:
• severe hepatic impairment or cardiovascular disease, bradycardia
• elderly patients
• pregnant patients.

Patient monitoring
• Monitor vital signs, especially for orthostatic hypotension. Also assess for peripheral edema.
• Assess neurologic status carefully; report severe adverse reactions.
• Monitor nutritional and hydration status.

Patient teaching
• Encourage patient to take drug with food if it causes nausea.
• Inform patient (and caregiver, as appropriate) that drug can cause serious

r

CNS reactions and tell him which ones to report; recommend appropriate home safety measures.

• Instruct patient to move slowly when sitting up or standing to avoid dizziness or light-headedness from sudden blood pressure decrease.

• Advise patient to report swelling of hands or feet.

• Instruct patient to avoid driving and other hazardous activities until he knows how drug affects concentration, vision, and alertness.

• As appropriate, review all other significant and life-threatening adverse reactions and interactions, especially those related to the drugs, tests, and herbs mentioned above.

ropivacaine hydrochloride
Naropin

Pharmacologic class: Amino amide
Therapeutic class: Local anesthetic
Pregnancy risk category B

Action
Blocks generation and conduction of nerve impulses, presumably by increasing nerve's threshold for electrical excitation, slowing nerve impulse propagation, and decreasing rate of rise of action potential

Availability
Injection: 0.2% (2 mg/ml), 0.5% (5 mg/ml), 0.75% (7.5 mg/ml), 1% (10 mg/ml)

Indications and dosages
➤ Lumbar epidural block
Adults: 15 to 30 ml (75 to 150 mg) I.V. of 0.5% solution, or 15 to 25 ml (113 to 188 mg) I.V. of 0.75% solution
➤ Lumbar epidural block during labor
Adults: 10 to 20 ml (20 to 40 mg) of

0.2% solution, then 6 to 14 ml/hour (12 to 28 mg/hour) as a continuous I.V. infusion; or 10- to 15 ml/hour (20 to 30 mg/hour) of 0.2% solution as an incremental "top-up" injection
➤ Lumbar epidural block for cesarean section
Adults: 20 to 30 ml (100 to 150 mg) I.V. of 0.5% solution, or 15 to 20 ml (113 to 150 mg) of 0.75% solution
➤ Thoracic epidural block for postoperative pain relief
Adults: 5 to 15 ml (25 to 75 mg) I.V. of 0.5% solution
➤ Major nerve block (brachial plexus)
Adults: 35 to 50 ml (175 to 250 mg) I.V. of 0.5% solution

Off-label uses
• Ocular surgery

Contraindications
• Hypersensitivity to drug or other amide-type local anesthetics (such as bupivacaine, lidocaine, mepivacaine)
• Complete heart block
• Septicemia
• Severe hypotension

Administration
• Be aware that test dose (containing epinephrine) should be given.
• Use small, incremental doses for titration; avoid rapid I.V. infusion.

Route	Onset	Peak	Duration
I.V.	5-20 min	Unknown	2-8 hr

Adverse reactions
CNS: anxiety, restlessness, drowsiness, disorientation, tremor, shivering, paresthesia, rigors, **seizures, loss of consciousness**
CV: bradycardia, hypotension, hypertension, **myocardial depression, cardiac arrest, arrhythmias, fetal or neonatal bradycardia**
EENT: blurred vision, miosis, tinnitus
GI: nausea, vomiting
GU: oliguria, urinary retention

Hematologic: anemia
Musculoskeletal: back pain
Respiratory: status asthmaticus, respiratory arrest
Skin: pruritus, rash, urticaria, burning sensation, skin discoloration, tissue necrosis
Other: edema, fever, chills, allergic reactions including **anaphylaxis**

Interactions

Drug-drug. *Chloroprocaine:* decreased action of both drugs
CNS depressants: additive CNS depression
Enflurane, epinephrine, halothane: arrhythmias
Fluvoxamine, imipramine, theophylline, verapamil: competitive inhibition of ropivacaine
Monoamine oxidase inhibitors, phenothiazines, tricyclic antidepressants: hypertension
Other amide-type local anesthetics: prolonged ropivacaine effects
Drug-herb. *St. John's wort:* increased hypotension

Precautions

Use cautiously in:
• inflammation or sepsis in region where drug will be injected
• severe hepatic disease, hypotension, hypovolemia, impaired cardiovascular function, heart block
• elderly or acutely ill patients
• breastfeeding patients
• children.

Patient monitoring

• Monitor vital signs, ECG, and cardiovascular status continuously.
• Assess neurologic status; stay alert for signs and symptoms of impending seizures.
◀£ Watch carefully for warning signs of allergic reaction and respiratory distress.

Patient teaching

• Explain all procedures to patient to help reduce anxiety.
• Reassure patient that she'll be closely monitored.

rosiglitazone maleate
Avandia

Pharmacologic class: Thiazolidinedione
Therapeutic class: Hypoglycemic
Pregnancy risk category C

Action

Inhibits alpha-glucosidases, enzymes that convert oligosaccharides and disaccharides to glucose; inhibition of these enzymes lowers blood glucose level, especially in postprandial hyperglycemia

Availability

Tablets: 2 mg, 4 mg, 8 mg

🖉 Indications and dosages

➤ Adjunct to diet and exercise in management of type 2 diabetes mellitus (used alone); or given with metformin when combination of diet, exercise, and metformin or sulfonylurea therapy doesn't produce glycemic control
Adults: 4 mg P.O. once daily or 2 mg b.i.d.; after 12 weeks, may increase if necessary to 8 mg once daily or 4 mg b.i.d.

Off-label uses

• Polycystic ovary syndrome

Contraindications

• Hypersensitivity to drug or its components
• Diabetic ketoacidosis or type 1 diabetes mellitus

r

- Concurrent insulin therapy
- Breastfeeding
- Children younger than age 18

Administration

- Give drug with or without food.

Route	Onset	Peak	Duration
P.O.	Unknown	Unknown	12-24 hr

Adverse reactions

CNS: fatigue, headache
EENT: sinusitis
GI: diarrhea
Hematologic: anemia
Metabolic: increased total cholesterol, low-density lipoprotein (LDL), and high-density lipoprotein (HDL) levels; hyperglycemia; hypoglycemia
Musculoskeletal: back pain
Respiratory: upper respiratory tract infection
Other: edema, injury, weight gain

Interactions

Drug-diagnostic tests. *Free fatty acids, HDL, LDL, total cholesterol:* increased levels
Hematocrit, hemoglobin: decreased levels
Drug-herb. *Aloe, bitter melon, chromium, coenzyme Q10, fenugreek, glucomannan, gymnema sylvestre, psyllium, St. John's wort:* additive hypoglycemic effects
Glucosamine: poor glycemic control

Precautions

Use cautiously in:
- edema, heart failure, jaundice, hepatic impairment, hypertension
- patients with New York Heart Association Class III or IV cardiac status
- females of childbearing age.

Patient monitoring

- Monitor complete blood count, lipid panel, blood glucose, and glycosylated hemoglobin levels.

- Monitor patient's weight. Assess for fluid retention, which may lead to heart failure.
- Closely monitor liver function test results; drug is structurally related to troglitazone, which may cause hepatotoxicity.

Patient teaching

- Tell patient he may take drug with or without food.
- Advise patient to monitor blood glucose level regularly and report significant changes.
◀€ Inform patient that drug may increase fluid retention, causing or exacerbating heart failure. Encourage him to weigh himself regularly and report sudden weight gain, swelling, or shortness of breath.
- Tell patient that he'll undergo regular blood testing during therapy.
- As appropriate, review all other significant adverse reactions and interactions, especially those related to the tests and herbs mentioned above.

rosuvastatin calcium
Crestor

Pharmacologic class: HMG-CoA reductase inhibitor
Therapeutic class: Antilipemic
Pregnancy risk category X

Action

Selective and competitive inhibitor of HMG-CoA reductase, an enzyme that converts 3-hydroxy-3-methyl glutaryl coenzyme A to mevalonate, a cholesterol precursor. Increases number of hepatic low-density lipoprotein (LDL) receptors on cell surface, enhancing LDL uptake and catabolism; also inhibits hepatic synthesis of very-low-density lipoproteins (VLDLs), reducing total number of LDL and VLDL particles

Availability
Tablets: 5 mg, 10 mg, 20 mg, 40 mg

Indications and dosages
➤ Primary heterozygous hypercholesterolemia, mixed dyslipidemia (Fredrickson types IIa and IIb)
Adults: 10 mg/day P.O. For patients who require less aggressive cholesterol reduction or have predisposing factors for myopathy, initial dosage of 5 mg/day may be considered. Maintenance dosage ranges from 5 to 40 mg/day.
➤ Homozygous familial hypercholesterolemia
Adults: 20 mg/day P.O.; maximum recommended dosage is 40 mg/day.
➤ Hypertriglyceridemia
Adults: Usual recommended initial dosage is 10 mg/day P.O. Maintenance dosage ranges from 5 to 40 mg/day.

Off-label uses
• Acute coronary syndrome

Contraindications
• Hypersensitivity to drug
• Active hepatic disease or unexplained, persistent hepatic enzyme elevations
• Pregnancy or breastfeeding

Administration
• Give with or without food.
• Lipid levels should be measured within 2 to 4 weeks after therapy starts and after titration.
• Drug should be given as an adjunct to other lipid-lowering treatments such as diet.

Route	Onset	Peak	Duration
P.O.	Unknown	3-5 hr	Unknown

Adverse reactions
CNS: headache, dizziness, depression, insomnia, hypertonia, paresthesia, asthenia, tremor, anxiety, vertigo, neuralgia
CV: palpitations, tachycardia, chest pain, angina pectoris, hypertension, vasodilation, peripheral edema
EENT: rhinitis, sinusitis, periodontal abscess, pharyngitis
GI: nausea, vomiting, diarrhea, constipation, abdominal pain, dyspepsia, gastritis, gastroenteritis, flatulence
GU: urinary tract infection
Hematologic: anemia
Hepatic: elevated hepatic enzyme levels
Metabolic: hyperglycemia, hypoglycemia, hypokalemia
Musculoskeletal: myalgia; myopathy; arthritis; pathologic fractures; back, pelvic, neck, or joint pain
Respiratory: respiratory tract infection, bronchitis, increased cough, dyspnea, pneumonia, asthma
Skin: rash, pruritus, bruising
Other: flulike symptoms, infection

Interactions
Drug-drug. *Antacids:* decreased rosuvastatin blood level
Cyclosporine, gemfibrozil: increased rosuvastatin bioavailability
Hormonal contraceptives: increased contraceptive blood level
Warfarin: increased International Normalized Ratio
Drug-diagnostic tests. *Alanine aminotransferase, alkaline phosphatase, aspartate aminotransferase, bilirubin, creatine phosphokinase, glucose:* increased levels
Potassium: decreased level
Thyroid function tests: altered results
Drug-food. *Caffeine-containing foods and beverages:* increased stimulant effect
Oat bran, pectin: impaired drug absorption
Urine-acidifying foods: increased drug blood level

r

Drug-herb. *Caffeine-containing herbs (such as cola nut, guarana, yerba maté), ephedra (ma huang):* increased stimulant effect

Precautions
Use cautiously in:
• predisposing factors for myopathy (such as renal failure, advanced age, hypothyroidism)
• heavy alcohol use
• history of hepatic disease or hypersensitivity to other HMG-CoA reductase inhibitors (such as fluvastatin, pravastatin, simvastatin)
• patients of Japanese or Chinese descent
• children (safety and efficacy not established).

Patient monitoring
• Monitor blood glucose and electrolyte levels, liver function studies, and lipid panel.
• Assess vital signs and cardiovascular status, especially for tachycardia or palpitations.
• Monitor for signs and symptoms of respiratory tract infection.
• Stay alert for myalgia, tremor, and asthenia.

Patient teaching
• Tell patient he may take drug with or without food; if he's using antacids, instruct him to take them 2 hours after taking drug.
• Instruct patient to consume a standard cholesterol-lowering diet.
• Teach patient how to check blood or urine glucose level and how to recognize signs and symptoms of hypoglycemia and hyperglycemia.
• Inform patient that foods, beverages, and preparations containing caffeine or ephedra may increase drug's stimulant effects; encourage him to limit caffeine intake and avoid ephedra.

• As appropriate, review all other significant adverse reactions and interactions, especially those related to the drugs, tests, foods, and herbs mentioned above.

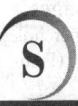

salmeterol xinafoate
Serevent, Serevent Diskus

Pharmacologic class: Beta$_2$-adrenergic receptor agonist (long-acting)
Therapeutic class: Bronchodilator
Pregnancy risk category C

Action
Stimulates intracellular adenylate cyclase, an enzyme that catalyzes conversion of adenosine triphosphate to cyclic-3',5'-adenosine monophosphate (cAMP). Increased cAMP levels relax bronchial smooth muscle and inhibit release of mediators of immediate hypersensitivity (especially from mast cells).

Availability
Aerosol for inhalation: 25 mcg/spray (per actuation) in 6.5-g (60-spray) or 13-g (120-spray) canister
Powder for inhalation: 50 mcg/blister

⏀ Indications and dosages
➤ Long-term treatment of asthma, treatment of bronchospasm in patients with chronic obstructive pulmonary disease, prevention of exercise-induced bronchospasm
Adults and children older than age 12: 50 mcg (two inhalations as aerosol or one as dry powder) b.i.d., approximately 12 hours apart. For exercise-

induced bronchospasm, 50 mcg (two inhalations as aerosol or one as dry powder) 30 to 60 minutes before exercise.

Off-label uses
• Cystic fibrosis
• High-altitude pulmonary edema
• Atopic asthma

Contraindications
• Hypersensitivity to drug or its components
• Acute asthma attack

Administration
• When using Serevent Diskus, activate device and hold it in horizontal position.
• Make sure patient doesn't exhale into device.
• Preferably give 12 hours apart in morning and evening.

Route	Onset	Peak	Duration
Inhalation	10-25 min	3-4 hr	12 hr

Adverse reactions
CNS: headache, nervousness, dizziness, tremor
CV: palpitations, hypertension, tachycardia, **arrhythmias**
GI: nausea, diarrhea, abdominal pain
Metabolic: hyperglycemia, hypokalemia
Musculoskeletal: muscle cramps and soreness
Respiratory: paradoxical bronchospasm
Skin: urticaria, angioedema, rash
Other: hypersensitivity reaction

Interactions
Drug-drug. *Diuretics (except potassium-sparing):* increased risk of hypokalemia
Monoamine oxidase inhibitors, tricyclic antidepressants: potentiation of salmeterol's action

Drug-diagnostic tests. *Glucose:* increased level
Potassium: decreased level
Drug-food. *Caffeine-containing foods and beverages:* increased stimulant effect
Urine-acidifying foods: increased drug blood level
Drug-herb. *Caffeine-containing herbs (such as cola nut, guarana, yerba maté), ephedra (ma huang):* increased stimulant effect

Precautions
Use cautiously in:
• cardiovascular disease, diabetes mellitus, hyperthyroidism
• pregnant or breastfeeding patients
• children under age 4.

Patient monitoring
• Assess pulmonary status and vital signs.
◀€ Stay alert for signs and symptoms of hypersensitivity reaction, particularly rash, urticaria, angioedema, and paradoxical bronchospasm.

Patient teaching
• Remind patient that drug isn't a rescue bronchodilator and won't provide immediate relief in emergencies.
• Teach patient proper technique for using inhaler or Diskus; instruct him not to exhale into device or use a spacer with Diskus.
• Instruct patient to keep Diskus dry and not to rinse or wash it.
• Advise patient to take regular doses 12 hours apart; tell him to take doses for exercise-induced bronchospasm 30 to 60 minutes before exercising.
• As appropriate, review all other significant and life-threatening adverse reactions and interactions, especially those related to the drugs, tests, foods, and herbs mentioned above.

S

Route	Onset	Peak	Duration
P.O.	5-30 min	1-3 hr	3-6 hr

salsalate
Amigesic, Anaflex 750, Disalcid, Marthritic, Mono-Gesic, Salflex, Salgesic, Salsitab

Pharmacologic class: Salicylate
Therapeutic class: Nonopioid analgesic, anti-inflammatory
Pregnancy risk category C

Action
Breaks down into salicylic acid, which lowers elevated body temperature by dilating peripheral vessels. Also reduces inflammation and relieves pain, probably by inhibiting prostaglandin synthesis.

Availability
Tablets: 500 mg, 750 mg

Indications and dosages
➤ Rheumatoid arthritis, nonarticular rheumatism, osteoarthritis, polyarthritis
Adults: Initially, 1 g P.O. t.i.d., titrated as needed

Contraindications
• Hypersensitivity to salicylates, other nonsteroidal anti-inflammatory drugs (NSAIDs), or tartrazine
• Hemophilia
• Bleeding ulcers
• Hemorrhagic states
• Blood coagulation defects
• Children and adolescents with viral infections

Administration
• Give drug with food to minimize GI upset.
◀€ Be aware that children and adolescents with viral infections shouldn't receive this drug because of increased risk of Reye's syndrome.

Adverse reactions
CNS: drowsiness, dizziness, confusion, headache, stimulation, hallucinations, depression, **seizures, coma**
CV: rapid pulse
EENT: hearing loss, tinnitus, laryngeal edema
GI: nausea, vomiting, dyspepsia, epigastric distress, heartburn, abdominal pain, anorexia, **GI bleeding**
Hematologic: increased bleeding, prothrombin, and activated partial thromboplastin times; reduced erythrocyte survival time; hemolytic anemia; **leukopenia; agranulocytosis; thrombocytopenia**
Hepatic: hepatitis, hepatotoxicity
Metabolic: hypoglycemia, hyponatremia, hypokalemia
Respiratory: wheezing, hyperpnea, **pulmonary edema**
Skin: rash, flushing, urticaria, bruising, angioedema
Other: salicylism, **Reye's syndrome, anaphylaxis**

Interactions
Drug-drug. *Activated charcoal:* decreased salsalate absorption
Angiotensin-converting enzyme inhibitors: decreased antihypertensive effect
Antacids, urinary alkalinizers: decreased salsalate efficacy
Beta-adrenergic blockers, probenecid, spironolactone, sulfinpyrazone, sulfonylureas: decreased effects of these drugs
Carbonic anhydrase inhibitors: increased risk of salicylism
Cefamandole, clopidogrel, eptifibatide, heparin, oral anticoagulants, plicamycin, thrombolytics, ticlopidine, tirofiban: increased bleeding
Corticosteroids: increased excretion and decreased blood level of salsalate
Insulin, oral hypoglycemics, penicillin,

phenytoin, sulfonamide, valproic acid: increased effects of these drugs
Methotrexate: increased methotrexate blood level and risk of toxicity
NSAIDs: decreased NSAID blood level, increased risk of adverse GI effects
Vancomycin: increased risk of ototoxicity

Drug-diagnostic tests. *Alanine aminotransferase, alkaline phosphatase, amylase, aspartate aminotransferase, carbon dioxide, coagulation studies, uric acid, urinary protein:* increased levels
Cholesterol, potassium, protein-bound iodine: decreased levels
Pregnancy test, protirelin-induced thyroid-stimulating hormone test, radionuclide thyroid imaging, uric acid, urine catecholamines, urine glucose, urine hydroxyindoleacetic acid, urine ketone tests using ferric chloride method, urine vanillylmandelic acid: interference with test results

Drug-food. *Urine-acidifying foods:* increased salsalate blood level

Drug-herb. *Anise, arnica, chamomile, clove, fenugreek, feverfew, garlic, ginger, ginkgo, ginseng, horse chestnut, kelp ware, licorice:* increased risk of bleeding

Drug-behaviors. *Alcohol use:* increased risk of GI bleeding

Precautions

Use cautiously in:
• severe renal disease, hepatic damage, asthma, rhinitis, nasal polyps, hypoprothrombinemia, vitamin K deficiency, chronic alcohol use or abuse
• history of GI bleeding or ulcer disease
• elderly patients
• pregnant patients (especially during third trimester) and breastfeeding patients.

Patient monitoring

• Monitor for signs and symptoms of anaphylaxis.
• Assess hearing and neurologic status.
• Monitor liver function test results, coagulation studies, and electrolyte and glucose levels.
• Assess for bleeding tendency and angioedema.

Patient teaching

◀€ Teach patient to recognize and immediately report signs or symptoms of severe hypersensitivity reaction.
◀€ Caution parents not to give drug to child with symptoms of viral illness.
• Instruct patient to report unusual bleeding or bruising.
• Inform patient that many common herbs increase risk of bleeding; advise him to discuss these with prescriber before using.
• Advise patient to avoid alcohol because it increases risk of GI bleeding.
• As appropriate, review all other significant and life-threatening adverse reactions and interactions, especially those related to the drugs, tests, foods, herbs, and behaviors mentioned above.

saquinavir
Fortovase

saquinavir mesylate
Invirase

Pharmacologic class: Protease inhibitor
Therapeutic class: Antiretroviral
Pregnancy risk category B

Action

Inhibits human immunodeficiency virus (HIV) protease, preventing cleavage of HIV polyproteins, blocking virus replication and maturation

Availability
saquinavir
Capsules (soft gelatin): 200 mg

saquinavir mesylate
Capsules: 200 mg

ⓘ Indications and dosages
➤ Advanced HIV infection in selected patients (given with other agents)
Adults: 600 mg (saquinavir mesylate) or 1,200 mg (saquinavir) t.i.d. in combination with an appropriate dose of a nucleoside analog

Contraindications
• Hypersensitivity to drug or its components
• Concurrent use of astemizole, cisapride, ergot derivatives, midazolam, terfenadine, or triazolam

Administration
• Give drug around the clock without missing doses and within 2 hours of a full meal.

Route	Onset	Peak	Duration
P.O.	Unknown	Unknown	Unknown

Adverse reactions
CNS: headache, dizziness, paresthesia, asthenia, depression, insomnia, anxiety, confusion, ataxia, **seizures, suicidal ideation, intracranial hemorrhage**
CV: chest pain, peripheral vasoconstriction, thrombophlebitis
EENT: buccal mucosal ulcers, altered taste
GI: nausea, vomiting, diarrhea, constipation, increased amylase level, abdominal pain, flatulence, dyspepsia, pancreatitis
GU: oliguria, urinary retention, nephrolithiasis, **acute renal insufficiency**
Hematologic: hemolytic anemia, **pancytopenia, thrombocytopenia, acute myeloblastic leukemia**
Hepatic: jaundice, portal hypertension, **exacerbation of chronic hepatic disease** (with grade 4 elevated liver function test results)
Metabolic: hypoglycemia, hyperglycemia, diabetes mellitus (exacerbation or new onset), hypercalcemia, hyperkalemia, increased creatinine phosphokinase level, decreased phosphate level
Musculoskeletal: musculoskeletal pain
Respiratory: bronchitis, cough
Skin: rash
Other: drug fever, **Stevens-Johnson syndrome**

Interactions
Drug-drug. *Astemizole, cisapride, ergot derivatives, midazolam, terfenadine, triazolam:* elevated blood level of these drugs, life-threatening arrhythmias, prolonged and life-threatening sedation
Carbamazepine, dexamethasone, nevirapine, phenobarbital, phenytoin, rifabutin, rifampin: reduced saquinavir steady-state level
Clarithromycin, delavirdine, indinavir, ketoconazole, nelfinavir, ritonavir: increased saquinavir blood level
Sildenafil: increased sildenafil blood level
Drug-diagnostic tests. *Alanine aminotransferase (ALT), amylase, aspartate aminotransferase (AST), bilirubin, calcium, creatinine phosphokinase, potassium:* increased levels
Blood glucose: increased or decreased level
Phosphate: decreased level
Platelets, red blood cells, white blood cells: decreased counts
Drug-food. *Any food:* increased drug absorption
Grapefruit juice: elevated drug blood level, increased pharmacologic and adverse effects
Drug-herb. *St. John's wort:* 50% reduction in drug blood level

Precautions
Use cautiously in:
• hepatic disease, hemophilia types A and B, diabetes mellitus

- pregnant or breastfeeding patients
- children under age 16.

Patient monitoring

- Monitor platelet count; complete blood count; liver function studies; and electrolyte, uric acid, and bilirubin levels. Watch for signs and symptoms of life-threatening blood dyscrasias and portal hypertension.
- Assess nutritional status and hydration.
- Monitor neurologic status; stay alert for depression, suicidal ideation, seizures, and signs or symptoms of intracranial hemorrhage.

Patient teaching

- Teach patient to take drug with food (but not grapefruit juice) or within 2 hours of a complete meal. Emphasize importance of taking doses around the clock on a regular schedule.
- ◀€ Inform patient (and significant others as appropriate) that drug may cause depression and suicidal thoughts, which should be reported immediately.
- Advise patient to notify prescriber if rash occurs.
- ◀€ Teach patient to recognize and immediately report signs and symptoms of liver disorder or bleeding tendency.
- As appropriate, review all other significant and life-threatening adverse reactions and interactions, especially those related to the drugs, tests, foods, and herbs mentioned above.

sargramostim (GM-CSF)
Leukine

Pharmacologic class: Granulocyte-macrophage colony stimulating factor

Therapeutic class: Hematopoietic agent

Pregnancy risk category C

Action

Stimulates proliferation and differentiation of hematopoietic cells that activate mature granulocytes and macrophages of target cells

Availability

Liquid: 500 mcg/ml
Powder for injection: 250 mcg, 500 mcg

✔️ Indications and dosages

➢ Postperipheral blood progenitor cell (PBPC) transplantation
Adults: 250 mcg/m²/day I.V. over 24 hours or S.C. daily, starting immediately after infusion of progenitor cells
➢ Mobilization of PBPCs into peripheral blood for collection by leukapheresis
Adults: 250 mcg/m²/day I.V. over 24 hours or S.C. daily, continued throughout harvesting
➢ Neutrophil recovery after chemotherapy in acute myelogenous leukemia
Adults: 250 mcg/m²/day I.V. over 4 hours, starting 4 days after completion of chemotherapy induction
➢ Bone marrow transplantation failure or engraftment delay
Adults: 250 mcg/m²/day as a 2-hour I.V. infusion for 14 days; if engraftment doesn't occur, may repeat after 7 days of drug hiatus
➢ Myeloid reconstitution after autologous bone marrow transplantation
Adults: 250 mcg/m²/day as a 2-hour I.V. infusion for 21 days, starting 2 to 4 hours after autologous bone marrow infusion and at least 24 hours after last chemotherapy or radiotherapy dose

Off-label uses

- Crohn's disease
- Melanoma
- Wound healing
- Mucositis
- Stomatitis
- Vaccine adjuvant

S

Contraindications
• Hypersensitivity to drug or yeast products
• Excessive leukemic myeloid blasts in bone marrow or peripheral blood (10% or more)
• Within 24 hours before or after chemotherapy or radiotherapy

Administration
◀€ Don't give within 24 hours of chemotherapy or radiotherapy.
• Add 1 ml of sterile water to powder for injection by directing stream of water against side of vial and swirling vial gently to disperse contents.
• Avoid shaking or agitating solution.
• For a final drug concentration of less than 10 mcg/ml, add human albumin 0.1% to saline solution; then dilute drug in normal saline solution.
• Infuse as soon as possible after reconstituting but no more than 6 hours after mixing.
• Don't add other drugs to infusion; don't use in-line filter.

Route	Onset	Peak	Duration
I.V.	Immediate	2 hr	3-6 hr
S.C.	15 min	1-3 hr	6 hr

Adverse reactions
CNS: malaise, asthenia
CV: peripheral edema, tachycardia, hypotension, transient supraventricular tachycardia, **pericardial effusion**
GI: nausea, vomiting, diarrhea, anorexia, stomatitis, **GI hemorrhage**
GU: urinary tract disorder, abnormal renal function
Hematologic: blood dyscrasias, hemorrhage
Hepatic: hepatic damage
Musculoskeletal: joint pain, myalgia, bone pain
Respiratory: dyspnea
Skin: rash, alopecia

Other: fever, chills, first-dose reaction (respiratory distress, hypoxia, syncope, tachycardia, hypotension, flushing)

Interactions
Drug-drug. *Corticosteroids, lithium:* potentiation of myeloproliferative effects
Vincristine: severe peripheral neuropathy

Precautions
Use cautiously in:
• renal or hepatic insufficiency, fluid retention, pulmonary disorders, pulmonary infiltrates, heart failure, leukocytosis, transient supraventricular arrhythmia
• cancer patients undergoing sargramostim-mobilized PBPC collection
• patients receiving purged bone marrow or previously exposed to intensive chemotherapy or radiotherapy
• pregnant or breastfeeding patients
• children.

Patient monitoring
• Monitor for dyspnea; halve dosage and contact prescriber if it occurs.
• Assess complete blood count with white cell differential; check for presence of blast cells and watch for signs and symptoms of blood dyscrasias.
• Closely monitor vital signs and fluid intake and output; stay alert for signs and symptoms of fluid overload.
• Monitor liver function test results; watch for signs and symptoms of hepatic damage and bleeding (especially GI hemorrhage).

Patient teaching
• Inform patient that sargramostim is a powerful drug that can cause significant adverse reactions; teach him to recognize and report serious reactions at once.
◀€ Instruct patient to immediately report yellowing of skin or eyes.

- Tell patient drug may cause weakness and musculoskeletal pain.
- Instruct patient to report unusual bleeding or bruising.
- Inform patient that he'll undergo regular blood testing during therapy.
- As appropriate, review all other significant and life-threatening adverse reactions and interactions, especially those related to the drugs mentioned above.

scopolamine (hyoscine)
Transderm-Scop

scopolamine hydrobromide (hyoscine hydrobromide)

Pharmacologic class: Antimuscarinic, belladonna alkaloid

Therapeutic class: Antiemetic, antivertigo agent, anticholinergic

Pregnancy risk category C

Action
Acts as a competitive inhibitor at postganglionic muscarinic receptor sites of parasympathetic nervous system and on smooth muscles that respond to acetylcholine but lack cholinergic innervation; may block cholinergic transmission from vestibular nuclei to higher CNS centers and from reticular formation to vomiting center

Availability
Injection: 0.3 mg/ml and 1 mg/ml in 1-ml vials, 0.4 mg/ml in 0.5-ml ampules and 1-ml vials, 0.86 mg/ml in 0.5-ml ampules
Tablets: 0.4 mg
Transdermal system (Transderm-Scop): 1.5 mg/patch (releases 0.5 mg scopolamine over 3 days)

Indications and dosages
➤ Excessive GI motility and hypertonia in such conditions as irritable bowel syndrome, mild dysentery, diverticulitis, pylorospasm, and cardiospasm
Adults: 0.4 to 0.8 mg P.O. daily
➤ Preanesthetic sedation and obstetric amnesia (given with analgesics)
Adults: 0.3 to 0.6 mg I.M., I.V., or S.C. 45 to 60 minutes before anesthesia
➤ Prevention or treatment of postoperative nausea and vomiting
Adults: One transdermal patch placed behind ear on evening before surgery and kept in place for 24 hours after surgery; for cesarean section, one transdermal patch placed behind ear 1 hour before surgery
➤ Motion sickness
Adults: One transdermal patch placed behind ear 4 hours before anticipated need, replaced q 3 days if needed

Off-label uses
- Drooling

Contraindications
- Hypersensitivity to scopolamine or other belladonna alkaloids
- Hypersensitivity to bromides (injection only)
- Narrow-angle glaucoma
- Acute hemorrhage
- Myasthenia gravis
- Obstructive uropathy
- Obstructive GI disease
- Paralytic ileus or intestinal atony
- Reflux esophagitis
- Ulcerative colitis or toxic megacolon

Administration
- For I.V. use, give by direct injection at prescribed rate after diluting with sterile water.
- After removing protective strip from transdermal patch, avoid finger contact with exposed adhesive layer to prevent contamination.

S

Route	Onset	Peak	Duration
P.O., I.M., S.C.	30 min	1 hr	4-6 hr
I.V.	10 min	1 hr	2-4 hr
Transdermal	4 hr	Unknown	72 hr

Adverse reactions

CNS: drowsiness, dizziness, confusion, restlessness, fatigue
CV: tachycardia, palpitations, hypotension, transient heart rate changes
EENT: blurred vision, mydriasis, photophobia, conjunctivitis
GI: constipation, dry mouth
GU: urinary hesitancy or retention
Skin: decreased sweating, rash

Interactions

Drug-drug. *Antidepressants, antihistamines, disopyramide, quinidine:* additive anticholinergic effects
Antidepressants, antihistamines, opioid analgesics, sedative-hypnotics: additive CNS depression
Oral drugs: altered absorption of these drugs
Wax-matrix potassium tablets: increased GI mucosal lesions
Drug-herb. *Angel's trumpet, jimsonweed, scopolia:* increased anticholinergic effects
Drug-behaviors. *Alcohol use:* increased CNS depression

Precautions

Use cautiously in:
• suspected intestinal obstruction; prostatic hypertrophy; chronic renal, hepatic, pulmonary, or cardiac disease; tachyarrhythmia or tachycardia; open-angle glaucoma; pyloric or bladder neck obstruction; autonomic neuropathy; hypertension; hyperthyroidism; ileostomy or colostomy
• history of seizures or psychosis
• elderly patients
• pregnant or breastfeeding patients (safety not established)
• children.

Patient monitoring

• Assess vital signs and neurologic, cardiovascular, and respiratory status.
• Monitor patient for urinary hesitancy or retention.

Patient teaching

• Tell patient transdermal patch is most effective if applied to dry skin behind ear 4 hours before traveling.
• Instruct patient to avoid touching exposed adhesive layer of transdermal patch.
• Teach patient to wash and dry hands thoroughly before and after applying patch.
• If patch becomes dislodged, tell patient to remove it and apply new patch on a different skin site behind ear.
• Tell patient withdrawal symptoms (headache, nausea, vomiting, dizziness) may occur if he uses patch for more than 72 hours; encourage him to limit use when feasible.
• Inform patient that his eyes may be markedly sensitive to light during patch use; instruct him to wear sunglasses and use other measures to protect his eyes from light.
• Urge patient to avoid alcohol because it may increase CNS depression.
• As appropriate, review all other significant adverse reactions and interactions, especially those related to the drugs, herbs, and behaviors mentioned above.

selegiline hydrochloride
Apo-Selegiline✤, Carbex, Eldepryl, Gen-Selegiline✤, Novo-Selegiline✤, Nu-Selegiline✤, SD Deprenyl✤

Pharmacologic class: Monoamine oxidase (MAO) inhibitor (type B)
Therapeutic class: Antidyskinetic
Pregnancy risk category C

Action
Unknown; thought to increase dopaminergic activity by inhibiting MAO type B in nerve cells, increasing availability of dopamine to brain cells.

Availability
Capsules: 5 mg
Tablets: 5 mg

🖊 Indications and dosages
➤ Adjunctive treatment of Parkinson's disease in patients who show deterioration despite carbidopa-levodopa therapy
Adults: 10 mg P.O. daily in divided doses (5 mg with breakfast and 5 mg with lunch). After 2 to 3 days, attempt to reduce dosage (typically by 10% to 30%).

Off-label uses
• Initial therapy for Parkinson's disease
• Alzheimer's disease
• Narcolepsy
• Adjunctive therapy for schizophrenia

Contraindications
• Hypersensitivity to drug or its components
• Concurrent meperidine therapy

Administration
• Give with or without food, but restrict foods high in tyramine (such as aged cheese, red wine, yogurt, and smoked high-protein foods).

Route	Onset	Peak	Duration
P.O.	Unknown	0.5-2 hr	Unknown

Adverse reactions
CNS: agitation, anxiety, bradykinesia, chorea, confusion, delusions, depression, dizziness, dyskinesias, hallucinations, headache, increased akinetic involuntary movements, insomnia, lethargy, light-headedness, loss of balance, syncope, vivid dreams

CV: orthostatic hypotension, hypertension, new or increased angina, palpitations, **arrhythmias**
GI: nausea, diarrhea, abdominal pain, dry mouth
GU: urinary retention
Musculoskeletal: leg pain, low back pain
Other: generalized aches, weight loss

Interactions
Drug-drug. *Adrenergics:* increased pressor response
Levodopa: increased levodopa adverse reactions
Meperidine, other opioids: stupor, muscle rigidity, severe agitation, fever, death
Other MAO inhibitors: hypertensive crisis
Selective serotonin reuptake inhibitors (SSRIs), tricyclic antidepressants (TCAs): CNS toxicity, mental status changes
Drug-food. *Tyramine-rich foods (such as aged cheese, red wine, yogurt, smoked high-protein foods):* hypertensive crisis
Drug-herb. *Cacao:* vasopressor effects
Ginseng: headache, tremor, mania

Precautions
Use cautiously in:
• patients receiving TCAs, SSRIs, or opioids concurrently
• elderly patients
• pregnant or breastfeeding patients
• children.

Patient monitoring
• Monitor vital signs and cardiovascular status.
• Assess neurologic status and motor function; institute safety measures as needed to prevent injury.
• Monitor weight and fluid intake and output.
• Monitor complete blood count and liver and kidney function test results.

S

Patient teaching

• Tell patient he may take drug with or without food.

• Teach patient (and caregiver as appropriate) to monitor neurologic status and motor function and to institute safety precautions as needed to prevent injury.

• Instruct patient to move slowly when sitting up or standing to avoid dizziness or light-headedness from sudden blood pressure decrease.

• Advise patient to limit foods high in tyramine. Provide a list of these foods.

• As appropriate, review all other significant and life-threatening adverse reactions and interactions, especially those related to the drugs, foods, and herbs mentioned above.

senna, sennosides

Argoral✽, Black Draught, Dr. Caldwell, Dosalax, Ex-Lax Chocolate, Ex-Lax Gentle, Fletcher's Castoria, Maximum Relief Ex-Lax, Nature's Remedy, Senexon, Senna-Gen, Senokot, Senokot Granules, SenokotXTRA, Senolax, X-Prep Liquid✽

Pharmacologic class: Anthraquinone laxative

Therapeutic class: Laxative (stimulant)

Pregnancy risk category C

Action

Causes local irritation in colon, which promotes peristalsis and bowel evacuation; softens feces by increasing water and electrolytes in large intestine

Availability

Granules: 15 mg/5 ml, 20 mg/5 ml
Liquid: 3 mg/ml, 8.8 mg/5 ml, 33.3 mg/5 ml (concentrate)

Powder: 15 mg/3 g
Syrup: 8.8 mg/5 ml
Tablets: 6 mg, 8.6 mg, 15 mg, 17 mg, 25 mg
Tablets (chewable): 15 mg

⚕ Indications and dosages

➤ Acute constipation, preparation for bowel examination

Adults and children older than age 12: Two tablets of Black Draught or one-fourth to one-half level tsp of granules mixed with water, or 10 to 15 ml syrup at bedtime. Maximum dosage varies with preparation.

Contraindications

• Hypersensitivity to drug or its components

• GI bleeding or obstruction

• Suspected appendicitis

• Acute surgical abdomen

• Fecal impaction

Administration

• Give with a full glass of cold water.

• To prepare patient for bowel examination, give drug 12 to 14 hours before procedure, followed by a clear liquid diet.

Route	Onset	Peak	Duration
P.O.	6-24 hr	Variable	Variable

Adverse reactions

GI: nausea, vomiting, diarrhea, abdominal cramps, nutrient malabsorption, yellow or yellowish-green feces, loss of normal bowel function (with excessive use), dark pigmentation of rectal mucosa (with long-term use), protein-losing enteropathy

GU: reddish-pink discoloration of alkaline urine, yellowish-brown discoloration of acidic urine

Metabolic: electrolyte imbalances (such as hypokalemia)

Other: laxative dependence (with long-term or excessive use)

Interactions

Drug-diagnostic tests. *Calcium, potassium:* decreased levels

Precautions

Use cautiously in:
• pregnant or breastfeeding patients
• children.

Patient monitoring

• Assess bowel movements to determine laxative efficacy.
• In long-term use, monitor fluid balance, nutritional status, and electrolyte levels and watch for laxative dependence.

Patient teaching

• Teach patient using drug for constipation to take oral form at bedtime with a glass of water.
• In long-term use, advise patient to watch for and report signs and symptoms of nutritional deficiencies or fluid and electrolyte imbalance.
• If patient is to undergo bowel examination, advise him to take drug 12 to 14 hours before procedure, followed by a clear liquid diet.
• As appropriate, review all other significant adverse reactions and interactions, especially those related to the tests mentioned above.

sertraline hydrochloride
Zoloft

Pharmacologic class: Selective serotonin reuptake inhibitor (SSRI)
Therapeutic class: Antidepressant
Pregnancy risk category C

Action

Inhibits neuronal uptake of serotonin in CNS, potentiating serotonin activity; has little effect on norepinephrine or dopamine uptake

Availability

Capsules: 50 mg, 100 mg
Oral concentrate: 20 mg/ml
Tablets: 25 mg, 50 mg, 100 mg

🕖 Indications and dosages

➤ Depression, obsessive-convulsive disorder
Adults: Initially, 50 mg/day P.O. as a single dose in morning or evening; depending on response, may increase at weekly intervals to a maximum of 200 mg/day
➤ Panic disorder, post-traumatic stress disorder
Adults: Initially, 25 mg/day P.O.; after 1 week, may increase to 50 mg/day

Off-label uses

• Social phobia
• Premenstrual dysphoric disorder
• Premature ejaculation

Contraindications

• Hypersensitivity to drug or its components
• Monoamine (MAO) inhibitor use within 14 days

Administration

◀⟨ Don't use rubber dropper when giving concentrate to patients with latex allergy.
• Don't administer within 14 days of MAO inhibitors.

Route	Onset	Peak	Duration
P.O.	Unknown	4.5-8.5 hr	Unknown

Adverse reactions

CNS: dizziness, drowsiness, fatigue, headache, insomnia, agitation, anxiety, confusion, emotional lability, poor concentration, mania, nervousness, weakness, yawning, tremor, hypertonia, hypoesthesia, paresthesia
CV: chest pain, palpitations

S

EENT: vision abnormalities, tinnitus, rhinitis, pharyngitis

GI: nausea, vomiting, diarrhea, constipation, dyspepsia, flatulence, abdominal pain, dry mouth, anorexia, altered taste

GU: urinary disorders, urinary frequency, sexual dysfunction, menstrual disorders

Hepatic: increased alanine aminotransferase (ALT) and aspartate aminotransferase (AST) levels

Musculoskeletal: back pain, myalgia

Skin: diaphoresis, rash

Other: increased appetite, fever, thirst, hot flashes

Interactions

Drug-drug. *Adrenergics:* increased adrenergic sensitivity, increased risk of serotonin syndrome

Cimetidine: increased sertraline blood level and effects

Clozapine, most benzodiazepines, phenytoin, tricyclic antidepressants, tolbutamide, warfarin: increased blood levels and effects of these drugs

Disulfiram: disulfiram reaction (nausea, vomiting, flushing, throbbing headache, diaphoresis, chest pain, palpitations, dyspnea, hyperventilation, tachycardia, hypotension, syncope, weakness, vertigo; in severe cases, respiratory depression, cardiovascular collapse, myocardial infarction, acute heart failure, seizures and death) with oral concentrate

Drugs metabolized by CYP450-2DC or CYP450-3A4: increased blood levels of these drugs

MAO inhibitors: potentially fatal reaction (hyperthermia, rigidity, myoclonus, autonomic instability with fluctuating vital signs and extreme agitation, which may proceed to delirium and coma)

Pimozide: increased pimozide blood level

Sumatriptan: weakness, hyperreflexia, incoordination

Drug-diagnostic tests. *ALT, AST:* increased levels

Drug-herb. *S-adenosylmethionine (SAM-e), St. John's wort:* increased risk of serotonergic side effects, including serotonin syndrome

Drug-behaviors. *Alcohol use:* increased CNS effects

Precautions

Use cautiously in:
• seizures disorders, severe hepatic or renal impairment
• history of mania
• patients at increased risk for suicide
• pregnant or breastfeeding patients
• children.

Patient monitoring

◀≦ Monitor patient's mental status carefully; stay alert for mood changes and any indications of suicidal ideation.

• Evaluate neurologic status regularly; institute safety measures as appropriate to prevent injury.

• Monitor temperature; stay alert for fever and other signs or symptoms of infection.

Patient teaching

• Advise patient to take drug once a day, either in morning or night, with or without food.

• If the evening dose causes insomnia, recommend switching to a morning dose.

• Instruct patient to mix oral concentrate with 4 oz of recommended liquid only. Advise him to swallow diluted drug immediately after mixing.

◀≦ Caution patient not to stop taking drug suddenly; dosage must be tapered.

• Tell patient drug may cause serious interactions with common drugs. Instruct him to tell all prescribers he's taking it.

◀≦ Teach patient (and significant other as appropriate) to monitor his men-

---

tal status carefully and to immediately report increased depression or suicidal thoughts or behavior.

• Instruct patient to avoid driving and other hazardous activities until he knows how drug affects concentration and alertness.

• As appropriate, review all other significant adverse reactions and interactions, especially those related to the drugs, tests, herbs, and behaviors mentioned above.

sildenafil citrate
Viagra

Pharmacologic class: Phosphodiesterase type 5 (PDE5) inhibitor
Therapeutic class: Anti-impotence agent
Pregnancy risk category B

Action
Enhances effects of nitric oxide released during sexual stimulation by inhibiting PDE5; this inhibition causes inactivation of cyclic guanosine monophosphate (cGMP). In corpus cavernosum, increased cGMP level causes smooth muscle relaxation, which promotes increased blood flow and subsequent erection.

Availability
Tablets: 25 mg, 50 mg, 100 mg

Indications and dosages
➤ Erectile dysfunction
Adults: 50 mg P.O., preferably taken 1 hour before anticipated sexual activity. Dosage range is 25 to 100 mg taken 30 minutes to 4 hours before sexual activity, not to exceed one dose daily.
Dosage adjustment
• Hepatic or renal impairment
• Concurrent use of hepatic isoenzyme

inhibitors (such as as cimetidine, erythromycin, itraconazole, ketoconazole)
• Elderly patients

Contraindications
• Hypersensitivity to drug
• Concurrent use of nitrates (nitroglycerin, isosorbide mononitrate or dinitrate)

Administration
◀€ Don't give concurrently with nitrates.
• Administer 30 minutes to 4 hours before sexual activity.

Route	Onset	Peak	Duration
P.O.	Within 1 hr	Unknown	Up to 4 hr

Adverse reactions
CNS: headache, dizziness, anxiety, drowsiness, vertigo, **seizures, cerebrovascular hemorrhage, transient ischemic attack**
CV: hypertension, **myocardial infarction (MI), cardiovascular collapse, ventricular arrhythmias, sudden death**
EENT: transient vision loss, blurred or color-tinged vision, increased light sensitivity, ocular redness, retinal bleeding, vitreous detachment or traction, photophobia, nasal congestion
GI: diarrhea, dyspepsia
GU: hematuria, urinary tract infection, priapism
Skin: flushing, rash

Interactions
Drug-drug. *Antihypertensives, nitrates:* increased risk of hypotension
Enzyme inducers, rifampin: reduced sildenafil plasma levels
Hepatic isoenzyme inhibitors (such as cimetidine, erythromycin, itraconazole, ketoconazole), protease inhibitors (such as indinavir, nelfinavir, ritonavir, saquinavir): increased sildenafil blood level and effects

S

Drug-food. *High-fat diet:* reduced drug absorption, decreased peak level

Precautions

Use cautiously in:
• serious cardiovascular disease (such as history of MI, cerebrovascular accident, or serious arrhythmia within past 6 months); heart failure or history of heart failure; coronary artery disease (or history of) with unstable angina; renal or hepatic impairment; anatomic penile deformity; bleeding disorders or active peptic ulcers; retinitis pigmentosa; conditions associated with priapism (sickle cell anemia, multiple myeloma, leukemia); resting blood pressure below 90/50 mmHg or above 170/110 mmHg
• history of uncontrolled hypertension or hypotension or resting blood pressure below 90/50 mmHg or above 170/110 mmHg
• concurrent use of antihypertensives, erythromycin, ketoconazole, itraconazole, or saquinavir
• patients older than age 65.

Patient monitoring

• Monitor cardiovascular status carefully.
• Evaluate patient's vision.
• Assess for drug efficacy.
• Monitor for priapism or erections lasting more than 4 hours, which may permanently damage penile tissue.

Patient teaching

• Advise patient to take drug 30 minutes to 4 hours before sexual activity.
• Tell patient not to exceed prescribed dosage or take more than one dose daily.
◀≋ Instruct patient to stop sexual activity and contact prescriber immediately if chest pain, dizziness, or nausea occurs.
◀≋ Teach patient to recognize and immediately report serious cardiac and vision problems.

• Tell patient drug can cause serious interactions with many common drugs; instruct him to tell all prescribers he's taking it.
◀≋ Caution patient never to take drug along with nitrates because of risk of potentially fatal hypotension.
• Teach patient that high-fat diet may interfere with drug efficacy.
• Instruct patient to avoid driving and other hazardous activities until he knows how drug affects concentration and alertness.
• As appropriate, review all other significant and life-threatening adverse reactions and interactions, especially those related to the drugs and foods mentioned above.

simethicone

Alka-Seltzer Gas Relief Maximum Strength, Gas-X, Gas-X Extra Strength, Genasyme, Maalox Anti-Gas, Maalox Anti-Gas Extra Strength, Maximum Strength Mylanta Gas, Mylanta Gas, Mylicon, Mylicon Infant Drops, Ovol♣, Phazyme, Phazyme Infant Drops

Pharmacologic class: Methylated linear siloxane mixture
Therapeutic class: Antiflatulent, antifoam agent
Pregnancy risk category NR

Action

Causes coalescence of gas bubbles and allows gas to pass through GI tract by belching or passing of flatus; silicone antifoam spreads on surface of aqueous liquids, forming a film of low surface tension that causes collapse of foam bubbles.

Availability

Capsules: 95 mg, 125 mg
Capsules (liquid-filled): 125 mg, 166 mg
Drops: 40 mg/0.6 ml, 40 mg/1 ml, 95 mg/1.425 ml
Suspension: 40 mg/0.6 ml, 50 mg/5 ml
Tablets: 60 mg, 62.5 mg, 80 mg, 95 mg
Tablets (chewable): 40 mg, 80 mg, 125 mg, 150 mg, 166 mg

Indications and dosages

➤ Excess gas in GI tract postoperatively or from air swallowing, dyspepsia, peptic ulcer, or diverticulitis
Adults and children older than age 12: 40 to 125 mg P.O. q.i.d. after meals and at bedtime, up to 500 mg/day
Children ages 2 to 12: 40 mg P.O. q.i.d., up to 240 mg/day
Children younger than age 2: 20 mg P.O. q.i.d.

Contraindications

• Hypersensitivity to drug

Administration

• Give as needed after meals and at bedtime.

Route	Onset	Peak	Duration
P.O.	Immediate	Unknown	3 hr

Adverse reactions

None significant

Interactions

None significant

Precautions

Use cautiously in:
• abdominal pain of unknown cause (especially when accompanied by fever).

Patient monitoring

• Monitor GI status to assess drug efficacy.

Patient teaching

• Teach patient to take drug after meals and at bedtime as needed.
• Caution patient not to take higher dose than indicated on package, unless prescriber approves.

simvastatin
Zocor

Pharmacologic class: HMG-CoA reductase inhibitor
Therapeutic class: Antihyperlipidemic
Pregnancy risk category X

Action

Inhibits hepatic enzyme HMG-CoA reductase, interrupting cholesterol synthesis and low-density lipoprotein (LDL) consumption, resulting in reduction of total cholesterol and serum triglycerides

Availability

Tablets: 5 mg, 10 mg, 20 mg, 40 mg, 80 mg

Indications and dosages

➤ Coronary artery disease, hyperlipidemia
Adults: 20 mg P.O. daily in evening, with dosage adjusted q 4 weeks based on response. Range is 5 to 80 mg/day.
Dosage adjustment
• Severe renal impairment
• Concurrent use of amiodarone, fibrates, niacin, or verapamil
• Elderly patients

Contraindications

• Hypersensitivity to drug
• Active hepatic disease or unexplained persistent serum transaminase elevations
• Pregnancy or breastfeeding

Administration

• Give with evening meal, but not with large amounts of grapefruit juice.

Route	Onset	Peak	Duration
P.O.	Unknown	Unknown	Unknown

Adverse reactions

CNS: headache, asthenia

GI: nausea, vomiting, diarrhea, abdominal pain or cramps, flatulence, dyspepsia, constipation

Hepatic: increased alanine aminotransferase (ALT) and aspartate aminotransferase (AST) levels

Musculoskeletal: myalgia

Respiratory: upper respiratory infection

Interactions

Drug-drug. *Amiodarone, verapamil:* increased risk of severe myopathy or rhabdomyolysis

Digoxin: increased digoxin blood level and possible toxicity

Other lipid-lowering drugs (such as fibrates, gemfibrozil, nicotinic acid): myopathy

Potent CYP3A4 inhibitors (clarithromycin, cyclosporine, erythromycin, itraconazole, ketoconazole, nefazodone, protease inhibitors): increased risk of severe myopathy or rhabdomyolysis

Propranolol: decreased bioavailability of both drugs

Warfarin: increased anticoagulant effects

Drug-diagnostic tests. *ALT, AST:* increased levels

Drug-food. *Grapefruit juice (more than 1 qt/day):* increased drug blood level, greater risk of adverse reactions

Drug-herb. *Red yeast rice:* increased risk of adverse reactions

Drug-behaviors. *Alcohol use:* increased risk of hepatotoxicity

Precautions

Use cautiously in:

• cross-sensitivity with other drugs that can affect steroid levels

• renal impairment; severe acute infection; hypotension; severe metabolic, endocrine, or electrolyte problems; uncontrolled seizures; visual disturbances; myopathy; major surgery; trauma; alcoholism

• history of hepatic disease

• concurrent use of amiodarone, clarithromycin, cyclosporine, digoxin, erythromycin, gemfibrozil and other fibrates, itraconazole, ketoconazole, nefazodone, nicotinic acid, protease inhibitors, verapamil, or warfarin

• women of childbearing age

• children younger than age 18 (safety not established).

Patient monitoring

• Watch for myositis and other adverse musculoskeletal reactions.

• Monitor liver function tests, complete blood count, and lipid levels.

• In patients receiving warfarin concurrently, closely monitor prothrombin time and International Normalized Ratio.

Patient teaching

• Teach patient to take drug with evening meal, but not with large amounts of grapefruit juice.

• Tell patient that drug may take up to 4 weeks to be effective.

◀ Caution patient to stop taking drug and contact prescriber if she suspects she is pregnant.

• Teach patient to recognize and report signs and symptoms of myopathy.

• Instruct patient to avoid alcohol and red yeast rice.

• As appropriate, review all other significant adverse reactions and interactions, especially those related to the drugs, tests, foods, herbs, and behaviors mentioned above.

---

sirolimus
Rapamune

Pharmacologic class: Macrocyclic lactone
Therapeutic class: Immunosuppressant
Pregnancy risk category C

Action
Inhibits early activation and proliferation of T lymphocytes and inhibits cell cycle progression at a later stage

Availability
Oral solution: 1 mg/ml
Tablets: 1 mg

Indications and dosages
➤ To prevent organ rejection in patients with kidney transplants
Adults and adolescents older than age 13 who weigh more than 40 kg (88 lb):
Initially, 6 mg P.O. as a single dose as soon as possible after transplantation, followed by a maintenance dosage of 2 mg P.O. once daily. Usually given with cyclosporine and corticosteroids.
Dosage adjustment
• Mild to moderate hepatic failure

Off-label uses
• Psoriasis

Contraindications
• Hypersensitivity to drug or its components

Administration
• Wait 4 hours after cyclosporine dose (if prescribed) before giving sirolimus.
• Administer either with or without food.
• Dilute oral solution in a glass or plastic (not Styrofoam) cup that contains at least 2 oz of water or orange juice.

Don't use other fluids, especially grapefruit juice.
• Swirl cup to mix drug thoroughly; discard syringe. Administer diluted drug right away. Then fill cup with 4 oz of water or orange juice, and have patient drink this fluid right away.
◀€ If solution touches your skin or mucous membranes, immediately wash affected area with soap and water.

Route	Onset	Peak	Duration
P.O.	Unknown	1-3 hr	Unknown

Adverse reactions
CNS: headache, drowsiness, paresthesia, hypesthesia, hypertonia, hypertonia, emotional lability, dizziness, confusion, syncope, malaise, asthenia, depression, anxiety, tremor, insomnia
CV: hypertension, hypotension, tachycardia, chest pain, edema, palpitations, vasodilation, peripheral edema, peripheral vascular disorders, thrombophlebitis, thrombosis, **heart failure, atrial fibrillation, hemorrhage**
EENT: abnormal vision, cataract, conjunctivitis, hearing loss, ear pain, otitis media, tinnitus, epistaxis, rhinitis, sinusitis, gingivitis, gum hyperplasia, pharyngitis
GI: nausea, vomiting, diarrhea, constipation, abdominal pain, dyspepsia, hernia, enlarged abdomen, ascites, esophagitis, eructation, flatulence, gastritis, gastroenteritis, dysphagia, stomatitis, mouth ulcers, oral candidiasis, anorexia, **peritonitis**
GU: dysuria, urinary frequency or incontinence, urinary retention, hematuria, albuminuria, urinary tract infection, nocturia, oliguria, pyuria, pelvic pain, kidney or bladder pain, hydronephrosis, impotence, scrotal edema, testes disorders, **GU hemorrhage, renal tubular necrosis, toxic nephropathy**
Hematologic: anemia, bruising, leukocytosis, polycythemia, **thrombocyto-**

S

penia, leukopenia, thrombotic thrombocytopenia

Metabolic: glycosuria, hyperglycemia, diabetes mellitus, hypercholesterolemia, hyperlipidemia, hypokalemia, hypophosphatemia, hypovolemia, acidosis, dehydration, hypercalcemia, Cushing's syndrome

Respiratory: dyspnea, cough, atelectasis, upper respiratory tract infection, asthma, bronchitis, hypoxia, pulmonary edema, pleural effusion, pneumonia

Skin: skin ulcers, skin hypertrophy, pruritus, fungal dermatitis, hirsutism, rash, acne, cellulitis

Other: weight changes, neck pain, fever, abscess, chills, facial edema, flu-like symptoms, infection, lymphadenopathy, abnormal healing, **sepsis**

Interactions

Drug-drug. *Aminoglycosides, amphotericin, other nephrotoxic drugs:* increased risk of nephrotoxicity
Bromocriptine, cimetidine, clarithromycin, danazol, erythromycin, fluconazole, indinavir, itraconazole, metoclopramide, nicardipine, ritonavir, verapamil, other CYP3A4 inhibitors: decreased sirolimus metabolism and increased blood level
Carbamazepine, phenobarbital, phenytoin, rifabutin, rifampin, other CYP3A4 inducers: decreased sirolimus blood level
Cyclosporine, diltiazem: increased sirolimus blood level
Live-virus vaccines: reduced vaccine efficacy

Drug-diagnostic tests. *Blood urea nitrogen, cholesterol, creatinine, hepatic enzymes, lipids, red blood cells:* increased levels
Calcium, glucose, phosphate, white blood cells: increased or decreased levels
Hemoglobin, magnesium, platelets, sodium: decreased levels

Drug-food. *Grapefruit juice:* decreased sirolimus metabolism and increased blood level

Drug-herb. *Astragalus, echinacea, melatonin, St. John's wort:* decreased immunosuppressant efficacy

Precautions

Use cautiously in:
• renal or hepatic disease, cancer, diabetes mellitus, hyperlipidemia, infectious complications
• patients with liver transplants
• pregnant or breastfeeding patients
• children younger than age 13.

Patient monitoring

• Watch closely for signs and symptoms of infection and lymphoma.
• Monitor renal function tests, lipid panels, electrolyte levels, blood chemistry studies, and sirolimus blood level.
• Evaluate all body systems carefully, especially cardiovascular and renal.
• Assess neurologic status closely; implement safety precautions as needed to prevent injury.

Patient teaching

• Teach patient correct procedure for taking drug.
• Advise patient to take drug consistently either with or without food, but not with grapefruit juice.
• Instruct patient to wait 4 hours after cyclosporine dose (if prescribed) before taking sirolimus.
• Teach patient to wash affected area with soap and water immediately if drug touches his skin or mucous membranes.
• Inform patient that drug affects almost every body system; advise him to report significant adverse reactions.
◀≣ Inform patient that drug lowers resistance to infection. Instruct him to immediately report fever, cough, breathing problems, sore throat, or other signs and symptoms of infection.

• Teach patient to avoid driving and other hazardous activities until he knows how drug affects concentration and alertness.

• Instruct patient to report unusual bleeding or bruising.

◀€ Advise female patient to report suspected pregnancy right away.

• As appropriate, review all other significant and life-threatening adverse reactions and interactions, especially those related to the drugs, tests, foods, and herbs mentioned above.

sodium bicarbonate
Arm & Hammer Baking Soda, Bell/ans, Citrocarbonate, Neut, Soda Mint

Pharmacologic class: Fluid and electrolyte agent
Therapeutic class: Alkalinizer, antacid
Pregnancy risk category C

Action
Restores body's buffering capacity; neutralizes excess acid

Availability
Injection (powder): 4% (2.4 mEq/5 ml), 4.2% (5 mEq/10 ml), 5% (297.5 mEq/500 ml), 7.5% (8.92 mEq/10 ml and 44.6 mEq/50 ml), 8.4% (10 mEq/10 ml and 50 mEq/50 ml)
Oral solution: sodium 30.46 mEq/3.9g and sodium citrate 1.82 g/3.9 g (Citrocarbonate)
Tablets: 325 mg, 650 mg

🕖 Indications and dosages
➤ Metabolic acidosis
Adults and children: Generally, 2 to 5 mEq/kg I.V. infusion over 4 to 8 hours; however, dosage is highly individualized depending on patient's condition

and blood's carbon dioxide content and pH.
➤ Cardiac arrest
Adults: 1 mEq/kg I.V.; may give repeat doses of 0.5 mEq/kg I.V. at 10-minute intervals during continued cardiac arrest.
Children younger than age 2: 1 mEq/kg I.V. given over 1 minute; may repeat at 10-minute intervals during continued cardiac arrest. Don't exceed 8 mEq/kg/day.
➤ Urinary alkalinization
Adults: Initially, 4 g P.O.; then 1 to 2 g P.O. q 4 hours
➤ Antacid
Adults: 300 mg to 2 g P.O. up to q.i.d., given with a glass of water

Contraindications
• Hypertension
• Peptic ulcer
• Renal disease
• Hypocalcemia
• Metabolic or systemic alkalosis
• Seizures
• Vomiting resulting in chloride loss
• Diuretic use resulting in hypochloremic alkalosis
• Acute ingestion of mineral acids (with oral form)

Administration
• For I.V. use, infuse at prescribed rate using controlled infusion device.

◀€ Don't give concurrently with catecholamines (such as norepinephrine, dobutamine, dopamine) or calcium. If patient is receiving both sodium bicarbonate and one or more of these drugs, flush I.V. line thoroughly after each dose to prevent contact between drugs.

Route	Onset	Peak	Duration
P.O.	Unknown	Unknown	Unknown
I.V.	Immediate	Immediate	Unknown

Adverse reactions

CNS: headache, irritability, confusion, stimulation, tremors, twitching, hyperreflexia, weakness, **seizures of alkalosis, tetany**

CV: irregular pulse, edema, **cardiac arrest**

GI: gastric distention, belching, flatulence, acid reflux, **paralytic ileus**

GU: renal calculi

Metabolic: hypokalemia, fluid retention, hypernatremia, hyperosmolarity (with overdose), **metabolic alkalosis**

Respiratory: slow and shallow respirations, cyanosis, **apnea**

Other: weight gain, pain and inflammation at I.V. site

Interactions

Drug-drug. *Anorexiants, flecainide, mecamylamine, methenamine, quinidine, sympathomimetics:* increased urinary alkalinization, decreased renal clearance of these drugs

Chlorpropamide, lithium, methotrexate, salicylates, tetracycline: increased renal clearance and decreased efficacy of these drugs

Enteric-coated tablets: premature gastric release of these drugs

Drug-diagnostic tests. *Lactate, potassium, sodium:* increased levels

Drug-herb. *Oak bark:* decreased sodium bicarbonate action

Precautions

Use cautiously in:
• renal insufficiency, heart failure, cirrhosis, toxemia
• pregnant patients.

Patient monitoring

• When giving I.V., closely monitor arterial blood gas results and electrolyte levels.

◀︎ Watch closely for signs and symptoms of metabolic alkalosis and electrolyte imbalances.

• Monitor fluid intake and output; assess for fluid overload.

◀︎ Avoid rapid infusion, which may cause tetany.

• Watch for inflammation at I.V. site.

Patient teaching

• Inform patient taking drug as antacid that too much sodium bicarbonate can cause systemic problems; encourage him to limit use to amount approved by prescriber.

• Advise patient not to take oral form with milk; also teach him to avoid the herb oak bark.

• Tell patient that sodium bicarbonate interferes with action of many common drugs; advise him to notify all prescribers if he's taking oral sodium bicarbonate on a regular basis.

• As appropriate, review all other significant and life-threatening adverse reactions and interactions, especially those related to the drugs, tests, and herbs mentioned above.

sodium chloride

Minims Sodium Chloride✤, Slo-Salt, Slow Sodium

Pharmacologic class: Electrolyte supplement
Therapeutic class: Sodium replacement
Pregnancy risk category C

Action

Replaces deficiencies of sodium and chloride and maintains these electrolytes at adequate levels

Availability

Injection: 0.45% sodium chloride— 25 ml, 50 ml, 150 ml, 250 ml, 500 ml, 1,000 ml; 0.9% sodium chloride— 2 ml, 3 ml, 5 ml, 10 ml, 20 ml, 25 ml, 30 ml, 50 ml, 100 ml, 150 ml, 250 ml, 500 ml, 1,000 ml; 3% sodium chloride—500 ml; 5% sodium chloride—

500 ml; 14.6% sodium chloride—
20 ml, 40 ml, 200 ml; 23.4% sodium
chloride—30 ml, 50 ml, 100 ml, 200 ml
Tablets: 650 mg, 1 g, 2.25 g
Tablets (slow-release): 600 mg

Indications and dosages

➤ Water and sodium chloride replacement; metabolic alkalosis; to dilute or dissolve drugs for I.V., I.M., or
S.C. use; to flush I.V. catheters; as a
priming solution in hemodialysis; to
initiate or terminate blood transfusions
Adults: Dosage individualized; 0.9%
sodium chloride (isotonic solution)
➤ Hydrating solution, treatment of
hyperosmolar diabetes
Adults: Dosage individualized; 0.45%
sodium chloride (hypotonic solution)
➤ Rapid fluid and electrolyte replacement in hyponatremia and hypochloremia; severe sodium depletion; drastic
body water dilution after excessive water intake
Adults: Dosage individualized; 3% or
5% sodium chloride (hypertonic solution) given only by slow I.V. when electrolyte levels are monitored closely
➤ Heat cramps caused by excessive
perspiration
Adults: See product label for dosing
guidelines.

Contraindications

• Normal or above-normal electrolyte
levels (with 3% and 5% solutions)
• Fluid retention

Administration

• Dilute I.V. doses per product label;
infuse slow I.V. to minimize risk of
pulmonary edema.
◀℥ Don't confuse normal saline solution for injection with concentrates
meant for use in total parenteral nutrition.
• Avoid salt tablets for heat cramps because they may pass through GI tract

undigested and may cause vomiting
and potassium loss.

Route	Onset	Peak	Duration
P.O.	Unknown	Unknown	Unknown
I.V.	Immediate	Immediate	Unknown

Adverse reactions

CV: thrombophlebitis, edema (when
given too rapidly or in excess), **heart
failure exacerbation**
Metabolic: fluid and electrolyte disturbances (such as hypernatremia and hyperphosphatemia), aggravation of existing metabolic acidosis (with excessive infusion)
Respiratory: pulmonary edema
Other: pain, swelling, local tenderness,
abscess, or tissue necrosis at I.V. site

Interactions

Drug-diagnostic tests. *Phosphate,
potassium, sodium:* increased levels

Precautions

Use cautiously in:
• renal impairment, heart failure, edema or sodium-retention, hypoproteinemia
• surgical patients.

Patient monitoring

• Monitor electrolyte levels and blood
chemistry results.
◀℥ Watch for signs and symptoms of
pulmonary edema or worsening heart
failure.
• Monitor vital signs, fluid balance,
weight, and cardiovascular status carefully.
• Assess injection site closely to help
prevent tissue necrosis and thrombophlebitis.

Patient teaching

• Teach patient to recognize and immediately report serious adverse reactions, such as breathing problems or
swelling.

S

• Instruct patient to report pain, tenderness, or swelling at injection site.
• As appropriate, review all other significant and life-threatening adverse reactions and interactions, especially those related to the tests mentioned above.

sodium iodide 131I
Iodotope, Sodium Iodide 131I
Therapeutic

Pharmacologic class: Radiopharmaceutical
Therapeutic class: Antithyroid drug
Pregnancy risk category X

Action
After being trapped by thyroid, drug is incorporated into iodoamino acids and deposited in follicular colloid, from which it's slowly released. Destructive beta particles in follicle act on thyroid's parenchymal cells, minimizing damage to surrounding tissue.

Availability
Iodotope
Capsules: radioactivity ranging from 1 to 130 millicuries (mCi)/capsule at time of calibration
Oral solution: radioactivity of 7.05 mCi/ml at time of calibration, in vials containing approximately 7, 14, 28, 70, or 106 mCi at time of calibration
Sodium Iodide 131I Therapeutic
Capsules: radioactivity ranging from 0.75 to 100 mCi/capsule at time of calibration
Oral solution: radioactivity ranging from 3.5 to 150 mCi/vial at time of calibration

Indications and dosages
➤ Thyroid cancer
Adults: Dosages highly individualized.

Usual dosage for ablation of normal thyroid tissue is 50 mCi P.O., with subsequent dosages of 100 to 150 mCi P.O.
➤ Hyperthyroidism
Adults: 4 to 10 mCi P.O. (This dosage usually achieves clinical remission without destroying thyroid.)

Contraindications
• Vomiting and diarrhea
• Known or suspected pregnancy
• Breastfeeding

Administration
◀ Don't administer drug if you're pregnant.
• Make sure all antithyroid drugs and thyroid preparations are discontinued 7 days before radioactive iodine therapy begins. Otherwise, consult prescriber about giving thyroid-stimulating hormone for 3 days.
• Tell patient to fast for 12 hours before therapy starts.
• Know that all doses must be measured by suitable radioactivity calibration system immediately before use.
• For female patients of childbearing age, give drug the week of or week after menstruation.
• Be aware that drug rarely is used to treat hyperthyroidism in patients under age 30.

Route	Onset	Peak	Duration
P.O.	Unknown	1-1.5 hr	Unknown

Adverse reactions
CV: chest pain, tachycardia
EENT: pain on swallowing, sore throat
GI: nausea, vomiting, severe salivary gland inflammation
Hematologic: anemia, **leukopenia, thrombocytopenia, acute leukemia, bone marrow depression**
Metabolic: hypothyroidism, transient thyroiditis, **acute thyroid crisis**
Respiratory: cough

Skin: temporary hair thinning, rash, hives, urticaria

Other: chromosomal abnormalities, neck tenderness and swelling, lymphedema, increase in clinical symptoms, **radiation sickness**

Interactions

Drug-drug. *Other antithyroid drugs (such as methimazole), iodine, thyroid agents:* altered uptake of sodium iodide ^{131}I

Drug-diagnostic tests. *Hemoglobin, platelets, white blood cells:* decreased levels

Precautions

Use cautiously in:
• hypersensitivity to sulfites (with some products)
• children (safety and efficacy not established).

Patient monitoring

◀◊ Monitor patient to make sure he's following full radiation precautions, including proper disposal of body fluids.

◀◊ If you're pregnant, don't provide care to patient who has received this drug.

• When monitoring patient who has received drug for thyroid cancer, limit patient contact to 30 minutes per shift on first day; increase as required to 60 minutes on second day and longer on subsequent days.

• Monitor thyroxine and thyroid-stimulating hormone blood levels, along with complete blood count with white cell differential.

• Assess fluid intake and output 48 hours after administration; encourage high fluid intake.

• Watch for signs and symptoms of hypothyroidism, including fatigue, cold intolerance, depression, and sudden weight gain.

• Monitor for signs and symptoms of radiation sickness (vomiting, dehydra-tion, skin lesions, and fatigue) and bleeding tendency.

Patient teaching

• Instruct patient to fast for 12 hours before therapy starts and to drink as much liquid as possible for 48 hours after administration.

• Teach patient and significant others how to follow full radiation exposure precautions.

• If patient is receiving drug for thyroid cancer, advise him to avoid contact with small children. Tell him not to sleep in same room with anyone else for 7 days after receiving dose.

• Teach patient to recognize and report signs and symptoms of hypothyroidism and radiation sickness.

• Advise patient to report unusual bleeding or bruising.

• As appropriate, review all other significant and life-threatening adverse reactions and interactions, especially those related to the drugs and tests mentioned above.

sodium phosphates

Fleet Enema, Fleet Pediatric Enema, Fleet Phospho-Soda, Visicol

Pharmacologic class: Phosphoric acid salt

Therapeutic class: Saline laxative
Pregnancy risk category NR

S

Action

Promotes hyperosmotic effect in small intestine and increases water retention, which indirectly stimulates peristalsis

Availability

Enema: 160 mg/ml sodium phosphate and 60 mg/ml dibasic sodium phosphate

Liquid: 2.4 g/5 ml monobasic sodium phosphate and 900 mg/5 ml dibasic sodium phosphate
Tablets: 1.102 g sodium phosphate and 0.398 g dibasic sodium phosphate

Indications and dosages

➤ To empty the bowel before colonoscopy
Adults: On night before procedure, three tablets P.O. with 240 ml of clear liquid q 15 minutes; repeat dose until patient has received 7.96 g dibasic sodium phosphate and 22.04 g sodium phosphate (20 tablets). On day of procedure, repeat dose 3 to 5 hours before procedure.
➤ Constipation
Adults and children older than age 12: 20- to 30-ml solution mixed with 120 ml cold water P.O.; or 60 to 135 ml P.R. as an enema

Contraindications

• Hypertension
• Signs or symptoms of appendicitis (nausea, vomiting, abdominal pain)
• Acute surgical abdomen
• Renal impairment
• Megacolon
• Intestinal obstruction or perforation
• Edema
• Heart failure
• Sodium-restricted diet

Administration

• Mix oral solution as indicated on label; have patient drink it right away.

Route	Onset	Peak	Duration
P.O.	0.5-3 hr	Variable	Variable
P.R.	5-10 min	Variable	Variable

Adverse reactions

CV: hypotension, widened QRS complex, **arrhythmias, cardiac arrest**
GI: nausea, diarrhea, cramps

Metabolic: fluid and electrolyte disturbances (such as hypernatremia and hyperphosphatemia)
Other: laxative dependence

Interactions

Drug-diagnostic tests. *Electrolytes:* decreased levels (with prolonged use)
Phosphate, sodium: increased levels

Precautions

Use cautiously in:
• anal excoriation or large hemorrhoids
• pregnant patients.

Patient monitoring

• Monitor fluid balance, electrolyte levels, and cardiovascular status if patient is using drug on a regular basis.
• Monitor bowel habits; watch for indications of laxative dependence.

Patient teaching

• Teach patient to mix oral solution as indicated on label and to drink it right after mixing.
• For enema use, instruct patient (or caregiver as appropriate) to use water-based lubricant to coat tip of applicator bottle.
• Teach patient to recognize and report signs or symptoms of fluid and electrolyte imbalances.
• Inform patient that drug can cause significant cardiovascular and metabolic effects; instruct him to use it only for short-term therapy.
• Tell patient that long-term use can cause laxative dependence; encourage him to increase dietary fiber and fluid intake (unless otherwise contraindicated) to help prevent constipation.
• As appropriate, review all other significant and life-threatening adverse reactions and interactions, especially those related to the tests mentioned above.

sodium polystyrene sulfonate

Kayexalate, K-Exit Poudre ✤, Kionex, SPS Sodium Polystyrene Sulfonate

Pharmacologic class: Cation exchange resin

Therapeutic class: Potassium-removing resin

Pregnancy risk category C

Action

Releases sodium ions in exchange for potassium ions in intestines; potassium is then eliminated in feces, resulting in decreased serum potassium levels

Availability

Oral or rectal powder for suspension: 1.25 g/5 ml
Suspension: 15 g/60 ml

🕖 Indications and dosages

➤ Hyperkalemia

Adults: 15 g P.O. one to four times daily in water or syrup, or 30 to 50 g P.R. q 6 hours; may instill through nasogastric tube as necessary

Contraindications

• Hypersensitivity to drug
• Severe hyperkalemia
• Hypokalemia or other electrolyte imbalances

Administration

• Know that drug may take hours to days to lower serum potassium level; thus, it shouldn't be used alone for severe hyperkalemia.
• For rectal use, mix resin in water or sorbitol only; never use mineral oil. Insert #28F rubber tube 20 cm into sigmoid colon, and tape it in place. Or use indwelling urinary catheter with a 30-ml balloon inflated distal to anal sphincter. Keep rectal solution at room temperature; swirl gently while administering. After giving dose, flush tubing with approximately 100 ml of sodium-free fluid; then flush rectum to remove drug residue.
• In elderly patients prone to fecal impaction, give cleansing enema before sodium polystyrene enema.

Route	Onset	Peak	Duration
P.O.	2-12 hr	Unknown	Unknown
P.R.	Unknown	Unknown	Unknown

Adverse reactions

GI: nausea, vomiting, constipation, fecal impaction, gastric irritation, anorexia
Metabolic: hypokalemia, sodium retention, other electrolyte abnormalities

Interactions

Drug-drug. *Antacids, laxatives:* systemic alkalosis
Drug-diagnostic tests. *Calcium, magnesium, potassium:* decreased levels
Sodium: increased level

Precautions

Use cautiously in:
• renal or heart failure, severe edema or hypertension
• pregnant patients.

Patient monitoring

• Monitor electrolyte levels; watch for signs and symptoms of electrolyte imbalances (particularly sodium overload).
• Monitor bowel movements; initiate measures to prevent or correct constipation or diarrhea, as needed.

Patient teaching

• Tell patient that drug may cause constipation (or diarrhea, if given with sorbitol); instruct him to report these problems.

S

• Teach patient about recommended diet (generally, low in sodium and potassium).
• For oral use, instruct patient to mix drug only with water, syrup, or sorbitol—never with orange juice.
• Advise patient to refrigerate oral solution to improve taste.
• As appropriate, review all other significant adverse reactions and interactions, especially those related to the drugs and tests mentioned above.

somatropin

Genotropin, Genotropin Miniquick, Humatrope, Norditropin, Nutropin, Nutropin AQ, Nutropin Depot, Saizen, Serostim

Pharmacologic class: Posterior pituitary hormone
Therapeutic class: Growth hormone (GH)
Pregnancy risk category C, B (Genotropin, Saizen, Serostim)

Action

Stimulates linear and skeletal growth, increases number and size of muscle cells, and influences internal organ size

Availability

Genotropin injection: 1.5 mg (about 4 IU/vial), 5.8 mg (about 15 IU/vial), 13.8 mg (about 41.4 IU/vial)
Genotropin Miniquick injection: 0.2 mg/vial, 0.4 mg/vial, 0.6 mg/vial, 0.8 mg/vial, 1 mg/vial, 1.2 mg/vial, 1.4 mg/vial, 1.6 mg/vial, 1.8 mg/vial, 2 mg/vial
Humatrope injection: 2 mg (about 6 IU/vial), 5 mg (about 15 IU/vial), 6 mg (about 18 IU/vial), 12 mg (about 36 IU/vial), 24 mg (about 72 IU/vial)
Norditropin injection: 4 mg (12 IU/vial), 8 mg (24 IU/vial)

Norditropin injection cartridge: 5 mg/1.5 ml, 10 mg/1.5 ml, 15 mg/1.5 ml
Nutropin AQ injection: 10 mg
Nutropin Depot: 13.5-mg, 18-mg, or 22.5-mg single-use vials; 13.5-mg, 18-mg, or 22.5-mg kits
Nutropin injection: 5 mg (about 15 IU/vial), 10 mg (about 30 IU/vial)
Saizem injection: 5 g (15 IU/vial)
Serostim injection: 5 mg (about 15 IU/vial), 6 mg (about 18 IU/ml)

Indications and dosages

➤ Long-term treatment of growth failure in children with inadequate secretion of endogenous GH
Children: 0.16 to 0.24 mg/kg (Genotropin) S.C. weekly in six or seven divided doses. Or 0.18 mg/kg/week (Humatrope) S.C. or I.M. divided equally and given on three alternate days six times weekly (or daily if epiphyseal closure hasn't occurred). Or 0.024 to 0.034 mg/kg (Norditropin) S.C. six or seven times weekly using NordiPen injection pen. Or 0.3 mg/kg/week (Nutropin or Nutropin AQ) S.C. in equally divided daily doses. Or 1.5 mg/kg (Nutropin Depot) S.C. monthly on same day each month or 0.75 mg/kg S.C. twice monthly on same days each month. Or 0.06 mg/kg (Saizen) S.C. or I.M. three times weekly.
➤ Replacement of endogenous GH in adults with GH deficiency
Adults: 0.04 mg/kg/week (Genotropin) S.C. in six or seven divided doses. Or 0.006 mg/kg/day (Humatrope) S.C. Or initially, no more than 0.006 mg/kg/day (Nutropin or Nutropin AQ) S.C.; may increase to a maximum of 0.025 mg/kg daily in patients under age 35 or 0.0125 mg/kg daily in patients over age 35.
➤ Long-term treatment of short stature related to Turner's syndrome
Children: 0.375 mg/kg/week (Humatrope) S.C. divided into equal doses given on 3 alternate days or daily. Or up to 0.375 mg/kg/week (Nutropin or

Nutropin AQ) S.C. divided into equal doses given three or seven times weekly.

➤ Long-term treatment of growth failure in children with Prader-Willi syndrome (confirmed by genetic testing)

Children: 0.24 mg/kg/week (Genotropin) S.C. in six or seven divided doses

➤ Infants born small for gestational age

Children: 0.48 mg/kg/week (Genotropin) S.C. in six or seven divided doses

➤ AIDS wasting or cachexia

Adults and children weighing more than 55 kg (121 lb): 6 mg (Serostim) S.C. at bedtime

Adults and children weighing 45 to 55 kg (99 to 121 lb): 5 mg (Serostim) S.C. at bedtime

Adults and children weighing 35 to 45 kg (77 to 99 lb): 4 mg (Serostim) S.C. at bedtime

Adults and children weighing less than 35 kg (77 lb): 0.1 mg/kg/day (Serostim) S.C. at bedtime

➤ Children with growth failure secondary to chronic renal insufficiency (up to time of renal transplantation)

Children: Up to 0.35 mg/kg/weekly (Nutropin or Nutropin AQ) S.C. divided in daily doses

Contraindications
• Hypersensitivity to drug, benzyl alcohol, glycerin, or metacresol (with some diluents)
• Active neoplasia
• Acute, critical illness after open-heart surgery, acute respiratory failure, or multiple trauma
• Children with closed epiphyses

Administration
• Reconstitute by injecting supplied diluent through rubber top of vial and aiming liquid stream at side of vial. Swirl vial gently to mix; don't shake.
• Inspect reconstituted solution; don't use if it has visible particles or is cloudy.

• Keep diluted drug refrigerated; use within 14 days.
• When using prefilled cartridges, follow manufacturer's instructions carefully.

Route	Onset	Peak	Duration
I.M., S.C.	Unknown	3-5 hr	12-48 hr

Adverse reactions
CNS: headache, weakness
CV: mild and transient edema
GU: hypercalciuria
Hematologic: leukemia
Metabolic: fluid retention, mild hyperglycemia, hypothyroidism, **ketosis**
Musculoskeletal: localized muscle pain, tissue swelling, joint pain
Skin: rash, urticaria
Other: pain, inflammation at injection site

Interactions
Drug-drug. *Androgens, thyroid hormone*: epiphyseal closure
Corticotrophin, corticosteroids: inhibited growth response (with long-term use)
Drug-diagnostic tests. *Alkaline phosphatase, glucose, inorganic phosphorus, parathyroid hormone*: increased levels

Precautions
Use cautiously in:
• hypothyroidism
• diabetes mellitus.

Patient monitoring
• Monitor patient's height, X-ray and blood chemistry results, blood glucose level, and thyroid function studies.
• Monitor for signs and symptoms of leukemia.

Patient teaching
• Advise patient and parents that regular check-ups and blood tests are needed to detect adverse reactions.
• Teach parents how to reconstitute and administer drug. Stress impor-

S

tance of following manufacturer's instructions carefully when using pre-filled cartridges.

• As appropriate, review all significant and life-threatening adverse reactions and interactions, especially those related to the drugs and tests mentioned above.

sotalol hydrochloride
Betapace, Betapace AF, Sotacor✽

Pharmacologic class: Beta-adrenergic blocker (nonselective)
Therapeutic class: Antiarrhythmic (classes II and III)
Pregnancy risk category B

Action
Blocks stimulation of cardiac beta$_1$-adrenergic and pulmonary, vascular, and uterine beta$_2$-adrenergic receptor sites; this action reduces cardiac output and blood pressure, depresses sinus heart rate, and prolongs refractory period of atrial and ventricular muscles.

Availability
Tablets: 80 mg, 120 mg, 160 mg, 240 mg
Tablets (Betapace AF): 80 mg, 120 mg, 160 mg

⭕ Indications and dosages
➤ Ventricular arrhythmias
Adults: 80 mg P.O. b.i.d. (Betapace); may increase dosage gradually. Usual maintenance dosage is 160 to 320 mg/day in two to three divided doses; some patients may require 480 to 640 mg/day in divided doses.
➤ Atrial fibrillation or atrial flutter
Adults: 80 mg P.O. b.i.d. (Betapace AF); with careful monitoring, may increase dosage to 120 mg b.i.d. as needed, to a maximum of 160 P.O. b.i.d.

Dosage adjustment
• Renal impairment

Contraindications
• Hypersensitivity to drug
• Heart failure
• Bronchial asthma, chronic obstructive pulmonary disease
• Congenital or acquired long-QT syndrome
• Sinus bradycardia, second- or third-degree atrioventricular (AV) block (unless patient has functioning pacemaker)

Administration
• Give drug 1 hour before or 2 hours after meals or antacids.
• Keep in mind that Betapace and Betapace AF are used for different indications and are not interchangeable or therapeutically equivalent.

Route	Onset	Peak	Duration
P.O.	Unknown	2-4 hr	8-12 hr

Adverse reactions
CNS: fatigue, weakness, anxiety, dizziness, drowsiness, insomnia, memory loss, depression, mental status changes, nervousness, paresthesia, nightmares
CV: orthostatic hypotension, peripheral vasoconstriction, bradycardia, **arrhythmias, heart failure, AV block**
EENT: blurred vision, dry eyes, nasal stuffiness
GI: nausea, constipation, diarrhea
GU: impotence, decreased libido
Metabolic: hyperglycemia, hypoglycemia
Musculoskeletal: joint pain, back pain, muscle cramps
Respiratory: wheezing, **bronchospasm**
Skin: itching, rashes
Other: lupus syndrome, hypersensitivity reaction

Interactions
Drug-drug. *Amphetamines, ephedrine, epinephrine, norepinephrine, phenyle-*

phrine, pseudoephedrine: unopposed alpha-adrenergic stimulation, causing excessive hypotension and bradycardia
Beta-adrenergic bronchodilators, theophylline: decreased efficacy of these drugs
Calcium channel blockers: increased risk of adverse cardiovascular reactions
Class IA antiarrhythmics (such as amiodarone, procainamide, quinidine): increased risk of arrhythmias
Clonidine: excessive rebound hypertension with clonidine discontinuation
Ergot alkaloids: peripheral ischemia or gangrene
General anesthetics, phenytoin (I.V.), verapamil: additive myocardial depression
Lidocaine: increased lidocaine blood level, resulting in toxicity
Sulfonylureas: increased hypoglycemic effect
Drug-diagnostic tests. *Antinuclear antibody:* increased titer
Blood urea nitrogen, glucose, lipoproteins, potassium, triglycerides, uric acid: increased levels
Drug-food. *Any food:* decreased drug absorption

Precautions

Use cautiously in:
• renal or hepatic impairment, hypokalemia, diabetes mellitus, hyperthyroidism
• history of severe allergic reactions
• elderly patients
• pregnant or breastfeeding patients
• children (safety not established).

Patient monitoring

• Monitor ECG, electrolyte levels, and vital signs closely for first 3 days of therapy.
• Evaluate closely for signs and symptoms of heart failure.
• In long-term use, watch for signs and symptoms of drug-induced lupus syndrome.

Patient teaching

• Tell patient that drug may cause significant cardiac effects; explain need for ECG monitoring during first few days of therapy.
◀€ Teach patient to recognize and immediately report signs or symptoms of heart failure and electrolyte imbalances.
• Inform patient that drug can cause serious interactions with many common drugs; instruct him to tell all prescribers he's taking it.
• Teach patient to recognize and promptly report signs and symptoms of drug-induced lupus syndrome.
• Advise patient that drug may cause CNS effects that increase his injury risk. Encourage him to use appropriate safety precautions.
• As appropriate, review all other significant and life-threatening adverse reactions and interactions, especially those related to the drugs, tests, foods, and behaviors mentioned above.

spironolactone
Aldactone, Novo-spiroton ✤

Pharmacologic class: Aldosterone inhibitor
Therapeutic class: Potassium-sparing diuretic
Pregnancy risk category D

S

Action

Inhibits the aldosterone effects in distal renal tubule, promoting sodium and water excretion and potassium retention

Availability

Tablets: 25 mg, 50 mg, 100 mg

✤ Canada   ◀€ Clinical alert   Reactions in **bold** are life-threatening

ⓘ Indications and dosages

➤ Edema associated with heart failure, hepatic cirrhosis, or nephrotic syndrome

Adults: As sole diuretic, initially 100 mg/day P.O. (range of 25 to 200 mg), continued for 5 or more days and then adjusted to optimal level

Children: 3.3 mg/kg/day P.O. as a single dose or in divided doses

➤ Essential hypertension

Adults: Initially, 50 to 100 mg/day P.O. as a single dose or in divided doses, continued for 2 weeks or more

Children: 1 to 2 mg/kg P.O. b.i.d.

➤ Diuretic-induced hypokalemia

Adults: 25 to 100 mg/day P.O.

➤ To diagnose primary hyperaldosteronism

Adults: 400 mg/day P.O. for 4 days (in short test) or for 3 to 4 weeks (in long test); or 400 mg/day P.O. for 3 to 4 weeks (in long test) after supplemental potassium therapy and normal diet for 5 days. If hypokalemia and hypertension resolve, a diagnosis of primary hyperaldosteronism is confirmed.

Off-label uses

• Acne vulgaris
• Familial male precocious puberty (with short-term combination therapy with testolactone)
• Premenstrual syndrome

Contraindications

• Hypersensitivity to drug
• Anuria
• Acute or chronic renal insufficiency
• Hyperkalemia
• Concurrent use of other potassium-sparing diuretics (such as amiloride, triamterene) or potassium supplements
• Pregnancy or breastfeeding

Administration

• Give the first dose of the day with breakfast. If patient takes two daily doses, give second with food in mid-afternoon.

Route	Onset	Peak	Duration
P.O.	Unknown	1-2 hr	2-3 days

Adverse reactions

CNS: headache, drowsiness, lethargy, ataxia, confusion

GI: vomiting, diarrhea, cramping, GI bleeding or ulcers, gastritis

GU: elevated blood urea nitrogen (BUN), gynecomastia, irregular menses or amenorrhea, postmenopausal bleeding, erectile dysfunction, **breast cancer**

Hematologic: agranulocytosis

Metabolic: hyponatremia, **hyperchloremic metabolic acidosis**, **hyperkalemia**

Skin: rash, pruritus, hirsutism

Other: deepening of voice, drug fever

Interactions

Drug-drug. *Angiotensin-converting enzyme inhibitors, potassium-sparing diuretics, potassium supplements, other potassium-containing drugs:* increased risk of hyperkalemia

Anticoagulants, heparin: decreased hypoprothrombinemic effects of these drugs

Digoxin: increased digoxin blood level

Salicylates: decreased diuretic effect

Drug-diagnostic tests. *BUN, potassium:* increased levels

Digoxin assays: false digoxin elevation

Granulocytes: decreased count

Drug-food. *Potassium-containing salt substitutes:* increased risk of hyperkalemia

Drug-herb. *Licorice:* potassium loss

Precautions

Use cautiously in:
• hepatic dysfunction, diabetes mellitus, fluid and electrolyte imbalances
• elderly or debilitated patients
• children (safety not established).

Patient monitoring

• Monitor electrolyte levels (especially potassium); watch for signs and symptoms of imbalances and metabolic acidosis.

• Monitor weight and fluid intake and output; stay alert for indications of fluid imbalance.

• Monitor complete blood cell count with white cell differential.

Patient teaching

• Teach patient to take daily dose with breakfast. If he takes two daily doses, advise him to take second with food in mid-afternoon.

• Advise patient to restrict intake of high-potassium foods and to avoid licorice and salt substitutes containing potassium.

• Tell male patient that drug may cause breast enlargement.

• Instruct patient to avoid driving and other hazardous activities until he knows how drug affects concentration and alertness.

• As appropriate, review all other significant and life-threatening adverse reactions and interactions, especially those related to the drugs, tests, foods, and herbs mentioned above.

stavudine (d4T)
Zerit, Zerit XR

Pharmacologic class: Nucleoside reverse transcriptase inhibitor
Therapeutic class: Antiretroviral
Pregnancy risk category C

Action

Inhibits replication of human immunodeficiency virus (HIV) by interfering with enzyme reverse transcriptase, which terminates the DNA chain

Availability

Capsules: 15 mg, 20 mg, 30 mg, 40 mg
Capsules (extended-release): 37.5 mg, 50 mg, 75 mg, 100 mg
Powder for oral solution: 1 mg/ml

Indications and dosages

➢ HIV-1 infection (given with other antiretrovirals)
Adults weighing 60 kg (132 lb) or more: 40 mg P.O. q 12 hours or 100 mg (extended-release) P.O. once daily
Adults weighing less than 60 kg (132 lb): 30 mg P.O. q 12 hours or 75 mg (extended-release) P.O. once daily
Children weighing 30 kg (66 lb) or more: 30 mg P.O. q 12 hours
Children older than 14 days who weigh less than 30 kg (66 lb): 1 mg/kg P.O. q 12 hours
Dosage adjustment
• Renal impairment
• Elderly patients

Contraindications

• Hypersensitivity to drug or its components

Administration

• Give with or without food.

Route	Onset	Peak	Duration
P.O.	Variable	60-90 min	Unknown
P.O. (extended)	Unknown	3 hr	Unknown

Adverse reactions

CNS: headache, insomnia, peripheral neuropathy
GI: nausea, vomiting, diarrhea, abdominal pain, anorexia, increased amylase and lipase levels, **pancreatitis**
Hematologic: anemia, **leukopenia, thrombocytopenia**
Hepatic: increased alanine aminotransferase (ALT), aspartate aminotransferase (AST), bilirubin, and gamma-glutamyl transferase (GGT) levels; **hepatic steatosis; hepatitis; hepatic failure**

S

Metabolic: increased glucose tolerance, **lactic acidosis**
Musculoskeletal: myalgia
Skin: rash
Other: chills, fever, allergic reaction

Interactions

Drug-drug. *Chloramphenicol, dapsone, didanosine, ethambutol, hydralazine, hydroxyurea, lithium, phenytoin, vincristine, zalcitabine:* increased risk of peripheral neuropathy
Doxorubicin, ribavarin, zidovudine: inhibition of stavudine's absorption and metabolism
Myelosuppressants: increased bone marrow depression
Drug-diagnostic tests. *Amylase, AST, ALT, bilirubin, GGT, lipase:* increased levels
Neutrophils, platelets: decreased counts

Precautions

Use cautiously in:
• bone marrow depression, renal or hepatic failure, advanced HIV infection, peripheral neuropathy
• pregnant or breastfeeding patients.

Patient monitoring

◀€ Monitor closely for signs and symptoms of lactic acidosis; consult prescriber about discontinuing therapy if these occur.
• Watch for and report onset and worsening of peripheral neuropathy.
• Monitor complete blood cell count; report signs and symptoms of bone marrow depression.
• Monitor liver function tests and blood chemistry results.

Patient teaching

• Tell patient he may take drug with or without food.
◀€ Teach patient to recognize and promptly report signs and symptoms of lactic acidosis (such as fatigue, GI distress, or difficult or rapid breathing).

• Instruct patient to report numbness or tingling in arms, legs, hands, or feet.
• As appropriate, review all other significant and life-threatening adverse reactions and interactions, especially those related to the drugs and tests mentioned above.

streptokinase
Streptase

Pharmacologic class: Group C beta-hemolytic streptococcal nonenzymatic protein
Therapeutic class: Thrombolytic
Pregnancy risk category C

Action

Converts plasminogen to plasmin, an enzyme that degrades fibrin clots and lyses thrombi and emboli; exerts activity at site of clot

Availability

Powder for injection: 250,000 IU/vial, 750,000 IU/vial, 1.5 million IU/vial

🛈 Indications and dosages

➤ Acute evolving transmural myocardial infarction
Adults: 1.5 million IU by I.V. infusion over 60 minutes as soon as possible after symptom onset. For intracoronary infusion, 20,000 IU bolus via coronary catheter followed by 2,000 IU/minute infusion for 60 minutes (total dosage of 140,000 IU).
➤ Deep-vein thrombosis (DVT)
Adults: Loading dose of 250,000 IU by I.V. infusion over 30 minutes, followed by 100,000 IU/hour I.V. for 72 hours. Begin therapy as soon as possible after thrombotic symptoms begin (preferably within 7 days).
➤ Pulmonary emboli
Adults: Loading dose of 250,000 IU by I.V. infusion over 30 minutes, followed

by 100,000 IU/hour I.V. for 24 hours (or for 72 hours if concurrent DVT is suspected). Begin therapy as soon as possible after onset of thrombotic symptoms (preferably within 7 days).

➤ Arterial thrombosis or emboli

Adults: Loading dose of 250,000 IU by I.V. infusion over 30 minutes, followed by 100,000 IU/hour I.V. for 24 to 72 hours. Begin therapy as soon as possible after onset of thrombotic symptoms (preferably within 7 days).

Contraindications

• Hypersensitivity to drug or anistreplase
• Use of drug within past 2 years
• Active bleeding
• Active peptic ulcer
• Acute pericarditis
• Aortic dissection
• Atrioventricular malformation or aneurysm
• Suspected thrombus in left side of heart
• Infectious endocarditis
• Intracranial neoplasm or vascular disease
• Organ biopsy
• Septic thrombophlebitis or occluded arteriovenous cannula at seriously infected site
• Severe hepatic or renal disease
• Severe, uncontrolled hypertension
• History of cerebrovascular disease
• Previous puncture of noncompressible blood vessels
• Recent major surgery or trauma
• Obstetric delivery
• Concurrent anticoagulant use
• Patients ages 75 and older

Administration

◀ Before giving drug, make sure hydrocortisone is available to treat allergic reaction and aminocaproic acid is available to treat excessive bleeding.

◀ As ordered, give test dose of 100 IU intradermally to check for hypersensitivity. Wheal-and-flare response

within 20 minutes indicates probable allergy.

• To reconstitute, add 5 ml of normal saline solution or dextrose 5% in water to each vial, then dilute again to 45 ml. Roll vial gently between hands; don't shake.
• If necessary, dilute drug further to 50 ml in plastic container or 500 ml in glass bottle.
• When filtering I.V. solution, use filter with pores of 0.8 micron or larger; use solution within 8 hours of reconstitution. (Refrigerate solution if it's not used right away.)
• Don't mix with other drugs or give other drugs through same I.V. line.

Route	Onset	Peak	Duration
I.V.	Immediate	1 hr	4 hr
Intra-coronary	Unknown	Unknown	Unknown

Adverse reactions

CNS: headache, **intracranial hemorrhage**
CV: hypotension, **arrhythmias**
EENT: periorbital swelling
GI: nausea, vomiting, **GI hemorrhage**
GU: hematuria
Hematologic: anemia, **bleeding tendency**
Musculoskeletal: musculoskeletal pain
Respiratory: minor breathing difficulties, **bronchospasm, apnea**
Skin: urticaria, itching, flushing
Other: bleeding at puncture sites, delayed hypersensitivity reaction

Interactions

Drug-drug. *Anticoagulants, aspirin, dipyridamole, indomethacin, phenylbutazone:* increased risk of bleeding
Drug-diagnostic tests. *Hemoglobin:* decreased value
International Normalized Ratio, transaminases: increased values
Partial thromboplastin time (PTT), prothrombin time (PT): prolonged

Precautions
Use cautiously in:
• conditions in which bleeding may prove difficult to manage
• pregnant or breastfeeding patients.

Patient monitoring
• Monitor vital signs and neurologic status carefully after giving test dose and then throughout therapy.
◄€ Watch for signs and symptoms of hypersensitivity reaction; stop drug if these occur.
• Check for bleeding every 15 minutes for first hour, then every 30 minutes for next 7 hours, and then every 4 hours.
◄€ Stop therapy and contact prescriber immediately if excessive bleeding occurs.
• Assess neurologic status closely; watch for indications of intracranial bleeding.
• Handle patient gently and sparingly; if necessary, pad bed rails to prevent injury.
• Monitor pulse hourly; also monitor distal circulation and sensation to extremities.
• Monitor PTT, PT, plasma thrombin time, hemoglobin, hematocrit, and platelet level.
• Avoid giving I.M. injections.

Patient teaching
• Teach patient why he's receiving drug.
◄€ Teach patient to recognize and immediately report signs or symptoms of hypersensitivity reaction or excessive bleeding.
• Instruct patient to report unusual bruising or bleeding. Teach him safety measures to avoid bruising and bleeding.
• Tell patient he'll undergo regular blood testing during therapy.
• As appropriate, review all other significant and life-threatening adverse reactions and interactions, especially those related to the drugs and tests mentioned above.

streptomycin sulfate

Pharmacologic class: Aminoglycoside
Therapeutic class: Anti-infective
Pregnancy risk category D

Action
Binds to 30S ribosomal subunits inhibiting protein synthesis in bacterial cells; causing misreading of genetic code and ultimately, bacterial death

Availability
Injection: 400 mg/ml in 2.5-ml ampules, 200 mg/ml in 1-g vials

💊 Indications and dosages
➤ Adjunct in tuberculosis and other mycobacterial infections
Adults: 15 mg/kg/day I.M., up to 1 g/day, given with other antituberculotics.
Children: 20 to 40 mg/kg I.M. daily, up to 1 g/day
➤ Enteroccocal or streptococcal infections
Adults: 1 g I.M. b.i.d. for 1 week, followed by 500 mg I.M. b.i.d. for 1 week. For enterococcal endocarditis, 1 g I.M. b.i.d. given with penicillin for 1 week, followed by 500 mg I.M. b.i.d. for 4 weeks.
➤ Brucellosis
Adults: 1 g I.M. once or twice daily with tetracycline or doxycycline for 1 week, then once daily for at least one additional week
➤ Tularemia
Adults: 1 to 2 g I.M. daily in divided doses for 7 to 14 days until patient is afebrile for 5 to 7 days. For tularemia caused by *Francisella tularensis* (as from bioterrorism or biologic warfare), 1 g I.M. b.i.d. for 10 days or 7.5 to 10 mg/kg I.M. b.i.d. for 10 to 14 days.

➤ Plague caused by *Yersinis pestis* (as from bioterrorism or biologic warfare)
Adults: 1 g I.M. b.i.d. for 10 to 14 days
Dosage adjustment
• Renal impairment
• Elderly patients

Off-label uses
• *Mycobacterium avium-intracellulare* complex in AIDS patients

Contraindications
• Hypersensitivity to drug, other aminoglycosides, or bisulfites
• Labyrinthine disease
• Pregnancy or breastfeeding

Administration
• Inject I.M. deep into upper outer quadrant of buttock.
• Alternate injection sites.
• Know that streptomycin will be discontinued after several months or when bacteriologic smears are negative and other antituberculars are continued for 1 year.

Route	Onset	Peak	Duration
I.M.	Rapid	30-90 min	Unknown

Adverse reactions
CNS: vertigo, myasthenia gravis–like syndrome, numbness and tingling, peripheral neuropathy, **neuromuscular blockade, seizures**
CV: myocarditis
EENT: amblyopia, ototoxicity
GI : nausea, vomiting
GU: azotemia, **nephrotoxicity**
Hematologic: eosinophilia, hemolytic anemia, **pancytopenia, leukopenia, thrombocytopenia**
Hepatic: hepatic necrosis
Musculoskeletal: muscle weakness, twitching
Respiratory: apnea
Skin: rash, urticaria, exfoliative dermatitis, toxic epidermal necrolysis, angioedema

Other: fever, superinfection, serum sickness, **anaphylaxis**

Interactions
Drug-drug. *Acyclovir, amphotericin B, cephalosporins, cisplatin, potent diuretics, vancomycin:* increased risk of ototoxicity and nephrotoxicity
Depolarizing and nondepolarizing neuromuscular junction blockers, general anesthetics: potentiation of neuromuscular blockade
Dimenhydrinate: masking of ototoxicity symptoms
Indomethacin: increased streptomycin peak and trough blood levels
Parenteral penicillins (ampicillin, ticarcillin): streptomycin inactivation
Drug-diagnostic tests. *Bilirubin, blood urea nitrogen, creatinine, lactate dehydrogenase, nonprotein nitrogen:* increased levels
Granulocytes, hemoglobin, platelets, white blood cells: decreased levels

Precautions
Use cautiously in:
• renal impairment, hearing impairment, neuromuscular disease (such as myasthenia gravis)
• elderly patients
• infants and neonates (safety not established).

Patient monitoring
• Evaluate peak drug level 1 hour after I.M. injection; draw blood for trough level just before next dose.
• Monitor liver and kidney function tests; watch for signs and symptoms of hepatotoxicity and nephrotoxicity.
• Monitor temperature; stay alert for fever and other signs and symptoms of superinfection.
• Assess neurologic status and sensory function carefully; especially watch for neurotoxicity, neuromuscular blockade, and seizures.
• Assess for signs and symptoms of ototoxicity.

S

• Monitor complete blood count; watch for indications of blood dyscrasias.

Patient teaching

• Instruct patient to report unusual bleeding or bruising.

◀℥ Inform patient that drug can be toxic to many body systems; teach him to recognize and immediately report serious adverse reactions.

◀℥ Tell patient that drug may promote growth of certain organisms; instruct him to immediately report signs and symptoms of superinfection.

• Tell patient drug may impair cognitive, motor, and sensory function. Advise him to use caution during driving and other hazardous activities.

• Tell patient he'll undergo regular blood testing during therapy.

• As appropriate, review all other significant and life-threatening adverse reactions and interactions, especially those related to the drugs and tests mentioned above.

succimer
Chemet

Pharmacologic class: Chelating agent
Therapeutic class: Antidote
Pregnancy risk category C

Action
Increases urinary elimination of lead while decreasing blood lead level and reducing target organ damage in lead poisoning

Availability
Capsules: 100 mg

🕖 Indications and dosages
➤ Lead poisoning in children with blood lead levels above 45 mcg/dl

Children: 10 mg/kg P.O. or 350 mg/m^2 P.O. q 8 hours for 5 days; then decrease to 10 mg/kg P.O. or 350 mg/m^2 P.O. q 12 hours for 2 weeks. Treatment lasts 19 days; repeated courses should follow 2-week rest period.

Off-label uses
• Prophylaxis of renal calculi in patients with homozygous cystinuria or mercury intoxication

Contraindications
• Hypersensitivity to drug

Administration
• Don't give succimer with other chelating drugs.
• For young children who can't swallow capsule, open capsule and sprinkle contents onto soft food or have them take it with fruit juice.

Route	Onset	Peak	Duration
P.O.	Rapid	2-4 hr	Unknown

Adverse reactions
CNS: dizziness, drowsiness, fatigue, headache, paresthesia, sensorimotor neuropathy
CV: arrhythmias
EENT: watery eyes, cloudy film in eye, otitis media, plugged-ear sensation, nasal congestion, rhinorrhea, sore throat
GI: nausea, vomiting, diarrhea, abdominal cramps, hemorrhoidal symptoms, metallic taste, anorexia
GU: oliguria, proteinuria, voiding difficulty
Hematologic: eosinophilia, thrombocytosis
Hepatic: elevated liver function test results
Musculoskeletal: back, rib, flank, or leg pain
Respiratory: cough
Skin: mucocutaneous eruptions, pruritus, rash

Other: chills, fever, flulike symptoms, moniliasis

Interactions
Drug-drug. *Chelating agents:* increased risk of adverse reactions to succimer
Drug-diagnostic tests. *Alkaline phosphatase, cholesterol, eosinophils, platelets, transaminases:* elevated levels
Creatine phosphokinase, uric acid: false decrease
Urine ketones measured with Ketostix: false-positive result

Precautions
Use cautiously in:
• renal failure
• pregnant or breastfeeding patients
• children younger than age 1 (safety not established).

Patient monitoring
• Monitor lead blood level weekly, and compare with baseline level. After therapy ends, monitor lead level initially for rebound increase.
• Assess ongoing response to therapy.
• Evaluate transaminase levels before therapy starts, and then weekly.
• Monitor vital signs, especially for arrhythmias.
◀€ Monitor complete blood count with white cell differential. Stop drug and contact prescriber if neutrophil count drops below 1,200/mm³.
• Watch for rash and other signs and symptoms of allergic reaction.
• Monitor fluid intake and output and nutritional status.

Patient teaching
• Tell parents to give capsules with or without food. If child can't swallow capsule, advise them to open capsule and sprinkle onto soft food or to have him take it with fruit juice.
• Emphasize importance of adequate fluid intake; teach parents to check that child's urinary output is appropriate for amount of fluid intake.

• Teach patient and parents to recognize and report rash and other signs and symptoms of allergic reaction.
• Advise parents that drug may cause CNS effects, such as dizziness and drowsiness; recommend appropriate safety measures.
• Refer parents to appropriate authorities to help them locate and remove environmental lead.
• Tell parents that child must undergo regular blood testing during therapy and for a period afterward.
• As appropriate, review all other significant and life-threatening adverse reactions and interactions, especially those related to the drugs and tests mentioned above.

succinylcholine chloride
Anectine, Anectine Flo-Pack, Quelicin

Pharmacologic class: Depolarizing neuromuscular blocker
Therapeutic class: Skeletal muscle relaxant
Pregnancy risk category C

Action
Produces skeletal muscle relaxation by decreasing response of nerve impulse transmission at cholinergic receptor sites and decreasing action of acetylcholine

Availability
Injection: 20 mg/ml, 50 mg/ml, 100 mg/ml, 500-mg vial, 1-g vial

Indications and dosages
➤ Adjunct to anesthesia to produce skeletal muscle relaxation during short surgical procedures; endotracheal intubation with mechanical ventilation; electrically induced convulsive therapy
Adults: 0.6 mg/kg I.V. given over 10 to 30 seconds; or give by continuous I.V.

infusion at 0.5 to 10 mg/minute; or give 0.04 to 0.07 mg/kg I.V. intermittently p.r.n.

Contraindications
• Hypersensitivity to drug or its components
• Genetic plasma pseudocholinesterase disorders
• Acute closed-angle glaucoma
• Myopathies associated with creatine kinase elevation
• Penetrating eye injury
• Personal or family history of malignant hyperthermia

Administration
◀€ Make sure patient has received sedatives or general anesthesia before administering.
◀€ Ensure that emergency resuscitation equipment is at hand before giving drug.
• As ordered, give test dose of 5 to 10 mg I.V. after anesthesia administration. Drug may be given if patient experiences no respiratory depression or if respiratory depression is transient (up to 5 minutes). Don't give drug if patient experiences respiratory paralysis sufficient to necessitate endotracheal intubation.
• For I.V. use, reconstitute with dextrose 5% in water or normal saline solution; administer via intermittent or continuous I.V. infusion. Don't mix with alkaline solutions, such as sodium bicarbonate, barbiturates, or thiopental sodium.
• Although I.V. route is preferred, drug may be given by deep I.M. injection into deltoid muscle in children if vein isn't accessible.

Route	Onset	Peak	Duration
I.V.	0.5-1 min	1-2 min	4-10 min
I.M.	2-3 min	Unknown	10-30 min

Adverse reactions
CV: flushing, tachycardia, hypertension, hypotension, bradycardia, **arrhythmias, cardiac arrest**
EENT: increased intraocular pressure
GI: excessive salivation
Hematologic: myoglobulinemia
Musculoskeletal: muscle fasciculations, postoperative muscle pain
Respiratory: prolonged respiratory depression, apnea, bronchoconstriction
Skin: rash, flushing, pruritus, urticaria
Other: hypersensitivity reaction, **anaphylaxis, malignant hyperthermia**

Interactions
Drug-drug. *Aminoglycosides (such as amikacin, gentamicin, kanamycin, streptomycin), anticholinesterases (such as echothiophate, edrophonium, neostigmine, physostigmine, pyridostigmine), general anesthetics (such as enflurane, halothane, isoflurane), polymyxin antibiotics (such as colistin, polymyxin B sulfate):* increased neuromuscular blockade
Amphotericin B, thiazide diuretics: increased succinylcholine effects
Cardiac glycosides: arrhythmias
Cyclophosphamide, lithium, monoamine oxidase inhibitors: prolonged apnea
Diazepam: prolonged neuromuscular blockade
Magnesium sulfate (given parenterally), methotrimeprazine, opioid analgesics: enhanced neuromuscular blockade leading to skeletal muscle relaxation and possible respiratory paralysis
Opioid analgesics: increased risk of bradycardia and sinus arrest
Drug-diagnostic tests. *Myoglobin, potassium:* increased levels
Drug-herb. *Melatonin:* potentiation of neuromuscular blockade

Precautions
Use cautiously in:
• renal, hepatic, or pulmonary impair-

ment; severe burns or trauma; electrolyte imbalances; spinal injury; cerebrovascular accident; neuromuscular disease; myasthenic syndrome related to lung cancer; dehydration; thyroid disorders; collagen disease; porphyria; pheochromocytoma; eye surgery; cesarean section
• elderly or debilitated patients
• breastfeeding patients
• children younger than age 2.

Patient monitoring
◀€ Watch for potentially fatal adverse reactions, including anaphylaxis, malignant hyperthermia, and hypersensitivity reactions.
• Monitor ECG and vital signs (especially respirations) until patient recovers fully from neuromuscular blockade.
• Assess recovery from neuromuscular blockade by checking hand grip, head lift, and voluntary cough response.

Patient teaching
• Teach patient why he'll receive drug; reassure him that he'll be monitored closely until he recovers fully from neuromuscular blockade.

sucralfate
Carafate, Sulcrate✢,
PMS-Sucralfate✢, Nu-Sucralfate✢

Pharmacologic class: GI protectant
Therapeutic class: Antiulcer agent
Pregnancy risk category B

Action
Reacts with gastric acid to form a protective coating on the surface of the ulcer, inhibiting gastric acid secretion, pepsin, and bile salts

Availability
Oral suspension: 500 mg/5 ml
Tablets: 1 g

⏣ Indications and dosages
➢ Active duodenal ulcer
Adults: 1 g P.O. q.i.d. 1 hour before meals and at bedtime for 4 to 8 weeks; maintenance dosage is 1 g P.O. b.i.d.

Off-label uses
• Gastroesophageal reflux
• GI symptoms caused by nonsteroidal anti-inflammatory drugs (including aspirin)
• Prevention of stress ulcers and GI bleeding in critically ill patients
• Oral and esophageal ulcers caused by radiation, chemotherapy, or sclerotherapy (oral suspension)

Contraindications
• Hypersensitivity to drug

Administration
• When giving through nasogastric tube, reconstitute drug and flush tube with water after administration.

Route	Onset	Peak	Duration
P.O.	Unknown	Unknown	6 hr

Adverse reactions
EENT: rhinitis
GI: constipation
Respiratory: respiratory difficulty
Skin: pruritus, rash
Other: facial swelling, hypersensitivity reaction

Interactions
Drug-drug. *Aluminum-containing antacids:* increased total body burden of aluminum
Anticoagulants: decreased hypoprothrombinemic effect
Diclofenac: decreased pharmacologic effects of diclofenac
Digoxin, quinidine: reduced blood levels and efficacy of these drugs

S

Histamine$_2$-receptor antagonists (such as cimetidine, ranitidine), fluoroquinolones, ketoconazole, tetracyclines, theophylline: decreased bioavailability of these drugs

Levothyroxine, penicillamine: decreased efficacy of these drugs

Phenytoin: decreased phenytoin absorption

Precautions

Use cautiously in:
- renal failure
- pregnant or breastfeeding patients
- children.

Patient monitoring

- Monitor bowel pattern; report severe, ongoing constipation.
- Assess for rash and itching.

Patient teaching

- Teach patient to take drug 1 hour before meals and again at bedtime.
- Caution patient not to take drug within 30 minutes of antacids or other drugs.
- Explain importance of completing entire course of therapy as prescribed, even after pain and other ulcer symptoms improve.
- As appropriate, review all other significant adverse reactions and interactions, especially those related to the drugs mentioned above.

sufentanil
Sufenta

Pharmacologic class: Opioid agonist

Therapeutic class: Narcotic agonist, analgesic

Controlled substance schedule II

Pregnancy risk category C

Action

Acts on selective opioid receptors, causing respiratory and CNS depression

Availability

Injection: 50 mcg/ml

Indications and dosages

➤ Adjunct to general anesthesia and oxygen therapy

Adults: Initially, 1 to 2 mcg/kg I.V.; maintenance dosage is 10 to 25 mcg/kg. Don't exceed 1 mcg/hour of expected surgical time.

➤ Epidural analgesia in labor and delivery

Adults: 10 to 15 mcg given epidurally with bupivacaine, with or without epinephrine; may repeat twice at intervals of more than 1 hour, to a total of three doses

Contraindications

- Hypersensitivity to drug or other opioids
- Acute or severe bronchial asthma
- Upper airway obstruction
- Significant respiratory depression
- During labor when delivery of premature neonate is anticipated
- Premature neonates

Administration

- Know that drug should be given only by health care professionals specifically trained in using I.V. and epidural anesthetics and managing respiratory effects of potent opioids.
- Keep resuscitative and intubation equipment and oxygen at hand.

Route	Onset	Peak	Duration
I.V.	Immediate	Unknown	Unknown

Adverse reactions

CNS: sedation, headache, vertigo, floating feeling, dizziness, lethargy, confusion, light-headedness, nervousness, unusual dreams, agitation, euphoria, hallucinations, delirium, insomnia,

anxiety, fear, disorientation, impaired mental and physical performance, coma, mood changes, weakness, tremor
CV: palpitations, circulatory depression, blood pressure changes, tachycardia, bradycardia, **arrhythmias, cardiac arrest, shock**
EENT: diplopia, blurred vision
GI: nausea, vomiting, constipation, biliary tract spasm, dry mouth, anorexia, elevated amylase and lipase levels
GU: urinary retention, oliguria, ureteral spasm, vesical sphincter spasm, antidiuretic effect, reduced libido or potency
Hepatic: abnormal liver function test results
Musculoskeletal: intraoperative muscle movement
Respiratory: slow and shallow respirations, suppressed cough reflex, **apnea, laryngospasm, bronchospasm**
Skin: clamminess, sweating, erythema
Other: hypersensitivity reaction

Interactions

Drug-drug. *Barbiturate anesthetics:* enhanced barbiturate effects
Beta-adrenergic blockers, calcium channel blockers: increased risk of hypotension, bradycardia
CNS depressants: additive CNS depression
Drug-diagnostic tests. *Amylase, lipase:* increased levels
Liver function tests: abnormal results

Precautions

Use cautiously in:
• hepatic disease, head injury, diabetes mellitus, arrhythmias, renal or pulmonary disease, obesity
• pregnant or breastfeeding patients
• children (safety and efficacy not established).

Patient monitoring

◀€ Monitor ECG and vital signs; stay alert for signs and symptoms of shock or impending cardiac arrest.

• Assess airway patency carefully; watch for respiratory depression and airway spasms.
• Monitor neurologic status during and after administration; institute safety measures as needed to prevent injury.
• Monitor fluid intake and output; watch for oliguria or urinary retention.

Patient teaching

• Explain use of drug; reassure patient he'll be monitored closely.

---

sumatriptan succinate
Imitrex

Pharmacologic class: Selective 5-hydroxytryptamine$_1$ (5-HT$_1$) agonist
Therapeutic class: Vascular headache suppressant
Pregnancy risk category C

Action

Selectively activates vascular 5-HT$_1$ receptor sites, causing vasoconstriction in intracranial arteries

Availability

Injection: 6 mg/0.5-ml prefilled syringes, 0.6 mg/0.5-ml vials, SELF dose injection kit (containing two prefilled syringes)
Nasal spray: 5 mg in 100-mcl unit dose spray device (package of six), 20 mg in 100-mcl unit dose spray device (package of six)
Tablets: 25 mg, 50 mg, 100 mg

⚕ Indications and dosages
➤ Acute migraine
Adults: Initially, 25 mg P.O.; if response is inadequate after 2 hours, may give up to 100 mg P.O. If migraine recurs, repeat dose q 2 hours, not to exceed 200 mg/day. Or 6 mg S.C., repeated as needed after 1 hour, not to exceed

S

12 mg in 24 hours. If P.O. therapy will follow S.C. injection, additional P.O. sumatriptan may be given q 2 hours, not to exceed 100 mg/day. Or a single dose of 5, 10, or 20 mg intranasally in one nostril, repeated as needed in 2 hours, not to exceed 40 mg in 24 hours or treatment of more than five episodes per month.

Dosage adjustment
• Hepatic impairment

Contraindications
• Hypersensitivity to drug
• Ischemic heart disease (or signs and symptoms of such), Prinzmetal's angina, uncontrolled hypertension
• Monoamine (MAO) inhibitor use within 14 days
• Ergotamine use within 24 hours

Administration
◀€ If patient has risk factors for coronary artery disease, know that first dose should be given in medical setting with emergency equipment available.

Route	Onset	Peak	Duration
P.O.	Within 30 min	2-2.5 hr	Unknown
S.C.	10-20 min	Unknown	Unknown
Intranasal	Unknown	Unknown	Unknown

Adverse reactions
CNS: dizziness, vertigo, anxiety, drowsiness, fatigue, headache, malaise, tight feeling in head, numbness
CV: angina, chest pressure or tightness, transient hypertension, ECG changes, **coronary vasospasm, myocardial infarction**
EENT: vision changes, nasal sinus discomfort, throat discomfort
GI: abdominal discomfort, dysphagia
Musculoskeletal: jaw discomfort, muscle cramps, myalgia, neck pain or stiffness
Skin: tingling; warm, cool or, burning sensation; flushing

Other: injection site reaction; feeling of heaviness or tightness

Interactions
Drug-drug. *Dihydroergotamine, ergotamine, methysergide:* increased risk of vasospastic reaction
Lithium, MAO inhibitors, selective serotonin reuptake inhibitors: weakness, hyperreflexia, incoordination
Drug-herb. *Horehound:* enhanced serotonergic effects

Precautions
Use cautiously in:
• patients with cardiovascular risk factors (hypertension, hypercholesterolemia, smoking, obesity, diabetes, family history of cardiovascular disease, men over age 40, menopausal women)
• elderly patients
• women of childbearing age
• pregnant or breastfeeding patients
• children younger than age 18 (safety not established).

Patient monitoring
• Monitor cardiovascular status closely.
• Watch for neurologic and vision changes; institute safety measures as needed to prevent injury.
• Monitor patient's response to drug; assess need for repeat doses.
• Watch for injection site reaction, which should subside within 1 hour.

Patient teaching
• Instruct patient to take drug as soon as possible after onset of migraine symptoms.
◀€ Teach patient to recognize and immediately report serious cardiovascular reactions.
• Teach patient proper drug use. Emphasize that drug is effective only in treating diagnosed migraine, not other headache types; stress that it doesn't prevent migraine.
• With S.C. use, teach patient to inject dose using spring-loaded injector sys-

tem included in package. If headache recurs after dose, tell him he may take second dose, but should wait at least 1 hour after initial dose and shouldn't exceed two 6-mg injections in 24-hour period. Instruct him to report injection site reactions that don't subside within 1 hour.

• With oral use, tell patient he may take second dose 2 hours after first dose if migraine recurs. Tell him he may repeat oral doses every 2 hours as needed, up to 200 mg in a 24-hour period.

• With intranasal use, teach patient to spray 5, 10, or 20 mg into one nostril, as prescribed. Tell him he may repeat dose after 2 hours but shouldn't exceed 40 mg in a 24-hour period.

• Advise patient to avoid driving and other hazardous activities until he knows how drug affects concentration and alertness.

• As appropriate, review all other significant and life-threatening adverse reactions and interactions, especially those related to the drugs and herbs mentioned above.

tacrine hydrochloride
Cognex

Pharmacologic class: Cholinergic (cholinesterase inhibitor)
Therapeutic class: Anti-Alzheimer's agent
Pregnancy risk category C

Action
Inhibits acetylcholine breakdown in cerebral cortex, thereby increasing acetylcholine levels

Availability
Capsules: 10 mg, 20 mg, 30 mg, 40 mg

Indications and dosages
➤ Mild to moderate dementia associated with Alzheimer's disease
Adults: 10 mg P.O. q.i.d. for 4 weeks. If alanine aminotransferase (ALT) level remains unchanged, increase to 20 mg q.i.d. As tolerated, increase incrementally at 4-week intervals, up to 160 mg/day (30 to 40 mg P.O. q.i.d.).
Dosage adjustment
• Elevated transaminase levels

Contraindications
• Hypersensitivity to drug or other acridine derivatives
• Jaundice related to previous tacrine therapy
• Bilirubin level above 3 mg/dl
• Hypersensitivity symptoms accompanied by transaminase elevations

Administration
• Preferably, give drug 1 hour before or 2 hours after meals. However, if GI upset occurs, drug can be given with meals (although food slows its absorption).

Route	Onset	Peak	Duration
P.O.	Unknown	1-2 hr	Unknown

Adverse reactions
CNS: dizziness, headache, confusion, insomnia, tremor, ataxia, drowsiness, anxiety, agitation, depression, hallucinations, hostility, abnormal thinking, fatigue, malaise
CV: hypotension, hypertension, chest pain, peripheral edema
EENT: conjunctivitis, rhinitis, sinusitis, pharyngitis
GI: nausea, vomiting, diarrhea, constipation, dyspepsia, abdominal pain, anorexia
GU: urinary frequency or incontinence, urinary tract infection
Hepatic: elevated hepatic enzyme levels

Musculoskeletal: back pain, myalgia
Respiratory: upper respiratory infection, cough, bronchitis, pneumonia, dyspnea
Skin: rash, flushing, purpura
Other: chills, fever

Interactions
Drug-drug. *Anticholinergics:* interference with anticholinergic action
Cholinergics (including bethanecol), succinylcholine: synergistic effects
Cimetidine: increased tacrine blood level
Theophylline: increased theophylline blood level, greater risk of toxicity
Drug-diagnostic tests. *ALT:* increased level
Drug-food. *Any food:* decreased tacrine bioavailability

Precautions
Use cautiously in:
• sick sinus syndrome, hepatic or renal disease, bladder obstruction, asthma, seizure disorders, bradycardia, prostatic hyperplasia
• history of ulcers or increased risk of GI bleeding (as from concurrent use of nonsteroidal anti-inflammatory drugs)
• pregnant or breastfeeding patients
• children.

Patient monitoring
• Monitor neurologic status to assess drug efficacy and determine optimal dosage.
• Check ALT level weekly for first 18 weeks. If level hasn't changed markedly by end of this period, monitor level every 3 months. Otherwise, continue weekly monitoring.

Patient teaching
• Tell patient or caregiver that drug should be taken 1 hour before or 2 hours after meals.

• Advise caregiver to monitor patient's neurologic status carefully and to use safety measures at home as needed to prevent injury.
• Recommend small, frequent servings of healthy food and adequate fluid intake to minimize GI upset.
• Explain that drug doesn't change underlying dementia, but may improve symptoms or slow further deterioration.
◀€ Stress importance of taking drug as prescribed; caution against sudden dosage decreases or abrupt drug withdrawal.
• Tell patient or caregiver that if drug is stopped for 4 weeks or longer, dosage adjustment and monitoring schedule should be discussed with prescriber before restarting.
• As appropriate, review all other significant adverse reactions and interactions, especially those related to the drugs, tests, foods, and behaviors mentioned above.

tacrolimus
Prograf

Pharmacologic class: Macrolide
Therapeutic class: Immunosuppressant
Pregnancy risk category C

Action
Unknown; thought to inhibit T-lymphocyte activation

Availability
Capsules: 0.5 mg, 1 mg, 5 mg
Injection: 5 mg/ml

⦿ Indications and dosages
➣ To prevent organ rejection in patients with allogeneic liver or kidney transplants

---

Adults: 0.03 to 0.05 mg/kg/day I.V. by continuous infusion. Or initially for liver transplantation, 0.1 to 0.15 mg/kg/day P.O. in two dived doses q 12 hours. Or initially, for renal transplantation, 0.2 mg/kg/day P.O. in two divided doses q 12 hours.

Dosage adjustment
• Hepatic or renal impairment

Contraindications
• Hypersensitivity to drug or its components (including castor oil derivatives)

Administration
• Start therapy within 24 hours of renal transplantation and no earlier than 6 hours after liver transplantation. Switch to oral dosing as soon as tolerable, starting 8 to 12 hours after I.V. dosing is discontinued.

🔈 Before giving I.V., ensure that epinephrine 1:1,000 and oxygen are readily available in case of emergency.
• For I.V. use, dilute in normal saline solution or dextrose 5% in water to a concentration of 0.004 to 0.02 mg/ml. (Diluted drug may be refrigerated for up to 24 hours in glass or polyethylene container.) Give by infusion only.

Route	Onset	Peak	Duration
P.O.	Unknown	1.5-3.5 hr	Unknown
I.V.	Rapid	1-2 hr	Unknown

Adverse reactions
CNS: tremor, headache, insomnia, paresthesia, delirium, asthenia, **coma**
CV: hypertension, peripheral edema
GI: nausea, vomiting, diarrhea, constipation, abdominal pain, ascites, anorexia
GU: abnormal renal function, urinary tract infection, albuminuria, hematuria, proteinuria, oliguria, increased blood urea nitrogen (BUN) and creatinine levels, **renal failure**

Hematologic: anemia, leukocytosis, **thrombocytopenia**
Metabolic: hyperkalemia, hypokalemia, hyperglycemia, hypomagnesemia
Musculoskeletal: back pain
Respiratory: dyspnea, **pleural effusion, atelectasis**
Skin: rash, flushing, pruritus, alopecia, pruritus
Other: pain, fever, chills, **anaphylaxis**

Interactions
Drug-drug. *Bromocriptine, chloramphenicol, cimetidine, clarithromycin, clotrimazole, cyclosporine, danazol, diltiazem, erythromycin, fluconazole, itraconazole, ketoconazole, methylprednisolone, metoclopramide, metronidazole, nicardipine, omeprazole, protease inhibitors, verapamil:* increased tacrolimus blood level
Cyclosporine: increased risk of nephrotoxicity
CYP450 inducers (such as carbamazepine, phenobarbital, phenytoin, rifampin): decreased tacrolimus metabolism
Immunosuppressants (except adrenocorticosteroids): immunologic oversuppression
Live-virus vaccines: interference with immune response to vaccine
Mycophenolate mofetil: increased mycophenolate blood level
Nephrotoxic drugs (such as aminoglycoside, amphotericin B, cisplatin, cyclosporine): additive or synergistic effects
Drug-diagnostic tests. *BUN, creatinine, glucose:* increased levels
Hemoglobin, magnesium, platelets, white blood cells: decreased levels
Liver function tests: abnormal values
Potassium: increased or decreased level
Drug-food. *Any food:* inhibited drug absorption
Grapefruit juice: increased drug blood level
Drug-herb. *Astragalus, echinacea, melatonin:* decreased immunosuppression

t

St. John's wort: decreased tacrolimus blood level

Precautions
Use cautiously in:
- severe hepatic disease, renal impairment, diabetes mellitus, hypertension, hyperkalemia, hyperuricemia, lymphoma
- pregnant or breastfeeding patients
- children younger than age 12.

Patient monitoring
◀€ After I.V. infusion starts, watch closely for signs and symptoms of anaphylaxis.
- Monitor liver and kidney function test results; watch for signs and symptoms of nephrotoxicity and hepatic dysfunction.
- Assess neurologic status for indications of neurotoxicity.
- Monitor potassium level closely; watch for signs and symptoms of hyperkalemia.
- Monitor blood glucose; watch for indications of hyperglycemia.
- Evaluate respiratory status regularly.

Patient teaching
◀€ Teach patient to recognize and immediately report serious adverse reactions.
- Tell diabetic patient to expect increased blood glucose level, which may warrant further antidiabetic therapy. Teach him to monitor glucose level carefully.
- As appropriate, review all other significant and life-threatening adverse reactions and interactions, especially those related to the drugs, tests, foods, and herbs mentioned above.

tadalafil
Cialis

Pharmacologic class: Phosphodiesterase type 5 (PDE5) inhibitor
Therapeutic class: Anti-impotence agent
Pregnancy risk category B

Action
Inhibits PDE5, increasing cyclic guanosine monophosphate (cGMP) level and enhancing erectile function

Availability
Tablets: 5 mg, 10 mg, 20 mg

🖉 Indications and dosages
➤ Erectile dysfunction
Adults: Initially, 10 mg P.O. 30 minutes to 12 hours before anticipated sexual activity; may increase up to 20 mg or decrease to 5 mg based on patient response and tolerance. For most patients, maximum recommended dosing frequency is once daily.
Dosage adjustment
- Mild to moderate hepatic impairment or renal insufficiency

Contraindications
- Hypersensitivity to drug or its components
- Concurrent use of organic nitrates (regularly or intermittently)
- Concurrent use of alpha-adrenergic agonists (except tamsulosin 0.4 mg/day)

Administration
- Know that patient should take drug with or without food, 30 minutes to 12 hours before anticipated sexual activity.

Route	Onset	Peak	Duration
P.O.	Rapid	30 min-6 hr	Up to 36 hr

Adverse reactions

CNS: headache, fatigue, dizziness, hyperesthesia, insomnia, paresthesia, drowsiness, vertigo, asthenia

CV: angina pectoris, chest pain, hypertension, hypotension, orthostatic hypotension, palpitations, syncope, tachycardia, **myocardial infarction**

EENT: blurred vision, color vision changes, conjunctivitis, eye pain, increased lacrimation, eyelid swelling, epistaxis, nasal congestion, pharyngitis

GI: nausea, vomiting, diarrhea, dyspepsia, esophagitis, gastroesophageal reflux, gastritis, upper abdominal pain, dysphagia, dry mouth

GU: increased or spontaneous erection

Hepatic: abnormal liver function tests, elevated lactate dehydrogenase (LD) and uric acid levels

Musculoskeletal: myalgia; back, neck, limb, and joint pain

Respiratory: dyspnea

Skin: pruritus, rash, sweating

Other: facial edema, pain

Interactions

Drug-drug. *Alpha-adrenergic blockers (except tamsulosin 0.4 mg/day):* markedly decreased blood pressure
Angiotensin receptor blockers, enalapril, metoprolol: decreased blood pressure
CYP450-3A4 inducers (such as carbamazepine, phenobarbital, phenytoin, rifampin): decreased tadalafil blood level
CYP450-3A4 inhibitors (such as erythromycin, itraconazole, ketoconazole, ritonavir): increased tadalafil blood level
Theophylline: slight increase in heart rate

Drug-diagnostic tests. *Alanine aminotransferase, alkaline phosphatase, aspartate aminotransferase, LD, uric acid:* increased levels

Drug-food. *Grapefruit juice:* increased drug blood level

Precautions

Use cautiously in:
• cardiac risk that makes sexual activity inadvisable, renal insufficiency, hepatic impairment, left ventricular outflow obstruction, erectile dysfunction not evaluated for underlying cause, conditions that increase risk of priapism
• concurrent use of potent CYP450-3A4 inhibitors.

Patient monitoring

• Monitor for priapism or erections lasting more than 4 hours, which may permanently damage penile tissue.

Patient teaching

• Advise patient to take drug 30 minutes to 12 hours before anticipated sexual activity.

◀€ Caution patient never to take tadalafil concurrently with nitrates.

◀€ Instruct patient to stop sexual activity and contact prescriber immediately if chest pain, dizziness, or nausea occurs.

• Tell patient drug can cause serious interactions with many common drugs; instruct him to tell all prescribers he's taking it.

• Advise patient to avoid driving and other hazardous activities until he knows how drug affects concentration and alertness.

• Tell patient that drug may cause temporary blood pressure drop, leading to light-headedness if he stands up suddenly. Teach him to rise slowly and carefully.

• As appropriate, review all other significant and life-threatening adverse reactions and interactions, especially those related to the drugs, tests, and foods mentioned above.

t

Route	Onset	Peak	Duration
P.O.	Unknown	5 hr	Unknown

tamoxifen citrate
Nolvadex, Nolvadex-D♣,
Novo-Tamoxifen♣, Tamofen♣

Pharmacologic class: Nonsteroidal
antiestrogen
Therapeutic class: Antineoplastic
Pregnancy risk category D

Action
Competes with estrogen receptors in
tumor cells for binding to target tissues
(such as breast); reduces DNA synthesis and estrogen response

Availability
Tablets: 10 mg, 20 mg
Tablets (enteric-coated): 20 mg

⏏ Indications and dosages
➤ Adjunctive treatment of breast
cancer
Adults: 20 to 40 mg P.O. daily for 5
years. Daily dosages of 20 mg may be
taken as a single dose; daily doses
above 20 mg should be divided and
taken b.i.d. (morning and evening).
➤ To reduce breast cancer incidence
in high-risk women; treatment of duc-
tal carcinoma in situ
Adults: 20 mg P.O. daily for 5 years

Off-label uses
• Mastalgia
• Ovulation stimulation

Contraindications
• Hypersensitivity to drug
• Concurrent warfarin use
• Women with a history of deep-vein
thrombosis or pulmonary embolism
• Pregnancy or breastfeeding

Administration
• Don't break or crush enteric-coated
tablets.

Adverse reactions
CNS: confusion, depression, headache,
weakness, fatigue, light-headedness
CV: chest pain, **deep-vein thrombosis**
EENT: blurred vision, ocular lesion,
retinopathy, corneal opacity
GI: nausea, vomiting, abdominal
cramps, altered taste, anorexia
GU: vaginal bleeding, discharge, or
dryness; irregular menses; amenorrhea;
oligomenorrhea; ovarian cyst; pruritus
vulvae; increased creatinine level; **endometrial or uterine cancer**
**Hematologic: leukopenia, thrombo-
cytopenia**
Hepatic: increased aspartate aminotransferase and bilirubin levels
Metabolic: hypercalcemia, fluid retention
Musculoskeletal: bone pain
Respiratory: cough, **pulmonary embolism**
Skin: skin changes, hair thinning or
partial hair loss
Other: weight loss, tumor flare, tumor
pain, hot flashes, edema

Interactions
Drug-drug. *Aminoglutethimide, estrogens:* decreased tamoxifen effects
Antineoplastics: increased risk of
thromboembolic events
Bromocriptine: increased tamoxifen
blood level
Warfarin: increased anticoagulant effect
Drug-diagnostic tests. *Bilirubin,
calcium, creatinine, hepatic enzymes:*
increased levels
Platelets, white blood cells: decreased
counts

Precautions
Use cautiously in:
• decreased bone marrow reserve,

leukopenia, thrombocytopenia, cataracts, hyperlipidemia
• women of childbearing age.

Patient monitoring
• Monitor lipid panel, calcium level, mammography results, and gynecologic examination results.
• Watch for signs and symptoms of thromboembolic events, including cerebrovascular accident and pulmonary embolism.
• Monitor menstrual cycle pattern for changes that may signal endometrial or uterine cancer.

Patient teaching
• Teach patient to swallow enteric-coated tablets whole without breaking or crushing.
◀€ Instruct patient to immediately report leg or calf pain, swelling, or tenderness; unexpected shortness of breath; sudden chest pain; coughing up blood; new breast lumps; vaginal bleeding; menstrual irregularities; changes in vaginal discharge; pelvic pain or pressure; and vision changes.
• Inform patient that increase in bone or tumor pain usually means that drug will be effective; advise her to discuss pain management with prescriber.
• Teach patient importance of having regular blood tests, mammograms, and gynecologic exams to identify early signs of serious adverse reactions.
• As appropriate, review all other significant and life-threatening adverse reactions and interactions, especially those related to the drugs and tests mentioned above.

tamsulosin hydrochloride
Flomax

Pharmacologic class: Alpha-adrenergic blocker
Therapeutic class: Anti-adrenergic
Pregnancy risk category B

Action
Decreases smooth muscle contractions of prostate by binding preferentially to alpha$_1$-adrenergic receptors; this action increases urine flow and reduces symptoms of benign prostatic hyperplasia (BPH).

Availability
Capsules: 0.4 mg

⏀ Indications and dosages
➢ BPH
Adults: 0.4 mg/day P.O. after a meal; after 2 to 4 weeks, may increase to 0.8 mg/day

Contraindications
• Hypersensitivity to drug

Administration
• Give 30 minutes after same meal each day.

Route	Onset	Peak	Duration
P.O.	Unknown	4-5 hr	9-15 hr

Adverse reactions
CNS: dizziness, headache, asthenia, insomnia, drowsiness, syncope, vertigo
CV: orthostatic hypotension, chest pain
EENT: rhinitis, amblyopia, pharyngitis, sinusitis, tooth disorder
GU: retrograde or diminished ejaculation, decreased libido
Musculoskeletal: back pain

Respiratory: increased cough
Other: infection

Interactions

Drug-drug. *Cimetidine:* increased tamsulosin blood level, greater risk of toxicity
Doxazosin, prazosin, terazosin: increased risk of hypotension
Drug-behaviors. *Alcohol use:* increased risk of hypotension

Precautions

Use cautiously in:
• patients at increased risk for prostate cancer.

Patient monitoring

• Monitor blood pressure; stay alert for orthostatic hypotension.

Patient teaching

• Teach patient to take drug 30 minutes after same meal each day.
• Caution patient not to chew or open capsule; advise him to swallow it whole.
• Instruct patient to move slowly when sitting up or standing to avoid dizziness or light-headedness from sudden blood pressure decrease.
• Caution patient not to perform hazardous activities on first day of therapy.
• Tell patient drug may cause abnormal ejaculation; advise him to discuss this problem with prescriber.
• As appropriate, review all other significant adverse reactions and interactions, especially those related to the drugs and behaviors mentioned above.

tegaserod maleate
Zelnorm

Pharmacologic class: Partial serotonin type 4 (5-HT$_4$) receptor agonist
Therapeutic class: Serotonin agonist
Pregnancy risk category B

Action

Unknown; activates 5-HT$_4$ receptors in GI tract; this action normalizes intestinal peristalsis reflex and relieves abdominal pain and discomfort.

Availability

Tablets: 2 mg, 6 mg

⚠ Indications and dosages

➢ Irritable bowel syndrome in women with constipation
Adults: 6 mg P.O. b.i.d. before meals for 4 to 6 weeks; patients who respond may receive 4 to 6 more weeks of therapy.

Contraindications

• Hypersensitivity to drug or its components
• Severe renal disease
• Moderate to severe hepatic disease
• Gallbladder disease
• Abdominal adhesions
• Sphincter of Oddi dysfunction
• Diarrhea or history of frequent diarrhea
• History of bowel obstruction
• Breastfeeding

Administration

• Give 1 hour before or 2 hours after meals.

Route	Onset	Peak	Duration
P.O.	1 hr	1-1.3 hr	Unknown

Adverse reactions
CNS: headache, dizziness, migraine, depression
GI: nausea, vomiting, diarrhea, abdominal pain, flatulence
Musculoskeletal: joint, back, or leg pain
Other: facial edema, accidental trauma

Interactions
Drug-drug. *Digoxin, hormonal contraceptives:* decreased effects of these drugs
Drug-diagnostic tests. *Alanine aminotransferase, amylase, aspartate aminotransferase, blood and urine glucose, creatinine kinase, triglycerides:* increased levels
Drug-food. *Any food:* decreased drug absorption

Precautions
Use cautiously in:
• pregnant patients.

Patient monitoring
◀€ Assess for abdominal pain; stop therapy if patient develops new or sudden exacerbation of abdominal pain (especially with severe diarrhea).
• Monitor patient for depression.

Patient teaching
• Instruct patient to take drug 1 hour before or 2 hours after meals.
◀€ Teach patient to report severe diarrhea; diarrhea accompanied by severe abdominal pain, cramping, or dizziness; or sudden increase in abdominal pain.
• Advise patient (and significant other as appropriate) to report depression.
• Instruct patient to report suspected pregnancy to prescriber.
• As appropriate, review all other significant adverse reactions and interactions, especially those related to the drugs, tests, and foods mentioned above.

telmisartan
Micardis

Pharmacologic class: Angiotensin II receptor antagonist
Therapeutic class: Antihypertensive
Pregnancy risk category C (first trimester), *D* (second and third trimesters)

Action
Inhibits vasoconstricting and blocks aldosterone-producing effects of angiotensin II at various receptor sites, including vascular smooth muscle and adrenal glands

Availability
Tablets: 20 mg, 40 mg, 80 mg

⚡ Indications and dosages
➤ Hypertension
Adults: 40 P.O. daily, given alone or with other agents

Contraindications
• Hypersensitivity to drug or its components
• Pregnancy (second and third trimesters), breastfeeding

Administration
• Don't remove tablet from blister pack until just before giving dose.

Route	Onset	Peak	Duration
P.O.	Unknown	0.5-1 hr	24 hr

Adverse reactions
CNS: dizziness, headache, fatigue
CV: chest pain, peripheral edema, hypertension
EENT: sinusitis, pharyngitis
GI: nausea, vomiting, diarrhea, dyspepsia, abdominal pain
GU: urinary tract infection, slightly increased creatinine level

Musculoskeletal: myalgia, back and leg pain
Respiratory: cough, upper respiratory infection
Other: pain, flu or flulike symptoms

Interactions
Drug-drug. *Antihypertensives, diuretics:* increased risk of hypotension
Digoxin: increased digoxin blood level
Warfarin: decreased warfarin blood level
Drug-diagnostic tests. *Creatinine:* slight elevation
Drug-food. *Any food:* slightly reduced drug bioavailability

Precautions
Use cautiously in:
• heart failure, impaired renal function secondary to primary renal disease or renal stenosis, obstructive biliary disorders, hepatic impairment, volume or sodium depletion
• patients receiving high-dose diuretics
• pregnant patients in first trimester
• women of childbearing age
• children younger than age 18 (safety not established).

Patient monitoring
• Watch for signs and symptoms of hypotension.
• Correct deficits in volume-depleted patients as appropriate before starting therapy; monitor fluid intake and output and creatinine level.

Patient teaching
• Teach patient to take drug 1 hour before or 2 hours after meals.
• Caution patient not to remove tablet from blister pack until just before he takes dose.
• Teach patient to report swelling or chest pain.
• Instruct patient to measure blood pressure regularly and report significant changes.

• As appropriate, review all other significant adverse reactions and interactions, especially those related to the drugs, tests, and foods mentioned above.

temazepam
Restoril, Temaz

Pharmacologic class: Benzodiazepine
Therapeutic class: Sedative-hypnotic
Controlled substance schedule IV
Pregnancy risk category X

Action
Depresses CNS at limbic, thalamic, and hypothalamic levels; enhances effects of gamma-aminobutyric acid, resulting in sedation, hypnosis, skeletal muscle relaxation, and anticonvulsant and anxiolytic activity

Availability
Capsules: 7.5 mg, 15 mg, 30 mg

Indications and dosages
➤ Short-term management of insomnia
Adults: 15 to 30 mg P.O. at bedtime when needed
Dosage adjustment
• Elderly or debilitated patients

Contraindications
• Hypersensitivity to drug or other benzodiazepines
• Pregnancy or breastfeeding

Administration
• Give with or without food at bedtime.

Route	Onset	Peak	Duration
P.O.	30 min	1.2-1.6 hr	Unknown

Adverse reactions

CNS: hangover, headache, dizziness, drowsiness, lethargy, fatigue, paradoxical stimulation, light-headedness, talkativeness, irritability, nervousness, confusion, euphoria, relaxed feeling, tremor, incoordination, impaired memory, nightmares, paresthesia

CV: chest pain, palpitations, tachycardia

EENT: eye irritation, pain, and swelling; photophobia; tinnitus

GI: nausea, vomiting, constipation, diarrhea, heartburn, abdominal pain, taste alteration, dry mouth, anorexia

Musculoskeletal: joint pain

Other: body pain, physical or psychological drug dependence, drug tolerance

Interactions

Drug-drug. *Antidepressants, antihistamines, opioid analgesics, other sedative-hypnotics:* additive CNS depression

Digoxin: increased digoxin blood level, greater risk of toxicity

Probenecid: faster temazepam onset and prolonged effects

Theophylline: antagonism of temazepam's sedative effects

Drug-herb. *Chamomile, hops, kava, skullcap, valerian:* increased CNS depression

Drug-behaviors. *Alcohol use:* additive CNS depression

Smoking: increased drug metabolism

Precautions

Use cautiously in:

• chronic pulmonary insufficiency, hepatic dysfunction, renal disease, psychoses, drug abuse

• history of suicide attempt or drug abuse

• elderly or debilitated patients

• children younger than age 15.

Patient monitoring

• Monitor neurologic status carefully; check for paradoxical reactions, especially in elderly patients.

• Watch for signs and symptoms of physical and psychological drug dependence; stay alert for drug hoarding.

Patient teaching

• Instruct patient to avoid driving and other hazardous activities on day after taking drug until he knows how it affects concentration and alertness.

• Teach patient to establish effective bedtime routine to help prevent or minimize insomnia.

• Instruct patient not to drink alcohol.

• Advise patient not to smoke or use herbs without consulting prescriber.

• Inform patient (and significant other if appropriate) that drug may cause psychological and physical dependence and should be used only as prescribed and needed.

• As appropriate, review all other significant adverse reactions and interactions, especially those related to the drugs, herbs, and behaviors mentioned above.

temozolomide
Temodal✤, Temodar

Pharmacologic class: Alkylating agent
Therapeutic class: Antineoplastic
Pregnancy risk category D

Action

Rapidly converts to monomethyl triazeno imidazole carboxamide, an active compound that prevents DNA transcription

Availability

Capsules: 5 mg, 20 mg, 100 mg, 250 mg

🖊 Indications and dosages

➣ Refractory anaplastic astrocytoma that has progressed despite treatment with a regimen containing nitrosurea and procarbazine

Adults: 150 mg/m² P.O. daily for 5 consecutive days of each 28-day treatment cycle; adjust dosage as appropriate based on blood counts.

Contraindications
• Hypersensitivity to drug, its components, or dacarbazine
• Pregnancy or breastfeeding

Administration
• Give drug daily with a full glass of water, either consistently with or without food.
• Be aware that dosages in 28-day cycle depend on nadir neutrophil and platelet counts.

Route	Onset	Peak	Duration
P.O.	Rapid	1 hr	Unknown

Adverse reactions
CNS: fatigue, headache, dysphasia, abnormal coordination, ataxia, anxiety, depression, dizziness, drowsiness, confusion, amnesia, insomnia, mental status changes, weakness, paresis, hemiparesis, paresthesias, **seizures**
CV: peripheral edema
EENT: abnormal vision, diplopia, pharyngitis, sinusitis
GI: nausea, vomiting, constipation, diarrhea, abdominal pain, anorexia
GU: urinary incontinence or frequency, urinary tract infection, breast pain (in women)
Hematologic: anemia, **leukopenia, thrombocytopenia**
Metabolic: adrenal hypercorticism
Musculoskeletal: abnormal gait, back pain, myalgia
Respiratory: cough, upper respiratory infection
Skin: pruritus, rash
Other: fever, viral infection, weight gain

Interactions
Drug-drug. *Antineoplastics:* additive bone marrow depression

Live-virus vaccines: decreased antibody response to vaccine, greater risk of adverse reactions
Valproic acid: decreased oral clearance of temozolomide
Drug-diagnostic tests. *Neutrophils, platelets:* decreased counts

Precautions
Use cautiously in:
• severe hepatic or renal impairment, active infection, decreased bone marrow reserve, other chronic debilitating illness
• elderly patients
• patients with childbearing potential
• children (safety not established).

Patient monitoring
• Monitor complete blood count with white cell differential; stay alert for bone marrow depression.
• Assess neurologic status carefully.
• Monitor fluid intake and output; weigh patient regularly.

Patient teaching
• Teach patient to take drug consistently with or without food, and with a full glass of water.
• Advise patient to take drug 1 hour before or 2 hours after a meal if it causes nausea and vomiting.
• Inform patient that drug may cause abnormal gait and dizziness.
• Teach patient to report unusual bleeding or bruising.
• Caution patient to avoid live-virus vaccines.
• Instruct patient to avoid driving and other hazardous activities until he knows how drug affects concentration, alertness, and vision
• As appropriate, review all other significant and life-threatening adverse reactions and interactions, especially those related to the drugs and tests mentioned above.

tenecteplase
TNKase

Pharmacologic class: Tissue plasminogen activator
Therapeutic class: Thrombolytic enzyme
Pregnancy risk category C

Action
Binds to fibrin and converts plasminogen to plasmin, which breaks down fibrin clots and lyses thrombi and emboli; causes systemic fibrinolysis

Availability
Powder for injection: 50 mg/vial with 10-ml syringe and TwinPak Dual Cannula Device and 10-ml vial of sterile water for injection

Indications and dosages
➤ To reduce mortality associated with acute myocardial infarction
Adults weighing 90 kg (198 lb) or more: 50 mg I.V. bolus administered over 5 seconds
Adults weighing 80 kg to 89 kg (176 to 197 lb): 45 mg I.V. bolus administered over 5 seconds
Adults weighing 70 kg to 79 kg (154 to 175 lb): 40 mg I.V. bolus administered over 5 seconds
Adults weighing 60 to 69 kg (132 to 153 lb): 35 mg I.V. bolus administered over 5 seconds
Adults weighing less than 60 kg (132 lb): 30 mg I.V. bolus administered over 5 seconds

Contraindications
• Hypersensitivity to drug or other tissue plasminogen activators
• Active internal bleeding
• Bleeding diathesis

• Recent intracranial or intraspinal surgery or trauma
• Severe uncontrolled hypertension
• Intracranial neoplasm
• Arteriovenous malformation or aneurysm
• History of cerebrovascular accident (CVA)

Administration
• Reconstitute by mixing contents of prefilled syringe with 10 ml of sterile water for injection. Swirl gently; don't shake. Draw up prescribed dosage from vial; then discard remainder of drug. Administer I.V. over 5 seconds through designated line.
• Don't give solution if it contains visible particles.
◀⏵ Don't administer in same I.V. line as dextrose solutions; flush I.V. line with normal saline solution before giving drug if patient has been receiving dextrose.
◀⏵ Give with heparin if ordered, but not through same I.V. line.

Route	Onset	Peak	Duration
I.V.	Immediate	Unknown	Unknown

Adverse reactions
CNS: intracranial hemorrhage, CVA
CV: hypotension, **arrhythmia, myocardial rupture, myocardial reinfarction, cardiogenic shock, atrioventricular block, cardiac arrest, cardiac tamponade, heart failure, pericarditis, pericardial effusion, mitral regurgitation, thrombosis, embolism, hemorrhage**
EENT: epistaxis, minor pharyngeal bleeding
GI: nausea, vomiting, **hemorrhage**
GU: hematuria
Hematologic: anemia, **bleeding tendency**
Respiratory: respiratory depression, **pulmonary edema, apnea**
Skin: bleeding at puncture sites, hematoma

t

Interactions
Drug-drug. *Anticoagulants, aspirin, dipyridamole, indomethacin, phenylbutazone:* increased bleeding risk
Drug-diagnostic tests. *Coagulation tests:* fibrinogen degradation in blood sample

Precautions
Use cautiously in:
• previous puncture of noncompressible vessels, organ biopsy, hypertension, acute pericarditis, high risk of left ventricular thrombosis, subacute bacterial endocarditis, hemostatic defects, diabetic hemorrhagic retinopathy, septic thrombophlebitis, obstetric delivery
• patients over age 75
• breastfeeding patients.

Patient monitoring
◀€ Monitor ECG; stay alert for reperfusion arrhythmias.

◀€ Monitor vital signs carefully; watch for respiratory depression and reinfarction.

◀€ Evaluate all body systems closely for signs and symptoms of bleeding; if bleeding occurs, stop drug and give antiplatelet agents as ordered.

• Monitor coagulation studies and complete blood cell count; however, be aware that tenecteplase can skew coagulation results.

Patient teaching
◀€ Inform patient that drug increases risk of bleeding; advise him to report signs and symptoms of bleeding immediately.

• Teach patient safety measures to avoid bruising and bleeding.
• Tell patient he'll undergo regular blood tests during therapy.
• As appropriate, review all other significant and life-threatening adverse reactions and interactions, especially those related to the drugs and tests mentioned above.

tenofovir disoproxil fumarate
Viread

Pharmacologic class: Nucleoside analog reverse transcriptase inhibitor
Therapeutic class: Antiretroviral
Pregnancy risk category B

Action
Inhibits the activity of human immunodeficiency virus (HIV) by competing with the natural substrate deoxyadenosine 5'-triphosphate; once incorporated into cellular DNA by HIV reverse transcriptase, causes DNA chain termination

Availability
Tablets: 300 mg

🖊 Indications and dosages
➤ HIV-1 infection
Adults: 300 mg P.O. daily with a meal (usually given with other antiretrovirals)
Dosage adjustment
• Renal impairment

Contraindications
• Hypersensitivity to drug
• Renal insufficiency
• Lactic acidosis
• Breastfeeding

Administration
• If patient is also receiving didanosine, give tenofovir at least 2 hours before or 1 hour after didanosine.

Route	Onset	Peak	Duration
P.O.	Rapid	45-75 min	Unknown

Adverse reactions
CNS: headache, asthenia
CV: creatine kinase (CK) elevation

GI: nausea, vomiting, diarrhea, abdominal pain, flatulence, anorexia, amylase elevation

GU: glycosuria

Hematologic: decreased neutrophil count

Hepatic: severe hepatomegaly with steatosis

Metabolic: hyperglycemia; triglyceride, aspartate aminotransferase (AST), and alanine aminotransferase (ALT) elevations; **lactic acidosis**

Other: body fat redistribution

Interactions

Drug-drug. *Acyclovir, cidofovir, didanosine, ganciclovir, indinavir, iopinavir, probenecid, ritonavir, valacyclovir, valganciclovir, other drugs eliminated by active tubular secretion:* increased blood level of either drug

Drug-diagnostic tests. *ALT, amylase, AST, blood and urine glucose, CK, triglycerides:* increased levels

Neutrophils: decreased count

Drug-food. *Any food:* decreased drug bioavailability and efficacy

Precautions

Use cautiously in:
• hepatic impairment, renal disease
• elderly patients
• pregnant patients
• children.

Patient monitoring

• Watch for and report signs and symptoms of lactic acidosis.
• Monitor kidney and liver function test results.
• Assess nutritional status and hydration in light of adverse GI reactions and underlying disease.

Patient teaching

• Teach patient to take drug once daily with a meal.
• If patient is also receiving didanosine, instruct him to take tenofovir at least 2 hours before or 1 hour after didanosine.

• Tell patient drug may cause weakness and headache; instruct him to avoid driving and other hazardous activities until he knows how drug affects performance.

• As appropriate, review all other significant and life-threatening adverse reactions and interactions, especially those related to the drugs, tests, and foods mentioned above.

terazosin hydrochloride
Hytrin

Pharmacologic class: Anti-adrenergic (peripherally acting)

Therapeutic class: Antihypertensive

Pregnancy risk category C

Action

Blocks postsynaptic alpha$_1$-adrenergic receptors, causing vasodilation and decreasing contractions of smooth muscle in the bladder neck and prostate

Availability

Tablets: 1 mg, 2 mg, 5 mg, 10 mg

🥼 Indications and dosages

➤ Hypertension

Adults: Initially, 1 mg P.O.; increase dosage slowly up to 5 mg/day. Usual range is 1 to 5 mg/day, not to exceed 20 mg/day; may give as a single dose or in two divided doses.

➤ Benign prostatic hyperplasia

Adults: 1 mg P.O. at bedtime; may increase gradually to 2 mg/day, then to 5 mg/day, and then to a maximum of 10 mg/day

Contraindications

• Hypersensitivity to drug or other quinazoline derivatives

t

Administration

◀€ Don't stop therapy suddenly; dosage must be tapered.

Route	Onset	Peak	Duration
P.O.	15 min	2-3 hr	24 hr

Adverse reactions

CNS: dizziness, headache, weakness, drowsiness, nervousness, paresthesia, vertigo, fatigue, syncope
CV: orthostatic hypotension (with first dose), rebound hypertension, chest pain, palpitations, peripheral edema, tachycardia, **arrhythmias**
EENT: blurred vision, conjunctivitis, amblyopia, nasal congestion, sinusitis
GI: nausea, vomiting, diarrhea, abdominal pain, dry mouth
GU: urinary frequency or incontinence, impotence, priapism
Musculoskeletal: joint, back, and extremity pain; arthritis
Respiratory: dyspnea
Skin: pruritus
Other: fever, weight gain, flulike symptoms

Interactions

Drug-drug. *Estrogens, nonsteroidal anti-inflammatory drugs (NSAIDs), sympathomimetics:* decreased antihypertensive effects
Midodrine: antagonism of terazosin's action
Nitrates, other antihypertensives: additive hypotension
Drug-herb. *Ephedra (ma huang):* antagonism of terazosin's action
Drug-behaviors. *Alcohol use:* additive hypotension

Precautions

Use cautiously in:
• prostate cancer, hepatic disease, dehydration, volume or sodium depletion
• pregnant or breastfeeding patients
• children (safety not established).

Patient monitoring

• Monitor blood pressure; stay alert for orthostatic hypotension (first dose effect) when therapy begins.
• Assess cardiovascular status; report chest pain, peripheral edema, palpitations, and other significant effects.

Patient teaching

• Teach patient to take drug at same time every day, with or without food.
◀€ Caution patient not to stop therapy abruptly; dosage must be tapered.
◀€ Advise patient to immediately report swelling, palpitations, chest pain, breathing difficulty, and other adverse cardiovascular reactions.
• Inform patient that drug may cause erectile dysfunction, priapism, and other sexual problems. Encourage him to discuss these issues with prescriber.
• Caution patient not to use NSAIDs or drink alcohol.
• Instruct patient to move slowly when sitting up or standing to avoid dizziness or light-headedness from sudden blood pressure decrease.
• As appropriate, review all other significant and life-threatening adverse reactions and interactions, especially those related to the drugs, herbs, and behaviors mentioned above.

terbinafine hydrochloride
Desenex Max, Lamisil

Pharmacologic class: Synthetic allylamine derivative
Therapeutic class: Antifungal
Pregnancy risk category B

Action

Unclear; interferes with sterol biosynthesis of fungal cell membrane permeability by selectively inhibiting the key enzymes responsible for normal fungal growth and maturation, resulting in cell death

Availability
Cream: 1%
Tablets: 250 mg

⏀ Indications and dosages
➤ Tinea cruris, tinea corporis, tinea pedis; onychomycosis of toenail or fingernail
Adults and children: Massage cream onto affected area and surrounding area once or twice daily; continue for 7 to 14 days, not to exceed 4 weeks. For fingernail infection, administer 250 mg P.O. daily for 6 weeks; for toenail infection, administer 250 mg P.O. daily for 12 weeks.

Contraindications
• Hypersensitivity to drug or its components
• Renal impairment
• Chronic active hepatic disease
• Pregnancy (with tablets) or breast-feeding

Administration
• Give drug with or without food, but not with coffee, cola, or tea.

Route	Onset	Peak	Duration
P.O.	Unknown	≤ 2 hr	Unknown
Topical	Unknown	Unknown	Unknown

Adverse reactions
CNS: headache
EENT: visual disturbances
GI: nausea, diarrhea, dyspepsia, abdominal pain, flatulence, taste disturbances
Hematologic: neutropenia
Hepatic: elevated hepatic enzyme levels, **hepatic failure**
Skin: burning, stinging, dryness, itching, and local irritation (with topical form); rash; pruritus; urticaria; erythema multiforme

Other: Stevens-Johnson syndrome

Interactions
Drug-drug. *Cimetidine:* decreased terbinafine clearance
Cyclosporine: increased cyclosporine clearance
Dextromethorphan: increased dextromethorphan blood level
Rifampin: increased terbinafine clearance
Warfarin: altered warfarin efficacy
Drug-diagnostic tests. *Hepatic enzymes:* increased levels
Neutrophils: decreased count
Drug-food. *Caffeine-containing foods and beverages:* decreased caffeine clearance
Drug-herb. *Chaparral, comfrey, germander, jin bu huan, kava, pennyroyal:* increased risk of hepatotoxicity
Cola nut, guarana, yerba maté: decreased clearance of these herbs

Precautions
Use cautiously in:
• pregnant patients (topical form)
• children (safety and efficacy not established).

Patient monitoring
• Monitor complete blood count and liver function test results.
• Watch for signs and symptoms of erythema multiforme; report early indications before they progress to Stevens-Johnson syndrome.

Patient teaching
• Tell patient he may take drug with or without food.
• Instruct patient to avoid coffee, tea, and colas because they can worsen adverse drug reactions.
• Inform patient that drug may take 4 weeks to be effective in fingernail infections and 10 weeks in toenail infections. Encourage him to continue taking it even though symptoms won't improve right away.

t

◀◣ Teach patient to immediately report rash, sore throat, cough, mouth sores, fever, or yellowing of skin or eyes.

• As appropriate, review all other significant and life-threatening adverse reactions and interactions, especially those related to the drugs, tests, foods, and herbs mentioned above.

terbutaline sulfate
Brethair, Brethine, Bricanyl

Pharmacologic class: Selective beta$_2$ agonist

Therapeutic class: Bronchodilator

Pregnancy risk category B

Action
Relaxes bronchial smooth muscle by stimulating beta$_2$-adrenergic receptors; stimulates adenylcyclase, which causes accumulation of cyclic 3′, 5′ adenosine monophosphate. Net effect is bronchial smooth muscle relaxation and inhibited release of mediators of immediate hypersensitivity, especially from mast cells.

Availability
Inhaler: 0.2 mg/inhalation
Injection: 1 mg/ml
Tablets: 2.5 mg, 5 mg

Indications and dosages
➤ Bronchospasm in reversible obstructive airway disease
Adults and children older than age 12: 0.25 mg S.C.; may repeat in 15 to 30 minutes p.r.n., up to a maximum of 0.5 mg in 4 hours. Or 2.5 to 5 mg P.O. q 6 hours t.i.d. while awake, up to a maximum of 15 mg/day in adults; or 2.5 mg P.O. q 6 hours t.i.d. while awake, up to a maximum of 7.5 mg/day in children.

Or 0.2 to 0.5 mg (one to two inhalations) q 4 to 6 hours.
Dosage adjustment
• Renal impairment

Off-label uses
• Tocolytic in preterm labor

Contraindications
• Hypersensitivity to drug, its components, or sympathomimetic amines

Administration
• Inject S.C. dose into lateral deltoid muscle.

Route	Onset	Peak	Duration
P.O.	30 min	2-3 hr	4-8 hr
S.C.	15 min	30 min	1.5-4 hr
Inhalation	Unknown	Unknown	Unknown

Adverse reactions
CNS: tremors, anxiety, insomnia, headache, dizziness, drowsiness, stimulation, nervousness
CV: palpitations, chest discomfort, tachycardia
GI: nausea, vomiting
Skin: diaphoresis, flushing

Interactions
Drug-drug. *Beta-adrenergic blockers:* blocked bronchodilating effects
Monoamine oxidase inhibitors, tricyclic antidepressants: potentiation of terbutaline's cardiovascular reactions
Other sympathomimetic amines: additive adverse cardiovascular reactions

Precautions
Use cautiously in:
• cardiovascular disorders, hyperthyroidism, diabetes mellitus, seizure disorders, hypertension, glaucoma, arrhythmias
• elderly patients
• breastfeeding patients.

Patient monitoring
• Monitor vital signs.
• Assess neurologic status.

Patient teaching
• Advise patient to take drug with or without food.
• Teach patient or parents to establish an effective bedtime routine to minimize insomnia.
• Instruct patient or parents to space doses evenly during waking hours to avoid taking drug at bedtime.
• As appropriate, review all other significant adverse reactions and interactions, especially those related to the drugs mentioned above.

teriparatide (recombinant)
Forteo

Pharmacologic class: Biosynthetic fragment of human parathyroid hormone
Therapeutic class: Parathyroid hormone
Pregnancy risk category C

Action
Stimulates new bone growth by binding to specific high-affinity cell-surface receptors

Availability
Injection: 750 mcg/3 ml (controlled pen device)

Indications and dosages
➤ Postmenopausal women with osteoporosis; men with primary or hypogonadal osteoporosis who are at high risk for bone fracture
Adults: 20 mcg/day S.C. for up to 2 years

Contraindications
• Hypersensitivity to drug
• Conditions that increase osteosarcoma risk (such as Paget's disease, unexplained alkaline phosphatase elevation, open epiphyses, skeletal radiation therapy)
• Bone cancer metastases or history of bone cancer
• Metabolic bone disease (other than osteoporosis)
• Hypercalcemia

Administration
• Give S.C. injection into thigh or abdominal wall while patient is lying down.
• Be aware that prefilled injection pen delivers 20 mcg/dose of drug per actuation and may be reused for up to 28 days after first injection. Discard pen in protected container after 28 days, even if it's not empty.

Route	Onset	Peak	Duration
S.C.	Rapid	Rapid	Unknown

Adverse reactions
CNS: dizziness, headache, insomnia, depression, vertigo, asthenia
CV: hypertension, angina, syncope
EENT: rhinitis, pharyngitis
GI: nausea, vomiting, diarrhea, dyspepsia, anorexia
Metabolic: hyperuricemia
Musculoskeletal: joint pain, cramps
Respiratory: cough, pneumonia, dyspnea
Skin: rash, sweating
Other: pain

Interactions
Drug-drug. *Digoxin:* increased digoxin toxicity
Drug-diagnostic tests. *Calcium:* increased level

Precautions
Use cautiously in:
• urolithiasis, hypotension

t

- concurrent use of cardiac glycosides
- pregnant or breastfeeding patients.

Patient monitoring
- Monitor respiratory and neurologic status; assess patient's mood.
- Monitor bone mineral density test results and calcium level.

Patient teaching
- Teach patient to promptly report such adverse reactions as cough and difficulty breathing.
- Inform patient that prefilled injection pen delivers 20 mcg/dose of drug per actuation. Tell him he may reuse it for up to 28 days after first injection. Instruct him to discard it in appropriate receptacle after 28 days, even if it's not empty.
- Teach patient to establish effective bedtime routine to minimize insomnia.
- Instruct patient to avoid driving and other hazardous activities he knows how drug affects strength and balance.
- As appropriate, review all other significant adverse reactions and interactions, especially those related to the drugs and tests mentioned above.

testosterone
Androderm, AndroGel, Testamone 100, Testaqua, Testim, Testoderm, Testoderm TTS, Testopel Pellets

testosterone enanthate
Andro La, Delatestryl, Everone 200

Pharmacologic class: Hormone
Therapeutic class: Androgenic and anabolic steroid, antineoplastic
Controlled substance schedule III
Pregnancy risk category X

Action
Responsible for normal growth and development of male sex organs and maintenance of secondary sex characteristics, including maturation; also decreases estrogen activity needed in treatment of breast cancer

Availability
testosterone
Gel: 1% (50 mg)
Injection aqueous suspension: 100 mg/ml
Pellets (S.C. implant): 75 mg
Transdermal system: 2.5, 4 mg, 5 mg, 6 mg
testosterone enanthate
Injection (in oil): 100 mg/ml, 200 mg/ml

🖊 Indications and dosages
➤ Male hypogonadism
Adult males: 10 to 25 mg (testosterone) I.M. two to three times weekly or 50 to 400 mg (enanthate) I.M. q 2 to 4 weeks for 3 to 4 years. Or 150 to 450 mg (pellet) implanted S.C. q 3 to 6 months. Or 5 mg daily transdermal (nonscrotal) system; may be increased up to 7.5 mg daily (Androderm); or 5 mg daily (Testoderm TTS), adjusted after 3 to 4 weeks; may be increased to 10 mg daily. Or 4 to 6 mg daily transdermal scrotal system (Testoderm with or without adhesive), adjusted after 3 to 4 weeks. Or 50 mg of testosterone gel (AndroGel 1%) applied topically daily, adjusted up to 75 mg daily within 14 days, with subsequent dosages up to 100 mg daily.
➤ Inoperable breast cancer in women 1 to 5 years post menopause
Adult females: 100 mg (testosterone) I.M. three times weekly or 200 to 400 mg (enanthate) I.M. q 2 to 4 weeks

Contraindications
- Hypersensitivity to drug, its components, or tartrazine (with some products)

- Serious cardiac, hepatic, or renal disease
- Males with breast cancer or suspected prostate cancer
- Enhancement of athletic performance or physique
- Females (with transdermal system or gel)
- Pregnancy or breastfeeding

Administration

- Inspect aqueous solution for injection; if crystals are visible, warm bottle and shake contents to dissolve crystals.
- Rotate I.M. injection sites among upper outer quadrant of gluteal maximus; inject deep into muscle.
- Apply gel once daily (preferably in morning) to clean, dry, intact skin on shoulders, upper arms, or abdomen.

Route	Onset	Peak	Duration
I.M.	Unknown	10-100 min	Unknown
S.C.	Unknown	Unknown	3-4 mo
Topical gel	30 min	Unknown	Unknown
Transdermal	Unknown	2-4 hr	Unknown

Adverse reactions

CNS: headache, depression, emotional lability, nervousness, anxiety, asthenia, memory loss, dizziness, vertigo, **cerebrovascular accident**
CV: edema, peripheral edema, **deep-vein phlebitis, heart failure**
GI: bleeding
GU: hematuria, urinary tract infection, impaired urination, scrotal cellulitis, benign prostatic hyperplasia, scrotal papilloma (with transdermal use), prostatitis, elevated prostate-specific antigen (PSA) level (with topical use), libido changes, breast pain or tenderness, gynecomastia, decreased creatinine and creatine excretion, increased 17-ketosteroid excretion, virilization in females, excessive hormonal effects in males

Hematologic: polycythemia, **leukopenia, suppressed clotting factors**
Hepatic: abnormal bilirubin level and liver function test results, **hepatic adenoma** (with long-term enanthate use)
Metabolic: hyperphosphatemia, hypernatremia, hypercalcemia, hypercholesterolemia, hyperkalemia, hypoglycemia, decreased thyroxine-binding globulin
Musculoskeletal: myalgia
Respiratory: sleep apnea
Skin: acne; rash, itching, burning, discomfort, irritation, burn-like blister, erythema (with transdermal use); pain, local edema, and induration at injection site
Other: hypersensitivity reaction, accidental injury, flulike symptoms

Interactions

Drug-drug. *Corticosteroids:* increased risk of edema
Hepatotoxic drugs: increased risk of hepatotoxicity
Insulin, oral hypoglycemics: decreased blood glucose level
Oral anticoagulants: increased anticoagulant effect
Oxyphenbutazone: increased oxyphenbutazone blood level
Propranolol: increased propranolol clearance
Drug-diagnostic tests. *Calcium, cholesterol, hematocrit, hemoglobin, liver function tests, potassium, phosphate, PSA, sodium:* increased levels
Clotting factors, glucose, thyroxine, thyroxine-binding globulin: decreased levels
Urine creatine and creatinine: decreased excretion
Urine 17-ketosteroids: increased excretion
Drug-herb. *Chaparral, comfrey, germander, jin bu huan, kava, pennyroyal:* increased risk of hepatotoxicity

t

Precautions

Use cautiously in:
• diabetes mellitus, cardiovascular or hepatic disease, sleep apnea, or hypercalcemia.

Patient monitoring

• Monitor electrolyte levels, liver function test results, blood and urine calcium levels, lipid panels, complete blood count with white cell differential, and semen studies.
• Assess diabetic patients carefully for hypoglycemia.
• Closely monitor neurologic status; stay alert for sleep apnea.
• Watch for excessive sexual stimulation or priapism in males.
• Assess for early signs of excessive hormonal effects in females (virilization); if these occur, drug withdrawal may be indicated because some effects (such as voice changes) may be irreversible.

Patient teaching

◀≋ Instruct patient to immediately report signs and symptoms of liver problems, including nausea, vomiting, yellowing of skin or eyes, and ankle swelling.
• Teach prepubertal males about signs and symptoms of excessive hormonal effects, such as acne, priapism, increased body and facial hair, and penile enlargement.
• Teach postpubertal males about signs and symptoms of excessive adverse hormonal effects, such as impotence, gynecomastia, epididymitis, testicular atrophy, and infertility.
◀≋ Instruct female patient to immediately report signs of masculinization, such as excessive body or facial hair, deepening of voice, clitoral enlargement, and menstrual irregularities.
• Advise females of childbearing age to use barrier contraceptives.
• Teach patient which patches can or can't be applied to scrotum.

• Instruct patient to apply transdermal patch daily to clean, dry skin (application area varies with product) after removing protective liner to expose drug-containing film. To prevent irritation, instruct him to apply each patch to a different site, waiting at least 1 week before reusing same site.
• Teach patient to apply topical gel once daily (preferably in morning) to clean, dry skin on shoulder, upper arm, or abdomen; advise him to wait until gel dries before getting dressed. Instruct him that after opening packet, he should squeeze entire contents into palm and apply immediately. Instruct him to wash hands with soap and water after applying gel.
• As appropriate, review all other significant and life-threatening adverse reactions and interactions, especially those related to the drugs, tests, and herbs mentioned above.

tetracycline hydrochloride

Achromycin, Actisite, Apo-Tetra✤, Bristacycline, Novotetra✤, Nu-Tetra✤, Sumycin, Sumycin Syrup

Pharmacologic class: Tetracycline
Therapeutic class: Anti-infective
Pregnancy risk category D, B (topical form)

Action

Unknown; thought to inhibit bacterial protein synthesis at level of 30S and 50S bacterial ribosomes and to alter cytoplasmic membrane of susceptible organisms

Availability

Capsules: 100 mg, 250 mg, 500 mg
Ointment: 3%
Oral suspension: 125 mg/5 ml

✔ Indications and dosages

➤ Mild to moderate infections caused by susceptible organisms

Adults: 500 mg P.O. b.i.d. or 250 mg P.O. q.i.d.

➤ Severe infections caused by susceptible organisms

Adults: 500 mg P.O. q.i.d.

Children over age 8: 25 to 50 mg/kg P.O. q.i.d.

➤ Syphilis in penicillin-allergic patients

Adults: 500 mg P.O. q.i.d. for 14 days

➤ Late syphilis (except neurosyphilis)

Adults: 500 mg P.O. q.i.d. for 28 days

➤ Leptospirosis when penicillin is contraindicated or ineffective

Adults: 1 to 2 g P.O. daily in two to four divided doses for 5 to 7 days

➤ Yaws

Adults: 1 to 2 g P.O. daily in two to four divided doses for 10 to 14 days

➤ Gonorrhea (in patients allergic to penicillin)

Adults: Initially, 1.5 g P.O., followed by 500 mg P.O. q 6 hours for 4 days, to a total of 9 g

➤ Uncomplicated urethral, endocervical, or rectal infections caused by *Chlamydia trachomatis*

Adults: 500 mg P.O. q.i.d for 7 days

➤ Rickettsial and mycoplasmal infections

Adults: 1 to 2 g P.O. daily in two to four divided doses for 7 days

➤ *Helicobacter pylori* infection

Adults: In patients with active duodenal ulcer, 500 mg P.O. q.i.d. at meals and bedtime for 14 days, given with other drugs (such as metronidazole, bismuth subsalicylate, amoxicillin, or omeprazole)

➤ Brucellosis

Adults: 500 mg P.O. q.i.d. for 3 weeks, given with streptomycin I.M. b.i.d. during first week and streptomycin once daily during second week

➤ Granuloma inguinale caused by *Calymmatobacterium granulomatis,*

chancroid caused by *Haemophilus ducreyi*

Adults: 1 to 2 g P.O. daily in two to four divided doses for 2 to 4 weeks

➤ Cholera

Adults: 500 mg P.O. q 6 hours for 48 to 72 hours

➤ Plague (when streptomycin is contraindicated or ineffective)

Adults: 2 to 4 g P.O. q.i.d. for 10 days

Children older than age 8: 30 to 40 mg/kg P.O. q.i.d. for 10 to 14 days

➤ Tularemia (as an alternative to streptomycin)

Adults: 1 to 2 g P.O. daily in two to four divided doses for 1 to 2 weeks

➤ *Campylobacter* infection

Adults: 1 to 2 g P.O. daily in two to four divided doses for 10 days

➤ Relapsing fever caused by *Borrelia recurrentis*

Adults: 1 to 2 g P.O. daily in two to four divided doses for 7 days or until patient is afebrile

➤ Adjunctive treatment of inflammatory acne

Adults and adolescents: 500 mg to 1 g P.O. q.i.d. for 1 to 2 weeks, then decreased gradually to 125 to 500 mg P.O. daily

➤ Acne vulgaris

Adults and children older than age 11: Apply 3% ointment to affected area b.i.d. (morning and evening) until skin is thoroughly wet.

Dosage adjustment

• Renal impairment

Off-label uses

• Rosacea
• Anthrax
• Arthritis
• Lyme disease
• Sclerosing agent to control pleural effusions

Contraindications

• Hypersensitivity to drug, other tetracyclines, bisulfites, or alcohol (with some products)

• Pregnancy or breastfeeding (except in anthrax treatment or with topical form)
• Children under age 11 (with topical form)
• Children under age 8 (except in anthrax treatment)

Administration

• Give with 8 oz of water at least 1 hour before or 2 hours after meals (especially meals containing milk or other dairy products), antacids, laxatives, or antidiarrheal drugs.

Route	Onset	Peak	Duration
P.O.	Rapid	2-3 hr	6-12 hr
Topical	Unknown	Unknown	Unknown

Adverse reactions

CNS: benign intracranial hypertension, paresthesia
CV: pericarditis
EENT: abnormal conjunctival pigmentation, black hairy tongue, glossitis, hoarseness, pharyngitis, permanent tooth discoloration (in children under age 8), tooth enamel defects
GI: nausea, vomiting, diarrhea, loose bulky stools, esophageal ulcers, epigastric distress, enterocolitis, oral and anogenital candidiasis, stomatitis, anorexia, **pancreatitis**
GU: anogenital lesions, dark yellow or brown urine, elevated blood urea nitrogen (BUN), vaginal candidiasis
Hematologic: eosinophilia, hemolytic anemia, **neutropenia, thrombocytopenia, thrombocytopenia purpura**
Hepatic: fatty liver, increased hepatic enzyme levels
Musculoskeletal: retarded bone growth, polyarthralgia
Respiratory: pulmonary infiltrates
Skin: stinging and yellowing of skin (with topical form), photosensitivity, maculopapular or erythematous rash, increased pigmentation, urticaria, onycholysis

Other: superinfection, exacerbation of systemic lupus erythematosus, serum sickness-like reaction, hypersensitivity reactions including **anaphylaxis**

Interactions

Drug-drug. *Adsorbent antidiarrheals, antacids, calcium, cholestyramine, cimetidine, colestipol, iron, magnesium, sodium bicarbonate:* decreased tetracycline absorption
Digoxin: increased digoxin blood level, greater risk of toxicity
Hormonal contraceptives: decreased contraceptive efficacy
Insulin: reduced insulin requirement
Lithium: increased or decreased lithium blood level
Methoxyflurane: increased risk of nephrotoxicity
Penicillin: decreased penicillin activity
Sucralfate: prevention of tetracycline absorption from GI tract
Warfarin: enhanced warfarin effects
Drug-diagnostic tests. *Alanine aminotransferase, alkaline phosphatase, amylase, aspartate aminotransferase, bilirubin, BUN:* increased levels
Hemoglobin, neutrophils, platelets, white blood cells: decreased values
Urinary catecholamines: false elevation
Drug-food. *Dairy products, foods containing calcium:* decreased drug absorption
Drug-behaviors. *Alcohol use:* decreased drug efficacy
Sun exposure: increased risk of photosensitivity

Precautions

Use cautiously in:
• renal disease, hepatic impairment, nephrogenic diabetes insipidus
• cachectic or debilitated patients.

Patient monitoring

• Monitor for signs and symptoms of superinfection and hypersensitivity reaction.

• With long-term use, monitor complete blood count, liver function tests, and (in prepubertal patients) bone growth.

• Assess neurologic status; stay alert for benign intracranial hypertension (especially in children).

Patient teaching

• Teach patient to take oral form with 8 oz of water at least 1 hour before or 2 hours after eating a meal, consuming dairy products, or taking antacids, laxatives, or antidiarrheal drugs. Advise him to take last daily dose at least 1 hour before bedtime.

• Remind patient to complete entire course of therapy as ordered, even after symptoms improve.

◀€ Caution patient not to use outdated tetracycline because it may cause serious kidney disease.

• Teach patient to recognize and report signs and symptoms of yeast infection and other infections.

• With long-long therapy, tell patient he'll need to undergo regular blood testing; teach parents that prepubertal children should have periodic bone X-rays.

• Instruct patient using topical form not to let drug touch eyes, nose, and mouth. Caution him that drug may cause skin yellowing.

• Advise patient to avoid alcohol.

• As appropriate, review all other significant and life-threatening adverse reactions and interactions, especially those related to the drugs, tests, foods, and behaviors mentioned above.

thalidomide
Thalomid

Pharmacologic class: Synthetic glutamic acid derivative

Therapeutic class: Immunomodulator, angiogenesis inhibitor

Pregnancy risk category X

Action

Suppresses excess levels of tumor necrosis factor-alpha in patients with erythema nodosum leprosum (ENL); alters leukocyte migration by changing cell surface characteristics

Availability

Capsules: 50 mg

🕖 Indications and dosages

➤ Acute treatment of cutaneous manifestations of moderate to severe ENL; maintenance treatment to prevent and suppress recurrent ENL

Adults weighing 50 kg (110 lb) or more: 100 to 300 mg P.O. daily with 8 oz of water at bedtime or 1 hour after evening meal. May give up to 400 mg P.O. daily, depending on disease severity or previous response. Therapy should continue until signs and symptoms of active reaction subside (usually after 2 weeks). Dosage may then be tapered in 50-mg decrements q 2 to 4 weeks.

Adults weighing less than 50 kg (110 lb): Initially, 100 mg P.O. daily with 8 oz of water at bedtime or 1 hour after evening meal. May give up to 400 mg P.O. daily, depending on disease severity or previous response. Therapy should continue until signs and symptoms of active reaction subside (usually after 2 weeks). Dosage may then be tapered in 50-mg decrements q 2 to 4 weeks.

t

Off-label uses

- Aphthous stomatitis
- Wasting syndrome associated with human immunodeficiency virus (HIV)
- Multiple myeloma
- Refractory Crohn's disease

Contraindications

- Hypersensitivity to drug
- Pregnancy or breastfeeding

Administration

◀€ Follow all instructions provided by System for Thalidomide Education and Prescribing Safety (S.T.E.P.S.™) program, accessible at http://www.steps-info.com.

- Give drug with 8 oz of water just before bedtime, at least 1 hour after evening meal.
- Know that patients who require prolonged maintenance therapy to prevent cutaneous ENL recurrence and those who have flares during tapering should be maintained on minimum effective dosage, with tapering attempted every 3 to 6 months. To taper, decrease dosage in 50-mg decrements every 2 to 4 weeks.

Route	Onset	Peak	Duration
P.O.	48 hr	1-2 mo	Unknown

Adverse reactions

CNS: drowsiness, peripheral neuropathy, dizziness, vertigo, sedation, tremor, asthenia
CV: bradycardia, orthostatic hypotension, peripheral edema
EENT: rhinitis, sinusitis, pharyngitis, tooth pain
GI: nausea, constipation, diarrhea, oral moniliasis, abdominal pain
GU: impotence
Hematologic: neutropenia
Hepatic: increased lactate dehydrogenase (LD) and lipid levels; elevated liver function test results
Musculoskeletal: back pain

Skin: exfoliative, purpuric, bullous, or maculopapular rash; pruritus; fungal dermatitis; nail disorder; photosensitivity; toxic epidermal necrolysis
Other: chills, accidental injury, hypersensitivity reactions, increased HIV viral load, **severe birth defects, fetal death, Stevens-Johnson syndrome**

Interactions

Drug-drug. *Barbiturates, chlorpromazine, reserpine, sedative-hypnotics, other CNS depressants:* increased sedation
Drugs linked to peripheral neuropathy: increased risk of peripheral neuropathy
Drug-diagnostic tests. *Alanine aminotransferase, aspartate aminotransferase, LD, lipids:* increased levels
Hemoglobin, neutrophils, white blood cells: decreased levels
Drug-food. *High-fat meal:* interference with drug absorption
Drug-behaviors. *Alcohol use:* increased sedation

Precautions

Use cautiously in:
- children under age 12 (safety not established).

Patient monitoring

◀€ Monitor for signs and symptoms of hypersensitivity reaction; if rash occurs, discontinue drug and contact prescriber immediately. If Stevens-Johnson syndrome, toxic epidermal necrolysis, or exfoliative, purpuric, or bullous rash occurs, don't restart drug.
- Watch for and report signs and symptoms of peripheral neuropathy.
- Assess complete blood count with white cell differential.
- Carefully monitor patient's reproductive status.

Patient teaching

- Instruct patient to take drug with 8 oz of water just before bedtime, at least 1 hour after dinner.

◀€ Teach patient to immediately report signs and symptoms of hypersensitivity reaction—especially rash.

• Teach patient about risks of fetal exposure to drug; carefully review relevant portions of S.T.E.P.S.™ program with patient.

• Instruct females of childbearing age to use two highly effective birth control methods simultaneously, from 1 month before first thalidomide dose until 1 month after last dose.

• Explain mandatory pregnancy testing schedule to female patients; encourage compliance.

• Advise female patient to contact prescriber immediately if she suspects she's pregnant.

• Instruct male patient to use latex condoms during every sexual encounter.

• Tell patient to avoid alcohol while taking this drug.

• As appropriate, review all other significant and life-threatening adverse reactions and interactions, especially those related to the drugs, tests, foods, and behaviors mentioned above.

theophylline

Accurbron, Aerolate, Apo-Theo LA✤, Aquaphyllin, Bronkodyl, Elixomin, Elixophyllin, Lanophyllin, Pulmophyllin ELX✤, Quibron-T, Slo-bid, Sustaire, Theobid, Theochron, Theoclear, Theolair, Theospan, Theo-24, Theovent, T-Phyl, Uni-Dur, Uniphyl

Pharmacologic class: Xanthine derivative

Therapeutic class: Bronchodilator, spasmolytic

Pregnancy risk category C

Action

Causes bronchodilation by relaxing bronchial smooth muscles and suppressing airway response to stimuli; inhibits phosphodiesterase and release of slow-reacting substance of anaphylaxis and histamine

Availability

Capsules (immediate-release): 100 mg, 200 mg
Capsules (timed-release, 8 to 12 hours): 50 mg, 60 mg, 65 mg, 75 mg, 100 mg, 125 mg, 130 mg
Capsules (timed-release, 12 hours): 50 mg, 125 mg, 130 mg, 250 mg, 260 mg
Capsules (timed-release, 24 hours): 100 mg, 200 mg, 300 mg
Elixir: 80 mg/15 ml
Injection (with dextrose): 0.4 mg/ml, 0.8 mg/ml, 1.6 mg/ml, 2 mg/ml, 3.2 mg/ml, 4 mg/ml
Solution: 80 mg/15 ml, 150 mg/15 ml
Syrup (cherry): 80 mg/15 ml, 150 mg/15 ml
Tablets (immediate-release): 100 mg, 125 mg, 200 mg, 250 mg, 300 mg
Tablets (timed-release, 8 to 12 hours): 100 mg, 200 mg, 250 mg, 300 mg, 500 mg
Tablets (timed-release, 8 to 24 hours): 100 mg, 200 mg, 300 mg, 450 mg
Tablets (timed-release, 12 to 24 hours): 100 mg, 200 mg, 300 mg
Tablets (timed-release, 24 hours): 200 mg, 250 mg, 260 mg, 400 mg, 600 mg

⚡ Indications and dosages

➤ Acute bronchospasm (in patients not receiving theophylline)
Adults (otherwise healthy non-smokers): Initially, 6 mg/kg P.O., followed in next 12 to 16 hours by 3 mg/kg P.O. q 6 hours for two doses, and then a maintenance dosage of 3 mg/kg P.O. q 8 hours
Children ages 9 to 16, young adult smokers: Initially, 6 mg/kg P.O., followed in next 12 to 16 hours by 3 mg/kg P.O. q 4 hours for three doses, then a

maintenance dosage of 3 mg/kg P.O. q 6 hours

Children age 1 to 9: Initially, 6 mg/kg P.O., followed in next 12 to 16 hours by 4 mg/kg P.O. q 4 hours for three doses, then a maintenance dosage of 4 mg/kg P.O. q 6 hours

➤ Acute bronchospasm (in patients receiving theophylline)

Adults and children: Loading dose determined partly by time, amount, and administration route of last dose and based on expectation that each 0.5 mg/kg of drug will result in 1 mcg/ml increase in theophylline blood level. In significant respiratory distress, loading dose may be 2.5 mg/kg P.O. or I.V. to increase theophylline level by approximately 5 mcg/ml.

➤ Chronic bronchospasm

Adults and children: *Immediate-release forms*—16 mg/kg P.O. daily or 400 mg P.O. daily (whichever is less) given in three to four divided doses q 6 to 8 hours. *Timed-release forms*—12 mg/kg P.O. daily or 400 mg P.O. daily (whichever is less) given in three to four divided doses q 8 to 12 hours. May increase dosage of either immediate- or timed-release form at 2- to 3-day intervals, to a maximum of 13 mg/kg or 900 mg daily (whichever is less) in patients over age 16, 18 mg/kg daily in children ages 12 to 16, 20 mg/kg daily in children ages 9 to 12, or 24 mg/kg daily in children up to age 9.

Dosage adjustment
• Cor pulmonale or heart failure
• Elderly patients
• Young adults (smokers and non-smokers)

Off-label uses
• Essential tremor
• Apnea and bradycardia in premature infants

Contraindications
• Hypersensitivity to drug or other xanthines (such as coffee, theobromine)

• Active peptic ulcer
• Seizure disorder

Administration
• For I.V. administration, use infusion solution designed for drug, or mix with dextrose 5% in water. Deliver by controlled infusion pump.
• Know that for treatment of acute bronchospasm, theophylline (often given as aminophylline) preferably is given I.V. as 20 mg/ml of theophylline (25 mg/ml of aminophylline).
• Don't administer timed-release forms to patient with acute bronchospasm.

Route	Onset	Peak	Duration
P.O.	Rapid	1-2 hr	6 hr
P.O. (timed)	Delayed	4-8 hr	8-24 hr
I.V.	Rapid	End of infusion	6-8 hr

Adverse reactions
CNS: irritability, dizziness, nervousness, restlessness, headache, insomnia, reflex hyperexcitability, **seizures**
CV: palpitations, marked hypotension, sinus tachycardia, extrasystole, **circulatory failure, ventricular arrhythmias**
GI: nausea, vomiting, diarrhea, hematemesis, gastroesophageal reflux
GU: increased diuresis, proteinuria
Metabolic: hyperglycemia, syndrome of inappropriate antidiuretic hormone secretion
Musculoskeletal: muscle twitching
Respiratory: tachypnea, **respiratory arrest**
Skin: urticaria, rash, alopecia, flushing
Other: fever, hypersensitivity reaction

Interactions
Drug-drug. *Allopurinol, calcium channel blockers, cimetidine, corticosteroids, disulfiram, ephedrine, hormonal contraceptives, influenza virus vaccine, interferon, macrolides, mexiletine, nonselective beta blockers, quinolones, thiaben-*

---

dazole: increased theophylline blood level, greater risk of toxicity

Aminoglutethimide, barbiturates, keto-conazole, rifampin, sulfinpyrazone, sym-pathomimetics: decreased theophylline blood level and effects

Carbamazepine, isoniazid, loop diuret-ics: increased or decreased theophylline blood level

Halothane: increased risk of arrhythmias

Hydantoins: decreased hydantoin blood level

Lithium: decreased therapeutic effect of lithium

Nondepolarizing muscle relaxants: reversal of neuromuscular blockade

Propofol: antagonism of sedative effects of propofol

Tetracyclines: increased risk of adverse reactions to theophylline

Drug-diagnostic tests. *Glucose:* increased level

Drug-food. *Any food:* altered bioavailability and absorption of some timed-release theophylline forms, causing rapid release and possible toxicity

Caffeine- or xanthine-containing foods and beverages: increased theophylline blood level and greater risk of adverse CNS and cardiovascular reactions

Diet high in protein and charcoal-broiled beef and low in carbohydrates: increased theophylline elimination and decreased efficacy

High-carbohydrate, low-protein diet: decreased theophylline elimination and increased risk of adverse reactions

Drug-herb. *Caffeine-containing herbs (such as cola nut, guarana, maté):* increased theophylline blood level, greater risk of adverse CNS and cardiovascular reactions

Ephedra (ma huang): increased stimulant effects

St. John's wort: decreased theophylline blood level and efficacy

Drug-behaviors. *Nicotine (as in ciga-rettes, gum, transdermal patches):* in-creased theophylline metabolism and decreased efficacy

Precautions

Use cautiously in:
• alcoholism; heart failure or other cardiac or circulatory impairment; renal or hepatic disease; COPD; hyperthyroidism; diabetes mellitus; glaucoma; peptic ulcer disease; hypoxemia; hypertension
• elderly patients
• children under age 1.

Patient monitoring

• Monitor for signs and symptoms of hypersensitivity reaction, including rash and fever.
• Assess respiratory status; monitor pulmonary function tests to gauge drug efficacy and identify adverse effects.
• Monitor cardiovascular and neurologic status carefully.
• Assess glucose level in diabetic patients.

Patient teaching

• Teach patient to take oral form 1 hour before or 2 hours after meals, along with 8 oz of water.
• Tell patient not to crush or chew timed-release forms.
• Advise patient not to use different drug brands interchangeably.
• Instruct patient to report worsening dyspnea and other respiratory problems.
• Teach patient to recognize and report adverse neurologic reactions.
• Tell patient that all nicotine forms (including cigarettes, patches, and gum) decrease drug efficacy; discourage nicotine use.
• Teach patient to avoid a diet high in protein and charcoal-broiled beef and low in carbohydrates because it makes drug less effective.
• Tell patient that high-carbohydrate, low-protein diet increases risk of ad-

t

verse reactions, as do products containing caffeine.

• Caution patient to avoid herbs, especially ephedra and St. John's wort.

• Advise patient not to take over-the-counter drugs without prescriber's approval. Tell him to inform all prescribers he's taking this drug because it interacts with many other drugs.

• As appropriate, review all other significant and life-threatening adverse reactions and interactions, especially those related to the drugs, tests, foods, herbs, and behaviors mentioned above.

thiopental sodium
Pentothal

Pharmacologic class: Barbiturate
Therapeutic class: Anesthetic
Controlled substance schedule III
Pregnancy risk category C

Action
Inhibits ascending nerve impulse transmission in reticular formation and depresses CNS; may enhance or mimic inhibitory action of gamma-amino butyric acid, causing sedation, hypnosis, and anticonvulsant effect. Increases cerebrovascular resistance, which reduces intracranial pressure (ICP).

Availability
Powder for injection: 2% (400 mg), 2.5% (500 mg)

⚕ Indications and dosages
➤ Slow induction and maintenance of anesthesia
Adults: 50 to 75 mg I.V. given slowly at 20- to 40-second intervals, based on patient response. May give additional doses of 25 to 50 mg I.V. p.r.n.

➤ Rapid induction and maintenance of anesthesia before other general anesthetics are given
Adults: 210 to 280 mg (3 to 4 mg/kg) I.V. in two to four divided doses
➤ Maintenance of anesthesia without other general anesthetics for short procedures
Adults: 0.2% or 0.4% solution intermittent I.V. injection or continuous I.V. infusion
➤ Seizures associated with anesthesia or other causes in mechanically ventilated patients
Adults: 75 to 125 mg I.V. infusion as soon as possible after seizure onset
➤ Increased ICP
Adults: 1.5 to 3.5 mg/kg intermittent I.V. infusion
➤ To facilitate narcoanalysis or narcosynthesis in psychiatric patients
Adults: Give test dose of 25 to 75 mg, as ordered, after anticholinergic is administered (dosage based on patient's age, sex, and weight). Administer by slow I.V. injection at 100 mg/minute with patient counting backwards from 100. Just after patient becomes confused with counting but before he falls asleep, discontinue drug; this allows patient to return to semidrowsy state in which conversation is coherent.

Contraindications
• Hypersensitivity to drug, its components, or other barbiturates
• Hepatic or renal impairment
• Porphyria

Administration
• Know that drug should be given by health care professionals qualified in use of I.V. anesthetics. Have resuscitative equipment on hand.
• Reconstitute drug according to manufacturer's directions.
• Give test dose of 25 to 75 mg I.V. as ordered; assess tolerance and monitor for hypersensitivity reaction for 1 minute.

• Administer I.V. injection over 20 to 30 seconds or by continuous I.V. infusion using infusion pump.
• Avoid extravasation to prevent severe tissue reaction (necrosis, sloughing). If extravasation occurs, stop infusion immediately, contact prescriber, apply moist heat, and inject 1% procaine hydrochloride, as prescribed.

Route	Onset	Peak	Duration
I.V.	10-40 sec	Unknown	10-30 min

Adverse reactions

CNS: anxiety, agitation, prolonged drowsiness, confusion, amnesia, headache, myoclonus, postoperative shivering
CV: venous thrombosis, phlebitis, and thrombophlebitis at I.V. site; bradycardia; tachycardia
Musculoskeletal: twitching
Respiratory: wheezing, cough, **laryngospasm, apnea, respiratory depression**
Skin: rash, hives
Other: pain at I.V. site, hiccups, hypersensitivity reaction

Interactions

Drug-drug. *Aminophylline (low-dose I.V. use):* partial reversal of sedation during early recovery phase
Clonidine, metoclopramide: enhanced thiopental effects
CNS depressants: additive CNS depression
Highly protein-bound drugs (such as diazoxide): hypotension
Protein-bound drugs (such as aspirin, meprobamate, probenecid, sulfisoxazole): potentiation of thiopental's hypnotic effects
Drug-herb. *Valerian:* increased sedation
Drug-behaviors. *Alcohol use:* additive CNS depression
Chronic alcohol use: decreased thiopental efficacy, necessitating dosage increase

Precautions

Use cautiously in:
• severe cardiovascular disease, hypotension, shock, status asthmaticus, conditions that could prolong hypnotic effect (such as excessive premedication, Addison's disease, myxedema, myasthenia gravis, increased blood urea concentration, severe anemia)
• pregnant patients.

Patient monitoring

• Monitor vital signs and ECG carefully.
• Closely monitor respiratory status, particularly for respiratory depression.
◀ Assess patient carefully to detect early signs and symptoms of shock; stop drug and contact prescriber immediately if these occur.
• Monitor neurologic status; institute safety measures if seizures, agitation, or anxiety occurs.
• Assess injection site closely and frequently to prevent extravasation and detect thrombophlebitis.

Patient teaching

• Explain why drug is being used; reassure patient he'll be closely monitored.

thioridazine
Mellaril-S

thioridazine hydrochloride
Apo-Thioridazine✤, Mellaril, Novo-Ridazine✤, PMS Thioridazine✤

Pharmacologic class: Phenothiazine
Therapeutic class: Antipsychotic
Pregnancy risk category C

Action

Blocks dopamine receptors in CNS; exerts strong alpha-adrenergic and anticholinergic blocking activity. Also depresses cerebral cortex, hypothalamus, and limbic system.

Availability
Oral solution (concentrated): 30 mg/ml, 100 mg/ml
Oral suspension: 10 mg/5 ml, 25 mg/5 ml, 100 mg/5 ml
Tablets: 10 mg, 15 mg, 25 mg, 50 mg, 100 mg, 150 mg, 200 mg

Indications and dosages
➤ Psychotic disorders
Adults: Initially, 50 to 100 mg P.O. t.i.d.; may increase gradually to a maintenance dosage of up to 800 mg/day
Severely disturbed, hospitalized children ages 2 to 12: Initially, 0.5 mg/kg P.O. daily in divided doses; may increase gradually until optimal effects occur. Maximum daily dosage is 3 mg/kg.
➤ Psychoneurotic manifestations
Adults: 25 mg P.O. t.i.d. Dosing regimens range from 10 mg two to four times daily to 50 mg three to four times daily; total daily dosage ranges from 20 to 200 mg.
➤ Short-term treatment of major depression with associated anxiety, agitation, depressed mood, tension, sleep disturbances, and fears in elderly patients
Adults: Initially, 25 mg P.O. t.i.d. Dosage ranges from 25 to 200 mg daily, depending on severity of symptoms and patient's age and condition.
Dosage adjustment
• Renal or hepatic impairment
• Elderly patients

Contraindications
• Hypersensitivity to drug, its components, or other phenothiazines
• Alcohol intolerance (with concentrate only)
• Hypokalemia
• Bone marrow depression
• Severe cardiovascular disease

• Bradycardia
• Prolonged QTc interval
• History of arrhythmias
• Concurrent use of drugs that prolong the QTc interval, inhibit CYP450-2D6 (such as fluoxetine, paroxetine), or reduce phenothiazine clearance by other means (such as fluvoxamine, pindolol, propranolol)

Administration
• Keep liquid form away from skin to avoid contact dermatitis.
• Before starting therapy, correct hypokalemia as ordered.
• Discontinue drug at least 48 hours before myelography because of risk of seizures.

Route	Onset	Peak	Duration
P.O.	Unknown	Unknown	8-12 hr

Adverse reactions
CNS: sedation, extrapyramidal reactions, tardive dyskinesia, **neuroleptic malignant syndrome, seizures**
CV: orthostatic hypotension, tachycardia, prolonged QTc interval, **arrhythmias**
EENT: lens opacities, pigmentary retinopathy (decreased visual acuity, brownish vision, and impaired night vision with high doses), dry eyes
GI: constipation, ileus, dry mouth, anorexia
GU: urinary retention, dark urine, galactorrhea, gynecomastia
Hepatic: jaundice
Hematologic: agranulocytosis, leukopenia
Skin: rash, photosensitivity reaction, pigmentation changes
Other: allergic reactions, hyperthermia

Interactions
Drug-drug. *Anticholinergic and anticholinergic-like drugs (including antihistamines, antidepressants, atropine, disopyramide, haloperidol, other phe-*

nothiazines): additive anticholinergic effects

Antihypertensives, nitrates: additive hypotension

CNS depressants (including antihistamines, general anesthetics, opioid analgesics, sedative-hypnotics): additive CNS depression

Diuretics: increased risk of electrolyte imbalances and arrhythmias

Drugs that inhibit CYP450-2D6 (such as fluoxetine, paroxetine), prolong the QTc interval (such as arsenic trioxide, azole antifungals, floxin antibiotics, octreotide), or decrease phenothiazine clearance by other means (such as fluvoxamine, pindolol, propranolol): increased risk of life-threatening arrhythmias

Lithium: disorientation, loss of consciousness, increased risk of extrapyramidal reactions

Drug-diagnostic tests. *Alanine aminotransferase (ALT), alkaline phosphatase, aspartate aminotransferase (AST), bilirubin:* increased levels

Granulocytes, hematocrit, hemoglobin, platelets, white blood cells: decreased levels

Pregnancy tests, urine bilirubin: false-positive results

Drug-herb. *Kava:* increased adverse drug reactions

Drug-behaviors. *Alcohol use:* additive hypotension

Precautions

Use cautiously in:
• cardiovascular or respiratory disease, mitral insufficiency, hepatic or renal impairment, glaucoma, depression, seizure disorder, risk factors for electrolyte imbalance (such as dehydration or diuretic therapy)
• elderly or debilitated patients
• pregnant or breastfeeding patients.

Patient monitoring

• Monitor neurologic status; stay alert for signs and symptoms of neuroleptic malignant syndrome.
• Watch for tardive dyskinesia and extrapyramidal symptoms.
• Assess for urinary retention, constipation, and blurred vision.
• Monitor bilirubin level, complete blood count, liver function tests, and vision tests. Be aware that liver function abnormalities may warrant drug discontinuation.
• Closely monitor depressed patient for suicidal ideation.

Patient teaching

• Instruct patient to dilute concentrate with water or fruit juice and take dose right away, with or without food.
◀€ Caution patient not to stop therapy suddenly; dosage must be tapered.
◀€ Instruct patient or caregiver to watch for and immediately report signs and symptoms of serious CNS reactions, including high fever, sweating, unstable blood pressure, stupor, muscle rigidity, tongue protrusion, cheek puffing, mouth puckering, chewing movements, and involuntary leg or arm movements.
• Tell patient to keep liquid form away from skin; if it contacts skin, advise him to wash it off thoroughly and immediately.
• Teach patient to report urinary retention, blurred vision, or constipation.
• Instruct patient to avoid driving and other hazardous activities.
• Caution patient not to drink alcohol.
• Teach patient effective ways to counteract photosensitivity.
• As appropriate, review all other significant and life-threatening adverse reactions and interactions, especially those related to the drugs, tests, herbs, and behaviors mentioned above.

t

thyroid, desiccated
Armour Thyroid, Thyrar, Thyroid Strong, Westhroid

Pharmacologic class: Hormone supplement
Therapeutic class: Thyroid hormone
Pregnancy risk category A

Action
Regulates cell growth and differentiation and increases metabolic rate of body tissues; effects mediated at cellular level

Availability
Tablets: 15 mg, 30 mg, 60 mg, 90 mg, 120 mg, 180 mg, 240 mg, 300 mg

🟊 Indications and dosages
➤ Mild hypothyroidism
Adults: Initially, 60 mg/day P.O.; may increase by 60 mg q 30 days to desired response. Usual maintenance dosage is 60 to 180 mg/day.
➤ Severe hypothyroidism
Adults: Initially, 15 mg/day P.O. daily; may increase to 30 mg/day after 2 weeks and then to 60 mg/day 2 weeks later. Assess after 1 month, and again 1 month later at 60 mg-dose. If necessary, dosage may then be increased to 120 mg/day P.O. for 2 months, with assessment repeated. Subsequent assessments and dosage increases may occur up to a maximum dosage of 180 mg/day.
➤ Congenital or severe hypothyroidism
Children: Initially, 15 mg P.O. daily; may increase to 30 mg/day after 2 weeks, with subsequent increases at 2-week intervals. Maintenance doses may be higher in growing children than in hypothyroid adults.

Dosage adjustment
• Cardiovascular disease
• Elderly patients

Contraindications
• Hypersensitivity to drug or its components
• Myocardial infarction
• Adrenal insufficiency
• Thyrotoxicosis

Administration
• Give drug before breakfast each day.

Route	Onset	Peak	Duration
P.O.	Unknown	12-48 hr	Unknown

Adverse reactions
CNS: insomnia, tremors, headache
CV: palpitations, angina pectoris, hypertension, tachycardia, **arrhythmias, cardiac arrest**
GI: nausea, vomiting, diarrhea
GU: menstrual irregularities
Metabolic: heat intolerance, **thyroid storm**
Musculoskeletal: accelerated bone maturation in children
Skin: sweating
Other: weight loss, appetite changes, fever

Interactions
Drug-drug. *Anticoagulants, catecholamines, sympathomimetics:* increased effects of these drugs
Bile acid sequestrants: decreased thyroid hormone absorption
Digoxin, insulin, oral hypoglycemics: decreased effects of these drugs
Estrogen: decreased thyroid hormone effects
Oral anticoagulants: increased risk of bleeding
Drug-diagnostic tests. *Aspartate aminotransferase, creatine kinase, glucose, lactate dehydrogenase, protein-bound iodine:* increased levels
Thyroid function tests: decreased values

Drug-herb. *Bugleweed, soy:* increased adverse drug reactions

Precautions

Use cautiously in:
• cardiovascular disease
• elderly patients
• breastfeeding patients.

Patient monitoring

◀€ Monitor for chest pain; if it occurs, withhold drug and contact prescriber.
• Assess vital signs and temperature frequently.
◀€ Monitor thyroid function tests closely; report signs and symptoms of thyroid storm immediately.
• In diabetic patients, monitor blood glucose level closely.
• In children, monitor sleeping pulse rate and basal morning temperature.
• In females on long-term therapy, monitor bone density tests.

Patient teaching

• Teach patient to take drug each morning before breakfast.
◀€ Caution patient not to stop therapy abruptly; dosage must be tapered.
• Teach patient to immediately report chest pain or signs and symptoms of drug toxicity (fever, chest pain, rapid pulse, skipped heartbeats, heat intolerance, excessive sweating, nervousness, emotional instability).
• Advise patient to tell all prescribers he's taking this drug. Caution him not to take over-the-counter drugs without consulting prescriber.
• Tell diabetic patient that drug may alter blood glucose level; encourage frequent glucose self-monitoring.
• As appropriate, review all other significant and life-threatening adverse reactions and interactions, especially those related to the drugs, tests, and herbs mentioned above.

tiagabine hydrochloride
Gabatril Filmtabs

Pharmacologic class: Nipecotic acid derivative

Therapeutic class: Anticonvulsant

Pregnancy risk category C

Action

Unknown; thought to raise the seizure threshold by enhancing activity of gamma-aminobutyric acid (a major inhibitory neurotransmitter in CNS)

Availability

Tablets: 2 mg, 4 mg, 12 mg, 16 mg

ⓘ Indications and dosages

➤ Adjunctive treatment of partial seizures

Adults older than age 18: Initially, 4 mg P.O. once daily for 1 week; then may increase by 4 to 8 mg/day at weekly intervals, up to 56 mg/day in two to four divided doses

Dosage adjustment
• Hepatic impairment

Off-label uses

• Anxiety

Contraindications

• Hypersensitivity to drug

Administration

◀€ Don't stop therapy suddenly; dosage must be tapered.

Route	Onset	Peak	Duration
P.O.	Unknown	45 min	Unknown

Adverse reactions

CNS: dizziness, insomnia, drowsiness, nervousness, asthenia, confusion, poor concentration, impaired memory, depression, emotional lability, hostility,

---

agitation, ataxia, abnormal gait, tremors, paresthesia, speech disorder, language problems
CV: vasodilation
EENT: nystagmus, pharyngitis, epistaxis
GI: nausea, vomiting, diarrhea, abdominal pain, mouth ulcers
Musculoskeletal: myasthenia
Respiratory: increased cough
Skin: rash, pruritis
Other: increased appetite, weight change, pain, allergic reaction

Interactions
Drug-drug. *Carbamazepine, phenobarbital, phenytoin, primidone:* increased tiagabine clearance and decreased blood level

Precautions
Use cautiously in:
• hepatic impairment
• pregnant or breastfeeding patients
• children under age 12 (safety not established).

Patient monitoring
• Watch for depression and suicidal ideation.
• Assess vital signs and cardiovascular status.
• Monitor closely for severe generalized weakness; if present, consult prescriber regarding possible dosage reduction.

Patient teaching
• Teach patient to take drug on a regular schedule with food.
◀€ Caution patient not to stop therapy suddenly; dosage must be tapered.
• Instruct patient to report signs or symptoms of depression.
◀€ Teach patient to report adverse neurologic reactions; tell him to contact prescriber immediately if severe overall weakness occurs.
• Advise female patient to notify prescriber of suspected pregnancy.

• As appropriate, review all other significant adverse reactions and interactions, especially those related to the drugs mentioned above.

ticarcillin disodium
Ticar

Pharmacologic class: Penicillin (extended-spectrum)
Therapeutic class: Anti-infective
Pregnancy risk category B

Action
Inhibits cell wall synthesis and division during microorganism replication, causing osmotically unstable cells to lyse and die

Availability
Powder for injection: 1 g, 3 g, 6 g, 20 g, 30 g

⨀ Indications and dosages
➤ Complicated urinary tract infections (UTIs)
Adults and children: 150 to 200 mg/kg I.V. infusion in divided doses q 4 to 6 hours
➤ Uncomplicated UTIs
Adults and children weighing more than 40 kg (88 lb): 1 g I.M. or direct I.V. in divided doses q 6 hours
Children older than 1 month who weigh less than 40 kg (88 lb): 50 to 100 mg/kg I.M. or direct I.V. in divided doses q 6 hours to 8 hours, not to exceed adult dosage
Dosage adjustment
• Hepatic or renal impairment

Contraindications
• Hypersensitivity to drug or other penicillins

Administration

• For direct I.V. injection, dilute with sodium chloride solution, dextrose 5% in water, or lactated Ringer's solution as directed. Inject by slow I.V. into vein or I.V. tubing, preferably no faster than 50 mg/ml to reduce vein irritation.
• For intermittent or continuous I.V. infusion, reconstitute and dilute with compatible I.V. solution to a concentration of 10 to 100 mg/ml. Give by slow or intermittent I.V. infusion over 30 to 120 minutes (in adults).
• Change I.V. site every 2 days.
• For I.M. use, reconstitute 1-g vial with 2 ml of sterile water for injection, sodium chloride injection, or 1% lidocaine solution without epinephrine. Solution will contain approximately 385 mg of ticarcillin per ml. Inject I.M. dose deep into large muscle, such as gluteus maximus; don't exceed 2 g per injection.
• Give ticarcillin at least 1 hour before aminoglycosides (such as amikacin, gentamicin, or tobramycin).

Route	Onset	Peak	Duration
I.V.	Rapid	End of infusion	Unknown
I.M.	Rapid	30-75 min	Unknown

Adverse reactions

CNS: lethargy, fatigue, hyperreflexia, neuromuscular excitability, asterixis, hallucinations, stupor, headache, giddiness, dizziness, **seizures**
GI: nausea, vomiting, diarrhea, flatulence, unpleasant taste, **pseudomembranous colitis**
Hematologic: eosinophilia, prolonged bleeding time, transient **neutropenia** and **leukopenia** (with high doses)
Hepatic: transient increases in liver function test results
Skin: urticaria, rash
Other: pain, vein irritation, erythema, phlebitis, and thrombophlebitis at I.V. site; pain, induration, and erythema at I.M. injection site; fever; overgrowth of nonsusceptible organisms; hypersensitivity reactions including **anaphylaxis**

Interactions

Drug-drug. *Aminoglycosides:* physically incompatible; aminoglycoside inactivation if mixed in same I.V. solution
Aminoglycosides, tetracyclines: additive activity against some bacteria
Lithium: altered lithium elimination
Probenecid: increased ticarcillin blood level
Drug-diagnostic tests. *Alanine aminotransferase, alkaline phosphatase, aspartate aminotransferase, eosinophils, lactate dehydrogenase, sodium:* increased levels
Granulocytes, hemoglobin, platelets, white blood cells: decreased levels
Urine glucose, urine protein: false-positive results

Precautions

Use cautiously in:
• cystic fibrosis, renal or hepatic disease
• pregnant or breastfeeding patients.

Patient monitoring

• Monitor complete blood count with white cell differential; also monitor liver function tests.
• Assess for superinfection and severe allergic reactions.
• Monitor neurologic status, especially for seizures.

Patient teaching

◀ᜒ Advise patient to report skin reactions promptly.
◀ᜒ Teach patient that drug may increase risk of other infections; instruct him to report signs and symptoms of new infection right away.
• Instruct patient to limit sodium intake.
• As appropriate, review all other significant and life-threatening adverse reactions and interactions, especially those related to the drugs and tests mentioned above.

t

ticarcillin disodium and clavulanate potassium
Timentin

Pharmacologic class: Penicillin (extended-spectrum)
Therapeutic class: Anti-infective
Pregnancy risk category B

Action
Ticarcillin disodium inhibits cell wall synthesis during microorganism replication; clavulic acid extends ticarcillin's antibiotic spectrum by inactivating beta-lactamase enzymes (which otherwise would degrade ticarcillin).

Availability
Injection: 3 g ticarcillin and 100 mg clavulanic acid in 3.1-g vials

🕖 Indications and dosages
➤ Systemic, urinary tract, and intra-abdominal infections caused by susceptible organisms
Adults weighing more than 60 kg (132 lb): 3.1 g (30:1 fixed-ratio combination of 3 g ticarcillin and 100 mg clavulanic acid) I.V. infusion q 4 to 6 hours
Adults and children ages 3 months to 16 years weighing less than 60 kg (132 lb): 200 mg/kg I.V. daily in divided doses q 6 hours
➤ Gynecologic infections caused by susceptible organisms
Adults weighing more than 60 kg (132 lb): For moderate infections, 200 mg/kg I.V. (30:1 fixed-ratio combination of 3 g ticarcillin and 100 mg clavulanic acid) daily in divided doses q 4 to 6 hours. For severe infections, 300 mg/kg I.V. (30:1 fixed-ratio combination) daily in divided doses q 4 hours by infusion.

➤ Mild to moderate or severe infections in children caused by susceptible organisms
Children ages 3 months to 16 years weighing less than 60 kg (132 lb): For mild to moderate infections, 200 mg/kg (30:1 fixed-ratio combination of 3 g ticarcillin and 100 mg clavulanic acid) I.V. daily in divided doses q 6 hours. For severe infections, 300 mg/kg (30:1 fixed-ratio combination) I.V. daily in divided doses q 4 hours.
Dosage adjustment
• Renal impairment

Contraindications
• Hypersensitivity to drug or other penicillins

Administration
• Add 13 ml of sterile water or normal saline solution to vial; shake gently. Dilute further to 10 to 100 mg/ml of ticarcillin; infuse I.V. over 30 minutes.
• Administer at least 1 hour before I.V. aminoglycosides (such as amikacin, gentamicin, or tobramycin).

Route	Onset	Peak	Duration
I.V.	Immediate	Immediate	Unknown

Adverse reactions
CNS: lethargy, fatigue, hyperreflexia, neuromuscular excitability, asterixis, hallucinations, stupor, headache, giddiness, dizziness, **seizures**
GI: nausea, vomiting, diarrhea, flatulence, unpleasant taste, **pseudomembranous colitis**
Hematologic: eosinophilia, prolonged bleeding time, transient **neutropenia** and **leukopenia** (with high doses)
Hepatic: transient increases in liver function test results
Skin: urticaria, rash
Other: pain, vein irritation, erythema, phlebitis, and thrombophlebitis at I.V. site; fever; overgrowth of nonsusceptible organisms; hypersensitivity reactions including **anaphylaxis**

Interactions

Drug-drug. *Aminoglycosides:* physical incompatibility, aminoglycoside inactivation if mixed in same I.V. solution
Aminoglycosides, tetracyclines: additive activity against some bacteria
Lithium: altered lithium elimination
Probenecid: increased ticarcillin blood level

Drug-diagnostic tests. *Alanine aminotransferase, alkaline phosphatase, aspartate aminotransferase, eosinophils, lactate dehydrogenase, sodium:* increased levels
Granulocytes, hemoglobin, platelets, white blood cells: decreased levels
Urine glucose, urine protein: false-positive results

Precautions

Use cautiously in:
• cystic fibrosis, renal or hepatic disease
• pregnant or breastfeeding patients.

Patient monitoring

• Monitor complete blood count with white cell differential; also assess liver function tests.
• Watch closely for signs and symptoms of superinfection and severe allergic reactions.
• Assess neurologic status; stay alert for seizures.

Patient teaching

◀€ Advise patient to report skin reactions right away.
◀€ Teach patient that drug may increase risk of other infections; advise him to promptly report signs and symptoms of new infection.
• Instruct patient to limit sodium intake; ticarcillin contains sodium.
• As appropriate, review all other significant and life-threatening adverse reactions and interactions, especially those related to the drugs and tests mentioned above.

ticlopidine hydrochloride
Ticlid

Pharmacologic class: Platelet aggregation inhibitor
Therapeutic class: Antiplatelet agent
Pregnancy risk category B

Action

Inhibits the release of first and second phases of adenosine diphosphate-induced effects on platelet aggregation, preventing thrombus formation

Availability

Tablets: 250 mg

Indications and dosages

➤ To prevent cerebrovascular accident (CVA) in patients with completed thrombotic CVA or CVA precursors when aspirin is ineffective or intolerable
Adults: 250 mg P.O. b.i.d. with meals
Dosage adjustment
• Renal impairment

Off-label uses

• Chronic arterial occlusion
• Coronary artery bypass graft
• Open-heart surgery
• Intermittent claudication
• Primary glomerulonephritis
• Sickle cell disease
• Subarachnoid hemorrhage
• Uremic patients with atrioventricular shunts or fistulas

Contraindications

• Hypersensitivity to drug
• Hematopoietic disorders
• Active bleeding
• Severe hepatic disease

Administration

• Give drug with meals.
• Don't give within 2 hours of antacids.

Route	Onset	Peak	Duration
P.O.	Within 4 days	8-11 days	2 wk

Adverse reactions

CNS: dizziness, headache, weakness, **intracerebral bleeding**

EENT: conjunctival hemorrhage, tinnitus, epistaxis

GI: nausea, vomiting, diarrhea, full sensation, GI pain, dyspepsia, flatulence, anorexia, **GI bleeding**

GU: hematuria

Hematologic: ecchymoses, eosinophilia, purpura, **thrombocytosis, neutropenia, agranulocytosis, thrombotic thrombocytopenic purpura, bone marrow depression**

Hepatic: abnormal liver function tests

Skin: rashes, bruising, pruritus, urticaria

Other: pain, posttraumatic or perioperative bleeding

Interactions

Drug-drug. *Antacids:* decreased ticlopidine blood level

Aspirin: potentiation of aspirin's effect on platelets

Cimetidine (long-term use): reduced ticlopidine clearance

Digoxin: slightly decreased digoxin blood level

Phenytoin: increased phenytoin blood level, greater risk of toxicity

Theophylline: decreased theophylline clearance, greater risk of toxicity

Vitamin A: altered anticoagulant effects

Drug-diagnostic tests. *Alanine aminotransferase, alkaline phosphatase, aspartate aminotransferase:* increased levels

Granulocytes, neutrophils, platelets, white blood cells: decreased counts

Drug-food. *Any food:* increased ticlopidine absorption

Drug-herb. *Alfalfa, anise, arnica, astragalus, bilberry, black current seed oil, bladderwrack, bogbean, boldo, borage oil, buchu, capsaicin, cat's claw, celery, chapparal, cinchona bark, clove oil, coenzyme Q10, dandelion, dong quai, evening primrose oil, fenugreek, feverfew, garlic, ginger, gingko, guggal, papaya extract, red clover, rhubarb, safflower oil, skullcap, St. John's wort, tan shen:* altered anticoagulant effects

Precautions

Use cautiously in:
• renal or hepatic impairment
• high risk for bleeding
• elderly patients
• pregnant or breastfeeding patients
• children under age 18 (safety not established).

Patient monitoring

• Monitor complete blood count with white cell differential.
• Monitor coagulation studies closely; watch for signs and symptoms of bleeding tendency.
• Assess neurologic status carefully; stay alert for indications of intracranial bleeding.
• Monitor liver function test results.

Patient teaching

• Teach patient to take drug with meals but not within 2 hours of antacids.
• Instruct patient to report diarrhea, easy bruising, and bleeding.
• Instruct patient to stop taking drug 10 to 14 days before elective surgery.
• Teach patient to inform all prescribers that he's taking this drug.
• Tell patient that aspirin-containing products and many herbs increase risk of bleeding; encourage him to consult prescriber before taking over-the-counter drugs or herbs.
• As appropriate, review all other significant and life-threatening adverse reactions and interactions, especially those related to the drugs, tests, foods, and herbs mentioned above.

timolol maleate
Apo-Timol✦, Blocadren,
Novo-Timol✦, Timoptic

Pharmacologic class: Beta-adrenergic
blocker (nonselective)

Therapeutic class: Antihypertensive,
vascular headache suppressant,
antiglaucoma agent

Pregnancy risk category C

Action
Blocks stimulation of beta$_1$-adrenergic
(myocardial) and beta$_2$-adrenergic
(pulmonary, vascular, and uterine)
receptor sites; may reduce aqueous
production, causing intraocular pressure (IOP) to decrease

Availability
Ophthalmic gel: 0.25%, 0.5%
Ophthalmic solution: 0.25%, 0.5%
Tablets: 5 mg, 10 mg, 20 mg

⚕ Indications and dosages
➤ Hypertension
Adults: Initially, 10 mg P.O. b.i.d., giv-
en alone or with a diuretic; may increase at 7-day intervals as needed.
Usual maintenance dosage is 10 to 20
mg daily in two divided doses, up to
60 mg/day.
➤ Acute myocardial infarction (MI)
Adults: 10 mg P.O. b.i.d. starting 1 to 4
weeks after MI
➤ To prevent vascular headaches
Adults: Initially, 10 mg P.O. b.i.d.; may
increase up to 10 mg in morning and
20 mg in evening. Maintenance dose
may be given as a single daily dose.
➤ Elevated IOP in patients with
open-angle glaucoma
Adults: One drop of 0.25% to 0.5%
ophthalmic solution in affected eye
b.i.d. or 0.25% to 0.5% ophthalmic gel
in affected eye once daily

Off-label uses
• Angina pectoris
• Supraventricular arrhythmias

Contraindications
• Hypersensitivity to drug or other
beta-adrenergic blockers
• Uncompensated heart failure
• Bradycardia or heart block
• Cardiogenic shock
• Pulmonary edema
• Bronchial asthma or chronic ob-
structive pulmonary disease

Administration
• Measure apical pulse before administering. If patient has significant bradycardia or tachycardia, withhold dose
and consult prescriber.

Route	Onset	Peak	Duration
P.O.	Unknown	1-2 hr	12-24 hr
Ophthalmic	≤ 30 min	1-2 hr	≤ 24 hr

Adverse reactions
CNS: fatigue, dizziness, asthenia, insomnia, headache, vertigo, nervousness, depression, paresthesia, hallucinations, memory loss, disorientation,
emotional lability, clouded sensorium
CV: hypotension, angina pectoris exacerbation, bradycardia, **atrioventricular
or sinoatrial block, arrhythmias,
heart failure**
EENT: visual disturbances, dry eyes,
tinnitus, nasal congestion
Respiratory: dyspnea, crackles, **bronchospasm**
GI: nausea, constipation, diarrhea, abdominal discomfort
GU: impotence, decreased libido, increased blood urea nitrogen (BUN)
Hematologic: decreased hemoglobin
and hematocrit
Hepatic: increased liver function test
results
Metabolic: hypoglycemia, hyperkalemia, hyperuricemia, decreased high-
density lipoprotein (HDL) level

t

Musculoskeletal: joint pain
Respiratory: pulmonary edema
Skin: itching, rash

Interactions
Drug-drug. *Antihypertensives, nitrates:*
additive hypotension
Insulin, oral hypoglycemics: altered efficacy of these drugs
Nonsteroidal anti-inflammatory drugs:
decreased antihypertensive effect of
timolol
Quinidine: inhibited timolol metabolism, leading to increased beta-adrenergic blockade and bradycardia
Reserpine: increased risk of hypotension and bradycardia
Theophylline: reduced effects of both
drugs
Drug-diagnostic tests. *Antinuclear
antibodies:* increased titer
BUN, potassium, uric acid: increased
levels
Glucose, HDLs, hematocrit, hemoglobin:
decreased levels
Drug-herb. *Ephedra (ma huang), St.
John's wort, yohimbine:* decreased timolol efficacy

Precautions
Use cautiously in:
• renal or hepatic impairment, diabetes
mellitus, thyrotoxicosis
• elderly patients
• pregnant or breastfeeding patients
• children (safety not established).

Patient monitoring
• Monitor vital signs, blood pressure,
cardiovascular status and ECG closely.
• Assess respiratory status; check
breath sounds for wheezing and bronchospasm.
• Monitor blood glucose levels in patients with diabetes mellitus.

Patient teaching
• Teach patient to take his pulse before
each dose; instruct him to contact pre-

scriber if pulse is outside the safe range
established by prescriber.
◀ Caution patient not to stop taking
drug abruptly; dosage must be tapered.
• Caution patient to administer eye
drops only as prescribed because they
are absorbed systemically.
• Teach patient to recognize and immediately report significant adverse
respiratory, cardiac, and neurologic reactions.
• Tell patient that many over-the-
counter drugs and herbs may decrease
timolol's efficacy. Advise him to consult prescriber before using these products.
• Tell diabetic patients that drug may
lower blood glucose; encourage regular
blood glucose monitoring.
• As appropriate, review all other significant and life-threatening adverse
reactions and interactions, especially
those related to the drugs, tests, and
herbs mentioned above.

tinzaparin sodium
Innohep

Pharmacologic class: Low-molecular-
weight heparin
Therapeutic class: Anticoagulant
Pregnancy risk category B

Action
Enhances inhibition of Factor Xa and
thrombi by binding to and accelerating
antithrombin III activity; has only
slight effect on thrombin and clotting
time

Availability
Injection: 20,000 anti-Xa IU/ml in 2-ml
vials

🖊 Indications and dosages
➤ Deep-vein thrombosis
Adults: 175 anti-Xa IU/kg S.C. once

daily for at least 6 days and until patient is adequately anticoagulated with warfarin sodium for 2 consecutive days.

Off-label uses
• Pulmonary embolism

Contraindications
• Hypersensitivity to drug, heparin, sulfites, benzyl alcohol, or pork products
• Active major bleeding
• History of heparin-induced thrombocytopenia

Administration
• Warfarin therapy usually begins within 1 to 3 days of the start of tinzaparin therapy.
• Give by deep S.C. injection into abdominal wall while patient is sitting or lying down.
◀̇ Don't give drug I.V. or I.M.
• Rotate injection sites among four quadrants of abdominal wall.
• Don't rub injection site after removing needle.
• Observe injection site closely for signs and symptoms of hematoma.

Route	Onset	Peak	Duration
S.C.	2-3 hr	4-5 hr	18-24 hr

Adverse reactions
CNS: dizziness, insomnia, confusion, headache, **cerebral or intracranial bleeding**
CV: hypotension, hypertension, angina pectoris, chest pain, tachycardia, dependent edema, **thromboembolism, arrhythmias, myocardial infarction (MI)**
EENT: ocular hemorrhage, epistaxis
GI: nausea, vomiting, constipation, flatulence, dyspepsia, melena, **GI hemorrhage, retroperitoneal or intra-abdominal bleeding**

GU: urinary tract infection, hematuria, urinary retention, dysuria, **vaginal hemorrhage**
Hematologic: anemia, **thrombocytopenia, granulocytopenia, agranulocytosis, pancytopenia, hemorrhage**
Hepatic: reversible elevations in aspartate aminotransferase (AST) and alanine aminotransferase (ALT)
Musculoskeletal: back pain, **intra-articular hemorrhage**
Respiratory: dyspnea, pneumonia, respiratory disorder, **pulmonary embolism**
Skin: pruritus, rash, bullous eruption, cellulitis, purpura, skin necrosis
Other: injection site hematoma and reactions, pain, fever, impaired healing, infection, hypersensitivity reaction, congenital anomaly, fetal distress, **fetal death**

Interactions
Drug-drug. *Oral anticoagulants, platelet inhibitors (such as dextran, dipyridamole, nonsteroidal anti-inflammatory drugs [NSAIDs], salicylate, sulfinpyrazone), thrombolytics:* increased risk of bleeding
Vitamin A: increased anticoagulant effect
Drug-diagnostic tests. *ALT, AST:* increased levels
Granulocytes, hemoglobin, platelets, red blood cells, white blood cells: decreased values
Drug-herb. *Alfalfa, anise, arnica, astragalus, bilberry, black currant seed oil, bladderwrack, bogbean, boldo (with fenugreek), borage oil, buchu, capsacin, cat's claw, celery, chaparral, chincona bark, clove oil, dandelion, dong quai, evening primrose oil, fenugreek, feverfew, garlic, ginger, ginkgo, guggul, papaya extract, red clover, rhubarb, safflower oil, skullcap, tan-shen:* increased anticoagulant effect

t

Precautions

Use cautiously in:

- renal impairment; bacterial endocarditis; uncontrolled hypertension; diabetic retinopathy; congenital or acquired bleeding disorders; hepatic failure and GI ulcers; recent brain, spinal, or ophthalmic surgery
- pregnant patients
- elderly patients.

Patient monitoring

- Monitor vital signs and ECG closely.
- ◀€ Assess neurologic status, particularly for indications of intracranial or intracerebral bleeding.
- Evaluate closely for signs and symptoms of bleeding in all body systems.
- ◀€ Monitor respiratory status carefully to detect pneumonia, pulmonary embolism, and other serious adverse reactions.
- Monitor cardiovascular status closely; stay alert for signs and symptoms of thrombophlebitis and edema.
- Monitor complete blood count, platelet count, and coagulation studies; assess stool for occult blood.

Patient teaching

- ◀€ Teach patient to immediately report unusual bleeding or bruising. Tell him drug can cause serious adverse reactions, especially bleeding; advise him to report new symptoms right away.
- Inform patient that aspirin products, NSAIDs, and many herbs increase the risk of bleeding; urge him to consult prescriber before taking these products.
- Tell patient he'll undergo regular blood tests during therapy.
- As appropriate, review all other significant and life-threatening adverse reactions and interactions, especially those related to the drugs, tests, and herbs mentioned above.

tirofiban hydrochloride

Aggrastat

Pharmacologic class: Glycoprotein (GP IIb/IIIa)-receptor inhibitor

Therapeutic class: Platelet aggregation inhibitor

Pregnancy risk category B

Action

Causes reversible platelet aggregation inhibition by binding to GP IIb/IIIa-receptor on platelets

Availability

Injection: 50-ml vials (250 mcg/ml), 250-ml and 500-ml premixed vials (50 mcg/ml)

🕖 Indications and dosages

➤ Acute coronary syndrome (given with heparin); patients undergoing percutaneous transluminal coronary angioplasty (PTCA) or atherectomy
Adults: Loading dose of 0.4 mcg/kg/minute I.V. for 30 minutes, followed by continuous I.V. infusion of 0.1 mcg/kg/minute for 48 to 108 hours in patients being medically managed. Continue infusion for 12 to 24 hours after PTCA or atherectomy.

Dosage adjustment
- Renal insufficiency

Contraindications

- Hypersensitivity to drug or its components
- Active internal bleeding or history of bleeding diathesis within past 30 days
- Cerebrovascular accident (CVA) within past 30 days, or history of hemorrhagic CVA
- History of intracranial hemorrhage, intracranial neoplasm, arteriovenous malformation, aneurysm, or thrombocytopenia after previous tirofiban use

• History, symptoms, or findings that suggest aortic dissection
• Major surgery or severe trauma within past 30 days
• Severe hypertension
• Concurrent use of other parenteral GP IIb/IIIa inhibitors
• Acute pericarditis
• Breastfeeding

Administration

◀≈ Know that drug comes in both premixed vials of 50 mcg/ml and in injection concentrate of 250 mcg/ml.
• Dilute injection concentrate to same concentration as premixed vials (50 mcg/ml) by withdrawing and discarding 50 ml of solution from 250-ml plastic bag of normal saline solution or dextrose 5% in water, or by withdrawing and discarding 100 ml of solution from 500-ml plastic bag of same solution and replacing with an equal volume of concentrated drug form.
• Mix I.V. solution well and inspect visually before administering.
• Squeeze plastic bag and check for leaks; discard bag if it has leaks.
• Don't use drug in series connections with other plastic bags; don't add other drugs to bag containing tirofiban.

Route	Onset	Peak	Duration
I.V.	Immediate	Immediate	4-6 hr

Adverse reactions

CNS: headache, dizziness, **spinal-epidural hematoma, intracranial hemorrhage**
CV: vasovagal reaction, bradycardia, **hemopericardium, coronary artery dissection**
GI: nausea, vomiting, occult bleeding, hematemesis, **retroperitoneal hemorrhage**
GU: pelvic pain, hematuria
Hematologic: bleeding, **thrombocytopenia**
Musculoskeletal: leg pain

Respiratory: pulmonary hemorrhage
Skin: diaphoresis
Other: infusion site bleeding, chills, fever, edema, allergic reactions, **anaphylaxis**

Interactions

Drug-drug. *Clopidogrel, dipyridamole, nonsteroidal anti-inflammatory drugs, oral anticoagulants (such as thrombolytics, ticlopidine, warfarin), other drugs affecting hemostasis:* increased risk of bleeding
Levothyroxine, omeprazole: increased renal clearance of tirofiban
Vitamin A: increased risk of bleeding
Drug-diagnostic tests. *Hematocrit, hemoglobin, platelets:* decreased values
Drug-herb. *Alfalfa, anise, arnica, astragalus, bilberry, black currant seed oil, bladderwrack, bogbean, boldo (with fenugreek), borage oil, buchu, capsaicin, cat's claw, celery, chaparral, chincona bark, clove oil, dandelion, dong quai, evening primrose oil, fenugreek, feverfew, garlic, ginger, ginkgo, guggul, papaya extract, red clover, rhubarb, safflower oil, skullcap, tan-shen:* increased risk of bleeding

Precautions

Use cautiously in:
• renal disease
• elderly patients
• pregnant patients
• children under age 18 (safety not established).

Patient monitoring

◀≈ Monitor complete blood count, platelet count, and coagulation studies; assess stool for occult blood.
• Watch for bleeding at puncture sites, especially at arterial site used for cardiac catheterization. Immobilize access site to reduce bleeding risk.
• Monitor for signs and symptoms of intracranial bleeding and bleeding in other body systems (especially respiratory, GI, and GU).

t

• Monitor vital signs and ECG.

◀€ Assess cardiovascular status; stay alert for signs and symptoms of coronary artery dissection or hemopericardium.

Patient teaching

◀€ Instruct patient to immediately report unusual bleeding or bruising.

• Teach patient to recognize and immediately report serious adverse reactions.

• Tell patient he'll undergo regular blood testing during therapy.

• As appropriate, review all other significant and life-threatening adverse reactions and interactions, especially those related to the drugs, tests, and herbs mentioned above.

---

tizanidine hydrochloride
Zanaflex

Pharmacologic class: Alpha-adrenergic agonist (centrally acting)

Therapeutic class: Skeletal muscle relaxant

Pregnancy risk category C

Action

Stimulates alpha$_2$-adrenergic agonist receptor sites; reduces spasticity by enhancing presynaptic inhibition of motor neurons

Availability

Tablets: 2 mg, 4 mg

⚕ Indications and dosages

➤ Management of increased muscle tone associated with spasticity in patients with multiple sclerosis or spinal cord injury

Adults: Initially, 4 mg P.O. q 6 to 8 hours (no more than three doses in 24 hours). Increase in increments of 2 to 4 mg, up to 8 mg/dose or 24 mg/day (not to exceed 36 mg/day).

Contraindications

• Hypersensitivity to drug or its components

Administration

• Give with or without food.

Route	Onset	Peak	Duration
P.O.	Unknown	1-2 hr	3-6 hr

Adverse reactions

CNS: drowsiness, asthenia, dizziness, speech disorder, dyskinesia, nervousness, anxiety, depression, paresthesia

CV: hypotension, bradycardia

EENT: blurred vision, pharyngitis, rhinitis

GI: vomiting, diarrhea, constipation, abdominal pain, dyspepsia, dry mouth

GU: urinary frequency, urinary tract infection

Hepatic: increased hepatic enzyme levels

Musculoskeletal: back pain, myasthenia

Skin: rash, skin ulcers, sweating

Other: fever, infection, flulike symptoms

Interactions

Drug-drug. *Alpha$_2$-adrenergic agonist antihypertensives:* increased risk of hypotension

CNS depressants (such as some antidepressants, antihistamines, opioids, sedative-hypnotics): additive CNS depression

Hormonal contraceptives: increased tizanidine blood level, greater risk of adverse reactions

Drug-diagnostic tests. *Alanine aminotransferase, alkaline phosphatase, aspartate aminotransferase, glucose:* increase levels

Drug-behaviors. *Alcohol use:* additive CNS depression

Precautions
Use cautiously in:
- renal or hepatic impairment
- elderly patients
- pregnant or breastfeeding patients
- children (safety not established).

Patient monitoring
- Monitor temperature and vital signs; stay alert for orthostatic hypotension, bradycardia, and fever or other signs and symptoms of infection.
- Assess liver function test results.

Patient teaching
- Advise patient he may take drug with or without food.
- Teach patient to report signs or symptoms of infection or depression.
- Instruct patient to move slowly when sitting up or standing to avoid dizziness or light-headedness from sudden blood pressure decrease.
- Caution patient not to drink alcohol.
- As appropriate, review all other significant adverse reactions and interactions, especially those related to the drugs, tests, and behaviors mentioned above.

tobramycin
AKtob, TOBI, Tobrex

tobramycin sulfate
Nebcin

Pharmacologic class: Aminoglycoside
Therapeutic class: Anti-infective
Pregnancy risk category D

Action
Interferes with protein synthesis in bacterial cell by binding to 30S ribosomal subunit

Availability
Injection: 10 mg/ml, 40 mg/ml, 1.2-g vial
Nebulizer solution: 300 mg/5 ml in 5-ml ampule
Ophthalmic ointment: 0.3%
Ophthalmic solution: 0.3%
Pediatric solution for injection: 20 mg/2 ml

Indications and dosages
➤ Serious infections caused by susceptible strains of *Escherichia coli* and *Proteus, Providencia,* and *Citrobacter* species
Adults: 3 mg/kg/day I.V. or I.M. in evenly divided doses q 8 hours. For life-threatening infections, may increase up to 5 mg/kg/day I.V. or I.M. in three or four evenly divided doses, then reduce to 3 mg/kg/day as soon as possible.
Children older than 1 week: 6 to 7.5 mg/kg/day in three or four evenly divided doses, such as 2 to 2.5 mg/kg I.V. or I.M. q 8 hours or 1.5 to 1.9 mg/kg I.V. or I.M. q 6 hours
Neonates less than 1 week old: Up to 4 mg/kg/day I.V. or I.M. in evenly divided doses q 12 hours
➤ *Pseudomonas aeruginosa* in cystic fibrosis patients
Adults and children over age 6: 300 mg inhalation b.i.d. (preferably q 12 hours but no less than 6 hours apart) for 28 days, then off for 28 days; then repeat cycle
➤ Ocular infections caused by susceptible organisms
Adults and children: For mild to moderate infections, apply a ribbon of ophthalmic ointment (approximately 1 cm) to infected eye two or three times daily, or instill one to two drops of ophthalmic solution into infected eye q 4 hours. For severe infections, initially apply ophthalmic ointment q 3 to 4 hours or instill two drops of ophthalmic solution into infected eye q 30 to 60 minutes; decrease dosing frequency

when improvement occurs. Therapy should continue for at least 48 hours after infection has been controlled.

Dosage adjustment
• Renal impairment

Contraindications

• Hypersensitivity to drug, other aminoglycosides, bisulfites (with some products), benzyl alcohol (in neonates, with some products)

Administration

• Dilute I.V. dose in 50 to 100 ml of normal saline solution or dextrose 5% in water; for child dosing, smaller volumes are needed.
• Infuse drug over at least 30 minutes. Flush line after administration.
• Give cephalosporins or penicillins 1 hour before or after tobramycin.
• Give inhalation doses by nebulizer over 10 to 15 minutes.

Route	Onset	Peak	Duration
I.V.	Rapid	15-30 min	Unknown
I.M.	Rapid	30-90 min	Unknown
Inhalation, ophthalmic	Unknown	Unknown	Unknown

Adverse reactions

CNS: confusion, lethargy, headache, delirium, dizziness, vertigo
EENT: eye stinging (with ophthalmic form), ototoxicity, hearing loss, roaring in ears, tinnitus
GI: nausea, vomiting, diarrhea, stomatitis
GU: oliguria, proteinuria, increased nonprotein nitrogen, **nephrotoxicity**
Hematologic: leukocytosis, anemia, eosinophilia, **leukopenia, thrombocytopenia, granulocytopenia**
Hepatic: increased alanine aminotransferase (ALT), aspartate aminotransferase (AST), and bilirubin levels
Metabolic: increased lactate dehydrogenase (LD), blood urea nitrogen (BUN), and creatinine levels; hypocal-

cemia; hyponatremia; hypokalemia; hypomagnesemia
Musculoskeletal: muscle weakness
Respiratory: apnea
Skin: rash, urticaria, itching
Other: superinfection, fever, pain and irritation at injection site

Interactions

Drug-drug. *Cephalosporins, vancomycin:* increased risk of nephrotoxicity
Dimenhydrinate: masking of ototoxicity symptoms
General anesthetics, neuromuscular blockers: increased neuromuscular blockade and respiratory depression
Indomethacin: increased tobramycin trough and peak levels
Loop diuretics: increased risk of ototoxicity
Penicillins: physical incompatibility; tobramycin inactivation when mixed in same I.V. solution
Polypeptide anti-infectives: increased risk of respiratory paralysis and renal dysfunction
Drug-diagnostic tests. *ALT, AST, bilirubin, BUN, creatinine, LD, nonprotein nitrogen, urine protein:* increased levels
Calcium, granulocytes, hemoglobin, magnesium, platelets, potassium, sodium, white blood cells: decreased levels

Precautions

Use cautiously in:
• renal or hearing impairment, neuromuscular diseases (such as myasthenia gravis), obesity
• elderly patients
• pregnant or breastfeeding patients
• neonates and premature infants.

Patient monitoring

• Draw blood sample for peak drug level 1 hour after I.M. or 30 minutes after I.V. administration; draw sample for trough level just before next dose.
• Assess liver and kidney function test results.

• Closely monitor patient's hearing.
• Monitor complete blood count with white cell differential.

Patient teaching

◀｡ Tell patient that drug may cause hearing impairment and other serious adverse reactions, such as unusual bleeding or bruising. Instruct him to report these reactions at once.
• Instruct patient to report new signs or symptoms of infection.
• With inhalation form, teach patient how to use nebulizer. Instruct him to administer dose over 10 to 15 minutes by breathing normally through mouthpiece while sitting or standing. Remind him to use only the hand-held nebulizer and compressor originally dispensed with drug. Advise him that a noseclip may help him breathe through his mouth. If he uses other inhaled drugs, instruct him to take tobramycin last.
• As appropriate, review all other significant and life-threatening adverse reactions and interactions, especially those related to the drugs and tests mentioned above.

tolbutamide sodium

Apo-Tolbutamide✣,
Novo-Butamide✣, Orinase

Pharmacologic class: Sulfonylurea (first-generation)
Therapeutic class: Hypoglycemic
Pregnancy risk category C

Action

Stimulates insulin release from pancreatic beta cells; increases peripheral tissue sensitivity to insulin, either by increasing the number of insulin receptors or enhancing insulin binding to cellular receptors

Availability
Tablets: 500 mg

🕖 Indications and dosages

➤ Adjunct in type 2 diabetes mellitus uncontrolled by diet and exercise
Adults: Initially, 1 to 2 g P.O. daily. Maintenance dosage is 250 mg to 2 g P.O. daily; maximum daily dosage is 3 g. May be given as a single dose in morning or in divided doses after meals.
Dosage adjustment
• Hepatic insufficiency

Contraindications
• Hypersensitivity to drug, its components, or other sulfonylureas
• Diabetic coma or ketoacidosis
• Sole therapy for type 1 diabetes mellitus

Administration
• Give as prescribed, either as a single dose in morning or in divided doses after meals, depending on GI tolerance.

Route	Onset	Peak	Duration
P.O.	1 hr	3-4 hr	6-12 hr

Adverse reactions
CNS: malaise, paresthesia, vertigo, headache, fatigue, dizziness
CV: increased risk of cardiovascular mortality
GI: nausea, heartburn, epigastric fullness, taste alteration
Metabolic: syndrome of inappropriate antidiuretic hormone secretion, **severe hypoglycemia**
Skin: transient rash, pruritis, erythema, urticaria, photosensitivity
Other: weight gain

Interactions
Drug-drug. *Androgens, anticoagulants, azole antifungals, chloramphenicol, clofibrate, fenfluramine, fluconazole, gemfibrozil, histamine$_2$ antagonists, magnesium salts, methyldopa, mono-*

t

*amine oxidase inhibitors, phenylbuta-
zone, probenecid, salicylates, sulfonamides, tricyclic antidepressants, urinary acidifiers:* increased hypoglycemia
*Beta-adrenergic blockers, calcium chan-
nel blockers, cholestyramine, corticosteroids, diazoxide, estrogens, hormonal
contraceptives, hydantoins, isoniazid,
nicotinic acid, phenothiazines, rifampin,
sympathomimetics, thiazide diuretics,
thyroid agents, urinary alkalinizers:* decreased hypoglycemic effects
Charcoal: decreased tolbutamide absorption
Digoxin: increased digoxin blood level
and risk of toxicity
Drug-diagnostic tests. *Glucose:* decreased level
Radioactive iodine: decreased thyroid
uptake
Urine albumin: false-positive reaction
Drug-herb. *Aloe, bitter melon, fenugreek, St. John's wort:* increased risk of
hypoglycemia
Drug-behaviors. *Alcohol use:* disulfiram-like effect

Precautions
Use cautiously in:
• stress caused by infection, fever, trauma, or surgery.

Patient monitoring
• Monitor blood glucose level frequently.
• Assess vital signs and cardiovascular
and neurologic status.
• Monitor nutritional status; report
significant problems.

Patient teaching
• Teach patient to take drug as prescribed, either as a single dose in morning or in divided doses after meals.
• Emphasize importance of adhering
to prescribed diet and exercise to aid
diabetes control.
• Teach patient to report significant
adverse reactions.

• Instruct patient to monitor blood
glucose level carefully.
• Caution patient not to drink alcohol.
• Tell patient that some herbs affect
blood glucose level; advise him to consult prescriber before taking any herbs.
• Teach patient effective ways to counteract photosensitivity.
• Tell patient he'll undergo regular
blood testing during therapy.
• As appropriate, review all other significant and life-threatening adverse
reactions and interactions, especially
those related to the drugs, tests, herbs,
and behaviors mentioned above.

tolcapone
Tasmar

Pharmacologic class: Catecholamine
inhibitor
Therapeutic class: Antiparkinsonian
Pregnancy risk category C

Action
Unknown; when administered with
levodopa-carbidopa, reversibly inhibits
catechol-O-methyltranferase, resulting
in increased levodopa bioavailability
and more constant dopaminergic stimulation in brain

Availability
Tablets: 100 mg, 200 mg

Indications and dosages
➤ Adjunct to levodopa-carbidopa in
patients with idiopathic Parkinson's
disease with fluctuating symptoms and
who don't respond adequately to other
adjunctive therapies
Adults: Initially, 100 mg P.O. t.i.d. giv-
en with levodopa-carbidopa. If beneficial, may increase dosage to 200 mg
P.O. t.i.d.; maximum dosage is 600 mg
daily. If response is inadequate after 3
weeks, stop therapy.

Dosage adjustment
• Moderate cirrhotic hepatic impairment

Contraindications
• Hypersensitivity to drug
• Nontraumatic rhabdomyolysis or hyperpyrexia
• Hepatic disease or increased alanine aminotransferase or aspartate aminotransferase level
• History of tolcapone-induced hepatocellular injury or drug-related confusion

Administration
◀𝄞 Before giving first dose, obtain patient's written informed consent for drug therapy.
• Know that levodopa dosage may be decreased to minimize dyskinesia.
• Check liver function test results before starting drug.
◀𝄞 Don't stop drug abruptly because this may cause a syndrome similar to neuroleptic malignant syndrome.

Route	Onset	Peak	Duration
P.O.	Unknown	2 hr	Unknown

Adverse reactions
CNS: asthenia, headache, fatigue, hypokinesia, mental deficiency, agitation, tremor, hyperactivity, paresthesia, irritability, syncope, depression, speech disorder, imbalance, confusion, sleep disorder, hallucinations, drowsiness, hypertonia, falling, hyperkinesias, dizziness, dystonia, dyskinesia, excessive dreaming
CV: hypotension, chest discomfort or pain, orthostatic complaints, palpitations
EENT: tinnitus, sinus congestion, pharyngitis
GI: nausea, vomiting, diarrhea, constipation, dyspepsia, abdominal pain, flatulence, dry mouth, anorexia
GU: impotence, hematuria, urinary tract infection (UTI), urinary incontinence, urine discoloration, micturition disorder
Hepatic: elevated hepatic enzyme levels, jaundice, **severe hepatocellular injury** including **fulminant liver failure** and **death**
Musculoskeletal: neck pain, arthritis, muscle cramps, stiffness, **rhabdomyolysis**
Respiratory: upper respiratory tract infection, dyspnea, bronchitis
Skin: rash, dermal bleeding, diaphoresis
Other: fever, influenza

Interactions
Drug-drug. *Desipramine:* increased risk of adverse tolcapone reactions
Warfarin: increased warfarin blood level

Precautions
Use cautiously in:
• renal or cardiac disease, hypertension, asthma
• pregnant or breastfeeding patients.

Patient monitoring
• Monitor parkinsonian symptoms during first 3 weeks of therapy; report improvement (or lack thereof) to help determine whether therapy should continue.
• Assess neurologic status closely.
◀𝄞 Monitor liver function test results; watch closely for signs and symptoms of hepatic impairment.
• Closely monitor temperature; watch for fever and other indications of infection, particularly upper respiratory infection, influenza, and UTI.

Patient teaching
• Teach patient to take drug with first levodopa-carbidopa dose each day.
◀𝄞 Advise patient to immediately report signs or symptoms of liver involvement (persistent nausea, fatigue, appetite loss, dark urine, itching, ten-

derness on right side of abdomen, and yellowing of skin or eyes).

• Teach patient to promptly report signs and symptoms of infection.

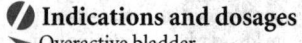 Advise female patient to immediately inform prescriber of suspected pregnancy.

• Tell patient that drug may cause involuntary movements, hallucinations, light-headedness, and other significant reactions. Encourage him to implement safety measures as needed.

• Caution patient to avoid driving and other hazardous activities until he knows how drug affects concentration and alertness.

• Advise patient to move slowly when sitting up or standing to avoid dizziness or light-headedness from sudden blood pressure decrease.

• As appropriate, review all other significant and life-threatening adverse reactions and interactions, especially those related to the drugs mentioned above.

tolterodine
Detrol, Detrol LA

Pharmacologic class: Anticholinergic
Therapeutic class: Urinary tract antispasmodic
Pregnancy risk category C

Action
Acts as a competitive muscarinic receptor antagonist, causing inhibition of bladder contractions, reducing urinary frequency

Availability
Capsules (extended-release): 2 mg, 4 mg
Tablets: 1 mg, 2 mg

Indications and dosages
➤ Overactive bladder
Adults: 2 mg (immediate-release) P.O.

b.i.d.; may decrease to 1 mg P.O. b.i.d. depending on response and tolerance. Or 4 mg (extended-release) P.O. daily; may be decreased to 2 mg P.O. daily, depending on response.

Dosage adjustment
• Hepatic impairment or disease
• Renal impairment
• Concurrent use of potent CYP3A4 inhibitors

Contraindications
• Hypersensitivity to drug or its components
• Urinary or gastric retention
• Uncontrolled narrow-angle glaucoma
• Breastfeeding

Administration
• Give with food to increase drug bioavailability.

Route	Onset	Peak	Duration
P.O.	Unknown	Unknown	12 hr

Adverse reactions
CNS: headache, dizziness, vertigo, drowsiness, paresthesia, fatigue, headache
CV: chest pain
EENT: vision abnormalities, xerophthalmia, pharyngitis
GI: diarrhea, constipation, abdominal pain, dyspepsia, dry mouth
GU: dysuria, urinary retention or frequency, urinary tract infection
Metabolic: weight gain
Musculoskeletal: joint pain
Skin: dry skin
Other: flulike symptoms, infection

Interactions
Drug-drug. *Clarithromycin, erythromycin, itraconazole, ketoconazole, miconazole:* inhibited metabolism and increased effects of tolterodine
Drug-food. *Any food:* increased drug bioavailability

Precautions
Use cautiously in
• GI obstructive disorders, significant bladder outflow obstruction, controlled narrow-angle glaucoma, significant hepatic impairment, renal impairment
• pregnant patients
• children (safety not established).

Patient monitoring
• Monitor bladder function.
• Assess blood pressure; stay alert for chest pain.
• Monitor neurologic status; report paresthesia or visual impairment.

Patient teaching
• Instruct patient to take drug with food.
• If patient is taking extended-release form, instruct him not to chew or crush it.
• Advise patient to use sugarless gum or hard candy to relieve dry mouth.
• Teach patient how drug works to improve bladder function; advise him to watch for improvement.
• As appropriate, review all other significant adverse reactions and interactions, especially those related to the drugs and foods mentioned above.

topiramate
Topamax

Pharmacologic class: Sulfamate-substituted monosaccharide derivative
Therapeutic class: Anticonvulsant
Pregnancy risk category C

Action
Blocks sodium channels, enhancing the action of gamma-amino butyrate, a neurotransmitter, and inhibits amino acid excitatory receptors

Availability
Sprinkle capsules: 15 mg, 25 mg
Tablets: 25 mg, 100 mg, 200 mg

Indications and dosages
➤ Adjunct in partial-onset seizures, primary generalized tonic-clonic seizures, and seizures associated with Lennox-Gastaut syndrome
Adults and children over age 17: Initially, 25 to 50 mg P.O. daily, increased by 25 to 50 mg weekly up to 200 mg b.i.d.
Children ages 2 to 16: Initially, less than 25 mg P.O. daily; increase at 1- or 2-week intervals in increments of 1 to 3 mg/kg/day given in two divided doses to achieve adequate response.
Dosage adjustment
• Renal impairment

Off-label uses
• Cluster headaches
• Infantile spasms
• Mood stabilization

Contraindications
• Hypersensitivity to drug
• Children under age 2

Administration
• Give drug with or without regard to meals.
• Don't break tablets because of their bitter taste.
• Administer sprinkle capsules whole or by carefully opening capsule and sprinkling entire contents into small amount of soft food. Instruct patient to swallow mixture immediately and not to chew sprinkles.
◀ Don't stop therapy suddenly; dosage must be tapered.

Route	Onset	Peak	Duration
P.O.	Unknown	2 hr	12 hr

Adverse reactions
CNS: dizziness, drowsiness, fatigue, malaise, poor memory and concentra-

tion, nervousness, psychomotor slowing, speech and language problems, aggressive reaction, agitation, anxiety, confusion, depression, irritability, ataxia, paresthesia, hyperesthesia, tremor, **suicide attempt, increased seizures**

EENT: abnormal vision, diplopia, nystagmus, acute myopia, secondary angle-closure glaucoma, decreased hearing, rhinitis, sinusitis, epistaxis, pharyngitis

GI: nausea, constipation, abdominal pain, dry mouth, gastroenteritis, altered taste, increased salivation (in children), anorexia

GU: renal calculi, urinary incontinence, leukorrhea, increased creatinine level

Hematologic: purpura, **leukopenia, thrombocytopenia**

Hepatic: elevated alanine aminotransferase (ALT), alkaline phosphatase (ALP), and aspartate aminotransferase (AST) levels

Metabolic: hypoglycemia, hypocalcemia, hyperchloremia, hypernatremia, hyponatremia, hypochlolesterolemia, hypophosphatemia

Musculoskeletal: myalgia, back pain, leg pain

Respiratory: pneumonia

Skin: rash, skin disorder, alopecia, dermatitis, hypertrichosis, eczema, seborrhea, skin discoloration

Other: weight loss, thirst, fever, flulike symptoms, hot flashes, infection, edema, allergic reaction

Interactions

Drug-drug. *Carbamazepine:* decreased topiramate blood level and effects
Carbonic anhydrase inhibitors (such as acetazolamide): increased risk of renal calculi
CNS depressants: increased risk of CNS depression and other adverse cognitive or neuropsychiatric reactions
Hormonal contraceptives: decreased contraceptive efficacy

Phenytoin: increased phenytoin blood level and effects, decreased topiramate blood level and effects
Valproic acid: decreased effects of both drugs

Drug-diagnostic tests. *ALP, ALT, AST, creatinine:* increased levels
Calcium, cholesterol, glucose, phosphate: decreased levels
Sodium: increased or decreased level

Drug-behaviors. *Alcohol use:* increased CNS depression

Precautions

Use cautiously in:
• renal or hepatic impairment, dehydration, urolithiasis, glaucoma, myopia
• pregnant or breastfeeding patients.

Patient monitoring

◀≶ Monitor seizure type and pattern; report new seizure types or worsening seizure pattern.
• Assess neurologic status closely; report significant adverse reactions.
◀≶ Watch for and immediately report signs and symptoms of depression or suicidal ideation.
• Monitor fluid intake and output; report indications of urinary tract infection, urinary incontinence, or renal calculi.
◀≶ Monitor vision; if patient becomes acutely nearsighted and has symptoms of secondary angle-closure glaucoma (such as cloudy vision and eye pain), stop drug and contact prescriber right away.

Patient teaching

• Tell patient he may take drug with or without food.
• Caution patient not to crush or break tablets.
• If patient is taking capsules, tell him he may open them, sprinkle contents onto small amount of soft food (such as applesauce), and consume it immediately. Tell him not to store this mixture.

◀€ Caution patient not to stop drug therapy suddenly; dosage must be tapered.

• Teach patient to drink plenty of fluids to reduce risk of kidney stones.

◀€ Teach patient that drug may cause new seizure types or worsen seizure pattern; instruct him to report these events immediately.

◀€ Instruct patient (and significant other as appropriate) to immediately report signs of depression or suicidal thoughts.

◀€ Advise patient to immediately report vision changes, especially nearsightedness, cloudy vision, or eye pain.

• Instruct patient not to drive or perform other hazardous activities.

• Tell patient not to drink alcohol.

• Advise female patients to notify prescriber of suspected pregnancy.

• As appropriate, review all other significant and life-threatening adverse reactions and interactions, especially those related to the drugs, tests, and behaviors mentioned above.

topotecan hydrochloride
Hycamtin

Pharmacologic class: DNA topoisomerase inhibitor
Therapeutic class: Antineoplastic
Pregnancy risk category D

Action
Regulates DNA replication and repair of broken DNA strands, relieving torsional strain; also exerts cytoxic effects during DNA synthesis

Availability
Injection: 4 mg in single-dose vial

Indications and dosages
➤ Metastatic ovarian carcinoma after chemotherapy failure; recurrent or progressive small-cell lung cancer in patients who initially responded to chemotherapy

Adults: 1.5 mg/m^2 I.V. infusion given over 30 minutes for 5 consecutive days, beginning on day 1 of 21-day cycle.

Dosage adjustment
• Renal impairment
• Neutropenia

Contraindications
• Hypersensitivity to drug or its components
• Severe bone marrow depression
• Pregnancy or breastfeeding

Administration
◀€ Before starting therapy, check blood counts. Patient must have baseline neutrophil count of more than 1,500 cells/mm^3 and platelet count of more than 100,000 cells/mm^3 to receive drug.

◀€ Prepare drug under vertical laminar flow hood, wearing gloves and protective clothing. Follow facility policy for discarding used drug containers and I.V. equipment.

• If skin comes into contact with drug, wash it off immediately with soap and water.

• To reconstitute drug, add 4 ml of sterile water to 4-mg vial. Dilute further in normal saline solution or dextrose 5% water; administer immediately over 30 minutes using infusion pump.

Route	Onset	Peak	Duration
I.V.	Unknown	Unknown	Unknown

Adverse reactions
CNS: asthenia, headache, fatigue, paresthesia

GI: nausea, vomiting, diarrhea, constipation, abdominal pain, stomatitis, anorexia

Hematologic: anemia, **leukopenia, thrombocytopenia, neutropenia**
Hepatic: elevated hepatic enzyme levels
Musculoskeletal: back pain, skeletal pain
Respiratory: coughing, dyspnea
Skin: erythematous or maculopapular rash, pruritus, urticaria, dermatitis, bullous eruption, alopecia
Other: fever, body pain, **sepsis**

Interactions
Drug-drug. *Cisplatin:* severe bone marrow depression
Granulocyte colony-stimulating factor: prolonged neutropenia
Live-virus vaccines: increased risk of infection from vaccine
Drug-diagnostic tests. *Alanine aminotransferase, aspartate aminotransferase, bilirubin:* increased levels

Precautions
Use cautiously in:
• children (safety and efficacy not established).

Patient monitoring
• Closely monitor complete blood count with white cell differential.
• Assess for signs and symptoms of bleeding tendency.
• Monitor closely for indications of sepsis, other infections, and hepatotoxicity.

Patient teaching
◀﹦ Advise patient to immediately report unusual bleeding or bruising, sore throat, fever, or chills.
• Teach patient to implement safety measures to avoid bruising and bleeding.
• Teach patient to minimize GI upset by eating small, frequent servings of healthy food and drinking plenty of fluids.

◀﹦ Advise female patient to notify prescriber of possible pregnancy.
• Inform patient that drug may cause hair loss.
• Tell patient he'll undergo regular blood testing during therapy.
• As appropriate, review all other significant and life-threatening adverse reactions and interactions, especially those related to the drugs and tests mentioned above.

torsemide
Demadex

Pharmacologic class: Loop diuretic
Therapeutic class: Diuretic, antihypertensive
Pregnancy risk category B

Action
Inhibits sodium and chloride reabsorption from ascending loop of Henle and distal renal tubule; increases renal excretion of water, sodium, chloride, magnesium, hydrogen, and calcium; may also exert renal and peripheral vasodilatory effects. Efficacy persists despite impaired renal function, resulting in natriuretic diuresis.

Availability
Injection: 10 mg/ml
Tablets: 5 mg, 10 mg, 20 mg, 100 mg

〽 Indications and dosages
➤ Heart failure
Adults: 10 to 20 mg P.O. or I.V. daily. If response is inadequate, titrate upward by doubling dosage until desired response occurs. Don't exceed 200 mg as a single dose.
➤ Hypertension
Adults: 5 mg P.O. daily. May increase to 10 mg once daily after 4 to 6 weeks;

if drug is still not effective, additional antihypertensive may be prescribed.

➤ Chronic renal failure

Adults: 20 mg P.O. or I.V. daily. If response is inadequate, titrate upward by doubling dosage until desired response occurs. Don't exceed 200 mg as a single dose.

➤ Hepatic cirrhosis

Adults: 5 or 10 mg P.O. or I.V. daily, given with aldosterone antagonist or potassium-sparing diuretic. Titrate upward by doubling dosage if response is inadequate. Don't exceed 40 mg as a single dose.

Contraindications

• Hypersensitivity to drug, thiazides, or sulfonylureas
• Anuria
• Hepatic coma

Administration

• Give I.V. by direct injection over at least 2 minutes, or by continuous I.V. infusion.
• Flush I.V. line with normal saline solution before and after administering drug.

Route	Onset	Peak	Duration
P.O.	Within 1 hr	1-2 hr	6-8 hr
I.V.	Within 10 min	Within 1 hr	6-8 hr

Adverse reactions

CNS: dizziness, headache, asthenia, insomnia, nervousness, syncope
CV: hypotension, ECG changes, chest pain, volume depletion, atrial fibrillation, **ventricular tachycardia, shunt thrombosis**
EENT: rhinitis, sore throat
GI: nausea, diarrhea, vomiting, constipation, dyspepsia, anorexia, rectal bleeding, **GI hemorrhage**
GU: excessive urination

Metabolic: hyperglycemia, hyperuricemia, hypokalemia
Musculoskeletal: joint pain, myalgia
Respiratory: increased cough
Skin: rash
Other: edema

Interactions

Drug-drug. *Aminoglycosides, cisplatin:* increased risk of ototoxicity
Amphotericin B, corticosteroids, mezlocillin, piperacillin, potassium-wasting diuretics, stimulant laxatives: additive hypokalemia
Antihypertensives, nitrates: additive hypotension
Lithium: increased lithium blood level and toxicity
Neuromuscular blockers: prolonged neuromuscular blockade
Nonsteroidal anti-inflammatory drugs, probenecid: inhibited diuretic response
Sulfonylureas: decreased glucose tolerance, hyperglycemia in patients with previously well-controlled diabetes
Drug-diagnostic tests. *Glucose, uric acid:* increased levels
Potassium: decreased level
Drug-herb. *Dandelion:* interference with diuresis
Ephedra (ma huang): reduced hypotensive effect of torsemide
Geranium, ginseng: increased risk of diuretic resistance
Licorice: rapid potassium loss
Drug-behaviors. *Acute alcohol ingestion:* additive hypotension

Precautions

Use cautiously in:
• severe hepatic disease accompanied by cirrhosis or ascites, preexisting uncorrected electrolyte imbalances, diabetes mellitus, worsening azotemia
• elderly patients
• pregnant or breastfeeding patients
• children under age 18.

t

Patient monitoring
• Monitor vital signs, especially for hypotension.
• Assess ECG for arrhythmias and other changes.
• Monitor weight and fluid intake and output to assess drug efficacy.
• Monitor electrolyte levels, particularly potassium; stay alert for signs and symptoms of hypokalemia.
• Assess hearing for indications of ototoxicity.
• Monitor blood glucose level carefully in diabetic patients; drug may cause hyperglycemia.

Patient teaching
• Advise patient to take drug in morning with or without food.
• Instruct patient to move slowly when sitting up or standing to avoid dizziness or light-headedness from sudden blood pressure decrease.
• Advise patient to monitor weight and report sudden increases.
• Teach diabetic patient to monitor blood glucose level carefully.
• Instruct patient to avoid alcohol.
• Advise patient to consult prescriber before using herbs.
• As appropriate, review all other significant and life-threatening adverse reactions and interactions, especially those related to the drugs, tests, herbs, and behaviors mentioned above.

tramadol hydrochloride
Ultram

Pharmacologic class: Opioid agonist
Therapeutic class: Analgesic
Pregnancy risk category C

Action
Inhibits reuptake of serotonin and norepinephrine in CNS

Availability
Tablets: 50 mg

⚡ Indications and dosages
➤ Moderate to moderately severe pain
Adults: In rapid titration, 50 to 100 mg P.O. q 4 to 6 hour (not to exceed 400 mg/day, or 300 mg/day in patients over age 75). In gradual titration, initially 25 mg P.O. daily; increase by 25 mg/day q 3 days to 100 mg/day, then increase by 50 mg/day q 3 days up to 200 mg/day.
Dosage adjustment
• Renal or hepatic impairment

Contraindications
• Hypersensitivity to drug, its components, or opioids
• Acute intoxication with alcohol, sedative-hypnotics, centrally acting analgesics, opioid analgesics, or psychotropic agents
• Physical opioid dependence

Administration
• Give as prescribed for pain, preferably before pain becomes severe.

Route	Onset	Peak	Duration
P.O.	1 hr	2-3 hr	4-6 hr

Adverse reactions
CNS: dizziness, vertigo, headache, drowsiness, anxiety, stimulation, confusion, incoordination, euphoria, nervousness, sleep disorder, asthenia, hypertonia, **seizures**
CV: vasodilation
EENT: visual disturbances
GI: nausea, vomiting, diarrhea, constipation, abdominal pain, dyspepsia, flatulence, dry mouth, anorexia
GU: urinary retention and frequency, proteinuria, menopausal symptoms
Hematologic: decreased hemoglobin
Metabolic: increase hepatic enzyme and creatinine levels

Respiratory: respiratory depression (with large doses, concomitant anesthetic use, or alcohol ingestion)
Skin: pruritus, sweating
Other: physical or psychological drug dependence, drug tolerance

Interactions

Drug-drug. *Anesthetics, antihistamines, CNS depressants, opioid analgesics, psychotropic agents, sedative-hypnotics:* increased risk of CNS depression
Carbamazepine: increased tramadol metabolism and decreased efficacy
Monoamine oxidase inhibitors: increased risk of serotonin syndrome and seizures
Drug-diagnostic tests. *Creatinine, hepatic enzymes:* increased levels
Hemoglobin: decreased level
Drug-herb. *Chamomile, hops, kava, skullcap, or valerian:* increased CNS depression
Drug-behaviors. *Alcohol use:* increased CNS depression

Precautions

Use cautiously in:
• seizure disorder or risk factors for seizures, renal or hepatic impairment, increased intracranial pressure, head trauma, acute abdomen
• history of opioid dependence or recent use of large opioid doses
• elderly patients
• children under age 16 (safety not established).

Patient monitoring

• Assess patient's response to drug 30 minutes after administration.
• Monitor respiratory status; withhold drug and contact prescriber if respirations become shallow or slower than 12 breaths/minute.
• Monitor for physical and psychological drug dependence; report signs to prescriber.

Patient teaching

• Tell patient that drug works best when taken before pain becomes severe.
• Teach patient (and significant other as appropriate) that drug may cause respiratory depression if used with alcohol; advise patient to avoid alcohol.
◀ Instruct patient to immediately report seizure.
• Tell patient that drug interacts with many common over-the-counter drugs and herbal remedies. Instruct him to consult prescriber before taking these.
• Inform patient that drug can cause physical and psychological dependence; emphasize that he should take it only as prescribed and needed.
• Caution patient to avoid driving and other hazardous activities until he knows how drug affects concentration and alertness.
• As appropriate, review all other significant and life-threatening adverse reactions and interactions, especially those related to the drugs, tests, herbs, and behaviors mentioned above.

trandolapril
Mavik

Pharmacologic class: Angiotensin-converting enzyme (ACE) inhibitor
Therapeutic class: Antihypertensive
Pregnancy risk category C (first trimester), *D* (second and third trimesters)

Action

Inhibits conversion of angiotensin I to the potent vasoconstrictor angiotensin II, promoting vasodilation. Also increases plasma renin and stimulates secretion of aldosterone, leading to diuresis.

Availability
Tablets: 1 mg, 2 mg, 4 mg

🔰 Indications and dosages
➤ Hypertension
Adults: For patients not receiving diuretics, 1 mg P.O. once daily in non-black patients or 2 mg P.O. once daily in black patients. If response is inadequate, may increase at weekly intervals up to 4 mg once daily. In patients receiving diuretics, start with 0.5 mg P.O. daily.
➤ Heart failure or left ventricular dysfunction after myocardial infarction
Adults: Initially, 1 mg P.O. daily; titrate up to 4 mg daily, if tolerated.
Dosage adjustment
• Renal or hepatic impairment

Contraindications
• Hypersensitivity to drug or other ACE inhibitors
• Angioedema with previous ACE inhibitor use
• Pregnancy (second and third trimesters)

Administration
• Give drug once or twice daily as prescribed, with or without food.

Route	Onset	Peak	Duration
P.O.	Within 1 hr	4-10 hr	Up to 24 hr

Adverse reactions
CNS: insomnia, paresthesia, dizziness, drowsiness, asthenia, syncope, **cerebrovascular accident**
CV: chest pain, hypotension, palpitations, intermittent claudication, bradycardia, first-degree atrioventricular block, **cardiogenic shock**
EENT: epistaxis, sinusitis, throat inflammation
GI: vomiting, diarrhea, constipation, abdominal pain or distention, gastritis, dyspepsia, **pancreatitis**
GU: urinary tract infection, impotence, decreased libido

Hematologic: agranulocytosis, neutropenia
Metabolic: hypocalcemia, hyperkalemia, gout
Musculoskeletal: muscle cramps, myalgia, extremity pain
Respiratory: cough, dyspnea, upper respiratory infection
Skin: rash, flushing, pruritus, angioedema
Other: edema

Interactions
Drug-drug. *Antacids:* decreased trandolapril absorption
Digoxin: increased digoxin blood level, greater risk of toxicity
Diuretics, general anesthetics, nitrates, other antihypertensives: additive hypotension
Indomethacin: reduced hypotensive effect of trandolapril
Lithium: increased lithium blood level, greater risk of toxicity
Phenothiazines: increased trandolapril effects
Potassium supplements, potassium-sparing diuretics, salt substitutes containing potassium: additive hyperkalemia
Drug-diagnostic tests. *Neutrophils, platelets:* decreased counts
Potassium: increased level
Drug-food. *Salt substitutes containing potassium:* hyperkalemia
Drug-herb. *Capsaicin:* increased incidence of cough
Ephedra (ma huang), yohimbine: antagonism of trandolapril effects
Drug-behaviors. *Acute alcohol ingestion:* additive hypotension

Precautions
Use cautiously in:
• renal or hepatic impairment, hypovolemia, hyponatremia, aortic stenosis or hypertrophic cardiomyopathy, cere-

brovascular or cardiac insufficiency, surgery and anesthesia, family history of angioedema, concurrent diuretic therapy, black patients with hypertension
• elderly patients
• pregnant patients (first trimester) or breastfeeding patients
• children (safety not established).

Patient monitoring
• Monitor vital signs, especially for hypotension and bradycardia when therapy begins.
• Assess complete blood count with white cell differential; watch for signs and symptoms of bleeding and infection.
• Monitor electrolyte levels, especially potassium; watch for indications of hyperkalemia.
• Assess renal function tests and fluid intake and output.

Patient teaching
• Tell patient drug may cause bleeding tendency or increase his risk of infection. Teach him which warning signs to report.
• Teach patient to recognize and report signs or symptoms of hyperkalemia.
• Instruct patient to move slowly when sitting up or standing to avoid dizziness or light-headedness from sudden blood pressure decrease.
• Caution patient not to exercise vigorously in hot environments.
• Advise patient not to use salt substitutes containing potassium and to avoid high-potassium foods.
• As appropriate, review all other significant and life-threatening adverse reactions and interactions, especially those related to the drugs, tests, foods, herbs, and behaviors mentioned above.

tranylcypromine sulfate
Parnate

Pharmacologic class: Monoamine oxidase (MAO) inhibitor
Therapeutic class: Antidepressant
Pregnancy risk category C

Action
Unknown; thought to increase concentrations of serotonin, epinephrine, and norepinephrine in CNS by inhibiting effects of MAO

Availability
Tablets: 10 mg

Indications and dosages
➤ Depression
Adults: 10 mg P.O. t.i.d.; increase by 10 mg P.O. daily at intervals of 1 to 3 weeks, to a maximum of 60 mg daily.

Contraindications
• Hypersensitivity to drug or other MAO inhibitors
• Pheochromocytoma
• Heart failure or other cardiovascular disease
• Confirmed or suspected cerebrovascular disorders
• Severe renal impairment
• Hypertension
• History of hepatic disease or elevated liver function test results
• History of headache
• Patients scheduled for elective surgery
• Concurrent use of other MAO inhibitors, dibenzazepine derivatives, CNS depressants, anesthetics, antihypertensives, bupropion, sympathomimetics, selective serotonin reuptake inhibitors (SSRIs), or dextromethorphan
• Consumption of caffeine, certain

t

cheeses, and other foods with high tryptophan or tyramine content

Administration

◀€ Don't stop therapy suddenly; dosage must be tapered.

Route	Onset	Peak	Duration
P.O.	Unknown	1-3.5 hr	10 days

Adverse reactions

CNS: dizziness, headache, hyperreflexia, tremor, mania, hypomania, confusion, impaired memory, hypersomnia or insomnia, weakness, fatigue, drowsiness, restlessness, increased anxiety, myoclonic movements, **suicidal ideation**
CV: orthostatic hypotension, tachycardia, palpitations, syncope, paradoxical hypertension, **hypertensive crisis**
EENT: blurred vision
GI: nausea, diarrhea, constipation, GI disturbances, abdominal pain, dry mouth, anorexia
GU: urinary retention, impaired ejaculation, impotence
Hematologic: anemia, **agranulocytosis, leukopenia, thrombocytopenia**
Hepatic: elevated transaminase levels
Musculoskeletal: muscle twitching
Other: weight gain, chills, edema

Interactions

Drug-drug. *Anesthetics, antihypertensives, bupropion, CNS depressants, dextromethorphan, dibenzazepine derivatives, other MAO inhibitors, SSRIs, sympathomimetics:* potentially fatal reactions
Beta-adrenergic blockers: bradycardia
Carbamazepine: hypertensive crisis, severe seizures, coma, circulatory collapse
Hypoglycemics: potentiation of hypoglycemic response
Levodopa: hypertensive reactions
Methylphenidate: increased risk of hypertensive crisis
Sulfonamides: sulfonamide or tranylcypromine toxicity
Thiazide diuretics: exaggerated hypotension
Drug-food. *Foods high in caffeine, tyramine, or tryptophan:* hypertension
Drug-herbs. *Cacao:* vasopressor effects
Ephedra (ma huang): severe reactions, including hypertensive crisis
Ginseng: tremor, headache, mania
Licorice: increased tranylcypromine activity
L-tryptophan: serotonin syndrome (overreactive reflexes, high body temperature, jaw clenching, sweating, drowsiness, euphoria, and even death)
Drug-behaviors. *Alcohol use:* increased CNS effects

Precautions

Use cautiously in:
• seizure disorders, diabetes mellitus, hyperactivity, schizophrenia, severe depression, suicidal attempt or ideation
• pregnant or breastfeeding patients
• children.

Patient monitoring

◀€ Monitor vital signs and cardiovascular status carefully; stay alert for indications of impending hypertensive crisis (palpitations, frequent headaches). Keep phentolamine available to lower blood pressure if needed.
• Monitor complete blood count and liver function test results.
• Observe patient closely for suicidal ideation and drug hoarding.

Patient teaching

◀€ Instruct patient and significant others to immediately report rapid heartbeat and frequent headaches (possible symptoms of hypertensive crisis).
• Advise patient to read food labels carefully and to avoid foods high in tyramine, tryptophan, or caffeine.
• Tell patient drug causes serious interactions with many common drugs; in-

struct him to tell all prescribers he's taking it.

• Advise patient to avoid alcohol and herbal remedies, because serious adverse effects can occur.

◀€ Caution patient not to stop therapy suddenly; dosage must be tapered.

• Instruct patient to move slowly when sitting up or standing to avoid dizziness or light-headedness from sudden blood pressure decrease.

• Teach patient to avoid driving and other hazardous activities until he knows how drug affects concentration, vision, and alertness.

• As appropriate, review all other significant and life-threatening adverse reactions and interactions, especially those related to the drugs, foods, herbs, and behaviors mentioned above.

trastuzumab
Herceptin

Pharmacologic class: Recombinant DNA-derived monoclonal antibody
Therapeutic class: Antineoplastic
Pregnancy risk category B

Action
Selectively binds to human epidermal growth factor receptor 2 (HER2), inhibiting proliferation of human tumor cells that overexpress HER2

Availability
Lyophilized powder: 440 mg

⚕ Indications and dosages
➤ Monotherapy for metastatic breast cancer in patients whose tumors overexpress HER2

Adults: Loading dose of 4 mg/kg I.V. infusion given over 90 minutes, followed by weekly maintenance dose of 2 mg/kg I.V. infusion given over 30 minutes. Don't give by I.V. push or bolus.

Contraindications
• Hypersensitivity to drug

Administration
• Follow facility policy for handling and disposal of carcinogenic, mutagenic, and teratogenic agents.

• Give antiemetic as prescribed before administering trastuzumab.

◀€ Administer by I.V. infusion only. Don't give by I.V. push or bolus.

• To reconstitute, add 20 ml of bacteriostatic water for injection to vial, pointing stream of diluent at lyophilized cake. Swirl vial gently; don't shake. Withdraw prescribed dose and add it to 250 ml of normal saline solution (don't use dextrose 5% in water).

• Infuse loading dose I.V. over 90 minutes; infuse weekly doses I.V. over 30 minutes.

• After reconstituting, immediately label vial in area marked "Do not use after:" with date that's 28 days from reconstitution date.

• If patient has benzyl alcohol hypersensitivity, reconstitute with sterile water for injection. Use drug immediately after reconstitution; discard unused portion.

◀€ Be aware that intrathecal administration causes death.

Route	Onset	Peak	Duration
I.V.	Unknown	Unknown	Unknown

Adverse reactions
CNS: dizziness, headache, depression, paresthesia, insomnia, ataxia, confusion, manic reaction, **seizures**
CV: peripheral edema, hypotension, tachycardia, syncope, **arrhythmias, shock, pericardial effusion, vascular thrombosis, heart failure, cardiotoxicity, cardiac arrest**
EENT: amblyopia, hearing loss
GI: nausea, vomiting, diarrhea, gastroenteritis, hematemesis, colitis, esophageal ulcer, stomatitis, ileus, anorexia, **intestinal obstruction, pancreatitis**

t

GU: urinary tract infection, hematuria, hemorrhagic cystitis, hydronephrosis, pyelonephritis, **renal failure**

Hematologic: coagulation disorder, pancytopenia, leukemia

Hepatic: ascites, **hepatitis, hepatic failure**

Metabolic: hypothyroidism, hypercalcemia, hyponatremia

Musculoskeletal: back, bone, or joint pain; myopathy; fractures; **bone necrosis**

Respiratory: upper respiratory infection, dyspnea, **acute respiratory distress syndrome**

Skin: cellulitis, rash, acne, herpes simplex, herpes zoster, skin ulcers

Other: weight loss, edema, infection, fever, chills, flulike syndrome, lymphangitis, hypersensitivity reactions including **anaphylaxis, infusion reaction**

Interactions

Drug-drug. *Anthracyclines, cyclophosphamide:* cardiotoxicity

Precautions

Use cautiously in
• cardiac disease, anemia, leukopenia
• elderly patients
• pregnant or breastfeeding patients
• children under age 18.

Patient monitoring

◀€ After administering, monitor closely for signs and symptoms of infusion reaction (including respiratory distress); discontinue infusion if these occur.
• Monitor vital signs, especially for hypotension and bradycardia.
• Assess cardiovascular status carefully; stay alert for indications of heart failure and peripheral edema.
• Assess neurologic status for depression and paresthesia.
• Inspect patient's mouth regularly for stomatitis; stop drug and contact prescriber if this reaction occurs.

• Monitor respiratory status; report increased dyspnea or flulike symptoms.
• Watch closely for signs and symptoms of infection, including herpes simplex.
• Monitor electrolyte levels and complete blood count with white cell differential.

Patient teaching

◀€ Instruct patient to immediately report difficulty breathing; fever, chills, and other signs and symptoms of infection (including herpes simplex); and flulike symptoms.

◀€ Advise patient to monitor weight and report sudden increase; also tell him to report swelling and other signs or symptoms of heart failure.
• Tell patient drug may cause depression; advise him (or significant other as appropriate) to contact prescriber if this occurs.
• As appropriate, review all other significant and life-threatening adverse reactions and interactions, especially those related to the drugs mentioned above.

trazodone hydrochloride
Desyrel, Trazorel✦, Trialodine

Pharmacologic class: Triazolopyridine derivative
Therapeutic class: Antidepressant
Pregnancy risk category C

Action
Unclear; thought to selectively inhibit serotonin and norepinephrine uptake in brain. Chemically and structurally unrelated to other antidepressants.

Availability
Tablets: 50 mg, 100 mg, 150 mg, 300 mg

⚕ Indications and dosages

➤ Major depression

Adults: 150 mg/day P.O. in three divided doses; may increase by 50 mg/day q 3 to 4 days until desired response occurs. Don't exceed 400 mg/day in outpatients or 600 mg/day in hospitalized patients.

Dosage adjustment

• Elderly patients

Off-label uses

• Alcohol dependence
• Anxiety neurosis
• Insomnia
• Cocaine withdrawal

Contraindications

• Hypersensitivity to drug
• Recovery period after myocardial infarction

Administration

• Give drug after meals or snacks.
• Know that drug is often used in conjunction with psychotherapy.

Route	Onset	Peak	Duration
P.O.	1-2 wk	2-4 wk	Wks

Adverse reactions

CNS: drowsiness, confusion, dizziness, fatigue, hallucinations, headache, insomnia, nightmares, slurred speech, syncope, weakness, tremor

CV: chest pain, hypotension, hypertension, palpitations, tachycardia, **arrhythmias**

EENT: blurred vision, tinnitus

GI: nausea, vomiting, diarrhea, constipation, excessive salivation, flatulence, dry mouth

GU: urinary frequency, hematuria, impotence, priapism

Hematologic: anemia, **leukopenia**

Musculoskeletal: myalgia

Skin: rash

Interactions

Drug-drug. *Antihypertensives, nitrates:* additive hypotension

Digoxin, phenytoin: increased blood levels of these drugs

Fluoxetine: increased trazodone blood level, greater risk of toxicity

Other CNS depressants (such as opioid analgesics, sedative-hypnotics): additive CNS depression

Drug-diagnostic tests. *Alkaline phosphatase, bilirubin, glucose:* increased levels

Urinary catecholamines: false increases

Urinary 5-hydroxyindole acetic acid, vanillylmandelic acid: decreased levels

Drug-herb. *Chamomile, hops, kava, skullcap, valerian:* increased CNS depression

S-adenosylmethionine (SAM-e), St. John's wort, increased risk of serotonergic adverse effects (including serotonin syndrome)

Drug-behaviors. *Alcohol use:* additive CNS depression and hypotension

Precautions

Use cautiously in:

• cardiovascular disease, severe hepatic or renal disease, suicidal behavior or ideation
• elderly patients
• pregnant or breastfeeding patients
• children (safety not established).

Patient monitoring

• Monitor vital signs and ECG.
• Monitor neurologic status; report significant adverse reactions.
• Assess patient's mood frequently; especially watch for worsening of depression and suicidal ideation.
• Watch for drug hoarding or overuse.

Patient teaching

• Advise patient to take drug with meals or snacks to improve drug absorption.

• Instruct patient to take drug only as prescribed; caution him not to overuse or hoard it.

• Teach patient (and significant other as appropriate) to monitor his mood; tell him drug should ease depression.

◀€ Caution patient (and significant other as appropriate) to immediately report suicidal thoughts or behavior.

• Tell patient that drug may cause significant adverse reactions; teach him to report priapism, hallucinations, syncope, and other serious problems.

• Instruct patient not to drink alcohol.

• Tell patient that many common herbs worsen drug's adverse reactions; tell him to consult prescriber before taking them.

• Teach patient to avoid driving and other hazardous activities until he knows how drug affects concentration, vision, and alertness. Reassure him that dizziness and drowsiness usually subside after first few weeks.

• As appropriate, review all other significant and life-threatening adverse reactions and interactions, especially those related to the drugs, tests, herbs, and behaviors mentioned above.

treprostinil sodium
Remodulin

Pharmacologic class: Synthetic prostacyclin analog

Therapeutic class: Antiplatelet agent, vasodilator

Pregnancy risk category B

Action

Causes direct vasodilation of pulmonary and systemic arterial vascular beds, thereby reducing right and left ventricular afterload and increasing cardiac output and stroke volume. Also inhibits platelet aggregation.

Availability
Injection: 1 mg/ml, 2.5 mg/ml, 5 mg/ml, 10 mg/ml

Indications and dosages
➤ To diminish exercise-induced symptoms in patients with pulmonary artery hypertension who have New York Heart Association Class II-IV symptoms

Adults: Initially, 1.25 ng/kg/minute by continuous S.C. infusion; for maintenance, may decrease infusion rate in increments of no more than 1.25 ng/kg/minute q week for first 4 weeks, and thereafter in increments of no more than 2.5 ng/kg/minute q week, if needed. Maximum dosage is 40 ng/kg/minute.

Dosage adjustment
• Hepatic insufficiency

Contraindications
• Hypersensitivity to drug, its components, or structurally related compounds

Administration
◀€ Give first dose in setting where resuscitation equipment is available and other health care personnel can assist if emergency arises.

• Administer by continuous S.C. infusion through S.C. catheter with infusion pump designed specifically for S.C. infusions.

• Expect to adjust dosage for first 6 to 12 weeks as prescriber balances symptomatic improvement against adverse reactions.

Route	Onset	Peak	Duration
S.C.	Unknown	Unknown	Unknown

Adverse reactions
CNS: dizziness, headache, anxiety, restlessness
CV: vasodilation, edema, hypotension
EENT: jaw pain
GI: nausea, vomiting, diarrhea

Skin: rash, pruritus
Other: infusion site pain or reaction (such as erythema, rash, induration)

Interactions

Drug-drug. *Anticoagulants:* increased risk of bleeding
Antihypertensives, diuretics, other vasodilators: increased risk of hypotension
Vitamin A: increased risk of bleeding
Drug-herb. *Alfalfa, anise, arnica, astragalus, bilberry, black currant seed oil, bladderwrack, bogbean, boldo (with fenugreek), borage oil, buchu, capsaicin, cat's claw, celery, chaparral, chincona bark, clove oil, dandelion, dong quai, evening primrose oil, fenugreek, feverfew, garlic, ginger, ginkgo, guggul, papaya extract, red clover, rhubarb, safflower oil, skullcap, tan-shen:* increased risk of bleeding

Precautions

Use cautiously in:
• renal disease
• history of hepatic disease
• elderly patients
• pregnant or breastfeeding patients
• children.

Patient monitoring

◄€ Especially after first dose, monitor closely for severe vasodilation resulting in chest pain and hypotension; these signs and symptoms call for emergency measures.
◄€ Monitor vital signs; assess carefully for indications of right ventricular failure.
• Assess neurologic status; institute safety measures as needed to prevent injury.
◄€ Watch for infusion site reaction.

Patient teaching

• Tell patient that therapy is a long-term measure to control pulmonary artery hypertension and requires a commitment to maintain infusion system.
◄€ Instruct patient to immediately report signs and symptoms of infusion site reaction (such as redness, rash, and hardened tissue).
• Teach patient which symptoms probably reflect underlying disease and which may reflect adverse reactions that he should report.
• As appropriate, review all other significant adverse reactions and interactions, especially those related to the drugs and herbs mentioned above.

tretinoin
Vesanoid

Pharmacologic class: Retinoid
Therapeutic class: Antineoplastic
Pregnancy risk category D

Action

Unknown; thought to cause differentiation of promyelocytic leukemic blast cells, leading to apoptosis (cell shrinkage and death) and remission induction

Availability

Capsules: 10 mg

🕖 Indications and dosages

➤ Acute promyelocytic leukemia (APL) classified M3 by French-American-British (FAB) system, when anthracycline chemotherapy fails or is contraindicated
Adults and children ages 1 and older: 45 mg/m²/day P.O. in two evenly divided doses. Discontinue after 90 days of therapy or 30 days after complete remission occurs, whichever comes first.

Contraindications

• Hypersensitivity to drug or parabens
• Pregnancy or breastfeeding

Administration

• Make sure female patient has had required pregnancy test before therapy starts.

Route	Onset	Peak	Duration
P.O.	Unknown	1-2 hr	Unknown

Adverse reactions

CNS: dizziness, headache, asthenia, paresthesia, confusion, agitation, hallucinations, anxiety, aphasia, depression, agnosia, insomnia, asterixis, cerebellar edema, hypotaxia, drowsiness, slow speech, facial paralysis, hemiplegia, hyporeflexia, dementia, hypotaxia, spinal cord disorder, tremors, dysarthria, **cerebrovascular accident (CVA), coma, seizures, intracranial hypertension, cerebral hemorrhage**

CV: heart murmur, chest discomfort, peripheral edema, hypertension, hypotension, phlebitis, edema, enlarged heart, ischemia, **arrhythmias, secondary cardiomyopathy, myocarditis, myocardial infarction (MI), heart failure, pericardial effusion, impaired myocardial contractility, progressive hypoxemia**

EENT: vision disturbances, visual acuity changes, visual field defect, absence of light reflex, hearing loss, earache, full sensation in ears

GI: nausea, vomiting, constipation, diarrhea, abdominal pain, GI disorders, mucositis, dyspepsia, ulcer, abdominal distention, anorexia, **GI hemorrhage**

GU: dysuria, urinary frequency, renal insufficiency, enlarged prostate, **renal tubular necrosis, acute renal failure**

Hematologic: leukocytosis, **disseminated intravascular coagulation (DIC), hemorrhage**

Hepatic: ascites, hepatosplenomegaly, **hepatitis**

Metabolic: fluid imbalance, acidosis, hypercholesterolemia, hypertriglyceridemia

Musculoskeletal: bone pain or inflammation, myalgia, flank pain

Respiratory: pneumonia, pulmonary hypertension, respiratory tract disorders, dyspnea, laryngeal edema, pulmonary infiltrates, expiratory wheezing, crackles, pleural effusion, bronchial asthma

Skin: rash, pallor, flushing, diaphoresis, alopecia, dry skin and mucous membranes, skin changes, pruritis, cellulitis

Other: weight changes, fever, lymphatic disorder, hypothermia, infections, facial edema, pain, **retinoic acid-APL syndrome, multisystem failure, septicemia**

Interactions

Drug-drug. *Ketoconazole:* enhanced tretinoin activity

Drug-food. *Any food:* enhanced tretinoin absorption

Drug-behaviors. *Sun exposure:* increased risk of photosensitivity

Precautions

Use cautiously in:
• eczema, sunburn.

Patient monitoring

◀❦ Monitor patient closely for septicemia, multisystem failure, and retinoic acid-APL syndrome (which manifests as pulmonary and pericardial effusion, fever, weight gain, and dyspnea).

◀❦ Assess closely for significant adverse CNS reactions, including CVA, seizures, and cerebral hemorrhage.

◀❦ Monitor cardiovascular status; stay alert for signs and symptoms of arrhythmias, MI, and heart failure.

◀❦ Closely monitor liver and kidney function tests; watch for signs and symptoms of hepatitis and renal failure.

◀❦ Monitor coagulation studies; watch carefully for DIC and hemorrhage.

• Evaluate respiratory status; stay alert for indications of pulmonary hypertension and respiratory insufficiency.

• Assess lipid panel and complete blood count with white cell differential.

Patient teaching
• Instruct patient to take doses with food.
• Teach patient to recognize and immediately report serious adverse reactions.
• Tell patient that he'll undergo regular blood testing during therapy.
• As appropriate, review all other significant and life-threatening adverse reactions and interactions, especially those related to the drugs, foods, and behaviors mentioned above.

triamcinolone
Aristocort, Kenacort, Nasacort AQ

triamcinolone acetonide
Aristocort, Aristocort A, Azmacort HFA, Azmacort Inhalation Aerosol, Flutex, Kenalog, Kenalog-10, Kenalog-40, Nasacort, Triacet, Triaderm✤, Triamonide 40, Tri-Kort, Trilog, Tri-Nasal Spray

triamcinolone diacetate
Amcort, Aristocort Forte, Aristocort Intralesional, Clinacort, Trilone

triamcinolone hexacetonide
Aristospan Intra-Articular, Aristospan Intralesional

Pharmacologic class: Synthetic corticosteroid
Therapeutic class: Anti-inflammatory (steroidal)
Pregnancy risk category C

Action
Unknown; thought to decrease inflammation primarily by inhibiting activities of mast cells, macrophages, and other mediators involved in allergic reactions. Also suppresses immune system by depressing lymphatic system activity.

Availability
Cream (acetonide): 0.025%, 0.1%, 0.5%
Inhalation aerosol, intranasal (acetonide): 55 mcg/inhalation (metered spray) in 20-g canister (240 metered inhalations)
Inhalation aerosol, oral (acetonide): 100 mcg/inhalation (metered spray)
Injectable suspension (acetonide): 3 mg/ml, 10 mg/ml, 40 mg/ml
Injectable suspension (diacetate): 25 mg/ml, 40 mg/ml
Injectable suspension (hexacetonide): 5 mg/ml, 20 mg/ml
Lotion (acetonide): 0.025%, 0.1%
Ointment (acetonide): 0.1%
Solution (acetonide): 50 mcg/metered spray
Suspension (acetonide): 55 mcg/metered spray
Syrup: 2 mg/5 ml, 4 mg/5 ml
Tablets: 1 mg, 2 mg, 4 mg, 8 mg

Indications and dosages
➤ Allergic rhinitis
Adults and children older than age 12: 8 to 12 mg (tablets) P.O. daily. Or 110 mcg (two sprays of inhalation aerosol or acetonide suspension) in each nostril once daily; may increase to 220 mcg (four sprays) in each nostril once daily (110 mcg b.i.d. or 55 mcg q.i.d.). Or 100 mcg (two sprays of acetonide solution) in each nostril once daily; may increase to 400 mcg (four sprays) in each nostril once daily or two sprays in each nostril b.i.d.
Children ages 6 to 12: 55 mcg (one spray of inhalation aerosol or acetonide suspension) in each nostril once daily

➣ Chronic asthma

Adults and children older than age 12:
Two metered inhalations three to four
times daily or four metered inhalations
b.i.d. (100 mcg/metered inhalation),
not to exceed 16 inhalations/day

Children ages 6 to 12: One to two metered inhalations three to four times
daily or two to four metered inhalations b.i.d. (100 mcg/metered inhalation), not to exceed 12 inhalations/day

➣ Severe inflammation; immunosuppression

Adults and children older than age 12:
4 to 48 mg (tablets) P.O. daily in one to
four divided doses. Or 60 mg (acetonide) I.M. at 6-week intervals; for intralesional or sublesional use, 1 mg at
each injection site, repeated one or
more times weekly; for intra-articular,
intrasynovial, or soft-tissue injection,
2.5 to 40 mg, repeated when signs and
symptoms recur. Or 200 mcg (two
sprays of acetonide inhalation aerosol)
three to four times daily. Or 40 mg (diacetate) I.M. weekly. Or 5 to 48 mg (diacetate) by intralesional or sublesional
injection, not to exceed 75 mg intralesionally. Or 2 to 40 mg (diacetate) by
intra-articular, intrasynovial, or soft-
tissue injection; may repeat at 1- to 8-
week intervals. Or 0.5 mg/square inch
of affected skin (hexacetonide) by intralesional or sublesional injection or 2
to 30 mg by intra-articular injection;
may repeat at 3- to 4-week intervals.

Children ages 6 to 12: 100 or 200 mcg
(one or two sprays of acetonide inhalation aerosol) three to four times daily,
or 0.03 to 0.2 mg/kg or 1 to 6.25 mg/
m² I.M. at intervals of 1 to 7 days

➣ Inflammatory and pruritic manifestations of corticosteroid-responsive
dermatoses

Adults and children older than age 12:
Apply cream, ointment, or lotion sparingly to affected areas two to four times
daily.

Contraindications

• Hypersensitivity to drug, tartrazine,
chlorofluorocarbon propellants, alcohol, propylene glycol, or polyethylene
glycol
• Acute asthma attacks, status asthmaticus
• Fungal infections
• Idiopathic thrombocytopenic purpura
• Administration of live-virus vaccines
(with immunosuppressant doses of triamcinolone)

Administration

◀€ Don't stop systemic corticosteroids
abruptly when patient begins inhalation steroid therapy. Be aware that patient will need additional steroids during times of stress or trauma.
• Use hand-held nebulizer supplied
with aerosol form.

◀€ Apply cream, lotion, or ointment
sparingly. Know that triamcinolone is
a high-potency steroid; it can be absorbed systemically and should not be
discontinued abruptly.

◀€ Avoid intralesional injection of
face or head because this may cause
blindness.
• Don't apply topical form near eyes.

Route	Onset	Peak	Duration
P.O.	Unknown	Unknown	2.25 days
I.M.	Unknown	Unknown	1-4 wk
Intra-lesional, sublesional, intra-articular	Slow	Unknown	Unknown
Inhalation	Immediate	Unknown	Unknown
Topical	Unknown	Unknown	Unknown

Adverse reactions

CNS: headache, vertigo, paresthesia,
syncope, personality changes, **pseudotumor cerebri, seizures**
CV: hypertension, thrombophlebitis,
**arrhythmias, thromboembolism,
heart failure**

EENT: cataract, glaucoma, increased intraocular pressure, exophthalmos, otitis, dry mucous membranes, nasal or sinus congestion, pharyngitis, rhinitis, epistaxis, throat discomfort, sneezing, toothache

GI: nausea, vomiting, dyspepsia, abdominal distention or pain, ulcerative esophagitis, oral candidiasis, dry mouth, peptic ulcers, **pancreatitis**

GU: cystitis, urinary tract infection, glycosuria, menstrual irregularities, vaginal candidiasis

Metabolic: fluid retention, hypernatremia, hypokalemia, hypokalemic alkalosis, hyperglycemia, hypocalcemia, hypercholesterolemia, decreased growth (in children), carbohydrate intolerance, exacerbation of latent diabetes mellitus, cushingoid appearance (moon face, buffalo hump), **acute adrenal insufficiency** (with abrupt withdrawal or acute stress in long-term use)

Musculoskeletal: muscle weakness; steroid myopathy; loss of muscle mass; myalgia; bursitis; tenosynovitis; osteoporosis; fractures; aseptic necrosis; osteonecrosis, tendon rupture, post-injection flare (with intra-articular injection)

Respiratory: cough, wheezing, chest congestion

Skin: delayed wound healing; thin and fragile skin; petechiae; bruising; with topical use—local eruptions, pruritus, hypopigmentation or hyperpigmentation, scarring, stinging, skin maceration, secondary infection, cutaneous or subcutaneous atrophy, diaphoresis, facial erythema

Other: weight gain, fever, pain, voice alteration, hypersensitivity reaction

Interactions

Drug-drug. *Erythromycin, indinavir, itraconazole, ketoconazole, ritonavir, saquinavir:* increased triamcinolone blood level and effects

Fluoroquinolones: increased risk of tendon rupture

Live-virus vaccines: decreased antibody response to vaccine

Nonsteroidal anti-inflammatory drugs (including aspirin): increased risk of adverse GI reactions

Potassium-wasting drugs (including amphotericin B, thiazide and loop diuretics, mezlocillin, piperacillin, ticarcillin): additive hypokalemia

Drug-diagnostic tests. *Skin tests:* suppressed reaction

Precautions

Use cautiously in:
• active untreated infection, systemic infection, immunosuppression, hypertension, osteoporosis, diabetes mellitus, glaucoma, renal disease, hypothyroidism, cirrhosis, diverticulitis, nonspecific ulcerative colitis, recent intestinal anastomoses, thromboembolic disorders, seizures, myasthenia gravis, heart failure, ocular herpes simplex, emotional instability
• pregnant or breastfeeding patients
• children younger than age 6 (safety not established).

Patient monitoring

• Monitor respiratory status; watch for worsening signs and symptoms.
• With long-term use, assess for adverse endocrine and musculoskeletal reactions.
• Monitor carefully for signs and symptoms of infection, which drug may mask.

Patient teaching

• Teach patient correct use of inhaled, oral, or topical drug form; make sure he has received manufacturer's patient information sheet.
• Instruct patient to rinse mouth after using oral syrup or solution.
◀€ Advise patient to contact prescriber immediately if acute asthma attack occurs; inhalation aerosol isn't meant for rapid relief of bronchospasm.

• Tell patient drug can affect many body systems; encourage him to report such effects promptly.

• Inform parents that drug may make child more vulnerable to childhood infections, such as chicken pox and measles.

• As appropriate, review all other significant and life-threatening adverse reactions and interactions, especially those related to the drugs and tests mentioned above.

triamterene
Dyrenium

Pharmacologic class: Potassium-sparing diuretic
Therapeutic class: Diuretic
Pregnancy risk category C

Action
Depresses resorption of sodium and excretion of potassium in renal distal tubule

Availability
Capsules: 50 mg, 100 mg

🚫 Indications and dosages
➤ Edema associated with heart failure, hepatic cirrhosis, nephrotic syndrome, secondary hyperaldosteronism, or steroid therapy; idiopathic edema
Adults: 100 mg P.O. b.i.d., not to exceed 300 mg/day
Dosage adjustment
• Concurrent antihypertensive drug therapy
• Elderly patients

Off-label uses
• Diabetes insipidus

Contraindications
• Hypersensitivity to drug
• Hyperkalemia

• Severe hepatic disease
• Anuria, severe renal dysfunction (except nephrosis)
• Concurrent use of other potassium-sparing diuretics or potassium supplements

Administration
• Know that drug may be used alone or as an adjunct to thiazide or loop diuretics.
• Make sure patient stops taking potassium supplements before starting triamterene.

Route	Onset	Peak	Duration
P.O.	2-4 hr	Unknown	12-16 hr

Adverse reactions
CNS: headache, fatigue, asthenia, dizziness
GI: nausea, vomiting, diarrhea, dry mouth
GU: azotemia, renal calculi, elevated blood urea nitrogen (BUN) and creatinine levels
Hematologic: megaloblastic anemia, **thrombocytopenia**
Hepatic: jaundice, elevated hepatic enzyme levels
Metabolic: hyperkalemia, hyperglycemia, metabolic acidosis
Skin: rash, photosensitivity
Other: anaphylaxis

Interactions
Drug-drug. *Amantadine:* increased amantadine blood level, greater risk of toxicity
Angiotensin-converting enzyme inhibitors, cyclosporine, indomethacin, potassium-sparing diuretics, potassium supplements, other potassium-containing preparations: increased risk of hyperkalemia
Antihypertensives, nondepolarizing muscle relaxants, other diuretics, preanesthetic and anesthetic agents: potentiated effects of these drugs

---

🍁 Canada   🔊 Clinical alert   Reactions in **bold** are life-threatening

Chlorpropamide: increased risk of hyponatremia

Cimetidine: increased bioavailability and decreased renal clearance of triamterene

Indomethacin: increased risk of acute renal failure

Lithium: decreased lithium clearance, greater risk of lithium toxicity

Drug-diagnostic tests. *Alkali reserves, hemoglobin, platelets:* decreased values

BUN, creatinine, glucose, potassium: increased levels

Liver function tests: increased values

Quinidine blood level: interference with fluorescent measurement

Drug-food. *Salt substitutes containing potassium:* increased risk of hyperkalemia

Drug-herb. *Gossypol, licorice:* increased risk of hypokalemia

Precautions

Use cautiously in:
• hepatic dysfunction, renal insufficiency, diabetes mellitus
• history of gout or renal calculi
• elderly or debilitated patients
• pregnant or breastfeeding patients
• children (safety not established).

Patient monitoring

• Monitor BUN, creatinine, and electrolyte levels; stay alert for hyperkalemia.
• Assess complete blood count with white cell differential.

Patient teaching

• Advise patient to take drug after meals to reduce nausea.
• Teach patient to take last daily dose in early evening to avoid nocturia.
• Teach patient to recognize and report signs and symptoms of electrolyte imbalances.
• As appropriate, review all other significant and life-threatening adverse reactions and interactions, especially those related to the drugs, tests, foods, and herbs mentioned above.

triazolam

Apo-Triazo✦, Gen-Triazolam✦, Halcion, Novo-Triolam✦

Pharmacologic class: Benzodiazepine
Therapeutic class: Sedative-hypnotic
Controlled substance schedule IV
Pregnancy risk category X

Action

Inhibits gamma-aminobutyric acid, a neurotransmitter that activates receptors at the limbic, thalamic, and hypothalamic levels of the CNS

Availability

Tablets: 0.125 mg, 0.25 mg, 0.5 mg

Indications and dosages

➤ Short-term management of insomnia

Adults: 0.125 to 0.5 mg P.O. at bedtime p.r.n.

Dosage adjustment
• Elderly or debilitated patients

Off-label uses

• Presurgical hypnotic

Contraindications

• Hypersensitivity to drug or other benzodiazepines
• Concurrent use of itraconazole, ketoconazole, or nefazodone
• Pregnancy
• Children under age 18

Administration

• Don't administer with grapefruit juice.

Route	Onset	Peak	Duration
P.O.	15-30 min	2 hr	Unknown

Adverse reactions

CNS: dizziness, excessive sedation, hangover, headache, anterograde or traveler's amnesia, confusion, incoordination, lethargy, depression, paradoxical excitation, light-headedness, psychological disturbance, euphoria

GI: nausea, vomiting

Other: physical or psychological drug dependence, drug tolerance, withdrawal symptoms (tremor, abdominal and muscle cramps, vomiting, diaphoresis, dysphoria, perceptual disturbances, insomnia)

Interactions

Drug-drug. *Antidepressants, antihistamines, chloral hydrate, opioid analgesics, other psychotropic drugs:* additive CNS depression

Cimetidine, disulfiram, fluconazole, hormonal contraceptives, isoniazid, itraconazole, ketoconazole, nefazodone, rifampin, and other drugs that inhibit CYP450-3A4–mediated metabolism: decreased oxidative metabolism and increased action of triazolam

Digoxin: increased digoxin blood level, greater risk of toxicity

Macrolide anti-infectives (such as azithromycin, clarithromycin, erythromycin): increased triazolam bioavailability

Probenecid: rapid onset and prolonged effects of triazolam

Ranitidine: increased triazolam blood level

Theophylline: decreased sedative effect of triazolam

Drug-food. *Grapefruit juice:* increased triazolam blood level and effects

Drug-herb. *Chamomile, hops, kava, skullcap, valerian:* increased CNS depression

Drug-behaviors. *Alcohol use:* increased CNS depression

Smoking: increased triazolam clearance

Precautions

Use cautiously in:
• sleep apnea, hepatic or renal dysfunction, respiratory compromise, psychosis
• history of suicide attempt or drug abuse
• elderly or debilitated patients
• breastfeeding patients.

Patient monitoring

• Monitor neurologic status; watch for paradoxical or rebound drug effects.
• Observe for signs of drug hoarding and drug abuse.

Patient teaching

• Teach patient to take drug at bedtime with a liquid other than grapefruit juice.
• Explain that drug is meant only for short-term use (7 to 10 days).
• Tell patient that rebound insomnia may occur for 1 to 2 nights after he discontinues drug.
• Instruct patient to avoid alcohol.
• Advise patient to avoid driving and other hazardous activities while under drug's influence.
• As appropriate, review all other significant adverse reactions and interactions, especially those related to the drugs, foods, herbs, and behaviors mentioned above.

trifluoperazine hydrochloride

Apo-Trifluoperazine✤, Novo-Fluorazine✤, PMS-Trifluoperazine✤, Solazine✤, Stelazine, Terfluzine

Pharmacologic class: Piperazine phenothiazine
Therapeutic class: Antipsychotic
Pregnancy risk category C

Action
Unknown; thought to act on the subcortical levels of the hypothalamic and limbic systems by producing antidopaminergic effects. Also exhibits varying degrees of adrenergic, muscarinic, and anticholinergic activity and lowers seizure threshold.

Availability
Injection: 2 mg/ml in 10-ml vials
Oral solution: 10 mg/ml in 60-ml bottles
Tablets: 1 mg, 2 mg, 5 mg, 10 mg

💊 Indications and dosages
➢ Schizophrenia
Adults: 2 to 5 mg P.O. b.i.d.; may increase gradually up to 40 mg/day. For prompt control of severe symptoms, 1 to 2 mg I.M. q 4 to 6 hours; patients may need more than 6 mg/day.
Children ages 6 to 12: Initially, 1 mg P.O. once or twice daily in hospitalized patients or those under close supervision; may increase gradually up to 15 mg/day P.O. until symptoms are controlled or adverse reactions become intolerable. For prompt control of severe symptoms, 1 mg I.M. once or twice daily.
➢ Short-term management of nonpsychotic anxiety
Adults: 1 to 2 mg P.O. b.i.d., not to exceed 6 mg/day or 12 weeks' duration
Dosage adjustment
• Hepatic disease
• Elderly or debilitated patients

Contraindications
• Hypersensitivity to drug, other phenothiazines, or bisulfites (with oral solution only)
• Severe hepatic disease
• Cerebral arteriosclerosis, coronary artery disease
• Severe hypotension or hypertension
• Myeloproliferative disorders
• Bone marrow depression
• Blood dyscrasias

• Coma
• Concomitant use of other CNS depressants in high doses

Administration
• Mix oral solution in at least 60 ml of liquid or semi-solid food before giving.
• Administer I.M. injection deep into muscle.
• Know that parenteral solution should be colorless to pale yellow; discard if it's markedly discolored.

Route	Onset	Peak	Duration
P.O.	Unknown	2-4 hr	12-24 hr
I.M.	Unknown	Unknown	4-6 hr

Adverse reactions
CNS: sedation, dizziness, drowsiness, insomnia, fatigue, extrapyramidal effects, **neuroleptic malignant syndrome**
CV: tachycardia, hypotension, orthostatic hypotension, peripheral edema, prolonged QT interval, torsades de pointes
EENT: dry eyes, blurred vision, miosis, mydriasis, epithelial keratopathy, pigmentary retinopathy
GI: constipation, cholestatic jaundice, adynamic ileus, biliary stasis, dry mouth, anorexia
GU: urinary retention, glycosuria, amenorrhea, ejaculatory disorders, galactorrhea, gynecomastia
Hematologic: leukopenia, agranulocytosis
Hepatic: elevated hepatic enzyme levels
Musculoskeletal: muscle weakness
Skin: photosensitivity, altered pigmentation, erythema, rash
Other: mild fever, weight gain, allergic reaction

Interactions
Drug-drug. *Alpha-adrenergic blockers:* additive effect

Antacids containing aluminum: decreased trifluoperazine absorption
Anticholinergics, anticholinergic-like drugs (including antidepressants, antihistamines, disopyramide, other phenothiazines, quinidine): additive anticholinergic effects
Anticonvulsants: decreased seizure threshold
Antihistamines, CNS depressants, general anesthetics, opioids, sedative-hypnotics: additive CNS depression
Barbiturates: decreased blood levels of both drugs
Guanethidine: decreased antihypertensive effect
Lithium: increased risk of extrapyramidal reactions, disorientation, and unconsciousness
Oral anticoagulants: decreased anticoagulant effect
Phenytoin: interference with phenytoin metabolism, causing phenytoin toxicity
Propranolol: increased blood levels of both drugs
Thiazide diuretics: additive orthostatic hypotension
Drug-diagnostic tests. *Phenylketonuria test:* false-positive result
Prolactin: increased level, causing interference with gonadotropin test results
Urine bilirubin: false-positive result
Drug-herb. *St. John's wort:* increased risk of photosensitivity
Drug-behaviors. *Alcohol use:* additive CNS depression and hypotension
Sun exposure: increased risk of photosensitivity

Precautions

Use cautiously in:
• seizure disorders, cardiovascular disorders, GI obstruction, glaucoma, retinopathy
• elderly or debilitated patients
• pregnant or breastfeeding patients.

Patient monitoring

• Monitor ECG and blood pressure; observe closely for hypotension.

• Assess complete blood count (including platelet count) and liver function studies; watch for signs and symptoms of hepatic damage and blood dyscrasias.
◀€ Monitor neurologic status, especially for indications of neuroleptic malignant syndrome (such as high fever, sweating, unstable blood pressure, stupor, muscle rigidity, and autonomic dysfunction).

Patient teaching

• Instruct patient taking oral solution to add solution to 60 ml or more of liquid (tomato or fruit juice, milk, carbonated beverage, coffee, tea, or water) or semisolid food (soup, pudding) just before taking.
• Tell patient that drug's full effect usually occurs in 1 to 2 weeks.
• Instruct patient to move slowly when sitting up or standing to avoid dizziness or light-headedness from sudden blood pressure decrease.
◀€ Teach patient to recognize and immediately report signs and symptoms of neuroleptic malignant syndrome.
• Caution patient to avoid driving and other hazardous activities until he knows how drug affects him.
• Tell patient to avoid alcohol and certain herbs.
• Advise patient to avoid sun exposure and to wear sunscreen and protective clothing when going outdoors.
• As appropriate, review all other significant and life-threatening adverse reactions and interactions, especially those related to the drugs, tests, herbs, and behaviors mentioned above.

trihexyphenidyl hydrochloride

Apo-Trihex✚, Artane, Artane Sequels, Novo-Hexidyl✚, PMS-Trihexyphenidyl✚, Trihexane, Trihexy

Pharmacologic class: Anticholinergic
Therapeutic class: Antidyskinetic
Pregnancy risk category C

Action

Inhibits the parasympathetic nervous system, relaxing smooth muscles and decreasing involuntary movements.

Availability

Capsules (sustained-release): 5 mg
Elixir: 2 mg/5 ml
Tablets: 2 mg, 5 mg

💊 Indications and dosages

➤ Adjunct in management of idiopathic, postencephalitic, or arteriosclerotic parkinsonism
Adults: 1 mg P.O. on first day; may increase in 2-mg increments q 3 to 5 days, up to a maximum of 6 to 10 mg/day. In postencephalitic parkinsonism, 12 to 15 mg P.O. daily. May give sustained-release form (Artane Sequels) in same dosage as conventional form, as a single dose or in two divided doses q 12 hours after daily dosage has been determined using conventional tablets or liquid.
➤ Drug-induced extrapyramidal symptoms
Adults: Initially, 1 mg P.O. daily, increased progressively if extrapyramidal symptoms aren't controlled within several hours. Usual dosage range is 5 to 15 mg/day P.O. given in divided doses.
Dosage adjustment
• Concurrent use of levodopa or other parasympathetic inhibitors
• Elderly patients

Off-label uses

• Dystonia

Contraindications

• Hypersensitivity to drug, its components, or alcohol (with elixir only)
• Narrow-angle glaucoma
• Pyloric or duodenal obstruction
• Stenosing peptic ulcer
• Megacolon
• Prostatic hypertrophy or bladder-neck obstruction
• Achalasia
• Myasthenia gravis

Administration

• Give with meals. However, if drug causes severe dry mouth, give before meals.
• Administer last dose at bedtime.

Route	Onset	Peak	Duration
P.O.	1 hr	2-3 hr	6-12 hr
P.O. (sustained)	Unknown	Unknown	12-24 hr

Adverse reactions

CNS: dizziness, nervousness, drowsiness, asthenia, headache
CV: orthostatic hypotension, tachycardia
EENT: blurred vision, mydriasis, increased intraocular pressure (IOP), narrow-angle glaucoma (with long-term use)
GI: nausea, vomiting, constipation, dry mouth
GU: urinary hesitancy or retention

Interactions

Drug-drug. *Amantadine, other anticholinergics (including disopyramide, phenothiazines, quinidine, tricyclic antidepressants):* additive anticholinergic effects
Other CNS depressants (such as antihistamines, opioids, sedative-hypnotics): additive CNS depression

t

Phenothiazines: decreased phenothiazine effects
Drug-herb. *Angel's trumpet, jimsonweed, scopolia:* increased anticholinergic effects
Drug-behaviors. *Alcohol use:* additive CNS depression

Precautions
Use cautiously in:
• chronic renal, hepatic, pulmonary, or cardiac disease; hypertension; tachycardia secondary to cardiac insufficiency; hyperthyroidism
• elderly patients
• pregnant or breastfeeding patients
• children (safety not established).

Patient monitoring
• With prolonged use, monitor vision and IOP regularly.
• Assess drug efficacy to help guide dosage titration.
• Monitor vital signs; watch for orthostatic hypotension.
• Closely monitor fluid intake and output; stay alert for urinary retention.

Patient teaching
• Teach patient to take drug with meals or, if severe dry mouth occurs, before meals.
• Tell patient drug has a bitter taste, which may be followed by numbness and tingling in mouth.
• Emphasize the need for follow-up eye examinations.
• Instruct patient to consult prescriber before taking over-the-counter preparations or herbs.
• Advise patient to avoid alcohol and all hazardous activities.
• Teach patient to move slowly when sitting up or standing to avoid dizziness or light-headedness from sudden blood pressure decrease.
• As appropriate, review all other significant adverse reactions and interactions, especially those related to the

drugs, herbs, and behaviors mentioned above.

trimethobenzamide hydrochloride
Arrestin, Benzacot, Brogan, Stemetic, Tebamide, Tegamide, T-Gen, Ticon, Tigan, Tiject-20, Triban, Tribenzagan, Trimazide

Pharmacologic class: Anticholinergic
Therapeutic class: Antiemetic
Pregnancy risk category C

Action
Unclear; thought to block dopamine receptors and emetic impulses in chemoreceptor trigger zone, preventing nausea and vomiting

Availability
Capsules: 100 mg, 250 mg, 300 mg
Injection: 100 mg/ml in 2-ml ampules and prefilled syringes and in 20-ml vials
Suppositories: 100 mg, 200 mg

ⓘ Indications and dosages
➤ Nausea and vomiting
Adults: 250 mg P.O. three to four times daily or 200 mg I.M. or P.R. three to four times daily
Children weighing 30 to 90 lb: 100 to 200 mg P.O. or P.R. three to four times daily
Children weighing less than 30 lb: 100 mg P.R. three to four times daily. Don't use in infants.

Contraindications
• Hypersensitivity to drug, benzocaine, or similar local anesthetics (with suppositories)
• Parenteral formulation in children
• Suppositories in infants

Administration

- In I.M. use, inject deep into upper outer quadrant of gluteus maximus.
- Withhold drug if child has signs or symptoms of Reye's syndrome.

Route	Onset	Peak	Duration
P.O., P.R.	10-40 min	Unknown	3-4 hr
I.M.	15-35 min	Unknown	2-3 hr

Adverse reactions

CNS: drowsiness, dizziness, headache, depression, disorientation, parkinsonian symptoms, **coma, seizures**
CV: hypotension
EENT: blurred vision
GI: diarrhea, rectal irritation (with suppositories)
Hematologic: blood dyscrasias
Hepatic: jaundice
Musculoskeletal: muscle cramps, opisthotonos
Skin: rash, urticaria, flushing
Other: pain and stinging at I.M. injection site, hypersensitivity reaction

Interactions

Drug-drug. *Antidepressants, antihistamines, CNS depressants, opioid analgesics, sedative-hypnotics:* additive CNS depression
Drug-behaviors. *Alcohol use:* additive CNS depression

Precautions

Use cautiously in:
- arrhythmias, encephalitis, gastroenteritis, dehydration, electrolyte imbalances
- elderly or debilitated patients
- pregnant or breastfeeding patients
- children with known or suspected viral illness.

Patient monitoring

- Monitor neurologic status, especially for parkinsonian symptoms and other serious adverse reactions.
- Assess complete blood count and liver function test results; watch for blood dyscrasias and jaundice.
- Evaluate injection site for pain and stinging.
- Monitor nutritional and hydration status closely; report continuing nausea.

Patient teaching

- Advise patient to take drug as needed for nausea and vomiting, but only as prescribed.
- Tell patient to contact prescriber promptly if nausea persists despite therapy.
- Instruct patient to minimize nausea and vomiting by eating small, frequent servings of healthy food and drinking plenty of fluids.
- Advise patient to avoid alcohol.
- Caution patient to avoid driving and other hazardous activities until effects of drug are known.
- As appropriate, review all other significant and life-threatening adverse reactions and interactions, especially those related to the drugs and behaviors mentioned above.

trimethoprim
Primsol, Proloprim, Trimpex

Pharmacologic class: Folate antagonist, dihydrofolate reductase inhibitor
Therapeutic class: Anti-infective
Pregnancy risk category C

Action

Prevents bacterial synthesis by binding to and reversibly inhibiting the required enzyme, dihydrofolate reductase

Availability

Oral solution: 50 mg/5 ml
Tablets: 100 mg, 200 mg

💊 Indications and dosages

➤ Urinary tract infection
Adults: 100 mg P.O. q 12 hours or 200 mg P.O. daily for 10 days
Dosage adjustment
• Renal impairment

Off-label uses

• *Pneumocystis jiroveci* (formerly *Pneumocystis carinii*) pneumonia

Contraindications

• Hypersensitivity to drug or its components
• Megaloblastic anemia caused by folate deficiency

Administration

• Administer drug with or without food.

Route	Onset	Peak	Duration
P.O.	Rapid	1-4 hr	Unknown

Adverse reactions

GI: nausea, vomiting, epigastric distress, glossitis
GU: elevated creatinine and blood urea nitrogen (BUN) levels
Hematologic: methemoglobinemia, **thrombocytopenia, leukopenia, neutropenia, megaloblastic anemia**
Hepatic: increased alanine aminotransferase (ALT), aspartate aminotransferase (AST), and bilirubin levels
Skin: rash, pruritus, **exfoliative dermatitis**
Other: fever

Interactions

Drug-drug. *Phenytoin:* increased phenytoin effects
Drug-diagnostic tests. *ALT, AST, bilirubin, BUN, creatinine:* increased levels
Creatinine (determined by Jaffe reaction): false elevation

Hemoglobin, platelets, white blood cells: decreased levels
Methotrexate assay: interference with results

Precautions

Use cautiously in:
• renal or hepatic disease, folate deficiency
• pregnant or breastfeeding patients.

Patient monitoring

• If patient is taking drug for a prolonged time, monitor complete blood count, including platelet count; drug may depress bone marrow.
• Assess kidney and liver function test results.

Patient teaching

• Explain drug therapy to patient; stress importance of taking entire amount prescribed, even if symptoms improve.
• Advise patient to drink at least 2 L of fluid daily, unless contraindicated.
• Instruct patient to promptly report adverse reactions or worsening signs and symptoms.
• As appropriate, review all other significant and life-threatening adverse reactions and interactions, especially those related to the drugs and tests mentioned above.

trimipramine maleate

Apo-Trimip✦, Novo-Tripramine✦, Rhotrimine✦, Surmontil

Pharmacologic class: Dibenzazepine derivative tricyclic

Therapeutic class: Tricyclic antidepressant

Pregnancy risk category C

Action
Unknown; thought to inhibit presynaptic norepinephrine and serotonin reuptake at CNS and peripheral receptors, causing increased synaptic concentrations of these neurotransmitters

Availability
Capsules: 25 mg, 50 mg, 100 mg

⚠ Indications and dosages
➤ Depression
Adults: In outpatients, 75 mg/day P.O. in divided doses, increased gradually p.r.n. to a maximum of 200 mg/day; maintenance dosage is 50 to 150 mg/day P.O. for approximately 3 months. In hospitalized patients, 100 mg/day P.O. in divided doses, increased over several days p.r.n. to 200 mg/day; if no improvement occurs in 2 to 3 weeks, may increase to a maximum of 300 mg/day.
Dosage adjustment
• Hepatic disease
• Elderly patients

Off-label uses
• Depression in adolescents

Contraindications
• Hypersensitivity to drug or other dibenzazepines
• Acute recovery phase after myocardial infarction (MI)
• Monoamine oxidase (MAO) inhibitor use within past 14 days

Administration
◀€ Wait at least 14 days after MAO inhibitor therapy ends before starting trimipramine.

Route	Onset	Peak	Duration
P.O.	Unknown	2 hr	Unknown

Adverse reactions
CNS: confusion, drowsiness, dizziness, asthenia, fatigue, headache, disorientation, hallucinations, delusions, restlessness, anxiety, agitation, insomnia, nightmares, hypomania, psychosis exacerbation, paresthesia, incoordination, ataxia, tremor, peripheral neuropathy, extrapyramidal symptoms, EEG changes, **seizures, cerebrovascular accident (CVA)**
CV: hypotension, hypertension, tachycardia, palpitations, **heart block, arrhythmias, MI**
EENT: blurred vision, mydriasis, abnormal accommodation, tinnitus
GI: nausea, vomiting, diarrhea, constipation, epigastric distress, abdominal cramps, abnormal taste, stomatitis, black tongue, dry mouth, **paralytic ileus**
GU: urinary retention or frequency, delayed micturition, urinary tract dilation, gynecomastia, galactorrhea, increased or decreased libido, impotence, testicular swelling
Hematologic: eosinophilia, purpura, **thrombocytopenia, agranulocytosis**
Hepatic: jaundice, hepatic dysfunction
Metabolic: syndrome of inappropriate antidiuretic hormone secretion, hypoglycemia, hyperglycemia
Skin: rash, petechiae, pruritus, urticaria, alopecia, diaphoresis, flushing, photosensitivity
Other: facial and tongue edema, weight changes, parotid gland swelling

Interactions
Drug-drug. *Anticholinergics (such as some antidepressants, antihistamines, atropine, disopyramide, haloperidol, phenothiazines, quinidine):* additive anticholinergic effects
Antihistamines, CNS depressants, opioid analgesics, sedative-hypnotics: additive CNS depression
Antithyroid drugs: increased risk of cardiotoxicity
Barbiturates: decreased trimipramine blood level, increased depressant effect
Cimetidine, flecainide, fluoxetine, paroxetine, phenothiazines, quinidine, sertra-

line: increased trimipramine blood level, greater risk of toxicity

Clonidine: increased risk of hypertensive crisis

Guanethidine: blocked effects of this drug

Local anesthetics containing epinephrine, local decongestants, sympathomimetic amines: increased effects of these drugs

MAO inhibitors: hypertension, hyperpyrexia, seizures, death

Drug-diagnostic tests. *Alanine aminotransferase, aspartate aminotransferase:* increased levels

Glucose: increased or decreased level

Drug-herb. *Angel's trumpet, belladonna, henbane, jimsonweed, scopolia:* increased anticholinergic effects

Chamomile, hops, kava, scopolia, skullcap, valerian: increased CNS depression

St. John's wort: decreased trimipramine blood level and efficacy

Drug-behaviors. *Alcohol use:* increased CNS depression

Sun exposure: increased risk of photosensitivity

Precautions

Use cautiously in:

• increased intraocular pressure, narrow-angle glaucoma, urinary retention, cardiac or hepatic disease, hyperthyroidism, urethral or ureteral spasm, seizure disorders, severe depression, suicidal ideation or behavior

• elderly patients

• pregnant or breastfeeding patients.

Patient monitoring

• Monitor neurologic status; watch for improvement in depression as well as signs and symptoms of CVA or seizures.

◀℥ Assess for suicide risk and drug hoarding.

• Monitor complete blood count and liver function studies; stay alert for

blood dyscrasias and hepatic dysfunction.

Patient teaching

• Tell patient he may take drug with or without food.

• Instruct patient to use drug only as prescribed.

• Caution patient against stopping drug therapy abruptly because doing so may cause nausea, headache, and malaise.

• Advise patient to avoid driving and other hazardous activities until effects of drug are known.

◀℥ Instruct patient (and significant other, as appropriate) to promptly report loss of consciousness, worsening depression, bleeding, bruising, or suicidal thoughts or behavior.

• Caution patient to avoid alcohol and herbs.

• Advise patient to avoid exposure to sun and to wear sunscreen and protective clothing when going outdoors.

• As appropriate, review all other significant and life-threatening adverse reactions and interactions, especially those related to the drugs, tests, herbs, and behaviors mentioned above.

triptorelin pamoate
Trelstar Depot, Trelstar LA

Pharmacologic class: Synthetic agonist analog of luteinizing hormone-releasing hormone (LHRH)

Therapeutic class: Antineoplastic

Pregnancy risk category X

Action

Initially causes transient surge in luteinizing hormone (LH), follicle-stimulating hormone (FSH), and testosterone levels; after chronic use or several weeks of therapy, LH and FSH secretion decrease, causing sustained testosterone reduction equivalent to pharmacologic castration.

Availability
Microgranules for injection: 3.75 mg (depot), 11.25 mg (long-acting)

⚕ Indications and dosages
➤ Palliative treatment of advanced prostate cancer
Adults: 3.75 mg (depot) I.M. monthly as a single injection or 11.25 mg (long-acting) I.M. q 84 days as a single injection

Off-label uses
• Infertility
• Endometriosis
• Uterine fibroids
• Precocious puberty

Contraindications
• Hypersensitivity to drug, other LHRH agonists, or LHRH

Administration
• Reconstitute with 2 ml of sterile water for injection, using accompanying syringe; don't use other diluents. Add syringe contents to vial containing particles; shake well. Withdraw vial contents and inject I.M. immediately.
• Inject deep I.M. into either buttock. Rotate injection sites.
◀ Keep epinephrine and emergency equipment at hand in case of anaphylactic reaction.

Route	Onset	Peak	Duration
I.M. (depot)	Slow	4 days	1 mo
I.M. (long-acting)	Slow	2-3 days	3 mo

Adverse reactions
CNS: insomnia, dizziness, headache, emotional lability, fatigue
CV: hypertension
GI: vomiting, diarrhea
GU: urinary retention, urinary tract infection, gynecomastia, impotence
Hematologic: anemia
Musculoskeletal: skeletal or leg pain
Skin: pruritus
Other: temporary worsening of disease, edema, hot flashes, pain at injection site, hypersensitivity reactions including **anaphylaxis**

Interactions
Drug-drug. *Metoclopramide and other drugs that can cause hyperprolactinemia:* increased prolactin production and risk of severe hyperprolactinemia
Drug-diagnostic tests. *Hemoglobin:* decreased value
Pituitary-gonadal function tests: misleading results (with continuous or long-term use)

Precautions
Use cautiously in:
• renal insufficiency
• prostate cancer with impending spinal cord compression or severe urinary tract disorder.

Patient monitoring
• Monitor serum testosterone and prostate-specific antigen levels periodically to assess drug efficacy.

Patient teaching
• Explain drug therapy to patient; emphasize need for follow-up laboratory tests.
• Tell patient that prostate cancer symptoms may worsen during first few weeks of therapy.
• Teach patient to monitor weight and report sudden weight gain or leg swelling.
• As appropriate, review all other significant and life-threatening adverse reactions and interactions, especially those related to the drugs and tests mentioned above.

t

tromethamine
Tham

Pharmacologic class: Protein substrate
Therapeutic class: Systemic alkalinizer
Pregnancy risk category C

Action
Corrects acidosis by combining with hydrogen ions to form bicarbonate and a buffer; also has some diuretic activity

Availability
Injection: 18 g/500 ml

Indications and dosages
➤ Metabolic acidosis associated with cardiac bypass surgery
Adults: 9 ml/kg (0.32 g/kg) by slow I.V. infusion; 500 ml (18 g) is usually adequate. Maximum individual dosage is 500 mg/kg infused over at least 1 hour.
➤ Metabolic acidosis associated with cardiac arrest
Adults: 3.6 to 10.8 g by I.V. injection into a large peripheral vein if chest isn't open, or 2 to 6 g I.V. directly into ventricular cavity if chest is open. After reversal of cardiac arrest, patient may need additional amounts to control persistent acidosis.
➤ To correct acidity of acid-citrate-dextrose (ACD) blood in cardiac bypass surgery
Adults: 0.5 to 2.5 g added to each 500 ml of ACD blood used for priming pump-oxygenator. Usual dosage is 2 g.
Dosage adjustment
• Elderly patients

Contraindications
• Hypersensitivity to drug
• Anuria
• Uremia

• Respiratory acidosis
• Salicylate toxicity

Administration
🔊 Make sure intubation equipment is close at hand in case respiratory depression occurs.
• For metabolic acidosis associated with cardiac bypass surgery, administer by slow I.V. infusion through large-bore I.V. catheter into a large antecubital vein. Elevate arm after infusion.
• If extravasation occurs, discontinue drug and infiltrate affected area with 1% procaine hydrochloride (containing hyaluronidase).
• Be aware that in cardiac arrest, drug is used in conjunction with standard resuscitative measures. When giving by direct I.V. injection into open chest, never inject drug into cardiac muscle.

Route	Onset	Peak	Duration
I.V.	Immediate	Immediate	Unknown

Adverse reactions
GU: oliguria
Hepatic: hemorrhagic hepatic necrosis
Metabolic: transient hypoglycemia, alkalosis, **fluid-solute overload, hyperkalemia**
Respiratory: respiratory depression
Other: fever; I.V. site infection; extravasation with venous thrombosis or phlebitis, inflammation, necrosis, and sloughing

Interactions
Drug-diagnostic tests. *Glucose:* decreased level
Potassium: increased level

Precautions
Use cautiously in:
• renal disease, severe respiratory disease, respiratory depression
• pregnant patients
• infants.

Patient monitoring

• Institute continuous cardiac monitoring.

• Monitor arterial blood gas levels; watch for alkalosis and signs and symptoms of respiratory depression.

• Assess liver function studies; stay alert for indications of hepatic impairment.

• Monitor glucose and potassium levels; watch for hypoglycemia and hyperkalemia.

• Closely monitor fluid intake and output; check for fluid and electrolyte imbalances and for oliguria related to hyperkalemia.

Patient teaching

• Explain drug therapy to patient; assure him he'll be monitored continuously.

• As appropriate, review all significant and life-threatening adverse reactions and interactions, especially those related to the tests mentioned above.

tubocurarine chloride
Tubocurarine

Pharmacologic class: Nondepolarizing neuromuscular blocker
Therapeutic class: Muscle relaxant
Pregnancy risk category C

Action
Blocks neuromuscular depolarization and contraction by preventing acetylcholine from binding to receptors on motor end-plate

Availability
Injection: 3 mg/ml (20 units/ml)

Indications and dosages
➤ Adjunct to anesthesia to relax skeletal muscles

Adults: 40 to 60 units (6 to 9 mg) I.V. when first incision is made, followed by 20 to 30 units in 3 to 5 minutes, if needed. Supplemental doses of 20 units may be required.
➤ Diagnosis of myasthenia gravis
Adults: 4 to 33 mcg/kg (0.004 to 0.033 mg/kg) I.V. as a single dose
Dosage adjustment
• Renal impairment
• Burns
• Concomitant use of the general anesthetics enflurane, isoflurane, methoxyflurane, halothane, or cyclopropane

Contraindications
• Hypersensitivity to drug
• Asthma and other conditions in which histamine release is hazardous

Administration
◀ Keep oxygen, airway management equipment, atropine, and neostigmine or edrophonium readily available.

• Assess renal function and electrolyte balance before giving drug.

• Administer I.V. over at least 1 minute.

• Be aware that if suitable vein isn't accessible, drug may be given I.M. in same dosage used in I.V. administration.

◀ When drug is used to diagnose myasthenia gravis, it may profoundly exaggerate myasthenic symptoms. If this occurs, give 1.5 to 2 mg of neostigmine I.V. 2 to 3 minutes after tubocurarine to terminate test.

Route	Onset	Peak	Duration
I.V.	1 min	2-5 min	25-90 min

Adverse reactions
CV: hypotension, bradycardia, **arrhythmias, cardiac arrest**
GI: decreased GI motility and tone
Musculoskeletal: profound and prolonged muscle relaxation, residual muscle weakness

Respiratory: prolonged apnea, bronchospasm, cyanosis, respiratory depression

Skin: rash, flushing, pruritus, urticaria

Other: increased salivation, hypersensitivity reaction

Interactions

Drug-drug. *Aminoglycosides, anticholinesterases, clindamycin, general anesthetics, polymyxin anti-infectives:* increased neuromuscular blockade and respiratory depression

Carbamazepine, hydantoins: decreased tubocurarine duration of action and efficacy

Corticosteroids: decreased tubocurarine action

Lithium: prolonged recovery from tubocurarine effects, possibly causing profound, severe respiratory depression

Loop diuretics: potentiation or antagonism of tubocurarine effects

Magnesium sulfate, nitrates: potentiation of tubocurarine effects, causing profound, severe respiratory depression

Drug-herb. *St. John's wort:* increased risk of cardiovascular collapse, delayed emergence from anesthesia

Precautions

Use cautiously in:
• renal, hepatic, or cardiac disease; electrolyte imbalance; respiratory or neuromuscular disease; peripheral neuropathy; dehydration; hypothermia; hypokalemia; respiratory acidosis; metabolic alkalosis; hypotension; sepsis; major burns
• pregnant or breastfeeding patients
• children under age 2.

Patient monitoring

• Monitor heart rhythm, blood pressure, and respiratory status.
• Assess muscle recovery using peripheral nerve stimulator and train-of-four monitoring.

🔊 Monitor patient's need for sedatives or analgesics. (Drug doesn't alter consciousness or relieve pain.)
• When drug is used to diagnose myasthenia gravis, assess for exaggerated muscle weakness, which signals positive result. Know that prolonged exaggerated symptoms must be reversed with tubocurarine antagonist (neostigmine) within 2 to 3 minutes.

Patient teaching

• Teach patient and family about purpose of drug therapy.
• Explain procedure to patient while he's still aware of surroundings.
• As appropriate, review all other significant and life-threatening adverse reactions and interactions, especially those related to the drugs and herbs mentioned above.

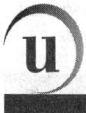

urea
Ureaphil

Pharmacologic class: Diamide salt of carbonic acid
Therapeutic class: Osmotic diuretic
Pregnancy risk category C

Action

Increases osmotic pressure of glomerular filtrate, inhibits tubular reabsorption of water and electrolytes, and elevates plasma osmolarity, causing increased water influx into extracellular fluid

Availability

Powder for reconstitution: 40 g/150 ml

✪ Indications and dosages
➤ To decrease intracranial pressure (ICP) or intraocular pressure (IOP)
Adults: 1 to 1.5 g/kg as 30% solution I.V. infused slowly over 1 to 2½ hours at a rate not exceeding 4 ml/minute; maximum dosage is 120 g/day.

Off-label uses
• Abortifacient

Contraindications
• Hypersensitivity to drug
• Severe renal impairment
• Marked dehydration
• Active intracranial bleeding
• Hepatic failure
• Infusion into lower leg veins in elderly patients

Administration
• Add dextrose 5% or 10% in water to container with 40 g of urea, to yield a final concentration of 300 mg/ml. Infuse no faster than 4 ml/minute.
• Infuse through large-bore catheter into large vein only.
◀︎﹦ Don't stop infusion abruptly.

Route	Onset	Peak	Duration
I.V.	30-45 min	1-2 hr	3-10 hr

Adverse reactions
CNS: headache, dizziness, agitation, confusion, disorientation, syncope, nervousness, drowsiness (with prolonged use in sickle cell patients), **subdural hemorrhage**
CV: hypotension, tachycardia, ECG changes, capillary bleeding, **cardiotoxicity**
GI: nausea, vomiting
GU: oliguria
Hematologic: hemolysis (with rapid administration)
Metabolic: hypervolemia, hyponatremia, hypokalemia, electrolyte imbalance

Skin: irritation or necrotic sloughing with extravasation
Other: pain, chemical phlebitis, thrombosis, or infection at injection site; fever; hyperthermia

Interactions
Drug-drug. *Lithium:* increased clearance and decreased efficacy of lithium
Drug-diagnostic tests. *Potassium, sodium:* decreased levels

Precautions
Use cautiously in:
• hepatic or renal disease, electrolyte imbalance, diabetes mellitus, sickle cell disease, membrane rupture, cervical stenosis, uterine fibroids
• pregnant or breastfeeding patients.

Patient monitoring
• Institute continuous cardiac monitoring.
• Closely monitor vital signs, ICP, and neurologic and cardiac status.
• Monitor electrolyte levels and kidney function test results.
• Assess fluid intake and output.
• If drug is used for IOP reduction, monitor IOP.

Patient teaching
• Explain drug therapy to patient.
◀︎﹦ Inform patient that drug may affect many body systems; instruct him to immediately report unusual symptoms—especially headache or confusion.
• As appropriate, review all significant and life-threatening adverse reactions and interactions, especially those related to the drugs and tests mentioned above.

u

urokinase
Abbokinase, Abbokinase Open-Cath

Pharmacologic class: Plasminogen
activator
Therapeutic class: Thrombolytic
enzyme
Pregnancy risk category B

Action
Promotes thrombolysis by directly
converting plasminogen to plasmin

Availability
Injection: 5,000 IU/vial, 250,000 IU/vial

🟋 Indications and dosages
➤ Pulmonary emboli
Adults: Loading dose of 4,400 IU/kg
I.V. administered at a rate of 90 ml/
hour over 10 minutes, followed by a
continuous infusion of 4,400 IU/kg/
hour at 15 ml/hour for 12 hours

Off-label uses
• Central venous catheter occlusion
• Myocardial infarction

Contraindications
• Hypersensitivity to drug
• Active bleeding
• Intraspinal surgery
• Severe hypertension
• Rheumatic valvular disease
• Cerebral embolism, thrombosis, or
hemorrhage
• CNS or intracranial neoplasm, arteri-
ovenous malformation, or aneurysm
• Bleeding diathesis
• History of cerebrovascular accident

Administration
◀€ Keep emergency equipment and
epinephrine readily available in case
anaphylaxis occurs.

• Before administering, check activated
partial thromboplastin time (APTT),
hematocrit, and platelet count. APTT
must be less than twice the normal
control value before drug can be given.
• Discontinue heparin as ordered before starting urokinase. (Heparin therapy may resume after urokinase therapy ends if APTT is less than twice the
normal control value.)
• Immediately before use, reconstitute
powder with preservative-free sterile
water for injection; reconstituted solution should be clear or a light straw
color. Solution may be filtered through
0.45-micron or smaller cellulose-mem-
brane filter. Dilute further with normal
saline solution or dextrose 5% in water
to yield a total volume not exceeding
195 ml.
• After infusion, make sure entire dose
is given by flushing (at a rate of 15 ml/
hour) any urokinase still in I.V. tubing
with a volume of compatible I.V. solution roughly equal to that of drug remaining in tubing.
◀€ Have blood products and aminocaproic acid available in case of serious
spontaneous bleeding.

Route	Onset	Peak	Duration
I.V.	Immediate	20 min-4 hr	12-24 hr

Adverse reactions
CNS: intracranial bleeding
CV: hypotension, hypertension, **reper-
fusion arrhythmias**
GI: GI or retroperitoneal bleeding
GU: GU bleeding
Hematologic: decreased hemoglobin
and hematocrit; bleeding at external
excision, I.V. puncture, or I.M. sites;
hemorrhage
Respiratory: altered respiration, **bron-
chospasm**
Skin: rash, urticaria, pruritus, flushing,
surface bleeding
Other: fever, phlebitis at I.V. injection
site, **anaphylaxis**

Interactions

Drug-drug. *Abciximab, anticoagulants, aspirin, cephalosporins (selected), clopidogrel, dipyridamole, eptifibatide, indomethacin, nonsteroidal anti-inflammatory drugs, phenylbutazone, plicamycin, ticlopidine, tirofiban, valproic acid, other drugs that affect platelet activity:* increased risk of bleeding

Drug-diagnostic tests. *Hematocrit, hemoglobin:* decreased values

Drug-herb. *Ginkgo:* increased risk of bleeding

Precautions

Use cautiously in:
• known or suspected left-sided thrombus, hypertension, acute pericarditis, subacute bacterial endocarditis, hemostatic defects, severe hepatic or renal dysfunction, diabetic hemorrhagic retinopathy or other hemorrhagic ophthalmic condition, septic thrombophlebitis, cerebrovascular disease
• recent GI or GU bleeding
• concurrent anticoagulant therapy
• elderly patients
• pregnant patients.

Patient monitoring

• Monitor vital signs and watch for reperfusion arrhythmias; check blood pressure manually.

◢€ Stay alert for other reperfusion reactions, such as fever, chills, hypotension or hypertension, nausea, vomiting, hypoxia, cyanosis, dyspnea, acidosis, or back pain. If any of these signs and symptoms occur, discontinue drug immediately and give antihistamines, adrenergics, or corticosteroids as prescribed.

• Monitor hemoglobin, hematocrit, prothrombin time, International Normalized Ratio, and APTT; watch for signs and symptoms of bleeding in all body systems.

• Monitor puncture sites. After needle puncture, apply pressure dressing for at least 30 minutes.

• Evaluate respiratory status closely, especially for bronchospasm.

Patient teaching

• Explain drug therapy to patient.
• Inform patient that drug can cause serious adverse reactions in many body systems. Instruct him to immediately report unusual symptoms.
• As appropriate, review all other significant and life-threatening adverse reactions and interactions, especially those related to the drugs, tests, and herbs mentioned above.

ursodiol
Actigall, Urso

Pharmacologic class: Bile acid
Therapeutic class: Digestive enzyme, gallstone solubilizer
Pregnancy risk category B

Action

Unknown; thought to suppress hepatic synthesis and inhibit intestinal reabsorption of cholesterol

Availability

Capsules: 300 mg
Tablets: 250 mg

⚕ Indications and dosages

➤ To dissolve radiolucent, noncalcified gallstones less than 20 mm in diameter when surgery is inadvisable
Adults: 8 to 10 mg/kg P.O. daily in two or three divided doses for no longer than 24 months

Off-label uses

• Biliary atresia or cirrhosis
• Caroli's syndrome

Contraindications
• Hypersensitivity to drug or other bile acids
• Calcified cholesterol, radiopaque, or radiolucent bile pigment stones
• Unremitting acute cholecystitis, cholangitis, biliary obstruction, chronic hepatic disease, or other compelling reasons for cholecystectomy

Administration
• Give drug with food; don't give with aluminum-containing antacids.

Route	Onset	Peak	Duration
P.O.	Unknown	1-3 hr	Unknown

Adverse reactions
CNS: headache, fatigue, anxiety, depression, sleep disorders
EENT: rhinitis
GI: nausea, vomiting, diarrhea, constipation, dyspepsia, flatulence, abdominal or biliary pain, cholecystitis, metallic taste, stomatitis
Musculoskeletal: joint pain, myalgia, back pain
Respiratory: cough
Skin: rash, dry skin, pruritus, urticaria, alopecia, diaphoresis

Interactions
Drug-drug. *Aluminum-containing antacids, cholestyramine, colestipol:* inhibited ursodiol absorption
Clofibrate, estrogens, hormonal contraceptives: increased hepatic cholesterol secretion, greater risk of cholesterol gallstones

Precautions
Use cautiously in:
• variceal bleeding, hepatic encephalopathy, ascites
• pregnant or breastfeeding patients
• children.

Patient monitoring
• Monitor gallbladder ultrasound results every 6 months for first year of therapy.

Patient teaching
• Instruct patient to take drug with food but not with aluminum-containing antacids.
• Tell patient he'll need months of therapy as well as periodic follow-up gallbladder ultrasound testing.
• Inform patient that drug doesn't completely dissolve gallstones in all patients and that gallstones may recur.
• As appropriate, review all other significant and adverse reactions and interactions, especially those related to the drugs mentioned above.

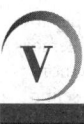

valacyclovir hydrochloride
Valtrex

Pharmacologic class: Acyclic purine nucleoside analog
Therapeutic class: Antiviral
Pregnancy risk category B

Action
Rapidly converts to acyclovir, which interferes with viral DNA synthesis and replication

Availability
Caplets: 500 mg, 1 g

Indications and dosages
➤ Herpes zoster (shingles)
Adults: 1 g P.O. t.i.d. for 7 days. Therapy should begin at the earliest sign or symptom of herpes zoster, within 48 hours of onset of zoster rash.
➤ Genital herpes
Adults: In initial episode, 1 g P.O. b.i.d.

for 10 days. In recurrent episodes, 500 mg P.O. b.i.d. for 3 days. For chronic suppression, 1 g P.O. daily for no more than 1 year; in patients with history of fewer than nine yearly recurrences, 500 mg P.O. daily for no more than 1 year.

Dosage adjustment
• Renal impairment

Off-label uses
• Prophylaxis of cytomegalovirus

Contraindications
• Hypersensitivity to drug, its components, or acyclovir

Administration
• Be aware that therapy may be ineffective if started more than 72 hours after initial genital herpes outbreak or more than 24 hours after symptom onset in genital herpes recurrence.

Route	Onset	Peak	Duration
P.O.	Unknown	1.5-2.5 hr	8-24 hr

Adverse reactions
CNS: headache, dizziness, depression
GI: nausea, vomiting, diarrhea, abdominal pain
GU: dysmenorrhea
Hematologic: anemia, **leukopenia, thrombocytopenia**
Hepatic: elevated hepatic enzyme levels
Musculoskeletal: joint pain
Other: hypersensitivity reaction

Interactions
Drug-drug. *Cimetidine, probenecid:* increased valacyclovir blood level
Drug-diagnostic tests. *Alanine aminotransferase, alkaline phosphatase, aspartate aminotransferase:* increased levels

Precautions
Use cautiously in:
• renal impairment
• pregnant or breastfeeding patients
• children.

Patient monitoring
• Monitor complete blood count; be alert for signs and symptoms of blood dyscrasias.
• Assess liver and kidney function test results.

Patient teaching
• Teach patient that herpes transmission can occur even when he's asymptomatic.
• Inform pregnant patient of risk of neonatal herpes infection.
• Instruct pregnant women and females of childbearing age to inform health care provider that they have herpes; after delivery, tell them to inform providers who care for neonate.
• Instruct patient to promptly report unusual bleeding or bruising, urinary changes, or serious adverse CNS reactions.
• As appropriate, review all other significant and life-threatening adverse reactions and interactions, especially those related to the drugs and tests mentioned above.

valdecoxib
Bextra

Pharmacologic class: Nonsteroidal anti-inflammatory drug (NSAID), selective cyclooxygenase-2 (COX-2) inhibitor
Therapeutic class: Anti-inflammatory
Pregnancy risk category C (first and second trimesters), *D* (third trimester)

Action
Inhibits prostaglandin synthesis by inhibiting COX-2, reducing inflammation

Availability
Tablets: 10 mg, 20 mg

V

⃠ Indications and dosages

➤ Osteoarthritis, adult rheumatoid arthritis
Adults: 10 mg P.O. daily
➤ Primary dysmenorrhea
Adults: 20 mg P.O. b.i.d. p.r.n.

Off-label uses

• Postoperative pain

Contraindications

• Hypersensitivity to drug, its components, other NSAIDs (including aspirin), iodides, or sulfonamides
• Third trimester of pregnancy

Administration

• Give drug with or without food.

Route	Onset	Peak	Duration
P.O.	Variable	2-3 hr	Unknown

Adverse reactions

CNS: headache, dizziness, asthenia, fatigue, depression, drowsiness, insomnia, tremor, confusion, vertigo, paresthesia, anxiety, migraine, hypertonia
CV: palpitations, hypotension, hypertension, tachycardia, peripheral edema, angina pectoris, **arrhythmias, myocardial infarction (MI), heart failure**
EENT: blurred vision, conjunctivitis, tinnitus, rhinitis, epistaxis, pharyngitis, sinusitis
GI: nausea, vomiting, diarrhea, constipation, abdominal pain or cramps, bloating, eructation, flatulence, dyspepsia, gastritis, gastroenteritis, melena, peptic ulcer, hematemesis, altered taste, stomatitis, dry mouth
GU: urinary frequency, polyuria, urinary tract infection, hematuria, albuminuria, cystitis, menstrual disorder, vaginal bleeding, impotence, elevated blood urea nitrogen (BUN) and creatinine levels
Hematologic: anemia, eosinophilia, **leukopenia, thrombocytopenia**
Hepatic: elevated hepatic enzyme levels, **hepatitis**

Metabolic: hyperglycemia, hypokalemia, hyperkalemia
Musculoskeletal: joint pain, myalgia, back pain
Respiratory: dyspnea, upper respiratory tract infection, bronchitis, cough, pneumonia, **bronchospasm**
Skin: diaphoresis, rash, pruritus, alopecia, eczema, bruising, photosensitivity
Other: appetite and weight changes, excessive thirst, chills, fever, edema, facial edema, lymphadenopathy, accidental injury, flulike symptoms, pain, allergic reaction

Interactions

Drug-drug. *Angiotensin-converting enzyme inhibitors, furosemide, thiazide diuretics:* decreased effects of these drugs
Antineoplastics, lithium: increased blood levels and risk of toxicity of these drugs
Dextromethorphan: increased dextromethorphan blood level
Fluconazole, ketoconazole: increased valdecoxib blood level
Glucocorticoids, NSAIDs: increased GI reactions, greater risk of bleeding
Oral anticoagulants: increased anticoagulant effect
Drug-diagnostic tests. *Alanine aminotransferase, alkaline phosphatase, aspartate aminotransferase, BUN, creatinine, eosinophils, glucose, potassium:* increased levels
Hematocrit, hemoglobin, platelets, potassium, white blood cells: decreased levels

Precautions

Use cautiously in:
• hypertension, bleeding, severe dehydration, heart failure, asthma, anemia
• history of hepatic or renal dysfunction; coagulation defects; GI ulcers, bleeding, or perforation
• pregnant women in first or second trimester, breastfeeding patients
• children under age 18.

Patient monitoring

• Monitor kidney and liver function studies, complete blood count, and electrolyte levels. Stay alert for signs and symptoms of organ dysfunction and blood dyscrasias.

Patient teaching

• Tell patient he may take drug with or without food.

• Explain risks and benefits of drug therapy; emphasize need for periodic follow-up laboratory tests.

◀ Teach patient to immediately report signs or symptoms of GI bleeding or ulcers, heart failure, or liver problems (such as fatigue, nausea, or yellowing of skin or eyes).

• Tell females of childbearing age to inform prescriber if they're pregnant or breastfeeding or plan to become pregnant or to breastfeed.

◀ Advise patient to stop taking drug and contact prescriber immediately if skin rash or other signs or symptoms of hypersensitivity reaction occur.

• As appropriate, review all other significant and life-threatening adverse reactions and interactions, especially those related to the drugs and tests mentioned above.

valganciclovir hydrochloride
Valcyte

Pharmacologic class: Synthetic guanine derivative

Therapeutic class: Antiviral

Pregnancy risk category C

Action

Rapidly converts to its active form, inhibiting activity of cytomegalovirus (CMV)

Availability

Tablets: 450 mg

Indications and dosages

➤ Active CMV retinitis in AIDS patients

Adults: For induction therapy, 900 mg P.O. b.i.d. for 21 days. Maintenance dosage is 900 mg P.O. daily.

Dosage adjustment

• Renal impairment

Contraindications

• Hypersensitivity to drug, its components, or ganciclovir

• Absolute neutrophil count below 500 cells/mm^3, platelet count below 25,000 cells/mm^3, or hemoglobin below 8 g/dl

Administration

• Avoid direct contact with broken or crushed tablets. If skin contact occurs, wash thoroughly with soap and water; if eye contact occurs, rinse eyes thoroughly with plain water.

Route	Onset	Peak	Duration
P.O.	Unknown	1-3 hr	Unknown

Adverse reactions

CNS: headache, insomnia, sedation, dizziness, peripheral neuropathy, paresthesia, hallucinations, confusion, agitation, psychosis, ataxia, **seizures**

EENT: retinal detachment

GI: nausea, vomiting, diarrhea, abdominal pain

GU: elevated creatinine level

Hematologic: anemia, **bone marrow depression, aplastic anemia, pancytopenia, thrombocytopenia, neutropenia**

Other: fever, catheter-related infection, local or systemic infection, hypersensitivity reaction, **sepsis**

Interactions

Drug-drug. *Cytotoxic drugs (such as adriamycin, amphotericin B, co-trimoxazole, dapsone, doxorubicin, flucytosine,*

V

pentamidine, vinblastine, vincristine): additive toxicity

Cilastatin, imipenem: seizures

Didanosine: increased didanosine blood level, decreased valganciclovir blood level

Nephrotoxic drugs (such as amphotericin B, cyclosporine): increased creatinine level

Probenecid: decreased renal clearance of valganciclovir

Zidovudine: increased risk of granulocytopenia and anemia

Drug-diagnostic tests. *Alanine aminotransferase, alkaline phosphatase, aspartate aminotransferase, creatinine:* increased levels

Creatinine clearance: decreased value

Granulocytes, hemoglobin, neutrophils, platelets, white blood cells: decreased levels

Drug-food. *Any food:* increased drug absorption

Precautions
Use cautiously in:
- cytopenia, impaired renal function
- myelosuppressive drug therapy or radiation therapy
- elderly patients
- pregnant or breastfeeding patients.

Patient monitoring
- Monitor complete blood count with white cell differential and platelet count; watch for signs and symptoms of blood dyscrasias.

◀≼ Stay alert for hypersensitivity reaction and signs and symptoms of infection.
- Closely monitor neurologic status; stay alert for signs of impending seizure.
- Assess creatinine level and creatinine clearance periodically.

Patient teaching
- Instruct patient to take drug with food.
- Explain drug therapy to patient; em-

phasize importance of taking drug exactly as prescribed to prevent overdose.

◀≼ Tell patient that drug can cause serious adverse reactions; teach him which ones to report immediately.
- Caution patient to avoid driving and other hazardous activities.
- Caution females of childbearing age to avoid pregnancy and breastfeeding.
- Advise male patients to use barrier contraception during therapy and for 90 days afterward.
- Discuss need for follow-up eye examinations every 4 to 6 weeks, as well as periodic laboratory testing.
- As appropriate, review all other significant and life-threatening adverse reactions and interactions, especially those related to the drugs, tests, and foods mentioned above.

valproate sodium
Depacon

valproic acid
Depakene

divalproex sodium
Depakote, Depakote ER, Depakote Sprinkle

Pharmacologic class: Carboxylic acid derivative

Therapeutic class: Anticonvulsant, mood stabilizer, antimigraine agent

Pregnancy risk category D

Action
Increases level of gamma-aminobutyric acid in brain, thereby reducing seizure activity

Availability
valproate sodium
Injection: 100 mg/ml in 5-ml vial
Syrup: 250 mg/5 ml

valproic acid
Capsules (liquid-filled): 250 mg
divalproex sodium
Capsules (containing coated particles or sprinkles): 125 mg
Tablets (delayed-release): 125 mg, 250 mg, 500 mg
Tablets (extended-release): 250 mg, 500 mg

🖉 Indications and dosages
➤ Complex partial seizures
Adults and children older than age 10: Initially, 10 to 15 mg/kg/day P.O. May increase by 5 to 10 mg/kg/day q week until therapeutic blood level is reached or adverse reactions occur; don't exceed 60 mg/kg/day. When daily dosage exceeds 250 mg, give in two divided doses.
➤ Simple or complex absence seizures
Adults and children older than age 10: Initially, 15 mg/kg/day P.O. May increase by 5 to 10 mg/kg/day at weekly intervals until therapeutic blood level is reached or adverse reactions occur; don't exceed 60 mg/kg/day. When daily dosage exceeds 250 mg, give in two divided doses.
➤ Mania
Adults: Initially, 750 mg (divalproex delayed-release) P.O. daily in divided doses; titrate rapidly to desired clinical effect or trough level of 50 to 125 mcg/ml. Don't exceed 60 mg/kg/day.
➤ To prevent migraine
Adults: 250 mg (divalproex delayed-release) P.O. b.i.d., up to 1 g/day. Or 500 mg (divalproex extended-release) P.O. daily for 1 week(up to 1 g/day).

Off-label uses
• Chorea
• Photosensitivity-related seizures
• Sedative-hypnotic withdrawal

Contraindications
• Hypersensitivity to drug or tartrazine (with some products)

• Hepatic impairment
• Posttraumatic seizures caused by head injury
• Urea cycle disorders
• Pregnancy

Administration
• Administer I.V. only when oral dosing isn't feasible.
• For I.V. use, dilute valproate sodium in at least 50 ml of dextrose 5% in water, lactated Ringer's solution, or normal saline solution. Infuse over 1 hour at a rate below 20 mg/minute.
• Know that I.V. and P.O. dosages and dosing frequencies are identical; however, patient should be switched to oral dosing as soon as possible.
• Administer oral forms with food.
• Be aware that divalproex extended-release and delayed-release forms are not bioequivalent.
• Make sure patient swallows divalproex extended-release tablets whole without chewing or crushing them.
• If patient can't swallow capsules containing coated particles, entire contents of capsule may be sprinkled on about 5 ml of semisolid food, such as pudding or applesauce, immediately before administration.
• Don't give syrup in carbonated beverages because it may irritate mouth and throat.

Route	Onset	Peak	Duration
P.O. (capsules)	Rapid	1-4 hr	6-24 hr
P.O. (delayed, extended)	Unknown	Unknown	Unknown
P.O. (syrup)	Rapid	15-120 min	6-24 hr
I.V.	Rapid	End of 1-hr infusion	Unknown

Adverse reactions
CNS: confusion, dizziness, headache, sedation, ataxia, paresthesia, asthenia, tremor, drowsiness, emotional lability, abnormal thinking, amnesia

EENT: amblyopia, blurred vision, nystagmus, tinnitus, pharyngitis
GI: nausea, vomiting, diarrhea, abdominal pain, dyspepsia, abnormal taste, anorexia, **pancreatitis**
Hematologic: prolonged bleeding time, **leukopenia, thrombocytopenia**
Hepatic: elevated hepatic enzyme levels, **hepatotoxicity**
Musculoskeletal: back pain
Respiratory: dyspnea
Skin: rash, alopecia, bruising
Other: increased appetite, weight gain, flulike symptoms, infection, pain, infusion site pain and reaction

Interactions

Drug-drug. *Activated charcoal, cholestyramine:* decreased valproate absorption
Antiplatelet agents (including abciximab, aspirin and other nonsteroidal anti-inflammatory drugs, eptifibatide, tirofiban), cefamandole, cefoperazone, cefotetan, heparin, thrombolytics, warfarin: increased risk of bleeding
Barbiturates, primidone: decreased metabolism and greater risk of toxicity of these drugs, decreased valproate efficacy
Carbamazepine: increased carbamazepine blood level, decreased valproate blood level, poor seizure control
Chlorpromazine: decreased valproate clearance and increased trough level
Cimetidine: decreased valproate clearance
Clonazepam: absence seizures in patients with history of these seizures
CNS depressants (such as antihistamines and antidepressants, monoamine oxidase inhibitors, opioid analgesics, sedative-hypnotics): additive CNS depression
Diazepam: displacement of diazepam from binding site, inhibited diazepam metabolism
Erythromycin, felbamate: increased valproate blood level, greater risk of toxicity

Ethosuximide: inhibited ethosuximide metabolism
Lamotrigine: decreased valproate blood level, increased lamotrigine blood level
Phenytoin: increased phenytoin effects and risk of toxicity, decreased valproate effects
Salicylates (large doses in children): increased valproate effects
Tricyclic antidepressants: increased blood levels of these drugs, greater risk of adverse reactions
Zidovudine: decreased zidovudine clearance in patients with human immunodeficiency virus
Drug-diagnostic tests. *Alanine aminotransferase, alkaline phosphatase, aspartate aminotransferase, bilirubin:* increased levels
Bleeding time: prolonged
Ketone bodies: false-positive results
Platelets, white blood cells: decreased counts
Thyroid function tests: interference with results
Drug-behaviors. *Alcohol use:* additive CNS depression

Precautions

Use cautiously in:
• bleeding disorders, organic brain disease, bone marrow depression, renal impairment
• history of hepatic disease
• breastfeeding patients
• children.

Patient monitoring

◀🔔 Closely monitor neurologic status; watch for seizures.
◀🔔 Evaluate GI status; stay alert for signs and symptoms of pancreatitis.
• Monitor I.V. infusion site for local reactions.
• Assess complete blood count (including platelet count), prothrombin time, International Normalized Ratio, and liver function studies.
• Monitor valproate blood level; therapeutic range is 50 to 100 mcg/ml.

Patient teaching

• Instruct patient to take drug with food to minimize GI upset.

• Tell patient taking extended-release tablets to swallow them whole without chewing or breaking them.

• Inform patient taking capsules that he may swallow them whole or open them and sprinkle contents on a teaspoon of semisolid food, such as pudding or applesauce.

• Tell patient (or parents) that valproate syrup shouldn't be taken with carbonated beverages.

◀◉ Teach patient to immediately report malaise, weakness, lethargy, appetite loss, vomiting, or discoloration of skin or eyes.

• If patient is taking drug for seizure control, tell him to avoid driving and other hazardous activities.

◀◉ Caution patient not to stop therapy abruptly.

• Instruct patient to avoid alcohol consumption.

• Inform patient of need for follow-up laboratory testing.

• As appropriate, review all other significant and life-threatening adverse reactions and interactions, especially those related to the drugs, tests, and behaviors mentioned above.

valrubicin
Valstar

Pharmacologic class: Anthracycline
Therapeutic class: Antibiotic antineoplastic
Pregnancy risk category C

Action

Inhibits DNA and RNA synthesis; penetrates into cells, inhibiting incorporation of nucleosides into nucleic acid, causing extensive chromosomal damage, and blocking cell in G2 phase

Availability

Solution for intravesical instillation: 200 mg/5 ml

🕖 Indications and dosages

➤ Urinary bladder cancer
Adults: 800 mg intravesically q week for 6 weeks

Off-label uses

• Gynecologic cancer

Contraindications

• Hypersensitivity to drug or other anthracyclines
• Perforated bladder or compromised bladder mucosa
• Small bladder capacity (intolerance of 75-ml instillation)
• Urinary tract infection
• Breastfeeding

Administration

◀◉ Follow facility protocol for handling, preparing, and administering chemotherapeutic drugs.

• For each instillation, slowly warm four vials of 200 mg/5 ml to room temperature. Withdraw solution and dilute with 55 ml of sodium chloride injection, for a total volume of 75 ml.

• Insert urinary catheter into patient's bladder, drain bladder, and slowly instill solution by gravity flow over several minutes; then remove catheter. Have patient retain solution for 2 hours before voiding.

Route	Onset	Peak	Duration
Intravesical	Unknown	Unknown	Unknown

Adverse reactions

CNS: asthenia, headache, malaise, dizziness
CV: vasodilation, chest pain, peripheral edema

GI: nausea, vomiting, diarrhea, abdominal pain, flatulence

GU: urinary frequency, urgency, retention, or incontinence; urinary tract infection; bladder spasms and pain; hematuria; cystitis; local burning; urethral or pelvic pain

Hematologic: anemia

Metabolic: hyperglycemia

Musculoskeletal: myalgia, back pain

Respiratory: pneumonia

Skin: rash

Other: fever

Interactions

Drug-diagnostic tests. *Glucose:* increased level

Hemoglobin: decreased level

Precautions

Use cautiously in:

• transurethral resection within past 2 weeks, concurrent use of antiplatelet drugs or anticoagulants, GI disorders, renal impairment, severe irritable bladder symptoms, significant bone marrow depression (especially leukopenia)

• history of bleeding disorders

• pregnant patients

• children (safety and efficacy not established).

Patient monitoring

• Monitor for disease recurrence or progression, including results of cystoscopy, bladder biopsy, and urine cytology every 3 months.

Patient teaching

• Tell patient he must retain solution in bladder for 2 hours.

• Encourage patient to drink plenty of fluid after each treatment.

• Inform patient that red-tinged urine is typical during first 24 hours; however, he should immediately report prolonged red-tinged urine or urinary urgency or frequency.

• Advise females of childbearing age to avoid pregnancy.

• Instruct male patients to use barrier contraception during therapy.

• As appropriate, review all other significant adverse reactions and interactions, especially those related to the tests mentioned above.

valsartan
Diovan

Pharmacologic class: Angiotensin II receptor antagonist

Therapeutic class: Antihypertensive

Pregnancy risk category C (first trimester), *D* (second and third trimesters)

Action

Blocks vasoconstrictive and aldosterone-producing effects of angiotensin II at various receptor sites, including vascular smooth muscle and adrenal glands

Availability

Tablets: 40 mg, 80 mg, 160 mg, 320 mg

🕖 Indications and dosages

➤ Hypertension

Adults: Initially, 80 to 160 mg P.O. daily; may increase as needed to a maximum of 320 mg P.O. daily, or a diuretic may be added

➤ Heart failure in patients intolerant of angiotensin-converting enzyme inhibitors

Adults: Initially, 40 mg P.O. b.i.d.; may increase to 160 mg P.O. b.i.d. as needed. Drug may be given alone or with other drugs.

Off-label uses

• Left ventricular hypertrophy

• Diabetic nephropathy

Contraindications

• Hypersensitivity to drug or its components

• Second or third trimester of pregnancy

Administration

• Give drug with or without food.

Route	Onset	Peak	Duration
P.O.	Within 2 hr	4-6 hr	24 hr

Adverse reactions

CNS: dizziness, fatigue, headache
CV: hypotension, palpitations
EENT: sinus disorders, dental pain
GI: nausea, diarrhea, constipation, abdominal pain, dry mouth
GU: renal impairment, albuminuria
Hematologic: neutropenia
Metabolic: hyperkalemia
Musculoskeletal: back pain, joint pain, muscle cramps
Skin: alopecia, angioedema
Other: fever, viral infection

Interactions

Drug-drug. *Other antihypertensives:* increased risk of hypotension
Potassium-sparing diuretics, potassium supplements: increased risk of hyperkalemia
Drug-diagnostic tests. *Urine albumin, urine potassium:* increased levels
Drug-food. *Salt substitutes containing potassium:* increased risk of hyperkalemia
Drug-herb. *Ephedra (ma huang):* reduced hypotensive effect of valsartan
Drug-behaviors. *Alcohol use:* increased CNS depression

Precautions

Use cautiously in:

• severe heart failure; volume or sodium depletion; hepatic impairment; renal impairment; obstructive biliary disorders; angioedema; aortic, mitral valve, or renal artery stenosis; hyperkalemia

• concurrent use of high-dose diuretics
• black patients
• females of childbearing age
• pregnant patients in first trimester
• children under age 18 (safety not established).

Patient monitoring

• Monitor blood pressure closely, especially during initial therapy and dosage adjustments.

• Assess potassium level; stay alert for hyperkalemia.

• Be aware that in black patients, drug may be ineffective when used alone; additional agents may be required.

Patient teaching

• Tell patient he may take drug with or without food.

◀€ Instruct females of childbearing age to report pregnancy immediately.

• Teach patient to avoid potassium-containing salt substitutes.

• Caution patient to avoid alcohol.

• As appropriate, review all other significant and life-threatening adverse reactions and interactions, especially those related to the drugs, tests, foods, herbs, and behaviors mentioned above.

vancomycin hydrochloride

Vancocin

Pharmacologic class: Tricyclic glycopeptide
Therapeutic class: Anti-infective
Pregnancy risk category C

V

Action

Binds to bacterial cell wall, producing immediate inhibition of cell wall synthesis and causing secondary damage to bacterial plasma membrane

---

Availability
Capsules: 125 mg, 250 mg
Powder for injection: 500-mg vial, 1-g vial, 5-g vial, 10 g-vial
Powder for oral solution: 1-g and 10-g bottles

🕖 Indications and dosages
➤ Severe, life-threatening infections when other anti-infectives fail or are contraindicated
Adults: 500 mg I.V. q 6 hours or 1 g I.V. q 12 hours
Children: 10 mg/kg I.V. q 6 hours
Infants and neonates: Initially, 15 mg/kg I.V., followed by 10 mg/kg I.V. q 8 hours in infants ages 8 days to 1 month or 10 mg/kg I.V. q 12 hours in neonates less than 8 days old
➤ To prevent endocarditis in penicillin-allergic patients at moderate risk who are scheduled for dental or upper respiratory tract procedures or certain GI, biliary tract, or GU tract procedures
Adults: 1 g I.V. slowly over 1 to 2 hours, with infusion completed 30 minutes before invasive procedure begins
Children: 20 mg/kg I.V. over 1 to 2 hours, with infusion completed 30 minutes before invasive procedure begins
➤ Enterocolitis caused by *S. aureus;* antibiotic-related pseudomembranous diarrhea caused by *Clostridium difficile*
Adults: 500 mg to 2 g P.O. daily in three or four divided doses for 7 to 10 days
Children: 40 mg/kg P.O. daily in three or four divided doses for 7 to 10 days, up to a maximum of 2 g/day
Dosage adjustment
• Renal impairment
• Elderly patients

Off-label uses
• Peritonitis
• Streptococcal infections
• Meningitis
• Intraocular infections
• Febrile neutropenia

Contraindications
• Hypersensitivity to drug

Administration
◀⧸ Know that I.V. therapy is ineffective against enterocolitis and pseudomembranous diarrhea.
• For intermittent I.V. infusion, dilute by adding 10 or 20 ml of sterile water for injection to vial containing 500 mg or 1 g of drug, respectively, to yield a concentration of 50 mg/ml. Dilute further by adding at least 100 ml or 200 ml, respectively, of dextrose 5% in water or normal saline solution; infuse over at least 1 hour.
• Don't give by I.M. route.
◀⧸ Keep emergency equipment and epinephrine on hand in case of anaphylaxis.

Route	Onset	Peak	Duration
P.O.	Unknown	Unknown	Unknown
I.V.	Immediate	Immediate	Unknown

Adverse reactions
CV: hypotension, **cardiac arrest, vascular collapse**
EENT: permanent hearing loss, ototoxicity, tinnitus
GI: nausea, vomiting, **pseudomembranous colitis**
GU: elevated blood urea nitrogen (BUN), creatinine, and albumin levels; **nephrotoxicity; severe uremia**
Hematologic: eosinophilia, **leukopenia, neutropenia**
Respiratory: wheezing, dyspnea
Skin: "red man" syndrome (nonallergic histamine reaction due to rapid I.V. infusion), rash, urticaria, pruritus, necrosis
Other: chills, fever, thrombophlebitis at injection site, **anaphylaxis**

Interactions
Drug-drug. *Aminoglycosides, amphotericin B, bacitracin, cephalosporins, cisplatin, colistin, nondepolarizing neuro-*

muscular blockers, pentamidine: increased risk of nephrotoxicity and ototoxicity

Warfarin: increased risk of bleeding

Drug-diagnostic tests. *BUN, creatinine:* increased levels

Eosinophils, neutrophils: decreased counts

Precautions

Use cautiously in:

• renal impairment, preexisting hearing loss

• concurrent use of anesthetics, immunosuppressants, or nephrotoxic or ototoxic drugs

• elderly patients

• pregnant or breastfeeding patients

• neonates.

Patient monitoring

• Monitor drug blood level weekly. Therapeutic peak ranges from 30 to 40 g/L; therapeutic trough, 5 to 10 mg/L.

• Assess BUN and creatinine levels every 2 days, or daily in patients with unstable renal function.

• Monitor urine output daily; weigh patient at least weekly.

• Assess hearing before and during therapy; stay alert for hearing loss. Patient may require baseline and weekly audiograms.

• Check I.V. site often for phlebitis.

• Watch for "red-man" syndrome, which can result from rapid infusion. Signs and symptoms include maculopapular rash on face, neck, trunk, and limbs; hypotension; and pruritus.

• Monitor complete blood count; watch for signs and symptoms of blood dyscrasias.

• Closely monitor respiratory status; stay alert for wheezing and dyspnea.

◀ Monitor vital signs and cardiovascular status, especially for vascular collapse and other signs of impending cardiac arrest.

Patient teaching

• Tell patient he may take drug with or without food.

• Instruct patient to take oral drug exactly as prescribed for as long as prescribed, even if symptoms improve.

• Explain importance of prophylactic I.V. therapy to patients at risk for endocarditis who are scheduled for invasive procedures.

◀ Teach patient to promptly report hearing loss, breathing problems, and signs and symptoms of "red-man" syndrome, nephrotoxicity, and blood dyscrasias.

• As appropriate, review all other significant and life-threatening adverse reactions and interactions, especially those related to the drugs and tests mentioned above.

vardenafil hydrochloride

Levitra

Pharmacologic class: Phosphodiesterase-5 (PDE5) inhibitor

Therapeutic class: Erectile dysfunction agent

Pregnancy risk category B

Action

Selectively blocks PDE5, which neutralizes cyclic guanosine monophosphate, resulting in enhanced erectile function

Availability

Tablets: 2.5 mg, 5 mg, 10 mg, 20 mg

Indications and dosages

➢ Erectile dysfunction

Adult males: 10 or 20 mg P.O. approximately 1 hour before anticipated sexual activity. Maximum dosing frequency is once daily.

Dosage adjustment

• Patients over age 65

• Concurrent use of CYP450-3A4 inhibitors
• Concurrent HIV therapy (except highly active antiretroviral therapy)

Contraindications
• Hypersensitivity to drug
• Concurrent use of nitrates or nitrate patches to treat angina
• Concurrent use of alpha-adrenergic blockers

Administration
• Instruct patient not to take more than one tablet daily.

Route	Onset	Peak	Duration
P.O.	Unknown	1 hr	4 hr

Adverse reactions
CNS: headache
CV: hypotension
EENT: blurred vision, altered color perception, light sensitivity, rhinitis
GI: dyspepsia
Musculoskeletal: increased creatine kinase level
Skin: flushing
Other: flulike symptoms

Interactions
Drug-drug. *Alpha-adrenergic blockers, nitrates:* hypotension
Erythromycin, itraconazole, ketoconazole, protease inhibitors: increased verdenafil blood level

Precautions
Use cautiously in:
• cardiovascular disease, retinitis pigmentosa, hepatic or renal impairment, reduced hepatic blood flow, increased risk of priapism (as from sickle-cell disease, leukemia, multiple myeloma, polycythemia, or history of priapism).

Patient monitoring
• Monitor blood pressure and heart rate, particularly if patient has cardiovascular disease.

Patient teaching
• Tell patient he may take drug with or without food.
• Teach patient to take one tablet about 1 hour before anticipated sexual activity. Caution him not to take more than one tablet daily.
• Tell patient to expect improvements in both erection hardness and ability to maintain an erection during sexual activity.
• Inform patient that he'll need to be sexually stimulated to have an erection after taking drug and that the erection should subside after orgasm.
• As appropriate, review all other significant adverse reactions and interactions, especially those related to the drugs mentioned above.

vecuronium bromide
Norcuron

Pharmacologic class: Nondepolarizing neuromuscular blocker (intermediate-acting)

Therapeutic class: Muscle relaxant

Pregnancy risk category C

Action
Inhibits neuromuscular depolarization by preventing acetylcholine from binding to receptors on motor end-plate

Availability
Injection: 10-mg and 20-mg vials

⚕ Indications and dosages
➤ Adjunct to anesthesia to facilitate endotracheal intubation
Adults and children over age 9: Initially, 0.08 to 0.1 mg/kg by I.V. bolus. During prolonged surgery, give maintenance dose of 0.01 to 0.015 mg/kg within 25 to 40 minutes of initial dose. In patients receiving balanced anesthe-

sia, maintenance dose may be given q 12 to 15 minutes.

Dosage adjustment
• Renal impairment
• Obesity
• Concurrent use of inhalation anesthetics
• Elderly patients

Contraindications
• Hypersensitivity to drug or other bromides

Administration
◀€ Know that drug should be given by specially trained personnel and only when respiratory support is available.
• When giving by I.V. bolus, administer over 1 to 2 minutes.
• When giving by continuous I.V. infusion, reconstitute by adding bacteriostatic water for injection to yield a concentration of 1 mg/ml. Dilute further with dextrose 5% in water, normal saline solution, or lactated Ringer's solution. Administer with infusion-control device.
◀€ Make sure patient's analgesic and sedative needs are met. (Drug doesn't relieve pain or provide sedation.)

Route	Onset	Peak	Duration
I.V.	1 min	3-5 min	15-25 min

Adverse reactions
CNS: musculoskeletal paralysis or weakness
Respiratory: respiratory paralysis, **prolonged apnea**
Other: anaphylaxis

Interactions
Drug-drug. *Aminoglycosides, anticholinesterases, general anesthetics, opioid analgesics, polymyxin anti-infectives:* enhanced neuromuscular blockade
Carbamazepine: decreased vecuronium duration of action
Fosphenytoin, phenytoin: altered vecuronium efficacy

Nicardipine, procainamide, verapamil: excessive neuromuscular blockade
Nitrous oxide: vecuronium toxicity
Drug-herb. *St. John's wort:* increased risk of cardiovascular collapse or delayed emergence from anesthesia

Precautions
Use cautiously in:
• neuromuscular, respiratory, hepatic, or cardiac disease; edema; severe obesity; dehydration; electrolyte imbalance
• elderly patients
• pregnant or breastfeeding patients
• children under age 2.

Patient monitoring
• Monitor heart rhythm, blood pressure, and pulse oximetry during and after administration.
• Assess sedation level.
• Monitor fluid intake and output; measure temperature.
• Assess muscle recovery using peripheral nerve stimulator and train-of-four monitoring.

Patient teaching
• Explain all procedures to patient while his hearing is still intact.
• As appropriate, review all significant and life-threatening adverse reactions and interactions, especially those related to the drugs and herbs mentioned above.

venlafaxine hydrochloride
Effexor, Effexor XR

Pharmacologic class: Phenethylamine derivative

Therapeutic class: Antidepressant, anxiolytic

Pregnancy risk category C

V

♣ Canada   ◀€ Clinical alert   Reactions in **bold** are life-threatening

Action
Inhibits neuronal serotonin and norepinephrine reuptake and weakly inhibits dopamine reuptake; lacks muscarinic, histaminergic, or alpha-adrenergic properties

Availability
Capsules (extended-release): 37.5 mg, 75 mg, 150 mg
Tablets: 25 mg, 37.5 mg, 50 mg, 75 mg, 100 mg

🕖 Indications and dosages
➤ Depression
Adults: In outpatients, 75 mg P.O. daily in two or three divided doses; may increase by up to 75 mg/day q 4 or more days to a maximum of 225 mg/day; extended-release form can be given as a single daily dose. In hospitalized patients, 75 mg P.O. daily in two or three divided doses; may increase in increments of 75 mg/day q 4 days to a maximum of 375 mg/day given in three divided doses.
➤ Generalized anxiety disorder
Adults: 37.5 to 75 mg (extended-release) P.O. daily given as a single dose; may increase in increments of 75 mg/day q 4 days to a maximum of 225 mg/day
Dosage adjustment
• Hepatic or renal impairment

Off-label uses
• Premenstrual dysphoric disorder

Contraindications
• Hypersensitivity to drug
• Monoamine oxidase (MAO) inhibitor use within past 2 weeks

Administration
◀ Know that at least 14 days should elapse between stopping MAO inhibitors and starting venlafaxine.

Route	Onset	Peak	Duration
P.O.	Within 2 wk	2-4 wk	Unknown

Adverse reactions
CNS: abnormal dreams, anxiety, dizziness, headache, insomnia, nervousness, abnormal thinking, agitation, confusion, depersonalization, drowsiness, emotional lability, worsening depression, twitching, tremor, asthenia, paresthesia, mania, hypomania, **suicidal ideation or behavior**
CV: chest pain, hypertension, palpitations, tachycardia, vasodilation
EENT: visual disturbances, blurred vision, mydriasis, tinnitus, rhinitis
GI: nausea, vomiting, diarrhea, constipation, abdominal pain, dyspepsia, flatulence, altered taste, dry mouth, anorexia
GU: urinary frequency or retention, sexual dysfunction, abnormal ejaculation, anorgasmia, impotence
Metabolic: hyponatremia, syndrome of inappropriate antidiuretic hormone secretion (SIADH)
Skin: bruising, pruritus, rash, diaphoresis, photosensitivity
Other: weight loss, chills, yawning

Interactions
Drug-drug. *Cimetidine:* increased venlafaxine effects
MAO inhibitors: potentially fatal reaction
Sumatriptan, trazodone: serotonin syndrome (including altered level of consciousness)
Drug-diagnostic tests. *Sodium:* decreased level
Drug-herb. *Chamomile, hops, kava, skullcap, valerian:* increased CNS depression
S-adenosylmethionine (SAM-e), St. John's wort: increased risk of sedative or hypnotic effects

Precautions
Use cautiously in:
• cardiovascular disease; hypertension; heart failure, recent myocardial infarction, and other conditions in which

increased heart rate poses a danger; hepatic or renal impairment; hyperthyroidism; glaucoma; hyponatremia; SIADH

• history of seizures, neurologic impairment, or drug abuse
• pregnant or breastfeeding patients
• children under age 18.

Patient monitoring

◀€ Monitor neurologic status, particularly for seizures, worsening depression, and suicidal ideation.

• Closely monitor vital signs and cardiovascular status; stay alert for hypertension and tachycardia.

• Monitor nutritional status, hydration, and weight.

Patient teaching

• Teach patient taking extended-release capsules to swallow them whole without chewing, breaking, dividing, or dissolving them.

◀€ Caution patient not to stop therapy abruptly.

◀€ Advise patient to promptly report seizures, worsening depression, or suicidal thoughts.

• Instruct patient to avoid driving and other dangerous activities until drug effects are known.

• As appropriate, review all other significant and life-threatening adverse reactions and interactions, especially those related to the drugs, tests, and herbs mentioned above.

verapamil hydrochloride

Apo-Verap✦, Calan, Calan SR, Covera-HS, Isoptin, Isoptin SR, Novo-Veramil✦, Nu-Verap✦, Verelan, Verelan PM

Pharmacologic class: Calcium channel blocker

Therapeutic class: Antianginal, antiarrhythmic (class IV), antihypertensive, vascular headache suppressant

Pregnancy risk category C

Action

Decreases conduction of the sinoatrial and atrioventricular (AV) nodes by inhibiting calcium influx into cardiac and vascular smooth muscle cells; also inhibits excitatory contraction. Effect is prolonged AV node refractoriness in conduction tissue, with reduced afterload and decreased myocardial oxygen consumption.

Availability

Capsules (extended-release): 100 mg, 120 mg, 180 mg, 200 mg, 240 mg, 300 mg, 360 mg
Capsules (sustained-release): 120 mg, 180 mg, 240 mg, 360 mg
Injection: 2.5 mg/ml in 2- and 4-ml vials, ampules, and syringes
Tablets (extended-release): 120 mg, 180 mg, 240 mg
Tablets (immediate-release): 40 mg, 80 mg, 120 mg

🕡 Indications and dosages

➢ Angina
Adults: Initially, 80 mg (immediate-release) P.O. t.i.d.; may titrate at daily or weekly intervals to 360 mg/day. Or initially, 180 mg (extended-release) P.O. once daily at bedtime, titrated up to 480 mg/day at bedtime.

V

➤ Supraventricular tachyarrhythmias
Adults: 5 to 10 mg (0.075 to 0.15 mg/kg) I.V. bolus over 2 minutes; may give an additional 10 mg after 30 minutes if response is inadequate. Or 240 to 480 mg (immediate-release) P.O. daily in three or four divided doses.

➤ To control ventricular rate in digitalized patients with chronic atrial flutter or atrial fibrillation
Adults: 240 to 320 mg P.O. daily in three or four divided doses

➤ Hypertension
Adults: Initially, 180 mg (extended-release tablet) or 200 mg (extended-release capsule) P.O. daily at bedtime. For maintenance, titrate up to 480 mg (extended-release tablet) or 400 mg (extended-release capsule) P.O. daily at bedtime. Or initially, 80 mg (immediate-release tablet) P.O. t.i.d.; may titrate at daily or weekly intervals up to 360 to 480 mg/day. Or initially, 240 mg (sustained-release capsule) P.O. q day in morning; for maintenance, may titrate up to 240 mg P.O. b.i.d. or 480 mg P.O. once daily in morning, based on response.

Dosage adjustment
• Renal or hepatic impairment
• Concurrent digoxin therapy

Off-label uses
• Ventricular tachycardia
• Migraine headache prophylaxis
• Neurogenic bladder
• Premature labor

Contraindications
• Hypersensitivity to drug or other calcium channel blockers
• Sick sinus syndrome
• Second- or third-degree AV block (unless artificial pacemaker is in place)
• Hypotension
• Heart failure, severe ventricular dysfunction, or cardiogenic shock (except when associated with supraventricular tachyarrhythmias)

• Atrial flutter or atrial fibrillation associated with accessory bypass tracts (for example, Wolff-Parkinson-White or Lown-Ganong-Levine syndrome)

Administration
• Give I.V. dose over at least 2 minutes.
• Discontinue disopyramide 48 hours before starting verapamil; don't restart for at least 24 hours after verapamil therapy ends.

Route	Onset	Peak	Duration
P.O. (immediate)	30 min	1-2 hr	3-7 hr
P.O. (extended)	Unknown	5-7 hr	24 hr
P.O. (sustained)	Unknown	Unknown	Unknown
I.V.	Immediate	3-5 min	2 hr

Adverse reactions
CNS: anxiety, confusion, dizziness, light-headedness, syncope, drowsiness, headache, jitteriness, abnormal dreams, disturbed equilibrium, psychiatric disturbances, asthenia, paresthesia, tremor, fatigue
CV: chest pain, hypotension, palpitations, peripheral edema, tachycardia, **arrhythmias, heart failure, bradycardia, AV block**
EENT: blurred vision, epistaxis, tinnitus, gingival hyperplasia
GI: nausea, vomiting, diarrhea, constipation, dyspepsia, dry mouth, anorexia
GU: dysuria, urinary frequency, nocturia, polyuria, sexual dysfunction, gynecomastia
Hematologic: anemia, **leukopenia, thrombocytopenia**
Hepatic: elevated hepatic enzyme levels
Metabolic: hyperglycemia
Musculoskeletal: joint stiffness, muscle cramps
Respiratory: cough, dyspnea, shortness of breath, **pulmonary edema**

Skin: dermatitis, flushing, diaphoresis, photosensitivity, pruritus, urticaria, rash, erythema multiforme
Other: edema, weight gain, **Stevens-Johnson syndrome**

Interactions

Drug-drug. *Antihypertensives:* additive hypotensive effect
Aspirin: increased risk of bleeding
Beta-adrenergic blockers, other antiarrhythmics: additive adverse cardiovascular reactions
Carbamazepine, cyclosporine: increased blood levels of these drugs
CYP450-3A4 inducers (such as rifampin): decreased verapamil blood level
CYP450-3A4 inhibitors (such as erythromycin, ritonavir): increased verapamil blood level
Digoxin: increased digoxin blood level, greater risk of toxicity
Lithium: increased or decreased lithium blood level
Neuromuscular blockers (succinylcholine, tubocurarine, vecuronium): prolonged neuromuscular blockade
Theophylline: decreased verapamil clearance, increased blood level, and possible toxicity
Drug-diagnostic tests. *Alanine aminotransferase, alkaline phosphatase, aspartate aminotransferase, blood urea nitrogen, glucose, lactate dehydrogenase:* increased levels
Granulocytes: decreased count
Drug-food. *Coffee, tea:* increased caffeine blood level
Grapefruit juice: increased verapamil blood level and effects
Drug-herb. *Black catechu:* increased drug effects
Cola nut, guarana: increased caffeine blood level
Ephedra (ma huang), St. John's wort: reduced hypotensive effect of verapamil
Yerba maté: decreased yerba maté clearance
Drug-behaviors. *Alcohol use:* additive hypotension

Precautions

Use cautiously in:
• renal or severe hepatic impairment; first-degree AV block; idiopathic hypertrophic cardiomyopathy; neuromuscular transmission defects (such as Duchenne's muscular dystrophy); respiratory depression; digital ulcers, ischemia, or gangrene
• elderly patients
• pregnant or breastfeeding patients.

Patient monitoring

• With I.V. use, monitor vital signs and ECG continuously.
• Assess blood pressure when therapy begins and when dosage is adjusted.
• Watch closely for signs and symptoms of heart failure.
◀℉ Monitor for signs and symptoms of erythema multiforme (fever, rash, sore throat, mouth sores, cough, iris lesions). Report early indications immediately before condition can progress to Stevens-Johnson syndrome.
• Assess complete blood count; watch for blood dyscrasias.
• Monitor blood glucose level; stay alert for hyperglycemia in diabetic patients.

Patient teaching

• Instruct patient to avoid chewing, breaking, or crushing extended-release forms.
◀℉ Advise patient to immediately report rash, unusual bleeding or bruising, fainting, and (in long-term use) fatigue, nausea, or yellowing of skin or eyes.
• Caution patient not to take drug with grapefruit juice.
• Instruct patient to limit caffeine intake and avoid alcohol.
• Advise patient to seek medical advice before taking over-the-counter medications or herbs.
• Teach patient to avoid sun exposure and to wear sunscreen and protective clothing when going outdoors.

V

• As appropriate, review all other significant and life-threatening adverse reactions and interactions, especially those related to the drugs, tests, foods, herbs, and behaviors mentioned above.

vinblastine sulfate (VLB)
Velban, Velbe✦

Pharmacologic class: Vinca alkaloid
Therapeutic class: Antineoplastic
Pregnancy risk category D

Action
Arrests mitosis in metaphase, blocks cell division, and interferes with nucleic acid synthesis; cell-cycle-phase specific

Availability
Lyophilized powder for injection: 10-mg vial

ⓘ Indications and dosages
➤ Hodgkin's disease, advanced testicular cancer, lymphoma, AIDS-related Kaposi's sarcoma, bladder cancer, non-small-cell lung cancer, melanoma, renal cancer, histiocytosis X, mycosis fungoides (advanced stages), breast cancer unresponsive to endocrine surgery and hormonal therapy, choriocarcinoma resistant to other chemotherapy
Adults: 3.7 mg/m^2 I.V. weekly; may increase to a maximum of 18.5 mg/m^2 I.V. weekly, based on response. Withhold weekly dose if white blood cell (WBC) count is below 4,000 cells/mm^3. May increase dosage in increments of 1.8 mg/m^2 if needed, but not after WBC count drops to approximately 3,000 cells/mm^3.
Dosage adjustment
• Hepatic impairment

Contraindications
• Hypersensitivity to drug
• Significant granulocytopenia from causes other than disease being treated
• Uncontrolled bacterial infections
• Intrathecal use
• Elderly patients with cachexia or skin ulcers
• Pregnancy or breastfeeding

Administration
◀❧ Follow facility protocol for handling and preparing chemotherapeutic drugs. Be especially careful to avoid eye contamination.
• Know that patient is usually premedicated with antiemetic.
◀❧ Give by I.V. route only; intrathecal injection is fatal.
• Reconstitute powder in 10-mg vial with 10 ml of normal saline solution for injection to a concentration of 1 mg/ml. Refrigerate solution and protect from light; discard after 28 days.
• Inject I.V. dose into tubing of running I.V. line, or inject directly into vein over about 1 minute.
• Avoid extravasation, which may cause tissue necrosis. If extravasation occurs, stop injection, inject hyaluronidase locally, and apply moderate heat.

Route	Onset	Peak	Duration
I.V.	Unknown	Unknown	Unknown

Adverse reactions
CNS: headache, malaise, depression, paresthesia, loss of deep tendon reflexes, peripheral neuropathy and neuritis, **cerebrovascular accident, seizures**
CV: hypertension, tachycardia, **myocardial infarction**
EENT: pharyngitis
GI: nausea, vomiting, diarrhea, constipation, bleeding ulcer, abdominal pain, stomatitis, anorexia, **paralytic ileus**
GU: aspermia
Hematologic: anemia, **thrombocytopenia, leukopenia**

Metabolic: hyperuricemia, syndrome of inappropriate antidiuretic hormone secretion

Musculoskeletal: bone pain, muscle pain and weakness

Respiratory: shortness of breath, **acute bronchospasm, pulmonary infiltrates**

Skin: alopecia, skin irritation

Other: weight loss; jaw pain; tumor site pain; phlebitis, cellulitis, and sloughing at I.V. site; tissue necrosis (with extravasation)

Interactions

Drug-drug. *Erythromycin, other CYP450 inhibitors:* increased vinblastine toxicity

Mitomycin: increased risk of bronchospasm and shortness of breath

Phenytoin: decreased phenytoin blood level

Precautions

Use cautiously in:
• hepatic or pulmonary dysfunction, renal disease with hypertension, malignant-cell infiltration of bone marrow, or neuromuscular disease.

Patient monitoring

• Assess respiratory status closely; drug may cause acute shortness of breath and bronchospasm, especially in patients previously treated with mitomycin

• Watch injection site closely for signs of extravasation.

• Monitor blood pressure.

• Assess complete blood count; stay alert for signs and symptoms of infection.

• Monitor closely for numbness and tingling of hands or feet and other adverse reactions.

Patient teaching

• Explain drug therapy to patient; stress need for follow-up laboratory testing.

• Teach patient to promptly report signs and symptoms of infection and to take his temperature daily.

• Instruct females of childbearing age to avoid pregnancy.

• Tell patient that drug may cause pain over tumor site.

• Teach patient to practice good oral hygiene to help prevent infected mouth sores.

• Inform patient that hair loss is a common side effect but typically reverses after treatment ends.

• As appropriate, review all other significant and life-threatening adverse reactions and interactions, especially those related to the drugs mentioned above.

vincristine sulfate (VCR)
Oncovin, Vincasar PFS

Pharmacologic class: Vinca alkaloid
Therapeutic class: Antineoplastic
Pregnancy risk category D

Action

Unknown; thought to block cell division and interfere with the synthesis of nucleic acid ; cell-cycle-phase specific

Availability

Solution for injection: 1 mg/ml in 1-, 2-, and 5-ml vials

Indications and dosages

➢ Acute leukemia, Hodgkin's disease, non-Hodgkin's lymphoma, rhabdomyosarcoma, Wilms' tumor

Adults: 0.4 to 1.4 mg/m^2 I.V. weekly, not to exceed 2 mg/dose

Dosage adjustment
• Hepatic impairment

V

Off-label uses

- Brain, hepatic, ovarian, testicular, and other cancers
- Neuroblastoma
- Kaposi's sarcoma
- Idiopathic thrombocytopenic purpura

Contraindications

- Hypersensitivity to drug
- Intrathecal use
- Demyelinating form of Charcot-Marie-Tooth disease
- Pregnancy or breastfeeding

Administration

◀€ Follow facility protocol for handling and preparing chemotherapeutic drugs. Be especially careful to avoid eye contamination.
- Be aware that patient is usually premedicated with antiemetic.

◀€ Give by I.V. route only; intrathecal injection is fatal.
- Inject into tubing of running I.V. line, or inject directly into vein over 1 minute.
- Avoid extravasation, which may cause tissue necrosis. If extravasation occurs, stop injection, inject hyaluronidase locally, and apply moderate heat.

Route	Onset	Peak	Duration
I.V.	Unknown	4 days	7 days

Adverse reactions

CNS: agitation, insomnia, depression, mental status changes, ascending peripheral neuropathy, transient cortical blindness, **seizures, coma**
EENT: diplopia
GI: nausea, vomiting, constipation, abdominal cramps, stomatitis, anorexia, **paralytic ileus**
GU: nocturia, oliguria, urinary retention, gonadal suppression
Hematologic: anemia, **leukopenia, thrombocytopenia** (mild and brief)

Metabolic: hyperuricemia, syndrome of inappropriate antidiuretic hormone secretion
Respiratory: bronchospasm
Skin: alopecia
Other: tissue necrosis (with extravasation), phlebitis at I.V. site

Interactions

Drug-drug. *Asparaginase:* decreased hepatic metabolism of vincristine
Live-virus vaccines: decreased antibody response to vaccine, increased risk of adverse reactions
Mitomycin: increased risk of bronchospasm and shortness of breath
Drug-diagnostic tests. *Platelets:* increased or decreased count
Uric acid: increased level
White blood cells: decreased count (slight leukopenia) 4 days after therapy, resolving within 7 days

Precautions

Use cautiously in:
- infections, decreased bone marrow reserve, hepatic impairment, acute uric acid nephropathy, neuromuscular disease, pulmonary dysfunction, other chronic debilitating illnesses
- females of childbearing age.

Patient monitoring

- Assess respiratory status; injection may cause bronchospasm, especially in patients previously treated with mitomycin.
- Monitor blood pressure.
- Evaluate neurologic status; neurotoxicity is a dose-limiting adverse reaction.
- Monitor complete blood count, including platelet count; watch for signs and symptoms of blood dyscrasias.
- Stay alert for signs and symptoms of infection.

Patient teaching

- Explain drug therapy to patient; stress need for follow-up laboratory testing.

• Advise patient to promptly report signs and symptoms of infection and to take his temperature daily.
• Teach patient to practice good oral hygiene to help prevent infected mouth sores.
• Instruct females of childbearing age to avoid pregnancy.
• Tell patient that hair loss is a common side effect but typically reverses after treatment ends.
• As appropriate, review all other significant and life-threatening adverse reactions and interactions, especially those related to the drugs and tests mentioned above.

vinorelbine tartrate
Navelbine

Pharmacologic class: Vinca alkaloid
Therapeutic class: Antineoplastic
Pregnancy risk category D

Action
Blocks cell division and interferes with nucleic acid synthesis; cell-cycle-phase specific

Availability
Injection: 10 mg/ml in 1-ml and 5-ml vials

💊 Indications and dosages
➤ Inoperable non-small-cell lung cancer in ambulatory patients
Adults: As monotherapy, 30 mg/m² I.V. weekly given over 6 to 10 minutes. In combination therapy, 30 mg/m² I.V. given with cisplatin on days 1 and 29, then q 6 weeks.
Dosage adjustment
• Hepatic impairment
• Neurotoxicity

Off-label uses
• Cervical, breast, or ovarian cancer

Contraindications
• Hypersensitivity to drug
• Pretreatment granulocyte count below 1,000 cells/mm³
• Pregnancy or breastfeeding

Administration
◀€ Follow facility protocols for handling and preparing chemotherapeutic drugs. Be especially careful to avoid eye contamination.
• Know that patient is usually premedicated with antiemetic.
◀€ Give by I.V. route only; intrathecal injection is fatal.
• Before use, dilute drug in syringe with dextrose 5% in water or normal saline solution to yield a concentration of 1.5 to 3 mg/ml. Or dilute in I.V. bag of compatible solution to yield a concentration of 0.5 to 2 mg/ml.
• Administer into tubing of running I.V. line or directly into vein over 6 to 10 minutes. Immediately after injection, flush line with 75 to 125 ml of compatible I.V. solution.

Route	Onset	Peak	Duration
I.V.	Unknown	7-10 days	7-15 days

Adverse reactions
CNS: fatigue, **neurotoxicity**
CV: chest pain, phlebitis
GI: nausea, vomiting, diarrhea, constipation, abdominal pain, intestinal obstruction, anorexia, **pancreatitis, paralytic ileus**
Hematologic: anemia, **bone marrow depression, severe granulocytopenia, neutropenia, thrombocytopenia**
Hepatic: transient hepatic enzyme elevation, increased alanine aminotransferase level
Metabolic: hyponatremia
Musculoskeletal: joint, back, or jaw pain; myalgia

V

Respiratory: acute respiratory distress syndrome, acute shortness of breath, bronchospasm, interstitial pulmonary changes
Skin: alopecia, rash, skin reactions
Other: tumor site pain; irritation, pain, and phlebitis at I.V. site; **sepsis**

Interactions

Drug-drug. *Cisplatin, other antineoplastics:* increased risk and severity of bone marrow depression
Mitomycin: increased risk of acute pulmonary reaction
Drug-diagnostic tests. *Bilirubin, liver function tests:* increased values
Granulocytes, hemoglobin, platelets, white blood cells: decreased levels

Precautions

Use cautiously in:
• hepatic impairment, decreased bone marrow reserve, past or present neuropathy
• history of radiation therapy
• females of childbearing age
• children (safety not established).

Patient monitoring

• Monitor vital signs closely.
• Assess liver function studies and complete blood count, including platelet count.
• Watch for signs and symptoms of infection.
• Observe injection site closely for reactions and extravasation.
• Closely monitor neurologic and respiratory status; drug may cause acute pulmonary changes, especially in patients previously treated with mitomycin.

Patient teaching

• Explain drug therapy to patient; stress importance of follow-up laboratory testing.
• Advise patient to promptly report signs and symptoms of infection and to take his temperature daily.

• Instruct females of childbearing age to avoid pregnancy.
• Teach patient to practice good oral hygiene to help prevent infected mouth sores.
• Tell patient that hair loss is a common side effect but typically reverses after treatment.
• As appropriate, review all other significant and life-threatening adverse reactions and interactions, especially those related to the drugs and tests mentioned above.

voriconazole
Vfend

Pharmacologic class: Triazole
Therapeutic class: Antifungal
Pregnancy risk category D

Action

Inhibits fungal cytochrome CYP450–mediated 14-alpha-lanosterol demethylation, thus preventing fungal biosynthesis and inactivating fungal cell

Availability

Lyophilized powder for injection: 200 mg
Tablets: 50 mg, 200 mg

🔹 Indications and dosages

➤ Invasive aspergillosis, serious fungal infections caused by *Scedosporium apiospermum* and *Fusarium* species (including *Fusarium solani*)
Adults and children older than age 12: Initially, 6 mg/kg I.V. q 12 hours for two doses (infused over 1 to 2 hours), followed by a maintenance dose of 4 mg/kg I.V. q 12 hours given no faster than 3 mg/kg/hour. Change to oral dosing as described below when patient can tolerate it.
Adults and children older than age 12 who weigh more than 40 kg (88 lb):

200 mg P.O. q 12 hours given 1 hour before or after a meal; may increase to 300 mg P.O. q 12 hours p.r.n.

Adults and children older than age 12 who weigh less than 40 kg (88 lb): 100 mg P.O. q 12 hours given at least 1 hour before or after a meal; may increase to 150 mg P.O. q 12 hours p.r.n.

Dosage adjustment
• Hepatic cirrhosis
• Renal impairment

Off-label uses
• Oropharyngeal candidiasis
• Febrile neutropenia (as empiric therapy)

Contraindications
• Hypersensitivity to drug or its components
• Concurrent use of long-acting barbiturates, ergot alkaloids, rifabutin, rifampin, CYP450-3A4 substrates (such as astemizole, cisapride, pimozide, quinidine, terfenadine), or carbamazepine

Administration
• Reconstitute powder with 19 ml of water for injection to yield a volume of 20 ml. Shake vial until powder dissolves. Withdraw prescribed dose, and dilute further in compatible I.V. solution for a final concentration of 0.5 to 5 mg/ml. Give I.V. over 1 to 2 hours at a rate not exceeding 3 mg/kg/hour.
• Don't give through same I.V. line with other drugs, blood products, or electrolytes.

Route	Onset	Peak	Duration
P.O.	1-2 hr	Unknown	Unknown
I.V.	Start of infusion	Unknown	Unknown

Adverse reactions
CNS: dizziness, hallucinations, headache
CV: hypotension, hypertension, tachycardia, chest pain, vasodilation, peripheral edema
EENT: photophobia, blurred vision, visual disturbances, eye hemorrhage, chromatopsia
GI: nausea, vomiting, diarrhea, abdominal pain, dry mouth
GU: increased creatinine level, renal dysfunction, **acute renal failure**
Hematologic: anemia, **pancytopenia, leukopenia, thrombocytopenia**
Hepatic: increased bilirubin, alanine aminotransferase (ALT), alkaline phosphatase (ALP), and aspartate aminotransferase (AST) levels; cholestatic jaundice; **hepatic failure**
Metabolic: hypomagnesemia, hypokalemia
Respiratory: respiratory disorders
Skin: pruritus, maculopapular rash, erythema multiforme, **toxic epidermal necrolysis**
Other: chills, fever, **sepsis, Stevens-Johnson syndrome, anaphylaxis**

Interactions
Drug-drug. *Barbiturates (long-acting), carbamazepine, phenytoin, rifampin:* decreased voriconazole blood level
Benzodiazepines: sedative effects
Calcium channel blockers, HMG-CoA reductase inhibitors (such as lovastatin, omeprazole): increased blood levels of these drugs
Cyclosporine, sirolimus, tacrolimus: increased blood levels of these drugs, greater risk of nephrotoxicity
CYP450-3A4 substrates: increased blood levels of these drugs, causing prolonged QT interval and risk of torsades de pointes
Ergot alkaloids: increased blood levels of these drugs, resulting in ergotism
Non-nucleoside reverse transcriptase inhibitors (such as delavirdine, efavirenz), protease inhibitors: inhibited voriconazole metabolism
Rifabutin: decreased voriconazole blood level, increased rifabutin blood level

V

Sulfonylureas: increased sulfonylurea blood level, greater risk of hypoglycemia

Vinca alkaloids: increased risk of neurotoxicity

Warfarin, other coumarin derivatives: increased partial thromboplastin time

Drug-diagnostic tests. *ALP, ALT, AST, creatinine:* increased levels

Drug-herb. *Gossypol:* increased risk of nephrotoxicity

Precautions

Use cautiously in:
• hypersensitivity to azoles
• renal disease, mild to moderate hepatic cirrhosis, galactose or lactose intolerance
• pregnant or breastfeeding patients.

Patient monitoring

• Monitor kidney and liver function studies; watch for signs and symptoms of organ toxicity.
• Assess electrolyte levels and complete blood count, including platelet count.
• Monitor ECG; stay alert for prolonged QT interval.
• Monitor for vision problems in therapy exceeding 28 days.

Patient teaching

• Explain therapy to patient; stress need for follow-up laboratory tests.
• Teach patient using oral form to take doses 1 hour before or after a meal.
• Emphasize importance of taking drug exactly as prescribed for duration prescribed.
• Instruct patient to promptly report adverse reactions.
• Instruct females of childbearing age to report pregnancy immediately.
• Caution patient to avoid driving and other hazardous activities because drug may cause visual disturbances.
• Advise patient to minimize GI upset by eating small, frequent servings of healthy food and drinking plenty of fluids.

• As appropriate, review all other significant and life-threatening adverse reactions and interactions, especially those related to the drugs, tests, and herbs mentioned above.

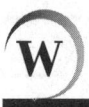

warfarin sodium
Coumadin, Warfilone ♣

Pharmacologic class: Coumarin derivative

Therapeutic class: Anticoagulant

Pregnancy risk category X

Action

Interferes with synthesis of vitamin K–dependent clotting factors (II, VII, IX, and X) in the liver and anticoagulant proteins C and S

Availability

Injection: 5 mg/vial
Tablets: 1 mg, 2 mg, 2.5 mg, 3 mg, 4 mg, 5 mg, 6 mg, 7.5 mg, 10 mg

Indications and dosages

➢ Venous thrombosis, pulmonary embolism, or atrial fibrillation; myocardial infarction (MI); thromboembolic complications of cardiac valve placement

Adults: Initially, 2.5 to 10 mg P.O. or I.V. daily for 2 to 4 days, then adjusted based on prothrombin time (PT) or International Normalized Ratio (INR). Usual maintenance dosage is 2 to 10 mg P.O. daily.

Dosage adjustment
• Elderly or debilitated patients

Off-label uses

• Acute coronary syndrome

- Intracoronary stent placement
- Prevention of catheter thrombosis

Contraindications

- Hypersensitivity to drug
- Uncontrolled bleeding
- Open wounds
- Severe hepatic disease
- Hemorrhagic or bleeding tendency
- Cerebrovascular hemorrhage
- Cerebral aneurysm or dissecting aorta
- Blood dyscrasias
- Pericarditis or pericardial effusion
- Bacterial endocarditis
- Recent brain, eye, or spinal cord injury or surgery
- Lumbar puncture and other procedures that may cause uncontrollable bleeding
- Major regional or lumbar block anesthesia
- Malignant hypertension
- Unsupervised senile, alcoholic, or psychotic patients
- Threatened abortion, eclampsia, preeclampsia
- Pregnancy

Administration

- Know that I.V. form is reserved for patients who can't tolerate oral form; I.V. and oral dosages are identical.
- For I.V. use, reconstitute vial with 2.7 ml of sterile water for injection; administer over 1 to 2 minutes. After reconstitution, drug is stable for 4 hours at room temperature.
- Warfarin's effects can be reversed with vitamin K; if major bleeding occurs, fresh frozen plasma may be given.
- When converting to warfarin from heparin, give both drugs concomitantly for 4 to 5 days until therapeutic effect of warfarin occurs.

Route	Onset	Peak	Duration
P.O.	Several hr	0.5-3 days	2-5 days
I.V.	Unknown	Unknown	Unknown

Adverse reactions

GI: nausea, vomiting, diarrhea, abdominal cramps, stomatitis, anorexia
GU: hematuria
Hematologic: eosinophilia, bleeding, **hemorrhage, agranulocytosis, leukopenia**
Hepatic: elevated hepatic enzyme levels, **hepatitis**
Skin: rash, dermatitis, urticaria, pruritus, alopecia, dermal necrosis
Other: fever, "purple toes" syndrome (bilateral painful, purple lesions on toes and sides of feet), hypersensitivity reaction

Interactions

Drug-drug. *Abciximab, acetaminophen (chronic use), androgens, aspirin, capecitabine, cefamandole, cefoperazone, cefotetan, chloral hydrate, chloramphenicol, clopidogrel, disulfiram, eptifibatide, fluconazole, fluoroquinolones, itraconazole, metronidazole (including vaginal use), nonsteroidal anti-inflammatory drugs, plicamycin, quinidine, quinine, sulfonamides, thrombolytics, ticlopidine, tirofiban, valproic acid:* increased response to warfarin, greater risk of bleeding
Barbiturates, hormonal contraceptives containing estrogen: decreased anticoagulant effect
Drug-diagnostic tests. *Alanine aminotransferase, aspartate aminotransferase, INR:* increased values
Partial thromboplastin time, PT: prolonged
Drug-food. *Vitamin K–rich foods (large amounts):* antagonism of anticoagulant effect
Drug-herb. *Angelica:* prolonged PT
Anise, arnica, asafetida, bromelain, chamomile, clove, danshen, devil's claw, dong quai, fenugreek, feverfew, garlic, ginger, ginkgo, ginseng, horse chestnut, licorice, meadowsweet, motherwort, onion, papain, parsley, passionflower, quassia, red clover, Reishi mushroom,

W

rue, sweet clover, turmeric, white willow, others: increased bleeding risk
Coenzyme Q10, green tea, St. John's wort: decreased anticoagulant effect
Drug-behaviors. *Alcohol use:* enhanced warfarin activity

Precautions

Use cautiously in:
• cancer, heparin-induced thrombocytopenia, moderate to severe renal impairment, moderate to severe hypertension, infectious GI disease, known or suspected deficiency in protein C–mediated anticoagulant response, polycythemia vera, vasculitis, severe diabetes mellitus
• indwelling catheter use
• history of poor compliance
• elderly or debilitated patients.

Patient monitoring

• Monitor PT, INR, and liver function test results.
• Watch for signs and symptoms of bleeding and hepatitis.

Patient teaching

◀€ Explain therapy to patient; stress importance of adhering to schedule for laboratory tests, which provide information that guides dosage adjustment.
◀€ Instruct patient to promptly report unusual bleeding or bruising.
• Caution patient to seek medical advice before taking over-the-counter preparations or herbs.
• Advise patient to inform other health care providers (including dentist) that he's taking warfarin.
• Teach patient not to vary his intake of foods containing vitamin K (such as leafy green vegetables, fish, pork, green tea, and tomatoes) to avoid alterations in drug's anticoagulant effect.
◀€ Instruct females of childbearing age to report pregnancy immediately.
• Advise patient to avoid contact sports and other activities that could cause injury and bleeding.

• Tell patient to avoid alcohol.
• As appropriate, review all other significant and life-threatening adverse reactions and interactions, especially those related to the drugs, tests, foods, herbs, and behaviors mentioned above.

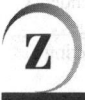

zafirlukast
Accolate

Pharmacologic class: Leukotriene receptor antagonist
Therapeutic class: Antiasthmatic, bronchodilator
Pregnancy risk category B

Action

Antagonizes activity of three leukotrienes at specific receptor sites on airway smooth muscle, thereby inhibiting inflammation

Availability

Tablets: 20 mg
Tablets (coated): 10 mg, 20 mg

🕖 Indications and dosages

➤ Long-term asthma management
Adults and children over age 12: 20 mg P.O. b.i.d.
Dosage adjustment
• Hepatic impairment

Off-label uses

• Exercise-induced bronchospasm
• Chronic urticaria

Contraindications

• Hypersensitivity to drug or its components
• Breastfeeding

Administration

• Give drug at least 1 hour before or 2 hours after a meal.

Route	Onset	Peak	Duration
P.O.	30 min	3.5 hr	12 hr

Adverse reactions

CNS: headache, dizziness, asthenia
GI: nausea, vomiting, diarrhea, abdominal pain, dyspepsia
Musculoskeletal: joint or back pain, myalgia
Other: fever, infection, pain

Interactions

Drug-drug. *Aspirin:* increased zafirlukast blood level
Erythromycin, theophylline: decreased zafirlukast blood level
Warfarin: increased warfarin effects, greater risk of bleeding
Drug-food. *Any food:* decreased rate and extent of zafirlukast absorption

Precautions

Use cautiously in:
• hepatic disease, acute asthma attacks
• patients over age 55
• pregnant patients
• children under age 7 (safety not established).

Patient monitoring

• Watch for and immediately report signs and symptoms of hepatic dysfunction, such as pain in right upper abdominal quadrant, nausea, fatigue, lethargy, itching, jaundice, and flulike symptoms.
• Assess patient's respiratory status to help evaluate drug efficacy.

Patient teaching

• Teach patient to take drug at least 1 hour before or 2 hours after a meal.
• Advise patient to take drug exactly as prescribed, even if he's symptom-free.
• Instruct patient to continue taking other asthma drugs unless prescriber directs otherwise.
◀€ Teach patient to immediately report asthma attack. Tell him not to use drug for rapid relief of bronchospasm.
• Advise female patient to consult prescriber if she plans to breastfeed.
• As appropriate, review all other significant adverse reactions and interactions, especially those related to the drugs and foods mentioned above.

zalcitabine (dideoxycytidine, ddC)
Hivid

Pharmacologic class: Nucleoside reverse transcriptase inhibitor
Therapeutic class: Antiretroviral
Pregnancy risk category C

Action

After conversion to active metabolite dideoxycytidine-5′-triphosphate, blocks activity of reverse transcriptase, thus inhibiting replication of human immunodeficiency virus (HIV)

Availability

Tablets: 0.375 mg, 0.75 mg

🕖 Indications and dosages

➤ Advanced HIV infection (CD4+ cell count of 300/mm³ or less), especially in patients intolerant of zidovudine or whose disease progresses during zidovudine therapy
Adults and children over age 13: 0.75 mg P.O. q 8 hours, given with other antiretrovirals
Dosage adjustment
• Renal impairment

Contraindications

• Hypersensitivity to drug or its components

- Concurrent lamivudine therapy
- Breastfeeding

Administration
- Give drug at least 1 hour before or 2 hours after a meal.

Route	Onset	Peak	Duration
P.O.	Unknown	1-2 hr	Unknown

Adverse reactions
CNS: headache, fatigue, dizziness, insomnia, depression, peripheral neuropathy, confusion, poor concentration, amnesia, tremor, hypertonia, anxiety, **seizures**
CV: chest pain, cardiomyopathy, **heart failure**
EENT: abnormal vision, eye pain, ototoxicity, nasal discharge, pharyngitis
GI: nausea, vomiting, diarrhea, constipation, abdominal pain, esophageal ulcer, glossitis, stomatitis, anorexia, **pancreatitis**
Hematologic: anemia, **leukopenia, thrombocytopenia, neutropenia**
Hepatic: abnormal liver function tests, **severe hepatomegaly with steatosis**
Metabolic: hypoglycemia, **lactic acidosis**
Musculoskeletal: myalgia, joint pain
Respiratory: cough
Skin: pruritus; urticaria; erythematous, maculopapular, or follicular rash
Other: night sweats, fever

Interactions
Drug-drug. *Aminoglycosides, amphotericin B, foscarnet, other drugs that can impair renal function:* increased risk of nephrotoxicity
Antacids containing aluminum or magnesium: decreased zalcitabine bioavailability
Chloramphenicol, cisplatin, dapsone, didanosine, disulfiram, ethionamide, glutethimide, gold salts, hydralazine, iodoquinol, isoniazid, metronidazole, phenytoin, other drugs that can cause peripheral neuropathy (such as rib-avirin, stavudine, vincristine): increased risk of peripheral neuropathy
Cimetidine, probenecid: increased zalcitabine blood level
Pentamidine: increased risk of pancreatitis
Drug-diagnostic tests. *Alanine aminotransferase, alkaline phosphatase, aspartate aminotransferase:* increased levels
Hemoglobin, platelets, white blood cells: decreased levels
Drug-food. *Any food:* decreased drug absorption

Precautions
Use cautiously in:
- HIV complications, lymphoma, renal or hepatic disease, peripheral neuropathy, heart failure, decreased CD4+ cell count
- known risk factors for, or history of, pancreatitis
- pregnant patients.

Patient monitoring
- Monitor CD4+ cell count, complete blood count, and electrolyte levels before and during therapy.
- Assess kidney function studies.
- Watch closely for signs and symptoms of peripheral neuropathy and worsening HIV infection.
- Monitor for signs and symptoms of pancreatitis.
◄€ Assess for hepatic dysfunction and lactic acidosis, which can be fatal.

Patient teaching
- Explain therapy to patient. Stress that drug doesn't cure HIV infection; teach him to practice safe sex.
- Instruct patient to take drug at least 1 hour before or 2 hours after a meal.
- Advise females of childbearing age to use effective contraception.
◄€ Teach patient to recognize and immediately report signs and symptoms of pancreatitis, lactic acidosis, or liver impairment.

• Emphasize importance of undergoing follow-up laboratory testing.
• As appropriate, review all other significant and life-threatening adverse reactions and interactions, especially those related to the drugs, tests, and foods mentioned above.

zaleplon
Sonata

Pharmacologic class: Pyrazolopyrimidine, nonbenzodiazepine hypnotic
Therapeutic class: Sedative-hypnotic
Controlled substance schedule IV
Pregnancy risk category C

Action
Binds to omega-1 receptor of gamma-aminobutyric acid receptor complex, relaxing smooth muscles, reducing anxiety, and producing sedation. Also has anticonvulsant effects.

Availability
Capsules: 5 mg, 10 mg

Indications and dosages
➢ Insomnia
Adults under age 65: 10 mg P.O. at bedtime; dosage range is 5 to 20 mg.
Dosage adjustment
• Hepatic impairment
• Elderly or debilitated patients

Contraindications
• Hypersensitivity to drug
• Severe hepatic impairment
• Breastfeeding

Administration
• Give drug at bedtime.
• Don't administer with high-fat meal.

Route	Onset	Peak	Duration
P.O.	Rapid	1 hr	3-4 hr

Adverse reactions
CNS: amnesia, anxiety, hallucinations, dizziness, drowsiness, depersonalization, headache, transient memory or psychomotor impairment, incoordination, malaise, vertigo, asthenia, hyperesthesia, paresthesia, tremor, lightheadedness
CV: peripheral edema
EENT: abnormal vision, eye pain, ear pain, hearing sensitivity, epistaxis, altered sense of smell
GI: nausea, abdominal pain, colitis, dyspepsia, anorexia
GU: dysmenorrhea
Musculoskeletal: myalgia
Skin: photosensitivity
Other: fever

Interactions
Drug-drug. *Cimetidine:* decreased metabolism and increased effects of zaleplon
CNS depressants (such as antihistamines, opioids, other sedative-hypnotics, phenothiazines, tricyclic antidepressants): additive CNS depression
CYP450-3A4 inducers (such as carbamazepine, phenobarbital, phenytoin, rifampin): decreased zaleplon effects
CYP450-3A4 inhibitors (such as erythromycin, ketoconazole): increased zaleplon blood level
Drug-food. *High-fat meal:* delayed drug absorption
Drug-herb. *Chamomile, hops, kava, skullcap, valerian:* increased CNS depression
Drug-behaviors. *Alcohol use:* increased CNS depression

Precautions
Use cautiously in:
• tartrazine sensitivity
• severe renal impairment, mild to moderate hepatic impairment, respiratory impairment, depression
• history of suicide attempt
• patients weighing less than 50 kg (110 lb)

Z

- patients over age 65
- pregnant patients
- children under age 18 (safety not established).

Patient monitoring
- Monitor drug efficacy; if insomnia persists after 7 to 10 days, patient should be reevaluated for underlying psychological or physical illness.
- Stay alert for adverse drug reactions.

Patient teaching
- Explain therapy to patient; emphasize importance of taking drug just before bedtime or after trying to sleep—but only if he'll be able to get at least 4 hours of sleep before he needs to be active.
- Caution patient to avoid driving and other hazardous activities while under drug's influence.
- Instruct patient to avoid alcohol.
- Inform patient that rebound insomnia may occur for 1 or 2 nights after he stops taking drug.
- Advise female of childbearing age to notify prescriber if she is or plans to become pregnant.
- As appropriate, review all other significant adverse reactions and interactions, especially those related to the drugs, foods, herbs, and behaviors mentioned above.

zanamivir
Relenza

Pharmacologic class: Neuraminidase inhibitor
Therapeutic class: Antiviral
Pregnancy risk category C

Action
Inhibits influenza virus enzyme, neuraminidase, essential for viral replication

Availability
Powder for inhalation: 5 mg/blister

Indications and dosages
➤ Uncomplicated acute illness caused by influenza virus A or B
Adults and children over age 7: Two oral inhalations (5 mg/inhalation) b.i.d. for 5 days, using Diskhaler device provided

Contraindications
- Hypersensitivity to drug or its components

Administration
- Give two doses on day 1, with doses spaced at least 2 hours apart. On subsequent days, space doses 12 hours apart, and give at about the same time each day.

Route	Onset	Peak	Duration
Inhalation	Rapid	1-2 hr	12 hr

Adverse reactions
CNS: headache, dizziness
EENT: sinusitis, EENT infections
GI: nausea, vomiting, diarrhea
Respiratory: bronchitis, cough
Other: allergic reaction

Interactions
None significant

Precautions
Use cautiously in:
- chronic obstructive pulmonary disease, asthma, lactose intolerance
- pregnant or breastfeeding patients
- children under age 7 (safety not established).

Patient monitoring
- Assess respiratory status; watch closely for signs and symptoms of declining respiratory function.

Patient teaching

• Explain therapy to patient; demonstrate how to use Diskhaler device.
• Teach patient to take drug exactly as prescribed for as long as directed, even if symptoms improve.
• If patient is also taking an inhaled bronchodilator, tell him to take bronchodilator before taking zanamivir.
• Emphasize that drug doesn't prevent spread of influenza to others.
• Teach patient to immediately report worsening respiratory symptoms.
• As appropriate, review other significant adverse reactions.

zidovudine

Apo-Zidovudine♣, Novo-AZT♣, Retrovir

Pharmacologic class: Nucleoside reverse transcriptase inhibitor
Therapeutic class: Antiretroviral
Pregnancy risk category C

Action

After conversion to its active metabolite, inhibits activity of human immunodeficiency virus (HIV) reverse transcriptase and terminates viral DNA growth

Availability

Capsules: 300 mg
Injection: 10 mg/ml in 20-ml vial
Syrup: 50 mg/5 ml
Tablets: 100 mg

⏀ Indications and dosages
➢ HIV infection
Adults and children older than age 12: 200 mg P.O. t.i.d. or 300 mg P.O. b.i.d. for a total daily dosage of 600 mg/day; or 1 mg/kg I.V. five to six times daily, given with other antiretrovirals
Children ages 6 weeks to 12 years: 160 mg/m² P.O. q 8 hours (480 mg/m²/day,

to a maximum of 200 mg q 8 hours), given with other antiretrovirals
➢ To prevent maternal-fetal transmission of HIV
Pregnant women: 500 mg P.O. daily in divided doses (usually as five 100-mg doses) until labor begins; then 2 mg/kg I.V. over 1 hour followed by a continuous infusion of 1mg/kg/hour until umbilical cord is clamped
Neonates: 2 mg/kg P.O. q 6 hours starting within 12 hours of delivery and continuing for 6 weeks
Dosage adjustment
• Hepatic or renal impairment

Off-label uses
• Occupational exposure to HIV

Contraindications
• Hypersensitivity to drug or its components
• Concomitant use of Combivir or Trizivir (zidovudine-containing products)

Administration
• For I.V. use, remove dose from vial and add to I.V. solution containing dextrose 5% in water, to yield a final concentration no greater than 4 mg/ml. Infuse over 1 hour.
• In adults, give by I.V. route only until patient can tolerate oral dose.

Route	Onset	Peak	Duration
P.O.	Variable	30-90 min	4 hr
I.V.	Rapid	End of infusion	4 hr

Adverse reactions
CNS: headache, paresthesia, malaise, insomnia, dizziness, drowsiness, asthenia, **seizures**
GI: nausea, vomiting, constipation, abdominal pain, dyspepsia, abnormal taste, anorexia, **pancreatitis**
Hematologic: severe anemia (necessitating transfusions), **agranulocytopenia, severe bone marrow depression**

Z

Musculoskeletal: myalgia, back pain, myopathy
Respiratory: dyspnea
Skin: diaphoresis, rash, altered nail pigmentation
Other: fever

Interactions

Drug-drug. *Acetaminophen, aspirin, indomethacin:* increased risk of zidovudine toxicity
Amphotericin B, dapsone, flucytosine, pentamidine: increased risk of nephrotoxicity and bone marrow depression
Cyclosporine: extreme drowsiness, lethargy
Cytotoxic drugs, myelosuppressants, nephrotoxic drugs (such as ganciclovir, interferon alfa): increased risk of hematologic toxicity
Fluconazole, methadone, probenecid, valproic acid: increased zidovudine blood level, greater risk of toxicity
Ribavirin: antagonism of zidovudine's antiviral activity
Drug-diagnostic tests. *Granulocytes, hemoglobin, platelets:* decreased values
Drug-herb. *St. John's wort:* decreased zidovudine efficacy

Precautions

Use cautiously in:
• renal or hepatic impairment, decreased bone marrow reserve, hemoglobin below 9.5 g/dl, or granulocyte count below 1,000 cells/mm^3
• pregnant or breastfeeding patients.

Patient monitoring

• Monitor neurologic status, especially for signs and symptoms of impending seizure.
• Periodically assess complete blood count and kidney and liver function studies. Be aware that drug can cause hepatotoxicity (rare).
• Watch for signs and symptoms of pancreatitis.

Patient teaching

• Explain therapy to patient; emphasize that drug doesn't cure HIV infection.
• Tell patient he may take drug with or without food.
• Instruct patient to remain upright after taking capsules and to take them with at least 4 oz of fluid.
• Teach patient to take drug exactly as prescribed.
• Advise females of childbearing age to use effective contraception.
◀€ Teach patient to recognize and immediately report signs and symptoms of serious side effects, such as seizures.
• Emphasize importance of follow-up laboratory testing.
• Inform pregnant HIV-infected patient that drug reduces risk of, but may not prevent, HIV transmission to neonate.
• As appropriate, review all other significant and life-threatening adverse reactions and interactions, especially those related to the drugs, tests, and herbs mentioned above.

zileuton

Zyflo

Pharmacologic class: 5-lipoxygenase inhibitor

Therapeutic class: Antiasthmatic
Pregnancy risk category C

Action

Blocks production, activity, and synthesis of leukotriene, an endogenous inflammatory mediator

Availability

Tablets: 600 mg

⬤Indications and dosages

➣ Prophylaxis and treatment of chronic asthma

Adults and children over age 12: 600 mg P.O. q.i.d.

Off-label uses
• Ulcerative colitis

Contraindications
• Hypersensitivity to drug or its components
• Active hepatic disease or transaminase levels at least three times the upper limit of normal

Administration
• Give drug with meals and at bedtime.
• Be aware that drug won't reverse bronchospasm in acute asthma attacks (including status asthmaticus); however, therapy can continue during attack.

Route	Onset	Peak	Duration
P.O.	30 min	1-5 hr	5-8 hr

Adverse reactions
CNS: headache, asthenia, dizziness, insomnia, nervousness, drowsiness, malaise
CV: chest pain
EENT: conjunctivitis
GI: nausea, vomiting, constipation, dyspepsia, abdominal pain, flatulence
GU: vaginitis, urinary tract infection (UTI)
Hematologic: leukopenia
Hepatic: elevated hepatic enzyme levels
Musculoskeletal: hypertonia, neck or joint pain, myalgia, rigidity
Skin: pruritus, urticaria
Other: fever, pain, accidental injury

Interactions
Drug-drug. *Astemizole, ergot derivatives, pimozide, terfenadine:* cardiotoxicity (prolonged QT interval, torsades de pointes, cardiac arrest)
Beta-adrenergic blockers: increased effects of these drugs
Theophylline: decreased theophylline clearance
Warfarin: increased prothrombin time

Precautions
Use cautiously in:
• acute asthmatic attack
• history of hepatic disease
• pregnant patients.

Patient monitoring
• Monitor respiratory status to help assess drug efficacy.
• Monitor liver function studies and complete blood count with white cell differential.
• Closely assess fluid intake and output; watch for signs and symptoms of UTI.

Patient teaching
• Explain therapy to patient; emphasize that drug's full effects may not appear for several days or weeks.
• Tell patient he may split tablet in half to ease swallowing.
• Caution patient not to take drug in larger doses or more often than prescribed.
• Suggest that patient take drug with meals and at bedtime to help him remember when to take doses.
• Explain that drug isn't a bronchodilator and shouldn't be used to treat acute asthma attacks.
◀€ Instruct patient to promptly report adverse reactions, especially yellowing of skin, itching, or dark urine.
• As appropriate, review all other significant and life-threatening adverse reactions and interactions, especially those related to the drugs mentioned above.

ziprasidone hydrochloride
Geodon

Pharmacologic class: Benzisoxazole derivative
Therapeutic class: Antipsychotic
Pregnancy risk category C

Z

Action

Unknown; may act by antagonizing dopamine$_2$ and serotonin$_2$ receptors

Availability

Capsules: 20 mg, 40 mg, 60 mg, 80 mg
Injection: 20 mg/ml

🖊 Indications and dosages

➤ Schizophrenia

Adults: Initially, 20 mg P.O. b.i.d. with food; may increase q 2 days up to 80 mg b.i.d. For maintenance, 20 to 80 mg P.O. b.i.d.; maximum recommended dosage is 80 mg b.i.d. For prompt control of acute agitation, 10 to 20 mg I.M. as a single dose; depending on patient's response, may repeat 10-mg I.M. dose q 2 hours or 20-mg I.M. dose q 4 hours to a maximum daily dosage of 40 mg.

Contraindications

• Hypersensitivity to drug
• History of arrhythmias, prolonged QT interval
• Recent myocardial infarction
• Uncompensated heart failure
• Concomitant use of arsenic trioxide, chlorpromazine, class IA or III antiarrhythmics, or other drugs that can prolong the QT interval

Administration

• Give drug with food.
• Know that oral therapy should replace I.M. therapy as soon as possible.

Route	Onset	Peak	Duration
P.O.	Several hr	1-3 days	Unknown
I.M.	Unknown	1 hr	Unknown

Adverse reactions

CNS: dizziness, drowsiness, dystonia, hypertonia, asthenia, akathisia, extrapyramidal reactions, agitation, headache, insomnia, personality disorder, paresthesia, speech disorder, **neuroleptic malignant syndrome, seizures, suicide attempt**

CV: orthostatic hypotension, hypertension, tachycardia, **arrhythmias** (secondary to prolonged QT interval)
EENT: abnormal vision, rhinitis
GI: nausea, vomiting, diarrhea, constipation, dyspepsia, dry mouth, anorexia
GU: dysmenorrhea, priapism
Musculoskeletal: myalgia
Respiratory: cough, cold symptoms
Skin: urticaria, rash, fungal dermatitis, diaphoresis, photosensitivity
Other: accidental injury, pain at I.M. injection site

Interactions

Drug-drug. *Antihypertensives:* additive hypotension
Carbamazepine: decreased ziprasidone blood level
Centrally acting drugs: additive CNS effects
Dopamine agonists, levodopa: antagonized effects of these drugs
Drugs that decrease potassium or magnesium level (such as diuretics) or prolong the QT interval (such as dofetilide, moxifloxacin, pimozide, quinidine, sotalol, sparfloxacin, thioridazine): increased risk of arrhythmias
Ketoconazole: increased ziprasidone blood level
Drug-herb. *Chamomile, hops, kava, skullcap, valerian:* increased CNS depression

Precautions

Use cautiously in:
• cardiovascular disorders, dysphagia, hyperprolactinemia, bradycardia, hypokalemia, hypomagnesemia
• adverse reactions with previous use of atypical antipsychotics (such as risperidone or clozapine)
• pregnant patients.

Patient monitoring

• Monitor ECG before and during therapy; stay alert for prolonged QT interval.

• Assess blood pressure for hypertension and orthostatic hypotension.

◀€ Monitor neurologic status, especially for seizures and signs or symptoms of neuroleptic malignant syndrome.

◀€ Watch for adverse reactions. Know that dizziness, syncope, or palpitations may signify life-threatening arrhythmias caused by prolonged QT interval.

◀€ Be aware that patients with bradycardia, hypokalemia, or hypomagnesemia are at greater risk for torsades de pointes and sudden death.

Patient teaching
• Explain therapy and need for follow-up laboratory testing.
• Teach patient to take drug with food.
◀€ Advise patient to promptly report fainting, seizures, high fever, sweating, unstable blood pressure, stupor, muscle rigidity, or suspected infection.
• Instruct patient to seek medical advice before taking over-the-counter preparations.
• Caution patient to avoid driving and other hazardous activities until effects of drug are known.
• Instruct patient to move slowly when sitting up or standing to avoid dizziness or light-headedness from sudden blood pressure decrease.
• Advise patient to avoid sun exposure and to wear sunscreen and protective clothing when going outdoors.
• As appropriate, review all other significant and life-threatening adverse reactions and interactions, especially those related to the drugs and herbs mentioned above.

zoledronic acid
Zometa

Pharmacologic class: Third-generation bisphosphonate
Therapeutic class: Calcium regulator
Pregnancy risk category D

Action
Inhibits osteoclast-mediated bone by blocking resorption of mineralized bone and cartilage, eventually causing cell death and thus limiting growth of tumors. Also limits calcium release produced by tumors.

Availability
Lyophilized powder for injection: 4 mg/vial

Indications and dosages
➤ Hypercalcemia caused by malignancy
Adults: 4 mg I.V. infused over 15 minutes. If albumin-corrected calcium level doesn't return to normal or stay normal, start retreatment with 4 mg I.V. no sooner than 7 days after initial treatment. For single dose, maximum recommended dosage is 4 mg.
➤ Multiple myeloma, bone metastasis from solid tumors
Adults: 4 mg I.V. infused over 15 minutes q 3 to 4 weeks; may continue treatment for 9 to 15 months, depending on clinical condition

Dosage adjustment
• Renal impairment

Off-label uses
• Paget's disease

Contraindications
• Hypersensitivity to drug, its components, or other bisphosphonates

Z

- Bone metastasis with severe renal impairment
- Pregnancy

Administration

- Before starting therapy, make sure patient is adequately hydrated.
- Reconstitute by adding 5 ml of sterile water for injection to 4-mg vial. Dilute further by adding reconstituted drug to 100 ml of normal saline solution or dextrose 5% in water.

◀℥ Give by I.V. infusion over no less than 15 minutes; faster infusion may cause renal failure.

- Know that patient usually receives oral calcium supplement of 500 mg and multivitamin containing 400 IU of vitamin D daily.

Route	Onset	Peak	Duration
I.V.	Unknown	Unknown	7-28 days

Adverse reactions

CNS: headache, agitation, confusion, insomnia, anxiety, drowsiness, fatigue, paresthesia
CV: hypotension
EENT: conjunctivitis
GI: nausea, vomiting, diarrhea, constipation, dysphagia, anorexia
GU: urinary tract infection, increased or decreased creatinine level, renal toxicity
Hematologic: anemia, **pancytopenia, granulocytopenia, thrombocytopenia**
Metabolic: dehydration, hypomagnesemia, hypercalcemia, hypophosphatemia
Musculoskeletal: myalgia, joint or bone pain
Respiratory: pleural effusion, dyspnea, cough
Other: infection, fever, chills, infusion site reactions

Interactions

Drug-drug. *Aminoglycosides, loop diuretics, thalidomide:* increased risk of renal toxicity

Drug-diagnostic tests. *Calcium, hemoglobin, magnesium, phosphorus, platelets, potassium, red blood cells, white blood cells:* decreased levels
Creatinine: increased or decreased level

Precautions

Use cautiously in:
- asthma, renal dysfunction, hepatic insufficiency, history of hypoparathyroidism
- breastfeeding patients.

Patient monitoring

- Monitor electrolyte levels (especially calcium); watch for signs and symptoms of electrolyte imbalance.
- Assess vital signs; stay alert for hypotension, dyspnea, and indications of pleural effusion.
- Closely monitor fluid intake and output and creatinine level; observe for signs and symptoms of renal toxicity.
- Monitor complete blood count, including platelet count.

Patient teaching

- Explain therapy to patient, including associated risk of renal failure and need for follow-up laboratory tests.
- Teach patient to report shortness of breath, unusual bleeding or bruising, decreased urine output, or other significant problems.
- Instruct patient to take a daily 500-mg oral calcium supplement and a multivitamin containing 400 IU of vitamin D, unless prescriber directs otherwise.
- Advise females of childbearing age to avoid pregnancy and breastfeeding.
- As appropriate, review all other significant and life-threatening adverse reactions and interactions, especially those related to the drugs and tests mentioned above.

zolmitriptan
Zomig, Zomig-ZMT

Pharmacologic class: Selective 5-hydroxytryptamine receptor agonist
Therapeutic class: Antimigraine agent
Pregnancy risk category C

Action
Blocks release of serotonin, causing selective constriction of inflamed and dilated cerebral and cranial blood vessels and reduction of nerve transmission in trigeminal pain pathways

Availability
Tablets (immediate-release): 2.5 mg, 5 mg
Tablets (orally disintegrating): 2.5 mg, 5 mg

Indications and dosages
➤ Acute migraine
Adults: 1.25 to 2.5 mg (immediate-release) P.O.; repeat dose if headache returns in 2 hours or less; usual dosage is 1.25 to 5 mg; maximum dosage is 10 mg in any 24-hour period. Or 2.5 mg (orally disintegrating tablet) P.O.; repeat dose if headache returns in 2 hours or less; usual dosage is 2.5 to 5 mg; maximum dosage is 10 mg in any 24-hour period.
Dosage adjustment
• Hepatic impairment

Contraindications
• Hypersensitivity to drug
• Hemiplegic or basilar migraine
• Ischemic heart disease or other significant cardiac disease
• Uncontrolled hypertension
• Cerebrovascular accident or transient ischemic attack
• Peripheral vascular disease, including ischemic bowel disease

• Ergot-containing drug use within 24 hours
• Monoamine oxidase (MAO) inhibitor use within past 14 days

Administration
• Place orally disintegrating tablet on patient's tongue, where it should dissolve.
• Don't break orally disintegrating tablets in half.

Route	Onset	Peak	Duration
P.O.	Unknown	2 hr	Unknown

Adverse reactions
CNS: paresthesia, asthenia, dizziness, insomnia, syncope, hyperesthesia, drowsiness, vertigo, agitation, depression, anxiety, emotional lability, fatigue, malaise
CV: chest pain, heaviness, or tightness; hypertension; palpitations; angina; **arrhythmias**
EENT: dry eyes, ear pain, tinnitus, epistaxis, altered sense of smell, laryngitis
GI: nausea, vomiting, dyspepsia, dysphagia, gastroenteritis, esophagitis, dry mouth
GU: urinary frequency, hematuria, polyuria, cystitis
Hepatic: hepatic dysfunction
Metabolic: hyperglycemia
Musculoskeletal: leg cramps, neck pain, tenosynovitis, myasthenia, myalgia, back pain
Respiratory: bronchitis, hiccups
Skin: pruritis, rash, diaphoresis, bruising, urticaria, photosensitivity
Other: fever, chills, excessive thirst, facial or tongue edema, pressure or tightness in throat or jaw, yawning, warm or cold sensation

Interactions
Drug-drug. *Cimetidine:* doubling of zolmitriptan's half-life
Ergot-containing drugs: vasospasms

Z

Fluoxetine, fluvoxamine, paroxetine, sertraline: weakness, incoordination, hyperreflexia
MAO inhibitors: increased zolmitriptan effects
Drug-diagnostic tests. *Blood glucose:* increased level
Drug-herb. *S-adenosylmethionine (SAM-e), St. John's wort:* serotonin syndrome

Precautions
Use cautiously in:
• hepatic or renal impairment
• risk factors for coronary artery disease (such as strong family history of disease, diabetes mellitus, obesity, cigarette smoking, high cholesterol levels, men over age 40, postmenopausal women)
• elderly patients
• pregnant or breastfeeding patients
• children.

Patient monitoring
• Assess patient's response, to help gauge drug efficacy.
• Watch for adverse cardiovascular and respiratory reactions, particularly dyspnea and chest pain or tightness.
• Assess blood glucose level in diabetic patients.

Patient teaching
• Explain that drug is intended to treat migraine, not prevent it.
• Teach patient to remove orally disintegrating tablet from blister pack just before taking it and then place it on his tongue and let it dissolve. Instruct him not to break it.
• Caution patient to avoid driving and other hazardous activities during severe migraine or if drug causes CNS side effects.
• Advise female of childbearing age not to take drug if she is, might be, or plans to become pregnant.
◀€ Tell patient to immediately report

shortness of breath or pain or tightness in chest or throat.
• Advise patient to avoid sun exposure and to wear sunscreen and protective clothing when going outdoors.
• As appropriate, review all other significant and life-threatening adverse reactions and interactions, especially those related to the drugs, tests, and herbs mentioned above.

zolpidem tartrate
Ambien

Pharmacologic class: Imidazopyridine
Therapeutic class: Sedative-hypnotic
Controlled substance schedule IV
Pregnancy risk category B

Action
Depresses CNS by binding to gamma-aminobutyric acid receptors

Availability
Tablets: 5 mg, 10 mg

⚠ Indications and dosages
➤ Short-term treatment of insomnia
Adults: 10 mg P.O. at bedtime
Dosage adjustment
• Hepatic impairment
• Elderly or debilitated patients

Off-label uses
• Long-term treatment of insomnia
• Insomnia related to selective serotonin reuptake inhibitors
• Postoperative sedation

Contraindications
• Hypersensitivity to drug

Administration
• Don't give drug with or immediately after a meal.

Route	Onset	Peak	Duration
P.O.	Rapid	30 min-2 hr	6-8 hr

Adverse reactions
CNS: amnesia, ataxia, confusion, euphoria, vertigo, daytime drowsiness, dizziness, drugged feeling
EENT: diplopia, abnormal vision
GI: nausea, vomiting, diarrhea, dry mouth
Other: hypersensitivity reaction, physical or psychological drug dependence, drug tolerance

Interactions
Drug-drug. *Antihistamines, opioid analgesics, phenothiazines, sedative-hypnotics, tricyclic antidepressants:* increased CNS depression
Ketoconazole, ritonavir: increased blood level and enhanced pharmacodynamic effects of zolpidem
Rifampin: decreased zolpidem efficacy
Drug-herb. *Chamomile, hops, kava, skullcap, valerian:* increased CNS depression
Drug-behaviors. *Alcohol use:* increased CNS depression

Precautions
Use cautiously in:
• pulmonary disease, hepatic or severe renal impairment
• history of psychiatric illness, suicide attempt, or substance abuse
• elderly or debilitated patients
• pregnant or breastfeeding patients
• children (safety not established).

Patient monitoring
• Monitor for physical and psychological drug dependence; watch for drug hoarding.
• Assess for adverse reactions, including confusion, ataxia, and amnesia.

Patient teaching
• Teach patient to take drug immediately before bedtime because it works quickly.
• Tell patient to take drug only when he's able to get a full night's sleep (7 to 8 hours) before he needs to be active.
• Explain that drug is meant for short-term use (7 to 10 days) only.
• Teach patient that rebound insomnia may occur for 1 to 2 nights after he discontinues drug.
• Tell patient drug may cause amnesia, drowsiness, and a drugged feeling the next day.
• Caution patient to avoid driving and other hazardous activities while under drug's influence.
• As appropriate, review all other significant adverse reactions and interactions, especially those related to the drugs, herbs, and behaviors mentioned above.

zonisamide
Zonegran

Pharmacologic class: Sulfonamide
Therapeutic class: Anticonvulsant
Pregnancy risk category C

Action
Raises seizure threshold and reduces seizure duration, probably by acting on sodium and calcium channels

Availability
Capsules: 25 mg, 50 mg, 100 mg

Indications and dosages
➤ Adjunctive treatment of partial seizures
Adults and children older than age 16: Initially, 100 mg P.O. daily for 2 weeks; then increased to 200 mg P.O. daily for at least 2 weeks. May be increased in increments of 100 mg at 2-week intervals as required. Daily dosage ranges from 100 to 600 mg.

Z

Dosage adjustment
- Hepatic or renal impairment
- Elderly patients

Off-label uses
- Infantile spasms
- Progressive myoclonic epilepsy
- Weight loss

Contraindications
- Hypersensitivity to drug or other sulfonamides

Administration
- Give drug with or without food.

Route	Onset	Peak	Duration
P.O.	Unknown	2-6 hr	24 hr

Adverse reactions
CNS: drowsiness, fatigue, agitation, irritability, depression, dizziness, psychomotor slowing, psychosis, asthenia, abnormal gait, hyperesthesia, incoordination, tremor, ataxia, headache, confusion, impaired memory, paresthesia, **seizures**

EENT: diplopia, amblyopia, nystagmus, tinnitus, rhinitis, pharyngitis

GI: nausea, vomiting, diarrhea, dyspepsia, abnormal taste, dry mouth, anorexia

GU: renal calculi, elevated blood urea nitrogen (BUN) and creatinine levels

Hematologic: anemia, **leukopenia**

Respiratory: cough

Skin: rash, pruritus, bruising

Other: weight loss, allergic reactions, oligohidrosis and hyperthermia (in pediatric patients), flulike symptoms, accidental injury, **Stevens-Johnson syndrome**

Interactions
Drug-drug. *Carbamazepine, phenobarbital, phenytoin, valproic acid:* decreased zonisamide blood level and effects

CYP450-3A4 inducers: decreased zonisamide half-life

CYP450-3A4 inhibitors: increased zonisamide blood level

Drug-diagnostic tests. *Platelets, white blood cells:* decreased counts

BUN, creatinine: increased levels

Precautions
Use cautiously in:
- hepatic or renal disease
- pregnant or breastfeeding patients
- children under age 16 (safety not established).

Patient monitoring
- Monitor complete blood count with white cell differential.
- Assess neurologic status; report significant adverse reactions.
- Monitor renal function studies; watch for signs and symptoms of renal calculi.

Patient teaching
- Explain therapy to patient; advise him to keep a seizure diary and show it to prescriber.
- Instruct patient to swallow capsules whole and drink 6 to 8 glasses of water daily to help prevent kidney stones.
- ◀€ Inform patient that stopping therapy abruptly may cause status epilepticus.
- Caution patient to avoid driving and other hazardous activities until he knows how drug affects him and until seizures are well controlled.
- ◀€ Tell patient to immediately report rash, fever, sore throat, sudden back pain, depression, speech or language problems, or painful urination.
- As appropriate, review all other significant and life-threatening adverse reactions and interactions, especially those related to the drugs and tests mentioned above.

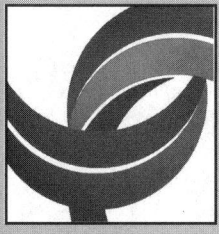

Part 2

Ophthalmic drugs
Drug classes
Vitamins and minerals
Herbs and supplements

Ophthalmic drugs

acetylcholine chloride
Miochol-E

Pregnancy risk category C

Action
Duplicates muscarinic effects of acetylcholine, causing pupillary constriction, stimulation of ciliary muscles, and increased aqueous humor outflow

Availability
Ophthalmic solution: 1% (after reconstitution)

⚡ Indications and dosages
➤ To produce miosis during ophthalmic surgery
Adults: Gently instill 0.5 to 2 ml of solution into anterior chamber.

Contraindications and precautions
• Contraindicated in hypersensitivity to drug and in certain inflammatory conditions (including iritis, uveitis, some secondary glaucoma forms, and anterior chamber inflammation)
• Use cautiously in acute heart failure, bronchial asthma, peptic ulcer, hyperthyroidism, GI spasm, urinary tract obstruction, Parkinson's disease, recent myocardial infarction, hypertension, hypotension, retinal detachment, retinal disease, miosis, corneal abrasion, breastfeeding patients, and children (safety and efficacy not established).

Administration
• Wash hands before and after administering; don't touch applicator tip to eye or surrounding skin.

Adverse reactions
Ophthalmic: corneal edema, clouding, decompensation
Other: bradycardia, hypotension, flushing, breathing difficulties, diaphoresis

atropine sulfate ophthalmic
Atropine-1, Isopto Atropine

Pregnancy risk category C

Action
Blocks response of iris and ciliary body to cholinergic stimulation, leading to pupillary dilation and paralysis of accommodation

Availability
Ophthalmic ointment: 1%
Ophthalmic solution: 0.5%, 1%, 2%

⚡ Indications and dosages
➤ Pupillary dilation in acute inflammatory conditions of the iris and uveal tract
Adults: Instill one or two drops of 0.5% or 1% solution into eye(s) up to q.i.d., or apply a small amount of ointment into conjunctival sac up to t.i.d.
Children: Instill one or two drops of 0.5% solution into eye(s) up to t.i.d.
➤ To produce mydriasis and cycloplegia for refraction
Adults: Instill one or two drops of 1% solution into eye(s) 1 hour before refraction.
Children: Instill one or two drops of 0.5% solution into eye(s) b.i.d. for 1 to 3 days before examination.

Contraindications and precautions

• Contraindicated in hypersensitivity to belladonna alkaloids or their components, primary glaucoma (current or previous), adhesions between iris and lens, and children with a history of severe systemic reaction to atropine

• Use with extreme caution in infants and small children.

Administration

• Apply pressure to lacrimal sac during instillation and for 1 to 2 minutes afterward.

Adverse reactions

Ophthalmic: increased intraocular pressure, blurred vision, photophobia, transient burning, visual hallucinations
Other: tachycardia; headache; parasympathetic stimulation; drowsiness; rash; hyperpyrexia; vasodilation; urinary retention; diminished GI motility; decreased secretions of salivary glands, sweat glands, pharynx, bronchi, and nasal passages

azelastine hydrochloride
Optivar

Pregnancy risk category C

Action
Suppresses release of histamine and other mediators from mast cells and other cells implicated in allergic response

Availability
Ophthalmic solution: 0.05%

Indications and dosages
➤ Itching of eye associated with allergic conjunctivitis

Adults and children ages 3 and older: Instill one drop of solution into each affected eye b.i.d.

Contraindications and precautions

• Contraindicated in hypersensitivity to drug or its components

Administration

• If patient wears contact lenses, remove them before instilling drops. Wait at least 10 minutes after instillation before reinserting lenses; however, if eyes are red, don't reinsert them.

Adverse reactions

Ophthalmic: pain, transient burning and blurred vision
Other: fatigue, headache, rhinitis, asthma, flulike symptoms, dyspnea, pruritus

bacitracin
AK-Tracin

Pregnancy risk category C

Action
Inhibits bacterial cell wall synthesis in gram-positive organisms

Availability
Ophthalmic ointment: 500 units/g

Indications and dosages
➤ Superficial ocular infections involving the conjunctiva or cornea
Adults: Administration and dosage vary. See manufacturer's insert.

Contraindications and precautions

• Contraindicated in hypersensitivity to drug and in atopy
• Use cautiously in deep-seated ocular

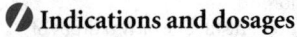

infections or infections likely to become systemic.

Administration
• Wash hands before and after applying; don't touch applicator tip to eye or surrounding skin.

Adverse reactions
Ophthalmic: burning, inflammation, corneal staining and itching
Other: hypersensitivity reactions (including swelling of lips and face), diaphoresis, chest tightness, hypotension, loss of consciousness, **apnea, cardiac arrest**

betaxolol hydrochloride
Betoptic, Betoptic S

Pregnancy risk category C

Action
Unknown; decreases elevated and normal intraocular pressure

Availability
Ophthalmic solution: 0.5%
Ophthalmic suspension: 0.25%

Indications and dosages
➤ Ocular hypertension and chronic open-angle glaucoma
Adults: Instill one or two drops in affected eye(s) b.i.d.
➤ Replacement therapy (single agent)
Adults: While continuing drug already being administered, instill one drop of betaxolol b.i.d. On following day, discontinue other drug and continue betaxolol.
➤ Replacement therapy (with multiple agents)
Adults: Adjust one drug at a time at weekly intervals. While continuing drugs already being administered, instill one drop of betaxolol b.i.d. On fol-

lowing day, discontinue one of the other drugs. Decrease dosage of or withdraw additional antiglaucoma drugs according to patient response.

Contraindications and precautions
• Contraindicated in hypersensitivity to drug, overt heart failure, or cardiogenic shock
• Use cautiously in asthma, chronic obstructive pulmonary disease, sinus bradycardia, or second- or third-degree atrioventricular block.

Administration
• If patient's receiving more than one topical ophthalmic drug, administer drugs at least 5 minutes apart.

Adverse reactions
Ophthalmic: keratitis, blepharoptosis, visual disturbances (including refractive changes), diplopia, ptosis, brief discomfort, occasional tearing
Other: syncope, headache, insomnia, depression, heart block, hypersensitivity (including localized and generalized rash), masking of hypoglycemia symptoms (in patients with insulin-dependent diabetes), nausea, abnormal taste and smell, glossitis, worsening of myasthenia gravis, urticaria, toxic epidermal necrolysis, alopecia, **cerebrovascular accident, heart failure, bronchospasm**

bimatoprost
Lumigan

Pregnancy risk category C

Action
Reduces intraocular pressure by increasing aqueous humor outflow through trabecular meshwork and uveoscleral route

Reactions in **bold** are life-threatening

Availability
Ophthalmic solution: 0.03% in 2.5 ml and 5 ml

🖊 Indications and dosages
➤ Ocular hypertension, open-angle glaucoma
Adults: One drop in affected eye(s) once daily in evening

Contraindications and precautions
• Contraindicated in hypersensitivity to drug or its components
• Use cautiously in bacterial keratitis, active intraocular inflammation, macular edema, aphakia, pseudophakia with torn posterior lens capsule, and known risk factors for macular edema.

Administration
• If patient wears contact lenses, remove them before instilling drug; may reinsert them 15 minutes later.

Adverse reactions
Ophthalmic: conjunctival edema or hyperemia, eyelash growth and darkening, itching, dryness, visual disturbances, burning and pain, foreign body sensation, periorbital pigmentation changes, blepharitis, cataract, superficial punctate keratitis, eyelid erythema, discharge, tearing, photophobia, allergic conjunctivitis, asthenopia, increased iris pigmentation
Other: colds, upper respiratory tract infection, headache, asthenia, hirsutism, abnormal liver function test results

brimonidine tartrate
Alphagan, Alphagan P

Pregnancy risk category B

Action
Reduces intraocular pressure by de-creasing aqueous humor production and increasing uveoscleral outflow

Availability
Ophthalmic solution: 0.15% and 0.2% in 5-ml, 10-ml, and 15-ml bottles

🖊 Indications and dosages
➤ To lower intraocular pressure in open-angle glaucoma; ocular hypertension
Adults: One drop in affected eye(s) t.i.d., with doses spaced approximately 8 hours apart. When used concomitantly with other ophthalmic drugs to reduce intraocular pressure, separate administration times by at least 5 minutes.

Contraindications and precautions
• Contraindicated in hypersensitivity to drug or its components and in concurrent monoamine oxidase inhibitor therapy
• Use cautiously in severe cardiovascular disease, cerebral or coronary insufficiency, Raynaud's phenomenon, orthostatic hypotension, thromboangiitis obliterans, and depression.

Administration
• Wash hands before administering; don't touch applicator tip to eye or surrounding skin.

Adverse reactions
Ophthalmic: burning, stinging, conjunctival hyperemia, allergic conjunctivitis, photophobia, corneal staining, foreign body sensation, ocular edema, blurred vision
Other: headache, drowsiness, hypertension, dry mouth, upper respiratory symptoms

carbachol
Carbastat, Miostat

Pregnancy risk category C

Action
Causes sphincter muscles of iris to contract, resulting in miosis; also causes ciliary muscle contraction, leading to accommodation. Miosis reduces outflow resistance, thereby increasing aqueous humor outflow and decreasing intraocular pressure.

Availability
Intraocular solution: 0.01% in 1.5-ml vials
Topical ophthalmic solution: 0.75%, 1.5%, 2.25%, 3%

Indications and dosages
➤ Miosis
Adults: Instill 0.5 ml of 0.01% solution into anterior chamber before or after sutures have been secured.
➤ Glaucoma
Adults: Instill one or two drops of 0.75% to 3% topical solution q 4 to 8 hours up to t.i.d., depending on patient response.

Contraindications and precautions
• Contraindicated in hypersensitivity to drug or when constriction is undesirable (as in acute iritis, acute uveitis, some secondary glaucoma forms, and acute inflammatory disease of anterior chamber)
• Use cautiously in acute heart failure, bronchial asthma, peptic ulcer, hyperthyroidism, GI spasm, urinary tract obstruction, Parkinson's disease, recent myocardial infarction, hypertension, and hypotension.

Administration
• Apply finger pressure to lacrimal sac for 1 to 2 minutes after instillation; remove excess solution around eye with a tissue. Wash hands immediately after instillation.

Adverse reactions
Ophthalmic: corneal edema, clouding, transient stinging and burning, bullous keratopathy, conjunctival vasodilation
Other: bradycardia, headache, hypotension, flushing, breathing difficulties, diaphoresis

cyclopentolate hydrochloride
AK-Pentolate, Cyclogyl, Pentolair

Pregnancy risk category C

Action
Anticholinergic activity blocks responses of iris's sphincter muscle and ciliary body muscle to cholinergic stimulation, leading to paralysis of accommodation and pupillary dilation

Availability
Ophthalmic solution: 0.5%, 1%, 2%

Indications and dosages
➤ Mydriasis and cycloplegia for refraction during diagnostic procedures
Adults: Instill one or two drops of 0.5%, 1%, or 2% ophthalmic solution into eye(s); repeat in 5 to 10 minutes, if necessary.
Children: Instill one or two drops of 0.5%, 1%, or 2% solution into eye(s); repeat in 5 to 10 minutes, as ordered, with a second application of 0.5% or 1% solution.

Contraindications and precautions

• Contraindicated in hypersensitivity to belladonna alkaloids or their components, narrow-angle glaucoma (current or previous), adhesions between iris and lens, and children with a history of severe systemic reaction to atropine

• Use cautiously in Down syndrome, sulfite sensitivity, and children with brain damage.

Administration

• To help prevent excessive systemic absorption, compress lacrimal sac with finger for 1 to 3 minutes after instillation.

Adverse reactions

Ophthalmic: increased intraocular pressure, transient stinging, irritation (with prolonged use), blurred vision, photophobia, corneal staining, visual hallucinations

Other: dry mouth and skin, tachycardia, headache, drowsiness, rash, psychotic reactions and behavioral disturbances in children

---

dexamethasone
Maxidex

dexamethasone sodium phosphate
Decadron Phosphate, Maxidex

Pregnancy risk category C

Action

Stimulates synthesis of enzymes responsible for easing the inflammatory response

Availability

dexamethasone
Ophthalmic suspension: 0.1%
dexamethasone sodium phosphate
Ophthalmic ointment: 0.05%
Ophthalmic solution: 0.1%

✇ Indications and dosages

➤ Inflammatory eye conditions, corneal injury

Adults: Initially, instill one or two drops of solution into conjunctival sac q hour during day and q 2 hours at night; after positive response, reduce dosage to one drop q 4 hours. In severe cases, instill one or two drops of suspension in conjunctival sac q hour. In mild cases, initially instill one or two drops of suspension four to six times daily or apply thin coating of ointment three to four times daily; if symptoms are controlled, reduce application to b.i.d. and then daily.

Contraindications and precautions

• Contraindicated in hypersensitivity to drug, dendritic keratitis, fungal diseases of ocular structures, vaccinia, varicella and most other viral diseases of cornea and conjunctiva, ocular tuberculosis, mycobacterial eye infection, acute or purulent untreated eye infections that steroids may mask or enhance, and after uncomplicated removal of superficial corneal foreign body

• Use cautiously in glaucoma and in potentially infected corneal abrasions.

Administration

• Wash hands before and after administering; don't touch applicator tip to eye or surrounding skin.

Adverse reactions

Ophthalmic: glaucoma, visual disturbances, posterior subcapsular cataract formation, delayed wound healing, secondary ocular infection, acute uveitis,

---

Reactions in **bold** are life-threatening

perforation of globe when corneal or scleral thinning exists, exacerbation of infection, transient burning, chemosis, dry eyes, keratitis, conjunctivitis, corneal ulcer, mydriasis, ptosis, pain, foreign body sensation, hyperemia, itching

Other: systemic effects and adrenal suppression (in long-term use)

diclofenac sodium
Voltaren Ophthalmic

Pregnancy risk category B

Action
Reduces inflammation by inhibiting an enzyme essential to prostaglandin biosynthesis

Availability
Ophthalmic solution: 0.1%

🕖 Indications and dosages
➤ Postoperative inflammation after cataract extraction
Adults: Instill one drop into affected eye q.i.d., starting 24 hours after surgery and continuing for 2 weeks after surgery.
➤ Corneal refractive surgery
Adults: Instill one or two drops into affected eye 1 hour before surgery, then within 15 minutes after surgery, then q.i.d. for up to 3 days.

Contraindications and precautions
• Contraindicated in hypersensitivity to drug or its components and in patients who wear soft contact lenses
• Use cautiously in surgical patients with bleeding tendencies and in patients receiving drugs known to cause bleeding.

Administration
• Wash hands before and after administering; don't touch applicator tip to eye or surrounding skin.

Adverse reactions
Ophthalmic: transient burning, keratitis, increased intraocular pressure, anterior chamber reaction, ocular allergy
Other: nausea, vomiting, viral infections

dorzolamide hydrochloride
Trusopt

Pregnancy risk category C

Action
Decreases intraocular pressure by inhibiting carbonic anhydrase in ciliary processes of eye, thereby decreasing aqueous humor secretion

Availability
Ophthalmic solution: 2%

🕖 Indications and dosages
➤ Open-angle glaucoma, ocular hypertension
Adults: One drop in affected eye(s) t.i.d. May be used concurrently with other topical ophthalmics to decrease intraocular pressure; if more than one ophthalmic drug is used, administer drugs at least 10 minutes apart.

Contraindications and precautions
• Contraindicated in hypersensitivity to drug or its components
• Use cautiously in Stevens-Johnson syndrome, toxic epidermal necrolysis, fulminant hepatic necrosis, agranulocytosis, aplastic anemia, and other blood dyscrasias.

Administration

• Remove patient's contact lenses before administration; may reinsert them 15 minutes later.

Adverse reactions

Ophthalmic: burning, superficial punctate keratitis, allergic reaction, blurred vision, lacrimation, dryness, photophobia
Other: headache, bitter taste, nausea, asthenia, fatigue, rash, urolithiasis

echothiophate iodide
Phospholine Iodide

Pregnancy risk category C

Action

Inhibits cholinesterase, an enzyme that potentiates acetylcholine's action on parasympathomimetic end organs; topical eye application produces intense miosis and muscle contraction. Also reduces intraocular pressure, which decreases resistance to aqueous humor outflow.

Availability

Ophthalmic powder for reconstitution: reconstitute to 0.03%, 0.06%, 0.125%, or 0.25% solution

Indications and dosages

➤ Open-angle glaucoma, glaucoma secondary to cataract surgery
Adults: Instill one drop of 0.03% solution b.i.d. at bedtime and in morning to maintain smooth diurnal tension curve. Once-daily or once-every-other-day dosing has been used with satisfactory results.
➤ To diagnose accommodative esotropia
Children: Instill one drop of 0.125% solution in both eyes once daily at bedtime for 2 to 3 weeks.

➤ Accommodative esotropia
Children: Instill one drop of 0.125% solution every other day or one drop of 0.06% solution daily. As appropriate, reduce dosage as treatment progresses.

Contraindications and precautions

• Contraindicated in hypersensitivity to drug, other cholinesterase inhibitors, or their components; active uveal inflammation or inflammatory disease of iris or ciliary body; and glaucoma associated with iridocyclitis
• Use cautiously in chronic narrow-angle glaucoma, narrow angles without glaucoma, marked vagotonia, bronchial asthma, spastic GI disturbances, peptic ulcer, pronounced bradycardia or hypotension, recent myocardial infarction, epilepsy, myasthenia gravis, parkinsonism, other disorders that may respond adversely to vagotonic effects, and history of quiescent uveitis.

Administration

• Wash hands before and after administering; don't touch applicator tip to eye or surrounding skin.

Adverse reactions

Ophthalmic: iritic cysts, burning, lacrimation, lid twitching, conjunctival and ciliary redness, latent iritis or uveitis activation, myopia with visual blurring, retinal detachment, lens opacities, conjunctival thickening, destruction of nasolacrimal canals
Other: nausea, vomiting, headache, abdominal cramps, diarrhea, urinary incontinence, syncope, diaphoresis, salivation, difficulty breathing, cardiac irregularities

---

Reactions in **bold** are life-threatening

epinephrine hydrochloride
Epifrin, Glaucon

Pregnancy risk category C

Action
Stimulates alpha- and beta-adrenergic receptors, causing conjunctival decongestion, transient mydriasis, and decreased intraocular pressure

Availability
Ophthalmic solution: 0.1%, 0.5%, 1%, or 2% (as base)

Indications and dosages
➤ Management of open-angle glaucoma
Adults: Instill one drop of 1% solution into affected eye(s) once or twice daily (frequency is determined by tonometry). May be used in combination with miotics, beta-adrenergic blockers, hyperosmotic agents, or carbonic anhydrase inhibitors; when giving with miotics, wait 10 minutes after miotic administration before instilling epinephrine.

Contraindications and precautions
• Contraindicated in hypersensitivity to epinephrine or its components, narrow-angle glaucoma, narrow angles without glaucoma, aphakia, and patients who wear soft contact lenses
• Use cautiously in hypertension (current or previous), diabetes mellitus, hyperthyroidism, heart disease, cerebral arteriosclerosis, asthma, and elderly patients.

Administration
• Administer at bedtime when possible.

Adverse reactions
Ophthalmic: transient burning, eye pain, brow ache, allergic eyelid reaction, conjunctival hyperemia, conjunctival or corneal pigmentation, ocular irritation (hypersensitivity), localized adrenochrome deposits in conjunctiva and cornea, reversible cystoid macular edema
Other: headache, palpitations, tachycardia, hypertension, syncope, **arrhythmias**

erythromycin
Ilotycin

Pregnancy risk category B

Action
Inhibits bacterial protein synthesis in susceptible organisms

Availability
Ophthalmic ointment: 0.5%

Indications and dosage
➤ Superficial ocular infections, including conjunctivitis, keratitis, keratoconjunctivitis, corneal ulcers, blepharitis, blepharoconjunctivitis, acute meibomianitis, and dacryocystitis
Adults: Apply a ribbon of ointment to affected eye(s) up to six times daily as prescribed.

Contraindications and precautions
• Contraindicated in hypersensitivity to drug, epithelial herpes simplex keratitis, vaccinia, varicella, mycobacterial infections, and fungal diseases of ocular structures

Administration
• Wash hands before and after applying; don't touch applicator tip to eye or surrounding skin.

Reactions in **bold** are life-threatening

Adverse reactions
Ophthalmic: burning, itching, inflammation, angioneurotic edema, urticaria
Other: dermatitis, urticaria

---

fluorometholone
Flarex, Fluor-Op, FML Forte, FML Liquifilm, FML S.O.P.

Pregnancy risk category C

Action
Stimulates synthesis of enzymes required to ease the inflammatory response

Availability
Ophthalmic ointment: 0.1%
Ophthalmic suspension: 0.1%, 0.25%

⚕ Indications and dosages
➤ Steroid-responsive inflammation of palpebral and bulbar conjunctiva, cornea, and anterior globe segment
Adults: Instill one or two drops of suspension into conjunctival sac two to four times daily; may increase dosage to two drops q 2 hours during first 24 to 48 hours. Or apply a small amount (½″ ribbon) of ointment to conjunctival sac one to three times daily; may increase frequency to once q 4 hours during first 24 to 48 hours.

Contraindications and precautions
• Contraindicated in hypersensitivity to drug; acute epithelial herpes simplex keratitis; fungal eye disease; vaccinia, varicella, and most other viral diseases of cornea and conjunctiva; ocular tuberculosis; mycobacterial eye infections; acute, purulent, untreated eye infections that steroids may mask or enhance; and after uncomplicated removal of superficial corneal foreign body

• Use cautiously in corneal abrasions that may be contaminated.

Administration
• Wash hands before and after administering; don't touch applicator tip to eye or surrounding skin.

Adverse reactions
Ophthalmic: glaucoma with optic nerve damage, blurred vision, visual acuity loss, visual field defects, cataract, delayed wound healing, secondary ocular infection, acute uveitis, globe perforation, exacerbation of corneal infections, transient burning, chemosis, dry eyes, epiphora, photophobia, keratitis, conjunctivitis, corneal ulcers, mydriasis, ptosis, eye discharge, ocular pain, foreign body sensation, hyperemia
Other: systemic effects (with extensive use)

---

flurbiprofen sodium
Ocufen

Pregnancy risk category C

Action
Inhibits cyclooxygenase, an enzyme essential to prostaglandin biosynthesis; exerts analgesic, antipyretic, and anti-inflammatory effects

Availability
Ophthalmic solution: 0.03%

⚕ Indications and dosages
➤ To inhibit intraoperative miosis
Adults: Instill one drop into affected eye q 30 minutes, starting 2 hours before surgery begins, for a total of four drops.

Contraindications and precautions

• Contraindicated in hypersensitivity to drug or its components

• Use cautiously in sensitivity to acetyl-salicylic acid and other nonsteroidal anti-inflammatory drugs, surgical patients with known bleeding tendencies, and patients taking drugs that can cause bleeding.

Administration

• Wash hands before and after instilling; don't touch applicator tip to eye or surrounding skin.

Adverse reactions

Ophthalmic: transient burning, ocular irritation, increased bleeding tendency of ocular tissues during surgery
Other: none

gentamicin sulfate
Garamycin, Genoptic Liquifilm, Genoptic S.O.P., Gentacidin, Gentak

Pregnancy risk category C

Action
Binds to bacterial ribosome subunit, inhibiting bacterial protein synthesis

Availability
Ophthalmic ointment: 3 mg/g
Ophthalmic solution: 3 mg/ml

Indications and dosages
➤ Superficial ocular infections caused by susceptible organisms
Adults: Administration and dosage vary with specific product. See manufacturer's insert.

Contraindications and precautions

• Contraindicated in hypersensitivity to drug or its components, epithelial herpes simplex keratitis, vaccinia, varicella, mycobacterial eye infections, fungal disease of ocular structures, and concurrent use of steroid combinations after uncomplicated removal of corneal foreign body

Administration

• Wash hands before and after instilling; don't touch applicator tip to eye or surrounding skin.

Adverse reactions

Ophthalmic: transient irritation, localized ocular toxicity and hypersensitivity, lid itching or swelling, conjunctival erythema, conjunctivitis, conjunctival epithelial defects, conjunctival hyperemia, corneal ulcers
Other: overgrowth of organisms (with long-term use)

homatropine hydrobromide
Isopto Homatropine

Pregnancy risk category C

Action
Blocks responses of sphincter muscle of iris and ciliary body muscle to cholinergic stimulation, causing pupillary dilation and paralysis of accommodation

Availability
Ophthalmic solution: 2%, 5%

Indications and dosages
➤ To produce mydriasis and cycloplegia for refraction
Adults: Instill one or two drops into

eye(s) immediately before procedure; repeat in 5 to 10 minutes if necessary.
Children: Instill one or two drops of 2% solution into eye(s) immediately before procedure; repeat at 10-minute intervals p.r.n.
➤ Uveitis
Adults: Instill one or two drops of 2% or 5% solution into eye(s) up to q 3 to 4 hours.
Children: Instill one drop of 2% solution into eye(s) two or three times daily.

Contraindications and precautions
• Contraindicated in hypersensitivity to drug, its components, or other belladonna alkaloids; primary glaucoma (current or previous); adhesions between iris and lens; and children with a history of severe systemic reaction to atropine
• Use cautiously in Down syndrome and children with brain damage.

Administration
• Compress lacrimal sac with finger for several minutes after instillation.

Adverse reactions
Ophthalmic: increased intraocular pressure, transient stinging, irritation (with prolonged use), blurred vision, photophobia with or without corneal staining
Other: dry mouth and skin; tachycardia; headache; parasympathetic stimulation; visual hallucinations; drowsiness; rash; abdominal distention (in infants); high fever; vasodilation; urinary retention; diminished GI motility; decreased secretions of salivary glands, sweat glands, pharynx, bronchi, and nasal passages; **medullary paralysis; coma; death**

ketorolac tromethamine
Acular, Acular LS

Pregnancy risk category C

Action
Inhibits an enzyme essential to biosynthesis of prostaglandins, which mediate intraocular inflammation

Availability
Ophthalmic solution: 0.5%

🕧 Indications and dosages
➤ Conjunctivitis
Adults: Instill one drop of 0.5% solution into affected eye(s) q.i.d.
➤ Postoperative or posttraumatic inflammation
Adults: Instill one drop of 0.5% solution into affected eye(s) q.i.d., starting 24 hours after surgery; continue for 2 weeks.
➤ Postoperative ocular pain and photophobia
Adults: Instill one drop of 0.5% solution into operative eye q.i.d. p.r.n. for up to 4 days after surgery.

Contraindications and precautions
• Contraindicated in hypersensitivity to drug or its components
• Use cautiously in sensitivity to acetylsalicylic acid and other nonsteroidal anti-inflammatory drugs, surgical patients with bleeding tendencies, and patients receiving drugs that can cause bleeding.

Administration
• Wash hands before and after instilling; don't touch applicator tip to eye or surrounding skin.

Reactions in **bold** are life-threatening

Adverse reactions

Ophthalmic: transient burning and stinging, ocular irritation, superficial keratitis, superficial ocular infections, dry eyes, corneal infiltrates, corneal ulcer, blurred vision

Other: headache, allergic reactions

ketotifen fumarate
Zaditor

Pregnancy risk category C

Action

Inhibits release of mediators from cells involved in hypersensitivity reactions; decreases chemotaxis and activation of eosinophils

Availability

Ophthalmic solution: 0.025%

Indications and dosages

➤ Prevention of ocular itching caused by allergic conjunctivitis

Adults and children ages 3 and older: Instill one drop into affected eye(s) q 8 to 12 hours.

Contraindications and precautions

• Contraindicated in hypersensitivity to drug or its components

Administration

• Wash hands before and after instilling; don't touch applicator tip to eye or surrounding skin.
• Remove patient's contact lenses before administration; wait at least 10 minutes before reinserting.

Adverse reactions

Ophthalmic: conjunctivitis; ocular burning, itching, pain, discharge, or dryness; eyelid disorder; keratitis; lacrimation disorder; mydriasis; photophobia

Other: headache, rhinitis, allergic reactions, rash, flulike symptoms, pharyngitis

latanoprost
Xalatan

Pregnancy risk category C

Action

Unclear; thought to reduce intraocular pressure by increasing aqueous humor outflow

Availability

Ophthalmic solution: 0.005%

Indications and dosages

➤ Open-angle glaucoma, ocular hypertension

Adults: One drop (1.5 mcg) in affected eye(s) once daily in evening. Don't administer more than once daily; more frequent dosing may limit drug's effect on intraocular pressure (IOP). If patient's receiving other topical ophthalmic drugs to reduce IOP, separate administration times by at least 5 minutes.

Contraindications and precautions

• Contraindicated in hypersensitivity to drug or its components
• Use cautiously in increased risk of macular edema, absence of intact posterior capsule, and history of intraocular inflammation.

Administration

• Remove contact lenses before each dose; wait 15 minutes before reinserting.

Reactions in **bold** are life-threatening

Adverse reactions

Ophthalmic: blurred vision; diplopia; ocular burning, itching, pain, dryness, or discharge; conjunctival hyperemia; foreign body sensation; increased iris pigmentation; punctate epithelial keratopathy; excessive tearing; eyelid edema and erythema; eyelid darkening; eyelash changes; photophobia; conjunctivitis; retinal artery embolus; retinal detachment; intraocular inflammation; macular edema

Other: upper respiratory tract infection; muscle, joint, back, or chest pain; allergic skin reaction

levobunolol hydrochloride
Betagan

Pregnancy risk category C

Action

Reduces intraocular pressure by decreasing aqueous production

Availability

Ophthalmic solution: 0.25%, 0.5%

⚕ Indications and dosages

➤ Chronic open-angle glaucoma, ocular hypertension
Adults: Instill one or two drops of 0.5% solution in affected eye(s) once daily or one to two drops of 0.25% solution in affected eye(s) b.i.d.

Contraindications and precautions

• Contraindicated in hypersensitivity to drug or its components, asthma, history of asthma or severe chronic obstructive pulmonary disease, sinus bradycardia, heart block, overt heart failure, and cardiogenic shock

• Use cautiously in diabetes mellitus, hyperthyroidism, and myasthenia gravis.

Administration

• Wash hands before and after instilling; don't touch applicator tip to eye or surrounding skin.

Adverse reactions

Ophthalmic: keratitis, blepharoptosis, blepharoconjunctivitis, visual disturbances, ptosis, transient burning, decreased corneal sensitivity

Other: syncope, headache, depression, hypersensitivity reaction (including localized or generalized rash), masking of hypoglycemia symptoms in patients with insulin-dependent diabetes, nausea, diarrhea, respiratory failure, ataxia, dizziness, exacerbation of myasthenia gravis, urticaria, alopecia, localized or generalized rash, impotence, decreased libido, **bronchospasm, arrhythmias, cerebrovascular accident, heart failure**

levocabastine hydrochloride
Livostin

Pregnancy risk category C

Action

Competes with histamine for histamine$_1$-receptor sites; suppresses allergic symptoms triggered by histamine

Availability

Ophthalmic suspension: 0.05%

⚕ Indications and dosages

➤ Temporary symptomatic relief of seasonal allergic conjunctivitis
Adults and children ages 12 and older: Instill one drop into affected eye(s) q.i.d. for up to 2 weeks.

Contraindications and precautions
• Contraindicated in hypersensitivity to drug or its components and in patients who wear soft contact lenses

Administration
• Wash hands before and after instilling; don't touch applicator tip to eye or surrounding skin.

Adverse reactions
Ophthalmic: mild, transient stinging; visual disturbances; pain; dryness; red eyelids; discharge; eyelid edema
Other: headache, dyspnea, dry mouth, fatigue, pharyngitis, cough, nausea, rash, drowsiness

levofloxacin
Quixin

Pregnancy risk category C

Action
Suppresses bacterial DNA gyrase, preventing DNA replication and transcription in susceptible organisms

Availability
Ophthalmic solution: 0.5%

⟁ Indications and dosages
➤ Bacterial conjunctivitis caused by susceptible organisms
Adults and children ages 1 and older: Instill one or two drops into affected eye(s) q 2 hours while awake (up to eight times daily) for 2 days, then q 4 hours while awake (up to q.i.d.) for the next 5 days.

Contraindications and precautions
• Contraindicated in hypersensitivity to drug or its components, epithelial herpes simplex keratitis, vaccinia, varicella, mycobacterial eye infections and fungal eye diseases

Administration
• Wash hands before and after instilling; don't touch applicator tip to eye or surrounding skin.

Adverse reactions
Ophthalmic: transient irritation, inflammation, white crystalline precipitates, lid margin crusting, conjunctival hyperemia, corneal staining, keratopathy, keratitis, lid edema, tearing, photophobia, corneal infiltrates, decreased vision, chemosis
Other: allergic reactions, headache, fever, vesicular or maculopapular dermatitis, abnormal taste, nausea

lodoxamide tromethamine
Alomide

Pregnancy risk category B

Action
May prevent calcium influx into mast cells when antigen stimulation occurs

Availability
Ophthalmic solution: 0.1%

⟁ Indications and dosages
➤ Vernal keratoconjunctivitis, vernal conjunctivitis, and vernal keratitis
Adults and children ages 2 and older: Instill one to two drops in affected eye(s) q.i.d. for up to 3 months.

Contraindications and precautions
• Contraindicated in hypersensitivity to drug or its components
• Patients shouldn't wear contact lenses during therapy.

Administration

- Wash hands before and after instilling; don't touch applicator tip to eye or surrounding skin.

Adverse reactions

Ophthalmic: transient discomfort, itching, blurred vision, dry eyes, discharge, hyperemia, crystalline deposits, corneal erosion, scales on lid or lashes, edema, chemosis, corneal abrasion, keratopathy, keratitis, blepharitis, sticky sensation, epitheliopathy
Other: allergic reactions, headache, dizziness, drowsiness, nausea, GI discomfort, sneezing, dry nose, rash

medrysone
HMS Liquifilm

Pregnancy risk category C

Action
Stimulates synthesis of enzymes needed to ease the inflammatory response

Availability
Ophthalmic suspension: 1%

⬤ Indications and dosages
➤ Allergic conjunctivitis, vernal conjunctivitis, episcleritis, and epinephrine sensitivity
Adults: Instill one drop into conjunctival sac up to q 4 hours.

Contraindications and precautions

- Contraindicated in hypersensitivity to drug; iritis; uveitis; acute epithelial herpes simplex keratitis; fungal eye diseases; vaccinia, varicella, and most other viral diseases of cornea and conjunctiva; ocular tuberculosis; mycobacterial eye infection; acute untreated purulent eye infections; and after uncomplicated

removal of superficial corneal foreign body

Administration

- Wash hands before and after instilling; don't touch applicator tip to eye or surrounding skin.

Adverse reactions

Ophthalmic: glaucoma with optic nerve damage, visual acuity loss, visual field defects, posterior subcapsular cataract formation, secondary ocular infection, acute uveitis, perforated globe, exacerbation of corneal infection, transient stinging, chemosis, dry eyes, epiphora, photophobia, keratitis, conjunctivitis, corneal ulcers, mydriasis, ptosis, blurred vision, eye discharge and discomfort, hyperemia
Other: adrenal suppression (in excessive or long-term use)

moxifloxacin hydrochloride
Vigamox

Pregnancy risk category C

Action
Inhibits both DNA gyrase (involved in bacterial DNA replication, transcription, and repair) and topoisomerase IV (critical to partitioning of chromosomal DNA during bacterial cell division)

Availability
Ophthalmic solution: 0.5%

⬤ Indications and dosages
➤ Conjunctivitis caused by susceptible organisms
Adults and children ages 1 and older: Instill one drop in affected eye(s) t.i.d. for 7 days.

Contraindications and precautions

• Contraindicated in hypersensitivity to drug or its components, epithelial herpes simplex keratitis, vaccinia, varicella, mycobacterial eye infections, fungal diseases of eye structures, and use of steroid combinations after uncomplicated removal of corneal foreign body

Administration

• Wash hands before and after instilling; don't touch applicator tip to eye or surrounding skin.

Adverse reactions

Ophthalmic: conjunctivitis, decreased visual acuity, dry eyes, keratitis, ocular pain or discomfort, itching, tearing, hyperemia, subconjunctival hemorrhage

Other: fever, increased cough, infection, otitis media, pharyngitis, rash, rhinitis

naphazoline hydrochloride

20/20 Eye Drops, AK-Con, Albalon, All Clear AR, Allerest Eye Drops, Clear Eyes, Clear Eyes ACR, Comfort Eye Drops, Nafazair, Naphcon, Naphcon Forte, VasoClear

Pregnancy risk category C

Action

Stimulates alpha-receptors of sympathetic nervous system, causing vasoconstriction and temporary relief of conjunctival congestion

Availability

Ophthalmic drops: 0.02%
Ophthalmic solution: 0.012%, 0.1%

⏧ Indications and dosages

➤ Conjunctivitis, itching, pruritus
Adults: Instill one or two drops into conjunctival sac of affected eye(s) q 3 to 4 hours, up to q.i.d.

Contraindications and precautions

• Contraindicated in hypersensitivity to drug or its components, narrow-angle glaucoma, narrow angles without glaucoma, and patients scheduled for peripheral iridectomy whose eyes are capable of angle closure
• Use cautiously in hypertension, diabetes mellitus, hyperthyroidism, cardiovascular abnormalities, and arteriosclerosis.

Administration

• Wash hands before and after instilling; don't touch applicator tip to eye or surrounding skin.

Adverse reactions

Ophthalmic: transitory stinging, blurred vision, mydriasis, increased redness, irritation, discomfort, punctate keratitis, lacrimation, increased intraocular pressure

Other: palpitations, hypertension, headache, brow ache, blanching, tremor, diaphoresis, dizziness, nervousness, drowsiness, weakness, hyperglycemia, nausea, **coronary occlusion, arrhythmias, pulmonary embolism, subarachnoid hemorrhage, myocardial infarction, cerebrovascular accident**

natamycin

Natacyn

Pregnancy risk category C

Action

Bind to sterols in fungal cell membrane, allowing vital cellular components to escape through membrane

Availability

Ophthalmic suspension: 5%

Indications and dosages

➤ Fungal keratitis

Adults: Initially, instill one drop into conjunctival sac of infected eye(s) q 1 or 2 hours for 3 to 4 days; then reduce to one drop q 3 to 4 hours. Continue therapy for 14 to 21 days or until active fungal keratitis resolves.

➤ Fungal blepharitis and conjunctivitis

Adults: Instill one drop into conjunctival sac of infected eye(s) q 4 to 6 hours.

Contraindications and precautions

• Contraindicated in hypersensitivity to drug or its components and in concurrent use of topical corticosteroids

Administration

• Wash hands before and after instilling; don't touch applicator tip to eye or surrounding skin.

Adverse reactions

Ophthalmic: conjunctival chemosis, hyperemia

Other: none

olopatadine hydrochloride
Patanol

Pregnancy risk category C

Action

Blocks histamine release from mast cells, inhibiting type 1 immediate hypersensitivity reaction

Availability

Ophthalmic solution: 0.1%

Indications and dosages

➤ Allergic conjunctivitis

Adults and children ages 3 and older: One drop in affected eye(s) b.i.d. at intervals of 6 to 8 hours

Contraindications and precautions

• Contraindicated in hypersensitivity to drug or its components

Administration

• Remove patient's contact lenses before administering; may reinsert them 10 minutes later.

Adverse reactions

Ophthalmic: burning or stinging, dry eyes, foreign body sensation, hyperemia, keratitis, eyelid edema, itching
Other: headache, asthenia, pharyngitis, rhinitis, sinusitis, abnormal taste

oxymetazoline hydrochloride
OcuClear, Visine L.R.

Pregnancy risk category C

Action

Stimulates alpha-adrenergic receptors in conjunctival arterioles, causing vasoconstriction that temporarily relieves conjunctival congestion

Availability

Ophthalmic solution: 0.025%

Indications and dosages

➤ Eye redness caused by minor irritation

Adults and children ages 6 and older: Instill one or two drops into affected eye(s) q 6 hours.

Reactions in **bold** are life-threatening

Contraindications and precautions

• Contraindicated in hypersensitivity to drug or its components, narrow-angle glaucoma, narrow angles without glaucoma, and patients scheduled for peripheral iridectomy whose eyes are capable of angle closure

• Use cautiously in hypertension, diabetes mellitus, hyperthyroidism, cardiovascular abnormalities, and arteriosclerosis.

Administration

• Wash hands before and after instilling; don't touch applicator tip to eye or surrounding skin.

Adverse reactions

Ophthalmic: mydriasis, increased redness, discomfort, blurring, punctate keratitis, lacrimation, increased intraocular pressure
Other: palpitations, hypertension, headache, blanching, tremor, diaphoresis, dizziness, nervousness, drowsiness, weakness, hyperglycemia, nausea, **coronary occlusion, arrhythmias, myocardial infarction, pulmonary embolism, subarachnoid hemorrhage, cerebrovascular accident**

---

pilocarpine hydrochloride
Akarpine, Isopto Carpine, Ocu-Carpine, Ocusert Pilo-20, Pilocar

Pregnancy risk category C

Action

Exerts cholinergic action, which causes iris sphincter muscle to contract. Resulting miosis promotes aqueous outflow, thereby decreasing intraocular pressure.

Availability

Ocular system: 20 mcg/hour for 7 days, 40 mcg/hour for 7 days
Ophthalmic gel: 4%
Ophthalmic solution: 0.25%, 0.5%, 1%, 2%, 3%, 4%, 6%, 8%, 10%

Indications and dosages

➢ Primary open-angle glaucoma; emergency treatment of acute narrow-angle glaucoma; to counteract mydriatic effect of sympathomimetics
Adults: Administration and dosage vary with specific product. See manufacturer's insert.

Contraindications and precautions

• Contraindicated in hypersensitivity to drug or its components and when vasoconstriction is undesirable

• Use cautiously in acute heart failure, recent myocardial infarction, asthma, peptic ulcer, GI spasm, hyperthyroidism, urinary tract obstruction, Parkinson's disease, hypertension, and hypotension.

Administration

• Wash hands before and after applying; don't touch applicator tip to eye or surrounding skin.

Adverse reactions

Ophthalmic: corneal edema or clouding, decompensation
Other: bradycardia, hypotension, flushing, diaphoresis, breathing difficulties

---

polymyxin B sulfate
Polymyxin B Sulfate Sterile

Pregnancy risk category C

Action

Binds to lipids in bacterial cell mem-

---

brane, altering membrane's osmotic barrier and causing leakage of essential metabolites; bactericidal

Availability

Powder for solution: 500,000 units in 20-ml vials

⚕ Indications and dosages

➢ Superficial conjunctival or corneal infections caused by susceptible organisms

Adults: Administration and dosage vary depending on infection.

Contraindications and precautions

• Contraindicated in hypersensitivity to drug or its components, epithelial herpes simplex keratitis, vaccinia, varicella, mycobacterial eye infections, fungal eye diseases, and use of steroid combinations after uncomplicated removal of corneal foreign body

Administration

• Wash hands before and after applying; don't touch applicator tip to eye or surrounding skin.

Adverse reactions

Ophthalmic: transient irritation, burning, stinging, itching, inflammation
Other: hypersensitivity reaction

---

prednisolone acetate
Econopred, Econopred Plus, Pred Forte, Pred Mild

prednisolone sodium phosphate
AK-Pred, Inflamase Forte, Inflamase Mild, Predsol

Pregnancy risk category C

Action

Stimulates synthesis of enzymes required to ease the inflammatory response

Availability

prednisolone acetate
Ophthalmic suspension: 0.12%, 0.125%, 1%
prednisolone sodium phosphate
Ophthalmic solution: 0.125%, 1%

⚕ Indications and dosages

➢ Inflammatory disorders of conjunctiva, cornea, and anterior globe segment; corneal injury; graft rejection
Adults and children: Administration and dosage vary with specific product. See manufacturer's insert.

Contraindications and precautions

• Contraindicated in hypersensitivity to drug or its components; acute epithelial herpes simplex keratitis; fungal eye diseases; vaccinia, varicella, and most other viral eye diseases; ocular tuberculosis; mycobacterial eye infections; acute, purulent, untreated eye infections; and after uncomplicated removal of superficial corneal foreign body

Administration

• Wash hands before and after instilling; don't touch applicator tip to eye or surrounding skin.

Adverse reactions

Ophthalmic: glaucoma with optic nerve damage, visual acuity loss, visual field defects, posterior subcapsular cataract formation, secondary infection, acute uveitis, perforated globe, exacerbation of corneal infection, transient stinging, chemosis, dry eyes, epiphora, photophobia, keratitis, conjunctivitis, corneal ulcers, mydriasis, ptosis, blurring, discharge, pain, foreign body sensation, hyperemia

---

Reactions in **bold** are life-threatening

Other: adrenal suppression (with long-term use), delayed wound healing

scopolamine hydrobromide
Isopto Hyoscine

Pregnancy risk category C

Actions
Blocks responses of iris sphincter muscle and ciliary body muscle to cholinergic stimulation, causing pupillary dilation and paralysis of accommodation

Availability
Ophthalmic solution: 0.25%

🌡 Indications and dosages
➢ To produce cycloplegia and mydriasis in diagnostic procedures
Adults: Instill one or two drops into affected eye(s) 1 hour before procedure.
Children: Instill one drop into affected eye(s) b.i.d. for 2 days before procedure.
➢ Acute inflammatory conditions of iris and uveal tract
Adults: Instill one or two drops into affected eye(s) up to t.i.d.
Children: Instill one drop into affected eye(s) up to t.i.d.

Contraindications and precautions
• Contraindicated in hypersensitivity to drug, its components, or other belladonna alkaloids; primary glaucoma or history of glaucoma; adhesions between iris and lens; and children with a history of severe systemic reaction to atropine

Administration
• Apply pressure to lacrimal sac with finger for 1 to 2 minutes after instilling.

Adverse reactions
Ophthalmic: increased intraocular pressure, visual hallucinations, transient stinging, blurred vision, photophobia, irritation (with prolonged use)
Other: dry mouth; dry skin; tachycardia; headache; parasympathetic stimulation; drowsiness; rash; abdominal distention in infants; high fever; vasodilation; urinary retention; diminished GI motility; decreased secretions of salivary glands, sweat glands, pharynx, bronchi, and nasal passages; **coma; medullary paralysis; death**

silver nitrate
Silver Nitrate

Pregnancy risk category C

Action
Acts on bacterial surface, producing changes in bacterial cell wall and membrane

Availability
Solution: 1% in wax ampules

🌡 Indications and dosages
➢ Prevention of gonorrheal ophthalmia neonatorum
Children: After cleaning neonate's eyes with sterile water, instill two drops into lower conjunctival sac of each eye at angle of nasal bridge and eye.

Contraindications and precautions
• Contraindicated in hypersensitivity to drug or its components

Administration
• Separate eyelids and elevate them to allow solution to contact conjunctival sac and eye for at least 30 seconds. Remove excess solution around eyes.

Adverse reactions
Ophthalmic: mild chemical conjunctivitis, periorbital edema, temporary staining of eyelids and surrounding tissue
Other: none

suprofen
Profenal

Pregnancy risk category C

Action
Blocks cyclooxygenase, an enzyme responsible for synthesis of prostaglandins, which mediate the inflammatory response

Availability
Ophthalmic solution: 1%

Indications and dosages
➣ To inhibit intraoperative miosis
Adults: Instill two drops into conjunctival sac q 4 hours on day before surgery. On day of surgery, instill two drops into conjunctival sac 3 hours, 2 hours, and 1 hour before surgery.

Contraindications and precautions
• Contraindicated in hypersensitivity to drug or its components and in epithelial herpes simplex keratitis
• Use cautiously in bleeding disorders and in sensitivity to nonsteroidal anti-inflammatory drugs.

Administration
• Wash hands before and after instilling; don't touch applicator tip to eye or surrounding skin.

Adverse reactions
Ophthalmic: transient burning, irritation
Other: none

tetracaine
Tetracaine HCl

Pregnancy risk category C

Action
Stabilizes neuronal membrane, making neuron less permeable to ions; this effect prevents nerve impulse initiation and transmission, causing local anesthetic action

Availability
Ophthalmic solution: 0.5%

Indications and dosages
➣ Local anesthesia for tonometry, gonioscopy, removal of corneal foreign bodies or sutures, conjunctival and corneal scraping for diagnosis, anterior chamber paracentesis, and short corneal and conjunctival procedures
Adults: Instill one or two drops into affected eye(s) before procedure.

Contraindications and precautions
• Contraindicated in hypersensitivity to drug, its components, or other ester-type local anesthetics and in prolonged use
• Use cautiously in abnormal or reduced plasma esterase levels, history of allergies, cardiac disease, or hyperthyroidism.

Administration
• Wash hands before and after instilling; don't touch applicator tip to eye or surrounding skin.

Adverse reactions
Ophthalmic: corneal epithelial erosions, poor healing of corneal erosions, severe keratitis, permanent corneal damage, transient stinging, conjunctival redness, descemetitis, iritis

---

Other: CNS depression, hypotension, allergic reaction, **arrhythmias**

tetrahydrozoline hydrochloride

Collyrium Fresh, Geneye, Geneye Extra, Murine Plus, Optigene 3, Tetrasine, Tetrasine EX

Pregnancy risk category C

Action
Produces vasoconstriction through adrenergic action on conjunctival vessels

Availability
Ophthalmic solution: 0.05%

Indications and dosages
➤ Conjunctival congestion, irritation
Adults: Instill one or two drops into eye(s) up to q.i.d.

Contraindications and precautions
• Contraindicated in hypersensitivity to drug, narrow-angle glaucoma, narrow angles without glaucoma, and before peripheral iridectomy in eyes capable of angle closure
• Use cautiously in hypertension, diabetes mellitus, hyperthyroidism, cardiovascular disease, and arteriosclerosis.

Administration
• Wash hands before and after administering; don't touch applicator tip to eye or surrounding skin.

Adverse reactions
Ophthalmic: stinging, blurred vision, mydriasis, increased redness, discomfort, punctate keratitis, lacrimation, increased intraocular pressure

Other: headache, blanching, tremor, diaphoresis, dizziness, nausea, nervousness, drowsiness, weakness, hyperglycemia, palpitations, hypertension, **coronary occlusion, arrhythmias, myocardial infarction, pulmonary embolism, subarachnoid hemorrhage, cerebrovascular accident, death**

timolol maleate

Betimol, Timoptic, Timoptic-XE

Pregnancy risk category C

Action
Unknown; thought to decrease aqueous humor production

Availability
Ophthalmic solution: 0.25%, 0.5%
Ophthalmic solution (gel-forming): 0.25%, 0.5%

Indications
➤ Open-angle glaucoma, ocular hypertension
Adults: Administration and dosage vary with specific product. See manufacturer's insert.

Contraindications and precautions
• Contraindicated in hypersensitivity to drug or its components, heart block, overt heart failure, cardiogenic shock, asthma, or history of asthma or severe chronic obstructive pulmonary disease
• Use cautiously in myasthenia gravis, diabetes mellitus, and hyperthyroidism.

Administration
• Remove patient's contact lenses before administering; may reinsert them 15 minutes later.

Reactions in **bold** are life-threatening

Adverse reactions

Ophthalmic: keratitis, blepharoptosis, blepharitis, visual disturbances, ptosis, ocular irritation, keratitis, decreased corneal sensitivity

Other: palpitations, hypotension, headache, depression, dizziness, syncope, lethargy, hallucinations, confusion, masking of hypoglycemia symptoms in type 1 diabetes mellitus, nausea, dyspnea, alopecia, localized or generalized rash, exacerbation of myasthenia gravis, impotence, decreased libido, diarrhea, hypersensitivity reaction, **arrhythmias, heart failure, cerebrovascular accident, bronchospasm, respiratory failure**

tobramycin
AKTob, Defy, Tobrex

Pregnancy risk category B

Action

Inhibits protein synthesis in susceptible bacteria by binding to 30S ribosomal subunit

Availability

Ophthalmic ointment: 3 mg
Ophthalmic solution: 0.3%

🕭 Indications and dosages

➤ Superficial ocular infections caused by susceptible organisms
Adults: Administration and dosage vary with specific product. See manufacturer's insert.

Contraindications and precautions

• Contraindicated in hypersensitivity to drug or its components, epithelial herpes simplex keratitis, vaccinia, varicella, mycobacterial eye infections, fungal eye diseases, or use of steroid combinations after uncomplicated removal of corneal foreign body

Administration

• Wash hands before and after administering; don't touch applicator tip to eye or surrounding skin.

Adverse reactions

Ophthalmic: transient irritation, inflammation, eyelid itching or swelling, conjunctival erythema, corneal ulcers, conjunctivitis, conjunctival epithelial defects

Other: contact dermatitis, hypersensitivity reaction

travoprost
Travatan

Pregnancy risk category C

Action

Unknown; thought to decrease intraocular pressure by promoting aqueous humor outflow

Availability

Ophthalmic solution: 0.004%

🕭 Indications and dosages

➤ Open-angle glaucoma, ocular hypertension
Adults: Instill one drop into affected eye(s) once daily in evening.

Contraindications and precautions

• Contraindicated in hypersensitivity to drug or its components and in pregnancy
• Use cautiously in active intraocular inflammation.

Administration
• Remove patient's contact lenses before administering; may reinsert them 15 minutes later.

Adverse reactions
Ophthalmic: hyperemia, decreased visual acuity, foreign body sensation, pain, itching, tearing, visual disturbances, blepharitis, cataract, conjunctivitis, keratitis, dry eyes, iris discoloration, subconjunctival hemorrhage
Other: angina pectoris, bradycardia, hypertension, hypotension, anxiety, depression, headache, arthritis, back pain, bronchitis, hypercholesterolemia, infection, sinusitis, urinary incontinence, urinary tract infecttion

trifluridine
Viroptic

Pregnancy risk category C

Action
Unclear; thought to interfere with DNA synthesis, suppressing viral cell replication

Availability
Ophthalmic solution: 1%

Indications and dosages
➤ Herpes simplex keratitis or keratoconjunctivitis
Adults: Instill one drop into affected eye(s) q 2 hours while patient is awake (up to nine drops daily), until corneal ulcer reepithelialization occurs; then instill one drop q 4 hours (at least five drops daily) for 7 more days.

Contraindications and precautions
• Contraindicated in hypersensitivity to or chemical intolerance of drug or its components

Administration
• Wash hands before and after instilling; don't touch applicator tip to eye or surrounding skin.

Adverse reactions
Ophthalmic: transient burning, irritation, hyperemia, palpebral edema, epithelial or superficial punctate keratopathy, stromal edema, keratitis sicca, increased intraocular pressure
Other: hypersensitivity reaction

tropicamide
Mydriacyl, Tropicacyl

Pregnancy risk category C

Action
Blocks responses of iris sphincter muscle and ciliary body muscle to cholinergic stimulation, causing pupillary dilation and paralysis of accommodation

Availability
Ophthalmic solution: 0.5%, 1%

Indications and dosages
➤ To produce mydriasis for funduscopic examination
Adults: Instill one or two drops of 0.5% solution into eye(s) 15 to 20 minutes before examination.
➤ Cycloplegia for refraction
Adults: Instill one or two drops of 1% solution into eye(s); repeat in 5 minutes.

Contraindications and precautions
• Contraindicated in hypersensitivity to drug, its components, or other belladonna alkaloids; primary glaucoma or history of glaucoma; adhesions between iris and lens; and children with history of severe systemic reaction to atropine

---

Reactions in **bold** are life-threatening

• Use cautiously in young children with spastic paralysis or brain damage.

Administration
• Compress lacrimal sac with finger for 1 to 3 minutes after administering.

Adverse reactions
Ophthalmic: increased intraocular pressure, transient burning, irritation, blurred vision, photophobia, visual hallucinations

Other: dry mouth and skin; tachycardia; headache; parasympathetic stimulation; drowsiness; rash; abdominal distention in infants; high fever; vasodilation; urinary retention; diminished GI motility; decreased secretions of salivary glands, sweat glands, pharynx, bronchi, and nasal passages; **coma; medullary paralysis; death**

unoprostone isopropyl
Rescula

Pregnancy risk category C

Action
Unclear; thought to decrease elevated intraocular pressure by promoting aqueous humor outflow

Availability
Ophthalmic solution: 0.15%

⚠ Indications and dosages
➤ Open-angle glaucoma, ocular hypertension
Adults: Instill one drop into affected eye(s) b.i.d. If given with other ophthalmics to lower intraocular pressure, separate administration times by 5 minutes.

Contraindications and precautions
• Contraindicated in hypersensitivity to drug or its components
• Use cautiously in active intraocular inflammation.

Administration
• Remove patient's contact lenses before administering; may reinsert them 15 minutes later.

Adverse reactions
Ophthalmic: ocular burning, itching, pain, discharge, or dryness; corneal lesion, deposits, edema, or opacity; eyelid or iris hyperpigmentation; eyelid disorder; increased number of eyelashes; abnormal vision; foreign body sensation; hemorrhage; lacrimation; blepharitis; conjunctivitis; keratitis; iritis; photophobia; cataract; vitreous disorder; acute intraocular pressure elevation; optic atrophy; ptosis; retinal hemorrhage

Other: flulike symptoms, allergic reaction, back pain, bronchitis, increased cough, diabetes mellitus, dizziness, headache, hypertension, insomnia, pharyngitis, pain, rhinitis, sinusitis

vidarabine
Vira-A

Pregnancy risk category C

Action
Unknown; thought to impede viral DNA synthesis

Availability
Ophthalmic ointment: 3%

⚠ Indications and dosages
➤ Herpes simplex keratitis or keratoconjunctivitis

Reactions in **bold** are life-threatening

Adults: Apply ½" strip of ointment to lower conjunctival sac(s) fives times daily at 3-hour intervals.

Contraindications and precautions
• Hypersensitivity to drug or its components

Administration
• Wash hands before and after applying ointment; don't touch applicator tip to eye or surrounding skin.

Adverse reactions
Ophthalmic: lacrimation, foreign body sensation, conjunctival infection, burning, irritation, superficial punctate keratitis, pain, photophobia, punctal occlusion, sensitivity, uveitis, stromal edema, secondary glaucoma, trophic defects, hyphema, corneal vascularization
Other: none

Drug classes

alkylating agents

busulfan, carboplatin, carmustine, chlorambucil, cisplatin, cyclophosphamide, dacarbazine, ifosfamide, lomustine, mechlorethamine hydrochloride, melphalan hydrochloride, oxaliplatin

Pregnancy risk category D

Action

Crosslink double-stranded DNA and other biologically important macromolecules; this effect causes deactivation of these macromolecules and interferes with replication of cancer cells and other cells (especially those of bone marrow, intestinal epithelium, and hair follicles)

Indications

Leukemias, advanced or metastatic ovarian cancer, brain tumors, multiple myeloma, Hodgkin's disease and other lymphomas, metastatic testicular tumors, advanced bladder cancer, breast cancer, neuroblastoma

Contraindications and precautions

• Contraindicated in hypersensitivity to drug, chronic myelogenous leukemia, severe bone marrow depression, bleeding, radiation therapy, chemotherapy, pregnancy, and breastfeeding

• Use cautiously in chronic lymphocytic leukemia, hearing loss, electrolyte abnormalities, renal or hepatic impairment, active infection, decreased bone marrow reserve, impaired pulmonary function, obesity, severe edema, previous radiation therapy or chemotherapy, concurrent steroid therapy, elderly or debilitated patients, and patients with childbearing potential.

Adverse reactions

CNS: anxiety, depression, dizziness, drowsiness, headache, encephalopathy, mental status changes, asthenia, peripheral neuropathy, ataxia, cranial nerve dysfunction, **seizures, cerebrovascular accident, cerebral hemorrhage, coma**

CV: chest pain, hypotension, hypertension, tachycardia, thrombosis, atrial fibrillation, cardiomegaly, heart block, pericardial effusion, **left-sided heart failure, embolism, cardiac tamponade, arrhythmias**

EENT: retinal hemorrhage, cataract, visual disturbances, ototoxicity, epistaxis, pharyngitis

GI: nausea, vomiting, diarrhea, constipation, abdominal distention and pain, hematemesis, rectal discomfort, pancreatitis, dyspepsia, stomatitis, anorexia, altered taste, dry mouth

GU: oliguria, dysuria, hematuria, increased blood urea nitrogen and creatinine, bladder fibrosis, progressive azotemia, amenorrhea, gynecomastia, gonadal suppression, **nephrotoxicity, hemorrhagic cystitis**

Hematologic: anemia, **bone marrow depression, leukopenia, thrombocytopenia**

Hepatic: hepatomegaly, **hepatitis**

Metabolic: hypokalemia, hypomagnesemia, hypophosphatemia, hyperuricemia, hypocalcemia, hyponatremia, metabolic acidosis

Musculoskeletal: joint pain, back pain, myalgia

Respiratory: pulmonary infiltrates, **pulmonary fibrosis**

Skin: pruritus, rash, acne, alopecia, erythema nodosum, exfoliative dermatitis, hyperpigmentation, urticaria, epidermal necrolysis

---

◁€ Clinical alert   Reactions in **bold** are life-threatening

Other: chills, fever, infection, edema, inflammation at injection site, allergic reaction, **Stevens-Johnson syndrome**

Interactions

Drug-drug. *Allopurinol, cimetidine, thiazide diuretics:* increased bone marrow depression

Anticoagulants, aspirin, nonsteroidal anti-inflammatory drugs: increased risk of bleeding

Cardiotoxic drugs (such as cytarabine, daunorubicin, doxorubicin): additive cardiotoxicity

Digoxin, phenytoin: decreased blood levels of these drugs

Live-virus vaccines: decreased antibody response to vaccine, increased risk of adverse reactions

Nephrotoxic or ototoxic drugs (such as aminoglycosides, loop diuretics): additive nephrotoxicity or ototoxicity

Succinylcholine: prolonged neuromuscular blockade

Drug-diagnostic tests. *Alkaline phosphatase, aspartate aminotransferase, bilirubin, blood urea nitrogen, creatinine, nitrogenous compounds (urea):* increased levels

Electrolytes, hematocrit, hemoglobin, neutrophils, platelets, red blood cells, white blood cells: decreased levels

Drug-food. *Any food:* decreased oral absorption of alkylating agent

Drug-behaviors. *Smoking:* increased risk of pulmonary toxicity

Sun exposure: photosensitivity reaction

Patient monitoring

• Watch for unusual bleeding or bruising, fever, chills, sore throat, cough, shortness of breath, yellowing of skin or eyes, flank or stomach pain, and changes in bladder or bowel function.

alpha-adrenergic blockers

carvedilol, dihydroergotamine mesylate, doxazosin mesylate, ergotamine, phentolamine, prazosin hydrochloride, tamsulosin hydrochloride, terazosin hydrochloride

Pregnancy risk category C

Action

Selectively block postsynaptic alpha$_1$-adrenergic receptors, causing dilation of arterioles and veins, which in turn results in reduced supine and standing blood pressure

Indications

Hypertension, refractory heart failure, peripheral vascular disorders, benign prostatic hypertrophy

Contraindications and precautions

• Contraindicated in hypersensitivity to drug

• Use cautiously in renal insufficiency, angina pectoris, overt heart failure, pregnant or breastfeeding patients, and children (safety not established) and when adding diuretics to drug regimen.

Adverse reactions

CNS: dizziness, headache, asthenia, drowsiness, nervousness, paresthesia, vertigo, fatigue

CV: orthostatic hypotension (with first dose), rebound hypertension, chest pain, palpitations, peripheral edema, tachycardia, **arrhythmias**

EENT: blurred vision, conjunctivitis, nasal congestion, sinusitis

GI: nausea, vomiting, diarrhea, abdominal pain, dry mouth

GU: urinary frequency or incontinence, priapism, impotence

Musculoskeletal: joint, back, or extremity pain
Respiratory: dyspnea
Skin: pruritus
Other: fever, weight gain

Interactions
Drug-drug. *Antihypertensives, nitrates:* additive hypotension
Cimetidine: increased alpha blocker blood level, greater risk of toxicity
Nonsteroidal anti-inflammatory drugs: decreased antihypertensive effect
Drug-diagnostic tests. *Pheochromocytoma screening test:* false-positive result
Sodium, urinary vanillylmandelic acid: increased levels

Patient monitoring
• Monitor electrolyte levels, ECG, and vital signs.

aminoglycosides
amikacin sulfate, gentamicin sulfate, kanamycin, neomycin sulfate, streptomycin sulfate, tobramycin sulfate

Pregnancy risk category D

Action
Bind irreversibly to 30S ribosomal subunit, interfering with initiation complex between messenger RNA and 30S subunit. This results in production of nonfunctional proteins and inability of polyribosomes to synthesize protein.

Indications
Uncomplicated urinary tract infections caused by organisms that resist less toxic drugs, severe systemic or localized infections, infections of superficial skin burns, external ocular infections, endocarditis prophylaxis for GI or GU procedures, respiratory tract infections, *Pseudomonas aeruginosa* infections in cystic fibrosis patients, hepatic encephalopathy, infectious diarrhea, serious gram-negative bacillary infections and staphylococcal infections when penicillins or other less toxic drugs are contraindicated

Contraindications and precautions
• Contraindicated in hypersensitivity to aminoglycosides or bisulfites (found in parenteral products) and intestinal obstruction
• Use cautiously in renal impairment, hepatic disease, hearing impairment, neuromuscular diseases (such as myasthenia gravis), parkinsonism, elderly or obese patients, pregnant or breastfeeding patients, neonates, and premature infants.

Adverse reactions
CNS: dizziness, vertigo, tremor, numbness, depression, confusion, lethargy, nystagmus, headache, paresthesia, **neuromuscular blockade, seizures, neurotoxicity**
CV: hypotension, hypertension, palpitations
EENT: visual disturbances; eye stinging, redness, itching, or dryness; photophobia; tinnitus; hearing loss; ototoxicity; increased salivation
GI: nausea, vomiting, splenomegaly, stomatitis, anorexia
GU: polyuria, dysuria, azotemia, increased urinary excretion of casts, impotence, **nephrotoxicity**
Hematologic: purpura, leukemoid reaction, hemolytic anemia, altered reticulocyte count, eosinophilia, **aplastic anemia, neutropenia, agranulocytosis, leukopenia, thrombocytopenia, pancytopenia**
Hepatic: hepatomegaly; increased alanine aminotransferase (ALT), aspartate aminotransferase (AST), and bilirubin levels; **hepatic necrosis**
Musculoskeletal: joint pain
Respiratory: apnea

◀€ Clinical alert   Reactions in **bold** are life-threatening

Skin: rash, urticaria, pruritus, exfoliative dermatitis, alopecia

Other: weight loss, superinfection, pain, irritation at I.M. injection site

Interactions

Drug-drug. *Acyclovir, amphotericin B, cephalosporins, cisplatin, other aminoglycosides, potent diuretics, vancomycin:* increased nephrotoxicity and ototoxicity

Dimenhydrinate: masking of ototoxicity symptoms

General anesthetics, neuromuscular junction blockers: increased neuromuscular blockade

Indomethacin: increased aminoglycoside trough and peak levels

Parenteral penicillin (ampicillin, ticarcillin): aminoglycoside inactivation

Drug-diagnostic tests. *ALT, AST, bilirubin, blood urea nitrogen, creatinine, lactate dehydrogenase, nonprotein nitrogen:* increased levels

Calcium, granulocytes, hemoglobin, platelets, potassium, sodium, white blood cells: decreased levels

Patient monitoring

• Monitor vital signs and fluid intake and output; increase fluid intake to help prevent renal tubular irritation.

• Monitor drug blood level.

• Assess for ototoxicity by comparing current and baseline audiograms.

amphetamines
(CNS stimulants)

amphetamine, dexmethylphenidate hydrochloride, dextroamphetamine sulfate, methylphenidate hydrochloride, pemoline

Pregnancy risk category C

Action

Release norepinephrine from central adrenergic neurons and cause central stimulation, which increases motor activity and mental alertness, reduces appetite, and lifts mood

Indications

Attention deficit hyperactivity disorder, narcolepsy

Contraindications and precautions

• Contraindicated in hypersensitivity to drug or tartrazine, advanced arteriosclerosis, cardiovascular disease, moderate to severe hypertension, agitation, hyperexcitable states (including hyperthyroidism), suicidal or homicidal tendencies, glaucoma, history of Tourette syndrome or drug abuse, concurrent use of monoamine oxidase (MAO) inhibitors, breastfeeding, and children under age 6

• Use cautiously in mild hypertension, diabetes mellitus, depression, seizures, psychosis, long-term amphetamine use, elderly or debilitated patients, and pregnant patients.

Adverse reactions

CNS: nervousness, insomnia, dizziness, headache, dyskinesia, chorea, drowsiness, hyperactivity, restlessness, tremor, depression, Tourette syndrome, **toxic psychosis**

CV: tachycardia, angina, palpitations, hypertension, hypotension, **arrhythmias**

EENT: blurred vision, poor accommodation

GI: nausea, vomiting, diarrhea, constipation, abdominal pain and cramps, anorexia, dry mouth, metallic taste

GU: impotence, increased libido

Hematologic: anemia, **leukopenia, thrombocytopenia**

Hepatic: hepatic dysfunction, **hepatic coma**

Skin: rash, alopecia, exfoliative dermatitis

Other: fever, weight loss, psychological or physical drug dependence, drug tolerance, abnormal behavior (with abuse)

Interactions

Drug-drug. *Acetazolamide, sodium bicarbonate:* prolonged amphetamine effects

Adrenergics: additive adrenergic effects

Ammonium chloride, ascorbic acid (large doses), haloperidol: decreased amphetamine effects

Anesthetics (including general anesthetics): increased risk of arrhythmias

Antihypertensives, pressors (such as dopamine, epinephrine): decreased efficacy of these drugs

Beta-adrenergic blockers, tricyclic antidepressants (TCAs): increased risk of adverse cardiovascular effects

Coumarin anticoagulants, phenobarbital, phenytoin, primidone, some selective serotonin reuptake inhibitors, TCAs: increased amphetamine blood level

Furazolidone: increased risk of amphetamine toxicity

Insulin: altered insulin requirements

MAO inhibitors: severe hypertensive crisis

Drug-diagnostic tests. *Bilirubin, blood urea nitrogen, creatinine, glucose, hepatic enzymes, potassium, uric acid:* increased levels

Patient monitoring

• Watch for and report fever, diaphoresis, excitation, delirium, tremors, and twitching.

◀᷃ Assess vital signs; stay alert for arrhythmias, tachycardia, hypertension, and cardiovascular changes with psychotic syndrome.

• Stay alert for and report signs of drug abuse.

angiotensin-converting enzyme (ACE) inhibitors

benazepril hydrochloride, captopril, enalapril, fosinopril sodium, lisinopril, moexipril hydrochloride, perindopril erbumine, quinapril hydrochloride, ramipril, trandolapril

Pregnancy risk category C, D (second and third trimesters)

Action

Lower blood pressure by preventing conversion of angiotensin I to angiotensin II, a potent vasoconstrictor that decreases peripheral resistance and aldosterone secretion

Indications

Hypertension, heart failure, left ventricular dysfunction, multiple sclerosis, diabetic neuropathy

Contraindications and precautions

᷃ Contraindicated in hypersensitivity to drug

• Use cautiously in renal or hepatic impairment, hypovolemia, hyponatremia, aortic stenosis and hypertrophic cardiomyopathy, cerebrovascular or cardiac insufficiency, surgery and anesthesia, concurrent diuretic therapy, family history of angioedema, black patients with hypertension, elderly patients, pregnant or breastfeeding patients, and children (safety not established for most ACE inhibitors).

Adverse reactions

CNS: dizziness, fatigue, headache, insomnia, asthenia, drowsiness, vertigo

CV: hypotension, angina pectoris, tachycardia, **myocardial infarction**

EENT: sinusitis

◀᷃ Clinical alert   Reactions in **bold** are life-threatening

GI: nausea, diarrhea, taste disturbances, anorexia
GU: proteinuria, impotence, decreased libido, **renal failure**
Hematologic: bone marrow depression, agranulocytosis
Hepatic: cholestatic jaundice progressing to hepatic necrosis and death
Metabolic: hyperkalemia
Respiratory: cough, bronchitis, eosinophilic pneumonitis, asthma, dyspnea
Skin: rash, angioedema
Other: fever, **anaphylaxis**

Interactions

Drug-drug. *Allopurinol:* increased risk of hypersensitivity reaction
Antacids: decreased ACE inhibitor absorption
Antihypertensives, diuretics, general anesthestics, nitrates, phenothiazines: increased hypotension
Cyclosporine, indomethacin, potassium-sparing diuretics, potassium supplements: hyperkalemia
Digoxin, lithium: increased blood levels of these drugs, greater risk of toxicity
Nonsteroidal anti-inflammatory drugs: blunted response to ACE inhibitor
Drug-diagnostic tests. *Alanine aminotransferase, alkaline phosphatase, aspartate aminotransferase, bilirubin, blood urea nitrogen, creatinine, potassium:* increased levels
Antinuclear antibody: positive titer
Sodium: decreased level
Drug-food. *Salt substitutes containing potassium:* hyperkalemia
Drug-herb. *Capsaicin:* cough
Drug-behaviors. *Acute alcohol ingestion:* additive hypotension

Patient monitoring

• Monitor vital signs, including blood pressure in both arms while lying, standing, and sitting.

• Assess fluid intake and output, electrolyte levels, complete blood count, and kidney and liver function test results.

• Evaluate urine for protein.

• Watch for microalbuminuria, especially in diabetic patients.

anti-Alzheimer's agents (acetylcholinesterase inhibitors)

donepezil hydrochloride, galantamine hydrobromide, rivastigmine tartrate, tacrine hydrochloride

Pregnancy risk category C, B (some agents)

Action

Reversibly inhibit acetylcholinesterase hydrolysis in CNS, which increases acetylcholine level and promotes nerve impulse transmission

Indications

Mild to moderate Alzheimer's disease

Contraindications and precautions

• Contraindicated in hypersensitivity to drug, other carbamates, piperidine derivatives, or acridines; narrow-angle glaucoma; undiagnosed skin lesions; and jaundice associated with previous use of these drugs

• Use cautiously in moderate to severe renal or hepatic dysfunction, GI bleeding, seizures, cardiovascular disease, asthma or chronic obstructive pulmonary disease, impaired urinary outflow, sick sinus syndrome, diabetes mellitus, obesity, history of ulcer, postmenopausal patients, elderly patients, pregnant or breastfeeding patients, and children.

Adverse reactions

CNS: tremor, confusion, insomnia, psychosis, hallucinations, depression, dizziness, headache, anxiety, drowsi-

ness, fatigue, abnormal dreams, irritability, paresthesia, aggression, vertigo, ataxia, restlessness, abnormal crying, nervousness, syncope, aphasia, **seizures**
CV: chest pain, hypotension, hypertension, peripheral edema, vasodilation, atrial fibrillation
EENT: cataract, blurred vision, eye irritation, rhinitis, pharyngitis, toothache, sore throat
GI: nausea, vomiting, diarrhea, constipation, abdominal pain, flatulence, eructation, anorexia
GU: urinary tract infection, urinary incontinence or frequency, increased libido
Metabolic: dehydration, hot flashes
Musculoskeletal: back pain, joint pain, bone fracture, muscle cramps, arthritis
Respiratory: upper respiratory tract infection, cough, bronchitis, dyspnea, influenza
Skin: rash, pruritus, urticaria, diaphoresis, flushing
Other: weight loss, pain, accidental trauma, flulike symptoms

Interactions

Drug-drug. *Anticholinergics:* interference with anticholinergic action
Cholinergics (such as bethanechol): potentiation of anti-Alzheimer's agent
Cimetidine, hormonal contraceptives, isocarboxazid, monoamine oxidase (MAO) inhibitors (including nonselective MAO inhibitors), propranolol, tranylcypromine: increased action of anti-Alzheimer's agent
Ergot derivatives, serotonin receptor agonists: extended vasospastic effects
Nonsteroidal anti-inflammatory drugs (NSAIDs): increased risk of GI bleeding
Selective serotonin reuptake inhibitors: weakness, hyperreflexia, incoordination
Succinylcholine: potentiation of induced neuromuscular blockade during anesthesia

Theophylline: increased theophylline blood level, greater risk of toxicity
Drug-herb. *Jaborandi tree, pill-bearing spurge:* additive effects
S-adenosylmethionine (SAM-e), St. John's wort: serotonin syndrome
Drug-behaviors. *Smoking:* increased drug clearance, decreased drug blood level

Patient monitoring

• Assess for severe nausea, vomiting, and diarrhea (which may lead to dehydration and weight loss).

◀ Watch closely for adverse effects in patients with a history of GI bleeding, arrhythmias, seizures, pulmonary conditions, or NSAID use.

• Monitor alanine aminotransferase level weekly during first 18 weeks of therapy.

antianginals

amlodipine besylate, amyl nitrite, bepridil hydrochloride, diltiazem hydrochloride, isosorbide dinitrate, isosorbide mononitrate, nadolol, nicardipine hydrochloride, nifedipine, nitroglycerin, propranolol hydrochloride, verapamil, verapamil hydrochloride

Pregnancy risk category C

Action

Nitrate antianginals (such as amyl nitrate, isosorbide, and nitroglycerin) stimulate production of cyclic guanosine monophosphate within cells, causing skeletal muscle relaxation. Postcapillary vessels dilate, reducing venous return to heart; arteriolar relaxation reduces systemic vascular resistance and afterload. These changes decrease myocardial oxygen requirements and improve blood flow redistribution

---

through collateral channels in myocardial tissue.

Calcium channel blockers (such as amlodipine, bepridil, diltiazem, nadolol, nicardipine, propranolol, and verapamil) inhibit calcium influx through cell membranes, depressing automaticity and conduction velocity in cardiac muscle; this action in turn decreases myocardial contraction. These agents also reduce total peripheral resistance and decrease amplitude, depolarization rate, and conduction in atria.

Indications
Acute angina pectoris

Contraindications and precautions
• Contraindicated in hypersensitivity to drug, sick sinus syndrome, second- or third-degree atrioventricular (AV) block (unless artificial pacemaker is in place), systolic blood pressure below 90 mmHg, heart failure, severe ventricular dysfunction, cardiogenic shock (unless associated with supraventricular tachyarrhythmias), and concurrent use of I.V. beta-adrenergic blockers
• Use cautiously in severe renal or hepatic impairment; hypotension; pulmonary disease (including asthma); diabetes mellitus; thyrotoxicosis; history of serious ventricular arrhythmias, heart failure, porphyria, or severe allergic reactions; elderly patients; pregnant or breastfeeding patients; and children.

Adverse reactions
CNS: anxiety, confusion, dizziness, light-headedness, drowsiness, headache, nervousness, insomnia, abnormal dreams, psychiatric disturbances, asthenia, paresthesia, tremor, fatigue, depression, syncope, memory loss, mental status changes
CV: bradycardia, chest pain, hypotension, orthostatic hypotension, palpitations, peripheral edema, peripheral vasoconstriction, tachycardia, **arrhythmias, heart failure**
EENT: blurred vision, dry eyes, tinnitus, epistaxis, disturbed equilibrium, nasal stuffiness, gingival hyperplasia
GI: nausea, vomiting, diarrhea, constipation, dyspepsia, dry mouth, anorexia
GU: dysuria, nocturia, polyuria, sexual dysfunction, decreased libido, gynecomastia
Hematologic: anemia, **leukopenia, thrombocytopenia**
Hepatic: abnormal liver function studies
Metabolic: hyperglycemia, hypoglycemia
Musculoskeletal: joint stiffness and pain, muscle cramps, back pain
Respiratory: cough, dyspnea, wheezing, **bronchospasm, pulmonary edema**
Skin: dermatitis, erythema multiforme, flushing, diaphoresis, photosensitivity, pruritus, urticaria
Other: lupuslike syndrome, weight gain, **Stevens-Johnson syndrome**

Interactions
Drug-drug. *Amphetamines, ephedrine, epinephrine, norepinephrine, phenylephrine, pseudoephedrine:* unopposed alpha-adrenergic stimulation (excessive hypertension, bradycardia)
Antihypertensives, fentanyl, other nitrates, quinidine: additive hypotension
Beta-adrenergic blockers, digoxin, disopyramide, phenytoin: bradycardia, conduction defects, heart failure
Calcium, vitamin D: decreased antianginal efficacy
Carbamazepine, cyclosporine, prazosin, quinidine: decreased metabolism of these drugs, greater risk of toxicity
Clonidine: increased hypotension and bradycardia
Digoxin: additive bradycardia
Diltiazem, general anesthetics, phenytoin (I.V.): additive myocardial depression

Dobutamine, dopamine: reduced beneficial beta-cardiovascular effects of these drugs

Insulin, oral hypoglycemics: altered efficacy of these drugs

Lithium: altered lithium blood level

Monoamine oxidase (MAO) inhibitors: hypertension

Nondepolarizing neuromuscular blockers: increased muscle-paralyzing effects

Nonsteroidal anti-inflammatory drugs: decreased anti-inflammatory action

Rifampin, theophylline: decreased efficacy of these drugs

Drug-diagnostic tests. *Antinuclear antibody:* increased titer

Blood urea nitrogen, glucose, lipoproteins, potassium, triglycerides, uric acid: increased levels

Drug-food. *Caffeine-containing foods and beverages:* increased caffeine blood level

Grapefruit juice: increased drug blood level and effects

Drug-herb. *Black catechu:* additive effects

Caffeine-containing herbs (cola nut, guarana, yerba maté): increased caffeine blood level

Yerba maté: decreased yerba maté clearance

Drug-behaviors. *Alcohol use:* additive hypotension

Cocaine use: unopposed alpha-adrenergic stimulation (excessive hypertension, bradycardia)

Patient monitoring

• Monitor vital signs; assess for sensitivity to drug's hypotensive effects (indicated by nausea, vomiting, pallor, restlessness, and cardiovascular collapse).

◀€ In patients with severe obstructive coronary artery disease, monitor closely for increased frequency, duration, or severity of angina or acute myocardial infarction when calcium channel blocker therapy begins and when dosage is increased.

antiarrhythmics

adenosine, amiodarone hydrochloride, bretylium tosylate, digoxin, disopyramide phosphate, dofetilide, esmolol, flecainide acetate, lidocaine hydrochloride, mexiletine, moricizine hydrochloride, phenytoin, phenytoin sodium, procainamide hydrochloride, propafenone hydrochloride, propranolol hydrochloride, quinidine gluconate, quinidine polygalacturonate, quinidine sulfate, sotalol hydrochloride, tocainide hydrochloride, verapamil hydrochloride

Pregnancy risk category C

Action

Antiarrhythmics are classified based on their action on cardiac muscle. *Class I* antiarrhythmics decrease rate of sodium entry during depolarization, reduce rate of action potential, and lengthen effective refractory period of fast-response fibers. Class I antiarrhythmics fall into three subdivisions. *Class IA* drugs (such as disopyramide, procainamide, and quinidine) depress phase 0 and lengthen the action potential. *Class IB* drugs (such as lidocaine, phenytoin, and tocainide) somewhat depress phase 0 and shorten the action potential. *Class IC* drugs (such as flecainide and propafenone) greatly depress phase 0 and slow conduction. Moricizine shares properties of IA, IB, and IC antiarrhythmics.

Class II antiarrhythmics (such as propranolol) block beta-adrenergic receptors competitively and depress phase 4 depolarization.

Class III antiarrhythmics (such as amiodarone, bretylium, dofetilide, ibutilide, and sotalol) prolong the action potential duration but don't affect the polarization phase or resting membrane potential.

Class IV antiarrhythmics (calcium channel blockers, such as diltiazem and verapamil) slow conduction velocity and enhance atrioventricular (AV) node refractoriness.

Indications
Arrhythmias, premature ventricular tachycardia, atrial flutter, atrial fibrillation, AV heart block

Contraindications and precautions
• Contraindicated in hypersensitivity to drug, congenital or acquired long-QT syndrome, baseline QT or QTc interval above 440 msec, severe renal impairment, sick sinus syndrome, second- or third-degree AV block (unless artificial pacemaker is in place), systolic pressure below 90 mmHg, recent myocardial infarction or pulmonary congestion, pulmonary hypertension, aortic stenosis, digoxin toxicity, pregnancy, breastfeeding, and neonates
• Use cautiously in renal or hepatic impairment, enlarged prostate, myasthenia gravis, glaucoma, diabetes mellitus, conduction abnormalities, potassium imbalance, ventricular arrhythmias, ventricular tachycardia, history of serious ventricular arrhythmias or heart failure, elderly patients, and children (safety not established).

Adverse reactions
CNS: dizziness, agitation, depression, fatigue, headache, nervousness, acute psychosis, syncope, malaise, insomnia, ataxia, involuntary movements, paresthesia, peripheral neuropathy, incoordination, tremor, abnormal dreams, anxiety, confusion, light-headedness, drowsiness, jitteriness, psychiatric disturbances, tremor
CV: chest pain, bradycardia, palpitations, peripheral edema, tachycardia, hypotension, heart failure, heart block, arrhythmias or worsening of arrhythmias
EENT: blurred vision, narrow-angle glaucoma, corneal microdeposits, optic neuritis or neuropathy, photophobia, dry eyes, tinnitus, disturbed equilibrium, epistaxis, dry nose, altered smell perception, gingival hyperplasia
GI: nausea, vomiting, diarrhea, constipation, bloating, flatulence, abdominal pain, dry mouth, anorexia
GU: dysuria, nocturia, polyuria, urinary hesitancy, urinary retention, urinary frequency, impotence, decreased libido, epididymitis, sexual dysfunction
Hematologic: anemia, decreased hemoglobin and hematocrit, **leukopenia, thrombocytopenia, agranulocytosis**
Hepatic: jaundice, hepatic dysfunction
Metabolic: hypoglycemia, hypokalemia, hypothyroidism, hyperthyroidism
Musculoskeletal: muscle weakness, aches, or cramps; joint stiffness
Respiratory: cough, dyspnea, pneumonia, pulmonary fibrosis, **adult respiratory distress syndrome**
Skin: rash, pruritus, alopecia, flushing, dermatosis, photosensitivity, bluish skin discoloration, toxic epidermal necrolysis
Other: edema, weight gain, **Stevens-Johnson syndrome**

Interactions
Drug-drug. *Amiloride, azole antifungals, cimetidine, cyclosporine, dextromethorphan, erythromycin, inhibitors of renal cationic secretion (such as megestrol, prochlorperazine), ketoconazole, macrolide antibiotics, metformin, methotrexate, nefazodone, norfloxacin, phenytoin, protease inhibitors, quinine, ranitidine, selective serotonin reuptake inhibitors (SSRIs), sulfamethoxazole, theophylline, triamterene, trimethoprim, verapamil, zafirlukast:* increased blood levels of these drugs

Beta-adrenergic blockers: increased risk of bradyarrhythmias, sinus arrest, or AV heart block

Calcium, vitamin D: decreased efficacy of these drugs

Carbamazepine, cyclosporine: decreased antiarrhythmic metabolism and increased risk of toxicity

Cholestyramine, phenytoin, rifampin: decreased blood levels of these drugs

Digoxin: increased risk of digoxin toxicity

Fentanyl: additive hypotension

Lithium, theophylline: increased or decreased effects of these drugs

Metoprolol: increased risk of adverse cardiovascular effects

Neuromuscular blockers: increased muscle-paralyzing effects of these drugs

Nonsteroidal anti-inflammatory drugs: decreased antiarrhythmic effect

Volatile anesthetics: increased risk of myocardial depression

Warfarin: increased warfarin activity

Drug-diagnostic tests. *Blood urea nitrogen, creatinine, hepatic enzymes, lipids:* increased levels

Glucose, hemoglobin, hematocrit: decreased levels

Drug-food. *Caffeine-containing foods and beverages:* increased caffeine blood level

Grapefruit juice: increased drug blood level and effects

Drug-herb. *Aloe, buckthorn bark or berry, cascara sagrada bark, rhubarb root:* increased potassium loss, causing increased antiarrhythmic effects

Black catechu: additive effects

Caffeine-containing herbs (such as cola nut, guarana, yerba maté): increased caffeine blood level

Jimsonweed: adverse cardiovascular effects

Yerba maté: decreased yerba maté clearance

Drug-behaviors. *Alcohol use:* additive hypotension

Patient monitoring

• Monitor antiarrhythmic blood level.

• Assess blood pressure and pulse; report heart rate below 50 or above 120 beats/minute.

• Monitor blood glucose and electrolyte levels and liver and kidney function test results.

◀€ Closely monitor extent of palpitations; stay alert for fluttering or missed heartbeats, chest pain, and fainting episodes. Obtain ECG to document arrhythmias.

anticholinergics

atropine sulfate, benztropine mesylate, biperiden, dicyclomine hydrochloride, glycopyrrolate, hyoscyamine, hyoscyamine sulfate, ipratropium bromide, propantheline bromide scopolamine hydrobromide

Pregnancy risk category B

Action

Block action of acetylcholine in CNS and on autonomic effectors; also block vagal effects on sinoatrial and atrioventricular nodes, causing heart rate to increase. Small doses decrease salivary and bronchial secretions and reduce sweating; intermediate doses cause pupil dilation, inhibit accommodation, and increase heart rate; large doses decrease GI and GU motility; even higher doses reduce gastric acid secretion.

Indications

Bradyarrhythmias, symptomatic bradycardia, peptic ulcer disease, acute iritis, cycloplegic refraction, pylorospasm, small intestine hypertoxicity, colonic hypermotility, bronchial spasm, parkinsonism, spastic bladder, mild dysentery, diverticulitis, infant colic, biliary and renal colic, pancreati-

---

◀€ Clinical alert   Reactions in **bold** are life-threatening

tis, acute rhinitis, sialorrhea, hyperhidrosis, anticholinesterase poisoning,
cystitis, heart block caused by vagal activity. Also used to control gastric secretions and block cardiac vagal reflexes preoperatively, promote diagnostic
hypotonic duodenography, and increase radiologic visibility of kidney.

Contraindications and precautions

• Contraindicated in hypersensitivity
to drug, GI or GU tract obstruction,
reflux esophagitis, severe ulcerative colitis, glaucoma, myasthenia gravis, intestinal atony, unstable cardiovascular
status in acute hemorrhage, tachycardia secondary to cardiac insufficiency
or thyrotoxicosis, toxic megacolon, GI
infection, severe prostatic hypertrophy,
bladder neck obstruction, bronchial
asthma, chronic obstructive pulmonary disease, arrhythmias, breastfeeding, and infants under age 6 months
• Use cautiously in alcohol, sulfite, or
tartrazine intolerance; high environmental temperatures; hepatic or renal
impairment; autonomic neuropathy;
prostatic hypertrophy; hyperthyroidism; coronary disease; arrhythmias;
heart failure; hypertension; hiatal hernia; ulcerative colitis; brain damage;
Down syndrome; spasticity; phenylketonuria; elderly patients; pregnant patients (safety not established); neonates; and immature infants.

Adverse reactions

CNS: asthenia, nervousness, insomnia,
drowsiness, dizziness, headache, confusion, stimulation
CV: palpitations, tachycardia
EENT: dilated pupils, blurred vision,
photophobia, increased intraocular
pressure, loss of taste
GI: nausea, vomiting, constipation, abdominal distention, epigastric distress,
heartburn, gastroesophageal reflux, dry
mouth, **paralytic ileus**

GU: urinary hesitancy or retention,
impotence, lactation suppression
Skin: urticaria, decreased sweating
Other: fever, irritation at I.M. injection
site, allergic reaction, **anaphylaxis**

Interactions

Drug-drug. *Adsorbent antidiarrheals,
antacids:* decreased anticholinergic absorption
*Amantadine, antiarrhythmics, antidys-
kinetics, antihistamines, antiparkinsonian drugs, disopyramide, glutethimide,
meperidine, muscle relaxants, phenothiazines, quinidine, tricyclic antidepressants (TCAs):* increased anticholinergic
effects and additive adverse effects
Antimyasthenic drugs: decreased intestinal motility
Cyclopropane anesthetics: increased
risk of ventricular arrhythmias and
other adverse cardiovascular effects
Haloperidol: decreased antipsychotic
effect
Ketoconazole, levodopa: decreased absorption of these drugs
Methotrimeprazine: increased risk of
extrapyramidal effects
Metoclopramide: decreased effect on GI
motility
Potassium chloride (oral): increased GI
mucosal lesions
Oral drugs: altered absorption of these
drugs
Drug-herb. *Angel's trumpet, jimsonweed, scopolia:* increased anticholinergic effects
Jaborandi tree, pill-bearing spurge: de-
creased drug effects
Drug-behaviors. *Alcohol use:* increased
CNS depression
Sun exposure: photophobia

Patient monitoring

• Closely monitor vital signs and urine
output.

anticoagulants

argatroban, bivalirudin, dalteparin sodium, danaparoid sodium, enoxaparin sodium, heparin calcium, heparin sodium, tinzaparin sodium, warfarin sodium

Pregnancy risk category B

Action

Interfere with one or more parts of pathways that lead to formation of stable fibrin clot; may inhibit coagulation factors, bind to antithrombin, cause release of tissue factor pathway inhibitors, and prevent conversion of fibrinogen to fibrin

Indications

Treatment or prophylaxis of venous thrombosis, pulmonary embolism, atrial fibrillation with embolization, myocardial infarction, or thromboembolic events (including deep-vein thrombosis); prevention of thrombus formation and embolization after prosthetic valve placement; during cardiovascular surgery; after abdominal surgery or total hip or knee replacement surgery

Contraindications and precautions

• Contraindicated in hypersensitivity to drug, uncontrolled bleeding; active major bleeding, or thrombocytopenia caused by antiplatelet antibodies associated with low-molecular-weight heparins
• Use cautiously in severe hepatic or renal disease; hypertensive or diabetic retinopathy; untreated or severe uncontrolled hypertension; hemorrhagic stroke; severe thrombocytopenia; active GI bleeding or ulcers or recent history of ulcer disease; cancer; bacterial endocarditis; history of congenital or acquired bleeding disorder; recent brain, spinal, or ophthalmic surgery; spinal or epidural anesthesia; patients weighing less than 45 kg (99 lb); elderly patients; pregnant or breastfeeding patients; and children (safety not established).

Adverse reactions

CNS: headache, dizziness, insomnia, confusion, **spinal hematoma, cerebral or intracranial bleeding**
CV: hypotension, hypertension, tachycardia, angina pectoris, **arrhythmias, pulmonary embolism, thromboembolism, myocardial infarction**
EENT: ocular hemorrhage, rhinitis, epistaxis
GI: nausea, vomiting, constipation, anorectal bleeding, melena, flatulence, hematemesis, dyspepsia, retroperitoneal or intra-abdominal bleeding, **GI hemorrhage**
GU: dysuria, hematuria, urinary tract infection, urinary retention, **vaginal hemorrhage**
Hematologic: purpura, anemia, **granulocytopenia, thrombocytopenia, agranulocytosis, pancytopenia, hemorrhage**
Hepatic: hepatitis
Musculoskeletal: back pain
Respiratory: dyspnea, pneumonia, respiratory disorder
Skin: bulbous eruption, cellulitis, injection site or wound hematoma, pruritus, rash, skin necrosis, urticaria, alopecia
Other: hypersensitivity reaction, fever, pain, infection, dependent edema, impaired healing, **congenital anomalies, fetal distress, fetal death**

Interactions

Drug-drug. *Abciximab, acetaminophen (chronic use), androgens, aspirin, capecitabine, cefamandole, cefoperazone, cefotetan, chloral hydrate, chloramphenicol, clopidogrel, disulfiram, eptifibatide,* *fluconazole, fluoroquinolones, itraconazole, metronidazole (including vaginal use), nonsteroidal anti-inflammatory drugs, plicamycin, quinidine, quinine, sulfonamides, thrombolytics, ticlopidine, tirofiban:* increased response to anticoagulant, greater risk of bleeding

Antihistamines, barbiturates, digoxin, hormonal contraceptives containing estrogen, tetracyclines: decreased anticoagulant effect

Drugs that cause hypoprothrombinemia (such as cefamandole, cefmetazole, cefoperazone, cefotetan, plicamycin, quinidine, thrombolytics): increased risk of bleeding

Streptokinase: relative resistance to anticoagulant

Drug-diagnostic tests. *Alanine aminotransferase, aspartate aminotransferase, International Normalized Ratio, partial thromboplastin time, prothrombin time:* increased values

Drug-food. *Large intake of foods high in vitamin K:* antagonism of anticoagulant effect

Drug-herb. *Anise, arnica, asafetida, bromelain, chamomile, clove, danshen, devil's claw, dong quai, fenugreek, feverfew, garlic, ginger, ginkgo, ginseng, horse chestnut, licorice, meadowsweet, motherwort, mushroom, onion, papain, parsley, passionflower, quassia, red clover, reishi, rue, sweet clover, turmeric, white willow:* increased bleeding risk

Coenzyme Q10, green tea, St. John's wort: decreased anticoagulant effect

Drug-behaviors. *Alcohol use:* enhanced anticoagulant activity

Smoking: decreased anticoagulant effect

Patient monitoring

◄€ Watch for unusual bleeding or bruising and tarry stools.

• Assess baseline coagulation tests and complete blood count with white cell differential.

• Monitor venipuncture sites for bleeding, hematoma, and inflammation.

anticonvulsants

carbamazepine, clonazepam, clorazepate dipotassium, diazepam, divalproex sodium, fosphenytoin sodium, gabapentin, lamotrigine, levetiracetam, magnesium sulfate, oxcarbazepine, pentobarbital, phenobarbital sodium, phenytoin sodium, primidone, tiagabine hydrochloride, topiramate, valproate sodium, valproic acid, zonisamide

Pregnancy risk category C, A (magnesium sulfate), *D* (some anticonvulsants)

Action

Selectively depress hyperactive brain areas responsible for seizures

Indications

Prophylaxis and treatment of status epilepticus and generalized tonic-clonic, mixed, petit mal, petit mal variant, akinetic, complex-partial, and myoclonic seizures; management of panic disorder, trigeminal neuralgia, migraine, anxiety, psychoneurotic reactions, and alcohol withdrawal; skeletal muscle relaxation for endoscopy or cardioversion

Contraindications and precautions

• Contraindicated in hypersensitivity to drug or intolerance of alcohol, propylene glycol, tartrazine, or tricyclic antidepressants; bone marrow depression; severe hepatic disease; and monoamine oxidase (MAO) inhibitor use within 14 days

• Use cautiously in hepatic or renal disease, severe cardiac or respiratory disease, coma, acute or chronic pain, fever, hyperthyroidism, diabetes mellitus, severe anemia, uremia, narrow-angle glaucoma, CNS depression, sinus bradycardia, sinoatrial block, second- or third-degree heart block, Stokes-Adams syndrome, obesity, history of suicide attempt or drug abuse, elderly or debilitated patients, and pregnant or breastfeeding patients.

Adverse reactions

CNS: dizziness, drowsiness, lethargy, sedation, depression, apathy, fatigue, light-headedness, syncope, disorientation, anger, hostility, manic or hypomanic episodes, restlessness, confusion, crying, delirium, headache, slurred speech, dysarthria, stupor, rigidity, tremor, dystonia, vertigo, euphoria, nervousness, poor concentration, vivid dreams, psychomotor retardation, paresthesia, extrapyramidal symptoms, mild paradoxical stimulation during first 2 weeks of therapy

CV: hypertension, hypotension, aggravation of coronary artery disease, palpitations, bradycardia, tachycardia, **cardiovascular collapse, heart failure, arrhythmias, atrioventricular block**

EENT: blurred vision, diplopia, corneal opacities, nystagmus and other abnormal eye movements, conjunctivitis, pharyngeal dryness, increased salivation

GI: nausea, vomiting, diarrhea, constipation, abdominal pain, dysphagia, gastric disorders, stomatitis, glossitis, dry mouth, anorexia

GU: urinary hesitancy, retention, frequency, or incontinence; albuminuria; glycosuria; dysuria; nocturia; menstrual irregularities; libido changes; impotence; gynecomastia

Hematologic: eosinophilia, **leukopenia, agranulocytosis, aplastic anemia, thrombocytopenia**

Hepatic: hepatitis

Metabolic: syndrome of inappropriate antidiuretic hormone secretion

Musculoskeletal: muscle rigidity

Respiratory: pneumonitis

Skin: photosensitivity, rash, urticaria, diaphoresis, erythema multiforme

Other: chills, fever, hiccups, weight changes, edema, lymphadenopathy, physical and psychological drug dependence, drug tolerance, **Stevens-Johnson syndrome**

Interactions

Drug-drug. *Acetaminophen:* increased risk of hepatotoxicity

Amiodarone, benzodiazepines, chloramphenicol, cimetidine, disulfiram, estrogens, felbamate, fluconazole, fluoxetine, halothane, influenza vaccine, isoniazid, itraconazole, ketoconazole, methylphenidate, miconazole, omeprazole, phenothiazines, phenylbutazone, salicylates, sulfonamides, tolbutamide, trazodone: increased anticonvulsant blood level and effects

Antacids, calcium, sucralfate: decreased absorption of oral anticonvulsant

Antidepressants, antihistamines, opioids, sedative-hypnotics: additive CNS depression

Barbiturates, reserpine: decreased anticonvulsant blood level and effects

Carbamazepine, chloramphenicol, clonazepam, corticosteroids, cyclosporine, dacarbazine, felodipine, griseofulvin, hormonal contraceptives, metronidazole, quinidine, theophylline, tricyclic antidepressants, verapamil, warfarin: decreased efficacy of these drugs

Corticosteroids, cyclosporine, doxycycline, estrogens, felbamate, methadone, quinidine, rifampin, streptozocin, theophylline: altered effects of these drugs

Cyclophosphamide: increased risk of hematologic toxicity

Dopamine: additive hypotension

Lidocaine, propranolol: additive cardiac depression

MAO inhibitors: decreased anticonvulsant metabolism and increased effects

---

Other CNS depressants (such as antihistamines, opioids): additive CNS depression

Drug-diagnostic tests. *Alkaline phosphatase, gamma-glutamyltransferase, glucose:* increased levels

Dexamethasone suppression test, metyrapone: interference with test results

Potassium, thyroxine: decreased levels

Drug-food. *Enteral tube feedings:* decreased drug absorption

Folic acid: decreased folic acid absorption

Grapefruit juice: increased anticonvulsant blood level and effects

Drug-herb. *Chamomile, hops, kava, skullcap, valerian:* increased CNS depression

Plantain (psyllium seed): inhibited GI absorption of drug

St. John's wort: decreased drug effects

Drug-behaviors. *Acute alcohol ingestion:* increased anticonvulsant blood level and effects

Alcohol use: additive CNS depression

Chronic alcohol ingestion: decreased anticonvulsant blood level and effects

Sun exposure: photophobia

Patient monitoring

• Monitor complete blood count, glucose and uric acid levels, urinalysis, and kidney and liver function test results.

◀€ With I.V. use, watch closely for respiratory depression and cardiovascular collapse.

• Monitor for sore throat, easy bruising, bleeding, and epistaxis.

• Stay alert for oversedation.

antidepressants

amitriptyline hydrochloride, amitriptyline pamoate, amoxapine, bupropion hydrochloride, citalopram hydrobromide, clomipramine hydrochloride, desipramine hydrochloride, doxepin hydrochloride, escitalopram oxalate, fluoxetine hydrochloride, fluvoxamine maleate, imipramine hydrochloride, mirtazapine, nefazodone hydrochloride, nortriptyline hydrochloride, paroxetine hydrochloride, phenelzine, sertraline hydrochloride, tranylcypromine sulfate, trazodone hydrochloride, trimipramine maleate, venlafaxine hydrochloride

Pregnancy risk category C, B (some antidepressants), *D* (imipramine)

Action

Produce changes in serotonin or norepinephrine receptor systems that help regulate these systems

Indications

Endogenous and reactive depression, including depression associated with anxiety and sleep disturbances

Contraindications and precautions

• Contraindicated in hypersensitivity to drug

• Use cautiously in cardiovascular disease; hypertension; hepatic or renal impairment; severe depression; increased intraocular pressure; narrow-angle glaucoma; hyperthyroidism; prostatic hypertrophy; acute recovery phase after myocardial infarction (MI); suicidal tendencies; electroshock therapy; elective surgery; history of seizures, neurologic impairment, mania, or drug abuse; pregnant or breastfeeding patients; and children under age 18.

Adverse reactions

CNS: lethargy, sedation, hallucinations, delusions, disorientation, nervousness, EEG changes, fatigue, peripheral neuropathy, anxiety, insomnia, restlessness, drowsiness, dizziness, syncope, extrapyramidal effects, **neuroleptic malignant syndrome, seizures, coma, cerebrovascular accident (CVA)**

CV: hypotension, hypertension, ECG changes, tachycardia, palpitations, chest pain, **arrhythmias, MI**

EENT: visual disturbances, blurred vision, dry eyes, mydriasis, increased intraocular pressure, tinnitus, rhinitis, altered taste

GI: nausea, vomiting, diarrhea, constipation, epigastric or abdominal pain, dyspepsia, dry mouth, anorexia, **paralytic ileus**

GU: urinary frequency or retention, gynecomastia, sexual dysfunction

Hematologic: leukopenia, agranulocytosis, thrombocytopenia

Hepatic: hepatitis

Metabolic: blood glucose changes

Skin: rash, urticaria, diaphoresis, bruising, pruritus, photosensitivity

Other: edema, chills, yawning, increased appetite, weight changes, hypersensitivity reaction

Interactions

Drug-drug. *Adrenergics, anticholinergics, anticholinergic-like drugs:* additive adverse effects

Amiodarone, cimetidine, hormonal contraceptives, phenothiazines, quinidine, ritonavir: increased antidepressant blood level and risk of toxicity

Anticoagulants: increased hypoprothrombinemia

Antihistamines, atropine, disopyramide, haloperidol, quinidine: additive anticholinergic effects

Antithyroid agents: increased risk of agranulocytosis

Ascorbic acid: decreased antidepressant efficacy

Barbiturates: altered antidepressant blood level and effects

Carbamazepine, class IC antiarrhythmics, phenothiazines: altered effects of both drugs

Clonidine: hypertensive crisis

CNS depressants (such as antihistamines, opioids, sedative-hypnotics): additive CNS depression

Decongestants, vasoconstrictors: additive adrenergic effects

Levodopa: delayed or decreased levodopa absorption, hypertension

Lithium: additive serotonergic effects

Monoamine oxidase inhibitors: hypotension, tachycardia, death

Moxifloxacin, sparfloxacin: increased risk of adverse cardiovascular effects

Rifabutin, rifampin, rifapentine: decreased antidepressant blood level and effects

Drug-diagnostic tests. *Alanine aminotransferase, alkaline phosphatase, aspartate aminotransferase, bilirubin, blood urea nitrogen, cholesterol, creatinine, uric acid:* increased levels

Glucose, phosphate, potassium: increased or decreased levels

Sodium: decreased level

Drug-food. *Enteral tube feedings:* decreased drug absorption

Folic acid: decreased folic acid absorption

Grapefruit juice: increased antidepressant blood level and effects

Drug-herb. *Belladonna leaf:* additive cholinergic effects

Chamomile, hops, kava, skullcap, valerian: increased CNS depression

Evening primrose: exacerbation of temporal lobe epilepsy or schizophrenia

Henbane leaf: increased anticholinergic effects

S-adenosylmethionine (SAM-e), St. John's wort: increased risk of adverse

serotonergic effects (including serotonin syndrome)
Drug-behaviors. *Alcohol use:* increased CNS depression
Smoking: increased metabolism and altered effects of drug
Sun exposure: increased risk of photosensitivity reaction

Patient monitoring
• Monitor complete blood count, blood glucose level, and kidney and liver function test results.
◀€ Assess ECG and heart sounds. Watch for tachycardia and an increase in angina attacks (which may precede MI or CVA).
• Evaluate neurologic function.
• Monitor for sleep disturbances, lethargy, apathy, impaired thought processes, and lack of therapeutic response.
• Check results of periodic eye examinations; report vision changes, headache, halos, eye pain, dilated pupils, or nausea.

antifungals
amphotericin B, caspofungin acetate, fluconazole, flucytosine, griseofulvin, itraconazole, ketoconazole, miconazole, nystatin, terbinafine hydrochloride, voriconazole

Pregnancy risk category B

Action
Varies with specific drug. See individual monographs.

Indications
Meningitis, visceral leishmaniasis in immunocompetent patients, invasive fungal infections, oral and perioral candidal infections, GI tract infections caused by *Candida albicans*, systemic fungal infections (histoplasmosis, coccidioidomycosis, blastomycosis, cryptococcosis, phycomycosis, disseminated candidiasis, zygomycosis)

Contraindications and precautions
• Contraindicated in hypersensitivity to antifungals and concurrent use of cisapride or pimozide
• Use cautiously in renal, hepatic, or cardiac disease; achlorhydria; pregnant or breastfeeding patients; and children under age 2.

Adverse reactions
CNS: anxiety, confusion, headache, insomnia, asthenia, abnormal thinking, anxiety, agitation, depression, dizziness, hallucinations, hypertonia, psychosis, drowsiness, speech disorder, stupor, transient vertigo, malaise, **seizures**
CV: hypotension, orthostatic hypotension, hypertension, tachycardia, phlebitis, chest pain, vasodilation, bradycardia, supraventricular tachycardia, **cardiac arrest, asystole, atrial fibrillation, shock**
EENT: diplopia, amblyopia, blurred vision, eye hemorrhage, hearing loss, tinnitus, epistaxis, rhinitis, sinusitis, pharyngitis, gingivitis, oral candidiasis
GI: nausea, vomiting, diarrhea, abdominal pain, abdominal distention, melena, stomatitis, dry mouth, anorexia, **GI hemorrhage**
GU: hematuria, albuminuria, dysuria, glycosuria, oliguria, urinary incontinence or retention, abnormal renal function with hypokalemia, **renal failure**
Hematologic: eosinophilia, leukocytosis, anemia, **thrombocytopenia, leukopenia, agranulocytosis**
Hepatic: jaundice, hyperbilirubinemia, abnormal liver function tests, **acute hepatic failure, hepatitis**
Metabolic: dehydration, hypomagnesemia, hypokalemia, hypocalcemia, hy-

pernatremia, hyperglycemia, acidosis, hypoproteinemia, hyperlipidemia
Musculoskeletal: myalgia; joint, neck, or back pain
Respiratory: increased cough, wheezing, dyspnea, tachypnea, hypoxia, hyperventilation, asthma, hemoptysis, **pulmonary edema, pleural effusion, bronchospasm, respiratory failure**
Skin: pruritus, acne, alopecia, diaphoresis, skin discoloration, nodules, ulcers, urticaria, maculopapular rash
Other: weight changes, chills, fever, infection, peripheral or facial edema, pain or reaction at injection site, tissue damage (with extravasation), allergic reactions including **anaphylaxis, sepsis, multisystem failure**

Interactions

Drug-drug. *Alfentanil, benzodiazepines, buspirone, cyclosporine, losartan, nisoldipine, phenytoin, rifabutin, tacrolimus, theophylline, tricyclic antidepressants, zidovudine, zolpidem:* increased blood levels of these drugs, greater risk of toxicity
Antineoplastics, nephrotoxic drugs (such as some anti-infectives, pentamidine): nephrotoxicity
Cardiac glycosides: increased risk of digoxin toxicity in potassium-depleted patients
Corticosteroids: increased risk of hypokalemia
Cyclosporine, tacrolimus: increased creatinine level
Flucytosine: increased risk of flucytosine toxicity
Glipizide, glyburide, skeletal muscle relaxants, tolbutamide, warfarin: increased effects of these drugs
Thiazides: increased electrolyte depletion
Zidovudine: increased risk of myelotoxicity and nephrotoxicity
Drug-diagnostic tests. *Alanine aminotransferase, alkaline phosphatase, aspartate aminotransferase, blood urea nitrogen, bilirubin, creatinine, gamma-glutamyltransferase, lactate dehydrogenase, nitrogenous compounds (urea), uric acid:* increased levels
Calcium, hemoglobin, magnesium, platelets, potassium, protein: decreased levels
Eosinophils, glucose, prothrombin time, white blood cells: increased or decreased levels
Drug-food. *Grapefruit juice:* decreased antifungal blood level and therapeutic effects
Drug-herb. *Gossypol:* increased risk of nephrotoxicity
Drug-behaviors. *Alcohol use:* increased blood alcohol level

Patient monitoring
• Monitor vital signs and fluid intake and output.
• Assess electrolyte levels, complete blood count, and kidney and liver function test results.

antihyperlipidemic drugs
atorvastatin calcium, fluvastatin sodium, gemfibrozil, lovastatin, pravastatin sodium, rosuvastatin, simvastatin

Pregnancy risk category X

Action
Competitively inhibit HMG-CoA reductase (an enzyme that catalyzes the first step in cholesterol synthesis pathway). This inhibition decreases total cholesterol, low-density lipoprotein (LDL), very-low-density lipoprotein, apolipoprotein B, and triglyceride levels while increasing high-density lipoprotein levels.

Indications
Elevations of LDL, total cholesterol, apolipoprotein B, or triglyceride levels

in patients with primary hypercholesterolemia or mixed dyslipidemia (Fredrickson types IIa and IIb); primary dysbetalipoproteinemia (Fredrickson type III); adjunct to diet in hypertriglyceridemia (Fredrickson type IV)

Contraindications and precautions

• Contraindicated in hypersensitivity to drug; active hepatic disease; persistent, unexplained elevations in liver function test results; pregnancy; and breastfeeding

• Use cautiously in severe metabolic, endocrine, or electrolyte disorders; visual disturbances; uncontrolled seizures; myopathy; cerebral arteriosclerosis; coronary artery disease; severe hypotension or hypertension; history of hepatic disease, alcoholism, renal impairment, severe acute infection, major surgery, or trauma; females of childbearing age; and children under age 18 (safety not established).

Adverse reactions

CNS: amnesia, abnormal dreams, emotional lability, facial paralysis, headache, hyperkinesia, poor coordination, malaise, paresthesia, syncope, peripheral neuropathy, drowsiness, asthenia

CV: orthostatic hypotension, palpitations, phlebitis, vasodilation, **arrhythmias**

EENT: eye hemorrhage, amblyopia, glaucoma, altered refraction, dry eyes, hearing loss, tinnitus, epistaxis, sinusitis, gingival hemorrhage, glossitis, pharyngitis, loss of taste

GI: nausea, vomiting, diarrhea, constipation, abdominal or biliary pain, cramps, colitis, GI ulcers, flatulence, dyspepsia, gastroenteritis, dysphagia, esophagitis, pancreatitis, melena, tenesmus, dry mouth, stomatitis, anorexia, **rectal hemorrhage**

GU: dysuria, urinary frequency or urgency, urinary retention, nocturia, cystitis, renal calculi, nephritis, hematuria, abnormal ejaculation, decreased libido, epididymitis, impotence

Hematologic: anemia, **thrombocytopenia**

Hepatic: jaundice, **hepatic failure, hepatitis**

Metabolic: hypoglycemia, hyperglycemia

Musculoskeletal: joint pain, bursitis, back pain, gout, leg cramps, myalgia, myasthenia gravis, myositis, neck rigidity, torticollis

Respiratory: dyspnea, pneumonia, bronchitis

Skin: diaphoresis, acne, pruritus, rash, urticaria, alopecia, contact dermatitis, eczema, dry skin, skin ulcers, seborrhea, photosensitivity

Other: increased appetite, weight gain, flulike symptoms, infection, fever, allergic reaction

Interactions

Drug-drug. *Antacids, colestipol:* decreased antihyperlipidemic blood level
Antifungals, cyclosporine, erythromycin, niacin, other HMG-CoA reductase inhibitors: increased risk of myopathy
Digoxin: increased digoxin blood level
Hormonal contraceptives: increased contraceptive blood level

Drug-diagnostic tests. *Alanine aminotransferase, aspartate aminotransferase:* increased levels

Drug-food. *Grapefruit juice:* increased drug blood level, greater risk of adverse reactions

Drug-herb. *Red yeast rice:* increased risk of adverse reactions

Patient monitoring

• Monitor liver function test results and lipid panel.

antineoplastics

aldesleukin, alemtuzumab, amifostine, anastrozole, asparaginase, bicalutamide, bleomycin sulfate, busulfan, capecitabine, carboplatin, carmustine, chlorambucil, cisplatin, cyclophosphamide, cytarabine, dacarbazine, dactinomycin, daunorubicin, denileukin diftitox, docetaxel, doxorubicin hydrochloride, epirubicin hydrochloride, etoposide, exemestane, floxuridine, fluorouracil, flutamide, gemcitabine hydrochloride, gemtuzumab ozogamicin, goserelin acetate, hydroxyurea, idarubicin hydrochloride, ifosfamide, imatinib mesylate, interferon alfa-2a, interferon alfa-2b, irinotecan hydrochloride, letrozole, leuprolide acetate, lomustine, mechlorethamine hydrochloride, megestrol acetate, melphalan hydrochloride, mercaptopurine, methotrexate sodium, mitomycin, mitoxantrone hydrochloride, nilutamide, paclitaxel, pegaspargase, pentostatin, porfimer, procarbazine hydrochloride, rituximab, tamoxifen citrate, temozolomide, topotecan hydrochloride, trastuzumab, triptorelin pamoate, valrubicin, vinblastine sulfate, vincristine sulfate, vinorelbine tartrate

Pregnancy risk category D

Action

Varies with specific drug. Generally inhibit normal substrate utilization in tumor cells, forming dysfunctional macromolecules by inserting themselves into abnormal cells; intercalate between DNA strands and interfere with DNA templates. Also may modify growth of hormone-dependent tumors.

Indications

Hodgkin's lymphoma, non-Hodgkin's lymphoma, testicular teratomas, mycosis fungoides, breast cancer, ovarian cancer, prostate cancer, lung cancer, chronic lymphatic or chronic myeloid leukemia, head and neck cancer, colorectal cancer, pancreatic cancer, malignant melanoma, bronchogenic carcinoma, and other cancers

Contraindications and precautions

• Contraindicated in hypersensitivity to drug or its components
• Use cautiously in heart disease, renal or hepatic impairment, decreased bone marrow reserve, active infections, severe myocardial insufficiency, coagulation and bleeding disorders, active thrombophlebitis or thromboembolic disorders, shock, trauma, major surgery within previous month, elderly or debilitated patients, patients with childbearing potential, and pregnant or breastfeeding patients.

Adverse reactions

CNS: dizziness, mental status changes, sensory or motor dysfunction, malaise, headache, impaired memory, depression, sleep disturbances, hallucinations, rigors, peripheral neuropathy, paresthesia, tremor, confusion, agitation, ataxia, flaccid paresis, fatigue, lethargy, drowsiness, emotional lability, abnormal gait, vertigo, syncope, acute cerebellar dysfunction, asthenia, cranial nerve dysfunction, demyelinization, hemiparesis, **seizures, leukoencephalopathy, cerebrovascular accident, suicidal ideation**
CV: hypotension, hypertension, chest pain, peripheral edema, tachycardia, cardiomegaly, prolonged QT interval, **thromboembolic events, arrhythmias, cardiac tamponade, torsades de**

pointes, cardiac arrest, capillary leak syndrome, myocardial infarction, left-sided heart failure, pericardial effusion

EENT: retinal thrombosis, photophobia, diplopia, visual changes, nystagmus, lacrimation, lacrimal duct stenosis, stye, corneal opacity, epistaxis, oral candidiasis, dysphagia, pharyngitis, mucositis

GI: nausea, vomiting, diarrhea, constipation, fecal incontinence, abdominal pain, dyspepsia, GI ulcer, ascites, dry mouth, anorexia, intestinal perforation, paralytic ileus, GI bleeding

GU: hematuria, dysuria, urinary hesitation or retention, urinary obstruction, cystitis, bladder fibrosis, progressive azotemia, vaginitis, vaginal hemorrhage, breast swelling and tenderness, menstrual abnormalities, abortion, gynecomastia, libido loss, impotence, sterility, decreased testes size, reduced sperm count, hemolytic uremic syndrome, nephrotoxicity, proteinuria, oliguria or anuria, renal failure

Hematologic: anemia, eosinophilia, neutropenia, thrombocytopenia, leukopenia, leukocytosis, bone marrow depression, agranulocytosis, pancytopenia, coagulation disorders, hemorrhage

Hepatic: abnormal liver function test results, jaundice, hepatitis, hepatotoxicity

Metabolic: hyperglycemia, hyperkalemia, fluid retention

Musculoskeletal: muscle twitching, joint or bone pain, decreased bone density, carpal tunnel syndrome

Respiratory: tachypnea, dyspnea, pleural effusion, wheezing, pulmonary congestion, cough, interstitial pneumonitis, chronic obstructive pulmonary disease, upper respiratory tract infection, tracheoesophageal fistula, bronchospasm, pulmonary toxicity, pulmonary edema, respiratory failure, apnea, pulmonary fibrosis (or worsening of this condition)

Skin: erythema, pruritus, rash, diaphoresis, night sweats, dry skin, urticaria, alopecia, phlebitis at I.V. site, epidermal necrolysis, palmar-plantar erythrodysesthesia, nail loss, bruising, petechiae, exacerbation of postradiation erythema, painful plaque erosions, exfoliative dermatitis

Other: increased appetite, weight gain, fever, chills, pain, flulike symptoms, herpes simplex or other infection, tumor flare, hypersensitivity reaction, risk of second malignancy, anaphylaxis, sepsis, Stevens-Johnson syndrome, tumor lysis syndrome

Interactions

Drug-drug. Anticholinergics: additive anticholinergic effects

Antihypertensives: potentiation of hypotension

Digoxin: decreased digoxin blood level

Folic acid derivatives: antagonism of antineoplastic effects

Fosphenytoin, phenytoin, theophylline: decreased blood levels of these drugs

Glucocorticoids: reduced antineoplastic effects

Hepatotoxic drugs: increased risk of hepatotoxicity

Live-virus vaccines: decreased antibody response to vaccine, greater risk of adverse reactions

Metrizamide: increased risk of seizures

Myelosuppressants: increased hematologic toxicity

Nonsteroidal anti-inflammatory drugs, phenylbutazone, probenecid, salicylates, sulfonamides: increased antineoplastic toxicity

Warfarin: increased warfarin effects

Drug-diagnostic tests. Calcium, hemoglobin, magnesium, phosphates, platelets, potassium, red blood cells, sodium, white blood cells: decreased levels

Coombs' test: positive result

Hepatic enzymes, protein-bound iodine, uric acid: increased levels

Pregnancy tests: false-positive result

Drug-food. *Any food:* delayed drug absorption, reduced peak drug level

Drug-herb. *Astragalus, echinacea, melatonin:* interference with immunosuppressant effect

St. John's wort: decreased drug effects

Drug-behaviors. *Alcohol use:* increased risk of hepatotoxicity

Smoking: increased risk of pulmonary toxicity

Sun exposure: photosensitivity

Patient monitoring

◀€ Watch for bleeding; if platelet count is low, avoid giving I.M. injections and taking rectal temperature.

• Stay alert for bone marrow depression, neutropenia, and anemia.

• Monitor for GI upset; as necessary, give antiemetics.

• Monitor fluid intake and output.

antiparkinsonian drugs

anticholinergics (benztropine, biperiden, trihexyphenidyl hydrochloride), antivirals (amantadine hydrochloride), dopamine agents (bromocriptine mesylate, carbidopa-levodopa, entacapone, levodopa, pergolide mesylate, pramipexole, ropinirole hydrochloride, tolcapone) monoamine oxidase inhibitor (selegiline)

Pregnancy risk category C, B (some antiparkinsonian drugs)

Action

Block central cholinergic receptors or inhibit prolactin secretion; also may act as dopamine receptor agonists by activating postsynaptic dopamine receptors

Indications

Parkinson's disease

Contraindications and precautions

• Contraindicated in hypersensitivity to drug, narrow-angle glaucoma, tardive dyskinesia, stenosing peptic ulcer, achalasia, pyloric or duodenal obstruction, prostatic hypertrophy or bladder neck obstruction, myasthenia gravis, and children under age 3

• Use cautiously in seizure disorders, arrhythmias, tachycardia, hypertension, hypotension, hepatic or renal dysfunction, alcoholism, exposure to hot environments, elderly patients, and pregnant or breastfeeding patients (safety not established).

Adverse reactions

CNS: confusion, headache, dizziness, fatigue, mania, light-headedness, drowsiness, delusions, nervousness, insomnia, nightmares, **seizures, cerebrovascular accident**

CV: hypotension, palpitations, extrasystole, bradycardia, **arrhythmias, acute myocardial infarction**

EENT: diplopia, blurred vision, burning eyes, nasal congestion

GI: nausea, vomiting, diarrhea, constipation, abdominal cramps, dry mouth, anorexia, **GI hemorrhage**

GU: urinary incontinence, frequency, or retention; diuresis; difficulty maintaining an erection

Hepatic: hepatic failure

Musculoskeletal: leg cramps

Skin: urticaria; cool, pale fingers and toes; facial and arm rash; alopecia

Other: numb fingers, hyperthermia, **heat stroke**

Interactions

Drug-drug. *Anticholinergics:* decreased antiparkinsonian drug absorption

Antihypertensives: additive hypotension

Haloperidol, papaverine, phenothiazines, phenytoin, reserpine: reversal of antiparkinsonian drug effects

Inhalation hydrocarbon anesthetics: increased risk of arrhythmias

Methyldopa: altered antiparkinsonian drug efficacy, increased risk of adverse CNS effects

Monoamine oxidase inhibitors: hypertension

Pyridoxine: antagonism of antiparkinsonian drug effects

Selegiline: increased risk of adverse reactions

Drug-diagnostic tests. *Alanine aminotransferase, alkaline phosphatase, aspartate aminotransferase, bilirubin, lactate dehydrogenase, uric acid:* increased levels

Coombs' test: false-positive result

Granulocytes, hemoglobin, platelets, white blood cells: decreased levels

Urine glucose, urine ketones: interference with test results

Drug-food. *Pyridoxine-rich foods:* reversal of antiparkinsonian drug effects

Drug-herb. *5-hydroxytryptophan (5-HTP):* harmful skin changes

Kava: decreased drug efficacy

Octacosanol: worsened dyskinesias

Drug-behaviors. *Cocaine use:* increased risk of adverse reactions

Patient monitoring

• Monitor fluid intake and output and vital signs (especially blood pressure).

antipsychotics

aripiprazole, chlorpromazine hydrochloride, clozapine, fluphenazine, haloperidol, loxapine, mesoridazine besylate, olanzapine, perphenazine, pimozide, prochlorperazine, quetiapine fumarate, risperidone, thioridazine hydrochloride, thiothixene, trifluoperazine hydrochloride, ziprasidone

Pregnancy risk category C, B (some antipsychotics)

Action

Block postsynaptic mesolimbic and mesocortical dopamine receptors in brain, relieving hallucinations, delusions, and psychoses. Also thought to relieve anxiety by filtering internal arousal stimuli to brainstem reticular system.

Indications

Acute or chronic psychosis, nausea and vomiting, intractable hiccups, preoperative sedation, acute intermittent porphyria

Contraindications and precautions

• Contraindicated in hypersensitivity to drug, phenothiazines, sulfites (when injected), or benzyl alcohol (with sustained-release forms); narrow-angle glaucoma; bone marrow depression; blood dyscrasias; myeloproliferative disorders; subcortical brain damage; cerebral arteriosclerosis; hepatic damage; coronary artery disease; severe hypotension or hypertension; coma; and severe depression

• Use cautiously in diabetes mellitus; respiratory disease; prostatic hypertrophy; CNS tumors; seizure disorders; intestinal obstruction; elderly or debilitated patients; pregnant or breastfeeding patients (safety not established); and children with acute illnesses, infections, gastroenteritis, or dehydration.

Adverse reactions

CNS: sedation, extrapyramidal reactions, tardive dyskinesia, drowsiness, pseudoparkinsonism, **seizures, neuroleptic malignant syndrome**

CV: hypotension (increased with I.M. and I.V. use), tachycardia

EENT: blurred vision, dry eyes, lens opacities, nasal congestion

GI: constipation, anorexia, dry mouth, **paralytic ileus**

GU: urinary retention, menstrual irregularities, inhibited ejaculation, priapism, galactorrhea
Hematologic: eosinophilia, hemolytic anemia, **agranulocytosis, leukopenia, aplastic anemia, thrombocytopenia**
Hepatic: jaundice, **hepatitis**
Skin: photosensitivity, pigmentation changes, rash, sterile abscesses
Other: allergic reactions, hyperthermia, pain at injection site

Interactions

Drug-drug. *Adsorbent antidiarrheals, antacids:* decreased antipsychotic absorption
Antidepressants, antihistamines, general anesthetics, monoamine oxidase inhibitors, opioid analgesics, sedative-hypnotics: additive CNS depression
Antihypertensives: additive hypotension
Barbiturates: increased metabolism and decreased efficacy of both drugs
Bromocriptine: decreased bromocriptine efficacy
Epinephrine, norepinephrine: decreased pressor effects of these drugs
Guanethidine: inhibited antihypertensive effects of guanethidine
Lithium: disorientation, unconsciousness, extrapyramidal symptoms
Meperidine: excessive sedation and hypotension
Metrizamide (subarachnoid use): increased risk of seizures
Phenytoin: altered blood levels of both drugs
Pimozide: increased risk of serious cardiovascular effects
Propranolol: increased blood levels of both drugs
Tricyclic antidepressants (TCAs): increased TCA blood levels and effects, increased risk of anticholinergic effects
Valproic acid: decreased elimination and increased effects of valproic acid
Drug-diagnostic tests. *Alanine aminotransferase, alkaline phosphatase, aspartate aminotransferase, bilirubin:* increased levels

Granulocytes, hematocrit, hemoglobin, platelets, white blood cells: decreased levels
Pregnancy tests: false-positive or false-negative result
Urine bilirubin: false-positive result
Drug-herb. *Angel's trumpet, jimsonweed, scopolia:* increased anticholinergic effects
Chamomile, hops, kava, skullcap, valerian: increased CNS depression
St. John's wort: increased risk of photosensitivity
Yohimbe: toxicity
Drug-behaviors. *Alcohol use:* increased CNS depression
Sun exposure: increased risk of photosensitivity

Patient monitoring

• Monitor vital signs (especially blood pressure), ECG, complete blood count, liver and kidney function test results, urinalysis, and periodic eye examination results.

antituberculars

dapsone, ethambutol hydrochloride, isoniazid, pyrazinamide, rifabutin, rifampin, rifapentine, streptomycin sulfate

Pregnancy risk category C

Action

Unknown; may interfere with synthesis of one or more bacterial metabolites, altering RNA synthesis during cell division

Indications

Tuberculosis and atypical mycobacterial infections caused by *Mycobacterium tuberculosis*

Contraindications and precautions

• Contraindicated in hypersensitivity to drug (including drug-induced hepatitis)

• Use cautiously in severe renal impairment, malnutrition, diabetes mellitus, chronic alcoholism, diabetic retinopathy, cataracts, optic neuritis and other ocular defects, history of liver damage or chronic alcohol ingestion, patients over age 50, Black or Hispanic females, postpartal patients, pregnant or breastfeeding patients, and children under age 13.

Adverse reactions

CNS: confusion, dizziness, hallucinations, headache, malaise, peripheral neuritis

EENT: optic neuritis, blurred vision, decreased visual acuity, eye pain, red-green color blindness

GI: nausea, vomiting, abdominal pain, anorexia

Hematologic: thrombocytopenia

Hepatic: hepatitis

Metabolic: hyperuricemia

Musculoskeletal: joint pain, gouty arthritis

Respiratory: bloody sputum

Skin: rash, toxic epidermal necrolysis

Other: fever, **anaphylaxis**

Interactions

Drug-drug. *Aluminum-containing antacids:* decreased drug absorption

Bacillus Calmette-Guérin vaccine: vaccine inefficacy

Carbamazepine: increased carbamazepine blood level, greater risk of hepatotoxicity

Chloramphenicol, corticosteroids, disopyramide, efavirenz, estrogens, fluconazole, hormonal contraceptives, itraconazole, ketoconazole, nevirapine, opioid analgesics, oral hypoglycemics, phenytoin, quinidine, ritonavir, theophylline, tocainide, verapamil, warfarin: increased metabolism and decreased efficacy of these drugs

Delavirdine, indinavir, nelfinavir, saquinavir: decreased blood levels of these drugs

Disulfiram: psychotic reactions, incoordination

Hepatotoxic drugs (including isoniazid, ketoconazole, pyrazinamide): increased risk of hepatotoxicity

Other antituberculars: additive CNS toxicity

Phenytoin: inhibited phenytoin metabolism

Drug-diagnostic tests. *Alanine aminotransferase, alkaline phosphatase, aspartate aminotransferase, bilirubin, blood urea nitrogen, uric acid:* increased levels

Dexamethasone suppression test, folic acid and vitamin B assays, urine tests: interference with tests based on color reaction

Direct Coombs' test: false-positive result

Hepatic uptake and excretion of sulfobromophthalein: delayed

Drug-food. *Foods high in tyramine (such as beer, Chianti, cheese, sour cream, bananas, red plums, figs, raisins, avocados, eggplant, pickled herring, salami, smoked meats, yogurt, chocolate, soy sauce):* severe reactions

High-fat foods: slow drug absorption

Drug-behaviors. *Alcohol use:* increased risk of hepatotoxicity

Patient monitoring

• Monitor vital signs (especially blood pressure), ECG, complete blood count, liver and kidney function studies, urinalysis, and periodic eye examination results.

antiulcer drugs

cimetidine hydrochloride, esomeprazole magnesium, famotidine, lansoprazole, omeprazole, pantoprazole sodium, rabeprazole sodium, ranitidine hydrochloride, sucralfate

Pregnancy risk category B

Action

Reduce gastric acid either by blocking histamine$_2$-receptors or inhibiting proton pump

Indications

Short-term treatment of active duodenal ulcer or benign gastric ulcer; prophylaxis of duodenal ulcer (at lower doses); treatment of gastroesophageal reflux disease, heartburn, acid indigestion, and gastric hypersecretory states (such as Zollinger-Ellison syndrome); prevention and treatment of stress-induced upper GI bleeding in critically ill patients

Contraindications and precautions

• Contraindicated in hypersensitivity to any antiulcer drug and in alcohol intolerance
• Use cautiously in renal impairment, elderly patients, and pregnant or breastfeeding patients.

Adverse reactions

CNS: confusion, dizziness, drowsiness, hallucinations, headache, peripheral neuropathy, symptoms of brain stem dysfunction
CV: hypotension, **arrhythmias, cardiac arrest**
EENT: altered taste
GI: nausea, diarrhea, constipation
GU: decreased sperm count, impotence, gynecomastia
Hematologic: anemia, **neutropenia, thrombocytopenia, agranulocytosis, aplastic anemia**
Hepatic: hepatitis
Other: pain at I.M. injection site, hypersensitivity reaction

Interactions

Drug-drug. *Antacids, sucralfate:* decreased antiulcer drug absorption
Benzodiazepines (especially chlordiazepoxide, diazepam, midazolam), calcium channel blockers, carbamazepine, chloroquine, lidocaine, metformin, metronidazole, moricizine, pentoxifylline, phenytoin, propafenone, quinidine, quinine, some beta-adrenergic blockers (labetalol, metoprolol, propranolol), sulfonylureas, tacrine, tetracycline, theophylline, triamterene, tricyclic antidepressants, valproic acid, warfarin: increased blood levels of these drugs, greater risk of toxicity
Carmustine, flecainide, fluorouracil, procainamide, succinylcholine: increased effects of these drugs
Fluoroquinolones, ketoconazole: decreased absorption of these drugs
Theophylline: increased theophylline clearance
Drug-diagnostic tests. *Creatinine, transaminases:* increased levels
Skin tests using allergenic extracts: false-negative results
Drug-food. *Caffeine-containing foods and beverages:* increased drug blood level, greater risk of toxicity
High-fat foods: decreased drug absorption
Drug-herb. *Pennyroyal:* altered metabolism of herb
Yerba maté: decreased drug clearance
Drug-behaviors. *Alcohol use:* increased blood alcohol level

Patient monitoring

• Monitor for improving or worsening of GI symptoms.

◀€ Clinical alert

• Assess complete blood count and liver function studies.

antivirals

abacavir sulfate, acyclovir sodium, adefovir dipivoxil, amantadine hydrochloride, amprenavir, cidofovir, delavirdine mesylate, didanosine, efavirenz, famciclovir, foscarnet sodium, ganciclovir, indinavir sulfate, lamivudine, nelfinavir mesylate, nevirapine, oseltamivir phosphate, ribavirin, rimantadine hydrochloride, ritonavir, saquinavir, stavudine, tenofovir disoproxil fumarate, valacyclovir hydrochloride, valganciclovir hydrochloride, zalcitabine, zanamivir, zidovudine

Pregnancy risk category C

Action

Inhibit release of enzyme required for DNA synthesis, viral nucleic acid synthesis, viral DNA or protein synthesis, viral replication, or protease reaction. Viral cell death results.

Indications

Genital herpes, herpes simplex, varicella zoster, herpes zoster (shingles), influenza type A virus, hepatitis, human immunodeficiency virus, cytomegalovirus

Contraindications and precautions

• Contraindicated in hypersensitivity to drug or its components
• Use cautiously in renal or hepatic impairment; peripheral neuropathy; phenylketonuria; hyperuricemia; elevated amylase level; hypercholesterolemia; sodium-restricted diet; history of mental illness, substance abuse, or he-patic impairment (including hepatitis B or C infection); elderly or debilitated patients; pregnant or breastfeeding patients; and children.

Adverse reactions

CNS: dizziness, anxiety, abnormal thinking, hypoesthesia, agitation, confusion, coma, hypertonia, asthenia, **seizures**
CV: hypotension, pseudoaneurysm, palpitations, atrioventricular block, thrombophlebitis, bradycardia, weak pulse, **nodal arrhythmias, embolism, ventricular tachycardia**
EENT: ocular hypotony, iritis, retinal detachment, diplopia
GI: nausea, vomiting, diarrhea, abdominal distention, dyspepsia, gastroesophageal reflux, hematemesis, dysphagia, dry mouth, **paralytic ileus**
GU: urinary retention, frequency, or incontinence; dysuria; prostatitis; **nephrotoxicity**
Hematologic: leukocytosis, anemia, petechiae, **thrombocytopenia, neutropenia, bleeding**
Hepatic: hepatomegaly
Metabolic: diabetes mellitus, hyperkalemia
Musculoskeletal: muscle contractions
Respiratory: pneumonia, bronchitis, pleurisy, dyspnea, wheezing, **pleural effusion, pulmonary edema, bronchospasm, pulmonary embolism**
Skin: rash, diaphoresis, urticaria, pruritus, bullous eruptions, pallor
Other: pain, peripheral coldness, edema, drug toxicity

Interactions

Drug-drug. *Acetaminophen, aspirin, cimetidine:* reduced antiviral blood level
CNS depressants (including antihistamines, opioids, sedative-hypnotics), methotrexate, zidovudine: increased CNS depression
Hormonal contraceptives: altered contraceptive efficacy

🔊 Clinical alert   Reactions in **bold** are life-threatening

Nephrotoxic drugs: increased risk of nephrotoxicity
Sildenafil: increased sildenafil blood level, greater risk of adverse reactions
Drug-diagnostic tests. *Alanine aminotransferase, alkaline phosphatase, aspartate aminotransferase, blood urea nitrogen, creatinine, lactate dehydrogenase:* increased levels
Hemoglobin, neutrophils, platelets: decreased levels
Drug-food. *High-fat foods:* decreased drug absorption
Drug-herb. *St John's wort:* reduced antiviral blood level
Drug-behaviors. *Alcohol use:* decreased drug elimination and increased drug effects

Patient monitoring
• Monitor complete blood count and liver and kidney function test results.
• As indicated, monitor viral load and T-cell levels.

beta-adrenergic blockers
acebutolol hydrochloride, atenolol, bisoprolol fumarate, carteolol hydrochloride, esmolol hydrochloride, metoprolol, nadolol, pindolol, propranolol hydrochloride, sotalol hydrochloride, timolol maleate

Pregnancy risk category C

Action
Combine reversibly with beta-adrenergic receptors, blocking response to sympathetic nerve impulses, catecholamines, or adrenergic drugs. Beta$_1$ blockade decreases heart rate, myocardial contractility, and cardiac output while slowing atrioventricular (AV) conduction. Beta$_2$ blockade increases bronchiolar airway resistance and catecholamines' inhibitory effect on peripheral vessels.

Indications
Hypertension; angina pectoris; myocardial infarction (MI); stable, symptomatic (class II or III) heart failure of ischemic, hypertensive, or cardiomyopathic origin; ventricular arrhythmias or tachycardia; migraine prophylaxis; tremors; aggressive behavior; drug-induced akathisia; anxiety; chronic intraocular glaucoma

Contraindications and precautions
• Contraindicated in hypersensitivity to drug, heart failure (unless secondary to tachyarrhythmia treatable with specific beta-adrenergic blocker), shock, sinus bradycardia, and greater than first-degree heart block
• Use cautiously in renal or hepatic impairment, pulmonary disease (especially asthma), pulmonary edema, diabetes mellitus, thyrotoxicosis, history of severe allergic reactions, elderly patients, pregnant or breastfeeding patients, and children (safety not established).

Adverse reactions
CNS: insomnia, headache, hyperactivity, malaise, CNS stimulation, dizziness, tremor, restlessness, nervousness, apprehension, anxiety, hyperkinesia, asthenia, vertigo, drowsiness
CV: hypertension, hypotension, tachycardia, angina, chest pain, palpitations, **arrhythmias**
EENT: epistaxis, nasal congestion, sore throat (with inhaled drug), nasal dryness and irritation, hoarseness, bad or unusual taste
GI: nausea, vomiting, heartburn, anorexia
Metabolic: hypoglycemia, hypokalemia
Musculoskeletal: muscle cramps

◀€ Clinical alert   Reactions in **bold** are life-threatening

Respiratory: cough, wheezing, dyspnea, bronchitis, increased sputum, paradoxical airway resistance (with repeated, excessive use of inhaled drug), **pulmonary edema, bronchospasm**
Skin: pallor, flushing, diaphoresis
Other: increased appetite, hypersensitivity reaction

Interactions
Drug-drug. *Amphetamines, ephedrine, epinephrine, norepinephrine, phenylephrine, pseudoephedrine:* unopposed alpha-adrenergic stimulation (excessive hypertension, bradycardia)
Clonidine: increased hypotension and bradycardia
Digoxin: additive bradycardia
Dobutamine, dopamine: reduction in beneficial beta$_1$ cardiovascular effects
General anesthetics, phenytoin (I.V.), verapamil: additive myocardial depression
Insulin, oral hypoglycemics: altered efficacy of these drugs
Monoamine oxidase inhibitors, theophylline, thyroid hormone: reduced beta blocker efficacy
Nonsteroidal anti-inflammatory drugs: decreased antihypertensive action
Other antihypertensives, nitrates: additive hypotension
Drug-diagnostic tests. *Alanine aminotransferase, alkaline phosphatase, aspartate aminotransferase, blood urea nitrogen, glucose, lactate dehydrogenase, lipoproteins, potassium, triglycerides, uric acid:* increased levels
Antinuclear antibody: increased titer
Drug-herb. *Aloe, buckthorn bark or berry, cascara sagrada bark, rhubarb root, senna leaf or fruit:* increased antihypertensive effect
Ephedra (ma huang): decreased antihypertensive effect
Drug-behaviors. *Alcohol use:* additive hypotension
Cocaine use: unopposed alpha-adrenergic stimulation (excessive hypertension, bradycardia)

Sun exposure: photophobia

Patient monitoring
• Monitor ECG, blood glucose and electrolyte levels, complete blood count, and liver and kidney function test results.
• Assess vital signs, fluid intake and output, and weight.

bronchodilators
albuterol, aminophylline, ephedrine, epinephrine, ipratropium bromide, isoproterenol, levalbuterol hydrochloride, metaproterenol sulfate, oxtriphylline, pirbuterol acetate, salmeterol, terbutaline sulfate, theophylline

Pregnancy risk category C

Action
Inhibit phosphodiesterase, an enzyme that degrades cyclic adenosine monophosphate (cAMP) by stimulating cAMP release and inhibiting release of slow-reacting substance of anaphylaxis and histamine. These actions cause bronchodilation and CNS and cardiac stimulation, promote diuresis, and increase gastric acid secretion.

Indications
Prevention of exercise-induced bronchospasm, prevention and treatment of bronchospasm in reversible obstructive airway disease

Contraindications and precautions
• Contraindicated in hypersensitivity to drug, angina, arrhythmias associated with tachycardia, ventricular arrhythmias that warrant inotropic therapy, organic brain damage, local anesthesia of certain areas (such as toes or fin-

gers), cardiac dilatation or insufficiency, cerebral arteriosclerosis, narrow-angle glaucoma, and labor
• Use cautiously in heart failure or other cardiac or circulatory impairment, chronic obstructive pulmonary disease, renal or hepatic disease, hyperthyroidism, peptic ulcer, severe hypoxemia, diabetes mellitus, seizure disorders, hypertension, glaucoma, elderly patients, pregnant or breastfeeding patients, young children, and infants.

Adverse reactions

CNS: insomnia, headache, hyperactivity, asthenia, malaise, CNS stimulation, dizziness, apprehension, anxiety, restlessness, nervousness, hyperkinesia, vertigo, drowsiness, tremor
CV: hypertension, hypotension, tachycardia, angina, chest pain, palpitations, **arrhythmias**
EENT: epistaxis, nasal congestion, nasal dryness and irritation, sore throat (with inhaled drug), hoarseness, unusual or bad taste
GI: nausea, vomiting, heartburn, anorexia
Metabolic: hypoglycemia, hypokalemia
Musculoskeletal: muscle cramps
Respiratory: cough, wheezing, dyspnea, bronchitis, paradoxical airway resistance (with repeated, excessive use of inhaled drug), increased sputum, **bronchospasm, pulmonary edema**
Skin: pallor, flushing, diaphoresis
Other: increased appetite, hypersensitivity reaction

Interactions

Drug-drug. *Adrenergics (sympathomimetics):* additive adverse CNS and cardiovascular effects
Beta blockers: inhibition of cardiac, bronchodilating, and vasodilating effects
Diuretics: decreased vascular response
General anesthetics: increased risk of arrhythmias

Guanethidine: altered effects of both drugs
Methyldopa: increased pressor response
Monoamine oxidase inhibitors: hypertensive crisis
Oxytocics: severe hypotension
Theophylline: increased cardiotoxicity, decreased theophylline blood level
Tricyclic antidepressants: increased or decreased pressor effect
Drug-diagnostic tests. *Free fatty acids, glucose:* increased levels
Drug-food. *Charcoal-broiled foods:* decreased drug efficacy
Foods and beverages containing caffeine or xanthine: increased risk of adverse CNS and cardiovascular effects
Drug-herb. *Caffeine-containing herbs (such as cola nut, guarana, yerba maté):* increased risk of adverse CNS and cardiovascular effects
Ephedra (ma huang): increased stimulant effects
St. John's wort: decreased blood level and efficacy
Drug-behaviors. *Alcohol use:* additive CNS depression

Patient monitoring

• Monitor vital signs, ECG, and fluid intake and output.

calcium channel blockers

amlodipine, diltiazem hydrochloride, felodipine, isradipine, nicardipine hydrochloride, nifedipine, nimodipine, nisoldipine, verapamil hydrochloride

Pregnancy risk category C

Action

Inhibit calcium influx through cell membrane of cardiac and smooth-muscle cells; this action depresses automaticity and conduction velocity in

◀€ Clinical alert   Reactions in **bold** are life-threatening

cardiac muscle, which in turn reduces myocardial contractility. Also reduces total peripheral resistance, depolarization rate, and atrial conduction.

Indications

Hypertension, angina pectoris, vasospastic (Prinzmetal's) angina, supraventricular tachyarrhythmias, rapid ventricular rate in atrial flutter or fibrillation

Contraindications and precautions

• Contraindicated in hypersensitivity to drug, sick sinus syndrome, second- or third-degree atrioventricular block (unless artificial pacemaker is in place), and systolic pressure below 90 mmHg
• Use cautiously in severe renal or hepatic impairment, advanced aortic stenosis, cardiogenic shock (unless associated with supraventricular tachyarrhythmias), history of serious ventricular arrhythmias or heart failure, concurrent use of I.V. beta blockers, elderly patients, pregnant or breastfeeding patients, and children (safety not established).

Adverse reactions

CNS: headache, abnormal dreams, anxiety, confusion, dizziness, syncope, drowsiness, nervousness, paresthesia, tremor, asthenia, psychiatric disturbances
CV: peripheral edema, chest pain, hypotension, palpitations, bradycardia, tachycardia, **arrhythmias, heart failure**
EENT: blurred vision, disturbed equilibrium, tinnitus, epistaxis, gingival hyperplasia, altered taste
GI: nausea, vomiting, diarrhea, constipation, dyspepsia, dry mouth, anorexia
GU: dysuria, nocturia, polyuria, sexual dysfunction, gynecomastia
Hematologic: anemia, **leukopenia, thrombocytopenia**
Hepatic: abnormal liver function test results

Metabolic: hyperglycemia
Musculoskeletal: joint stiffness, muscle cramps
Respiratory: cough, dyspnea
Skin: rash, dermatitis, pruritus, urticaria, flushing, diaphoresis, photosensitivity, erythema multiforme
Other: weight gain, **Stevens-Johnson syndrome**

Interactions

Drug-drug. *Beta blockers, digoxin, disopyramide, phenytoin:* bradycardia, conduction defects, heart failure
Calcium, vitamin D: decreased efficacy of calcium channel blocker
Carbamazepine, cyclosporine, prazosin, quinidine: decreased metabolism of these drugs, increased risk of toxicity
Digoxin: increased digoxin blood level
Fentanyl, nitrates, other antihypertensives, quinidine: additive hypotension
Lithium: altered lithium blood level
Nondepolarizing neuromuscular blockers: increased muscle paralysis
Nonsteroidal anti-inflammatory drugs: decreased antihypertensive effect
Rifampin: decreased rifampin efficacy
Drug-diagnostic tests. *Alanine aminotransferase, alkaline phosphatase, aspartate aminotransferase, blood urea nitrogen, lactate dehydrogenase:* increased levels
Granulocytes: decreased count
Drug-food. *Caffeine-containing foods and beverages:* increased caffeine blood level
Grapefruit juice: increased drug blood level and effects
Drug-herb. *Black catechu:* additive effects
Caffeine-containing herbs (such as cola nut, guarana, yerba maté): increased caffeine blood level
Yerba maté: decreased yerba maté clearance
Drug-behaviors. *Alcohol use:* additive hypotension

◀≶ Clinical alert   Reactions in **bold** are life-threatening

Patient monitoring
• Monitor blood glucose and electrolyte levels, fluid intake and output, and liver and kidney function studies.
• Assess vital signs, ECG, weight, and blood pressure in both arms (with patient lying down, sitting, and standing).

cephalosporins
First generation: cefadroxil, cefazolin sodium, cephalexin hydrochloride, cephradine

Second generation: cefaclor, cefamandole, cefmetazole sodium, cefonicid sodium, cefotetan disodium, cefoxitin sodium, cefprozil, cefuroxime axetil, loracarbef

Third generation: cefdinir, cefditoren pivoxil, cefepime hydrochloride, cefixime, cefoperazone sodium, cefotaxime sodium, cefpodoxime proxetil, ceftazidime, ceftibuten, ceftizoxime sodium, ceftriaxone sodium

Pregnancy risk category B

Action
Bind to bacterial cell wall, causing leakage of cell contents and subsequent cell death

Indications
Skin and skin-structure infections (including burn wounds), pneumonia, otitis media, urinary tract infections, bone and joint infections, and septicemia (including endocarditis) caused by susceptible organisms

Contraindications and precautions
• Contraindicated in hypersensitivity to drug
• Use cautiously in hypersensitivity to penicillin; phenylketonuria; renal impairment; seizure disorders; bronchial asthma; coronary occlusion; history of GI disease (especially colitis); elderly, debilitated, or emaciated patients; and pregnant or breastfeeding patients.

Adverse reactions
CNS: headache, lethargy, paresthesia, **seizures**
CV: phlebitis, thrombophlebitis
EENT: hearing loss, oral candidiasis
GI: nausea, vomiting, diarrhea, cramps, **pseudomembranous colitis**
GU: elevated blood urea nitrogen, vaginal candidiasis, **renal failure, nephrotoxicity**
Hematologic: eosinophilia, hemolytic anemia, hypoprothrombinemia, lymphocytosis, **bone marrow depression, agranulocytosis, neutropenia, thrombocytopenia, bleeding**
Hepatic: hepatomegaly, **hepatic failure**
Musculoskeletal: joint pain
Respiratory: dyspnea
Skin: sterile abscess
Other: rash; urticaria; pain, induration, and phlebitis at I.V. site; superinfection; chills; fever; edema; serum sickness; **anaphylaxis**

Interactions
Drug-drug. *Aluminum- and magnesium-containing antacids, histamine₂-receptor antagonists:* increased cephalosporin absorption
Anticoagulants, antiplatelet drugs, plicamycin, thrombolytics, valproic acid: increased effects of these drugs, increased risk of bleeding
Iron supplements: decreased cephalosporin absorption
Loop diuretics, nephrotoxic drugs (including aminoglycosides): increased risk of nephrotoxicity

---

Nonsteroidal anti-inflammatory drugs: increased risk of bleeding

Probenecid: increased cephalosporin half-life and blood level

Drug-diagnostic tests. *Alanine aminotransferase, alkaline phosphatase, aspartate aminotransferase, bilirubin, blood urea nitrogen, creatinine, eosinophils, gamma-glutamyltransferase, lactate dehydrogenase:* increased levels

Hemoglobin, platelets, white blood cells: decreased levels

Urine protein: false-positive result

Drug-herb. *Angelica, anise, arnica, asafetida, bogbean, boldo, celery, chamomile, clove, danshen, fenugreek, feverfew, garlic, ginger, ginkgo, ginseng, horse chestnut, horseradish, licorice, meadowsweet, onion, papain, passionflower, poplar, prickly ash, quassia, red clover, turmeric, wild carrot, wild lettuce, willow:* increased risk of bleeding

Drug-behaviors. *Alcohol use:* disulfiram-like effect

Patient monitoring

• Monitor for signs and symptoms of overgrowth of resistant organisms.

• Assess kidney function and complete blood count.

◀€ Monitor International Normalized Ratio in prolonged therapy and in patients with malnutrition or high risk for renal or hepatic impairment.

cholinergics

bethanechol chloride, cevimeline hydrochloride, edrophonium chloride, neostigmine, pyridostigmine bromide

Pregnancy risk category C

Action

Stimulate cholinergic receptors, causing urinary bladder contraction, de-creased bladder capacity, more frequent ureteral peristaltic waves, increased GI tone and peristalsis, increased lower esophageal sphincter pressure, and increased gastric secretions

Indications

Postpartum or postoperative nonobstructive urinary retention, urinary retention caused by neurogenic bladder, diagnosis of myasthenia gravis (Tensilon test), antidote for curare (to reverse nondepolarizing neuromuscular blockade)

Contraindications and precautions

• Contraindicated in hypersensitivity to drug or sulfites, hyperthyroidism, peptic ulcer, latent or active bronchial asthma, pronounced bradycardia or atrioventricular (AV) conduction defects, vasomotor instability, coronary artery disease, coronary occlusion, hypotension, hypertension, seizure disorders, parkinsonism, GI or GU tract obstruction, impaired GI or GU wall integrity, spastic GI disturbances, acute inflammatory GI tract lesions, peritonitis, marked vagotonia, and when GI tract or urinary bladder activity could be harmful (for instance, postoperatively)

• Use cautiously in arrhythmias, toxic megacolon, poor GI motility, and pregnant patients.

Adverse reactions

CNS: asthenia, dysarthria, dysphonia, dizziness, drowsiness, headache, syncope, **loss of consciousness, seizures**

CV: hypotension, AV block, bradycardia, **cardiac arrest, thrombophlebitis** (with I.V. use)

EENT: diplopia, miosis, conjunctival hyperemia, excessive lacrimation and salivation

GI: nausea, vomiting, diarrhea, abdominal cramps, dysphagia

GU: urinary frequency or incontinence
Musculoskeletal: muscle cramps, fasciculations
Respiratory: dyspnea, **respiratory muscle paralysis, central respiratory paralysis, laryngospasm, bronchospasm, respiratory depression, respiratory arrest**
Skin: rash, diaphoresis, flushing
Other: anaphylaxis

Interactions
Drug-drug. *Aminoglycosides:* prolonged or enhanced muscle weakness
Anesthetics (local or general), corticosteroids, magnesium, procainamide, quinidine: antagonism of cholinergic effects
Cardiac glycosides: increased cardiac sensitivity to cholinergics
Depolarizing neuromuscular blockers: increased neuromuscular blockade, prolonged respiratory depression
Other cholinergics: increased cholinergic effects (mimicking myasthenia-like weakness)
Drug-food. *High-fat foods:* decreased drug absorption
Drug-herb. *Angel's trumpet, jimsonweed, scopolia:* antagonism of cholinergic effects
Jaborandi tree, pill-bearing spurge: additive drug effects

Patient monitoring
• Monitor ECG, glucose and electrolyte levels, urinalysis, and liver and kidney function test results.
◀€ Assess platelet count in long-term use. Report unusual bleeding or bruising, petechiae, other skin disorders, and signs or symptom of diabetes mellitus.

corticosteroids
beclomethasone dipropionate, betamethasone, budesonide, cortisone acetate, dexamethasone, fludrocortisone, hydrocortisone, methylprednisolone, mometasone, prednisolone, prednisone, triamcinolone

Pregnancy risk category C (prednisolone), *NR* (all others)

Action
Reduce the immune response by inhibiting prostaglandin synthesis, macrophage and leukocyte accumulation at the inflammation site, phagocytosis, and lysosomal enzyme release. Also reduce the number of T lymphocytes, monocytes, and eosinophils and interfere with binding of immunoglobulins to cell-surface receptors. Some corticosteroids regulate metabolic pathways involving protein, carbohydrate, and fat; others regulate electrolyte and water balance.

Indications
Adrenocortical insufficiency; adrenal, inflammatory, allergic, hematologic, neoplastic, and autoimmune disorders; asthma; cerebral edema; Crohn's disease; hypercalcemia; acute spinal cord injury; nausea and vomiting caused by chemotherapy; prevention of organ rejection in transplant patients; prevention of neonatal respiratory distress in women with high-risk pregnancies

Contraindications and precautions
• Contraindicated in hypersensitivity to drug or intolerance of alcohol, bisulfites, or tartrazine, as well as in active untreated infections
• Use cautiously in hypertension, osteoporosis, diabetes mellitus, glauco-

---

◀€ Clinical alert   Reactions in **bold** are life-threatening

ma, immunosuppression, seizure disorders, renal disease, hypothyroidism, cirrhosis, diverticulitis, active or latent peptic ulcer, inflammatory bowel disease, ulcerative colitis, thromboembolic disorder or tendency, myasthenia gravis, heart failure, metastatic cancer, emotional instability, recent GI surgery, pregnant or breastfeeding patients, and children under age 6 (safety not established).

Adverse reactions

CNS: headache, nervousness, restlessness, depression, euphoria, personality changes, psychosis, vertigo, paresthesia, insomnia, **increased intracranial pressure, seizures**

CV: hypotension, hypertension, thrombophlebitis, **heart failure** (secondary to fluid retention), **thromboembolism, fat embolism, arrhythmias, shock**

EENT: glaucoma (in long-term use), increased intraocular pressure, cataract, nasal congestion and irritation, perforated nasal septum, epistaxis, nasopharyngeal or oropharyngeal fungal infection, sneezing, dysphonia, hoarseness, throat irritation, bad taste

GI: nausea, vomiting, esophageal candidiasis or ulcer, pancreatitis, abdominal distention, anorexia, dry mouth, peptic ulcer

GU: amenorrhea, irregular menses

Metabolic: adrenal suppression, decreased growth (in children), diabetes mellitus, cushingoid state, hypothalamic-pituitary-adrenal suppression (with systemic use exceeding 5 days), sodium and fluid retention, hyperglycemia, hypokalemia, hypocalcemia, increased cholesterol level

Musculoskeletal: muscle wasting, muscle pain and weakness, myopathy, spontaneous fractures, aseptic joint necrosis, tendon rupture, osteoporosis, osteonecrosis

Respiratory: cough, wheezing, **bronchospasm**

Skin: rash, pruritus, contact dermatitis, acne, decreased wound healing, bruising, hirsutism, thin and fragile skin, petechiae, purpura, striae, atrophy of subcutaneous fat, injection site atrophy, angioedema

Other: increased appetite (in long-term use), weight gain, facial edema, Churg-Strauss syndrome, greater susceptibility to infection, aggravation or masking of infection, immunosuppression, hypersensitivity reaction

Interactions

Drug-drug. *Acetaminophen:* increased risk of hepatotoxicity

Aminoglutethimide: decreased adrenal response to corticotropin

Amphotericin B, mezlocillin, piperacillin, thiazide and loop diuretics, ticarcillin: additive hypokalemia

Anticholinergics: glaucoma exacerbation

Anticoagulants: decreased anticoagulant effect

Asparaginase: increased hyperglycemic effect

Carbonic anhydrase inhibitors: increased potassium depletion

Cholestyramine, colestipol: decreased corticosteroid effects

Cyclophosphamide, cyclosporine, hormonal contraceptives: increased corticosteroid effects

Digoxin: increased risk of digoxin toxicity

Erythromycin, indinavir, itraconazole, ketoconazole, ritonavir, saquinavir: increased corticosteroid blood level and effects

Fluoroquinolones: increased risk of tendon rupture

Insulin, oral hypoglycemics: increased requirements for these drugs

Live-virus vaccines: decreased antibody response to vaccine, greater risk of adverse reactions

Nonsteroidal anti-inflammatory drugs: increased risk of adverse GI reactions

---

Phenobarbital, phenytoin, rifampin: stimulated metabolism and decreased efficacy of corticosteroid

Ritodrine: increased risk of cerebral edema

Somatrem, somatropin: inhibited growth-promoting effect of these drugs

Streptozocin: increased risk of hyperglycemia

Theophyllines: increased theophylline effects

Tricyclic antidepressants: increased risk of mental disturbances

Drug-diagnostic tests. *Calcium, potassium, triiodothyronine, thyroxine:* decreased levels

Cholesterol, glucose: increased levels

Nitroblue-tetrazolium test for bacterial infection: false-negative result

Drug-food. *Potassium supplements:* decreased potassium level

Drug-herb. *Echinacea:* increased immune-stimulating effect

Ginseng: potentiation of immunomodulation

Licorice: increased corticosteroid blood level

Lily of the valley, pheasant's eye: increased drug efficacy and adverse effects (with long-term corticosteroid use)

Drug-behaviors. *Alcohol use:* increased risk of gastric irritation and GI ulcers

Patient monitoring

• Monitor ECG, blood glucose and electrolyte levels, urinalysis, and kidney and liver function test results.

◀︎≋ Assess platelet count in long-term therapy. Report unusual bleeding, bruising, petechiae, skin disorders, and signs and symptom of diabetes mellitus.

• Monitor appearance for changes typical of Cushing's syndrome.

diuretics

Loop diuretics: bumetanide, furosemide, torsemide

Osmotic diuretic: mannitol

Potassium-sparing diuretics: amiloride hydrochloride, spironolactone, triamterene

Thiazide and thiazide-like diuretics: chlorthalidone, chlorothiazide, hydrochlorothiazide, indapamide, metolazone

Pregnancy risk category C, B (some diuretics)

Action

Loop diuretics inhibit reabsorption of sodium and chloride (and therefore water) in proximal and distal tubules and loop of Henle. *Osmotic* diuretics increase plasma osmolality, drawing water from body tissues into extracellular fluid and then out through the kidney. *Potassium-sparing* diuretics inhibit sodium reabsorption in distal renal tubule, causing sodium and water loss. *Thiazide and thiazide-like* diuretics decrease rate of sodium and chloride reabsorption by distal renal tubule and increase water excretion.

Indications

Hypertension or edema secondary to heart failure or other causes, cerebral edema, hemolytic transfusion reaction, drug toxicity, prevention of oliguria or acute renal failure

Contraindications and precautions

• Contraindicated in hypersensitivity to drug, alcohol intolerance (with some liquid furosemide forms), anuria, renal decompensation, hepatic coma

---

◀︎≋ Clinical alert   Reactions in **bold** are life-threatening

or precoma, severe electrolyte depletion, severe pulmonary congestion or edema, active intracranial bleeding (except during craniotomy), and severe dehydration

• Use cautiously in severe hepatic disease accompanied by cirrhosis or ascites, electrolyte depletion, worsening azotemia, renal insufficiency (blood urea nitrogen above 30 mg/dl or creatinine clearance below 30 ml/minute), diabetes mellitus, elderly or debilitated patients, pregnant or breastfeeding patients, and children younger than age 18.

Adverse reactions

CNS: dizziness, headache, insomnia, nervousness, vertigo, asthenia, paresthesia, confusion, fatigue, drowsiness, **encephalopathy**

CV: hypotension, chest pain, volume depletion, thrombophlebitis, **arrhythmias**

EENT: blurred vision, nystagmus, hearing loss, tinnitus

GI: nausea, vomiting, diarrhea, constipation, dyspepsia, gastric irritation, dry mouth, anorexia, **acute pancreatitis**

GU: polyuria, nocturia, glycosuria, premature ejaculation, difficulty maintaining erection, nipple tenderness, **renal failure, oliguria**

Hematologic: leukopenia, other blood dyscrasias

Hepatic: jaundice

Metabolic: dehydration, hyperglycemia, hyperuricemia, hypokalemia, hypochloremic alkalosis, hypomagnesemia

Musculoskeletal: joint pain, muscle cramps, myalgia

Skin: photosensitivity, rash, pruritus, urticaria, diaphoresis

Other: weight gain

Interactions

Drug-drug. *Aminoglycosides, cisplatin:* increased risk of ototoxicity

Amphotericin B, corticosteroids, mezlocillin, other diuretics, piperacillin, stimulant laxatives: additive hypokalemia

Anticoagulants, thrombolytics, warfarin: increased anticoagulant effect

Antihypertensives, nitrates: additive hypotension

Digoxin: increased risk of digoxin toxicity

Neuromuscular blockers: prolonged neuromuscular blockade

Nonsteroidal anti-inflammatory drugs, probenecid: inhibited response to diuretic

Drug-diagnostic tests. *Calcium, magnesium, platelets, potassium, sodium:* decreased levels

Cholesterol, creatinine, glucose, nitrogenous compounds: increased levels

Drug-herb. *Dandelion:* interference with diuretic activity

Licorice: rapid potassium loss

Drug-behaviors. *Acute alcohol ingestion:* additive hypotension

Sun exposure: increased risk of photosensitivity

Patient monitoring

• Monitor fluid intake and output, weight, complete blood count, and levels of blood glucose, blood urea nitrogen, creatinine, carbon dioxide, and electrolytes (especially potassium).

• Assess vital signs during rapid diuresis.

fluoroquinolones

ciprofloxacin, enoxacin, gatifloxacin, levofloxacin, lomefloxacin hydrochloride, moxifloxacin hydrochloride, nalidixic acid, norfloxacin, ofloxacin

Pregnancy risk category C

Action

Interfere with DNA gyrase and topoisomerase IV (enzymes needed to synthesize bacterial DNA), thus preventing DNA replication, partitioning, transcription, and repair in susceptible bacteria

Indications

Infections of GU tract, respiratory tract, skin and skin structures, bones, and joints; complicated intra-abdominal infections; nosocomial pneumonia; postexposure treatment of inhalation anthrax

Contraindications and precautions

• Contraindicated in hypersensitivity to drug or other fluoroquinolones, tendinitis or tendon rupture associated with previous fluoroquinolone use, concurrent use of QTc-prolonging drugs or history of QT prolongation, inability or unwillingness to comply with safety measures regarding phototoxicity prophylaxis, pregnancy, and children under age 18 (except in postexposure inhalation or cutaneous anthrax)

• Use cautiously in CNS disease, bradycardia, acute myocardial ischemia, renal impairment, cirrhosis, elderly patients, dialysis patients, and breastfeeding patients (safety not established).

Adverse reactions

CNS: dizziness, drowsiness, headache, insomnia, acute psychosis, agitation, confusion, hallucinations, tremor, light-headedness, **seizures, increased intracranial pressure**
CV: vasodilation, prolonged QT interval, **arrhythmias**
EENT: altered taste
GI: nausea, diarrhea, abdominal pain, **pseudomembranous colitis**
GU: interstitial cystitis, vaginitis
Hepatic: hepatitis
Metabolic: blood glucose changes
Musculoskeletal: tendinitis, tendon rupture

Skin: rash, photosensitivity, phototoxicity
Other: phlebitis at I.V. site, hypersensitivity reactions including **anaphylaxis, Stevens-Johnson syndrome**

Interactions

Drug-drug. *Amiodarone, bepridil, disopyramide, erythromycin, pentamidine, phenothiazines, pimozide, procainamide, quinidine, sotalol, tricyclic antidepressants:* increased risk of serious adverse cardiovascular reactions
Antacids, bismuth subsalicylate, iron salts, sucralfate, zinc salts: decreased fluoroquinolone absorption
Antineoplastics: decreased fluoroquinolone blood level
Cimetidine, probenecid: decreased fluoroquinolone elimination
Corticosteroids: increased risk of tendon rupture
Digoxin: increased digoxin blood level
Foscarnet: increased risk of seizures
Nitrofurantoin: antagonism of fluoroquinolone's effect in urinary tract
Other fluoroquinolones: increased risk of nephrotoxicity
Theophylline: increased theophylline blood level, greater risk of toxicity
Warfarin: increased warfarin effects
Drug-diagnostic tests. *Alanine aminotransferase, alkaline phosphatase, aspartate aminotransferase, bilirubin, lactate dehydrogenase, platelets:* increased levels
Hematocrit, hemoglobin: decreased levels
Drug-food. *Concurrent tube feedings, milk and yogurt (but not other dietary calcium sources):* impaired drug absorption
Drug-herb. *Dong quai, St. John's wort:* increased risk of phototoxicity
Fennel: decreased drug absorption
Drug-behaviors. *Sun exposure:* increased risk of phototoxicity

---

◀€ Clinical alert   Reactions in **bold** are life-threatening

Patient monitoring

• Monitor vital signs, fluid intake and output, complete blood count, and liver and kidney function studies.

• Watch closely for signs and symptoms of superinfection.

• Monitor glucose level in diabetic patients.

hypoglycemics

acarbose, chlorpropamide, glimepiride, glipizide, glyburide, metformin hydrochloride, miglitol, nateglinide, pioglitazone hydrochloride, repaglinide, rosiglitazone maleate, tolazamide, tolbutamide sodium

Pregnancy risk category C, B (some hypoglycemics)

Action

Bind to plasma membrane of functional pancreatic beta cells, decreasing potassium permeability and membrane depolarization; this effect increases intracellular calcium transport and enhances release of insulin-containing secretory granules.

Indications

Type 2 diabetes mellitus

Contraindications and precautions

• Contraindicated in hypersensitivity to drug and in diabetes mellitus complicated by ketoacidosis or pregnancy

• Use cautiously in severe cardiovascular, hepatic, or renal disease; intestinal disorders; thyroid, pituitary, or adrenal dysfunction; malnutrition; high fever; prolonged nausea or vomiting; dehydration; hypoxemia; excessive alcohol ingestion (acute or chronic); heart failure; elderly patients; and pregnant or breastfeeding patients.

Adverse reactions

CNS: lethargy, sedation, hallucinations, delusions, disorientation, peripheral neuropathy, EEG changes, nervousness, restlessness, anxiety, fatigue, insomnia, drowsiness, dizziness, syncope, asthenia, extrapyramidal effects, **seizures, coma, cerebrovascular accident, neuroleptic malignant syndrome**

CV: hypotension, hypertension, ECG changes, tachycardia, palpitations, chest pain, **arrhythmias, myocardial infarction**

EENT: blurred vision, visual disturbances, mydriasis, dry eyes, increased intraocular pressure, tinnitus, rhinitis, altered taste

GI: nausea, vomiting, diarrhea, constipation, epigastric or abdominal pain, dyspepsia, dry mouth, anorexia, **paralytic ileus**

GU: urinary frequency or retention, gynecomastia, sexual dysfunction

Hematologic: leukopenia, agranulocytosis, thrombocytopenia

Hepatic: hepatitis

Metabolic: blood glucose changes

Skin: photosensitivity, rash, urticaria, pruritus, diaphoresis, bruising, photosensitivity

Other: weight changes, edema, increased appetite, chills, yawning, hypersensitivity reaction

Interactions

Drug-drug. *Activated charcoal, corticosteroids, digestive enzymes, diuretics, estrogen, hormonal contraceptives, isoniazid, nicotinic acid, phenothiazines, phenytoin, progestins, sympathomimetics, thyroid preparations:* decreased hypoglycemic efficacy

Amiloride, calcium channel blockers, digoxin, morphine, procainamide, quinidine, ranitidine, triamterene, trimethoprim, vancomycin: altered hypoglycemic effect

Androgens (such as testosterone), chloramphenicol, clofibrate, guanethidine, monoamine oxidase inhibitors, non-

steroidal anti-inflammatory drugs (except diclofenac), salicylates, sulfonamides, warfarin: increased risk of hypoglycemia

Beta-adrenergic blockers: altered response to hypoglycemic

Cimetidine, furosemide: increased hypoglycemic effect

Digoxin: decreased digoxin blood level and efficacy

Insulin: decreased blood levels of these drugs, increased risk of hypoglycemia

Iodinated contrast media: increased risk of lactic acidosis

Nifedipine: increased hypoglycemic absorption and effects

Propranolol, ranitidine: decreased absorption of these drugs

Drug-diagnostic tests. *Urine ketones:* false-positive result

Drug-herb. *Chromium, coenzyme Q10, fenugreek:* additive hypoglycemic effects

Glucosamine: poor glycemic control

Drug-behaviors. *Alcohol use:* disulfiram-like reaction, increased risk of hypoglycemia

Patient monitoring

• Monitor blood glucose level, especially during times of increased stress (such as infection, fever, surgery, and trauma).

• Assess weight and nutritional status.

immunosuppressants

azathioprine, basiliximab, chlorambucil, cyclophosphamide, cyclosporine, daclizumab, infliximab, methotrexate sodium, muromonab-CD3, mycophenolate mofetil, sirolimus, tacrolimus, thalidomide

Pregnancy risk category C, B (basiliximab), D (azathioprine)

Action

Inhibit binding of interleukin (IL)-I with IL-1 receptors; prevent proliferation and differentiation of activated B and T cells; inhibit lymphokine production and IL-2 release; react with T-lymphocyte membranes, depleting blood of CD3+ T cells; and bind to intracellular proteins to prevent T cell activation

Indications

Moderately to severely active rheumatoid arthritis, prevention of kidney transplant rejection

Contraindications and precautions

• Contraindicated in hypersensitivity to drug or its components, fluid overload, uncompensated heart failure, seizure disorders, and pregnant patients with rheumatoid arthritis

• Use cautiously in cancer, renal or hepatic disease, diabetes mellitus, hyperkalemia, hyperuricemia, infection, hypertension, pregnant or breastfeeding patients, and children under age 13.

Adverse reactions

CNS: headache, insomnia, paresthesia, dizziness, tremor, drowsiness, anxiety, confusion, agitation, rigors, asthenia, **coma, seizures**

CV: hypotension, hypertension, tachycardia, palpitations, chest pain, ECG abnormalities, torsades de pointes, **prolonged QT interval**

EENT: blurred vision, painful red eye, dry and irritated eyes, eyelid edema, earache, tinnitus, nasopharyngitis, epistaxis, postnasal drip, sinusitis, sore throat, oral blisters, oral candidiasis

GI: nausea, vomiting, diarrhea, constipation, fecal incontinence, dyspepsia, abdominal pain, dry mouth, anorexia, **GI hemorrhage**

GU: urinary incontinence, oliguria, breakthrough bleeding, renal impairment, **vaginal hemorrhage, renal failure**

Hematologic: anemia, **thrombocytopenia, neutropenia, hemorrhage, disseminated intravascular coagulation**

Hepatic: increased alanine aminotransferase and aspartate aminotransferase levels

Metabolic: hypokalemia, hypomagnesemia, hyperglycemia, hypoglycemia, acidosis, **hyperkalemia**

Musculoskeletal: myalgia; joint, bone, back, neck, and limb pain

Respiratory: dyspnea, cough, hypoxia, wheezing, tachypnea, decreased or abnormal breath sounds, hemoptysis, upper respiratory tract infection, **pleural effusion**

Skin: pruritus, dermatitis, bruising, dry skin, diaphoresis, night sweats, flushing, erythema, petechiae, hyperpigmentation, urticaria, skin lesions, pallor, local exfoliation

Other: weight changes, fever, lymphadenopathy, edema, facial edema, bacterial infection, herpes simplex infection, pain, hypersensitivity reaction, **sepsis**

Interactions

Drug-drug. *Aminoglycosides, amphotericin B, other nephrotoxic drugs:* increased risk of nephrotoxicity

Antifungals, bromocriptine, cimetidine, clarithromycin, danazol, diltiazem, erythromycin, fluconazole, indinavir, itraconazole, metoclopramide, nicardipine, ritonavir, verapamil: increased immunosuppressant blood level

Carbamazepine, phenobarbital, phenytoin, rifabutin, other CYP450-3A4 enzyme inducers: decreased immunosuppressant blood level

Live-virus vaccines: reduced vaccine efficacy

Drug-diagnostic tests. *Blood urea nitrogen, cholesterol, creatinine, hepatic enzymes, lipids, red blood cells:* increased levels

Calcium, glucose, phosphate, white blood cells: increased or decreased levels

Hemoglobin, magnesium, platelets, sodium: decreased levels

Drug-food. *Grapefruit juice:* decreased immunosuppressant metabolism

Drug-herb. *Astragalus, echinacea, melatonin, St. John's wort:* decreased immunosuppressant effect

Patient monitoring

• Assess for signs and symptoms of infection and injection site reaction.

• Monitor vital signs, complete blood count (including platelet count), fluid intake and output, electrolyte and blood glucose levels, and liver and kidney function test results.

inotropics
digoxin, inamrinone lactate, milrinone lactate

Pregnancy risk category C

Action

Inhibit sodium and potassium-activated adenosine triphosphatase phosphodiesterase, which raises intracellular and extracellular calcium levels. These effects strengthen myocardial contractility, prolong refractory period of atrioventricular (AV) node, decrease conduction through sinoatrial and AV nodes, and relax and dilate vascular smooth muscle to reduce preload and afterload.

Indications

Heart failure, tachyarrhythmias, atrial fibrillation or flutter, paroxysmal atrial tachycardia

Contraindications and precautions

• Contraindicated in hypersensitivity to drug, known alcohol intolerance (with elixir only), and ventricular fibrillation

• Use cautiously in electrolyte abnormalities (such as hypokalemia, hypercalcemia, hypomagnesemia), myocardial infarction, AV block, idiopathic hypertrophic subaortic stenosis, constrictive pericarditis, renal impairment, obesity, elderly patients, pregnant or breastfeeding patients, and children.

Adverse reactions

CNS: fatigue, headache, asthenia
CV: bradycardia, ECG changes, **arrhythmias**
EENT: blurred or yellow vision
GI: nausea, vomiting, diarrhea, anorexia
GU: gynecomastia
Hematologic: thrombocytopenia

Interactions

Drug-drug. *Amiodarone, amphotericin B, corticosteroids, cyclosporine, diclofenac, diltiazem, loop and thiazide diuretics, mezlocillin, piperacillin, propafenone, quinidine, quinine, ticarcillin, verapamil:* increased inotropic blood level, greater risk of toxicity
Antacids, cholestyramine, colestipol, kaolin and pectin: decreased inotropic absorption
Beta-adrenergic blockers, other antiarrhythmics (such as disopyramide, quinidine): additive bradycardia
Laxatives (excessive use): hypokalemia, increased risk of inotropic toxicity
Spironolactone: decreased inotropic effect, increased risk of digoxin toxicity
Thyroid hormones: decreased inotropic efficacy
Drug-diagnostic tests. *Creatine kinase:* increased level
Drug-food. *High-fiber meal:* decreased drug absorption
Drug-herb. *Cola seed, guarana seed, horsetail, licorice, natural stimulant products (such as aloe), yerba maté:* increased risk of hypokalemia

Ephedra (ma huang): arrhythmias
Hawthorn: cardiotoxicity
Indian snakeroot: bradycardia
Licorice: inotropic toxicity
Psyllium: decreased inotropic absorption
St. John's wort: decreased inotropic blood level and effects

Patient monitoring

• Monitor vital signs, weight, electrolyte levels, fluid intake and output, drug blood level, and kidney function test results.

laxatives

bisacodyl, calcium polycarbophil, castor oil, docusate, glycerin, lactulose, magnesium salts, methylcellulose, psyllium, senna, sodium phosphate

Pregnancy risk category NR, B (psyllium), *C* (docusate, senna)

Action

Stimulate smooth muscle of bowel, increasing contractions; increase stool bulk by causing water retention and inhibiting digestive process in stomach. Also soften hard feces, promoting their passage through lower intestine.

Indications

Constipation, prophylaxis of constipation in patients who shouldn't strain during defecation (for example, after anorectal surgery or myocardial infarction), colonic evacuation for rectal and bowel examination

Contraindications and precautions

• Contraindicated in hypersensitivity to drug or its components, intestinal obstruction, undiagnosed abdominal pain, suspected appendicitis, and fecal impaction

• Use cautiously in severe cardiovascular disease, anal or rectal fissures, enteritis, ulcerative colitis, diverticulitis, pregnant or breastfeeding patients, and children under age 2.

Adverse reactions

GI: nausea, vomiting, diarrhea; esophageal, gastric, small intestine, or rectal obstruction (with dry drug form); abdominal cramps in severe constipation; anorexia

GU: reddish-pink discoloration of alkaline urine, yellow-brown discoloration of acidic urine

Metabolic: alkalosis, fluid and electrolyte imbalances

Musculoskeletal: tetany

Other: laxative dependence (with excessive long-term use)

Interactions

Drug-drug. *Antacids:* gastric irritation, dyspepsia

Mineral oil: increased mineral oil absorption and toxicity

Tetracyclines: impaired tetracycline absorption

Drug-diagnostic tests. *Fluids, electrolytes:* fluid or electrolyte imbalances

Drug-food. *Milk:* gastric irritation

Drug-herb. *Lily of the valley, pheasant's eye, squill:* increased adverse laxative effects

Patient monitoring

• Monitor fluid and electrolyte balance.

■ ■ ■ ■ ■ ■ ■ ■
▩ ▩ ▩

macrolide anti-infectives

azithromycin, clarithromycin, dirithromycin, erythromycin

Pregnancy risk category B (azithromycin, erythromycin), *C* (clarithromycin, dirithromycin)

Action

Inhibit bacterial protein synthesis by combining with 50S ribosomal subunit of susceptible organisms

Indications

Infections caused by susceptible organisms, including upper and lower respiratory tract infections, otitis media, skin and skin-structure infections, pertussis, diphtheria, erythrasma, intestinal amebiasis, pelvic inflammatory disease, nongonococcal urethritis, syphilis, Legionnaires' disease, and rheumatic fever; as a penicillin substitute in patients with penicillin hypersensitivity

Contraindications and precautions

• Contraindicated in hypersensitivity to macrolides, alcohol intolerance (with most topical forms), tartrazine sensitivity (with some forms), neonates (with forms containing benzyl alcohol), hepatic dysfunction, and concurrent use of pimozide or sparfloxacin

• Use cautiously in severe hepatic impairment, renal impairment, pregnant or breastfeeding patients, and children under age 2 (safety not established).

Adverse reactions

CNS: dizziness, drowsiness, fatigue, headache, vertigo

CV: chest pain, palpitations

GI: nausea, diarrhea, abdominal pain, dyspepsia, flatulence, melena, **pseudomembranous colitis**

GU: nephritis, vaginitis, candidiasis
Hepatic: cholestatic jaundice
Metabolic: hyperglycemia, hyperkalemia
Skin: photosensitivity, rash, angioedema

Interactions

Drug-drug. *Alfentanil, alprazolam, bromocriptine, buspirone, carbamazepine, clozapine, cyclosporine, diazepam, disopyramide, ergot alkaloids, felodipine, methylprednisolone, midazolam, tacrolimus, theophylline, triazolam, vinblastine, warfarin:* increased blood levels of these drugs, greater risk of toxicity
Aluminum- and magnesium-containing antacids: decreased macrolide peak blood level
Clindamycin, lincomycin: decreased efficacy of these drugs
HMG-CoA reductase inhibitors: increased risk of myopathy and rhabdomyolysis
Pimozide, sparfloxacin: increased risk of serious arrhythmias
Rifabutin, rifampin: decreased macrolide effects, increased risk of adverse GI reactions
Theophylline: increased theophylline blood level
Zidovudine: altered zidovudine effects
Drug-diagnostic tests. *Alanine aminotransferase, alkaline phosphatase, aspartate aminotransferase, bilirubin:* increased levels
Urinary catecholamines: false elevations
Drug-food. *Any food:* decreased drug absorption (with multidoses of oral suspension forms)
Drug-behaviors. *Sun exposure:* photosensitivity

Patient monitoring

• Monitor patient for signs and symptoms of superinfection.
• Assess liver function test results.

neuromuscular blockers
atracurium besylate, cisatracurium besylate, doxacurium chloride, mivacurium chloride, pancuronium bromide, rocuronium bromide, succinylcholine chloride, tubocurarine chloride, vecuronium bromide

Pregnancy risk category C, B (some neuromuscular blockers)

Action

Nondepolarizing (competitive) neuromuscular blockers (all listed above except succinylcholine) bind competitively to cholinergic receptors on motor end-plate, preventing muscle contraction. *Depolarizing* neuromuscular blockers (succinylcholine) initially excite skeletal muscle, then prevent muscle contraction by prolonging the refractory period.

Indications

Adjunct to anesthesia to facilitate endotracheal intubation and relax skeletal muscles during surgery or mechanical ventilation, to facilitate orthopedic manipulation, to reduce muscle contractions during pharmacologically or electrically induced seizures, myasthenia gravis diagnosis

Contraindications and precautions

• Contraindicated in hypersensitivity to drug, low plasma pseudocholinesterase level, narrow-angle glaucoma, myopathy with elevated creatine kinase level, penetrating eye injury, and personal or family history of malignant hyperthermia
• Use cautiously in heart disease; electrolyte imbalance; dehydration; neuro-

muscular, respiratory, or hepatic disease; pregnant or breastfeeding patients, and children under age 2.

Adverse reactions
CV: hypotension, bradycardia, **arrhythmias, cardiac arrest**
Musculoskeletal: profound and prolonged muscle relaxation, residual muscle weakness
Respiratory: prolonged apnea, bronchospasm, cyanosis, respiratory depression
Skin: rash, flushing, pruritus, urticaria
Other: hypersensitivity reaction

Interactions
Drug-drug. *Acetylcholinesterase inhibitors, edrophonium, neostigmine, pyridostigmine:* reversal of neuromuscular blockade
Aminoglycosides, amphotericin B, anticholinesterases, corticosteroids, ethacrynic acid, furosemide, general anesthetics, lithium, loop and thiazide diuretics, methotrimeprazine, opioid analgesics, polymyxin antibiotics (such as colistin, polymyxin B sulfate), propranolol, quinidine, theophylline, verapamil: increased neuromuscular blockade
Carbamazepine, phenytoin, theophylline: resistance to or reversal of neuromuscular blockade
Other neuromuscular blockers: faster onset and depth of muscle relaxation

Patient monitoring
◄€ Monitor vital signs, pulmonary status, and temperature continuously.

nonopioid analgesics
celecoxib, diclofenac, diflunisal, etodolac, ibuprofen, indomethacin, ketoprofen, ketorolac tromethamine, meloxicam, nabumetone, naproxen, oxaprozin, piroxicam, rofecoxib, sulindac, valdecoxib

Pregnancy risk category C, B (some nonopioid analgesics)

Action
Inhibit cyclooxygenase, an enzyme needed for prostaglandin synthesis; this inhibition stimulates the anti-inflammatory response and blocks pain impulses

Indications
Inflammatory conditions (such as osteoarthritis, rheumatoid arthritis, ankylosing spondylitis), dysmenorrhea, actinic keratoses, fever

Contraindications and precautions
• Contraindicated in hypersensitivity to drug or sulfonamides and in history of asthma, urticaria, or allergic reaction to aspirin or other nonsteroidal anti-inflammatory drugs (NSAIDs)
• Use cautiously in severe cardiovascular, renal, or hepatic disease; GI disorders; cardiac decompensation; active GI bleeding or ulcer; asthma; history of ulcer disease; and chronic alcohol use or abuse.

Adverse reactions
CNS: dizziness, headache, insomnia, fatigue, paresthesia, tremor, vertigo, syncope, anxiety, confusion, depression, nervousness, drowsiness, malaise, **seizures**
CV: palpitations, tachycardia, angina pectoris, hypertension, hypotension,

arrhythmias, heart failure, myocardial infarction
EENT: abnormal vision, conjunctivitis, hearing loss, tinnitus, pharyngitis
GI: nausea, vomiting, diarrhea, constipation, abdominal pain, dyspepsia, flatulence, colitis, duodenal or gastric ulcer, gastritis, gastroesophageal reflux, esophagitis, dry mouth, **altered taste, GI hemorrhage, pancreatitis**
GU: albuminuria, hematuria, urinary frequency, urinary tract infection, **renal failure**
Hematologic: anemia, purpura, **leukopenia, thrombocytopenia, other blood dyscrasias**
Hepatic: hepatitis
Metabolic: dehydration
Musculoskeletal: myalgia, joint or back pain
Respiratory: dyspnea, cough, asthma, upper respiratory tract infection, **bronchospasm**
Skin: rash, urticaria, diaphoresis, pruritus, alopecia, bullous eruption, angioedema, photosensitivity
Other: flulike symptoms, edema, accidental injury, fever, increased appetite, weight changes, allergic reaction

Interactions

Drug-drug. *Acetaminophen:* increased risk of adverse renal reactions
Antineoplastics: increased risk of adverse hematologic reactions
Cefamandole, cefoperazone, cefotetan, plicamycin, thrombolytics, valproic acid, warfarin and other drugs that affect platelet function (such as abciximab, clopidogrel, eptifibatide, ticlopidine, tirofiban): increased risk of bleeding
Corticosteroids, NSAIDs: additive adverse GI effects
Cyclosporine: increased risk of nephrotoxicity
Digoxin: increased digoxin blood level
Diuretics, other antihypertensives: decreased efficacy of these drugs

Insulin, oral hypoglycemics: increased hypoglycemic effect
Lithium: increased lithium blood level and risk of toxicity
Methotrexate: increased risk of methotrexate toxicity
Probenecid: increased risk of toxicity (when taken with ibuprofen)
Drug-diagnostic tests. *Alanine aminotransferase, alkaline phosphatase, aspartate aminotransferase, blood urea nitrogen, creatinine, lactate dehydrogenase, potassium:* increased levels
Bleeding time: prolonged (for up to 4 days after therapy ends)
Creatinine clearance, glucose, hematocrit, hemoglobin, platelets, white blood cells: decreased levels
Urine 5-hydroxyindoleacetic acid, urine steroids: altered results
Drug-herb. *Anise, arnica, chamomile, clove, dong quai, fenugreek, feverfew, garlic, ginger, ginkgo, ginseng, licorice, white willow:* increased bleeding risk
Drug-behaviors. *Alcohol use:* increased risk of adverse GI effects
Smoking: GI irritation and bleeding
Sun exposure: phototoxicity

Patient monitoring

• Monitor complete blood count and liver and kidney function test results.

opioid analgesics

alfentanil, buprenorphine hydrochloride, butorphanol tartrate,
codeine, fentanyl citrate, hydrocodone, hydromorphone, meperidine
hydrochloride, methadone hydrochloride, morphine sulfate, nalbuphine hydrochloride, oxycodone,
oxymorphone hydrochloride, propoxyphene, remifentanil hydrochloride, sufentanil

Pregnancy risk category C, B (meperidine, nalbuphine), *D* (with long-term
use)

Action
Attach to specific CNS receptors, decreasing cell membrane permeability,
slowing pain impulse transmission,
and altering response to pain

Indications
Moderate to severe pain, intraoperative
anesthesia, labor, cough, diarrhea

Contraindications and precautions
• Contraindicated in hypersensitivity
to drug, diarrhea caused by poisoning,
acute bronchial asthma, and upper airway obstruction
• Use cautiously in severe cardiovascular, renal, or hepatic disease; cardiac
decompensation; GI disorders; history
of ulcer disease; chronic alcohol use or
abuse; elderly patients; and pregnant or
breastfeeding patients.

Adverse reactions
CNS: drowsiness, sedation, dizziness,
tremor, irritability, syncope, stimulation (in children)

CV: hypertension, hypotension, palpitations, bradycardia, tachycardia, extrasystole, **arrhythmias**
EENT: blurred vision, nasal dryness
and congestion, dry throat, sore throat
GI: nausea, vomiting, constipation, intestinal obstruction, epigastric distress,
dry mouth, anorexia
GU: urinary retention or hesitancy,
dysuria, early menses, decreased libido,
impotence
Hematologic: hemolytic or hypoplastic
anemia, **thrombocytopenia, agranulocytosis, leukopenia, pancytopenia**
Respiratory: thickened bronchial secretions, chest tightness, wheezing
Skin: urticaria, rash, diaphoresis
Other: hypersensitivity reaction (with
I.V. use), **anaphylactic shock**

Interactions
Drug-drug. *Antihistamines, barbitu-
rates, clomipramine, sedative-hypnotics,
tricyclic antidepressants:* additive CNS
depression
Cimetidine: decreased metabolism and
increased effects of opioid analgesic
Lithium, methotrexate: increased blood
levels of these drugs
Monoamine oxidase (MAO) inhibitors:
additive effects
Naloxone: opioid withdrawal symptoms
Oral anticoagulants: increased risk of
GI bleeding
Warfarin: increased anticoagulant ef-
fect
Drug-diagnostic tests. *Amylase, lipase:*
increased levels
Drug-food. *Grapefruit juice:* decreased
drug metabolism, increased risk of
drug toxicity
Drug-herb. *Chamomile, hops, kava,
skullcap, valerian:* increased CNS de-
pression
Drug-behaviors. *Alcohol use:* increased
CNS depression

Patient monitoring
• Assess vital signs and pulmonary
status.

◀€ Clinical alert   Reactions in **bold** are life-threatening

• Monitor complete blood count, electrolyte levels, and liver and kidney function test results.

skeletal muscle relaxants
baclofen, carisoprodol, chlorzoxazone, cyclobenzaprine hydrochloride, dantrolene sodium, diazepam, methocarbamol, tizanidine hydrochloride

Pregnancy risk category C

Action
Unknown; muscle relaxation may result from sedative properties and inhibition of activity in descending reticular formation and spine. These drugs also decrease muscle tone and involuntary movements.

Indications
Muscle spasms (as from trauma or inflammation), hyperreflexia and hypertonia (as from parkinsonism), tetanus, cerebral palsy, multiple sclerosis, tension headache

Contraindications and precautions
• Contraindicated in hypersensitivity to drug or polyethylene glycol (with parenteral forms), renal impairment (with parenteral forms), active hepatic disease, upper motor neuron disorder, and patients who use spasticity to maintain posture or balance
• Use cautiously in cardiac, hepatic, or renal dysfunction; history of allergies; seizure disorders (with parenteral forms); pregnant or breastfeeding patients; and children (safety not established).

Adverse reactions
CNS: dizziness, anxiety, abnormal thinking, hyperesthesia, agitation, confusion, hypertonia, **seizures, coma**
CV: pseudoaneurysm, palpitations, fistula, thrombophlebitis, hypotension, bradycardia, weak pulse, complete or incomplete atrioventricular block, **embolism, nodal arrhythmias, ventricular tachycardia**
EENT: diplopia
GI: nausea, vomiting, diarrhea, dyspepsia, gastroesophageal reflux, hematemesis, dysphagia, **paralytic ileus, GI bleeding**
GU: urinary frequency or incontinence, dysuria, renal dysfunction, cystalgia, prostatitis
Hepatic: hepatitis
Musculoskeletal: muscle rigidity
Respiratory: pneumonia, bronchitis, pleurisy, abnormal breath sounds, dyspnea, wheezing, **pleural effusion, pulmonary edema, pulmonary embolism, bronchospasm**
Skin: rash, urticaria, pruritus
Other: edema, chills, fever

Interactions
Drug-drug. *Anticholinergics and anticholinergic-like drugs (such as antihistamines, atropine, disopyramide, haloperidol, phenothiazines):* additive anticholinergic effects
CNS depressants (such as opioids, sedative-hypnotics): additive CNS depression
Monoamine oxidase inhibitors: hyperpyretic crisis, seizures, death
Drug-diagnostic tests. *Urinary 5-hydroxyindoleacetic acid, vanillylmandelic acid:* false elevations
Drug-herb. *Chamomile, hops, kava, skullcap, valerian:* increased CNS depression
Drug-behaviors. *Alcohol use:* additive CNS depression
Sun exposure: phototoxicity

Patient monitoring
• Monitor vital signs and liver function test results.

---

sulfonamides
sulfadiazine, sulfamethoxazole, sulfisoxazole

Pregnancy risk category C

Action
Interfere with bacterial DNA synthesis by inhibiting dihydropteroate synthetase (a bacterial enzyme)

Indications
Toxoplasmosis, chloroquine-resistant *Plasmodium falciparum* malaria, *Nocardia* infection, meningitis, asymptomatic meningococcal carrier state, urinary tract infection, chancroid, trachoma, otitis media, conjunctivitis, corneal ulcer and other superficial ocular infections, prophylaxis and treatment of rheumatic fever

Contraindications and precautions
• Contraindicated in hypersensitivity to sulfonamides, salicylates, bisulfites, furosemide, sulfonylureas, or carbonic anhydrase inhibitors; porphyria; pregnant patients at term; breastfeeding patients; and infants younger than 2 months
• Use cautiously in bronchial asthma, glucose-6-phosphate dehydrogenase deficiency, blood dyscrasias, severe hepatic or renal impairment, active peptic ulcer, GI or GU tract obstruction, porphyria, history of multiple allergies, and pregnant patients (until term).

Adverse reactions
CNS: headache, depression, hallucinations, insomnia, vertigo, fatigue, anxiety, **seizures**

CV: allergic myocarditis
GI: nausea, vomiting, abdominal pain, pancreatitis, stomatitis, glossitis, dry mouth, anorexia, **enterocolitis**
GU: yellow-orange urine, crystalluria, hematuria, increased blood urea nitrogen and creatinine levels, proteinuria, oligospermia, **renal failure, toxic nephrosis with oliguria and anuria**
Hematologic: megaloblastic anemia, **agranulocytosis, thrombocytopenia, leukopenia, aplastic anemia, hemolytic anemia**
Hepatic: jaundice, **hepatitis**
Skin: generalized skin eruption, photosensitivity, urticaria, pruritus, alopecia, exfoliative dermatitis, erythema multiforme, **toxic epidermal necrolysis**
Other: local irritation; extravasation; chills; hypersensitivity reactions, including serum sickness, drug fever, **anaphylaxis, Stevens-Johnson syndrome**

Interactions
Drug-drug. *Aspirin:* inhibited uricosuric effects of sulfonamides
Barbiturates, oral anticoagulants, tolbutamide, uricosurics: increased effects of these drugs
Cyclosporine: increased nephrotoxicity
Digoxin: reduced digoxin absorption
Folic acid: decreased sulfonamide absorption
Hepatotoxic agents: increased risk of hepatitis
Hormonal contraceptives: decreased contraceptive efficacy
Indomethacin, probenecid, salicylates: increased sulfonamide blood level
Iron: decreased sulfonamide blood level
Methenamine: increased crystalluria
Methotrexate, oral hypoglycemics, phenytoin, warfarin, zidovudine: enhanced action of these drugs, greater risk of toxicity
Other anti-infectives: altered action of these drugs

◀€ Clinical alert   Reactions in **bold** are life-threatening

Thiazide diuretics: increased risk of thrombocytopenia

Drug-diagnostic tests. *Alanine aminotransferase, aspartate aminotransferase, bilirubin, blood urea nitrogen, creatinine, eosinophils:* increased levels

Fibrinogen, granulocytes, hemoglobin, platelets, prothrombin time, white blood cells: decreased levels

Urine glucose: false-positive result

Drug-herb. *Dong quai, St. John's wort:* increased risk of photosensitivity

Drug-behaviors. *Sun exposure:* increased risk of photosensitivity

Patient monitoring

• Monitor complete blood count, blood glucose level, bleeding times, cultures, and liver and kidney function test results.

• Monitor fluid intake and output.

tetracyclines

demeclocycline hydrochloride, doxycycline, minocycline hydrochloride, tetracycline hydrochloride

Pregnancy risk category D

Action

Bind to 50S ribosomal subunit, interfering with bacterial protein synthesis; also block binding of aminoacyl-tRNA to messenger RNA–ribosome complex

Indications

Rocky Mountain spotted fever, typhoid fever, Q fever, tick fever, rickettsialpox, gonorrhea and syphilis (in penicillin-allergic patients), acne, periodontitis, chlamydia, brucellosis, urethral syndrome in women, *Helicobacter pylori* infection, cholera, malaria, respiratory and urinary tract infections, meningitis, acute intestinal amebiasis, prevention of chronic bronchitis exacerbation

Contraindications and precautions

• Contraindicated in hypersensitivity to drug, alcohol, or bisulfates

• Use cautiously in renal or hepatic impairment, nephrogenic diabetes insipidus, cachexia, debilitated patients, pregnant or breastfeeding patients, and children under age 8.

Adverse reactions

CNS: benign intracranial hypertension, paresthesia

CV: pericarditis, thrombophlebitis, phlebitis

EENT: vestibular reactions, oral candidiasis, pharyngitis, permanent tooth discoloration, tooth enamel defects, black hairy tongue, hoarseness

GI: nausea, vomiting, diarrhea, pancreatitis, epigastric distress, esophagitis, enterocolitis, anogenital inflammation and lesions, glossitis, anorexia

GU: dark yellow or brown urine, elevated blood urea nitrogen, vaginal candidiasis

Hematologic: eosinophilia, hemolytic anemia, **neutropenia, thrombocytopenia, other blood dyscrasias**

Hepatic: hepatoxicity

Musculoskeletal: bone growth retardation

Skin: maculopapular or erythematous rash, photosensitivity, increased pigmentation, urticaria, photosensitivity

Other: phlebitis at I.V. site, superinfection, hypersensitivity reactions including **anaphylaxis**

Interactions

Drug-drug. *Adsorbent antidiarrheals, bismuth salts, cholestyramine, colestipol, sodium bicarbonate, sucralfate:* decreased tetracycline absorption

Antacids containing aluminum, calcium, iron, or magnesium: chelate formation, causing decreased tetracycline absorption

Anticoagulants: increased thrombocytopenia

Barbiturates, carbamazepine, phenytoin: decreased tetracycline blood level
Bumetanide, diuretics, methoxyflurane: increased risk of nephrotoxicity
Digoxin: increased digoxin bioavailability
Hormonal contraceptives: decreased contraceptive efficacy
Insulin: decreased insulin requirement
Iron preparations: decreased tetracycline effects
Penicillin: decreased penicillin activity
Warfarin: enhanced warfarin effects
Drug-diagnostic tests. *Alanine aminotransferase, alkaline phosphatase, amylase, aspartate aminotransferase, bilirubin, blood urea nitrogen:* increased levels
Hemoglobin, neutrophils, platelets, white blood cells: decreased levels
Urinary catecholamines: false elevations
Drug-food. *Calcium-containing foods and beverages:* chelate formation, causing decreased drug absorption
Drug-herb. *Bromelain:* increased tetracycline blood level
Drug-behaviors. *Alcohol use:* decreased tetracycline effects
Sun exposure: increased risk of photosensitivity

Patient monitoring
• Monitor vital signs and fluid intake and output.

thrombolytics

alteplase, anistreplase, reteplase, streptokinase, tenecteplase, urokinase

Pregnancy risk category C

Action
Convert plasminogen to plasmin, an enzyme that degrades fibrin clots and lyses thrombi and emboli

Indications
Acute massive pulmonary embolism, acute ischemic cerebrovascular accident (CVA), thrombotic coronary arterial obstruction in acute myocardial infarction, deep-vein thrombosis, arterial emboli or thromboses, occlusion of venous access device

Contraindications and precautions
• Contraindicated in hypersensitivity to drug or other thrombolytics, active internal bleeding, bleeding diathesis, severe uncontrolled hypertension, intracranial neoplasm, arteriovenous malformation or aneurysm, recent CVA, or recent intracranial or intraspinal surgery or trauma
• Use cautiously in obstetric delivery, organ biopsy, GI or GU bleeding, trauma, major surgery, hypertension, left-sided cardiac thrombus (including mitral stenosis), acute pericarditis, subacute bacterial endocarditis, hemostatic defects, diabetic hemorrhagic retinopathy, septic thrombophlebitis, previous puncture of noncompressible vessels, patients over age 75, and pregnant or breastfeeding patients.

Adverse reactions
CNS: intracranial hemorrhage
CV: hypotension, **arrhythmias, cholesterol embolization, venous thrombosis**
GI: nausea, vomiting, **GI or retroperitoneal bleeding**
GU: hematuria
Hematologic: anemia, **bone marrow depression, hemorrhage, bleeding tendency**
Respiratory: respiratory depression, apnea
Skin: bruising, urticaria
Other: fever, edema, phlebitis or hemorrhage at I.V. site, hypersensitivity reactions including **anaphylaxis, sepsis**

◀€ Clinical alert   Reactions in **bold** are life-threatening

Interactions

Drug-drug. *Anticoagulants, aspirin, dipyridamole, drugs affecting platelets, indomethacin, phenylbutazone:* increased risk of bleeding

Drug-diagnostic tests. *Hemoglobin:* decreased value

International Normalized Ratio (INR), partial thromboplastin time (PTT), pro-thrombin time (PT): increased values

Patient monitoring

• Monitor vital signs and neurologic status closely.

◀€ Assess for signs and symptoms of unusual bleeding or bruising.

• Monitor INR, PT, and PTT.

thyroid hormones

levothyroxine sodium; liothyronine sodium; liotrix; thyroid, desiccated

Pregnancy risk category A

Action

Regulate growth and development by controlling protein synthesis; also stimulate normal metabolism by oxygenating body tissues

Indications

Hypothyroidism, euthyroid or multinodal goiter, subacute or chronic lymphocytic thyroiditis

Contraindications and precautions

• Contraindicated in hypersensitivity to drug, recent myocardial infarction, adrenal insufficiency, and thyrotoxicosis

• Use cautiously in cardiovascular disease, severe renal insufficiency, uncorrected adrenocortical disorders, angina pectoris, ischemia, diabetes mellitus, myxedema, elderly patients, and pregnant or breastfeeding patients.

Adverse reactions

CNS: insomnia, irritability, nervousness, tremor, headache

CV: tachycardia, angina pectoris, hypotension, hypertension, increased cardiac output, palpitations, **arrhythmias, cardiovascular collapse**

GI: vomiting, diarrhea, abdominal cramps

GU: menstrual irregularities

Metabolic: hyperthyroidism

Musculoskeletal: accelerated bone maturation in children

Skin: alopecia (in children), diaphoresis

Other: weight loss, appetite changes, heat intolerance

Interactions

Drug-drug. *Adrenergics, levarterenol:* increased adverse cardiovascular effects

Antidepressants: altered effects of both drugs

Beta-adrenergic blockers: decreased beta-blocker efficacy

Bile acid sequestrants: decreased absorption of oral thyroid preparations

Calcium salts: decreased thyroid hormone absorption from GI tract

Cardiac glycosides: decreased cardiac glycoside effect

Corticosteroids: increased tissue damage from corticosteroids

Digoxin: decreased digoxin effects

Estrogens: increased thyroid hormone requirements

Insulin, oral hypoglycemics: increased requirements for these drugs

Ketamine: severe hypertension

Phenytoin: increased thyroid hormone effects

Theophylline: decreased theophylline clearance

Warfarin: altered warfarin efficacy

Drug-diagnostic tests. *Aspartate aminotransferase, creatine kinase, glucose, lactate dehydrogenase, protein-bound iodine:* increased levels

Drug-herb. *Bugleweed:* increased adverse drug reactions

Horseradish: abnormal thyroid function

Lemon balm: antithyroid effects

Soy: decreased thyroid hormone level

Patient monitoring

• Monitor thyroid function test results, vital signs, weight, and ECG.

thyroid hormone antagonists

methimazole, potassium iodide, propylthiouracil, radioactive iodine

Pregnancy risk category D

Action

Rapidly inhibit iodine release and synthesis in thyroid gland, decreasing thyroid vascularity and preventing iodine uptake

Indications

Hyperthyroidism, thyroid cancer, thyrotoxicosis, control of hyperthyroidism in preparation for thyroidectomy or radioactive iodine therapy

Contraindications and precautions

• Contraindicated in hypersensitivity to thyroid hormone antagonists and in breastfeeding

• Use cautiously in bone marrow depression, tuberculosis, bronchitis, hyperkalemia, renal impairment, recent myocardial infarction, large nodular goiter, vomiting and diarrhea, patients under age 30, and pregnant patients.

Adverse reactions

CNS: headache, vertigo, paresthesia, neuritis, neuropathies, CNS stimulation, depression, drowsiness

CV: chest pain, tachycardia

EENT: pain on swallowing, sore throat, salivary gland enlargement, fullness in neck

GI: nausea, vomiting, diarrhea, constipation, epigastric distress, GI irritation, dry mouth, loss of taste, anorexia, **paralytic ileus**

GU: nephritis

Hematologic: anemia, eosinophilia, **bone marrow depression, leukopenia, thrombocytopenia, leukemia, agranulocytosis**

Hepatic: jaundice, hepatic dysfunction, **hepatitis**

Metabolic: hypothyroidism, thyroid hyperplasia, hyperkalemia

Musculoskeletal: joint pain, myalgia

Respiratory: cough

Skin: rash, urticaria, skin discoloration, pruritus, erythema nodosum, exfoliative dermatitis, alopecia, acneiform eruption

Other: fever, lupuslike syndrome, lymphadenopathy, lymphedema, radiation sickness (with radioactive iodine)

Interactions

Drug-drug. *Angiotensin-converting enzyme inhibitors, potassium-sparing diuretics, potassium supplements:* additive hyperkalemia (with potassium iodide use)

Anticoagulants: potentiation of anticoagulant effect

Antineoplastics: additive bone marrow depression

Digoxin: increased digoxin blood level

Lithium: hypothyroidism

Phenothiazines: increased risk of agranulocytosis

Drug-diagnostic tests. *Alanine aminotransferase, alkaline phosphatase, aspartate aminotransferase, bilirubin, lactate dehydrogenase, prothrombin time:* increased values

Patient monitoring

• Monitor complete blood count and thyroid function test results.

Vitamins and minerals

ascorbic acid (vitamin C)
Cecon, Cevi-Bid, Dull-C, Vita-C

Action
Water-soluble vitamin with antioxidant properties; stimulates collagen formation and enhances tissue repair

Availability
Capsules: 500 mg
Crystals: 1,000 mg/½ tsp
Injection: 250 mg/ml, 500 mg/ml
Liquid: 500 mg/5 ml
Powder: 60 mg/½ tsp, 1,060 mg/½ tsp
Solution: 100 mg/ml
Tablets: 250 mg, 500 mg, 1,000 mg, 1,500 mg
Tablets (timed-release): 500 mg, 1,000 mg, 1,500 mg

⚕ Indications and dosages
➢ Recommended dietary allowance (RDA)
Adults: 60 mg daily
➢ Chronic illness, infection, febrile states, hemovascular disorders, promotion of wound healing
Adults: 300 to 500 mg P.O., S.C., I.V., or I.M. daily for 7 to 10 days
Children: 100 to 300 mg P.O., S.C., I.V., or I.M. daily
➢ Scurvy
Adults: Initially, 300 mg to 1 g/day P.O., S.C., I.M. or I.V. depending on severity; then a maintenance dosage of 70 to 150 mg daily
Children: 100 to 300 mg P.O., S.C., I.M., or I.V. depending on severity; then a maintenance dosage of 30 mg daily

Contraindications and precautions
• Contraindicated in hypersensitivity to tartrazine or sulfites (with products containing these compounds) and before tests for occult blood in stool; prolonged use of excessive doses contraindicated in diabetes mellitus, sodium-restricted diet, concurrent anticoagulant use, and history of recurrent renal calculi
• Don't exceed recommended amount in pregnant patients. Use with caution in breastfeeding patients. Avoid rapid I.V. infusion.

Adverse reactions
Transient mild soreness at I.M. or S.C. injection site; transient light-headedness or dizziness (with rapid I.V. administration)

cholecalciferol (vitamin D₃)
Delta-D

Action
Biologically active vitamin D metabolite that controls intestinal absorption of dietary calcium, tubular reabsorption of calcium by the kidneys, and (in conjunction with parathyroid hormone [PTH]), mobilization of calcium from skeleton. Acts directly on bone cells to stimulate skeletal growth and on parathyroid glands to suppress PTH synthesis and secretion.

Availability
Tablets: 400 IU, 1,000 IU

⚕ Indications and dosages
➢ Recommended dietary allowance (RDA) as a dietary supplement
Adults: 400 to 1,000 IU/day

Reactions in **bold** are life-threatening

Children: 200 IU/day

➤ Prophylaxis or treatment of secondary hyperparathyroidism associated with chronic renal failure and other vitamin D deficiency conditions
Adults: Dosage individualized; typical initial dosage is 10,000 IU P.O. daily, increased to a maximum of 500,000 I.U. daily based on response.

Contraindications and precautions

• Contraindicated in hypercalcemia, vitamin D toxicity, malabsorption syndrome, abnormal sensitivity to vitamin D effects, and renal dysfunction
• Don't exceed RDA during normal pregnancy. Use cautiously in breast-feeding patients. Safety and efficacy of dosages above RDA in children haven't been established.

Adverse reactions

Nausea; vomiting; constipation; weakness; headache; drowsiness; dry mouth; metallic taste; muscle or bone pain; hypertension; polyuria; polydipsia; nocturia; anorexia; irritability; weight loss; mild acidosis; hypercalciuria; anemia; reversible azotemia; ectopic or generalized vascular calcification; nephrocalcinosis; conjunctivitis; photophobia; rhinorrhea; pruritus; hyperthermia; pancreatitis; decreased libido; albuminuria; hypercholesterolemia; elevated aspartate aminotransferase, alanine aminotransferase, and blood urea nitrogen levels; **arrhythmias**

chromium (chromic chloride)

Chroma-Pak

Action

Component in glucose tolerance factor, which activates insulin-mediated reactions; helps maintain normal glucose metabolism and peripheral nerve function

Availability

Injection: 4 mcg/ml (as 20.5 mcg chromic chloride hexahydrate), 20 mcg/ml (as 102.5 mcg chromic chloride hexahydrate)

🕖 Indications and dosages

➤ Supplement to I.V. solutions used in total parenteral nutrition
Adults: 10 to 15 mcg/day; for metabolically stable adults with intestinal fluid loss, 20 mcg/day
Children: 0.14 to 0.2 mcg/kg/day

Contraindications and precautions

• Contraindicated in pregnancy (unless clearly needed) and premature infants (some products contain benzyl alcohol, associated with fatal gasping syndrome)
• Adjust dosage or avoid use in patients with renal or GI dysfunction.
• Multiple trace element solutions may cause overdose if patient's requirement for one element exceeds that for other elements in formulation. Chromium may need to be given separately.

Adverse reactions

Toxicity is rare at recommended dosages; hypersensitivity reaction to iodide may occur.

copper

Cupric Sulfate

Action

Serves as cofactor for ceruloplasmin, an oxidase needed for proper formation of transferrin (an iron carrier protein); helps maintain normal rate of red and white blood cell formation

---

Availability
Injection: 0.4 mg/ml, 2 mg/ml

🥼 Indications and dosages
➤ Supplement to I.V. solutions used in total parenteral nutrition
Adults: 0.5 to 1.5 mg/day
Children: 20 mcg/kg/day

Contraindications and precautions
• Contraindicated in renal or GI dysfunction, Wilson's disease, pregnancy (unless clearly needed), and premature infants (some products contain benzyl alcohol, associated with fatal gasping syndrome)
• Be aware that giving copper without zinc (or vice versa) may decrease blood level of the other mineral; monitor levels before giving subsequent doses.
• Multiple trace element solutions may cause overdose if patient's requirement for one element exceeds that for other elements in formulation. Copper may need to be given separately.

Adverse reactions
Hypersensitivity reaction to iodides

---

cyanocobalamin (vitamin B$_{12}$)
Big Shot B-12, Cyanoject, Rubramin

hydroxocobalamin, crystalline (vitamin B$_{12}$)
Hydro-Cristi-12, LA-12

Action
Essential to growth, cell reproduction, hematopoiesis, and nucleoprotein and myelin synthesis; participates in nucleic acid synthesis. Plays a role in red blood cell formation through activation of folic acid coenzymes.

Availability
cyanocobalamin
Injection: 100 mcg/ml, 1,000 mcg/ml
Intranasal gel: 500 mcg/0.1 ml
Tablets: 100 mcg, 500 mcg, 1,000 mcg
hydroxocobalamin
Injection: 1,000 mcg/ml

🥼 Indications and dosages
➤ Recommended dietary allowance
Adults and children older than age 11: 2 mcg cyanocobalamin daily
➤ Vitamin B$_{12}$ deficiency
Adults: 30 mcg hydroxocobalamin S.C. or I.M. daily for 5 to 10 days, depending on cause and severity of deficiency; maintenance dosage is 100 to 200 mcg I.M. monthly.
Children: Total dosage of 1 to 5 mg hydroxocobalamin S.C. or I.M. given over 2 or more weeks in divided doses of 100 mcg; then a maintenance dosage of 30 to 50 mcg I.M. q 4 weeks

Contraindications and precautions
• Contraindicated in hypersensitivity to vitamin B$_{12}$, cobalt, or product components

Adverse reactions
Mild transient diarrhea; polycythemia vera; severe, rapid optic nerve atrophy; injection site pain, itching, or rash; with parenteral forms—**pulmonary edema, heart failure, peripheral vascular thrombosis, anaphylactic shock**

---

doxercalciferol
Hectorol

Action
Synthetic vitamin D analogue that acts directly on parathyroid gland to stimulate and suppress parathyroid hormone synthesis and secretion

---

Availability
Capsules: 0.5 mcg, 2.5 mcg
Injection: 2 and 4 mcg/vial

🗲 Indications and dosages
➤ To reduce elevated intact parathyroid hormone (iPTH) levels in management of secondary hyperparathyroidism due to chronic renal dialysis
Adults: Dosage individualized. Recommended initial dosage is 10 mcg P.O. three times weekly at dialysis (approximately every other day). Adjust dosage as needed to lower blood iPTH to 150 to 300 pg/ml. Maximum dosage is 20 mcg P.O. three times weekly.

Contraindications and precautions
• Contraindicated in hypercalcemia, evidence of vitamin D toxicity, abnormal sensitivity to vitamin D effects, malabsorption syndrome, and renal dysfunction
• Use cautiously in elderly patients with coronary disease, renal impairment, or arteriosclerosis.

Adverse reactions
Nausea; vomiting; constipation; weakness; headache; drowsiness; dry mouth; metallic taste, muscle or bone pain; hypertension; polyuria; polydipsia; nocturia; anorexia; irritability; weight loss; mild acidosis; hypercalciuria; anemia; reversible azotemia; ectopic or generalized vascular calcification; nephrocalcinosis; conjunctivitis; photophobia; rhinorrhea; pruritus; hyperthermia; pancreatitis; decreased libido; albuminuria; hypercholesterolemia; elevated aspartate aminotransferase, alanine aminotransferase, and blood urea nitrogen levels; **arrhythmias**

folic acid
Folvite

Action
Promotes production of red and white blood cells and platelets in some megaloblastic anemias

Availability
Injection: 5 mg/ml
Tablets: 0.4 mg, 0.8 mg, 1 mg

🗲 Indications and dosages
➤ Recommended dietary allowance
Adults and children older than age 14: 180 to 400 mcg
Children younger than age 14: 25 to 150 mcg
➤ Megaloblastic anemia related to folic acid deficiencies seen in sprue, nutritional deficiency, pregnancy, infancy, or childhood
Adults: Up to 1 mg/day P.O., I.M., I.V., or S.C. (given orally except in severe disease or severely impaired GI absorption). Higher dosages may be needed in severe cases, with a maintenance dosage of 0.4 mg/day. In pregnant and breastfeeding patients, 0.8 mg/day.
Children over age 4: Maintenance dosage of 0.4 mg/day P.O., I.M., or S.C. (given orally except in severe disease or severely impaired GI absorption)
Children under age 4: Maintenance dosage of up to 0.3 mg/day P.O., I.M., or S.C. (given orally except in severe disease or severely impaired GI absorption)

Contraindications and precautions
• Contraindicated in allergy to folic acid preparations and in pernicious, aplastic, and normocytic anemia
• Use cautiously in breastfeeding patients.

Adverse reactions

Altered sleep pattern, general malaise, poor concentration, impaired judgment, hyperactivity, anorexia, nausea, flatulence, bitter taste, allergic reaction (including rash, pruritus, erythema), **bronchospasm**

leucovorin calcium (citrovorum factor, folinic acid)

Action

Active, chemically reduced derivative of folic acid used as antidote to methotrexate and other drugs that act as folic acid antagonists; also enhances therapeutic effects of fluoropyrimidines used in cancer therapy

Availability

Injection: 3 mg/ml, 10 mg/ml
Powder for injection: 50 mg/vial, 100 mg/vial, 350 mg/vial
Tablets: 5 mg, 15 mg, 25 mg

Indications and dosages

➤ Advanced colorectal cancer
Adults: Usually given in one of the following regimens: Leucovorin 200 mg/m² slow I.V. injection over at least 3 minutes, followed by fluorouracil (5-FU) 370 mg/m² I.V. injection. Or leucovorin 20 mg/m² I.V. injection, followed by 5-FU 425 mg/m² I.V. injection. Repeat daily for 5 days. May repeat course at 4-week (28-day) intervals for two courses and then at 4- to 5-week (28- to 35-day) intervals if patient recovers completely from toxic effects of previous course.
➤ Leucovorin rescue after high-dose methotrexate therapy in osteosarcoma
Adults and children: 15 mg (10 mg/m²) P.O., I.M., or I.V. q 6 hours for 10 doses, beginning 24 hours after start of methotrexate infusion (based on

methotrexate dosage of 12 to 15 g/m² I.V. over 4 hours)
➤ To counteract hematologic toxicity from overdose of folic acid antagonists (such as methotrexate, pyrimethamine, trimethoprim)
Adults and children: 5 to 15 mg I.M. or I.V. daily
➤ Megaloblastic anemia secondary to folic acid deficiency
Adults and children: Maximum dosage of 1 mg I.M. daily

Contraindications and precautions

• Contraindicated in pregnancy (unless clearly needed)
• Use cautiously in breastfeeding patients.

Adverse reactions

Allergic reactions including anaphylactoid reactions and urticaria

manganese, chelated

manganese chloride

Action

Acts as a cofactor in various enzyme systems; stimulates hepatic cholesterol and fatty acid synthesis and influences mucopolysaccharide synthesis

Availability

Injection: 0.1 mg/ml (as 0.36 mg manganese chloride)
Tablets: 20 mg and 50 mg of chelated manganese

Indications and dosages

➤ Recommended dietary allowance
Adults: 20 to 50 mg daily
➤ Supplement to I.V. solutions used for total parenteral nutrition
Adults: 0.15 to 0.8 mg/day
Children: 2 to 10 mcg/kg/day

Contraindications and precautions

• Contraindicated in pregnancy (unless clearly needed) and in premature infants (some products contain benzyl alcohol, associated with fatal gasping syndrome)

• Reduce dosage in renal or GI dysfunction.

• Multiple trace element solutions may cause overdose if patient's requirement for one element exceeds that for other elements in formulation. Manganese may need to be given separately.

Adverse reactions

Hypersensitivity reactions to iodides

niacin (nicotinic acid, vitamin B₃)

Slo-Niacin

niacinamide (nicotinamide)

Action

Serves as a component of two coenzymes essential in oxidation-reduction reactions

Availability

Capsules (extended-release): 250 mg, 400 mg
Capsules (sustained-release): 125 mg, 500 mg
Capsules (timed-release): 250 mg, 500 mg
Tablets: 50 mg, 100 mg, 250 mg, 500 mg
Tablets (controlled-release): 250 mg, 500 mg, 750 mg
Tablets (sustained-release): 500 mg
Tablets (timed-release): 250 mg, 500 mg

Indications and dosages

➤ Recommended dietary allowance (RDA)

Adults: 15 to 20 mg P.O. daily in males, 13 to 15 mg P.O. daily in females
➤ Pellagra
Adults: Up to 500 mg daily
➤ Niacin deficiency
Adults: Up to 100 mg daily
➤ Hyperlipidemia
Adults: Initially, 250 mg P.O. daily; increase up to 1 or 2 g/day (given in divided doses) at 4- to 7-day intervals. Don't exceed 6 g/day.

Contraindications and precautions

• Contraindicated in hypersensitivity to niacin, hepatic dysfunction, active peptic ulcer, and arterial bleeding

• Use cautiously in heart disease (give only under doctor's supervision), regular consumption of large amounts of alcohol, history of hepatic disease, and pregnant or breastfeeding patients. Don't exceed RDA in children (safety and efficacy haven't been established).

Adverse reactions

Flushing, pruritus, rash, dry skin, tingling, acanthosis nigricans, GI distress, nausea, vomiting, diarrhea, dyspepsia, peptic ulcer, abdominal pain, fulminant hepatic necrosis, abnormal hepatic function tests, hyperuricemia, gout, decreased glucose tolerance, hypotension, transient headache, toxic amblyopia, cystoid macular edema, orthostasis, atrial fibrillation and other **arrhythmias, hepatotoxicity**

paricalcitol
Zemplar

Action
Synthetic vitamin D analog that suppresses parathyroid hormone in patients with chronic renal failure

Availability
Injection: 5 mcg/ml

🕖 Indications and dosages
➤ Hyperparathyroidism associated with chronic renal failure
Adults: 0.04 to 0.1 mcg/kg (2.8 to 7 mcg) I.V. as a single bolus dose given no more often than every other day during dialysis. Dosage may be increased by 2 to 4 mcg at 2- to 4-week intervals.

Contraindications and precautions
• Contraindicated in hypercalcemia, vitamin D toxicity, malabsorption syndrome, abnormal sensitivity to vitamin D effects, and decreased renal function
• Don't exceed recommended dietary allowance during normal pregnancy or in children (safety and efficacy not established). Use cautiously in breast-feeding patients.

Adverse reactions
Nausea; vomiting; constipation; weakness; headache; drowsiness; dry mouth; muscle pain; bone pain; metallic taste; polyuria; nocturia; polydipsia; anorexia; irritability; weight loss; mild acidosis; albuminuria; hypercalciuria; anemia; reversible azotemia; ectopic or generalized vascular calcification; hypertension; arrhythmias; nephrocalcinosis; pancreatitis; conjunctivitis; photophobia; rhinorrhea; pruritus; hyperthermia; decreased libido; hyper-

cholesterolemia; elevated aspartate aminotransferase, alanine aminotransferase, and blood urea nitrogen levels

phytonadione (vitamin K₁)
AquaMEPHYTON, Mephyton

Action
Promotes hepatic synthesis of active prothrombin, proconvertin, plasma thromboplastin component, and Stuart factor

Availability
Aqueous colloidal solution for injection: 2 mg/ml
Tablets: 5 mg

🕖 Indications and dosages
➤ Hypoprothrombinemia secondary to anticoagulant therapy
Adults: Initially, 2.5 to 10 mg P.O., I.M., or S.C.; repeat if needed within 12 to 48 hours after P.O. dose or within 6 to 8 hours of I.M. or S.C. dose. Subsequent dosages are determined by prothrombin time response or clinical condition.
➤ Hypoprothrombinemia secondary to other causes
Adults: 2.5 to 25 mg (rarely, up to 50 mg); dosage and administration route are based on severity of condition and response.
Children: 5 to 10 mg; dosage and administration route are based on severity of condition and response.
➤ Prevention and treatment of hemorrhagic disease of newborn
Neonates: For prevention, 0.5 to 1 mg P.O. or I.M. as a single dose within 1 hour of birth; repeat after 2 to 3 weeks if mother received anticoagulant, anticonvulsant, antibiotic, or antitubercolotic therapy during pregnancy. For treatment, 1 mg S.C. or I.M. if mother received oral anticoagulants.

Reactions in **bold** are life-threatening

Contraindications and precautions

• Contraindicated in hypersensitivity to drug or its components (life-threatening reactions resembling hypersensitivity or anaphylaxis have occurred during and immediately after I.V. injection), children, and neonates (if product contains benzyl alcohol)

• Use cautiously in pregnant or breastfeeding patients. Avoid oral route in disorders that may prevent adequate absorption.

Adverse reactions

Anaphylactoid reactions; hyperbilirubinemia (in infants); with parenteral administration—pain, swelling, tenderness at injection site; itchy rash after repeated injections; and transient flushing sensations and peculiar taste

pyridoxine hydrochloride (vitamin B₆)

Beesix, Doxine, Nestrex, Rodex

Action

Converts to physiologically active forms of vitamin B₆, pyridoxal phosphate and pyridoxamine phosphate, which promote metabolic functions affecting carbohydrate, protein, and lipid use

Availability

Injection: 100 mg/ml
Tablets: 25 mg, 50 mg, 100 mg, 250 mg, 500 mg
Tablets (enteric-coated): 20 mg

ⓘ Indications and dosages

➤ Recommended dietary allowance (RDA)

Adults: 1.7 to 2 mg daily in males; 1.4 to 1.6 mg daily in females. Requirement increases as dietary protein intake rises.

➤ Prophylaxis or treatment of pyridoxine deficiency, including drug-induced deficiency (as from isoniazid, hydralazine, or hormonal contraceptives)

Adults: For prophylaxis, 6 to 100 mg/day P.O., I.V., or I.M. For established neuropathy, 50 to 200 mg/day.

Contraindications and precautions

• Contraindicated in hypersensitivity to pyridoxine

• Don't exceed RDA in children (safety and efficacy not established).

• Use cautiously in breastfeeding patients.

• Be aware that drug abuse and dependence have occurred after withdrawal from dosage of 200 mg/day.

Adverse reactions

Sensory neuropathic syndrome (including unstable gait, ataxia, clumsiness of hands, pedal and perioral numbness, paresthesia, and decreased sensation to touch, temperature, and vibration), photoallergic reaction

retinol (vitamin A)

Aquasol A, Palmitate-A 5000

Action

Stimulates and supports retinal function, reproduction, bone growth, epithelial tissue differentiation and embryonic development

Availability

Capsules: 10,000 IU, 15,000 IU, 25,000 IU
Injection: 50,000 IU/ml
Tablets: 5,000 IU

ⓘ Indications and dosages

➤ Recommended dietary allowance (RDA)

Reactions in **bold** are life-threatening

Adults: 1,000 mcg retinol equivalents (RE) daily in males; 800 mcg RE daily in females
➤ Kwashiorkor in children
Children: 30 mg (as water-miscible palmitate) I.M., followed by intermittent P.O. retinoid therapy
➤ Xerophthalmia in children
Children older than age 1: 110 mg P.O. or 55 mg retinol palmitate I.M., plus an additional 110 mg P.O. on following day and an additional 110 mg P.O. before discharge
➤ Severe vitamin A deficiency
Adults: 100,000 IU I.M. daily for first 3 days, followed by 50,000 IU I.M. daily for 2 weeks
Children ages 1 to 8: 17,500 to 35,000 IU I.M. daily for 10 days
Infants: 7,500 to 15,000 IU I.M. daily for 10 days, followed by 5,000 to 10,000 IU/day P.O. of therapeutic multivitamin preparation

Contraindications and precautions
• Contraindicated in retinol hypersensitivity, hypervitaminosis A, and malabsorption syndrome (with P.O. use)
• Don't exceed RDA during normal pregnancy.
• Use cautiously in patients with renal failure and in I.V. use.

Adverse reactions
Increased intracranial pressure, headache, anorexia, cheilitis, facial dermatitis, dry mucous membranes, stratum corneum fragility, sticky skin, palmoplantar peeling, alopecia, pyogenic granuloma-like lesions in acne, paronychia, conjunctivitis, corneal opacities; **anaphylactic shock and death** (with I.V. use)

riboflavin (lactoflavin, vitamin B$_2$)

Action
Serves as two coenzymes that catalyze oxidation-reduction reactions, such as glucose oxidation, amino acid deamination, and fatty acid breakdown

Availability
Tablets: 50 mg, 100 mg

⊘ Indications and dosages
➤ Recommended dietary allowance (RDA)
Adults: 1.4 to 1.8 mg in males; 1.2 to 1.3 mg in females
➤ Riboflavin deficiency
Adults: 5 to 10 mg P.O. daily
➤ Supplement to I.V. solution used in total parenteral nutrition
Adults and children older than age 11: 3.6 mg/day
Children ages 1 to 11: 1.4 mg/day

Contraindications and precautions
• Use cautiously when giving more than RDA to pregnant or breastfeeding women.

Adverse reactions
None

selenium
Sele-Pak, Selepen

Action
Guards cell components against oxidative damage caused by peroxides generated during cellular metabolism

Availability
Injection: 40 mcg/ml

Ⓘ Indications and dosages

➤ Supplement to I.V. solutions used in total parenteral nutrition (TPN)
Metabolically stable adults: 20 to 40 mcg/day
➤ Recommended dietary allowance
Adults: 40 to 70 mcg in males; 45 to 55 mcg in females

Contraindications and precautions

• Contraindicated in pregnancy (unless clearly needed), premature infants (if product contains benzyl alcohol, associated with fatal gasping syndrome), and renal or GI dysfunction (in some cases)
• Dosage reduction may be required in renal or GI dysfunction.
• Multiple trace element solutions may cause overdose if patient's requirement for one element is appreciably higher than that for other elements in formulation. Selenium may need to be given separately.

Adverse reactions

Hypersensitivity reaction to iodides

thiamine (vitamin B₁)

Biamine, Thiamilate, Thiamine Hydrochloride

Action

Water-soluble vitamin that combines with adenosine triphosphate and thiamine diphosphokinase to form thiamine pyrophosphate, a coenzyme essential for normal aerobic metabolism, normal growth, nerve impulse transmission and acetylcholine synthesis

Availability

Injection: 100 mg/ml
Tablets: 50 mg, 100 mg, 250 mg
Tablets (enteric-coated): 20 mg

Ⓘ Indications and dosages

➤ Recommended dietary allowance
Adults: 1.2 to 1.5 mg/day in males; 1 to 1.1 mg/day in females
➤ Thiamine deficiency
Adults: Up to 100 mg/L I.V. as rapidly as possible until deficiency is corrected
➤ Beriberi
Adults: 10 to 20 mg I.M. t.i.d. for 2 weeks
➤ Neuritis of pregnancy
Adults: 5 to 10 mg/day I.M.
➤ Wernicke-Korsakoff syndrome
Adults: Initially, 100 mg I.V., followed by 50 to 100 mg/day I.M. until patient can consume a regular balanced diet.

Contraindications and precautions

• Contraindicated in thiamine hypersensitivity and in pregnant or breast-feeding women (unless clearly needed)

Adverse reactions

Warm sensation, pruritus, urticaria, weakness, diaphoresis, nausea, restlessness, throat tightness, angioneurotic edema, cyanosis, hypersensitivity reaction, tenderness and induration (with I.M. use), **pulmonary edema, hemorrhage into GI tract, cardiovascular collapse, anaphylactic shock, death**

tocopherols (alpha tocopherols, vitamin E)

Aquavit E, d'Apha E, Nutr-E-Sol, Vita-Plus E

Action

Guards cellular components against oxidation, prevents formation of toxic oxidation products, maintains integrity of red blood cell (RBC) wall, protects RBCs against hemolysis, stimulates steroid metabolism, suppresses prostaglandin production, and inhibits platelet aggregation

Availability
Capsules: 100 IU, 200 IU, 400 IU, 1,000 IU
Drops: 15 IU/0.3 ml
Liquid: 15 IU/30 ml
Tablets: 100 IU, 200 IU, 400 IU, 500 IU, 800 IU

✔ Indications and dosages
➤ Recommended dietary allowance
Adults: 15 IU in males; 12 IU in females

Contraindications and precautions
None

Adverse reactions
Hypervitaminosis E

---

zinc sulfate
Zinca-Pak

zinc chloride

zinc gluconate

Action
Serves as a cofactor for over 70 different enzymes; promotes wound healing and helps maintain normal growth rates, normal skin hydration, and taste and smell sensations

Availability
Capsules: 220 mg
Injection: 1 mg/ml (as 2.09 mg chloride)
Tablets (gluconate): 10 mg, 15 mg, 50 mg
Tablets (sulfate): 66 mg, 110 mg

✔ Indications and dosages
➤ Recommended dietary allowance
Adults: 12 to 15 mg
➤ Supplement to I.V. solution used in total parenteral nutrition (TPN)

Metabolically stable adults: 2.5 to 4 mg/day; may give additional 2 mg/day in acute catabolic states. In patients with fluid loss from small bowel, give an additional 12.2 mg/L of TPN solution.
➤ Dietary supplement
Adults: 25 to 50 mg zinc P.O. daily

Contraindications and precautions
• Contraindicated in pregnancy (unless clearly needed), in premature infants (if product contains benzyl alcohol, associated with fatal gasping syndrome), and in renal or GI dysfunction (in some cases)
• Dosage decrease may be required in renal or GI dysfunction.
• Multiple trace element solutions may cause overdose if patient's requirement for one element is appreciably higher than that for other elements in formulation. Zinc may need to be given separately.

Adverse reactions
Hypersensitivity reaction to iodides; nausea, vomiting

Herbs and supplements

The information provided in these monographs reflects commonly held assumptions about the actions and uses of common herbs and nutritional supplements. However, in many cases, these assumptions haven't been confirmed by clinical trials. Although herbal remedies have been used for thousands of years, few have undergone well-designed scientific studies to determine how they work, if they're safe, and whether they're effective in treating the medical conditions for which they're commonly used. Advise patients to consult a health care practitioner before using herbs to help determine if herb use may be safe for them.

aloe

Purported action
When used topically, causes a moisturizing effect in burns and wounds, which prevents air from drying the wound and increases blood flow to stimulate healing. When taken internally, may produce a laxative effect by stimulating the large intestine and increasing peristalsis.

Reported uses
Used topically (as a gel) to inhibit infection and promote healing of minor burns, abrasions, wounds, and frostbite and to treat certain skin diseases (such as psoriasis and seborrheic dermatitis). Used systemically (as liquid extract

concentrate, capsules, or dried aloe latex) as a strong laxative.

Contraindications and precautions
Internal use is contraindicated in inflammatory bowel disease, elderly patients with suspected intestinal obstruction, pregnant or breastfeeding women, and children under age 12.

Adverse reactions
• With topical use: redness, itching, and burning sensation in dermabraded skin
• With P.O. use: edema, cramps, diarrhea, electrolyte abnormalities, weight loss, **arrhythmias**

Interactions
Antiarrhythmics, thiazide diuretics: hypokalemia
Cardiac glycosides: increased effects of these drugs
Corticosteroids, licorice: increased potassium level

bilberry

Purported action
Relieves mild GI tract inflammation, easing diarrhea; reduces oral mucous membrane irritation; increases microcirculation by redistributing new capillary formation; strengthens capillary walls; promotes overall health of the circulatory system; and exerts a protective effect on stomach and liver (possibly through increased prostaglandin production)

Reported uses
Nonspecific diarrhea; mouth and throat irritation; to improve visual acuity and accommodation. Further studies are needed to confirm that bil-

berry promotes circulatory, GI, or hepatic health.

Contraindications and precautions
Contraindicated in bleeding disorders, pregnancy, and breastfeeding

Adverse reactions
• At typical dosages: GI distress, skin rash, drowsiness
• At higher dosages: unknown

Interactions
Anticoagulants, antiplatelet drugs, salicylates: potentiated effects, causing increased prothrombin time
Hypoglycemics: reduced blood glucose level

black cohosh

Purported action
Binds to estrogen receptors, directly or indirectly influencing luteinizing hormone release. Studies show black cohosh increases bone mineral density in rats but not in humans.

Reported uses
Management of some menopause symptoms (as an alternative to hormone replacement therapy), premenstrual syndrome, and dysmenorrhea; treatment of arthritis, kidney problems, malaria, and sore throat

Contraindications and precautions
Contraindicated in pregnancy (may cause premature birth or miscarriage)

Adverse reactions
• GI distress
• Headache, weight gain, nausea, vomiting, dizziness, nervous system and vi-

sual disturbances, reduced heart rate, increased perspiration

Interactions
Antihypertensives: additive hypotension
Docetaxel: increased docetaxel blood level

cat's claw

Purported action
Stimulates the immune system, enhances phagocytosis, dilates peripheral vessels, inhibits sympathetic nervous system activity, slows the heart rate, decreases the cholesterol level, promotes diuresis, inhibits urinary bladder contraction, relaxes smooth muscle, and exerts local anesthetic effects. Studies show cat's claw has some anticancer and immunostimulant properties.

Reported uses
Inflammation; GI disorders (including colitis, inflammatory bowel disease, Crohn's disease); AIDS; as an astringent, antiviral, anti-infective, and general tonic

Contraindications and precautions
Contraindicated in multiple sclerosis, tuberculosis, autoimmune disease, pregnancy, and breastfeeding. Use cautiously in GI disease (herb increases stomach acid secretion).

Adverse reactions
• Hypotension
• With decoction: few known risks

Interactions
Anticoagulants, antiplatelets: inhibited platelet aggregation, prolonged bleeding time
Antihypertensives: potentiation of antihypertensive effects

Food: enhanced absorption of herb
Immunosuppressants: negation of immunosuppressant effects

chamomile

Purported action
Reduces inflammation and fever, promotes healing of burns, and prevents ulcer formation. May also exert antispasmodic, anxiolytic, and sedative effects through action on CNS receptors.

Reported uses
Vomiting, flatulence, colic, fever, cystitis, parasitic worm infections, spasms, inflammation, anxiety; as an antibacterial, astringent, deodorant, or skin wash (to increase sloughing of necrotic tissue and promote granulation and epithelialization)

Contraindications and precautions
Contraindicated in ragweed allergy, hepatic or renal disease, pregnancy, and breastfeeding. Use cautiously in patients receiving anticoagulants.

Adverse reactions
Contact dermatitis, **anaphylaxis,** and other **severe hypersensitivity reactions** in patients allergic to ragweed, asters, chrysanthemums, or other members of Compositae family (such as arnica, feverfew, tansy, and yarrow)

Interactions
All concurrently administered drugs: delayed drug absorption
Anticoagulants: increased anticoagulant effect
Sedatives (such as benzodiazepines): enhanced sedative effects

dong quai

Purported action
Exerts antispasmodic effect on smooth muscles, including those of airway and uterus. Forms containing coumarin have anticoagulant effects.

Reported uses
Asthma, allergies, menstrual disorders, menopausal symptoms, rheumatic pain; as an antispasmodic, anti-inflammatory, and anticoagulant

Contraindications and precautions
Contraindicated in patients receiving warfarin concurrently and in pregnant or breastfeeding patients (may influence uterine contractions or cause unknown effects in fetus)

Adverse reactions
• With authentic dong quai: no known reactions
• With other dong quai forms: increased risk of phototoxicity, abortion, uterine stimulation, and altered menstrual cycle

Interactions
Anticoagulants: increased anticoagulation
Calcium channel blockers: synergistic effect

echinacea

Purported action
Stimulates the immune system; with topical use, may have mild antibacterial and antiviral properties

---

Reported uses

Urinary tract and yeast infections, promotion of wound healing, prevention and treatment of upper respiratory infections (including colds and flu)

Contraindications and precautions

Contraindicated in immunocompromised patients (because of immune-stimulating properties)

Adverse reactions

Nausea, mild GI upset, allergic reactions, **anaphylaxis**

Note: Adverse reactions may be more common in patients allergic to daisy-type plants.

Interactions

Corticosteroids: interference with chemotherapeutic effects of these drugs

Immunosuppressants: interference with immunosuppressant effects

evening primrose

Purported action

Contains essential fatty acids (EFAs) that may improve cellular structural elements and serve as precursors of prostaglandins, which help regulate metabolic functions (including cervical ripening)

Reported uses

Disorders caused by EFA deficiency or disturbed EFA metabolism, including cardiovascular disease, premenstrual syndrome, mastalgia and other breast disorders, rheumatoid arthritis, multiple sclerosis, atopic dermatitis and other dermatologic disorders, Raynaud's syndrome, Sjögren's syndrome, Alzheimer's disease, schizophrenia, and attention deficit hyperactivity disorder

Contraindications and precautions

Contraindicated in pregnancy, breast-feeding, and history of allergy or seizures

Adverse reactions

Headache, nausea, vomiting, diarrhea, flatulence, allergic reaction, abdominal pain, indigestion

Interactions

Anticoagulants: bleeding, bruising
Anticonvulsants: lowered seizure threshold, decreased anticonvulsant efficacy

feverfew

Purported action

Inhibits prostaglandin synthesis and serotonin release from platelets and polymorphonuclear leukocyte granules; extract may inhibit phagocytosis and platelet deposition on collagen surfaces. Exhibits antithrombotic potential and *in vitro* antibacterial activity, inhibits mast cell release of histamine, exerts cytotoxic activity, and suppresses enzyme release from white blood cells in inflamed joints and skin. May promote contraction and relaxation of vascular smooth muscle.

Reported uses

Menstrual pain, asthma, dermatitis, psoriasis, arthritis; prevention of migraine; as an antipyretic

Contraindications and precautions

Contraindicated in pregnancy, breast-feeding, and children under age 2

Adverse reactions

• Hypersensitivity reaction, increased heart rate, oral mucosa and tongue inflammation

• After withdrawal: cluster of CNS reactions (rebound migraine, anxiety, disturbed sleep pattern), muscle and joint stiffness

Interactions

Anticoagulants, aspirin: increased antithrombotic effect of these drugs

garlic

Purported action

Inactivates thiol enzymes (such as coenzyme A and HMG-CoA reductase) and oxidizes glutamate synthase complex, both of which are required for lipid synthesis. Also may exert mild antibacterial, antifungal, and hypotensive activity.

Reported uses

Reduction of blood lipid levels (transient effect); as an antibacterial, antiseptic, or antithrombotic. Insufficient data exist regarding effects of garlic on clinical cardiovascular conditions, such as claudication and myocardial infarction.

Contraindications and precautions

Pregnant and breastfeeding patients should avoid large amounts of garlic. Use cautiously in severe renal or hepatic disease and in children.

Adverse reactions

Allergic reaction, contact dermatitis, headache, insomnia, fatigue, vertigo, facial flushing, GI distress, shortness of breath

Interactions

Anticoagulants, antiplatelet agents, nonsteroidal anti-inflammatory drugs, other drugs and herbs with anticoagulant effects: increased prothrombin and bleeding times, increased International Normalized Ratio

Hypoglycemics: decreased blood glucose level in patients requiring stringent blood glucose control

ginger

Purported action

Inhibits prostaglandin and thromboxane biosynthesis and promotes platelet aggregation. Also possesses antiemetic, antithrombotic, antibacterial, antioxidant, antihepatotoxic, anti-inflammatory, antimutagenic, stimulant, cardiotonic, immunostimulant, diuretic, and spasmolytic properties.

Reported uses

To stimulate digestion, increase intestinal peristalsis, promote gastric secretions, reduce cholesterol level, raise blood glucose level, and stimulate peripheral circulation. To treat nausea and vomiting associated with motion sickness, hyperemesis gravidarum, and migraine; dyspepsia; colic; anorexia; bronchitis; and rheumatism.

Contraindications and precautions

Large amounts are controversial in pregnant patients. Avoid use in gallstones, bleeding disorders, hypertension, hypotension, and diabetes mellitus.

Adverse reactions

CNS depression, interference with cardiac function or anticoagulant activity

Interactions
Anticoagulants: increased bleeding time
Antihypertensives: interference with antihypertensive effect
Hypoglycemics: decreased blood glucose level

ginkgo

Purported action
Exerts antioxidant and neuroprotective activity, including arteriolar vasodilation, increased tissue perfusion and cerebral blood flow, decreased arterial spasm, and reduced platelet aggregation

Reported uses
Raynaud's disease, cerebral insufficiency, anxiety, stress, tinnitus, dementia, circulatory disorders, asthma, memory impairment, headache, depression, impotence; as an adjunct in schizophrenia therapy

Contraindications and precautions
Pregnant or breastfeeding patients should avoid ginkgo. Use cautiously in diabetes mellitus, hypertension, and in patients receiving antiplatelets or anticoagulants.

Adverse reactions
• Headache, dizziness, palpitations, GI and dermatologic disorders
• With excessive use: **seizures, subdural hematoma**
• Ginkgo pollen can be strongly allergenic; contact with fleshy fruit pulp causes allergic dermatitis similar to that caused by poison ivy.

Interactions
Antithrombolytics: increased effects of these drugs

ginseng

Purported action
Increases natural killer cell activity, stimulates interferon production, accelerates nuclear RNA synthesis, decreases blood glucose level, and increases high-density lipoprotein levels; also possesses depressant, anticonvulsant, and analgesic properties

Reported uses
Fatigue, poor concentration, nervousness, hypertension or hypotension, impotence, gastritis, cancer, certain CNS and endocrine conditions

Contraindications and precautions
Contraindicated in pregnant or breastfeeding patients. Patients taking monoamine oxidase inhibitors should avoid ginseng. Use cautiously in hypertension or diabetes mellitus.

Adverse reactions
Nervousness, stimulation, diffuse mammary nodules, vaginal bleeding, hypoglycemia, ginseng abuse

Interactions
Hypoglycemics: increased hypoglycemic effect
Loop diuretics: poor diuretic response
Stimulants: stimulant potentiation
Warfarin: subtherapeutic International Normalized Ratio

glucosamine

Purported action
Serves as a building block for cartilage glycosaminoglycans (GAG), thereby aiding treatment of osteoarthritis

(marked by progressive GAG degeneration). Also may possess chondroprotective, antireactive, and antiarthritic properties.

Reported uses
Osteoarthritis, joint pain and inflammation, protection of joint cartilage from damaging effects of some nonsteroidal anti-inflammatory drugs

Contraindications and precautions
Diabetic patients should consult health care provider before taking glucosamine because it may increase blood glucose level.

Adverse reactions
Gastric discomfort (such as heartburn, diarrhea, nausea, vomiting), headache, drowsiness, insomnia, tachycardia, pruritus

Interactions
Diuretics: decreased glucosamine effects

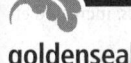

goldenseal

Purported action
Contains alkaloids (hydrastine and berberine) that exert modest antimicrobial activity. May have cardiostimulatory, anti-inflammatory, peripheral vasoconstrictive, antihemorraghic, and muscle relaxant effects.

Reported uses
Topical infections (such as wounds and herpes labialis lesions); conjunctivitis; inflamed mucous membranes (as an ingredient in cold and flu preparations); postpartum hemorrhage; as a diuretic or laxative

Contraindications and precautions
Contraindicated in hypertension, heart disease (especially arrhythmias), heart failure, and pregnancy

Adverse reactions
Skin rash, headache, insomnia, nausea, vomiting, abdominal pain, tachycardia, bradycardia, **seizures, respiratory depression** (with high doses)

Interactions
Anticoagulants: reduced anticoagulant effect
Antihypertensives: enhanced antihypertensive effect
Hypoglycemics, insulin: increased effects of these drugs

grapeseed

Purported action
Exerts antioxidant, anticarcinogenic, cytoprotective, and vascular activity; also inhibits proteolytic enzymes, causing collagen stabilization

Reported uses
Prevention of cancer, cardiovascular disease, and dental caries; treatment of venous insufficiency, edema, and allergic rhinitis

Contraindications and precautions
Contraindicated in known hypersensitivity to grapeseed. Use cautiously in hepatic disease. Safety during pregnancy hasn't been established.

Adverse reactions
Hepatotoxicity

Interactions
None reported

Reactions in **bold** are life-threatening

green tea

Purported action
Maintains significant plasma levels of catechin, which may exert antioxidant activity against lipoproteins. Delays lipid peroxidation, exerts antimicrobial effects against oral and diarrhea-causing bacteria, and contributes antimutagenic potential against dietary carcinogens.

Reported uses
Atherosclerosis, headache, wounds, stomach disorders, cancer, diarrhea, elevated lipid levels; dental caries prevention

Contraindications and precautions
Green tea should be avoided by pregnant or breastfeeding women and by women who may become pregnant (because of caffeine content). Use cautiously in cardiac disease, renal disease, and hyperthyroidism.

Adverse reactions
Asthma, nervousness, insomnia, tachycardia, constipation, diarrhea, increased blood glucose and cholesterol levels, impaired iron metabolism, **esophageal cancer** (with heavy consumption)

Interactions
Stimulants: increased stimulant effects
Warfarin: decreased International Normalized Ratio

hawthorn

Purported action
Increases coronary blood flow and heart rate; exerts antiarrhythmic and positive inotropic effects

Reported uses
Atherosclerosis, angina pectoris, blood pressure and heart rhythm regulation; as an antispasmodic or sedative

Contraindications and precautions
Contraindicated in severe renal or hepatic disease and in pregnancy and breastfeeding

Adverse reactions
• Agitation, dizziness, hypotension, sedation, nausea, sweating
• With high doses: toxicity

Interactions
Antiarrhythmics: enhanced antiarrhythmic action
Antihypertensives, nitrates: increased effects of these drugs
Cardiac glycosides: increased risk of cardiac glycoside toxicity

kava

Purported action
Produces mild anxiolytic and anticonvulsant effects; also may exert antithrombotic effects on platelets

Reported uses
Anxiety, stress, restlessness, seizure disorders, headache, infection, local anesthesia

---

Reactions in **bold** are life-threatening

Contraindications and precautions

Contraindicated in history of hepatic problems. Pregnant or breastfeeding patients should avoid kava. Use cautiously in neutropenia, renal disease, and thrombocytopenia.

Adverse reactions

Morning fatigue, headache, drowsiness, mydriasis, mild GI disturbances, diarrhea, hematuria, hypertension, shortness of breath, visual disturbances, scaly rash (with heavy use)

Interactions

Alcohol, benzodiazepines: potentiation of CNS effects
Antiplatelet drugs, monoamine oxidase inhibitors: additive effects of these drugs
Levodopa: reduced levodopa efficacy

licorice

Purported action

Licorice root derivative (carbenoxolone) soothes inflamed mucous membranes, increases life span of gastric epithelial cells by stimulating secretin release, and inhibits peptic and prostaglandin activity

Reported uses

GI complaints, cough, asthma, gastric and duodenal ulcers; used investigationally in lupus and inflammation

Contraindications and precautions

Contraindicated in renal, hepatic, and cardiovascular disease. Pregnant or breastfeeding women should avoid licorice.

Adverse reactions

• Headache, lethargy, water retention, hypokalemia, hypernatremia, visual disturbances, hypertension, **pulmonary edema**
• With prolonged, daily use of large amounts: reactions ranging from muscle weakness to quadriplegia

Interactions

Antihypertensives, corticosteroids, diuretics, procainamide, quinidine: increased effects of these drugs
Digoxin: increased risk of digoxin toxicity

melatonin

Purported action

Endogenous melatonin plays a role in circadian rhythms; light inhibits melatonin synthesis and darkness stimulates it. Exogenous melatonin increases melatonin blood levels without affecting endogenous melatonin production; also affects body temperature regulation, cardiovascular function, and reproduction.

Reported uses

Short-term sleep pattern regulation, jet lag, tinnitus, depression, cluster headaches, cancer, chemotherapy-induced thrombocytopenia

Contraindications and precautions

Contraindicated in hepatic insufficiency, cerebrovascular disease, depression, and neurologic disorders. Caution patient not to drive or perform other hazardous activities for 30 to 60 minutes after taking.

Adverse reactions

Headache, depression, confusion, tachycardia, pruritus

Interactions

Benzodiazepines: increased anxiolytic effects

Methamphetamines: increased monoaminergic effects of these drugs

Nifedipine: interference with antihypertensive effect

milk thistle

Purported action

Produces hepatoprotective effect, possibly by stimulating RNA and DNA synthesis. Thought to scavenge prooxidant free radicals and increase intracellular concentration of glutathione (a substance needed to detoxify hepatic cell reactions); alters outer membrane of hepatic cells. Also may exert anti-inflammatory effect on platelets.

Reported uses

Liver dysfunction (including damage caused by acute viral hepatitis or longterm phenothiazine or butyrophenone use); dyspepsia; gallbladder and spleen disorders; antidote for Amanita mushroom poisoning; reduction of increased total and high-density lipoprotein levels

Contraindications and precautions

Contraindicated in pregnancy and breastfeeding

Adverse reactions

Brief GI disturbances, diarrhea, cramping, mild allergic reactions, urticaria

Interactions

None known

saw palmetto

Purported action

Reduces enlarged prostate by inhibiting testosterone 5-alpha reductase (an enzyme that converts testosterone to 5-alpha-testosterone in prostate). Inhibits cell proliferation induced by prolactin and growth factor; also may exert anti-inflammatory, immunostimulant, antiandrogen, antiestrogenic, and astringent activity.

Reported uses

Symptomatic treatment of benign prostatic hyperplasia (BPH), including urinary frequency, reduced urinary flow, and nocturia; bronchitis; asthma

Contraindications and precautions

Contraindicated in pregnancy and in patients receiving concurrent hormone therapy (including contraceptives and hormone replacement therapy). Patients receiving drugs that may alter immunostimulant or anti-inflammatory activity should use saw palmetto cautiously.

Adverse reactions

Headache, hypertension, abdominal pain, constipation, diarrhea, nausea, GI upset, urine retention

Interactions

None known

shark cartilage

Purported action

Helps control cancer by inhibiting new blood vessel formation (angiogenesis)

Reactions in **bold** are life-threatening

in tumors; also may have anti-inflammatory effect

Reported uses
Prostate cancer, AIDS-associated Kaposi's sarcoma, arthritis, eczema

Contraindications and precautions
Contraindicated in pregnancy or breastfeeding and in children. Use cautiously in hepatic disease.

Adverse reactions
Hepatitis

Interactions
None known

soy

Purported action
Isoflavones (phytoestrogens found in soybean) produce effects similar to those of estradiol (a female hormone); they also bind to cholesterol, limiting cholesterol absorption in intestine. May enhance immune function, produce antioxidant effects, and exert beneficial effects on GI function.

Reported uses
Menopausal symptoms, osteoporosis and minor GI problems, reduction of total cholesterol and low-density lipoprotein levels. Also serves as source of fiber, protein, and minerals.

Contraindications and precautions
Contraindicated in estrogen-dependent tumors and peanut allergy (cross-sensitivity may occur)

Adverse reactions
Some experts are concerned that phytoestrogens in soy-based infant formulas may influence CNS and psychomotor development.

Interactions
None known

St. John's wort

Purported action
Inhibits postsynaptic serotonin reuptake or antagonizes monoamine oxidase

Reported uses
Depression, wounds, muscle pain, burns. Also used investigationally to treat human immunodeficiency virus and certain other viruses.

Contraindications and precautions
Contraindicated in concurrent use of prescription antidepressants, pregnancy, and males or females planning pregnancy

Adverse reactions
Abdominal pain, constipation, other GI symptoms, dry mouth, dizziness, confusion, fatigue, mania, photosensitivity

Interactions
Cyclosporine, digoxin, protease inhibitors, theophylline, warfarin: decreased efficacy of these drugs
Hormonal contraceptives: breakthrough bleeding
Selective serotonin reuptake inhibitors: sedative-hypnotic toxicity

---

Reactions in **bold** are life-threatening

valerian

Purported action
Binds to gamma-aminobutyric acid (GABA) and benzodiazepine receptors, stimulating release of these substances. Glutamine, a free amino acid in valerian extract, can cross the blood-brain barrier and may be metabolized to GABA, causing central sedation.

Reported uses
Nervousness, restlessness, sleep disorders; as an antispasmodic

Contraindications and precautions
Avoid use in hepatic dysfunction, pregnancy, and breastfeeding.

Adverse reactions
With overdose or prolonged use: excitability, headache, insomnia, nausea, blurred vision, cardiac dysfunction, **hepatotoxicity**

Interactions
Alcohol, CNS depressants: additive sedative effect

Part 3

Appendices
Selected references
Index

Normal laboratory values for blood tests

The table below shows normal laboratory values for commonly ordered blood tests. Results may vary slightly among laboratories.

Hematology

White blood cell count
4,100 to 10,900/mm^3
Red blood cell count
Men: 4.5 to 6.2 million/mm^3
Women: 4.2 to 5.4 million/mm^3
Hemoglobin
Men: 14 to 18 g/dl
Women: 12 to 16 g/dl
Hematocrit
Men: 42% to 54%
Women: 38% to 46%
Platelet count
140,000 to 400,000/mm^3
Red blood cell indices
MCH: 26 to 32 pg
MCHC: 32 to 36 g/dl
MCV: 80 to 95 μm^3
Reticulocyte count
0.5% to 2% of total red blood
cell count
White blood cell differential
Basophils: 0.3% to 2%
Eosinophils: 0.3% to 7%
Lymphocytes: 16.2% to 43%
Monocytes: 4% to 10%
Neutrophils: 47.6% to 76.8%

Coagulation studies

Partial thromboplastin time
60 to 70 seconds
Prothrombin time
10 to 14 seconds
International Normalized Ratio
2.0 to 3.0 in patients receiving
warfarin
Bleeding time
3 to 6 minutes (template and
Ivy methods)
1 to 3 minutes (Duke method)

Chemistry

Glucose
70 to 100 mg/dl
Blood urea nitrogen
8 to 20 mg/dl
Creatinine
Men: 0.8 to 1.2 mg/dl
Women: 0.6 to 1.1 mg/dl
Sodium
135 to 145 mEq/L
Potassium
3.5 to 5.0 mEq/L
Anion gap
8 to 16 mEq/L
Chloride
100 to 108 mEq/L
Carbon dioxide
22 to 34 mEq/L
Albumin
3.3 to 4.5 g/dl
Calcium
9 to 10.5 mg/dl
Magnesium
1.5 to 2.5 mEq/L
Phosphorus
2.5 to 4.5 mg/dl
Amylase
60 to 180 units/L
Lipase
0 to 110 units/L
**Alanine amino-
transferase**
Men: 10 to 35 units/L
Women: 9 to
24 units/L

Chemistry (continued)

Alkaline phosphatase
39 to 117 units/L
**Aspartate amino-
transferase**
Men: 8 to 20 units/L
Women: 5 to 40 units/L
Creatine kinase
Men: 52 to
170 units/L
Women: 38 to
135 units/L
Cardiac troponin
< 0.1 mcg/ml
Lactate dehydrogenase
48 to 115 IU/L

Arterial blood gases

pH
7.35 to 7.45 mmHg
Paco$_2$
35 to 45 mmHg
Pao$_2$
75 to 100 mmHg
HCO$_3$-
22 to 26 mEq/L
Sao$_2$
94% to 100%

KEY MCH: Mean corpuscular hemoglobin
MCHC: Mean corpuscular hemoglobin concentration
MCV: Mean corpuscular volume

Adult immunization schedule by age group

This 2004 schedule shows the recommended age groups for routine administration of vaccines for adults ages 19 and older. A person may receive a combination vaccine if any components of the combination are indicated (unless the vaccine's other components are contraindicated). Consult the package insert for detailed recommendations.

For more information about recommended vaccines and contraindications for immunization, visit www.cdc.gov/nip or call the National Immunization Hotline at 800-232-2522 (English) or 800-232-0233 (Spanish).

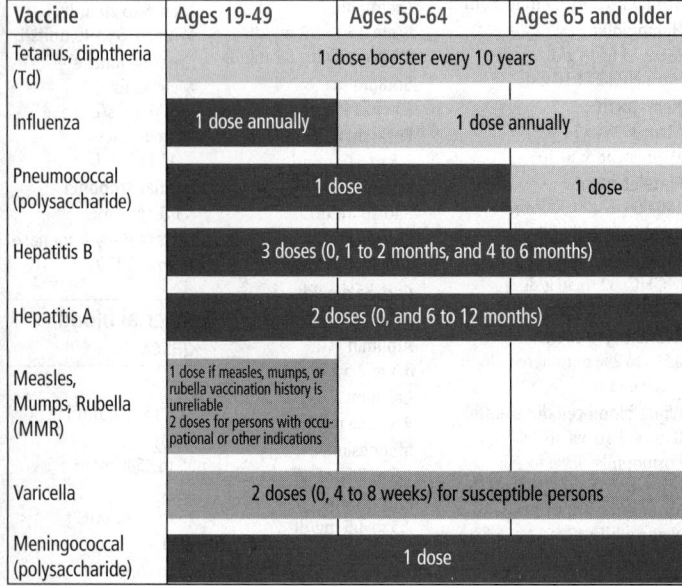

Vaccine	Ages 19-49	Ages 50-64	Ages 65 and older
Tetanus, diphtheria (Td)	1 dose booster every 10 years		
Influenza	1 dose annually	1 dose annually	
Pneumococcal (polysaccharide)	1 dose		1 dose
Hepatitis B	3 doses (0, 1 to 2 months, and 4 to 6 months)		
Hepatitis A	2 doses (0, and 6 to 12 months)		
Measles, Mumps, Rubella (MMR)	1 dose if measles, mumps, or rubella vaccination history is unreliable 2 doses for persons with occupational or other indications		
Varicella	2 doses (0, 4 to 8 weeks) for susceptible persons		
Meningococcal (polysaccharide)	1 dose		

KEY:

　　　For all persons in this age group

　　　Catch-up on childhood vaccinations

　　　For persons with medical or exposure indications

Approved by Advisory Committee on Immunization Practices; accepted by American College of Obstetricians and Gynecologists and American Academy of Family Physicians. Published by Advisory Committee on Immunization Practices, Department of Health and Human Services, Centers for Disease Control and Prevention.

Childhood and adolescent immunization schedule

This 2004 schedule shows recommended ages for routine administration of childhood vaccines for children through age 18. A child who doesn't receive a given dose at the recommended age should receive it at a subsequent visit. "Catch-up immunization" indicates ages at which children should receive the vaccine if they haven't previously received it. Consult the package insert for detailed recommendations.

For more information about vaccines (including precautions and contraindications for immunization and vaccine shortages), visit www.cdc.gov/nip or call the National Immunization Information Hotline at 800-232-2522 (English) or 800-232-0233 (Spanish).

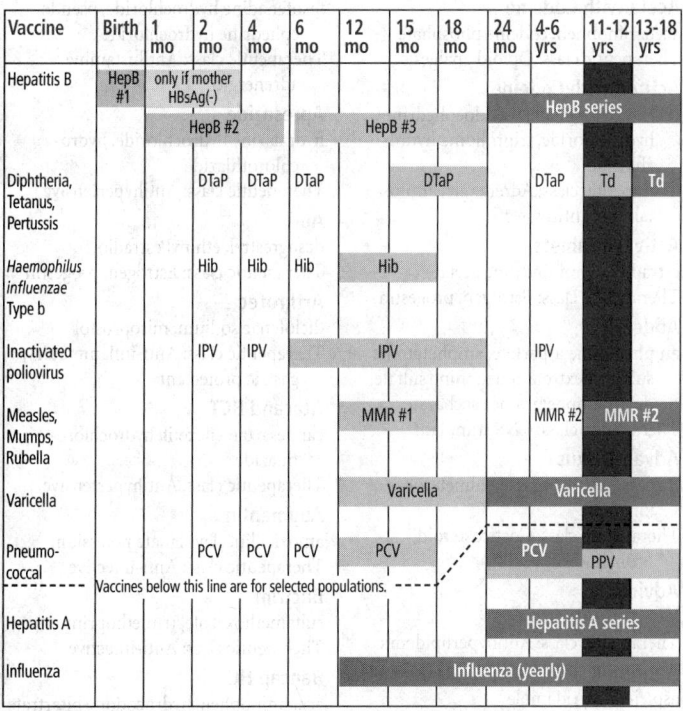

Vaccine	Birth	1 mo	2 mo	4 mo	6 mo	12 mo	15 mo	18 mo	24 mo	4-6 yrs	11-12 yrs	13-18 yrs
Hepatitis B	HepB #1	only if mother HBsAg(-)									HepB series	
			HepB #2			HepB #3						
Diphtheria, Tetanus, Pertussis			DTaP	DTaP	DTaP		DTaP			DTaP	Td	Td
Haemophilus influenzae Type b			Hib	Hib	Hib	Hib						
Inactivated poliovirus			IPV	IPV		IPV				IPV		
Measles, Mumps, Rubella						MMR #1				MMR #2	MMR #2	
Varicella						Varicella				Varicella		
Pneumococcal			PCV	PCV	PCV	PCV				PCV	PPV	
Hepatitis A										Hepatitis A series		
Influenza						Influenza (yearly)						

Vaccines below this line are for selected populations.

KEY:
- Range of recommended ages
- Catch-up immunization
- Preadolescent assessment

DTaP: Diphtheria, Tetanus, Pertussis
HBsAg(-): Hepatitis B surface antigen negative

HepB: Hepatitis B vaccine
HiB: Haemophilus influenzae type b
MMR: Measles, Mumps, Rubella
PCV: Pneumococcal vaccine
PPV: Pneumococcal polysaccharide vaccine
Td: Tetanus and diphtheria toxoids

Approved by Advisory Committee on Immunization Practices, American Academy of Pediatrics, and American Academy of Family Physicians. Published by Advisory Committee on Immunization Practices, Department of Health and Human Services, Centers for Disease Control and Prevention.

Common combination drug products

Many drugs (especially over-the-counter preparations) are combination products that contain several active ingredients and are sold under a discrete trade name. The combination products below are listed by trade name, followed by active ingredients and therapeutic class.

Accuretic
hydrochlorothiazide, quinapril hydrochloride
Therapeutic class: Antihypertensive

Aceta with Codeine
acetaminophen, codeine phosphate
Therapeutic class: Opioid analgesic

Actifed with Codeine
codeine phosphate, pseudoephedrine
hydrochloride, triprolidine hydrochloride
Therapeutic class: Adrenergic, antihistamine, antitussive

Activella Tablets
estradiol, norethindrone acetate
Therapeutic class: Estrogen, progestin

Adderall
amphetamine aspartate, amphetamine
sulfate, dextroamphetamine sulfate,
dextroamphetamine saccharate
Therapeutic class: CNS stimulant

Advair Diskus
fluticasone propionate, salmeterol
xinafoate
Therapeutic class: Corticosteroid,
bronchodilator

Advicor
lovastatin, niacin
Therapeutic class: Antihyperlipidemic

Aggrenox
aspirin, dipyridamole
Therapeutic class: Antiplatelet drug

Aldactazide
hydrochlorothiazide, spironolactone
Therapeutic class: Diuretic

Aldoclor
chlorothiazide, methyldopa
Therapeutic class: Antihypertensive

Aldoril
hydrochlorothiazide, methyldopa
Therapeutic class: Antihypertensive

Allegra-D
fexofenadine hydrochloride, pseudoephedrine hydrochloride
Therapeutic class: Antihistamine,
adrenergic

Apresazide
hydralazine hydrochloride, hydrochlorothiazide
Therapeutic class: Antihypertensive

Apri
desogestrel, ethinyl estradiol
Therapeutic class: Estrogen, progestin

Arthrotec
diclofenac sodium, misoprostol
Therapeutic class: Anti-inflammatory,
gastric protectant

Atacand HCT
candesartan cilexetil, hydrochlorothiazide
Therapeutic class: Antihypertensive

Augmentin
amoxicillin, clavulanate potassium
Therapeutic class: Anti-infective

Bactrim
sulfamethoxazole, trimethoprim
Therapeutic class: Anti-infective

Bancap HC
acetaminophen, hydrocodone bitartrate
Therapeutic class: Opioid analgesic

Caduet
amlodipine besylate, atorvastatin
calcium
Therapeutic class: Antihypertensive,
antihyperlipidemic

Capozide
captopril, hydrochlorothiazide
Therapeutic class: Antihypertensive

Ciprodex
ciprofloxacin, dexamethasone
Therapeutic class: Anti-infective, anti-inflammatory drug

Claritin-D
loratadine, pseudoephedrine sulfate
Therapeutic class: Antihistamine, adrenergic

Clindex
chlordiazepoxide hydrochloride, clidinium bromide
Therapeutic class: Anxiolytic, anticholinergic

Col-Probenecid
colchicine, probenecid
Therapeutic class: Antigout drug

CombiPatch
estradiol, norethindrone acetate
Therapeutic class: Estrogen, progestin

Combipres
chlorthalidone, clonidine hydrochloride
Therapeutic class: Antihypertensive

Combivent
albuterol sulfate, ipratropium bromide
Therapeutic class: Bronchodilator

Combivir
lamivudine, zidovudine
Therapeutic class: Antiviral

Corzide
bendroflumethiazide, nadolol
Therapeutic class: Antihypertensive

Cotazym
amylase, lipase, pancreatin, protease
Therapeutic class: Digestive enzyme

Demi-Regroton
chlorthalidone, reserpine
Therapeutic class: Antihypertensive

EMLA Cream
lidocaine, prilocaine
Therapeutic class: Anesthetic

Endocet
acetaminophen, oxycodone hydrochloride
Therapeutic class: Opioid analgesic

Enduronyl
deserpidine, methylclothiazide
Therapeutic class: Antihypertensive

Etrafon
amitriptyline hydrochloride, perphenazine
Therapeutic class: Antipsychotic, antidepressant

Fansidar
pyrimethamine, sulfadoxine
Therapeutic class: Antimalarial drug

femhrt
ethinyl estradiol, norethindrone acetate
Therapeutic class: Estrogen, progestin

Fioricet
acetaminophen, butalbital, caffeine
Therapeutic class: Barbiturate analgesic

Fiorinal
aspirin, butalbital, caffeine
Therapeutic class: Barbiturate analgesic

Glucovance
glyburide, metformin hydrochloride
Therapeutic class: Hypoglycemic

Helidac
bismuth subsalicylate, metronidazole, tetracycline hydrochloride
Therapeutic class: Anti-infective

Humulin 70/30
insulin suspension, isophane; insulin, recombinant human
Therapeutic class: Hypoglycemic

Hycodan
homatropine methylbromide, hydrocodone bitartrate
Therapeutic class: Opioid analgesic

Hydrocet
acetaminophen, hydrocodone bitartrate
Therapeutic class: Opioid analgesic

Hyzaar
hydrochlorothiazide, losartan potassium
Therapeutic class: Antihypertensive

Inderide
hydrochlorothiazide, propranolol hydrochloride
Therapeutic class: Antihypertensive

(continued)

Common combination drug products (continued)

Innovar
droperidol, fentanyl citrate
Therapeutic class: Opioid analgesic

Kaletra
lopinavir, ritonavir
Therapeutic class: Antiviral

Lexxel
enalapril maleate, felodipine
Therapeutic class: Antihypertensive

Librax
chlordiazepoxide hydrochloride,
clidinium bromide
Therapeutic class: Anxiolytic

Lomotil
atropine sulfate, diphenoxylate
hydrochloride
Therapeutic class: Antidiarrheal, anticholinergic

Lopressor HCT
hydrochlorothiazide, metoprolol tartrate
Therapeutic class: Antihypertensive

Lortab
acetaminophen, hydrocodone bitartrate
Therapeutic class: Opioid analgesic

Lotensin HCT
benazepril hydrochloride,
hydrochlorothiazide
Therapeutic class: Antihypertensive

Lotrel
amlodipine besylate, benazepril
hydrochloride
Therapeutic class: Antihypertensive

Macrobid
nitrofurantoin macrocrystals, nitrofurantoin monohydrate
Therapeutic class: Anti-infective

Maxzide
hydrochlorothiazide, triamterene
Therapeutic class: Antihypertensive,
diuretic

Minizide
polythiazide, prazosin hydrochloride
Therapeutic class: Antihypertensive

Moduretic
amiloride hydrochloride, hydrochlorothiazide
Therapeutic class: Diuretic

NuLYTELY
polyethylene glycol, potassium chloride,
sodium bicarbonate, sodium chloride
Therapeutic class: Laxative

Ortho-Cyclen
ethinyl estradiol, norgestimate
Therapeutic class: Contraceptive

Pediazole
erythromycin ethylsuccinate, sulfisoxazole acetyl
Therapeutic class: Anti-infective

Percocet
acetaminophen, oxycodone hydrochloride
Therapeutic class: Opioid analgesic

Percodan
aspirin, oxycodone hydrochloride, oxycodone terephthalate
Therapeutic class: Opioid analgesic

Premphase
conjugated estrogens, medroxyproges-
terone acetate
Therapeutic class: Contraceptive

Primaxin
cilastatin sodium, imipenem
Therapeutic class: Anti-infective

Quibron
guaifenesin, theophylline
Therapeutic class: Bronchodilator, expectorant

Rifamate
isoniazid, rifampin
Therapeutic class: Antitubercular

Rifater
isoniazid, pyrazinamide, rifampin
Therapeutic class: Antitubercular

Seasonale
ethinyl estradiol, levonorgestrel
Therapeutic class: Estrogen, progestin

Septra
sulfamethoxazole, trimethoprim
Therapeutic class: Anti-infective

Sinemet
carbidopa, levodopa
Therapeutic class: Antiparkinsonian

Solage
mequinol, tretinoin
Therapeutic class: Antineoplastic

Stalevo
carbidopa, entacapone, levodopa
Therapeutic class: Antiparkinsonian

Symbyax
fluoxetine hydrochloride, olanzapine
Therapeutic class: Mood stabilizer

Tenoretic
atenolol, chlorthalidone
Therapeutic class: Antihypertensive

Triavil
amitriptyline hydrochloride,
    perphenazine
Therapeutic class: Antipsychotic,
    antidepressant

Tylox
acetaminophen, oxycodone hydro-
    chloride
Therapeutic class: Opioid analgesic

Unasyn
ampicillin sodium, sulbactam sodium
Therapeutic class: Anti-infective

Vaseretic
enalapril maleate, hydrochlorothiazide
Therapeutic class: Antihypertensive,
    diuretic

Zestoretic
hydrochlorothiazide, lisinopril
Therapeutic class: Antihypertensive

Ziac
bisoprolol fumarate, hydrochloro-
    thiazide
Therapeutic class: Antihypertensive

Tablets and capsules *not* to crush

SAFETY
GUIDELINES

Crushing extended-release or other long-acting oral drug forms can cause the ingredients to be released all at once instead of gradually. Similarly, crushing can break the coating of enteric-coated drugs, leading to GI irritation. Other drugs may taste bad or have carcinogenic or teratogenic potential when crushed. Never crush the trade-name drugs listed below.

Aciphex	Dexedrine Spansule
Adalat CC	Diamox Sequels
Aerolate	Dilacor XR
Aggrenox	Dilatrate-SR
Allegra D	Disobrom
Artane Sequels	Ditropan XL
Arthrotec	Donnatal Extentabs
Asacol	Donnazyme
Bayer EC	Drixoral
Bellergal-S	Dulcolax
Betachron ER	DynaCirc CR
Biaxin XL	Easprin
Boniva	Ecotrin
Breonesin	Effexor XR
Calan SR	Efidac/24
Carbatrol	Entex LA
Carbiset-TR	Ergomar
Cardene SR	Erythromycin Base
Cardizem CD, LA, SR	Eskalith CR
Carter's Little Pills	Factive
Cartia XT	Flomax
Ceclor CD	Glucotrol XL
CellCept	Guaifed
Choledyl SA	Ilotycin
Claritin-D	Imdur
Colace	Inderal LA
Colestid	Inderide LA
Compazine Spansules	Indocin SR
Concerta	Isoptin SR
Cotazym-S	Isordil Sublingual, Tembids
Covera-HS	Isosorbide Dinitrate Sublingual
Creon	Kadian
Cytospaz M	Kaon-Cl
Cytovene	K-Dur
Cytoxan	Klor-Con
Deconamine SR	Klotrix
Depakene	K-Tab
Depakote	Levbid
Desoxyn Gradumets	Levsinex Timecaps

Lexxel
Lithobid
Lodine XL
Macrobid
Mestinon Timespans
Methylin ER
Micro-K Extencaps
Monafed
MS Contin
Naldecon
Naprelan
Nexium
Nia-Bid
Niaspan
Nicotinic Acid
Nitro-Bid
Nitroglyn
Nitrong
Nitrostat
Norflex
Norpace CR
Novafed A
Oramorph SR
OxyContin
Pancrease MT
PCE
Pentasa
Perdiem
Permital Chronotab
Phazyme
Phyllocontin
Plendil
Pneumomist
Prelu-2
Prevacid
Prilosec
Pro-Banthine
Procainamide HCL SR
Procardia
Proscar
Protonix
Proventil Repetabs
Prozac
Quibron-T/SR
Quinaglute Dura-Tabs
Quinidex Extentabs
Respaire SR
Respbid
Reyataz
Ritalin-SR

Roxanol SR
Ru-Tuss
Sinemet CR
Slo-bid Gyrocaps
Slo-Niacin
Slo-Phyllin GG, Gyrocaps
Slow FE
Slow-K
Sorbitrate SA
Striant
Sudafed 12 Hour
Sular
Sustaire
Tavist-D
Tegretol-XR
Teldrin
Tenuate Dospan
Tessalon Perles
Theobid Duracaps
Theochron
Theoclear LA
Theo-Dur
Theolair-SR
Theo-Sav
Theospan-SR
Theo-24
Theovent
Theo-X
Thorazine Spansules
Tiazac
Toprol XL
T-Phyl
Tranxene-SD
Trental
Triaminic
Trilafon Repetabs
Trinalin Repetabs
Tuss-Ornade Spansules
Tylenol Extended Relief
Ultrase MT
Uniphyl
Verelan
Volmax
Voltaren, XR
Wellbutrin SR, XL
Xanax-XR
ZORprin
Zyban
Zymase

Drug names that look or sound alike

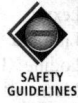

SAFETY
GUIDELINES

The drug names below can easily be confused, either verbally or in writing, because they either sound alike or have similar spellings. Generic names of these drugs appear in regular type; trade names are capitalized and in **boldface**.

Accupril, **Accutane**

Accutane, **Anturane**

acetazolamide, acetohexamide

acetylcholine, acetylcysteine

Aciphex, **Aricept**

Adderall, **Inderal**

albuterol, atenolol

Aldactazide, **Aldactone**

Aldomet, **Aldoril**

Aldoril, **Elavil**

alfentanil, fentanyl, **Sufenta**, sufentanil

Allegra, **Viagra**

alprazolam, lorazepam

Altace, alteplase

Alupent, **Atrovent**

amantadine, rimantadine

Ambien, **Amen**

Amicar, **Amikin**

amiloride, amlodipine

amitriptyline, nortriptyline

Anafranil, enalapril

Apresazide, **Apresoline**

Asacol, **Os-Cal**, **Oxytrol**

Atarax, **Ativan**

atenolol, timolol

Avinza, **Invanz**

azithromycin, erythromycin

baclofen, **Bactroban**

Benadryl, **Benylin**, **Betalin**

bepridil, **Prepidil**

Betagan, **BetaGen**

Bumex, **Buprenex**

bupivacaine, ropivacaine

bupropion, buspirone

Calan, **Colace**

calcifediol, calcitriol

Capitrol, captopril

Cardene, **Cardizem**

Cardene, codeine

cefazolin, cefprozil

cefotaxime, ceftizoxime

cefuroxime, deferoxamine

Cefzil, **Kefzol**

Celebrex, **Celexa**

Celebrex, **Cerebyx**

chlorpromazine, chlorpropamide, promethazine

Ciloxan, **Cytoxan**

Clinoril, **Clozaril**

clofazimine, clonidine, clozapine

clomiphene, clomipramine

clonazepam, clorazepate

clonidine, quinidine

clotrimazole, co-trimoxazole

codeine, **Lodine**

Coreg, **Zomig**

Cozaar, **Zocor**

cyclobenzaprine, cyproheptadine

cycloserine, cyclosporine

dacarbazine, procarbazine

dactinomycin, daunorubicin

danazol, **Dantrium**

dapsone, **Diprosone**

Darvon, **Diovan**

daunorubicin, idarubicin

Decadron, **Percodan**

desipramine, imipramine

Desogen, desonide

desoximetasone, dexamethasone

Desoxyn, digitoxin, digoxin

diazepam, **Ditropan**

diazoxide, **Dyazide**

dimenhydrinate, diphenhydramine

Diprivan, **Ditropan**

dipyridamole, disopyramide

dobutamine, dopamine

doxapram, doxazosin, doxepin, doxycycline

Doxil, Paxil, Plavix

dronabinol, droperidol

dyclonine, dicyclomine

Dynacin, DynaCirc

Echogen, Epogen

Elavil, Equanil, Mellaril

Eldepryl, enalapril

Elmiron, Imuran

eloxatin, **Exelon**

enalapril, ramipril

Entex, Tenex, Xanax

ephedrine, epinephrine

esmolol, **Osmitrol**

Estraderm, Estratab, Estratest

Estraderm, Testoderm

ethosuximide, methsuximide

etidronate, etretinate

Eurax, Urex

Evista, E-vista

Femara, FemHRT

fenoprofen, flurbiprofen

Fioricet, Fiorinal

Flaxedil, Flexeril

Flomax, Fosamax

flunisolide, fluocinonide

fluoxetine, fluvastatin, fluvoxamine

flurazepam, temazepam

folic acid, folinic acid

Foradil, Toradol

fosinopril, lisinopril, **Risperdal**

fosphenytoin, phenytoin

furosemide, torsemide

glimepiride, glipizide, glyburide

Granulex, Regranex

guaifenesin, guanfacine

Haldol, Stadol

heparin, **Hepsera, Hespan**

Hycodan, Vicodin

hydralazine, hydroxyzine

hydromorphone, morphine

Hyperstat, Nitrostat

imipenem, **Omnipen**

imipramine, **Norpramin**

Inderal, Inderide, Isordil

Intropin, Isoptin

Lamasil, Lomotil

Lamictal, Lamisil

lamivudine, lamotrigine

Lanoxin, Lasix, Lonox

Levatol, Lipitor

Levbid, Lithobid

Levitra, Raptiva

Librax, Librium

Loniten, Lotensin, lovastatin

Lorabid, Slo-bid

losartan, valsartan

Mandol, nadolol

Maxidex, Maxzide

Mazicon, Mevacor, Mivacron

mebendazole, methimazole

meclizine, memantine

melphalan, **Mephyton**

meperidine, meprobamate

Mesantoin, Mestinon

metaproterenol, metoprolol

methicillin, mezlocillin

methotrexate, metolazone

metoprolol, misoprostol

minoxidil, **Monopril**

mithramycin, mitomycin

naloxone, naltrexone

Naprelan, Naprosyn

Navane, Nubain

nelfinavir, nevirapine

Neurontin, Noroxin

niacinamide, nicardipine

nicardipine, nifedipine, nimodipine

Norpace, Norpramin

Ocufen, Ocuflox

olanzapine, olsalazine

Orinase, Ornade

oxaprozin, oxazepam

oxycodone, **OxyContin**

paclitaxel, paroxetine

Panadol, pindolol, **Plendil**

pancuronium, pipecuronium

Parlodel, pindolol

paroxetine, pralidoxime, pyridoxine

Pelamine, pemoline

pentobarbital, phenobarbital

(continued)

Drug names that look or sound alike (continued)

pentosan, pentostatin
Percocet, Percodan
Phenaphen, Phenergan
phenelzine, **Phenylzin**
phentermine, phentolamine
pioglitazone, rosiglitazone
Pitocin, Pitressin
Pravachol, Prevacid
Pravachol, propranolol
prednisolone, prednisone, primidone
Premarin, Primaxin
Prilosec, Prinivil, Proventil
Prilosec, Prozac
ProAmatine, protamine
probenecid, **Procanbid**
promazine, promethazine
Proscar, Prozac
protamine, **Protopam, Protropin**
Quarzan, Questran
quinidine, quinine
ranitidine, rimantadine
Relpax, Revex, Revia
Reminyl, Robinul
reserpine, **Risperdal**
Restoril, Vistaril
Retrovir, ritonavir
ribavirin, riboflavin
rifabutin, rifampin
Rifadin, Rifamate, Rifater
Rifadin, Ritalin, ritodrine
Roxanol, Roxicet
Salbutamol, salmeterol
saquinavir, **Sinequan**
selegiline, **Stelazine**
Septa, Septra
Serentil, Serevent
Seroquel, Serzone
Solu-Cortef, Solu-Medrol
somatropin, sumatriptan
Spiriva, Stalevo
Sufenta, Survanta
sulfadiazine, sulfasalazine, sulfisoxazole
sumatriptan, zolmitriptan
Tambocor, tamoxifen

tegaserod, **Tegretol, Toradol**
Tequin, Ticlid
terbinafine, terbutaline, terfenadine
terbutaline, tolbutamide
terconazole, tioconazole
testolactone, testosterone
thiamine, **Thorazine**
tiagabine, tizanidine
Ticar, Tigan
Timoptic, Vioptic
Tobradex, Tobrex
tolazamide, tolbutamide
tolnaftate, **Tornalate**
Trandate, Tridate
Trendar, Trental
tretinoin, trientine
triamcinolone, **Triaminicin,
    Triaminicol**
triaminic, **Triaminicin**
triamterene, trimipramine
trifluoperazine, triflupromazine
Urised, Urispas
valacyclovir, valganciclovir
Vancenase, Vanceril
Vanceril, Vansil
VePesid, Versed
verapamil, **Verelan**
Verelan, Virilon
vinblastine, vincristine, vindesine,
    vinorelbine
Wellbutrin, Wellcovorin, Wellferon
Xanax, Zantac
Zantac, Zyrtec
Zestril, Zostrix
Zocor, Zoloft
Zofran, Zosyn
Zymar, Zyprexa, Zyrtec

Understanding the Needlestick Safety and Prevention Act

SAFETY GUIDELINES

The Needlestick Safety and Prevention Act of 2000 updated a 30-year-old blood-borne pathogens standard enforced under the Occupational Safety and Health Act. Key revisions mandate the use of safer medical equipment (such as needleless systems and sharps with injury protectors) to reduce or eliminate health care workers' exposure to bloodborne pathogens.

Under the 2000 law, employers must:
• keep a log of sharps injuries, with brief details of each injury, including the department where it occurred and the type and brand of device used
• regularly evaluate exposure plans and revise them if necessary to incorporate new, safer medical devices—and then document use of these devices
• ask frontline health care workers for ideas on how to avoid sharps injuries and make the workplace safer.

Ensuring facility compliance
To help determine if your facility is complying with the Needlestick Safety and Prevention Act, answer the questions below.
Drawing blood
• Does your facility use blood-drawing equipment with safety features designed to prevent needlesticks?
• Does your facility use plastic (rather than glass) blood collection tubes?
• Has your facility replaced all unnecessary needles with needleless devices?
• Does your facility use lancets that automatically retract?
• Has the facility's staff been warned not to remove needles from blood-drawing devices by hand and not to recap needles manually?
Giving injections
• When possible, does your facility use prefilled syringes with built-in safety features?
• Does your facility use devices for I.M or S.C. injections that have retracting needles and other safety features?
Administering I.V. infusions
• Has your facility replaced old I.V. infusion systems with needleless ones?
Inserting peripheral I.V. lines
• Does your facility use vascular access devices that protect you from the stylet as you withdraw it from the patient?
Safeguarding specialized areas
• Does your facility have safety alternatives in place for specialized areas, such as the blood bank, operating room, dialysis area, and laboratories?

Evaluating the exposure control plan
Every health care facility should have a written exposure control plan that lists all jobs and duties that expose a healthcare worker to bloodborne pathogens. The plan should be assessed and updated yearly to incorporate new, safer medical equipment and to include ideas from nonmanagerial employees who perform direct patient care.

Keeping a sharps injury log
Your facility must keep a log of any needlesticks that occur. The log should include how the exposure occurred, exactly where it occurred, and what brand and type of device was involved. The log should be documented and maintained in a way that ensures employee confidentiality.

Monitoring blood levels

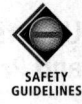

SAFETY
GUIDELINES

The table below shows therapeutic and toxic blood levels for selected drugs. Keep in mind that such levels may vary slightly among laboratories.

Drug	Therapeutic blood level	Toxic blood level
amikacin	Peak: 25 to 35 mcg/ml	> 35 mcg/ml
	Trough: 5 to 10 mcg/ml	> 10 mcg/ml
aminophylline	10 to 20 mcg/ml	> 20 mcg/ml
amiodarone	1 to 2.5 mcg/ml	> 2.5 mcg/ml
amitriptyline	120 to 250 ng/ml	> 500 ng/ml
bepridil	1 to 2 ng/ml	> 2 ng/ml
calcium	9 to 10.5 mg/dl	> 12 mg/dl
carbamazepine	4 to 14 mcg/ml	> 15 mcg/ml
clonazepam	10 to 80 ng/ml	> 100 ng/ml
creatinine	0.6 to 1.2 mg/dl	> 4 mg/dl
cyclosporine	50 to 300 ng/ml	> 400 ng/ml
desipramine	115 to 300 ng/ml	> 400 ng/ml
diazepam	0.5 to 2 mcg/ml	> 3 mcg/ml
digoxin	0.8 to 2 ng/ml	> 2 ng/ml
disopyramide	2 to 8 mcg/ml	> 8 mcg/ml
ethosuximide	40 to 100 mcg/ml	>100 mcg/ml
flecainide	0.2 to 1 mcg/ml	>1 mcg/ml
gentamicin	Peak: 4 to 12 mcg/ml	> 12 mcg/ml
	Trough: 1 to 2 mcg/ml	> 2 mcg/ml
glucose	70 to 110 mg/dl	> 300 mg/dl
haloperidol	5 to 20 ng/ml	> 20 ng/ml
imipramine	225 to 300 ng/ml	> 500 ng/ml
lidocaine	1.5 to 6 mcg/ml	> 6 mcg/ml
lithium	0.6 to 1.2 mEq/L	> 1.5 mEq/L
meperidine	100 to 550 ng/ml	> 1,000 ng/ml
mezlocillin	35 to 45 mcg/ml	> 45 mcg/ml
milrinone	150 to 250 ng/ml	> 250 ng/ml
nifedipine	0.025 to 0.1 mcg/ml	> 0.1 mcg/ml
nortriptyline	50 to 140 ng/ml	> 300 ng/ml
phenobarbital	10 to 40 mcg/ml	> 40 mcg/ml
phenytoin	10 to 20 mcg/ml	> 20 mcg/ml

Drug	Therapeutic blood level	Toxic blood level
potassium	3.5 to 5.0 mEq/L	> 6 mEq/L
primidone	4 to 12 mcg/ml	> 12 mcg/ml
procainamide	4 to 8 mcg/ml	> 10 mcg/ml
propranolol	50 to 200 ng/ml	> 200 ng/ml
quinidine	2 to 5 mcg/ml	> 5 mcg/ml
salicylates	100 to 300 mcg/ml	> 300 mcg/ml
sodium	135 to 145 mEq/L	> 160 mEq/L
streptomycin	25 mcg/ml	> 25 mcg/ml
theophylline	10 to 20 mcg/ml	> 20 mcg/ml
tobramycin	Peak: 4 to 12 mcg/ml	> 12 mcg/ml
	Trough: 1 to 2 mcg/ml	> 2 mcg/ml
tocainide	4 to 10 mcg/ml	Not established
valproic acid	50 to 100 mcg/ml	> 100 mcg/ml
vancomycin	Peak: 20 to 40 mcg/ml	> 40 mcg/ml
	Trough: 5 to 15 mcg/ml	> 15 mcg/ml
verapamil	0.08 to 0.3 mcg/ml	Not established

Effects of dialysis on drug therapy

SAFETY GUIDELINES

A patient receiving a drug that's removed by hemodialysis will need supplemental doses of that drug. The chart below shows which drugs are removed by dialysis and therefore will necessitate supplemental dosing during or after dialysis. Drugs listed as "unlikely" haven't been studied; however, because of their chemical properties, dialysis is unlikely to remove them.

Generic drug	Removed by hemodialysis	Generic drug	Removed by hemodialysis
acetaminophen	Yes	diphenhydramine	Unlikely
acyclovir	Yes	drotrecogin alfa	Unlikely
adenosine	Unlikely	edetate calcium	Yes
albumin	Unlikely	enalapril	Yes
allopurinol	Yes	epinephrine	No data
amikacin	Yes	epoetin alfa	No
amiodarone	No	erythromycin	No
amoxicillin	Yes	esmolol	Yes
amphotericin B	No	ethacrynic acid	No
ampicillin	Yes	famciclovir	Yes
ascorbic acid	Yes	famotidine	No
aspirin	Yes	fluconazole	Yes
atenolol	Yes	flucytosine	Yes
aztreonam	Yes	foscarnet	Yes
bleomycin	No	furosemide	No
bumetanide	No	gabapentin	Yes
captopril	Yes	ganciclovir	Yes
carboplatin	Yes	gentamicin	Yes
carmustine	No	haloperidol	No
cefaclor	Yes	heparin	No
cefadroxil	Yes	hydralazine	No
cefazolin	Yes	hydrochlorothiazide	No
cefepime	Yes	hydrocodone	No data
cefmetazole	Yes	hydromorphone	No data
cefoxitin	Yes	hydroxyzine	No
cefuroxime	Yes	ibuprofen	No
cephalexin	Yes	ibutilide	No data
chloramphenicol	Yes	imipenem	Yes
ciprofloxacin	No	imipramine	No
cyclophosphamide	Yes	insulin	No
desipramine	No	isoniazid	No
dexamethasone	No	isosorbide dinitrate	No
diazepam	No	isosorbide mononitrate	Yes
diazoxide	Yes	ketoconazole	No
digoxin	No	ketoprofen	Unlikely
diltiazem	No	labetalol	No

Generic drug	Removed by hemodialysis	Generic drug	Removed by hemodialysis
lansoprazole	No	octreotide	Yes
levetiracetam	Yes	ofloxacin	Yes
levofloxacin	Unlikely	omeprazole	Unlikely
lisinopril	Yes	ondansetron	Unlikely
lithium	Yes	oxycodone	No data
loracarbef	Yes	paclitaxel	No
loratadine	No	pancuronium	No data
lorazepam	No	paroxetine	No
lovastatin	Unlikely	penicillin	Yes
loxapine	No data	phenobarbital	Yes
mannitol	Yes	phenytoin	No
maprotiline	No	piperacillin	Yes
melphalan	No	pravastatin	No
meperidine	No	prednisone	No
mercaptopurine	Yes	procainamide	Yes
meropenem	Yes	propofol	Unlikely
mesalamine	Yes	propranolol	No
mesna	No data	quinapril	No
metformin	Yes	ramipril	No
methadone	No	ranitidine	No
methicillin	No	reteplase	No data
methotrexate	Yes	rifampin	No
methyldopa	Yes	risperidone	No data
methylprednisolone	Yes	ritodrine	Yes
metoprolol	Yes	ritonavir	Unlikely
metronidazole	Yes	simvastatin	Unlikely
mexiletine	Yes	sotalol	Yes
mezlocillin	Yes	stavudine	Yes
miconazole	No	streptomycin	Yes
midazolam	No	sulbactam	Yes
minoxidil	Yes	sulfamethoxazole	Yes
morphine	No data	sulfisoxazole	Yes
nadolol	Yes	tamoxifen	No data
nafcillin	No	tazobactam	Yes
nalbuphine	No data	temazepam	No
naloxone	No data	theophylline	Yes
naltrexone	No data	ticarcillin	Yes
neomycin	Yes	tobramycin	Yes
nicardipine	No	trimethoprim	Yes
nifedipine	No	valacyclovir	Yes
nilutamide	No data	vancomycin	No
nimodipine	No	warfarin	No
nitroglycerin	No	zalcitabine	No data
nitroprusside	Yes	zolpidem	No

Managing poisonings and overdoses

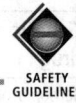

SAFETY
GUIDELINES

This chart serves as a quick reference for managing poisonings and drug overdoses. For more detailed instructions, consult your local poison control center. To find your local center, call the American Association of Poison Control Centers at 1-800-222-1222 or visit http://www.aapcc.org/findyour.htm.

Poison or drug	Antidote and dosage
acetaminophen	**acetylcysteine** Give orally as 5% solution by diluting with carbonated diet beverage. Loading dose: One-time dose of 140 mg/kg. Repeat dose if patient vomits within 1 hour of administration. Maintenance dose: 70 mg/kg q 4 hours, starting 4 hours after loading dose for 17 doses. Repeat any dose if patient vomits within 1 hour of administration.
alpha$_2$-adrenergic agonists opiates	**naloxone** *Adults:* 0.4 to 2 mg I.V.; may repeat q 2 to 3 minutes. If no response occurs after patient has received maximum dosage of 10 mg, reevaluate diagnosis of narcotic-induced toxicity. *Children:* Initially, 0.01 mg/kg I.V.; if desired response doesn't occur, give subsequent dose of 0.1 mg/kg I.V. *Neonates:* Initially, 0.01 mg/kg I.V., repeated q 2 to 3 minutes p.r.n. **nalmefene** Initially, 0.5 mg/70 kg I.V., followed by a second dose of 1 mg/70 kg I.V. 2 minutes later, if necessary
anticholinergic agents antihistamines atropine	**physostigmine** *Adults:* 0.5 to 2 mg slow I.V. injection (not to exceed 1 mg/minute). May repeat if coma, arrhythmia, or seizure occurs. *Children:* 0.02 mg/kg I.M. or slow I.V. injection (not to exceed 0.5 mg/minute). May repeat q 5 to 10 minutes until therapeutic response occurs or maximum dosage of 2 mg is given.
benzodiazepines	**flumazenil** *Adults:* Initially, 0.2 mg I.V. injected over 30 seconds; follow with 0.3 mg if desired level of consciousness isn't reached. May give further doses of 0.5 mg at 60-second intervals until therapeutic response occurs or maximum dosage of 3 mg is given. If sedation recurs, repeat dose at 20-minute intervals. Maximum dosage is 3 mg/hour.
digoxin	**digoxin immune Fab** Calculate dosage as number of vials, using this formula: Digoxin level (in ng) × patient's weight (in kg) divided by 100. Usual dosage range is four to six vials. If ingested amount of digoxin is unknown, give 10 to 20 vials (380 to 800 mg) I.V. over 30 minutes through a 0.22-micron filter. May give bolus dose if cardiac arrest is imminent.

Poison or drug	Antidote and dosage
ethylene glycol	**fomepizole** Loading dose: 15 mg/kg I.V. over 30 minutes, followed by 10 mg/kg I.V. over 30 minutes q 12 hours for four doses Maintenance dose: 15 mg/kg I.V. over 30 minutes q 12 hours until ethylene glycol level falls below 20 mg/dl
heparin	**protamine sulfate** Dosage is based on partial thromboplastin time; usually, 1 mg for each 100 units of heparin. Give I.V. over 10 minutes in doses not exceeding 50 mg.
iron	**deferoxamine** *Acute iron intoxication:* Initially, 1 g I.M., followed by 500 mg q 4 hours for two doses depending on clinical response, and then 500 mg q 4 to 12 hours. May give I.V. infusion of 10 to 15 mg/kg/hour for first 1 g. Subsequent doses shouldn't exceed 125 mg/hour. Maximum dosage is 6 g in 24 hours. *Chronic iron intoxication:* In adults, 1 to 2 g/day S.C. In children, maximum dosage of 6 g/24 hours or 2 g/dose S.C.
organophosphate insecticides	**pralidoxime** *Adults:* 1 to 2 g in 100 ml of normal saline solution infused over 15 to 30 minutes. If pulmonary edema occurs, may give as 5% solution I.V. over 5 minutes. May repeat dose in 1 hour if muscle weakness persists; may give additional doses cautiously if muscle weakness continues. *Children:* 20 to 40 mg/kg (up to 1 g) in 250 ml normal saline solution I.V. over 30 minutes
warfarin	**phytonadione** *Adults:* 2.5 to 10 mg S.C. based on prothrombin time/International Normalized Ratio; may repeat in 6 to 8 hours as needed In emergency, 10 to 50 mg slow I.V. (no faster than 1 mg/minute); may repeat q 4 hour, as needed
miscellaneous drug overdose	**activated charcoal** *Adults:* 25 to 100 g mixed in 120 to 240 ml of water and given P.O. or through nasogastric tube if patient can't have oral intake; may give multiple doses in severe overdose

Reporting adverse events

SAFETY GUIDELINES

A vaccine adverse event reporting form should be completed whenever an adverse reaction to a vaccine occurs. The information submitted provides valuable information to the Centers for Disease Control and Prevention and may enhance the understanding of adverse reactions to vaccines.

WEBSITE: www.vaers.org   E-MAIL: info@vaers.org   FAX: 1-877-721-0366

VAERS

VACCINE ADVERSE EVENT REPORTING SYSTEM
24 Hour Toll-Free Information 1-800-822-7967
P.O. Box 1100, Rockville, MD 20849-1100
PATIENT IDENTITY KEPT CONFIDENTIAL

For CDC/FDA Use Only

VAERS Number _____

Date Received _____

Patient Name:	Vaccine administered by (Name):	Form completed by (Name):
Last First M.I.	Responsible Physician _____	Relation ☐ Vaccine Provider ☐ Patient/Parent to Patient ☐ Manufacturer ☐ Other
Address	Facility Name/Address	Address (if different from patient or provider)
City State Zip	City State Zip	City State Zip
Telephone no. (___)	Telephone no. (___)	Telephone no. (___)

| 1. State | 2. County where administered | 3. Date of birth mm dd yy | 4. Patient age | 5. Sex ☐ M ☐ F | 6. Date form completed mm dd yy |

7. Describe adverse events(s) (symptoms, signs, time course) and treatment, if any

8. Check all appropriate:
☐ Patient died   (date ___/___/___ mm dd yy)
☐ Life threatening illness
☐ Required emergency room/doctor visit
☐ Required hospitalization (_____days)
☐ Resulted in prolongation of hospitalization
☐ Resulted in permanent disability
☐ None of the above

9. Patient recovered   ☐ YES ☐ NO ☐ UNKNOWN

10. Date of vaccination mm dd yy   Time ____ AM PM

11. Adverse event onset mm dd yy   Time ____ AM PM

12. Relevant diagnostic tests/laboratory data

13. Enter all vaccines given on date listed in no. 10

Vaccine (type)	Manufacturer	Lot number	Route/Site	No. Previous Doses
a.				
b.				
c.				
d.				

14. Any other vaccinations within 4 weeks prior to the date listed in no. 10

Vaccine (type)	Manufacturer	Lot number	Route/Site	No. Previous doses	Date given
a.					
b.					

| 15. Vaccinated at: ☐ Private doctor's office/hospital ☐ Public health clinic/hospital ☐ Military clinic/hospital ☐ Other/unknown | 16. Vaccine purchased with: ☐ Private funds ☐ Military funds ☐ Public funds ☐ Other/unknown | 17. Other medications |

| 18. Illness at time of vaccination (specify) | 19. Pre-existing physician-diagnosed allergies, birth defects, medical conditions (specify) |

| 20. Have you reported this adverse event previously? ☐ No ☐ To doctor ☐ To health department ☐ To manufacturer | **Only for children 5 and under** |
| | 22. Birth weight _____ lb. _____ oz. | 23. No. of brothers and sisters |

21. Adverse event following prior vaccination (check all applicable, specify)	**Only for reports submitted by manufacturer/immunization project**
Adverse Event / Onset Age / Type Vaccine / Dose no. in series	24. Mfr./imm. proj. report no.	25. Date received by mfr./imm.proj.
☐ In patient		
☐ In brother or sister	26. 15 day report? ☐ Yes ☐ No	27. Report type ☐ Initial ☐ Follow-Up

Health care providers and manufacturers are required by law (42 USC 300aa-25) to report reactions to vaccines listed in the Table of Reportable Events Following Immunization. Reports for reactions to other vaccines are voluntary except when required as a condition of immunization grant awards.

Form VAERS-1(FDA)

The Food and Drug Administration (FDA) requires that all deaths and serious injuries related to a drug or medical device be reported using the MedWatch form shown below. This mandatory two-page form is designed for use by facilities, distributors, importers, applicants, and manufacturers.

Page 1

Reporting adverse events (continued)

Medication and Device Experience Report
(Continued)

Submission of a report does not constitute an admission that medical personnel, user facility, importer, distributor, manufacturer or product caused or contributed to the event.

U.S. DEPARTMENT OF HEALTH AND HUMAN SERVICES
Public Health Service • Food and Drug Administration

FDA USE ONLY

Refer to guidelines for specific instructions.   Page ____ of ____

F. FOR USE BY USER FACILITY/IMPORTER (Devices Only)

1. Check One
   - [ ] User Facility
   - [ ] Importer

2. UF/Importer Report Number

3. User Facility or Importer Name/Address

4. Contact Person

5. Phone Number

6. Date User Facility or Importer Became Aware of Event (mo/day/yr)

7. Type of Report
   - [ ] Initial
   - [ ] Follow-up #

8. Date of This Report (mo/day/yr)

9. Approximate Age of Device

10. Event Problem Codes (Refer to coding manual)
    - Patient Code ___ - ___
    - Device Code ___ - ___

11. Report Sent to FDA?
    - [ ] Yes
    - [ ] No   (mo/day/yr)

12. Location Where Event Occurred
    - [ ] Hospital
    - [ ] Home
    - [ ] Nursing Home
    - [ ] Outpatient Treatment Facility
    - [ ] Outpatient Diagnostic Facility
    - [ ] Ambulatory Surgical Facility
    - [ ] Other: _____ (Specify)

13. Report Sent to Manufacturer?
    - [ ] Yes
    - [ ] No   (mo/day/yr)

14. Manufacturer Name/Address

G. ALL MANUFACTURERS

1. Contact Office - Name/Address (and Manufacturing Site for Devices)

2. Phone Number

3. Report Source (Check that apply)
   - [ ] Foreign
   - [ ] Study
   - [ ] Literature
   - [ ] Consumer
   - [ ] Health Professional
   - [ ] User Facility
   - [ ] Company Representative
   - [ ] Distributor
   - [ ] Other:

4. Date Received by Manufacturer (mo/day/yr)

5.
   (A)NDA #_____
   IND #_____
   PLA #_____
   Pre-1938 [ ] Yes
   OTC Product [ ] Yes

6. If IND, Give Protocol #

7. Type of Report (Check all that apply)
   - [ ] 5-day
   - [ ] 10-day
   - [ ] Initial
   - [ ] 15-day
   - [ ] Periodic
   - [ ] Follow-up #

8. Adverse Event Term(s)

9. Manufacturer Report Number

H. DEVICE MANUFACTURERS ONLY

1. Type of Reportable Event
   - [ ] Death
   - [ ] Serious Injury
   - [ ] Malfunction
   - [ ] Other:

2. If Follow-up, What Type?
   - [ ] Correction
   - [ ] Additional Information
   - [ ] Response to FDA Request
   - [ ] Device Evaluation

3. Device Evaluated by Manufacturer?
   - [ ] Not Returned to Manufacturer
   - [ ] Yes [ ] Evaluation Summary Attached
   - [ ] No (Attach page to explain why not) or provide code:

4. Device Manufacture Date (mo/yr)

5. Labeled for Single Use?
   - [ ] Yes   [ ] No

6. Evaluation Codes (Refer to coding manual)
   - Method ___ - ___ - ___
   - Results ___ - ___ - ___
   - Conclusions ___ - ___ - ___

7. If Remedial Action Initiated, Check Type
   - [ ] Recall
   - [ ] Repair
   - [ ] Replace
   - [ ] Relabeling
   - [ ] Other:
   - [ ] Notification
   - [ ] Inspection
   - [ ] Patient Monitoring
   - [ ] Modification/Adjustment

8. Usage of Device
   - [ ] Initial Use of Device
   - [ ] Reuse
   - [ ] Unknown

9. If action reported to FDA under 21 USC 360i(f), list correction/removal reporting number:

10. [ ] Additional Manufacturer Narrative   and / or   11. [ ] Corrected Data

---

The public reporting burden for this collection of information has been estimated to average one hour per response, including the time for reviewing instructions, searching existing data sources, gathering and maintaining the data needed, and completing and reviewing the collection of information. Send comments regarding this burden estimate or any other aspect of this collection of information, including suggestions for reducing this burden to:

FORM FDA 3500A (9/03) (Back)

Department of Health and Human Services
Food and Drug Administration
MedWatch; HFD-410
5600 Fishers Lane
Rockville, MD 20857
Please DO NOT RETURN this form to this address.

OMB Statement:
"An agency may not conduct or sponsor, and a person is not required to respond to, a collection of information unless it displays a currently valid OMB control number."

The voluntary form below is designed for use by healthcare professionals and consumers who wish to report adverse events and other problems with drugs, medical devices, special nutritional products, and other FDA-regulated items. Use of this form promotes rapid detection of problems.

U.S. Department of Health and Human Services

Form Approved: OMB No. 0910-0291, Expires: 03/31/05
See OMB statement on reverse.

MEDWATCH

The FDA Safety Information and Adverse Event Reporting Program

For VOLUNTARY reporting of adverse events and product problems

Page ____ of ____

FDA USE ONLY

Triage unit sequence #

A. PATIENT INFORMATION

1. Patient Identifier ____ In confidence
2. Age at Time of Event: ____ or Date of Birth: ____
3. Sex ☐ Female ☐ Male
4. Weight ____ lbs or ____ kgs

B. ADVERSE EVENT OR PRODUCT PROBLEM

1. ☐ Adverse Event and/or ☐ Product Problem (e.g., defects/malfunctions)
2. Outcomes Attributed to Adverse Event (Check all that apply)
   - ☐ Death: ____ (mo/day/yr)
   - ☐ Life-threatening
   - ☐ Hospitalization - initial or prolonged
   - ☐ Disability
   - ☐ Congenital Anomaly
   - ☐ Required Intervention to Prevent Permanent Impairment/Damage
   - ☐ Other: ____
3. Date of Event (mo/day/year)
4. Date of This Report (mo/day/year)
5. Describe Event or Problem
6. Relevant Tests/Laboratory Data, Including Dates
7. Other Relevant History, Including Preexisting Medical Conditions (e.g., allergies, race, pregnancy, smoking and alcohol use, hepatic/renal dysfunction, etc.)

PLEASE TYPE OR USE BLACK INK

C. SUSPECT MEDICATION(S)

1. Name (Give labeled strength & mfr/labeler, if known) #1 ____ #2 ____
2. Dose, Frequency & Route Used #1 ____ #2 ____
3. Therapy Dates (If unknown, give duration) from/to (or best estimate) #1 ____ #2 ____
4. Diagnosis for Use (Indication) #1 ____ #2 ____
5. Event Abated After Use Stopped or Dose Reduced?
   #1 ☐ Yes ☐ No ☐ Doesn't Apply
   #2 ☐ Yes ☐ No ☐ Doesn't Apply
6. Lot # (if known) #1 ____ #2 ____
7. Exp. Date (if known) #1 ____ #2 ____
8. Event Reappeared After Reintroduction?
   #1 ☐ Yes ☐ No ☐ Doesn't Apply
   #2 ☐ Yes ☐ No ☐ Doesn't Apply
9. NDC# (For product problems only) - -
10. Concomitant Medical Products and Therapy Dates (Exclude treatment of event)

D. SUSPECT MEDICAL DEVICE

1. Brand Name
2. Type of Device
3. Manufacturer Name, City and State
4. Model # ____ Lot # ____ Catalog # ____ Expiration Date (mo/day/yr) ____ Serial # ____ Other # ____
5. Operator of Device ☐ Health Professional ☐ Lay User/Patient ☐ Other: ____
6. If Implanted, Give Date (mo/day/yr)
7. If Explanted, Give Date (mo/day/yr)
8. Is this a Single-use Device that was Reprocessed and Reused on a Patient? ☐ Yes ☐ No
9. If Yes to Item No. 8, Enter Name and Address of Reprocessor
10. Device Available for Evaluation? (Do not send to FDA) ☐ Yes ☐ No ☐ Returned to Manufacturer on: ____ (mo/day/yr)
11. Concomitant Medical Products and Therapy Dates (Exclude treatment of event)

E. REPORTER (See confidentiality section on back)

1. Name and Address ____ Phone # ____
2. Health Professional? ☐ Yes ☐ No
3. Occupation
4. Also Reported to: ☐ Manufacturer ☐ User Facility ☐ Distributor/Importer
5. If you do NOT want your identity disclosed to the manufacturer, place an "X" in this box: ☐

Mail to: MEDWATCH 5600 Fishers Lane Rockville, MD 20852-9787 -or- FAX to: 1-800-FDA-0178

FORM FDA 3500 (12/03) Submission of a report does not constitute an admission that medical personnel or the product caused or contributed to the event.

Drug imprint codes

SAFETY
GUIDELINES

A patient may bring a prescription drug into the hospital that the staff can't identify by sight. In some cases, identification may be crucial to accurate assessment and treatment. Drug imprint codes, such as those shown below, can help you identify individual tablets and capsules that might otherwise be unrecognizable. To access additional drug imprint codes, visit www.nursesdrughandbook.com.

Code	Drug	Color & form	Strength	Manufacturer
0822;4060	chlordiazepoxide hydrochloride	Green and yellow capsule	5 mg	Watson
0822;4065	chlordiazepoxide hydrochloride	Black and green capsule	10 mg	Watson
0822;4070	chlordiazepoxide hydrochloride	Green and white capsule	25 mg	Watson
0822;5	diphenoxylate hydrochloride with atropine	White tablet	0.025 mg	Pfizer
0822;5	diphenoxylate hydrochloride with atropine	White tablet	2.5 mg	Pfizer
10	isoxsuprine hydrochloride	White tablet	10 mg	Sandoz
10;LL;C21	chlorpromazine hydrochloride	Light-brown coated tablet	10 mg	Lederle Laboratories
17;TRIANGLE	Theokin	Yellow tablet	448 mg	
17;TRIANGLE	Theokin	Yellow tablet	450 mg	
18;895	Biphetamine	White capsule	3.75 mg	Fisons Pharmaceuticals
18;899	Biphetamine-T	Green and black capsule	6.25 mg	Fisons Pharmaceuticals
18;899	Biphetamine-T	Green and black capsule	40 mg	Fisons Pharmaceuticals
18;900	Biphetamine-T	Red and black capsule	10 mg	Fisons Pharmaceuticals
18;900	Biphetamine-T	Red and black capsule	40 mg	Fisons Pharmaceuticals
25;LL;C22	chlorpromazine hydrochloride	Tan coated tablet	25 mg	Lederle Laboratories
50;LL;C23	chlorpromazine hydrochloride	Tan coated tablet	50 mg	Lederle Laboratories

Code	Drug	Color & form	Strength	Manufacturer
54;023	meprobamate	Tablet	200 mg	Roxane Laboratories
54;132	meprobamate	Tablet	400 mg	Roxane Laboratories
54;160	niacin	White tablet	100 mg	Roxane Laboratories
54;652	chlordiazepoxide hydrochloride	Opaque white capsule	25 mg	Roxane Laboratories
54;729	sulfisoxazole	Tablet	500 mg	Roxane Laboratories
54;863	chlordiazepoxide hydrochloride	Opaque green capsule	10 mg	Roxane Laboratories
75	Manoplax	White coated tablet	75 mg	Boots Pharmaceuticals
78 212;10	Metaprel	White tablet	10 mg	Novartis Pharmaceuticals
78 213;20	Metaprel	White tablet	20 mg	Novartis Pharmaceuticals
78;57	Plexonal	White tablet	0.08 mg	Novartis Pharmaceuticals
78;57	Plexonal	White tablet	0.16 mg	Novartis Pharmaceuticals
78;57	Plexonal	White tablet	45 mg	Novartis Pharmaceuticals
100	dicumarol	Tablet	100 mg	Abbott Laboratories
100;LL;C24	chlorpromazine hydrochloride	Tan coated tablet	100 mg	Lederle Laboratories
160	Dolonil	Maroon tablet	0.3 mg	
160	Dolonil	Maroon tablet	15 mg	
160	Dolonil	Maroon tablet	150 mg	
200 000	penicillin G potassium	White tablet	200,000 units	
200;LL;C25	chlorpromazine hydrochloride	Tan coated tablet	200 mg	Solvay Pharmaceuticals
200;ZPP	Rescaps-D SR	Clear white capsule with blue and white beads	40 mg	Searle
200;ZPP	Rescaps-D SR	Clear white capsule with blue and white beads	75 mg	Searle

Most commonly used drugs in nursing specialties

Nurses are often required to float to units they're not accustomed to working in, where they might have to administer unfamiliar drugs. If you know ahead of time which drugs are most commonly used in the various nursing specialties, you'll be able to acquaint yourself with these drugs—and reduce the chance of making a drug error. The table below shows the 10 most commonly used drugs in nine nursing specialties.

Specialty	Top 10 drugs
Critical care nursing	amiodarone hydrochloride diltiazem hydrochloride dopamine hydrochloride epinephrine hydrochloride furosemide insulin lorazepam metoprolol tartrate morphine sulfate nitroglycerin
Emergency care nursing	acetaminophen aspirin diltiazem diphtheria and tetanus toxoids famotidine ketorolac ibuprofen levofloxacin metoclopramide nitroglycerin
Home care nursing	acetaminophen acetaminophen/oxycodone acetaminophen/propoxyphene napsylate digoxin diltiazem hydrochloride docusate sodium furosemide metformin hydrochloride potassium chloride warfarin
Long-term care nursing	carbidopa/levodopa digoxin docusate sodium donepezil hydrochloride enalapril maleate furosemide metoprolol tartrate mirtazapine pantoprazole sodium potassium chloride

Specialty	Top 10 drugs
Medical-surgical nursing	acetaminophen diltiazem hydrochloride enalapril maleate furosemide heparin sodium insulin levofloxacin metoprolol tartrate morphine sulfate potassium chloride
Obstetric nursing	acetaminophen/codeine acetaminophen/oxycodone dinoprostone ibuprofen magnesium sulfate nalbuphine hydrochloride oxytocin penicillin promethazine hydrochloride terbutaline sulfate
Pediatric nursing	albuterol amoxicillin/clavulanate potassium amoxicillin trihydrate cetirizine hydrochloride co-trimoxazole fluticasone propionate gentamicin sulfate hydrocortisone (topical) methylphenidate hydrochloride montelukast sodium
Post-anesthesia care nursing	bupivacaine hydrochloride fentanyl citrate hydromorphone hydrochloride lidocaine hydrochloride lorazepam meperidine hydrochloride metoclopramide hydrochloride midazolam hydrochloride morphine sulfate ondansetron hydrochloride
Psychiatric nursing	carbamazepine clonazepam divalproex sodium escitalopram oxalate lithium carbonate olanzapine paroxetine hydrochloride risperidone sertraline hydrochloride venlafaxine hydrochloride

Wholesale cost per year of therapy for the top 50 drugs used by the elderly

The table below shows the wholesale annual cost per year of therapy in 2003 of the 50 most commonly prescribed drugs for the elderly. The drugs are ranked by the number of claims per year.

Brand or generic drug name	Dosage strength and form	Annual cost (2003)
1. Lipitor	10-mg tablet	$ 871
2. Norvasc	5-mg tablet	$ 549
3. Fosamax	70-mg tablet	$ 894
4. Plavix	75-mg tablet	$1,539
5. Prilosec	20-mg capsule (CR)	$1,684
6. Celebrex	200-mg capsule	$2,102
7. furosemide*	40-mg tablet	$ 59
8. Zocor	20-mg tablet	$1,674
9. Prevacid	30-mg capsule (CR)	$1,690
10. Norvasc	10-mg tablet	$ 794
11. Lipitor	20-mg tablet	$1,330
12. Klor-Con M20*	20-mEq tablet (CR)	$ 386
13. Toprol XL	50-mg tablet (CR)	$ 277
14. Xalatan	0.005% solution	$ 186
15. Vioxx	25-mg tablet	$1,050
16. Lanoxin*	0.125-mg tablet	$ 88
17. Synthroid*	0.1-mg tablet	$ 153
18. Synthroid*	0.05-mg tablet	$ 136
19. metoprolol tartrate*	50-mg tablet	$ 405
20. isosorbide mononitrate*	30-mg tablet (CR)	$ 407
21. Digitek*	0.125-mg tablet	$ 69
22. isosorbide mononitrate*	60-mg tablet (CR)	$ 429
23. metoprolol tartrate*	50-mg tablet	$ 405
24. Synthroid*	0.075-mg tablet	$ 150
25. Zoloft	50-mg tablet	$ 966
26. Protonix	40-mg tablet	$1,282

* Generic or co-marketed versions of this drug product are available.
CR = controlled-release

Wholesale cost per year of therapy for the top 50 drugs used by the elderly (continued)

Brand or generic drug name	Dosage strength and form	Annual cost (2003)
27. Cozaar	50-mg tablet	$ 553
28. atenolol*	25-mg tablet	$ 298
29. Premarin	0.625-mg tablet	$ 324
30. furosemide*	20-mg tablet	$ 52
31. Zocor	40-mg tablet	$ 1,674
32. Evista	60-mg tablet	$ 895
33. Nexium	40-mg capsule	$ 1,614
34. Zocor	10-mg tablet	$ 959
35. Combivent	1 mg aerosol	$10,868
36. Miacalcin	200 IU/activation spray	$ 7,132
37. atenolol*	50-mg tablet	$ 304
38. Pravachol	20-mg tablet	$ 1,124
39. Paxil	20-mg tablet	$ 1,031
40. Toprol XL	100-mg tablet (CR)	$ 416
41. Celexa	20-mg tablet	$ 880
42. hydrochlorothiazide*	25-mg tablet	$ 29
43. Glucotrol XL	10-mg tablet (CR)	$ 308
44. Klor-Con 10*	10-mEq tablet (CR)	$ 342
45. furosemide*	40-mg tablet	$ 57
46. potassium chloride*	10-mEq capsules (CR)	$ 221
47. Lanoxin*	0.25-mg tablet	$ 88
48. Claritin	10-mg tablet	$ 1,178
49. Diovan	80-mg tablet	$ 567
50. HCTZ/triamterene*	37.5-mg/25-mg capsules	$ 137

* Generic or co-marketed versions of this drug product are available.
CR = controlled-release

Source: "Wholesale Cost Per Year of Therapy for Top 50 Drugs (by number of claims) Used by the Elderly" (Table 3). *Out of Bounds: Rising Prescription Drug Prices for Seniors*. Adapted and reprinted with permission from Families USA Foundation, 2003.

Top 200 most commonly prescribed drugs

The table below lists the top 200 most commonly prescribed drugs in the United States in 2002, based on more than 3.05 billion prescriptions written. Drugs are listed by generic name or brand name (capitalized).

1. hydrocodone/APAP
2. Lipitor
3. atenolol
4. Synthroid
5. Premarin
6. Zithromax
7. furosemide
8. amoxicillin
9. Norvasc
10. hydrochlorothiazide
11. alprazolam
12. Albuterol Aerosol
13. Zoloft
14. Paxil
15. Zocor
16. Prevacid
17. ibuprofen
18. triamterene/HCTZ
19. Toprol-XL
20. cephalexin
21. Celebrex
22. Zyrtec
23. Levoxyl
24. Allegra
25. Ortho Tri-Cyclen
26. Celexa
27. prednisone
28. Prilosec
29. Vioxx
30. Claritin
31. fluoxetine
32. acetaminophen/codeine
33. Ambien
34. metoprolol tartrate
35. lorazepam
36. Fosamax
37. propoxyphene N/APAP
38. metformin
39. ranitidine hydrochloride
40. amitriptyline
41. Viagra
42. Prempro
43. Trimox
44. Neurontin
45. Wellbutrin SR
46. Pravachol
47. Augmentin
48. Nexium
49. Accupril
50. lisinopril
51. Effexor XR
52. Singulair
53. Zestril
54. potassium chloride
55. clonazepam
56. naproxen
57. warfarin
58. trazodone
59. Cipro
60. Flonase
61. cyclobenzaprine
62. verapamil hydrochloride
63. enalapril
64. albuterol sulfate
65. isosorbide mononitrate
66. Levaquin
67. diazepam
68. Glucotrol XL
69. Coumadin
70. Plavix

71. Diflucan	113. Flomax
72. Advair Diskus	114. temazepam
73. Protonix	115. Ultram
74. Lotrel	116. Hyzaar
75. Amoxil	117. Oxycontin
76. Diovan	118. Humulin N
77. glyburide	119. Depakote
78. carisoprodol	120. Concerta
79. Altace	121. Klor-Con
80. allopurinol	122. Glucovance
81. estradiol	123. Imitrex Oral
82. Avandia	124. Terazosin
83. Actos	125. Claritin D 24 Hour
84. Lotensin	126. Cartia XT
85. Clarinex	127. Amaryl
86. medroxyprogesterone	128. spironolactone
87. oxycodone/APAP	129. Tricor
88. doxycycline hyclate	130. Ortho-Novum
89. Lanoxin	131. hydroxyzine hydrochloride
90. Cozaar	132. Monopril
91. Nasonex	133. Combivent
92. diltiazem hydrochloride	134. meclizine
93. clonidine	135. triamcinolone acetonide
94. Prinivil	136. Klor-Con M20
95. Digitek	137. metoclopramide
96. methylprednisolone	138. minocycline
97. Evista	139. bisoprolol/HCTZ
98. folic acid	140. propranolol
99. Glucophage XR	141. Glucophage
100. penicillin VK	142. Propacet
101. Flovent	143. Valtrex
102. Risperdal	144. Remeron
103. Cotrim	145. famotidine
104. promethazine	146. metronidazole
105. Diovan HCT	147. Bextra
106. Aciphex	148. Avapro
107. Zyprexa	149. glipizide
108. Allegra-D	150. buspirone
109. Levothroid	151. nystatin
110. doxazosin	152. Skelaxin
111. Xalatan	153. Serevent
112. gemfibrozil	154. Dilantin

(continued)

Top 200 most commonly prescribed drugs (continued)

155. promethazine/codeine
156. Necon
157. captopril
158. clindamycin
159. aspirin
160. Seroquel
161. acyclovir
162. macrobid
163. Claritin D 12 Hour
164. amoxicillin/clavulanate
165. Adderall XR
166. Biaxin XL
167. Trivora-28
168. Ortho-Cyclen
169. Cefzil
170. Humulin 70/30
171. Detrol LA
172. Coreg
173. Tiazac
174. Biaxin
175. tramadol
176. Nasacort AQ
177. Humalog
178. Ultracet
179. Endocet
180. Bactroban
181. Veetids
182. trimethoprim/sulfamethoxazole
183. timolol maleate
184. Rhinocort Aqua
185. Claritin Reditabs
186. nortriptyline
187. Aviane
188. Actonel
189. Topamax
190. Microgestin Fe
191. tamoxifen
192. Mircette
193. nifedipine
194. ditropan XL
195. tetracycline
196. Apri
197. Zestoretic
198. diclofenac
199. Augmentin ES-600
200. carbidopa/levodopa

Adapted with permission from "The Top 200 Prescriptions for 2002 by Number of U.S. Prescriptions Dispensed" accessed on www.rxlist.com/top200/htm.

Selected references

Blumenthal, M., et al, eds. *The Complete German Commission E Monographs: Therapeutic Guide to Herbal Medicines.* Newton, Mass.: Integrative Medicine Communications, 1999.

Drug Facts and Comparisons 2004, 58th ed. St. Louis: Facts and Comparisons, 2004.

Drug Information for the Health Care Professional (USP DI), vol. 1. Greenwood Village, Colo.: Micromedex Thomson Healthcare, 2004.

Hansten, P.D., and Horn, J.R. *Hansten and Horn's Drug Interactions Analysis and Management.* St Louis: Facts and Comparisons, 1999 (plus quarterly updates).

Hardman, J.G., et al, eds. *Goodman & Gilman's The Pharmacological Basis of Therapeutics,* 10th ed. The McGraw Hill Companies, Inc., 2001.

King Guide to Parenteral Admixtures, Summer 2003 ed. Napa, Calif.: King Guide Publications, Inc., 2003.

McEvoy, G. K., et al, eds. *AHFS Drug Information 2003.* Bethesda, Md.: American Society of Health-System Pharmacists, American Hospital Formulary Service, 2003.

Mosby's Drug Consult 2004, 14th ed. St Louis: Mosby, Inc., 2004.

PDR for Herbal Medicines, 2nd ed. Montvale, N.J.: Thomson Healthcare, 2000.

Physicians' Desk Reference 2004, 58th ed. Montvale, N.J.: Thomson Healthcare, 2003.

Physicians' Desk Reference Companion Guide 2004, 58th ed. Montvale, N.J.: Thomson Healthcare, 2003.

RxFACTS: Natural Products. St. Louis: Facts and Comparisons, 2002.

Sweetman, S.C. *Martindale: The Complete Drug Reference,* 33rd ed. London: Pharmaceutical Press, 2004.

Websites

Drugs@FDA (catalog of FDA-approved drugs): www.accessdata.fda.gov/scripts/cder/drugsatfda/

Health Canada (Canadian drug product database): www.hc-sc.gc.ca/hpb/drugs-dpd

National Library of Medicine and National Institutes of Health (drug information): www.nlm.nih.gov/medlineplus/druginformation.html

Physician's Desk Reference: www.drugs.com

RxList: www.rxlist.com

U.S. Food and Drug Administration: www.fda.gov/cder/index.html

Index

    Boldface: Color section

T: Table

Boldface: Color section

Boldface: Color section

T: Table **Boldface: Color section**

Boldface: Color section

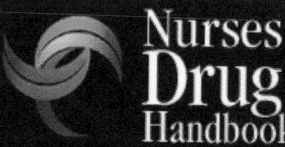

Nurses Drug Handbook

Home

SEARCH	

Search includes commonly used monographs, drug news, approvals and indications —

HOME

Safe drug administration for oral, I.M., and I.V. routes —

SAFE DRUG ADMINISTRATION

IDENTIFYING DRUGS

Photogallery and imprint codes —

MOST COMMONLY USED DRUGS

DRUG APPROVALS & UPDATES

FEDERAL GUIDELINES

Fully customizable patient teaching aids that can be printed and given to patients —

PATIENT TEACHING AIDS

REPORTING INCIDENTS

CONTINUING EDUCATION

Ten FREE hours of drug-specific CE —

MORE...

Calcu	
Paren	
Emer	
Monit	
Drugs	

NEWS

Summaries of recent drug news —

Warning: Atypical Antipsychotic Hyperglycemia Warnings

First in a Strong New Antibiotic Class

Spiriva — New Once-a-Day Inhaler for COPD

Bar Codes for Medications — New Requirements from HHS

Herbal Version of Ecstasy Causes Adverse Events

More News...

From the Publishers of

Nursing Spectrum

Hom

Fede

© Nu